Prenatal and Postnatal Care

A Person-Centered Approach

Prenatal and Postnatal Care

A Person-Centered Approach

THIRD EDITION

Edited By

Karen Trister Grace

Cindy L. Farley

Noelene K. Jeffers

Tanya Tringali

WILEY Blackwell

Registered Offices
John Wiley & Sons, Inc., 111 River Street, Hoboken, NJ 07030, USA
John Wiley & Sons Ltd, The Atrium, Southern Gate, Chichester, West Sussex, PO19 8SQ, UK

For details of our global editorial offices, customer services, and more information about Wiley products visit us at www.wiley.com.

Wiley also publishes its books in a variety of electronic formats and by print-on-demand. Some content that appears in standard print versions of this book may not be available in other formats.

Library of Congress Cataloging-in-Publication Data
Names: Grace, Karen Trister, editor. | Farley, Cindy L., editor. | Jeffers, Noelene K., editor. | Tringali, Tanya, editor.
Title: Prenatal and postnatal care : a person-centered approach / edited by Karen Trister Grace, Cindy L. Farley, Noelene K. Jeffers, Tanya Tringali.
Description: Third edition. | Hoboken, NJ : Wiley-Blackwell, 2024. | Includes bibliographical references and index.
Identifiers: LCCN 2023012164 (print) | LCCN 2023012165 (ebook) | ISBN 9781119852698 (paperback) | ISBN 9781119852704 (adobe pdf) | ISBN 9781119852711 (epub)
Subjects: MESH: Maternal-Child Nursing | Pregnancy Complications–nursing | Pregnancy–physiology
Classification: LCC RJ254 (print) | LCC RJ254 (ebook) | NLM WY 157.3 | DDC 618.92/01–dc23/eng/20230705
LC record available at https://lccn.loc.gov/2023012164
LC ebook record available at https://lccn.loc.gov/2023012165

Cover Design: Wiley
Cover Image: Courtesy of Robin G. Jordan

Set in 10.5/11.5pt MinionPro by Straive, Pondicherry, India

SKY10076942_060624

We dedicate the third edition to the lead editor of the first and second editions of this book, Robin G. Jordan, feminist scholar and lifelong advocate for women and their families.
Thank you for trusting us with its legacy.

To my awesome and supportive husband and
kids, Peter, Jeremy, and Mara.
~Karen~

To Nell L. Tharpe, who first invited me on the book writing and editing journey; to Robin G. Jordan, who joined me along the way; and to my family, for their love and support—my mother, Carol Farley, my sister and her husband, Becky and Mike Doherty, and to my children, Kyle and Katy McEvoy—all my love.
~Cindy~

To my loving husband, Ebbed. And to the joyful, curious, and attached little one who made me a mother, Xavi.
~Noelene~

To my husband, Pablo, and my mother, Miriam, for their endless love and support. And of course, to Gabriella, my daughter, for the gifts of motherhood and midwifery.
~Tanya~

Contents

About the Editors

Karen Trister Grace, PhD, MSN, CNM, FACNM has been a practicing midwife since 2000. She received a BA in sociology from Barnard College, a BSN and MSN from the University of Pennsylvania, and a PhD from Johns Hopkins University School of Nursing. She completed a postdoctoral fellowship at Johns Hopkins Bloomberg School of Public Health. Her research focuses on pregnancy intention and reproductive coercion. She has been a nursing and midwifery educator since 2007. She is currently an Assistant Professor at George Mason University's School of Nursing. She practices clinically at Mary's Center, a federally qualified health center in metropolitan Washington, DC, USA.

Cindy L. Farley, PhD, MSN, CNM, FACNM, studied midwifery at Emory University. She received her BSN and PhD from The Ohio State University and her MSN from Emory University. She is a Professor at Georgetown University in the WHNP and Nurse-Midwifery/WHNP programs. She serves as a board member of the Cincinnati Birth Center. She works as a legal expert on selected cases involving midwifery regulatory issues and clinical care. She is coeditor/author of *Clinical Practice Guidelines for Midwifery and Women's Health* and this text. She has been instrumental in organizing groups of midwifery students to visit their federal legislators and advocate for positive change in important maternal health policies and legislation. She held a faculty residency at the University of Oxford, Oxford, England. She is active in international research on midwifery student confidence for supporting physiologic birth. She has participated in global health initiatives in collaboration with local community health and education leaders, most recently in Liberia and Tanzania.

Noelene K. Jeffers, PhD, CNM, IBCLC has served Washington, DC families as a Certified Nurse-Midwife since 2012. She received a BS in Foreign Services from Georgetown University, a MSN from the Yale School of Nursing, and a PhD from Johns Hopkins University School of Nursing. She completed a postdoctoral fellowship in Maternal and Child Health at the Johns Hopkins Bloomberg School of Public Health. She is an Assistant Professor at the Johns Hopkins University School of Nursing. Her research mission is to promote the health, well-being, and thriving of Black birthing people. She examines the impact of systems of oppression (e.g., racism, sexism, ableism, etc.) on the structural and social determinants of Black perinatal health. She also explores the role of Black midwifery, through culturally affirming and community-based care, in combating Black maternal morbidity and mortality. She serves on the board of directors of the National Association to Advance Black Birth, a national organization that exists to combat the impact of racism on Black maternal health, and led NAABB's development of the Black Birthing Bill of Rights.

Tanya Tringali, MS, CNM, FACNM received a BSN from New York University in 2003 and her MS in Midwifery from Philadelphia University in 2007 where she joined the faculty a year later. She is currently adjunct faculty at New York University and Georgetown University. She practiced full-scope midwifery in and around New York City until 2018 when she created Mother Wit Maternity & Consulting Services providing virtual midwifery care and wellness options to people navigating the perinatal period. She is a National Academy of Sports Medicine certified personal trainer, CrossFit Level 1, and Pregnancy and Postpartum Athleticism Coach, working diligently to provide clients and clinicians with the information, evidence, and tools needed to help people stay active during pregnancy and return to physical activity postpartum.

Contributors

Kathlyn Albert, DNP, FNP-BC, CNM
Director, Nurse-Midwifery Program
Clinical Assistant Professor
Marquette University College of Nursing
Milwaukee, WI

Tia P. Andrighetti, DNP, CNM, CNE, CHSE-A
Associate Professor
Frontier Nursing University
Madbury, NH

Aishwarya Arjunan, MS, MPH, CGC, CPH
Certified Genetic Counselor
Senior Medical Science Liaison
GRAIL LLC
Menlo Park, CA

Rhonda Arthur, DNP, CNM, WHNP-BC, FNP-BC, CNE
Associate Professor
Frontier Nursing University
Floyd, VA

Melissa D. Avery, PhD, CNM, FACNM, FAAN
Editor-in-Chief
Journal of Midwifery & Women's Health
Professor Emeritus
School of Nursing
University of Minnesota
Minneapolis, MN

Jenna Benyounes, DNP, CNM, WHNP, NCMP
Adjunct Faculty
Nurse-Midwifery/WHNP and WHNP Programs
Georgetown University School of Nursing
Washington, DC

Esther Ellsworth Bowers, MSN, MS, MEd, CNM/WHNP
Adjunct Instructor
Nurse-Midwifery/WHNP and WHNP Programs
Georgetown University School of Nursing
Flagstaff, AZ

Heather M. Bradford, PhD, CNM, FACNM
Assistant Program Director
Nurse-Midwifery/WHNP and WHNP Programs
Georgetown University School of Nursing
Seattle, WA

Victoria H. Burslem, MSN, CNM, CNE(cl), FACNM
Senior Instructor
Department of Midwifery and Women's Health
Frontier Nursing University
Nicholasville, KY

Judith M. Butler, DNP, CNM, CNE, WHNP
Assistant Professor
Frontier Nursing University
Tucson, Arizona

Joyce D. Cappiello, PhD, FNP, FAANP
Associate Professor of Nursing Emeritus
College of Health and Human Services
University of New Hampshire
Durham, NH

Emma Clark, MHS, MSN, CNM, FACNM
Adjunct Faculty
Nurse-Midwifery/WHNP and WHNP Programs
Georgetown University School of Nursing
Washington, D.C.

Anne Z. Cockerham, PhD, CNM, WHNP-BC, CNE, FACNM
Professor
Frontier Nursing University
Pinehurst, NC

Katie Daily, CNM, MSN
Adjunct Faculty
Nurse-Midwifery/WHNP and WHNP Programs
Georgetown University School of Nursing
Washington, DC

Katie DePalma, DNP, CNM, WHNP-BC, FACNM
Instructor
Nurse-Midwifery/WHNP and WHNP Programs
Georgetown University School of Nursing
Washington, DC

Debora M. Dole, PhD, CNM, FACNM
Vice Dean, Academic Affairs
Associate Professor
Georgetown University School of Nursing
Washington, DC

Mary Broderick Donnelly, DBE, HCEC-C, RN
Clinical Assistant Professor, Marcella Niehoff School of Nursing
Loyola University of Chicago
Clinical Ethics Consultant, Loyola University Medical Center
Maywood, IL

Janet L. Engstrom, PhD, APRN, CNM, WHNP-BC, CNE
Faculty, Frontier Nursing University
Versailles, KY

Melicia Escobar, DNP, CNM, WHNP-BC, FACNM
Program Director, Assistant Professor
Nurse-Midwifery/WHNP and WHNP Programs
Georgetown University School of Nursing
Philadelphia, PA

Jenifer Fahey, MSN, PhD, CNM, FACNM
Assistant Professor and Director, Division of Midwifery
University of Maryland
School of Medicine
Department of Obstetrics, Gynecology and Reproductive Science
Baltimore, MD

Cindy L. Farley, PhD, MSN, CNM, FACNM
Professor, Nurse-Midwifery/WHNP and WHNP Programs
Senior Advisor to the Dean on Research and Scholarship
Georgetown University School of Nursing
Yellow Springs, OH

Gina M. Fullbright, DNP, WHNP-BC
Infectious Disease Clinician, New Mexico Department of Health
Adjunct Faculty
Nurse-Midwifery/WHNP and WHNP Programs
Georgetown University School of Nursing
Las Cruces, NM

Raven Fulton, CNM, WHNP, MS
Atlanta, GA

Elizabeth Gabzdyl, DNP, CNM, ARNP
Assistant Professor
Program Director, Nurse-Midwifery Education Program
College of Nursing
Seattle University
Seattle, WA

Meghan Garland, PhD, CNM, FACNM
Faculty
Frontier Nursing University
Forest Park, IL

Karen Trister Grace, PhD, MSN, CNM, FACNM
Assistant Professor
School of Nursing
George Mason University
Bethesda, MD

Lisa Hachey, DNP, APRN-CNM
Associate Professor
Program Director, Nurse-Midwifery
University of Cincinnati
Cincinnati, OH

Susan Hancock, MS, CGC
Certified Genetic Counselor
Staff Genetic Counselor
Illumina, Inc
Foster City, CA

Lisa Hanson, PhD, CNM, FACNM
Klein Professor and Associate Director, Midwifery Program
Marquette University
College of Nursing
Milwaukee, WI

Lise Hauser, DNP, RN
Assistant Clinical Professor, Marcella Niehoff School of Nursing
Loyola University Chicago
Chicago, IL

Ella T. Heitzler, PhD, WHNP-BC, FNP-BC, RNC-OB
Associate Professor
Georgetown University School of Nursing
Washington, DC

Katie Huffling, DNP, RN, CNM, FAAN
Executive Director
Alliance of Nurses for Healthy Environments
Mount Rainier, MD

Sascha James-Conterelli, DNP, CNM, FACNM, FAAN, FNYAM
Assistant Professor
Yale University
School of Nursing
Orange, CT

Noelene K. Jeffers, PhD, CNM, IBCLC
Assistant Professor
Johns Hopkins School of Nursing
Baltimore, MD

Cecilia M. Jevitt, RM, CNM, ARNP, PhD, FACNM
Associate Professor
Midwifery Program Director
The University of British Columbia
Vancouver, British Columbia, Canada

Robin G. Jordan, PhD, CNM, FACNM
Editor Emeritus
Prenatal and Postnatal Care: A Woman-Centered Approach, first and second editions
Petoskey, MI

Deborah Brandt Karsnitz, DNP, CNM, FACNM, CNE
Professor
Frontier Nursing University
Simpsonville, KY

Julia Lange-Kessler, DNP, CM, FACNM
Certified Somatic Therapist: Pregnancy and Birth
Westtown, New York

Melissa Kitzman, MSN, CNM, WHNP-BC
Lead Certified Nurse-Midwife
M Health Fairview
Adjunct Faculty and Clinical Faculty Advisor
Nurse-Midwifery/WHNP and WHNP Programs
Georgetown University School of Nursing
Minneapolis, MN

Ebony Marcelle, DNP, CNM, FACNM
Adjunct faculty
Nurse-Midwifery/WHNP and WHNP Programs
Georgetown University School of Nursing
Washington, DC

Emily Malloy, PhD, CNM
Staff Nurse-Midwife and Director of Midwifery Research
Advocate Aurora UW Medical Group
Milwaukee, WI
Participating Faculty
Marquette University College of Nursing
Milwaukee, WI

Clinical Adjunct Associate Professor
University of Wisconsin School of Medicine and Public Health
Madison, WI

Amy Marowitz, DNP, CNM, CNE
Associate Professor
Frontier Nursing University
Maple City, MI

Latrice Martin, DNP, CNM, FNP-C, PMHNP-BC
Instructor
Frontier Nursing University
Versailles, Kentucky

LuVerda Sayles Martin, DNP, CNM
Staff Midwife
Advocate Aurora Health
Milwaukee, WI

Katie McDevitt, MSN, CNM, WHNP-BC
Staff Midwife
Mary's Center
Washington, DC

Linda McDaniel, DNP, CNM, FACNM, RNFA
Assistant Professor
Frontier Nursing University
Versailles, KY

Carrie E. Neerland, PhD, CNM, FACNM
Assistant Professor
School of Nursing
University of Minnesota
Minneapolis, MN

Lisa Noguchi, PhD, CNM, FACNM, CPPS
Director, Maternal Newborn Health, Jhpiego
Associate, Department of Epidemiology
Johns Hopkins Bloomberg School of Public Health
Washington, DC

Cynthia Nypaver, PhD, CNM, WHNP-BC, FACNM
Associate Professor of Clinical
College of Nursing
University of Cincinnati
Cincinnati, OH

Signey Olson, DNP, CNM, WHNP-BC, FACNM
Assistant Professor
Nurse-Midwifery/WHNP and WHNP Programs
Georgetown University School of Nursing
Washington, DC

Nancy Pesta Walsh, DNP, PMHNP, FNP
Assistant Professor
Frontier Nursing University
Belgrade, MN

Catherine Ruhl, DNP, CNM
Certified Nurse-Midwife
Presbyterian Hospital
Albuquerque, New Mexico

Jenna Shaw-Battista, PhD, PHN, NP, CNM, FACNM
Certified Nurse-Midwife, Sutter Health
Women's Health Nurse Practitioner, Elica Health Centers
Yolo County, California

Nell L. Tharpe, MS, CNM, FACNM, CRNFA (E)
Perinatal Consultant
Perinatal Quality Collaborative for Maine
Midwifery Educator
Midwife Workshops
East Boothbay, ME

Signy Toquinto, MSN, CNM, WHNP, MA
(she/her/ella)
OB Program Manager
Marin Community Clinic
MarinHealth Medical Center
San Francisco, CA

Tanya Tringali, MS, CNM, FACNM
Adjunct Faculty
New York University, Rory Meyers College of Nursing
Georgetown University School of Nursing
Plantation, FL

Kimberly K. Trout, PhD, CNM, FACNM, FAAN
Associate Professor
M. Louise Fitzpatrick College of Nursing
Villanova University
Villanova, PA

Marsha Walker, RN, IBCLC
Vice President
National Lactation Consultant Alliance
International Board Certified Lactation Consultant
Weston, MA

Holly White, CNM, PMHNP
Brooklyn, NY

Rhea Williams, PhD(c), CNM, FACNM
Nutrition Specialist
Instructor
Nurse-Midwifery/WHNP and WHNP Programs
Georgetown University School of Nursing
Columbia, MD

Jennifer Wolfe, DNP APRN WHNP-BC
Clinical Assistant Professor of Practice
The Ohio State University College of
Nursing in Columbus
Ohio

Preface

Pregnancy and the birth of a baby are significant life-changing events. Optimal care not only focuses on the physical process but also on the emotional experience of pregnancy and the postpartum period. The context of culture, life experiences, social roles, and physical and mental health status on the childbearing experience influence options, choices, and outcomes.

This book both describes and challenges current prenatal and postnatal care practices. Prenatal care visits within the current pathology-centered model of care are brief and focused on testing, legalities, and reimbursement. Too often this approach emphasizes the needs of the provider within the office setting rather than the person's needs during pregnancy. Postnatal care is often limited in scope and connection at a time when the new family needs guidance and support from professionals as well as family members. This is a disservice to clients and their families. Opportunities to promote health and well-being during pregnancy, birth, and beyond are being lost in contemporary practice. These missed opportunities are reflected in the rising maternal mortality rate in the United States.

The pregnant person and their unique needs are the rightful focus of prenatal and postnatal care. *Person-centered care* is the term used to describe a philosophy of maternity care that is based on the needs and preferences of the pregnant person. This care emphasizes the importance of informed choice, continuity of care, active participation, best care practices, provider responsiveness, and accessibility. Pregnancy, childbirth, and the postpartum period are the start of family life. A full account of the meaning and values that each person brings to the experience of pregnancy and parenting should be included in care.

The fundamental principles of person-centered care encompass the following tenets:

- Co-creation of perinatal care with healthcare providers, incorporating the individual's preferences and meaningful cultural traditions.
- The right to informed choice to accept or decline the options available during pregnancy, labor, birth, and the postnatal period, including the place of birth, who provides care, and where care is provided.
- Authority over the key decisions that affect the content and progress of care.
- The moral and legal right to decisions regarding bodily integrity and autonomy.
- The right to care that supports optimal health.

Prenatal and postnatal care provided within the context of the person's own experience, focused on both the life-changing nature of the pregnancy experience as well as physical adaptations and needs, leads to improved maternal and infant outcomes. The views, beliefs, and values of the pregnant person, their partner, and their family in relation to care are sought and respected at all times. Adequate time is spent in providing optimal prenatal and postnatal care with kindness, respect, and dignity.

The Need for This Text

A growing body of scientific evidence supports the benefits of physiologic childbearing for the birthing person and their baby. Several decades of escalating pregnancy and birth medicalization have shown that interventions applied on a large scale and without medical indication lead to significant negative iatrogenic consequences. However, care supporting physiologic labor and birth does not begin with the first contraction; rather, it begins in the preconception or interconception period and continues into the postpartum period. Too much faith is placed in technology and too little faith is placed in human connection. This book brings balance to the fore; it adds a holistic framework from which to enter into dialogue with the person who presents for care. Midwives, nurse practitioners, physicians, physician assistants and other prenatal and postnatal healthcare providers, and students with common practice foundations in providing holistic care, emphasizing patient education and health maintenance in the context of an ongoing relationship, will find this book useful.

The editors of this book are experienced clinicians and educators of midwives, nurse practitioners, nurses, medical students, and other healthcare providers. We have found that many available obstetric and maternity care texts offer limited content on prenatal and postnatal care. Additionally, an appreciation of the effects of the mind–body connection and the background social dynamics of the pregnant person and their family on overall health and childbearing experience has been lacking. This appreciation, in addition to a solid understanding of normal childbearing processes, will increase healthcare providers' competency in supporting the normal and recognizing the abnormal. This text provides a breadth and depth of knowledge on pregnancy and postpartum processes and care not found in other texts.

New in the Third Edition

Since the publication of the second edition of this book, the world has changed in previously unimaginable ways. Work on this edition began in 2021, while isolating in our homes from a global pandemic that has affected countless families and individuals and altered many aspects of healthcare. Content in some chapters has been updated to address COVID-19 and the realities of care during a pandemic, but this disease is rapidly evolving. As the body of knowledge grows in this area, changes in clinical practice can be expected. As work on this text was nearing completion in June of 2022, the Dobbs v. Jackson Women's Health Organization decision was handed down by the Supreme Court of the United States, reversing the constitutional right to abortion and threatening the reproductive and bodily autonomy of people across the country. Several chapters had to undergo additional revisions to reflect the rapidly changing landscape of human rights in the United States, and some of this content may become obsolete. Readers are advised to be aware of legislative changes that may affect this area of clinical practice.

The editors shared with chapter authors the vision that we had for this edition. We envisioned a book that would:

- Describe health disparities and inequities that exist in perinatal healthcare and outcomes.
- Identify the ways that racism, bias, and the social determinants of health generate health disparities and inequities during pregnancy, birth, postpartum, breastfeeding, and early parenting.
- Highlight ways that healthcare clinicians can work to disrupt racism, bias, and discrimination in the healthcare setting at an individual and a systems level.
- Utilize language that is respectful, inclusive, and strives to be free of bias.

We asked authors of every chapter to integrate evidence around health disparities and inequities and to highlight this content in a new section of each chapter called *Health Equity Key Points*. We asked authors to report health disparities data across social identities, such as race, ethnicity, socioeconomic status, age, location, gender, disability status, and sexual orientation. This included a discussion of the root causes of inequities, and explicitly naming the dynamic (e.g., racism, sexism, classism, ableism, or homophobia) implicated in generating the health inequity. An intersectional approach was encouraged, examining how multiple forms of oppression may interact and amplify to further marginalize specific groups. And finally, wherever possible, a strength-based discussion was included, discussing individual, cultural, and community factors that may enhance health outcomes and resilience among individuals and communities.

Throughout the book, we have edited language to reflect our recognition that not all women have the capacity for pregnancy, and that some pregnant people do not identify as women. We wish to state, in unequivocal terms, our unwavering support for pregnant people of all genders. To this end, we edited the subtitle of this book to "A person-centered approach." In addition, the editorial team asked authors to utilize gender-inclusive and bias-free language. Examples of gender-inclusive language include words like client, person, people, parent, and individual. This has challenged all of us to reflect on our biases and our gendered assumptions and interpretations of pregnancy and birth. The interested reader can find the guidelines we used in the following publications: APA bias-free language guide (American Psychological Association, 2021) Academy of Breastfeeding Medicine (Bartick et al., 2021; Eidelman, 2021), *Journal of Human Lactation* (Bamberger et al., 2021), *Journal of Midwifery & Women's Health* (Likis, 2021), and *Obstetrics & Gynecology* (Moseson et al., 2020).

Even with such guidance noted above, there are a number of language choices that the editors and authors needed to consider. Most published research includes only sex assigned at birth, although increasingly studies are capturing data that include self-identified gender identity as well. Gendered language is used in some of the statements and guidelines by national organizations and certifying bodies cited in this book. Some gender-inclusive terms do not fully reflect the words they replace. For example, chestfeeding may be used although anatomically, the breast is the organ of lactation. And neither chestfeeding nor breastfeeding captures human milk feeding from donor or stored sources. The editors and authors made decisions in line with language guidelines current at the time this edition goes to press; however, language will evolve over time. It is our intent to use language that communicates deep respect of each individual's humanity and autonomy, and we strongly urge clinicians to inquire about and use terminology that is preferred by each individual patient.

This edition has been updated in all chapters to reflect current standards and care recommendations. The following new chapters have been added:

- Health Equity
- Ethics in Perinatal Care
- Physical Activity and Exercise in the Perinatal Period
- Sexuality
- Culture and Community
- Preconception, Pregnancy, and Postpartum Care of LGBTQ+ Individuals
- Violence and Trauma in the Perinatal Period
- Occupational and Environmental Health in Pregnancy

We are pleased that the first and second editions of this book have been well received by clinicians and faculty of various health professions involved in prenatal and postnatal care. The first edition was honored with the 2015 Book of the Year award from the American College of Nurse-Midwives. We are extremely fortunate to have many highly regarded contributors to the third edition and to mentor some talented new writers. Contributing authors have a background in clinical practice, and many are established content experts in their field. Most of our contributors are also educators, bringing an understanding of the needs of students to the text. We want to acknowledge the coeditors of the first edition, Julie A. Marfel and Janet L. Engstrom, and their work in launching the first edition.

We also acknowledge and owe a deep debt of gratitude to the lead editor of the first and second editions, Robin G. Jordan. This book was born under her leadership in the first two editions, and we are honored to carry on its legacy.

The current editorial team includes Karen Trister Grace who has stepped into the lead editor position after serving as coeditor in the second edition, and Cindy L. Farley who has served as coeditor in all editions of this book. They provided background and experience in finding a balance of continuity and change for this edition while remaining true to its vision. Noelene K. Jeffers and Tanya Tringali are welcomed to the editorial team for the third edition. They each brought their talent, experience, and knowledge to bear in shaping this edition of the book.

This book was written as a resource for all those interested in providing person-centered prenatal and postnatal care. While aspects of this care are timeless and do not change, certain elements of prenatal and postnatal care are refined as new evidence is incorporated into existing bodies of knowledge. Healthcare providers are responsible for their ongoing learning in the field and should read critically and widely among the many resources available to them. Evidence-based healthcare encompasses psychosocial and cultural aspects of care applied in a mutual dialogue and determination with each individual.

The authors, editors, and publisher have made every effort to assure the accuracy of information as this book goes to press. Nevertheless, they are not responsible for errors, omissions, or outcomes related to the application of this information in the clinical setting. This is at the healthcare provider's own discretion.

Karen Trister Grace
Cindy L. Farley
Noelene K. Jeffers
Tanya Tringali

References

American Psychological Association. (2021). *Inclusive language guidelines.* https://www.apa.org/about/apa/equity-diversity-inclusion/language-guidelines.pdf

Bamberger, E. T., JHL Editorial Team, & Farrow, A. (2021). Gendered and inclusive language in the preparation of manuscripts: Policy statement for the *Journal of Human Lactation. Journal of Human Lactation, 37*(2), 227–229. https://doi.org/10.1177/0890334421995103

Bartick, M., Stehel, E. K., Calhoun, S. L., Feldman-Winter, L., Zimmerman, D., Noble, L., Rosen-Carole, C., Kair, L. R., & The Academy of Breastfeeding Medicine. (2021). Academy of Breastfeeding Medicine position statement and guideline: Infant feeding and lactation-related language and gender. *Breastfeeding Medicine, 16*(8), 587–590. https://doi.org/10.1089/bfm.2021.29188.abm

Eidelman, A. I. (2021). Breastfeeding Medicine publication policy and ABM's statement regarding infant feeding and lactation-related language and gender. *Breastfeeding Medicine, 16*(8), 585–586. https://doi.org/10.1089/bfm.2021.29189.aie

Likis, F. E. (2021). Inclusive language promotes equity: The power of words. *Journal of Midwifery & Women's Health, 66*(1), 7–9. https://doi.org/10.1111/jmwh.13225

Moseson, H., Zazanis, N., Goldberg, E., Fix, L., Durden, M., Stoeffler, A., Hastings, J., Cudlitz, L., Lesser-Lee, B., Letcher, L., Reyes, A., & Obedin-Maliver, J. (2020). The imperative for transgender and gender nonbinary inclusion: Beyond women's health. *Obstetrics & Gynecology, 135*(5), 1059–1068. https://doi.org/10.1097/AOG.0000000000003816

About the Companion Website

Do not forget to visit the companion website for this book:

www.wiley.com/go/grace/prenatal

There you will find MCQs and other self-test material designed to enhance your learning:

- Multiple choice questions
- Case studies

Part I

Foundational Approaches to Prenatal and Postnatal Care

1

Health Equity

Noelene K. Jeffers and Karen Trister Grace

The editors gratefully acknowledge Nena Harris, Cindy L. Farley, and Michal Wright, who authored portions of the previous edition of this chapter.

Relevant Terms

Ableism—a set of beliefs or practices that devalue and discriminate against people with disabilities and often rests on the assumption that disabled people need to be "fixed"

Bias—prejudgments in favor of or against a particular thing, person, or group, typically in a manner considered to be unfair

Classism—the systematic assignment of characteristics of worth and ability based on social class; the systematic oppression of subordinated class groups to advantage and strengthen dominant class groups

Cisgenderism—societal assumptions about gender expression matching sex assignment at birth

Critical race theory—an academic and legal framework that denotes that structural racism is part of American society—from education and housing to employment and healthcare; racism is embedded in laws, policies, and institutions that uphold and reproduce racial inequalities

Disability—any condition of the body or mind that makes it more difficult for the person with the condition to do certain activities and interact with the world around them

Discrimination—the unfair or prejudicial treatment of people because of their actual or perceived group membership (e.g., membership based on identities such as race, gender, age, sexual orientation, ability, and more); may include both overt and covert behaviors, such as microaggressions or indirect or subtle behaviors that reflect negative attitudes or beliefs typically toward an individual of a group that has been minoritized

Eugenics—the scientifically erroneous theory of "racial improvement" and "planned breeding," which gained popularity during the early twentieth century; eugenicists use methods such as involuntary sterilization, segregation, and social exclusion to rid society of individuals deemed by them to be unfit

Food apartheid—an analytic framework to understand and address the structural causes of inequitable access to food

Food desert—an area with limited or no access to fresh, healthful foods; often found in impoverished urban areas or geographically remote areas

Food insecurity—uncertainty about the availability of adequate and safe nutrition

Health disparity—a difference in the incidence, prevalence, and burden of disease in a specified population as compared with the general population

Health equity—a commitment to give every person the opportunity to attain their full health potential with no one disadvantaged from achieving this potential due to social position or other socially determined circumstances

Health inequity—systematic differences in opportunities groups have to achieve optimal health because of their social position or other socially determined circumstance

Heterosexism—the assumption that all people are or should be heterosexual; excludes the needs, concerns, and life experiences of lesbian, gay, bisexual, and queer people while giving advantages to heterosexual people

Internalized racism—the acceptance of stereotypes and discriminatory beliefs that casts one's own racial group as inferior, less capable, and less intelligent than that of the racial majority group

Interpersonal racism—racism that occurs between two individuals; prejudice and discrimination that may be intentional or unintentional

Intersectionality—a critical theoretical framework that describes how intersecting systems of oppression such as racism, ableism, sexism, cisgenderism, heterosexism, and classism structure individual-level experiences, particularly for people marginalized at multiple intersections

Lifecourse—an approach that acknowledges that current health is shaped by exposures to physical, environmental, and psychosocial factors from pregnancy onward

Maternity care desert—areas where there is low or no access to maternity care, no hospitals or birth centers offering pregnancy and birth care, and no perinatal providers

---

Prenatal and Postnatal Care: A Person-Centered Approach, Third Edition. Edited by Karen Trister Grace, Cindy L. Farley, Noelene K. Jeffers, and Tanya Tringali.
© 2024 John Wiley & Sons Ltd. Published 2024 by John Wiley & Sons Ltd.
Companion website: www.wiley.com/go/grace/prenatal

Medical mistrust—lack of confidence in healthcare providers and the healthcare system; a rational or expected response to distinct historical experiences of mistreatment and discrimination in the healthcare and research settings linked to group identity, personal experience, vicarious experiences, and oral histories

Microaggressions—verbal, nonverbal, and environmental slights, snubs, or insults, whether intentional or unintentional, which communicate hostile, derogatory, or negative messages to target persons based solely on their membership in a marginalized group

Poverty—an annual income less than the US federal poverty threshold, which is based on family size and composition

Prejudice—a preconceived opinion that is not based on reason or actual experience, typically negative in nature

Race—a social construct primarily based on phenotype (physical characteristics), ethnicity, and other indicators of social differentiation that results in varying access to power and social and economic resources

Racism—a system of structuring opportunity and assigning value based on physical (phenotypical) characteristics such as skin color and hair texture

Reproductive justice—a cross-disciplinary critical feminist theory, framework, and movement rooted in the lived experience of Black women that upholds the human rights to maintain personal bodily autonomy, have children, not have children, and parent children in safe and sustainable communities

Stereotype—oversimplified attitudes people hold toward those outside one's own experience who are different

Structural competency—awareness of forces that influence health outcomes at levels beyond individual interactions

Structural racism—the totality of ways in which societies foster racial discrimination through mutually reinforcing systems of housing, employment, healthcare, and criminal justice

Introduction

Health and well-being during the pregnancy continuum is not experienced equally among all populations in the United States. Some communities and populations experience significant and persistent **health disparities,** defined as differences in the incidence, prevalence, or burden of disease in a subgroup when compared to a larger population. It is important to recognize that the root causes of these disparities have no easy, quick solution. Healthcare providers will not be able to resolve the deep-seated societal and historical factors shaping these disparities during their brief interactions with the client. So, why is there a need to understand them? It is necessary for healthcare providers to understand the structural and social factors that impact a person's **lifecourse** and which subsequently affect the course of the pregnancy and present risks to the pregnant person and their fetus (Crear-Perry et al., 2021; Jones et al., 2019). Healthcare providers play a role in decreasing the nation's health disparities and promoting **health equity** by providing respectful, holistic care that addresses structural and social determinants of health. Comprehensive, multilevel assessment and intervention that involves a team of committed personnel and knowledge of local social services is necessary. A team-based approach to assisting the person to access available resources is a beginning step in optimizing health for the client, their child, and their family. Additionally, all healthcare providers can promote structural change through advocacy for equitable public policies and institutional practices, and by leading the way for new, respectful cultural norms around healthcare.

Key Conceptual Frameworks and Theories

This edition of this text highlights health disparities across a range of populations, explores the root causes of these disparities, and identifies potential solutions to achieve health equity. This chapter introduces current theories underlying the differences in health outcomes. All chapters that follow draw attention to the inequities specific to the content of the chapter in a text box titled *Health Equity Key Points*.

Reproductive Justice

Reproductive justice is a cross-disciplinary critical feminist framework, social movement, and theory that upholds the human right to maintain personal bodily autonomy, have children, not have children, and parent children in safe and sustainable communities. The reproductive justice framework is rooted in the lived experience of reproductive oppression experienced by Black women in historical and contemporary forms.

Origins of the reproductive justice movement

The concept of Reproductive Justice began to take shape when members of a women of color delegation returned from the 1994 International Conference on Population and Development in Cairo, Egypt. Shortly after, a group of African-American women caucused at the Illinois Pro-Choice Alliance Conference in Chicago. The group became known as Women of African Descent for Reproductive Justice. They decided to devise a strategy to challenge the proposed healthcare reform campaign by the Clinton Administration that did not include guaranteeing access to abortion. They integrated the concepts of reproductive rights, social justice, and human rights to launch the term "Reproductive Justice"—Loretta Ross

(Source: Graham, 2015).

Whereas the reproductive rights movement was originally framed around individualism related to the legal right to privacy, choice, and access and was primarily concerned with the right to abortion, the reproductive justice movement is centered on the lived experience of reproductive oppression of Black women (Ross & Solinger, 2017). For Black women, reproductive oppression has included abortion restriction as well as other forms of reproductive control, rooted in **eugenics**, that were designed to limit childbearing (e.g., forced sterilization; Ko, 2016). Additionally, structural racism, economic marginalization, and exploitation have generated communities with low resources that are not always safe or sustainable environments for having and raising children. Chronic disinvestment and deprivation of Black neighborhoods have led to decreased opportunities in education and employment, increased policing and surveillance, and high levels of crime (Krivo et al., 2015). Implementing the reproductive justice framework includes implementing **intersectionality**, centering the most marginalized, working to achieve human rights, and working to dismantle racism (Ross & Solinger, 2017). Centering the most marginalized means prioritizing the needs of those that are disproportionately impacted by intersecting systems of oppression (e.g., racism, ableism, sexism, **heterosexism**, cisgenderism, and classism). The reproductive justice movement is grounded in a human rights framework, which recognizes that every person, regardless of identity or social group membership, has a set of inalienable rights, and it is the responsibility of governments and healthcare institutions to guarantee these rights and to ensure a system of accountability.

Intersectionality

Intersectionality describes how intersecting systems of oppression, such as racism, sexism, ableism, heterosexism, and classism, structure individual-level experiences, particularly for people marginalized at multiple intersections (Bowleg, 2012). For example, someone may experience marginalization at the intersection of their racial/ethnic *and* sexual *and* disability status) (Bowleg, 2012). This framework was developed by Kimberlé Crenshaw, a civil rights and **critical race theory** scholar (Crenshaw, 1989, 1991). She originally conceptualized intersectionality based on her observation that Black women stand at a "crossroads" or an intersection of marginalized identities. Black women faced hundreds of years of racism, but the civil rights movement focused primarily on the struggles of Black men. Similarly, the feminist movement and efforts to address sexism and gender **discrimination** were primarily concerned with the needs of White women and failed to advocate for the rights of Black women. Intersectionality calls us to think about how individuals and groups may be excluded or oppressed based on the marginalized identities that they hold and their relative distance from power.

> Intersectionality is a lens through which you can see where power comes and collides, where it interlocks and intersects. It's not simply a race problem here, a gender problem here, and a class or LGBTQ problem there. Many times, that framework erases what happens to people who are subject to all of these things.—Kimberlé Crenshaw
>
> (Source: Columbia Law School, 2017).

Systems of Oppression and Their Impact on Health

Racism

This section provides an overview of **racism** and its conceptual underpinnings, with the caveat that there are no universally accepted definitions of racism. The definitions and conceptualizations presented below are commonly used, but as racism is increasingly studied, the understanding and conceptualization of racism will evolve. It is critical for healthcare providers to approach this topic with humility and a commitment to continual self-education.

Racism occurs across multiple levels: individual, interpersonal, and structural (Ford & Airhihenbuwa, 2010; Bailey et al., 2017; Dean & Thorpe, 2022). **Internalized racism** is sometimes referred to as internalized racial oppression, and it is a form of individual-level racism that includes the acceptance of **stereotypes** and discriminatory beliefs that cast one's own racial group as inferior, less capable, and less intelligent than that of the racial majority group (Gale et al., 2020; Williams & Williams-Morris, 2000). **Interpersonal racism** occurs between two individuals. **Structural racism** is "the totality of ways in which societies foster racial discrimination through mutually reinforcing systems of housing, employment, healthcare, and criminal justice" (Bailey et al., 2017, p. 1453). There are multiple pathways through which racism is theorized to impact health outcomes (see the text box titled *Pathways Linking Racism to Health Outcomes*).

> ### Pathways linking racism to health outcomes
>
> Physiologic response to chronic stress caused by exposure to multilevel racism.
>
> 1. Results in overactivation of the hypothalamic–pituitary–adrenal axis and release of cortisol and other maternal stress hormones that produce uterine contractions may lead to preterm birth (PTB).
> 2. Chronic stress weakens the immune system, making a pregnant person more prone to illness and infection that can induce poor outcomes such as PTB and hypertensive disorders.
> 3. Chronic stress causes a hyperinflammatory state that contributes to the pathogenesis of preterm labor and birth. The body's response to stress as a result of racism leads to measurable increases in biological markers that propagate the pathophysiologic processes contributing to racial disparities in PTB.
>
> Differential exposure to social and environmental risks such as neighborhood safety and housing.
> Differential access to socioeconomic opportunities.
> Differential access to quality healthcare and health information.
>
> Source: Borders et al. (2015); Black et al. (2014); Williams & Mohammed (2013).

Internalized Racism

Internalized racism is often a result of exposure to racism at other levels (i.e., interpersonal and structural). There is a dearth of research specifically examining the relationship between internalized racism and perinatal health outcomes and experiences. However, internalized racism is associated with negative psychological and mental health impacts including depression, anxiety, and low self-esteem (Gale et al., 2020).

Interpersonal Racism

The vast majority of the research examining racism and perinatal health focuses on the experience of interpersonal racism (Bailey et al., 2017). Significant relationships are demonstrated between racial discrimination and preterm birth (PTB), small for gestational age, and low birth weight (Alhusen et al., 2016; Black et al., 2014; Bower et al., 2018). Additionally, the greater the exposure to racially discriminatory events, the greater the negative impact on birth outcomes (Black et al., 2014). Experiences of racial discrimination occur both inside and outside of healthcare settings.

Structural Racism

Structural racism is a key driver of **social determinants of health** and contributes to significant health disparities in maternal and infant morbidity and mortality that persist in the United States. The impact of structural racism occurs across the reproductive lifespan and is not just confined to pregnancy (Chambers et al., 2021). Black women in particular have noted that structural racism intersects in many ways, through negative cultural attitudes; housing discrimination and inaffordability; differential access to quality healthcare; **bias** in the law enforcement system; exclusion from hidden resources and opportunities; reduced employment opportunities; diminished education options and disinvestment in community infrastructure; and the policing of Black families (Chambers et al., 2021). Structural racism, measured through exposure to racial residential segregation, incarceration inequality, and income inequality are associated with race-associated disparities in PTB, low birth weight, stillbirth, and severe maternal morbidity (Chambers

et al., 2020, 2019, 2018; Janevic et al., 2021; Wallace et al., 2015; Williams et al., 2018).

Race-Associated Perinatal Health Disparities

It is critical for providers to understand the contributing factors to race-associated perinatal health disparities. Disparities and healthcare experiences are shaped by structural, not biological, factors. For many years, unacceptable theories that espoused a biologic definition of **race** blamed people of color for the poor health outcomes they experienced (Scott et al., 2019). These theories advanced the idea that there were intractable, biological differences between racial groups. The most accurate etiology of racial health disparities relies on an understanding of race as a social construct and the fact that racism, not race, causes and sustains these longstanding perinatal health disparities.

Inequities in perinatal healthcare, healthcare experiences, and outcomes across racial and ethnic populations must be addressed. A nation's maternal and infant mortality rates are indicative of the value and political will put toward safeguarding the health of its residents. In 2020, there were 23.8 maternal deaths for every 100,000 live births in the United States—a ratio more than double that of most other high-income countries (Hoyert, 2022; Organization for Economic Co-Operation and Development [OECD], 2022). In contrast, the maternal mortality ratio was 3 per 100,000 or fewer in the Netherlands, Norway, and New Zealand. In addition, whereas worldwide the maternal mo rate has decreased by 43% since 1990, the United States remains the only industrialized nation in which the maternal mortality has increased in recent years (see Figure 1.1; Centers for Disease Control and Prevention [CDC], 2022a; OECD, 2022).

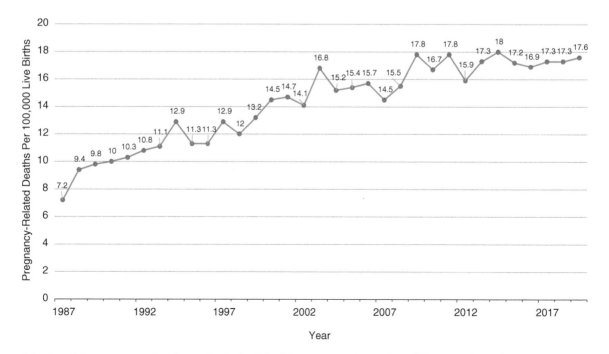

Figure 1.1 Trends in pregnancy-related mortality in the United States, 1987–2018. Adapted from CDC (2022a).

Table 1.1 Selected Maternal and Infant Outcomes by Race/Ethnicity

Outcomes	Total	White, Non-Hispanic, or Latinx	Black or African-American, not Hispanic or Latinx	American Indian or Alaska Native	Asian	Native Hawaiian or other Pacific Islander	Hispanic or Latinx
Preterm live births (percent, <37 weeks), 2020	10.1	9.1	14.4	11.6	8.5	12.1	9.8
Infant deaths, 2020 (number per 1,000 live births)	5.4	4.4	10.6	7.7	3.1	7.2	4.7
Maternal mortality (number per 100,000 live births through 42 days postpartum), 2020	23.8	19.1	55.3	[a]	[a]	[a]	18.2
Pregnancy-related deaths (number per 100,000 live births through one year postpartum), 2016–2018	17.3	13.7	41.4	26.5	14.1		11.3

[a] 2020 rates not reported by CDC due to low number of deaths in this group.
Source: Adapted from CDC (2022a); Ely and Driscoll (2022); Osterman et al. (2022); Organization for Economic Co-Operation and Development (2022).

Approximately 84% of these maternal deaths are preventable—a fact that simultaneously incites incredulity about our society's tacit acceptance of these deaths and also hope that change is possible (Trost et al., 2022). Black and Indigenous birthing people bear a disproportionate burden of this maternal mortality crisis with pregnancy mortality rates three to four times and almost twice, respectively, as high as White birthing people (CDC, 2022a). In addition to mortality, Black pregnant people also experience disparities in other key perinatal health outcomes including PTB, infant mortality, and severe maternal morbidity (Table 1.1).

Experiences of Care

In addition to experiencing persistent perinatal health outcome disparities, people of color also report that mistreatment, disrespect, racism, and discrimination are commonly experienced when receiving care during pregnancy, birth, and postpartum. In one recent study assessing mistreatment in pregnancy or birth in the United States, White women were the least likely to report being mistreated (14.1%; Vedam et al., 2019), while almost one-third of Native American reported being mistreated (32.8%); many Hispanic (25.0%) and Black (22.5%) women reported at least one form of mistreatment. Common forms of mistreatment included being shouted at, having their request declined or not responded to in a timely manner, having their physical privacy violated, and being threatened by their healthcare provider with withholding treatment (Vedam et al., 2019). Women of color consistently report that they are not listened to, are not provided with education needed to make an informed decision, or are excluded from decision-making during the perinatal period (Altman et al., 2019; Lori et al., 2011; Mclemore et al., 2018). Women of color also explicitly report experiencing differential treatment by healthcare providers or healthcare staff because of their race, class, insurance status, or other characteristics associated with membership in a group that has experienced marginalization (McLemore et al., 2018; Mehra et al., 2020; Okoro et al., 2020).

Strategies to Address Racism in Perinatal Health

In addition to identifying the effects of racism on perinatal health, it is imperative to implement sustainable and effective multilevel strategies to address racism. The perinatal healthcare provider should begin with intense and ongoing self-reflection of the internal attitudes and biases that might manifest in implicit and explicit ways in the client–provider interactions and through clinical decision-making (Koschmann et al., 2020). Clinicians who want to explore their biases around race and other salient domains, such as weight, gender, and disability, can take implicit association tests (https://implicit.harvard.edu/implicit/index.jsp) created by Project Implicit at Harvard University. This is a first step in becoming more aware of biases, and the healthcare provider can use their increased awareness as a jumping off point to foster internal change.

Healthcare providers can also work toward developing **structural competency**, an awareness of forces that influence health outcomes at levels beyond individual interactions (Metzl & Hansen, 2014). Viewing **health inequities** through a structural lens helps avoid placing blame on clients and sees health inequities not as individual but societal failings. This is a lens that requires continual refinement because our knowledge of how structural dynamics impact health is rapidly advancing. Being committed to developing this lens and growing in consciousness serves to empower the clinician to identify ways that they as individuals and as capable actors within the healthcare system can advocate for change and develop effective interventions.

Table 1.2 Culturally Affirming Models of Midwifery and Perinatal Support

Organization	Website
BeLovedBirth Black Centering in Oakland CA	https://www.alamedahealthsystem.org/family-birthing-center/black-centering
Changing Woman Initiative in New Mexico	https://cwi-health.org
CHOICES Center for Reproductive Health in Memphis, TN	https://yourchoices.org/midwifery-services
Community of Hope Family Health and Birth Center Washington, DC	https://www.communityofhopedc.org
Kindred Space in Los Angeles, CA	https://kindredspacela.com
Mamatoto Village in Washington, DC	https://www.mamatotovillage.org

There are also a number of promising strategies that can be implemented through policy and practice changes in the healthcare system to address racism by promoting healthy perinatal outcomes.

- *Expansion of postpartum Medicaid coverage:* Over two-thirds of maternal deaths occur in the postpartum period, and expanding postpartum Medicaid coverage from the first 60 days after birth through the first 12 months postpartum might help postpartum people remain connected to the healthcare system and provide opportunities to reduce preventable maternal mortality (Daw et al., 2020; Gordon et al., 2020; Kumar et al., 2021).
- *Restructuring and individualizing postpartum care beyond the six-week visit:* In 2018, the American College of Obstetricians and Gynecologists (ACOG) recommended that every person receive individualized postpartum care with multiple opportunities to engage with a healthcare provider (2021a). At a minimum, this includes a recommended contact with a healthcare provider in the first three weeks after birth (e.g., phone call, in-office visit, and home visit) and a comprehensive postpartum visit that occurs between 4 and 12 weeks. Additional visits such as blood pressure checks and other high-risk follow-up care are provided as indicated. The new guidelines emphasize that postpartum care is an ongoing process that should be individualized based on the person's health and social needs.
- *Integrating doulas into the perinatal health system:* Doulas provide information and health education, engage in advocacy, and provide practical and emotional support. Doula support is associated with reduced cesarean sections, increased vaginal births, decreased use of pain-relief medications, greater duration of breastfeeding, and improved satisfaction with birth (Bohren et al., 2017). National and state efforts to train, pay, and support doulas can help promote the sustainable integration of doulas into the healthcare system and normalize them as an integral part of the perinatal health team. As of publication, approximately half of all states provide Medicaid doula reimbursements or are in the process of implementing this coverage (Chen, 2022). Additionally, the US Department of Health and Human Services devoted $4.5 million dollars in 2022 to hire, train, and pay community doulas (2022).
- *Culturally affirming models of care:* The emergence of culturally affirming models of midwifery and perinatal support are increasingly seen as a promising intervention to transform the current landscape of perinatal care (see Table 1.2 for examples of Culturally Affirming Black and Indigenous Models of Care; Golden et al., 2022). These models prioritize racial/cultural concordance, incorporate cultural strengths, and emphasize social support, relationship-building, and culturally safety. Efforts to scale up and invest in these models of care are underway.

Ableism

Ableism is a set of beliefs and practices that devalue and discriminate against people with physical, intellectual, or psychiatric disabilities and often rests on the assumption that people with disabilities need to be "fixed" in some way (Smith, n.d.). Similar to racism, it is helpful to conceptualize ableism as a multilevel framework, including individual, interpersonal, and structural levels. Approximately one in four American adults has a disability (Okoro, 2018). Perinatal healthcare providers should anticipate that they will care for people with disabilities since about 12% of people with capacity for pregnancy have a disability (Courtney-Long et al., 2015) and people with disabilities are equally as likely to report a pregnancy as people without disabilities (Horner-Johnson et al., 2016). A **disability** is "any condition of the body or mind (impairment) that makes it more difficult for the person with the condition to do certain activities (activity limitation) and interact with the world around them (participation restriction)" (CDC, 2020). Disability categories include, but are not limited to, those disabilities that are acquired, congenital, intellectual, neurologic, sensory, mobility-related, psychiatric, and episodic. People with disabilities are not monolithic. Individuals may have one or multiple disabilities and not all disabilities are immediately visible. Additionally, one form of disability may impact two individuals in different ways.

Language considerations when caring for disabled people

The phrase "disabled people" is an example of identity first language. Disabled people who use identity first language prefer this approach because it posits "disabled" as a positive identity and affirms disability culture. Others prefer to use person-first language such as "people with disabilities." Person-first language puts the person before the disability, making sure not to reduce the person to their disability. However, this approach has been criticized because it implies that disability is negative. There is no one correct approach, and preferences for person-first or identify-first language will vary. This chapter uses both phrases interchangeably, as both are appropriate. Clients with disabilities may prefer one approach over another. Thus, healthcare providers should ask clients their preferred terminology.

Source: Andrews et al. (2022).

Perinatal health disparities exist among disabled pregnant and birthing people (Akobirshoev et al., 2019; Mitra et al., 2015; Ransohoff et al., 2022), and the causes are likely multifactorial. Some disparities may be related to medical complications associated with the individual's disability, but some may be due to implicit and explicit bias including negative attitudes around pregnancy among people with disabilities, and structural barriers. Disabled pregnant people report that their healthcare provider may have limited knowledge of their disability, appear unprepared to manage their pregnancy given this limited knowledge, and exhibit bias during clinical encounters (Mitra et al., 2016; Tarasoff, 2015). Structural barriers include inaccessibility of medical offices, examination rooms, scales, and other equipment during pregnancy (Mitra et al., 2016).

Perinatal disparities among disabled people

- There are increased rates of preterm birth and low birth among women with physical disabilities compared to women without disabilities.
- Black/African-American birthing people with intellectual and developmental disabilities experience higher risks of stillbirth and labor- and birth-related medical billing charges as compared to White birthing people with intellectual and developmental disabilities.
- Women with physical and intellectual disabilities are less likely to receive prenatal care in the first trimester than women without physical and intellectual disabilities.
- Infants born to women with disabilities were more likely to experience infant mortality and have a need for intensive care as compared to infants born to women without disabilities.
- Women with disabilities experience higher odds of experiencing early pregnancy loss than women without disabilities.

Source: Akobirshoev et al. (2019); Dissanayake et al. (2020); Mitra et al. (2015); Mwachofi Brodi (2017); Ransohoff et al. (2022).

Caring for Pregnant People with Disabilities

Healthcare providers should examine the assumptions, beliefs, and attitudes they have toward people with disabilities. Many healthcare providers operate within a framework called the medical model of disability, which frames disability as a problem (Andrews et al., 2022). However, the end of the twentieth century saw the rise of the social model of disability, which proposes that disability is actually socially constructed and that the exclusion of people with disabilities from full participation in society is based on and perpetuated by bias and prejudice toward disability. The diversity model builds on the social model of disability by acknowledging the impact of discrimination, racism, and bias and promoting disability pride that rebuffs internalized ableism and accepts disability as a natural part of human diversity.

Healthcare providers should engage in learning and be prepared to offer or to refer to relevant services and support. Doulas may also provide additional support to people with disabilities (Horton & Hall, 2020). Healthcare providers should also be aware of the landmark federal civil rights laws, which impact people with disabilities, and be knowledgeable about how these laws impact clinical practice (Table 1.3; Iezzoni et al., 2022).

Cisgenderism and Heterosexism

Cisgenderism, transphobia, homophobia, heterosexism, and heteronormativity all describe systems of oppression and discrimination against people who have gender identities and sexual orientations other than cisgender and/or heterosexual. A heteronormative and cisgenderist society makes assumptions about sexual desire only occurring between men and women, and gender expression matching sex assignment at birth. These assumptions exclude people with other identities, rendering them invisible and vulnerable to harm. There is ample evidence that the discrimination faced by people with these identities within and outside of the healthcare setting impacts health, including the experience of parenting and parenting stress (Appelgren Engström et al., 2022), inappropriate and unnecessary medical care (Hoffkling et al., 2017), and reduced screening and preventive care (Elk, 2021; Rosenberg et al., 2021). Health equity is supported by practitioners who provide inclusive care including use of correct names and pronouns, normalizing patient gender expression, efforts to educate themselves, and creation of accepting and respectful healthcare environments (Hoffkling et al., 2017); see Chapter 25, *Preconception, Pregnancy, and Postpartum Care of LGBTQ+ Individuals*.

Classism

Wealth distribution and unequal opportunities have broad implications for people's lives and health outcomes. The burden of health inequity is inequitably borne by people with lower socioeconomic status, due to lower quality healthcare resources, barriers to access, increased exposure to toxic environments and other

Table 1.3 Overview of Federal Civil Rights Laws for People with Disabilities

Year	Federal statutes	Major civil rights protections
1973	Section 504 of the Rehabilitation Act	Forbids organizations and employers from excluding or denying individuals with disabilities an equal opportunity to receive federal program benefits and services.
1990	Americans with Disabilities Act (ADA)	Landmark legislation that defined disability and empowered individuals to file suit for protection under the ADA. In the context of healthcare, it mandates that clinical practices must: • Provide equal access and "reasonable" accommodations" to people with disabilities. • Decisions about accommodation must take place within collaboration, incorporating both the healthcare provider's judgment about clinical appropriateness and the client's preferences and needs. • Not refuse to see a patient due to their disability. • Pay costs associated with providing reasonable accommodations. Patients cannot be required to provide their own accommodations. This law is enforced by the Department of Justice and the Office of Civil Rights in the Department of Health and Human Services.
2008	ADA Amendments Act (ADAAA)	Intended to clarify and expand the scope of the definition of disability which had previously been so narrowly defined that many people were excluded from the law's protections. Made it easier for individuals who were seeking protection of the ADA to establish that they have a disability that falls within the definition outlined in the statute.

Source: Adapted from ADA National Network (2017, 2020); Iezzoni et al. (2022).

health threats, and fewer sources of resilience, such as healthy food, safe outdoor green space, and mental health/wellness resources. In addition, overt discrimination is experienced by people based on their social class, both within the healthcare system, directly impacting care, and in everyday interactions, influencing stress and chronic health conditions. **Classism** has self-perpetuating aspects as well, when the experience of illness further impacts an individual's economic well-being (Fisher et al., 2021). Providers working with people who are economically marginalized must consider ways that their healthcare systems can promote respectful high-quality care regardless of ability to pay, which accommodates a variety of work schedules and transportation and childcare challenges among other barriers to healthcare. Supporting structural solutions to classist inequities in healthcare outcomes including universal healthcare coverage is another way providers can work to advance health equity.

Sexism

Individual-level misogyny and discrimination on the basis of sex assigned at birth is also an oppressive system impacting health equity. **Sexism**, the systematic privileging of people who identify as men, exists on a structural level as well, manifesting as wage and workforce participation gaps, restrictions on abortion access, patriarchal and conservative religions, and social policies (Homan, 2021). A "benevolent" sexism is experienced by pregnant people who receive paternalistic advice to avoid certain foods or activities or who are refused service in restaurants and bars, ultimately maintaining broader hostilities and social injustice (Sutton et al., 2011). The impact of sexism on health outcomes is greater for women who are also

people of color, reflecting the exacerbation of effects based on intersectional identities (Homan et al., 2021; Rapp et al., 2021).

Social Determinants of Perinatal Health

In this section, we explore some of the major **social determinants of health**, describe how they might impact health and well-being during pregnancy, and offer practical suggestions for addressing the social determinants of health in the context of prenatal care. Healthcare providers may want to incorporate routine or targeted screening for needs related to these social determinants of health. We have included resources for screening for social needs in the *Resources for Healthcare Providers* section.

Food

Lack of financial resources impacts the ability to obtain adequate nutrition, which is a significant factor in maintaining a healthy pregnancy (Cox & Phelan, 2008; Harnisch et al., 2012; Procter & Campbell, 2014). **Food insecurity**, or concerns about one's ability to obtain adequate and safe nutrition, can lead to underweight, overweight, or obesity (Koller et al., 2022; Sarlio-Lähteenkorva & Lahelma, 2001; Townsend et al., 2001). Food insecurity in pregnancy is also associated with disordered eating, variations in gestational weight gain dependent on initial weight, and decreased likelihood of breastfeeding (Laraia et al., 2022). Inadequate nutrition can be characterized by insufficient intake of calories as well as deficiencies of vitamins and minerals in spite of adequate or excessive caloric intake. The latter often occurs when people purchase foods that are less expensive but have low nutritional value (Sarlio-Lähteenkorva & Lahelma, 2001). These foods often contain high amounts of saturated fats, sodium, and calories but contain very little in the way of vitamins and minerals. Alternatively, people may experience cycles of food unavailability followed by availability, during which they overeat or indulge in energy-dense foods (Townsend et al., 2001). People with this type of eating pattern may be overweight, whereas those with a chronically insufficient caloric intake will likely be underweight or lose weight during pregnancy if the demands of the pregnancy outweigh intake. People with limited incomes are at risk of periods of no or low weight gain, followed by excessive weight gain, during pregnancy (Herring et al., 2012). In both cases, the pregnant person and fetus are not provided the nutrients and calories for optimal health. Food insecurity is a social determinant of health and is highly influenced by income and significant life events (e.g., death of a loved one, birth of a child, marriage, major illness, and job loss; Banks et al., 2021). Additionally, some groups may be more at risk for food insecurity including some racial and ethnic groups (e.g., Black, Latinx; Walker et al., 2021) and people with disabilities (Heflin et al., 2019). Structural factors, including racism and neighborhood segregation, can influence these relationships. Evidence of the impact of food insecurity on breastfeeding duration is mixed. One large study of the 2009–2014 National Health and Nutrition Examination Surveys found no relationship (Orozco et al., 2020), but other studies found decreased duration of breastfeeding (Dinour et al., 2020; Gross et al., 2019).

The availability of healthy food items, including fresh fruits and vegetables, is limited in low-income neighborhoods, causing them to historically be referred to as **food deserts** (Treuhaft & Karpyn, 2010). However, the term **food apartheid** is growing in popularity because it acknowledges that the inequitable distribution of good quality and healthful food options is not naturally occurring, like a desert, but rather is the consequence of intentional design through the structural factors designed to uphold racism such as racial residential segregation (Sbicca, 2012). Few grocery stores in low-income areas carry high-quality fresh food, while high-fat, high-calorie fast-food options are readily available. Clients trying to make healthier food choices may need to travel further to obtain these items, making the availability of transportation crucial to health status. For example, in Mississippi, the state with the highest level of adult and childhood obesity in the country, 70% of individuals eligible for food stamps travel at least 30 miles in order to find a grocery store that will accept food stamps. The presence of corner stores and liquor stores in low-income areas is 30% greater than in higher income neighborhoods and sheds light on what is readily available to low-income people in their home communities. The absence of vital healthy food options within certain communities is incongruous in a wealthy nation.

Addressing food security during the prenatal visit can be challenging due to stigma and fear. While there is no current recommendation for routine screening around food insecurity, prenatal care providers might consider adding it to their social history, especially when there are high rates of food insecurity in their clinical practice communities. Similar to other sensitive topics, routine screening might reduce barriers to disclosing, especially given that food insecurity might evoke shame, stigma, and fear of intrusive intervention by authorities. Healthcare providers should be prepared to provide relevant resources and referrals should their clients report food insecurity. In addition to the social services described in detail below, healthcare providers should be aware of community resources to deal with food insecurity, including soup kitchens, diaper banks, and food pantries (Belarmino et al., 2021).

Healthcare providers can refer clients to their local office of Women, Infants, and Children (WIC). The WIC program is federally funded and located in each state. Eligibility requirements are determined based on categorical, residential, financial, and nutritional risks. All pregnant people are eligible during pregnancy and up to six weeks after birth, early pregnancy loss, or pregnancy termination. Infants up to one year and children up to five years of age are also categorically eligible. Residential requirements are that the pregnant/postpartum person, infant, or child live in the state through which the benefit is administered. There is no requirement for the length of residency. Financial eligibility is determined by each state but must be between 100% and 185% of federal poverty requirements. Nutritional risk is determined either by the WIC office or by a healthcare provider. A preapplication assessment is available online to determine eligibility and lists the documentation needed as well as the address of the local WIC office (US Department of Agriculture, 2017).

Healthcare providers can also refer clients to apply for benefits through the Supplemental Nutrition Assistance Program (SNAP; formerly called the Food Stamp Program). The SNAP provides important nutritional support for low-income families and older adults and people with disabilities living on fixed incomes (Center on Budget and Policy Priorities, 2022). Persons may be eligible if their household income is at or below 130% of the federal poverty line; benefits may vary if they are disabled or elderly. Per-person SNAP benefits totaled approximately $127 per month (or about $4.16 a day) in 2021, although they were temporarily expanded due to the COVID-19 pandemic to $218 per month (or about $7.30 a day) (Center on Budget and Policy Priorities, 2022). Receiving SNAP benefits has been shown to reduce the likelihood of food insecurity by 30% (Mabli et al., 2013). SNAP benefits can be used in most grocery, convenience, large retail, and some online stores. Many farmers markets also accept SNAP benefits, and some may offer a matching program where clients can double some or all of their SNAP benefits.

Housing

Understanding the healthcare implications of poor housing compared to safe and sanitary housing is essential to providing comprehensive perinatal healthcare. Access to safe and comfortable shelter is significantly influenced and limited by poverty. Furthermore, housing that is crowded, unsanitary, with poor lighting and aeration, utilities not up to code, containing peeling, lead-based paint, surrounded by violence and drug use, or infested with insects and/or rodents creates unsafe and stressful conditions that expose the pregnant person and fetus to physical, environmental, and psychological threats to health (Chaudhuri, 2004; Raugh et al., 2008). In pregnancy, psychological distress caused by living conditions can lead to biophysical changes, such as increased cortisol levels, that adversely impact fetal intra-uterine growth and development (LeWinn et al., 2009; Obel et al., 2005).

Poverty plays a key role in the homelessness of families and individuals since the majority of persons experiencing homelessness cite the inability to afford housing and/or unemployment as the reasons behind their homelessness (National Alliance to End Homelessness, 2022). Rates of poverty have increased in recent years, and the homelessness rate continues to be a national crisis.

The healthcare needs of pregnant people experiencing homelessness can be varied and complex. Homeless women are more likely to have poorly managed chronic illness, communicable diseases, mental illness, substance abuse, chronic stress, and histories of physical and sexual abuse (ACOG, 2013). Unstable housing can result in delays or disruptions in healthcare for conditions that are easily prevented or managed; concerns about shelter, food, and safety often take priority over healthcare needs (McGeough et al., 2020). These concerns, along with barriers such as lack of transportation or childcare for other children, have historically interfered with the ability to obtain consistent prenatal care and continue to elude effective intervention. The cumulative effect of these stressors also places pregnant people experiencing homelessness at an increased risk for PTB (Cutts et al., 2015; DiTosto et al., 2021).

An assessment of a client's living arrangements should always be conducted during care, understanding that people experiencing homelessness might be hesitant to disclose. Some parents have been reported to child protective services and have had their children taken away because of homelessness (Smid et al., 2010). A punitive process such as this must be avoided; rather, clients should be assisted in obtaining safe and sanitary living arrangements. Building a trusting and compassionate relationship during prenatal care will increase the likelihood that clients will continue their care and enhance health outcomes. The healthcare provider should become familiar with available housing resources in order to educate clients of their options, in addition to making a referral to social services for further assistance.

Families in poverty are more likely to be headed by single mothers and are more vulnerable to experiencing homelessness. Single mothers who are also homeless experience compounded stress at a level higher than those dealing with either of the two conditions alone, creating significant concerns for health, fetal health, depression, lack of social support, unintended pregnancy, unemployment, or underemployment, low parenting satisfaction, and punitive parenting practices (Broussard, 2010; Crosier et al., 2007; Eamon & Wu, 2011; Finer & Henshaw, 2006; Wu & Eamon, 2011; Zhan, 2006).

Economic Stability

Pregnant clients with low income may experience challenges that affect the health of the individual and their fetus and place them at risk for poor outcomes. People with low income are likely to experience more stressors and hardship around the time of pregnancy than those with higher incomes; these life stressors can include job loss, homelessness, intimate partner violence, relationship dissolution, and incarceration (Braveman et al., 2010). Poverty is a risk factor in PTB and low birth weight (McHale et al., 2022). Furthermore, children who are born into impoverished environments are exposed to a variety of related stressors and have increased risk for poor behavioral, emotional, and physical outcomes including malnutrition, chronic disease, developmental delays, and low school performance (Engle & Black, 2008).

Clients with low income may benefit from referrals to a variety of social services. Insurance coverage for pregnancy care is a priority, so assistance to access Medicaid is an ideal starting point. Financial assistance for families with minor children is available under the Temporary Assistance to Needy Families program. An interdisciplinary approach that includes medical and social as well as legal services will provide the most comprehensive overview of available options. Since the breadth of many services is determined by income levels, it can be helpful for healthcare providers to help clients locate where they fall in respect to federal poverty thresholds. A basic understanding of how income will be defined by agencies offering medical, social, and legal assistance can help clients anticipate their eligibility. For example, the poverty threshold for families with two adults and one child is $21,811.00 whereas the threshold for one adult and three children is $27,575 (US Census Bureau, 2022).

Some clients may be single parents, and while adequate finances do not address all of the challenges that single parents face, they can relieve some of the burden of parenting alone. Obtaining child support from the other parent of the baby through legal means is another intervention that can alleviate some financial hardships (Huang & Han, 2012). The Office of Child Support Enforcement, a division of the US Department of Health and Human Services, exists to assist custodial parents in establishing paternity in cases of uncertainty or contest, determining the amount of support that is owed, and acquiring support from the noncustodial parent. Clients should be referred to their state Child Support Enforcement Office for information on the specific procedure and documentation required to initiate a case in that state. Links to information on collecting child support and contact information to state Child Support Enforcement Offices are available in the *Resources for Clients and Their Families* section.

Education

Education is touted by many to be an equalizer of inequity in multiple areas, but studies show that the impact of racism overshadows benefits of education on health outcomes for Black pregnant people (Homan et al., 2021). Nonetheless, education-based solutions are paramount to establishing health equity. Segregated school systems on racial and economic lines perpetuate systemic societal-level injustice that is reflected in health inequity. When students have health challenges, their education and ability to learn are compromised. Educational institutions are also important vehicles for educating people about health, health risks, and protective behaviors (Hahn & Truman, 2015). The relationship between a strong and just education system and public health is an essential component of achieving health equity.

Social and Community Context

Health equity and pregnancy and birth outcomes are strongly impacted by social and community support. Support may come from partners, family, friends, religious communities, professional networks, or cultural organizations. Higher social support may provide a buffering effect for some people against the impact of negative influences on health outcomes such as stress (Hetherington et al., 2015). Reporting inadequate social support is associated with being unpartnered, having economic challenges, and coping with mental health disorders, such as depression and anxiety (Bedaso et al., 2021), though many of these factors are interdependent and temporal associations are unclear. It is important to note that those who are unmarried but partnered may not have the same risk for poor outcomes as those who are unpartnered or partnered but in a bad relationship (Young & Declercq, 2010). Research also demonstrates that strong social support networks may override relationship status (Bilszta et al., 2008). Therefore, it is essential to assess client support networks and provide strategies for accessing that support when it is needed during pregnancy and postpartum. For example, a recent study showed that single parents drawing on informal childcare from members of their social networks had more positive employment trajectories than those without such support (Brady, 2016).

Healthcare Access and Quality

Access to high-quality healthcare is a critical component of health equity. In 2022, the March of Dimes report on **maternity care deserts** highlighted that approximately one out of every three people with the capacity for pregnancy and who are of reproductive age (35.6%) live in a maternity care desert. Maternity care deserts are counties in the United States that have zero hospitals or birthing centers and zero maternity care providers (see Table 1.4). Many individuals also live in areas with low (11.9%) or moderate (7.9%) maternity care access. While the vast majority of maternity care deserts are located in rural counties (81.4%), almost one in five maternity care deserts are urban (18.6%). Segregation of neighborhoods remains common in urban and rural communities in the United States (Arnett

Table 1.4   Definitions of Maternity Care Deserts and Access to Maternity Care

Definitions	Maternity care desert	Low access to maternity care	Moderate access to maternity care	Full access
Hospitals and birth centers in county offering pregnancy and birth care	Zero	<2	<2	≥2
Pregnancy and birth care providers in county (OB/GYNS, and CNM/CMs)	Zero	<60	<60	≥60
Proportion of women 18–64 in county without health insurance	N/A	≥10%	<10%	N/A

N/A = not applicable.
Source: March of Dimes (2022).

et al., 2016), limiting access to maternity care providers. For example, 2017 marked the closure of two labor and delivery units in Washington, DC, which mainly affected low-income communities. In 2014, only 75 labor and delivery units remained in Georgia out of 180 hospitals statewide. These closures represent a trend of declining access to maternity care for inner city and rural communities. The presence of maternity care deserts in the setting of poor maternal outcomes in the United States signals a critical need for investment in increasing a diversified perinatal healthcare workforce and expanding the number of facilities that provide obstetric care, including birth centers.

Healthcare in the United States is increasingly unaffordable, limiting access to care. Medicaid is the largest payer for pregnancy-related services, and it covers over 42% of births in the United States (CDC, 2022a; Ranji et al., 2022). The expansion of the Affordable Care Act in 2014 was associated with a number of positive outcomes including greater continuity of insurance coverage in the preconception, pregnancy, and postpartum periods and decreased disparities between Black and White infants in PTB and low birth weight (Bellerose et al., 2022). Medicaid eligibility is generally income based, but variations by state exist and may be based on other characteristics such as immigration status. Providers should be aware of the insurance coverage options available in their state for pregnant people and aware of the insurance options accepted by prenatal care and birth settings. There can be a mismatch in the payment methods accepted by providers and payment methods used by clients, leaving many pregnant people unable to access prenatal healthcare (Arnett et al., 2016).

Healthcare quality varies widely in the United States, and poor perinatal health quality is a major contributor to adverse outcomes and health disparities. Racial residential segregation shapes the quality of care delivered in the hospital setting. Black individuals giving birth in segregated hospitals (i.e., hospitals which serve a disproportionately high number of Black individuals) are at increased risk for severe maternal morbidity (Howell et al., 2016). Other factors shaping the quality of care provided during the birth hospitalization include the on-site availability of anesthesiology, implementation (or lack thereof) of structured approaches to improve processes of care and outcomes, staffing, and more (Howell & Zeitlin, 2017). These factors vary widely by hospital, and efforts to improve the quality of hospital-based perinatal care is an area of emerging research. Research on factors that influence the quality of care in community birth settings (i.e., home birth or birth center practices) is lacking but much needed.

Incarceration and Criminal Justice Involvement

It is estimated that approximately 4% of incarcerated people assigned female at birth (AFAB) are pregnant, but 80% have children (Wang, 2021; Kajstura, 2019). Incarceration has been rapidly increasing among people who are AFAB, rising from 26,378 in 1980 to 222,455 in 2019, representing an increase of more than 700% (Carson, 2021). Most are incarcerated for nonviolent crimes, such as drug possession, sex work, and property offenses (Carson, 2021).

There are disparities in women's rates of imprisonment; Black women were almost twice as likely to be imprisoned in 2015 as White women (Carson & Anderson, 2016). These disparities are rooted in structural racism and bias in the criminal justice system including arrests, pretrial detention and bail decisions, prosecutorial conduct, and sentencing (ACOG, 2021b; The Sentencing Project, 2021). In many cases, drug use and drug-related activities are precipitated by a relationship with a partner who is involved in drugs. Incarcerated women experience disease and mental illness at higher rates than women in the general population (ACOG, 2021b). Healthcare providers working in jails and prisons provide a vital service to this vulnerable population with complex healthcare needs.

Incarcerated people have an increased likelihood of having a history of substance use disorder, exposure to sexually transmitted infections, and intimate partner violence (ACOG, 2021b). People who have been incarcerated at any point in their pregnancy are also at risk for exposure to communicable diseases that are prevalent in places with close living arrangements, such as influenza, tuberculosis, and COVID-19, all of which have increased risks for people who are pregnant. Prenatal care can be the avenue by which incarcerated people receive comprehensive assessment and access treatment and interventions and can enable pregnant people to receive adequate screening, treatment, education, and referrals for problems that might otherwise go unattended (Dooley & Ringler, 2012). However, prenatal care is likely to be initiated later in the pregnancy with inconsistent and inadequate subsequent care (Testa & Jackson, 2020). For clients who are incarcerated, their pregnancies likely occurred in the midst of challenging life circumstances, and attention to the pregnancy may not be an urgent need compared to other hardships that require immediate attention. Managing stressful life circumstances often presents barriers to obtaining the prenatal care and the benefits that it can offer for this high-risk population. Clients with drug-related incarcerations can face barriers to federal programs such as WIC and housing assistance, which exacerbates the financial barriers that might interfere with timely and consistent prenatal care. The impact of criminal justice system involvement is not just limited to the incarcerated person; evidence shows that having a partner who is incarcerated also impacts pregnancy and birth outcomes, including PTB, low birth weight, small for gestational age, and neonatal intensive care unit admission (Yi et al., 2021).

Substance use that leads to incarceration can negatively impact fetal and maternal health. For those who are using drugs during their pregnancy, the fear of detection and punishment may play a role in the lack of timely and sufficient prenatal care. This prevents possible entry into drug rehabilitation to minimize fetal exposure to drugs and alcohol and maximize maternal health. Caring for a person who has been incarcerated should include a thorough assessment of the reasons for their incarceration, with an understanding that a history of substance use is a significant possibility. The healthcare provider must be familiar with the laws guiding local practice since some states require reporting of cases in which a fetus is being exposed to substances during the pregnancy or at birth. For clients who will give birth while incarcerated, anticipatory guidance as to the policies that will affect their care during labor is necessary (see Chapter 18, *Substance Use during Pregnancy*).

While organizations such as the American College of Nurse-Midwives (ACNM) (2016), the ACOG (2021b), the Association of Women's Health, Obstetric and Neonatal Nurses (AWHONN, 2011), and the National Commission on Correctional Health Care (2020) have taken a stance opposing the practice of shackling incarcerated people during labor, many state correction agencies still enforce this policy (Poehlmann & Shlafer, 2016). Healthcare providers not working within a jail or prison system may only rarely encounter an incarcerated client; providers of labor and birth services might, on occasion, attend the birth of a person who is incarcerated. Nonetheless, healthcare providers treat pregnant and postpartum people who have a history of incarceration, who are currently incarcerated, or who are at risk for future incarceration. Those working in a jail or prison system will likely be required to follow strict protocols for prenatal care services developed by prison administration officials. Early prenatal care for people who are at risk for incarceration is essential; the health education and counseling that is a hallmark of quality prenatal care has the potential to influence positive social and health-related changes (Dooley & Ringler, 2012; Hotelling, 2008). Doula care is an underutilized but effective model of care to provide compassionate support for labor and birth among pregnant people who are incarcerated (Shlafer et al., 2015, 2021). Examples of

---

Guidelines to consider for pregnant people experiencing incarceration

1. Recognize that a person's effort to attain prenatal care is a step toward caring for themselves and their baby and that they have likely overcome significant barriers to attend the appointment. Acknowledge efforts to prioritize their and their baby's health.
2. Develop a plan for assessment based on common risk factors.
3. Approach care through a trauma-informed lens and with awareness of gender-related needs.
4. Assess for the following:
   - reasons for incarceration
   - nature of life circumstances leading up to and following the period of incarceration
   - history of childhood and adult exposure to violence, including sexual, physical, and intimate partner violence (IPV)
   - thoughts about the pregnancy, including circumstances surrounding pregnancy, whether the pregnancy was planned or unplanned, plans for pregnancy, parenting, and child placement, involvement of the partner and family members, concerns about parenting, and structure of family and living arrangements
   - depression, anxiety, and emotional distress
   - sexually transmitted infections, including human immunodeficiency virus; provide treatment as needed according to practice guidelines

   - substance use, including last use, drugs used, and attempts at rehabilitation; refer to a specialist for initiation of opioid therapy for people with opioid use disorder
   - maternal attachment and role development in the prenatal and postnatal periods
5. Obtain permission to access any medical records for previous prenatal visits at other clinics.
6. Encourage timely follow-up and assist with removing any identified barriers to attending appointments, such as lack of transportation, lack of childcare for other children, and lack of insurance.
7. Provide education about breastfeeding and assist with needed arrangements for breastfeeding or pumping after birth.
8. Be aware of community options for doula support and refer as necessary.
9. Provide anticipatory education on the circumstances of labor and birth while incarcerated. Advocate for ceasing use of shackles to ensure freedom of movement during labor and birth.
10. Advocate for clients to be kept with their infants after birth.

Source: ACNM (2016); ACOG (2021b); AWHONN (2011); Clarke and Adashi (2011); National Commission on Correctional Health Care (2020).

---

longstanding doula programs that serve incarcerated pregnant people include the Minnesota Prison Doula Project (http://www.mnprisondoulaproject.org) and Birth Behind Bars (https://www.birthbehindbars.com/). Pregnant people with a history of incarceration may be especially motivated during pregnancy to make positive changes and can benefit from support.

Medical Mistrust

Medical mistrust contributes to healthcare disparities (Arnett et al., 2016; Ho et al., 2022). The vast majority of the research around medical mistrust centers on the perspectives and experiences of Black/African-American individuals, but Latinx and Indigenous individuals also report higher levels of mistrust in healthcare providers and institutions as compared to their White counterparts (Benkert et al., 2019). Among immigrants and people with economic challenges, financial constraints or lack of insurance increases susceptibility to care practices that limit patient autonomy, such as relegation to certain hospitals that accept uninsured clients and operate within certain parameters, based on either biased policy or the **prejudices** of the providers accustomed to working with the population. Medical mistrust can lead to underutilization of primary care services and overuse of emergency department services (Arnett et al., 2016; Benkert et al., 2019).

Medical mistrust is a response to historical and ongoing injustices that are rooted in racism and other systems of oppression. Federally funded forced sterilization took place in the twentieth century across the United States, particularly in the South and in Puerto Rico (Ko, 2016). The United States government also has a history of medical exploitation and experimentation on Black Americans. One well-known example is the Tuskegee Study of Untreated Syphilis in the Negro Male, a research study conducted between 1932 and 1972 to observe the natural progression of the disease among Black men (CDC, 2022b). Study participants were informed that they were receiving treatment for the disease, but researchers withheld treatment and actively discouraged them from seeking medical treatment. The study was eventually halted, and it precipitated the creation of national regulations and procedures to provide the ethical oversight of research. However, the Tuskegee study left behind a legacy of mistrust that continues to shape contemporary patterns of healthcare access and utilization. The mistrust continues in present day with a higher proportion of Black women reporting that they do not feel a connection with their providers and that they experience discrimination and **microaggressions** in the prenatal care setting (Lori et al., 2011). Ultimately, it is the responsibility of the healthcare system and healthcare providers to demonstrate trustworthiness and gain the trust of clients through respectful, dignified, and trauma-informed care (Jaiswal, 2019).

Affirming Individual, Family, and Community Strengths

A holistic approach to perinatal health equity promotion calls us to acknowledge that our clients and their families and communities embody unique strengths. Discussions around health equity often inadvertently advance narratives that portray marginalized groups through a predominantly risk-based lens. A common pitfall when discussing health disparities is to advance a deficit-based approach in which groups that have experienced marginalization are viewed solely as products of oppressive structural dynamics. Healthcare providers should avoid reducing clients to risk factors but rather utilize a strength- or asset-based approach to understanding all of the ways that clients, in relation to their families, communities, and wider structural factors, are able to cultivate and build these strengths to nurture their health and well-being.

Summary

The healthcare provider plays a key role in promoting perinatal health equity. Acknowledging the role of racism and other systems of oppression in shaping the structural and social determinants of health as well as reflecting on one's own biases and prejudices is an important first step in taking ownership of one's role in promoting health equity. In the exam room, the healthcare provider should prioritize relationship-building, person-centered care, listening, and believing the client, honoring them as the expert of their experience and partnering with them in identifying and achieving the health goals that matter to them. The clinical encounter is also a unique opportunity to identify how social needs may impact client health and to address those needs. A familiarity with local community, state, and federal agencies that exist to provide aid to individuals in vulnerable circumstances is essential. Finally, the healthcare provider can also be an advocate for policies needed to make structural changes. Sexual and reproductive health providers and people with privilege need to join with people of color and with other groups that continue to be marginalized in fighting for social justice.

Resources for Clients and their Families

Disabled Parenting Project: An online space for sharing experiences, advice, and conversations among disabled parents as well as those considering parenthood. https://disabledparenting.com

How to obtain child support: Child support handbook. https://www.acf.hhs.gov/css/outreach-material/handbook-child-support-enforcement

Local food pantries. Assist people in locating local food banks or pantries using the link: http://feedingamerica.org/foodbank-results.aspx

Medicaid. Learn how to apply for coverage. https://www.medicaid.gov/about-us/beneficiary-resources/index.html

Temporary Assistance for Needy Families (TANF). A program that helps families transition from public assistance to work by providing financial support, work opportunities, and childcare assistance. For details about the program and eligibility, visit: http://www.acf.hhs.gov/programs/ofa/programs/tanf

Child Care Aware America. Find a Child Care Resource & Referral Agency (CCR&R). https://www.childcareaware.org/

The National Association of Free and Charitable Clinics. Organization for clinics providing free healthcare for uninsured or underinsured individuals across the country. https://www.nafcclinics.org/

The Special Supplemental Nutrition Program for WIC. https://www.fns.usda.gov/wic

US Department of Housing and Urban Development. public housing assistance is offered in the form of public housing or housing choice vouchers (section 8). https://www.hud.gov/topics/rental_assistance

Resources for Healthcare Providers

American Association of Family Physician. Social determinants of health: Guide to social needs screening. https://www.aafp.org/dam/AAFP/documents/patient_care/everyone_project/hops19-physician-guide-sdoh.pdf

American College of Nurse-Midwives (ACNM). Position statement: Provision of Health Care for Women in the Criminal Justice System. https://www.midwife.org/acnm/files/ACNMLibraryData/UPLOADFILENAME/000000000304/Provision-of-Healthcare-for-Women-in-the-Criminal-Justice-System-Dec-2016.pdf

American College of Nurse-Midwives (ACNM). Position statement: Racism and racial bias. https://www.midwife.org/acnm/files/acnmlibrarydata/uploadfilename/000000000315/PS-Racism%20and%20Racial%20Bias%20FINAL%20to%20ACNM%2026-Oct-19.pdf

American College of Obstetricians and Gynecologists. Committee opinion: Reproductive healthcare for incarcerated pregnant, postpartum, and nonpregnant individuals. https://www.acog.org/-/media/project/acog/acogorg/clinical/files/committee-opinion/articles/2021/07/reproductive-health-care-for-incarcerated-pregnant-postpartum-and-nonpregnant-individuals.pdf

American College of Obstetricians and Gynecologists. Committee opinion: Optimizing postpartum care. https://www.acog.org/clinical/clinical-guidance/committee-opinion/articles/2018/05/optimizing-postpartum-care

Black Mamas Matter Alliance. Issue Briefs, Reports, and Publications. https://blackmamasmatter.org/literature

National Association to Advance Black Birth. The Black Birthing Bill of Rights. https://thenaabb.org/black-birthing-bill-of-rights

National Commission on Correctional Health Care. Women's Health Care in Correctional Settings (Position Statements on Breastfeeding in Correctional Settings, Transgender and Gender Diverse Health Care in Correctional Settings, and Women's Health Care in

Correctional Settings). https://www.ncchc.org/position-statements

National Health Care for the Homeless Council. Reproductive Health Care for Homeless Patients: Summary of Recommended Practice Adaptations: https://nhchc.org/wp-content/uploads/2019/08/Reproductive-Health-Care.pdf

Project Implicit. Implicit Association Tests: https://implicit.harvard.edu/implicit/index.jsp

Women's Prison Association. A summary of jail and prison nursery programs: https://www.prisonpolicy.org/scans/wpa/Mothers_Infants_and_Imprisonment_2009.pdf

References

ADA National Network. (2017). Accessible health care. https://adata.org/sites/adata.org/files/files/Accessible_Health_Care_final2019.pdf

ADA National Network. (2020). *Health care and the Americans with Disabilities Act.* https://adata.org/sites/adata.org/files/files/Health%20Care%20and%20the%20ADA%20FINAL%202-11-2020.pdf

Akobirshoev, I., Mitra, M., Parish, S. L., Simas, T. A. M., Dembo, R., & Ncube, C. N. (2019). Racial and ethnic disparities in birth outcomes and labour and delivery-related charges among women with intellectual and developmental disabilities. *Journal of Intellectual Disability Research, 63*(4), 313–326. https://doi.org/10.1111/jir.12577

Alhusen, J. L., Bower, K. M., Epstein, E., & Sharps, P. (2016). Racial discrimination and adverse birth outcomes: An integrative review. *Journal of Midwifery & Women's Health, 61*(6), 707–720. https://doi.org/10.1111/jmwh.12490

Altman, M. R., Oseguera, T., McLemore, M. R., Kantrowitz-Gordon, I., Franck, L. S., & Lyndon, A. (2019). Information and power: Women of color's experiences interacting with health care providers in pregnancy and birth. *Social Science & Medicine, 238*, 112491. https://doi.org/10.1016/j.socscimed.2019.112491

American College of Nurse-Midwives (ACNM). (2016). *Position statement: Provision of Health Care for Women in the Criminal Justice System.* https://www.midwife.org/acnm/files/ACNMLibraryData/UPLOADFILENAME/000000000304/Provision-of-Healthcare-for-Women-in-the-Criminal-Justice-System-Dec-2016.pdf

American College of Obstetricians & Gynecologists (ACOG). (2013). Health care for homeless women. Committee opinion no. 576. *Obstetrics and Gynecology, 122*(4), 936–940.

American College of Obstetricians & Gynecologists (ACOG). (2021a). Optimizing postpartum care. Committee opinion no. 736. *Obstetrics and Gynecology, 131*(5), e140–e150.

American College of Obstetricians & Gynecologists (ACOG). (2021b). Reproductive health care for incarcerated pregnant, postpartum, and nonpregnant individuals. Committee opinion no. 830. *Obstetrics and Gynecology, 138*(1), e24–e34.

Andrews, E. E., Powell, R. M., & Ayers, K. (2022). The evolution of disability language: Choosing terms to describe disability. *Disability and Health Journal, 15*(3), 101328. https://doi.org/10.1016/j.dhjo.2022.101328

Appelgren Engström, H., Borneskog, C., Loeb, C., Häggström-Nordin, E., & Almqvist, A. (2022). Associations between heteronormative information, parental support and stress among same-sex mothers in Sweden—A web survey. *Nursing Open, 9*(6), 2826–2835. https://doi.org/10.1002/nop2.986

Arnett, M., Thorpe, R., Gaskin, D., Bowie, J., & LaVeist, T. (2016). Race, medical mistrust, and segregation in primary care as usual source of care: Findings from the exploring health disparities in integrated communities study. *Journal of Urban Health, 93*(3), 456–467.

Association of Women's Health, Obstetric and Neonatal Nurses (AWHONN). (2011). Shackling incarcerated women (position statement). *Journal of Obstetric, Gynecologic, & Neonatal Nursing, 40*(6), 817–818.

Bailey, Z., Krieger, N., Agénor, M., Graves, J., Linos, N., & Bassett, M. (2017). Structural racism and health inequities in the USA: Evidence and interventions. *The Lancet, 389*(10077), 1453–1463. http://10.0.3.248/S0140-6736(17)30569-X

Banks, A. R., Bell, B. A., Ngendahimana, D., Embaye, M., Freedman, D. A., & Chisolm, D. J. (2021). Identification of factors related to food insecurity and the implications for social determinants of health screenings. *BMC Public Health, 21*(1), 1410. https://doi.org/10.1186/s12889-021-11465-6

Bedaso, A., Adams, J., Peng, W., & Sibbritt, D. (2021). Prevalence and determinants of low social support during pregnancy among Australian women: A community-based cross-sectional study. *Reproductive Health, 18*(1), 158. https://doi.org/10.1186/s12978-021-01210-y

Belarmino, E. H., Malinowski, A., & Flynn, K. (2021). Diaper need is associated with risk for food insecurity in a statewide sample of participants in the special supplemental nutrition program for women, infants, and children (WIC). *Preventive Medicine Reports, 22*, 101332.

Bellerose, M., Collin, L., & Daw, J. R. (2022). The ACA Medicaid expansion and perinatal insurance, health care use, and health outcomes: A systematic review. *Health Affairs, 41*(1), 60–68. https://doi.org/10.1377/hlthaff.2021.01150

Benkert, R., Cuevas, A., Thompson, H. S., Dove-Medows, E., & Knuckles, D. (2019). Ubiquitous yet unclear: A systematic review of medical mistrust. *Behavioral Medicine, 45*(2), 86–101. https://doi.org/10.1080/08964289.2019.1588220

Bilszta, J., Tang, T., Meyer, D., Milgrom, J., Ericksen, J., & Buist, A. (2008). Single motherhood versus poor partner relationship: Outcomes for antenatal mental health. *The Australian and New Zealand Journal of Psychiatry, 42*(1), 56–65.

Bohren, M. A., Hofmeyr, G. J., Sakala, C., Fukuzawa, R. K., & Cuthbert, A. (2017). Continuous support for women during childbirth. *Cochrane Database of Systematic Reviews, 7*. https://doi.org/10.1002/14651858.CD003766.pub6

Borders, A. E. B., Wolfe, K., Qadir, S., Kim, K.-Y., Holl, J., & Grobman, W. (2015). Racial/ethnic differences in self-reported and biologic measures of chronic stress in pregnancy. *Journal of Perinatology, 35*, 580–584.

Bower, K. M., Geller, R. J., Perrin, N. A., & Alhusen, J. (2018). Experiences of racism and preterm birth: Findings from a pregnancy risk assessment monitoring system, 2004 through 2012. *Women's Health Issues, 28*(6), 495–501. https://doi.org/10.1016/j.whi.2018.06.002

Bowleg, L. (2012). The problem with the phrase women and minorities: Intersectionality—an important theoretical framework for public health. *American Journal of Public Health, 102*(7), 1267–1273. https://doi.org/10.2105/AJPH.2012.300750

Brady, M. (2016). Gluing, catching, and connecting: How informal childcare strengthens single mothers' employment trajectories. *Work, Employment, and Society, 30*(5), 821–837. https://doi.org/10.1177/0950017016630259

Braveman, P., Marchi, K., Egerter, S., Kim, S., Metzler, M., Stancil, T., & Libet, M. (2010). Poverty, near-poverty, and hardship around the time of pregnancy. *Maternal and Child Health Journal, 14*, 20–35.

Broussard, C. A. (2010). Research regarding low-income single mothers' mental and physical health: A decade in review. *Journal of Poverty, 14*, 443–451.

Carson, E.A. (2021). *Prisoners in 2020.* US Department of Justice, Bureau of Justice Statistics (NCJ250229). https://bjs.ojp.gov/content/pub/pdf/p20st.pdf

Carson, E.A. & Anderson, E. (2016). *Prisoners in 2015.* US Department of Justice, Bureau of Justice Statistics (NCJ250229). https://www.bjs.gov/content/pub/pdf/p15.pdf

Center on Budget and Policy Priorities. (2022). *The supplemental nutrition assistance program (SNAP).* Policy Basics. https://www.cbpp.org/sites/default/files/policybasics-SNAP-6-9-22.pdf

Centers for Disease Control and Prevention [CDC]. (2020). *Disability and health overview* https://www.cdc.gov/ncbddd/disabilityand-health/disability.html

Centers for Disease Control and Prevention [CDC]. (2022a). *Pregnancy mortality surveillance system.* https://www.cdc.gov/reproductivehealth/maternalinfanthealth/pmss.html

Centers for Disease Control and Prevention [CDC]. (2022b). *The U.S. Public Health Service Syphilis Study at Tuskegee.* https://www.cdc.gov/tuskegee/about.html

Chambers, B. D., Arabia, S. E., Arega, H. A., Altman, M. R., Berkowitz, R., Feuer, S. K., Franck, L. S., Gomez, A. M., Kober, K., Pacheco-Werner, T., Paynter, R. A., Prather, A. A., Spellen, S. A., Stanley, D., Jelliffe-Pawlowski, L. L., & McLemore, M. R. (2020). Exposures to structural racism and racial discrimination among pregnant and early post-partum Black women living in Oakland, California. *Stress and Health*, 36(2), 213–219. https://doi.org/10.1002/smi.2922

Chambers, B. D., Arega, H. A., Arabia, S. E., Taylor, B., Barron, R. G., Gates, B., Scruggs-Leach, L., Scott, K. A., & McLemore, M. R. (2021). Black women's perspectives on structural racism across the reproductive lifespan: A conceptual framework for measurement development. *Maternal and Child Health Journal*, 25(3), 402–413. https://doi.org/10.1007/s10995-020-03074-3

Chambers, B. D., Baer, R. J., McLemore, M. R., & Jelliffe-Pawlowski, L. L. (2019). Using index of concentration at the extremes as indicators of structural racism to evaluate the association with preterm birth and infant mortality—California, 2011–2012. *Journal of Urban Health: Bulletin of the New York Academy of Medicine*, 96(2), 159–170. https://doi.org/10.1007/s11524-018-0272-4

Chambers, B. D., Erausquin, J. T., Tanner, A. E., Nichols, T. R., & Brown-Jeffy, S. (2018). Testing the association between traditional and novel indicators of county-level structural racism and birth outcomes among Black and White women. *Journal of Racial and Ethnic Health Disparities*, 5(5), 966–977. https://doi.org/10.1007/s40615-017-0444-z

Chaudhuri, N. (2004). Interventions to improve children's health by improving the housing environment. *Reviews on Environmental Health*, 19, 197–222.

Chen, A. (2022). *Current state of doula Medicaid implementation efforts in November 2022*. https://healthlaw.org/resource/current-state-of-doula-medicaid-implementation-efforts-in-november-2022

Clarke, J., & Adashi, E. (2011). Perinatal care for incarcerated patients: A 25-year-old woman pregnant in jail. *Journal of the American Medical Association*, 305(9), 923–929.

Columbia Law School. (2017, June 8) *Kimberlé Crenshaw on intersectionality, more than two decades later*. www.law.columbia.edu/news/archive/kimberle-crenshaw-intersectionality-more-two-decades-later

Courtney-Long, E. A., Carroll, D. D., Zhang, Q. C., Stevens, A. C., Griffin-Blake, S., Armour, B. S., & Campbell, V. A. (2015). Prevalence of disability and disability type among adults—United States, 2013. *Morbidity and Mortality Weekly Report*, 64(29), 777–783.

Cox, J. T., & Phelan, S. T. (2008). Nutrition during pregnancy. *Obstetrics and Gynecology Clinics of North America*, 35, 369–383.

Crear-Perry, J., Correa-de-Araujo, R., Lewis Johnson, T., McLemore, M. R., Neilson, E., & Wallace, M. (2021). Social and structural determinants of health inequities in maternal health. *Journal of Women's Health*, 30(2), 230–235. https://doi.org/10.1089/jwh.2020.8882

Crenshaw, K. (1989). Demarginalizing the intersection of race and sex: A Black feminist critique of antidiscrimination doctrine, feminist theory and antiracist politics. *University of Chicago Legal Forum*, 1989(1), 8. https://chicagounbound.uchicago.edu/cgi/viewcontent.cgi?article=1052&context=uclf

Crenshaw, K. (1991). Mapping the margins: Intersectionality, identity politics, and violence against women of color. *Stanford Law Review*, 43(6), 1241–1299. https://doi.org/10.2307/1229039

Crosier, T., Butterworth, P., & Rodgers, B. (2007). Mental health problems among single and partnered mothers: The role of financial hardship and social support. *Social Psychiatry and Psychiatric Epidemiology*, 42(1), 6–13.

Cutts, D. B., Coleman, S., Black, M. M., Chilton, M. M., Cook, J. T., de Cuba, S. E., Heeren, T. C., Meyers, A., Sandel, M., Casey, P. H., & Frank, D. A. (2015). Homelessness during pregnancy: A unique, time-dependent risk factors of birth outcomes. *Maternal Child Health Journal*, 19(6), 1276–1283.

Daw, J. R., Winkelman, T. N. A., Dalton, V. K., Kozhimannil, K. B., & Admon, L. K. (2020). Medicaid expansion improved perinatal insurance continuity for low-income women: Study examines the impact of state Medicaid expansions on continuity of insurance coverage for low-income women across three time points: Preconception, delivery, and postpartum. *Health Affairs*, 39(9), 1531–1539. https://doi.org/10.1377/hlthaff.2019.01835

Dean, L. T., & Thorpe, R. J., Jr. (2022). What structural racism is (or is not) and how to measure it: Clarity for public health and medical researchers. *American Journal of Epidemiology*, kwac112. https://doi.org/10.1093/aje/kwac112

Dinour, L. M., Rivera Rodas, E. I., Amutah-Onukagha, N. N., & Doamekpor, L. A. (2020). The role of prenatal food insecurity on breastfeeding behaviors: Findings from the United States pregnancy risk assessment monitoring system. *International Breastfeeding Journal*, 15(1), 30. https://doi.org/10.1186/s13006-020-00276-x

Dissanayake, M. V., Darney, B. G., Caughey, A. B., & Horner-Johnson, W. (2020). Miscarriage occurrence and prevention efforts by disability status and type in the United States. *Journal of Women's Health*, 29(3), 345–352. https://doi.org/10.1089/jwh.2019.7880

DiTosto, J. D., Holder, K., Soyemi, E., Beestrum, M., & Yee, L. M. (2021). Housing instability and adverse perinatal outcomes: A systematic review. *American Journal of Obstetrics & Gynecology MFM*, 3(6), 100477. https://doi.org/10.1016/j.ajogmf.2021.100477

Dooley, E. K., & Ringler, R. L. (2012). Prenatal care: Touching the future. *Primary Care*, 39(1), 17–37.

Eamon, M. K., & Wu, C. F. (2011). Effects of unemployment and underemployment on material hardship in single-mother families. *Children and Youth Services Review*, 33, 233–241.

Elk, R. (2021). The intersection of racism, discrimination, bias, and homophobia toward African American sexual minority patients with cancer within the health care system. *Cancer*, 127(19), 3500–3504. https://doi.org/10.1002/cncr.33627

Ely, D. M., & Driscoll, A. K. (2022). Infant mortality in the United States, 2020: Data from the period linked birth/infant death file. *National Vital Statistics Report*, 71(5). https://www.cdc.gov/nchs/data/nvsr/nvsr71/nvsr71-05.pdf

Engle, P. L., & Black, M. M. (2008). The effect of poverty on child development and educational outcomes. *Annals of the New York Academy of Sciences*, 1136(1), 243–256. https://doi.org/10.1196/annals.1425.023

Finer, L. B., & Henshaw, S. K. (2006). Disparities in rates of unintended pregnancy in the United States, 1994 and 2001. *Perspectives on Sexual and Reproductive Health*, 38(2), 90–96.

Fisher, M., Scanlon, C., Deojee, B., Hutton, V., & Sisko, S. (2021). Classism. In V. Hutton & S. Sisko (Eds.), *Multicultural responsiveness in counselling and psychology* (pp. 103–124). Palgrave Macmillan. https://doi.org/10.1007/978-3-030-55427-9

Ford, C. L., & Airhihenbuwa, C. O. (2010). Critical race theory, race equity, and public health: Toward antiracism praxis. *American Journal of Public Health*, 100(Suppl 1), S30–S35. https://doi.org/10.2105/AJPH.2009.171058

Gale, M. M., Pieterse, A. L., Lee, D. L., Huynh, K., Powell, S., & Kirkinis, K. (2020). A meta-analysis of the relationship between internalized racial oppression and health-related outcomes. *The Counseling Psychologist*, 48(4), 498–525. https://doi.org/10.1177/0011000020904454

Golden, B., Asiodu, I. V., Franck, L. S., Ofori-Parku, C. Y., Suárez-Baquero, D. F. M., Youngston, T., & McLemore, M. R. (2022). Emerging approaches to redressing multi-level racism and reproductive health disparities. *npj Digital Medicine*, 5(1), Article 1. https://doi.org/10.1038/s41746-022-00718-2

Gordon, S. H., Sommers, B. D., Wilson, I. B., & Trivedi, A. N. (2020). Effects of Medicaid expansion on postpartum coverage and outpatient utilization. *Health Affairs (Project Hope)*, 39(1), 77–84. https://doi.org/10.1377/hlthaff.2019.00547

Graham, J. (Host)(2015). *Trusting Black women: Building sustainable respect with Loretta. J. Ross. (No. 159)* [Audio podcast episode]. Our Common Ground. Our Common Ground Radio. https://podcastaddict.com/episode/https%3A%2F%2Fwww.blogtalkradio.com%2Focg%2F2015%2F11%2F08%2Ftrusting-black-women-building-sustainable-respect-with-loretta-j-ross.mp3&podcastId=1628319

Gross, R. S., Mendelsohn, A. L., Arana, M. M., & Messito, M. J. (2019). Food insecurity during pregnancy and breastfeeding by low-income Hispanic mothers. *Pediatrics*, 143(6), e20184113. https://doi.org/10.1542/peds.2018-4113

Hahn, R. A., & Truman, B. I. (2015). Education improves public health and promotes health equity. *International Journal of Health Services*, 45(4), 657–678. https://doi.org/10.1177/0020731415585986

Harnisch, J. M., Harnisch, P. H., & Harnisch, D. R. (2012). Family medicine obstetrics: Pregnancy and nutrition. *Primary Care, 39*, 39–35.

Heflin, C. M., Altman, C. E., & Rodriguez, L. L. (2019). Food insecurity and disability in the United States. *Disability and Health Journal, 12*(2), 220–226. https://doi.org/10.1016/j.dhjo.2018.09.006

Herring, S. J., Nelson, D. B., Davey, A., Klotz, A. A., Dibble, L., Oken, E., & Foster, G. D. (2012). Determinants of excessive gestational weight gain in urban, low-income women. *Women's Health Issues, 22–5,* e439–e446. https://doi.org/10.1016Zj.whi.2012.05.004

Hetherington, E., Doktorchik, C., Premji, S. S., McDonald, S. W., Tough, S. C., & Sauve, R. S. (2015). Preterm birth and social support during pregnancy: A systematic review and meta-analysis. *Paediatric and Perinatal Epidemiology, 29*(6), 523–535. https://doi.org/10.1111/ppe.12225

Ho, I. K., Sheldon, T. A., & Botelho, E. (2022). Medical mistrust among women with intersecting marginalized identities: A scoping review. *Ethnicity & Health, 27*(8), 1733–1751. https://doi.org/10.1080/13557858.2021.1990220

Hoffkling, A., Obedin-Maliver, J., & Sevelius, J. (2017). From erasure to opportunity: A qualitative study of the experiences of transgender men around pregnancy and recommendations for providers. *BMC Pregnancy and Childbirth, 17*(S2), 332. https://doi.org/10.1186/s12884-017-1491-5

Homan, P. (2021). Sexism and health: Advancing knowledge through structural and intersectional approaches. *American Journal of Public Health, 111*(10), 1725–1727. https://doi.org/10.2105/AJPH.2021.306480

Homan, P., Brown, T. H., & King, B. (2021). Structural intersectionality as a new direction for health disparities research. *Journal of Health and Social Behavior, 62*(3), 350–370. https://doi.org/10.1177/00221465211032947

Horner-Johnson, W., Darney, B. G., Kulkarni-Rajasekhara, S., Quigley, B., & Caughey, A. B. (2016). Pregnancy among US women: Differences by presence, type, and complexity of disability. *American Journal of Obstetrics and Gynecology, 214*(4), 529.e1–529.e9. https://doi.org/10.1016/j.ajog.2015.10.929

Horton, C., & Hall, S. (2020). Enhanced doula support to improve pregnancy outcomes among African American women with disabilities. *The Journal of Perinatal Education, 29*(4), 188–196. https://doi.org/10.1891/J-PE-D-19-00021

Hotelling, B. A. (2008). Perinatal needs of pregnant, incarcerated women. *The Journal of Perinatal Education, 17*(2), 37–44. https://doi.org/10.16%2024/105812408X298372

Howell, E. A., Egorova, N. N., Balbierz, A., Zeitlin, J., & Hebert, P. L. (2016). Site of delivery contribution to black-white severe maternal morbidity disparity. *American Journal of Obstetrics & Gynecology, 215*(2), 143–152. https://doi.org/10.1016/j.ajog.2016.05.007

Howell, E. A., & Zeitlin, J. (2017). Improving hospital quality to reduce disparities in severe maternal morbidity and mortality. *Seminars in Perinatology, 41*(5), 266–272. https://doi.org/10.1053/j.semperi.2017.04.002

Hoyert, D. L. (2022). *Maternal mortality rates in the United States, 2020.* NCHS Health E-Stats. https://www.cdc.gov/nchs/data/hestat/maternal-mortality/2020/maternal-mortality-rates-2020.htm

Huang, C.-C., & Han, K.-Q. (2012). Child support enforcement in the United States: Has policy made a difference? *Children and Youth Services Review, 34*, 622–627.

Iezzoni, L. I., McKee, M. M., Meade, M. A., Morris, M. A., & Pendo, E. (2022). Have almost fifty years of disability civil rights laws achieved equitable care? *Health Affairs, 41*(10), 1371–1378. https://doi.org/10.1377/hlthaff.2022.00413

Jaiswal, J. (2019). Whose responsibility is it to dismantle medical mistrust? Future directions for researchers and health care providers. *Behavioral Medicine, 45*(2), 188–196. https://doi.org/10.1080/08964289.2019.1630357

Janevic, T., Zeitlin, J., Egorova, N. N., Hebert, P., Balbierz, A., Stroustrup, A. M., & Howell, E. A. (2021). Racial and economic neighborhood segregation, site of delivery, and morbidity and mortality in neonates born very preterm. *The Journal of Pediatrics, 235*, 116–123. https://doi.org/10.1016/j.jpeds.2021.03.049

Jones, N. L., Gilman, S. E., Cheng, T. L., Drury, S. S., Hill, C. V., & Geronimus, A. T. (2019). Life course approaches to the causes of health disparities. *American Journal of Public Health, 109*(S1), S48–S55. https://doi.org/10.2105/AJPH.2018.304738

Kajstura, A. (2019). *Women's mass incarceration: The whole pie 2019.* Prison Policy Initiative. https://www.prisonpolicy.org/reports/pie2019women.html

Ko, L. (2016). *Unwanted sterilization and eugenics programs in the United States.* Independent Lens. http://www.pbs.org/independentlens/blog/unwanted-sterilization-and-eugenics-programs-in-the-united-states

Koller, E. C., Egede, L. E., Garacci, E., & Williams, J. S. (2022). Gender differences in the relationship between food insecurity and body mass index among adults in the USA. *Journal of General Internal Medicine.* https://doi.org/10.1007/s11606-022-07714-y

Koschmann, K. S., Jeffers, N. K., & Heidari, O. (2020). "I can't breathe": A call for antiracist nursing practice. *Nursing Outlook, 68*(5), 539–541.

Krivo, L. J., Byron, R. A., Calder, C. A., Peterson, R. D., Browning, C. R., Kwan, M.-P., & Lee, J. Y. (2015). Patterns of local segregation: Do they matter for neighborhood crime? *Social Science Research, 54*, 303–318. https://doi.org/10.1016/j.ssresearch.2015.08.005

Kumar, N. R., Borders, A., & Simon, M. A. (2021). Postpartum Medicaid extension to address racial inequity in maternal mortality. *American Journal of Public Health, 111*(2), 202–204. https://doi.org/10.2105/AJPH.2020.306060

Laraia, B. A., Gamba, R., Saraiva, C., Dove, M. S., Marchi, K., & Braveman, P. (2022). Severe maternal hardships are associated with food insecurity among low-income/lower-income women during pregnancy: Results from the 2012–2014 California maternal infant health assessment. *BMC Pregnancy and Childbirth, 22*(1), 138. https://doi.org/10.1186/s12884-022-04464-x

LeWinn, K. Z., Stroud, L. R., Molnar, B. E., Ware, J. H., Koenen, K. C., & Buka, S. L. (2009). Elevated maternal cortisol levels during pregnancy are associated with reduced childhood IQ. *International Journal of Epidemiology, 38*(6), 1700–1710.

Lori, J., Hwa Ya, C., & Martyn, K. (2011). Provider characteristics desired by African-American women in prenatal care. *The Journal of Transcultural Nursing, 22*(1), 71–76.

Mabli, J., Ohls, J., Dragoset, L., Castner, L., & Santos, B. (2013). *Measuring the effect of Supplemental Nutrition Assistance Program (SNAP) participation on food security.* https://www.mathematica.org/publications/measuring-the-effect-of-supplemental-nutrition-assistance-program-snap-participation-on-food-security

March of Dimes. (2022). *Maternity care deserts across The U.S.* https://www.marchofdimes.org/sites/default/files/2022-10/2022_Maternity_Care_Report.pdf

McGeough, C., Walsh, A., & Clyne, B. (2020). Barriers and facilitators perceived by women while homeless and pregnant in accessing antenatal and or postnatal healthcare: A qualitative evidence synthesis. *Health & Social Care in the Community, 28*(5), 1380–1393. https://doi.org/10.1111/hsc.12972

McHale, P., Maudsley, G., Pennington, A., Schlüter, D. K., Barr, B., Paranjothy, S., & Taylor-Robinson, D. (2022). Mediators of socioeconomic inequalities in preterm birth: A systematic review. *BMC Public Health, 22*(1), 1134. https://doi.org/10.1186/s12889-022-13438-9

McLemore, M. R., Altman, M. R., Cooper, N., Williams, S., Rand, L., & Franck, L. (2018). Health care experiences of pregnant, birthing and postnatal women of color at risk for preterm birth. *Social Science & Medicine, 201*, 127–135. https://doi.org/10.1016/j.socscimed.2018.02.013

Mehra, R., Boyd, L. M., Magriples, U., Kershaw, T. S., Ickovics, J. R., & Keene, D. E. (2020). Black pregnant women "get the most judgment": A qualitative study of the experiences of Black women at the intersection of race, gender, and pregnancy. *Women's Health Issues, 30*(6), 484–492. https://doi.org/10.1016/j.whi.2020.08.001

Metzl, J. M., & Hansen, H. (2014). Structural competency: Theorizing a new medical engagement with stigma and inequality. *Social Science & Medicine, 103*, 126–133. https://doi.org/10.1016/j.socscimed.2013.06.032

Mitra, M., Clements, K. M., Zhang, J., Iezzoni, L. I., Smeltzer, S. C., & Long-Bellil, L. M. (2015). Maternal characteristics, pregnancy complications and adverse birth outcomes among women with disabilities. *Medical Care, 53*(12), 1027–1032. https://doi.org/10.1097/MLR.0000000000000427

Mitra, M., Long-Bellil, L. M., Iezzoni, L. I., Smeltzer, S. C., & Smith, L. D. (2016). Pregnancy among women with physical disabilities: Unmet needs and recommendations on navigating pregnancy. *Disability and Health Journal, 9*(3), 457–463. https://doi.org/10.1016/j.dhjo.2015.12.007

Mwachofi Brody, A. K. (2017). A comparative analysis of pregnancy outcomes for women with and without disabilities. *Journal of Health Disparities Research & Practice, 10*(1), 28–48.

National Alliance to End Homelessness. (2022). *State of homelessness: 2022 edition.* https://endhomelessness.org/wp-content/uploads/2023/05/StateOfHomelessness_2022.pdf

National Commission on Correctional Health Care. (2020). *Nonuse of restraints for pregnant and postpartum incarcerated individuals.* https://www.ncchc.org/nonuse-of-restraints-for-pregnant-and-postpartum-incarcerated-individuals-2020

Obel, C., Hedegaard, M., Henriksen, T. B., Secher, N. J., Olsen, J., & Levine, S. (2005). Stress and salivary cortisol during pregnancy. *Psychoneuroendocrinology, 30,* 647–656. https://doi.org/10.1016/j.psyneuen.2004.11.006

Okoro, C. A. (2018). Prevalence of disabilities and health care access by disability status and type among adults—United States, 2016. *MMWR. Morbidity and Mortality Weekly Report, 67.* https://doi.org/10.15585/mmwr.mm6732a3

Okoro, O. N., Hillman, L. A., & Cernasev, A. (2020). "We get double slammed!": Healthcare experiences of perceived discrimination among low-income African-American women. *Women's Health, 16,* 1745506520953348. https://doi.org/10.1177/1745506520953348

Organization for Economic Co-Operation and Development. (2022). Health status: Maternal and infant mortality (OECD Stat) [Data set]. ICPSR. https://stats.oecd.org

Orozco, J., Echeverria, S., Armah, S., & Dharod, J. (2020). Household food insecurity, breastfeeding, and related feeding practices in US infants and toddlers: Results from NHANES 2009–2014. *Journal of Nutrition Education and Behavior, 52.* https://doi.org/10.1016/j.jneb.2020.02.011

Osterman, M. J. K., Hamilton, B. E., Martin, J. A., Driscoll, A. K., & Valenzuela, C. P. (2022). Births: Final data for 2020. *National Vital Statistics Report, 70*(17). https://www.cdc.gov/nchs/data/nvsr/nvsr70/nvsr70-17.pdf

Poehlmann, J., & Shlafer, R. J. (2016). Perinatal experiences of low-income and incarcerated women. In A. Wenzel (Ed.), *The Oxford handbook of perinatal psychology* (pp. 602–617). Oxford University Press.

Procter, S. B., & Campbell, C. G. (2014). Position of the Academy of Nutrition and Dietetics: Nutrition and lifestyle for a healthy pregnancy outcome. *The Journal of the Academy of Nutrition and Dietetics, 114*(7), 1099–1103.

Ranji, U., Gomez, I., Rosenzweig, C., Kellenberg, R., May 19, K. G. P., & 2022. (2022, May 19). *Medicaid coverage of pregnancy-related services: Findings from a 2021 state survey.* Women's Health Policy. https://www.kff.org/womens-health-policy/report/medicaid-coverage-of-pregnancy-related-services-findings-from-a-2021-state-survey

Ransohoff, J. I., Sujin Kumar, P., Flynn, D., & Rubenstein, E. (2022). Reproductive and pregnancy health care for women with intellectual and developmental disabilities: A scoping review. *Journal of Applied Research in Intellectual Disabilities, 35*(3), 655–674. https://doi.org/10.1111/jar.12977

Rapp, K. S., Volpe, V. V., & Neukrug, H. (2021). State-level sexism and women's health care access in the United States: Differences by race/ethnicity, 2014–2019. *American Journal of Public Health, 111*(10), 1796–1805. https://doi.org/10.2105/AJPH.2021.306455

Raugh, V. A., Landrigan, P. J., & Claudio, L. (2008). Housing and health: Intersection of poverty and environmental exposures. *Annals of the New York Academy of Sciences, 1136,* 276–288.

Rosenberg, S., Callander, D., Holt, M., Duck-Chong, L., Pony, M., Cornelisse, V., Baradaran, A., Duncan, D. T., & Cook, T. (2021).

Cisgenderism and transphobia in sexual health care and associations with testing for HIV and other sexually transmitted infections: Findings from the Australian trans & gender diverse sexual health survey. *PLoS One, 16*(7), e0253589. https://doi.org/10.1371/journal.pone.0253589

Ross, L., & Solinger, R. (2017). *Reproductive justice: An introduction.* University of California Press.

Sarlio-Lähteenkorva, S., & Lahelma, E. (2001). Food insecurity is associated with past and present economic disadvantage and body mass index. *The Journal of Nutrition, 131,* 2880–2884.

Sbicca, J. (2012). Growing food justice by planting an anti-oppression foundation: Opportunities and obstacles for a budding social movement. *Agriculture and Human Values, 29*(4), 455–466. https://doi.org/10.1007/s10460-012-9363-0

Scott, K. A., Britton, L., & McLemore, M. R. (2019). The ethics of perinatal care for Black women: Dismantling the structural racism in "mother blame" narratives. *The Journal of Perinatal & Neonatal Nursing, 33*(2), 108–115. https://doi.org/10.1097/JPN.0000000000000394

Shlafer, R., Davis, L., Hindt, L., & Pendleton, V. (2021). The benefits of doula support for women who are pregnant in prison and their newborns. In J. Poehlmann-Tynan & D. Dallaire (Eds.), *Children with incarcerated mothers: Separation, loss, and reunification* (pp. 33–48). Springer International Publishing. https://doi.org/10.1007/978-3-030-67599-8_3

Shlafer, R. J., Hellerstedt, W., Secor-Turner, M., Gerrity, E., & Baker, R. (2015). Doulas' perspectives about providing support to incarcerated women: A feasibility study. *Public Health Nursing, 32*(4), 316–326. https://doi.org/10.1111/phn.12137

Smid, M., Bourgois, P., & Auerswald, C. L. (2010). The challenge of pregnancy among homeless youth reclaiming a lost opportunity. *Journal of Health Care for the Poor and Underserved, 21,* 140–156.

Smith. (n.d.). *#Ableism.* Center for Disability Rights. https://cdrnys.org/blog/uncategorized/ableism/#:~:text=Ableism%20is%20a%20set%20of,one%20form%20or%20the%20other.

Sutton, R. M., Douglas, K. M., & McClellan, L. M. (2011). Benevolent sexism, perceived health risks, and the inclination to restrict pregnant women's freedoms. *Sex Roles, 65*(7–8), 596–605. https://doi.org/10.1007/s11199-010-9869-0

Tarasoff, L. A. (2015). Experiences of women with physical disabilities during the perinatal period: A review of the literature and recommendations to improve care. *Health Care for Women International, 36*(1), 88–107. https://doi.org/10.1080/07399332.2013.815756

Testa, A., & Jackson, D. B. (2020). Incarceration exposure and barriers to prenatal care in the United States: Findings from the pregnancy risk assessment monitoring system. *International Journal of Environmental Research and Public Health, 17*(19), 7331. https://doi.org/10.3390/ijerph17197331

The Sentencing Project. (2021). *The color of justice: Racial and ethnic disparity in state prisons.* https://www.sentencingproject.org/app/uploads/2022/08/The-Color-of-Justice-Racial-and-Ethnic-Disparity-in-State-Prisons.pdf

Townsend, M. S., Peerson, J., Love, B., Achterberg, C., & Murphy, S. P. (2001). Food insecurity is positively related to overweight in women. *The Journal of Nutrition, 131,* 1738–1745.

Treuhaft, S., & Karpyn, A. (2010). *The grocery gap: Who has access to healthy food and why it matters.* PolicyLink. https://www.policylink.org/resources-tools/the-grocery-gap-who-has-access-to-healthy-food-and-why-it-matters

Trost, S., Beauregard, J., Chandra, G., Njie, F., Berry, J., Harvey, A. & Goodman, D.A. (2022). *Pregnancy-related deaths: Data from maternal mortality review committees in 36 US states, 2017–2019.* https://www.cdc.gov/reproductivehealth/maternal-mortality/docs/pdf/Pregnancy-Related-Deaths-Data-MMRCs-2017-2019-H.pdf

US Census Bureau. (2022). *Poverty: Poverty thresholds by size of family and number of children, 2021.* https://www.census.gov/data/tables/time-series/demo/income-poverty/historical-poverty-thresholds.html

US Department of Agriculture. (2017). *Special supplemental nutrition program for women, infants and children* (WIC). https://www.fns.usda.gov/wic

US Department of Health and Human Services. (April 1, 2022). *Health Resources and Services Administration announces availability of new funding to support community-based doulas.* https://www.hhs.gov/about/news/2022/04/01/hrsa-announced-the-availability-of-4-million-for-hiring-training-certifying-compensating-community-based-doulas.html

Vedam, S., Stoll, K., Taiwo, T. K., Rubashkin, N., Cheyney, M., Strauss, N., McLemore, M., Cadena, M., Nethery, E., Rushton, E., Schummers, L., & Declercq, E., & the GVtM-US Steering Council(2019). The giving voice to mothers study: Inequity and mistreatment during pregnancy and childbirth in the United States. *Reproductive Health*, *16*(1), 77. https://doi.org/10.1186/s12978-019-0729-2

Walker, R. J., Garacci, E., Dawson, A. Z., Williams, J. S., Ozieh, M., & Egede, L. E. (2021). Trends in food insecurity in the United States from 2011–2017: Disparities by age, sex, race/ethnicity, and income. *Population Health Management, 24*(4), 496–501. https://doi.org/10.1089/pop.2020.0123

Wallace, M. E., Mendola, P., Liu, D., & Grantz, K. L. (2015). Joint effects of structural racism and income inequality on small-for-gestational-age birth. *American Journal of Public Health, 105*(8), 1681–1688. https://doi.org/10.2105/AJPH.2015.302613

Wang, L. (2021). *Unsupportive environments and limited policies: Pregnancy, postpartum, and birth during incarceration.* Prison Policy Initiative. https://www.prisonpolicy.org/blog/2021/08/19/pregnancy_studies

Williams, A. D., Wallace, M., Nobles, C., & Mendola, P. (2018). Racial residential segregation and racial disparities in stillbirth in the United States. *Health & Place, 51*, 208–216. https://doi.org/10.1016/j.healthplace.2018.04.005

Williams, D. R., & Mohammed, S. A. (2013). Racism and health I: Pathways and scientific evidence. *The American Behavioral Scientist, 57*(8), 1152–1173. https://doi.org/10.1177/0002764213487340

Williams, D. R., & Williams-Morris, R. (2000). Racism and mental health: The African American experience. *Ethnicity & Health, 5*(3–4), 243–268. https://doi.org/10.1080/713667453

Wu, C. F., & Eamon, M. K. (2011). Patterns and correlates of involuntary unemployment and underemployment in single-mother families. *Children and Youth Services Review, 33*(6), 820–828.

Yi, Y., Kennedy, J., Chazotte, C., Huynh, M., Jiang, Y., & Wildeman, C. (2021). Paternal jail incarceration and birth outcomes: Evidence from New York City, 2010–2016. *Maternal and Child Health Journal, 25*(8), 1221–1241. https://doi.org/10.1007/s10995-021-03168-6

Young, R. L., & Declercq, E. (2010). Implications of subdividing marital status: Are unmarried mothers with partners different from unmarried mothers without partners? An exploratory analysis. *Maternal Child Health Journal, 14*(2), 209–214.

Zhan, M. (2006). Economic mobility of single mothers: The role of assets and human capital development. *Journal of Sociology and Social Welfare, 33*(4), 127–150.

2

Ethics in Perinatal Care

Mary Broderick Donnelly

Relevant Terms

Bioethics—a field of ethics that explores issues that arise in clinical care and in human subject research
Ethical dilemma—an event in which two or more ethics principles are in conflict and give rise to competing priorities
Ethics—a disciplined approach to studying and understanding morality
Ethics codes—a set of standards that describes acceptable actions by a profession and its members
Ethics consultation—a process by which a clinician consults with an expert in bioethics to identify and assess ethical dilemmas, and make recommendations as to how to move forward within accepted ethical standards (ASBH, 2011)
Morality—standards of good and harmful actions that humans should or should not do
Principlism—an approach to the examination of moral dilemmas that is based upon the application of ethical principles

Starting with a Case Study

Suzanne S. is a 20-year-old Black G1 P0000 cisgender woman who first presented to you for care at 9-weeks' gestational age. Suzanne graduated from high school but has not attended school since. She works at a local coffee shop and shares a two-bedroom apartment with one of her parents and two siblings. Paul, age 19, a White, cisgender man, is the father of Suzanne's baby. He works with Suzanne at the coffee shop. Paul and his mother, Eloise, accompany Suzanne to prenatal visits. Before her first prenatal visit, Suzanne had not received healthcare for four years because "it is just too expensive" but "Eloise is paying for my visits to you." At some visits, Suzanne appears withdrawn, seems reluctant to express opinions, and often acquiesces to Eloise's preferences. Now, at 40.4-week gestation, you discuss scheduling a nonstress test to assess fetal well-being, and you also discuss the option of labor induction if there is no spontaneous labor by 41 weeks

and the recommendation for labor induction if there is no spontaneous labor by 42 weeks. Eloise objects to any discussion of induction.

As you read further, consider what ethical dilemmas are presented in this case and how you might respond.

Ethics and the Healthcare Clinician

The explosion of biomedical technological innovation in the 1960s and 1970s caused an increase in clinical questions that could not have been imagined in the early part of the twentieth century. In the 1960s, questions arose in Seattle regarding the just allocation of clinical resources as the decision of who could have access to hemodialysis was debated (Jonsen, 1993). Egregious breaches of biomedical research ethics became public in the early 1970s when the decades-old research study referred to as the "Tuskegee Study of Untreated Syphilis in the Negro Male" was revealed (White, 2019). In the Tuskegee study, hundreds of Black men were studied for the effects of syphilis without consent; as part of the research, life-saving treatment was withheld from study subjects (White, 2019). Prolonged ventilator support, and the right to refuse it, was contemplated in the Karen Ann Quinlan matter (Jonsen, 1993). The ethical complexities of assisted reproductive technology came into consideration after Louise Brown, the first so-called test-tube baby, was born in the United Kingdom in 1978 (Franklin, 2013). These events made it clear that clinical ethics was no longer limited to the physician–patient relationship. Rather, rigorous academic study and the safeguards of public policy were required (Lee, 2017).

The torrent of technological advances and concomitant questions invigorated a response from academia and its philosophers and clinicians. **Ethics**, a disciplined approach to studying and understanding **morality**, had been studied for millennia (Chervenak & McCullough, 2017). **Bioethics**, a field of ethics that explores issues that arise in clinical care and in human subject research (Lee, 2017), was born amidst the 1960s' and 1970s' technological

Prenatal and Postnatal Care: A Person-Centered Approach, Third Edition. Edited by Karen Trister Grace, Cindy L. Farley, Noelene K. Jeffers, and Tanya Tringali.
© 2024 John Wiley & Sons Ltd. Published 2024 by John Wiley & Sons Ltd.
Companion website: www.wiley.com/go/grace/prenatal

boom (Jonsen, 1993). Beginning with that time period, normative guidelines and principles for clinical practice began to be studied, developed, and disseminated (Jonsen, 1993).

To the dedicated clinician working in today's fast-paced milieu of clinical care, the steps taken to provide care that meets ethics standards may be so innate that clinicians do not appreciate that they are also acting consistently with established ethics principles and guidelines. Also, a clinician can act with the primary goal of compliance with laws, statutes, and regulations. However, laws and ethics, at times, can either overlap or be at odds. It is important to be able to clearly identify **ethical dilemmas** in practice. Specific knowledge of ethics guidelines and the ability to articulate and to act upon this knowledge are necessary to provide optimal care to patients.

Health equity key points

- To practice in congruence with the established ethics principle of justice, clinicians must address racism in healthcare.
- Clinicians have an ethical obligation to address health inequities.
- Most ethics codes require addressing health disparities on local, national, and global levels.
- The history of health inequity for pregnant people from disadvantaged populations must be considered in addressing disparities from an ethics perspective.

Ethics Codes

The health sciences professions have, for decades, instituted various **ethics codes.** The codes are generally value based, concentrate on the population the profession serves, and describe mechanisms of self-regulation (Ozar, 1999). The individuality of each code supports professional identity. Healthcare institutions are also guided by organizational ethics, which form the basis for the institution's mission statements and which are embodied in their policies (Lahey et al., 2020).

Examples of ethics codes that are relevant to pre- and postnatal care include the International Code of Ethics for Midwives (International Confederation of Nurse Midwives, 2014), the Code of Ethics of the American College of Nurse-Midwives (ACNM; ACNM, 2015), the Code of Professional Ethics of the American College of Obstetricians and Gynecologists (ACOG; ACOG, 2018), and the Ethics and Professionalism Guidelines of the International Federation of Gynecology and Obstetrics (FIGO; FIGO, 2021), among others. Clinicians serving patients during the prenatal and postnatal periods share the goal of providing excellent care. Therefore, it is not surprising that the professional ethics codes supporting this care frequently overlap. Emphasis on the patient's dignity and autonomy, the ethical obligation to respect patients and to do good in caring for them, and the mandate to increase health access and equity are established ethical obligations that frequently appear in these codes.

Basic Principles

When the scandal of the decades-long Tuskegee research was revealed, it resulted in an onrush of public outrage, leading the US government to form a commission to determine appropriate ethics guidelines in biomedical research (Lee, 2017). This commission generated the Belmont Report in the late 1970s, articulating three basic bioethics principles: (a) respect for autonomy, (b) beneficence, and (c) justice (Lee, 2017). Though initially meant for the biomedical research arena, these principles were determined to be applicable to the clinical area as well. Academicians Tom Beauchamp and James Childress added nonmaleficence as a fourth principle, and, in their classic text *Principles of Biomedical Ethics* (Beauchamp & Childress, 2001), gave direction in the use of **principlism** to facilitate ethical action (Varkey, 2021; Lee, 2017). In particular, principlism is used to approach ethical dilemmas, defined as events in which two or more ethics principles are in conflict and give rise to competing priorities (Rainer et al., 2018).

The principle of **respect for autonomy** emphasizes the human dignity and worth of each person and the authority persons have in all aspects of their lives, including decisions around healthcare (Varkey, 2021). The principle of **beneficence** requires clinicians to ensure that the goal of recommended treatments and interventions is the best possible outcome for a patient (Varkey, 2021; Chervenak & McCullough, 2017). The principle of **nonmaleficence** directs the clinician to undertake a careful analysis of the burdens of a proposed intervention, so that there may be a minimization of any potential harm (Varkey, 2021). Finally, the principle of **justice** requires the clinician to protect populations that are disadvantaged and to work toward fair and equitable distribution of resources (Varkey, 2021). Each of these four principles has equal standing, and clinicians have obligations to uphold each of them equally, unless the principles are in conflict in a clinical situation and give rise to an ethical dilemma (Varkey, 2021).

Ethical Practice

Describing all clinical scenarios in the pre- and postnatal periods in which the need for ethics analysis arises is beyond the scope of this chapter, but a sampling of common issues is provided below.

Patient Privacy and Confidentiality

Privacy is defined as an individual's determination as to which information relevant to their life's circumstances will be shared with others. Confidentiality is defined as the safeguarding of the private information an individual shares (Anthony & Stablein, 2016). Keeping a patient's private health information confidential is an ethical obligation historically embodied in practice and in ethics codes (Anthony & Stablein, 2016). Certainly, the ethical obligation of privacy and confidentiality predates the well-known patient privacy law, the federal Health Information Portability and Accountability Act of 1996 (HIPAA).

Private information is often shared during the healthcare interface, including during the provision of pre- and postnatal care. A patient's reproductive decisions, some of the most private in any person's life, are the focus of clinical encounters in pregnancy. In addition, pregnancy care involves the physical examination of the most intimate parts of an essentially healthy patient's body. Though the pregnant person may have a partner, family members, or friends that wish to participate in their pre- and postnatal care, it cannot be assumed that the pregnant person has waived a privacy right. For example, it is common for pregnant persons to be accompanied to healthcare visits, and it may be that the pregnant person desires certain persons to do so. However, clinicians should be mindful that a patient's agreement to being accompanied may be limited and may not include having private health information discussed or a physical examination performed in the presence of the support person. Conferring with the patient to establish desired boundaries is necessary.

In addition, the need for confidentiality protection has been heightened by the advent of social media. As a function of their private lives, clinicians may post on social media sites on a regular basis. However, the clinician should be aware that allowing these actions to become second nature and entwined with the provision of patient care may place the patient's privacy and the obligation of confidentiality in jeopardy. Whether it is purposeful, or inadvertent as a result of habit, the dissemination of private health information such as photographs and any information that may identify a patient, without permission, is unethical.

Informed Consent and Informed Refusal

A thorough informed consent process, which is a clinician's ethical obligation, flows from the principle of respect for autonomy (Varkey, 2021). During this process, clinicians are required to discuss the details of an intervention, including benefits, risks, and alternatives (Varkey, 2021). Informed consent is undertaken as a shared process to ensure that patients receive the benefit of a clinician's expertise while being supported to act within their own value systems (Halpern, 2018). In order to make the process meaningful, the clinician must also be prepared to conduct the informed consent process through the lens of the pregnant person's age, cultural preferences, and family structure.

In pre- and postnatal care, there are a daunting number of decisions to be made by the pregnant person (Malek, 2017). The lives of the pregnant person and the fetus are "interconnected and interdependent," which increases the complexity of decision-making (Ali et al., 2016, p. 137). This interconnectedness gives rise to clinical situations in which a disease process and or a treatment decision may jeopardize the health of the pregnant person or the fetus or both (Ali et al., 2016). In these instances, the principles that most apply are respect for the autonomy of the pregnant person and the goal of beneficence for both the pregnant person and fetus.

Clinicians must also recognize that it is the right of the pregnant person to decline or refuse recommended treatment (Kidson-Gerber et al., 2016). Though this is a long-established right, clinicians do not always respond positively to such a refusal (Niles et al., 2021). Patients report instances of having to "fight" for their right to refuse; of being advised that their actions will harm them or their fetus; of an increase in tension; and of a sense of mistrust between clinician and patient (Niles et al., 2021, p. 1). Clinicians should be aware of the possibility of contributing to a negative atmosphere if a patient has made an informed refusal, and seek to affirmatively respect the pregnant person's decision in actions and words.

The Primacy of the Pregnant Person as Decision-Maker

In pregnancy, treatment decisions may be needed for the fetus as well as for the pregnant patient. When a partner, perhaps one who is also the parent of the fetus, or another support person or significant other demonstrates care and concern for both the pregnant person and for the fetus, should they be involved in the informed consent process?

Considering a pregnant person's right to privacy, and the need to respect autonomy, the primacy of the pregnant person must be at the forefront of the decision-making process. A "woman's right to determine what happens to her own body has such great moral weight" (Malek, 2017, p. 11) that no other opinion need be elicited as to the pregnancy care decision. Naturally, there will be times when the pregnant person may affirmatively state a preference to have supportive partners and others involved in decision-making. This stated preference should be honored, and excluding a pregnant person's support person from the informed consent process is not necessary or even desirable under these circumstances. However, including them must be verified with the pregnant individual.

Adolescents and Decision-Making

In order to enter into the shared decision-making process, the clinician must be certain that the patient has the capacity or the ability to make a choice and to fully understand it consequences. A patient may lack capacity due to illness, loss of consciousness, or pharmaceutical intervention (Fishman et al., 2020). A patient will also lack capacity from a legal standpoint if they have not yet reached the age of majority, defined in most jurisdictions in the United States as 18 years of age (Fishman et al., 2020).

However, in the care of a pregnant adolescent who has not reached the age of capacity, the laws of most US states waive the requirement of age-related capacity in consent (Salter, 2017). Because of this, it is legally and ethically acceptable for clinicians to enter into the shared decision-making process with a pregnant person who has not reached the age of majority, and to not share details of clinical encounters with the adolescent's parents (Salter, 2017). This exception is made not because it is assumed that pregnancy confers the ability to fully understand the consequences of choices. Rather, it is made because public policy and health principles dictate that it is desirable for an adolescent to be able to seek and consent to treatment, and they may be more likely to do so if they may act independently (Salter, 2017). Certain attributes of the adolescent must still be considered when entering into a shared decision-making process. There is variability in maturity within the adolescent population, and studies have demonstrated that an adolescent's capacity may be affected by highly emotional states and the influence of peers (Salter, 2017). The informed consent process must consider these attributes in full.

Abortion

The question of the morality of induced abortion has played a prominent role in American culture as well as in the American legal system at least since the US Supreme Court case of *Roe v. Wade* (1973). Nearly 50 years later, as this chapter goes to press, the legal aspects of abortion are being examined in the US Supreme Court. Just as there are differing views among the general populace as to the morality of abortion, there are differing views among clinicians (Edvardsson et al., 2015). In particular, opinions about the point during gestation when the fetus becomes a separate person from the pregnant person vary from as early as the moment of conception to the time in the pregnancy when fetal viability is established (Edvardsson et al., 2015). Clinicians that consider abortion to be a moral act may believe that participation in the intervention is ethical. Conversely, if a clinician considers abortion to be immoral, the same clinician may believe that participation in the intervention is unethical. Further, healthcare institutions vary in whether they allow abortion: some forbid it, and others offer abortion to the full extent that standards of practice and laws allow.

To render beneficent care, and to respect the patient's autonomy, the clinician will fully counsel and advise the pregnant person of all options and respect the pregnant person's decision once it is made (ACNM, reviewed and revised, 2016a; ACOG, reaffirmed, 2020). All options should be discussed with the pregnant person, including parenting, abortion, and adoption (ACNM, 2016b; ACOG, reaffirmed 2020). ACOG asserts the clinician "should not seek to impose their personal beliefs upon their patients nor allow personal beliefs to compromise patient health, access to care, or informed consent" (ACOG, reaffirmed 2020). If the patient's choice causes ethical conflict and moral distress to the clinician, a transfer of the patient to another provider may be appropriate (ACNM, 2016c; ACNM, 2016a) and ethically acceptable.

Labor and Birth Choices

Historically, pregnant persons gave birth to their newborns in the home, accompanied by family, friends, and, often, a midwife. In the last part of the nineteenth century and in the twentieth century, physicians and others have discredited midwives and promoted hospital birth (Dawley, 2000). As a result, childbirth moved from the home setting to the clinical setting of the hospital, with physicians and hospital staff in control of the labor and birth process (Zielinski et al., 2015). In fact, this evolution has continued to the point that "in most developed nations, the choice of where to give birth is not really a consideration, because birthing in a hospital is the cultural norm" (Zielinski et al., 2015, p. 361). Today, however, there are many reasons that a community birth setting, such as a home or a freestanding birth center, is chosen by pregnant individuals, such as an experience of a previous traumatic hospital birth and the desire to make choices unsupported by hospital policies. Home birth is seen by some providers as an unsafe choice, but it should be placed in context. Pregnancy and birth are not risk free in any environment. Birth choices and interventions have potential benefits and harms to consider. Risk is not destiny; it is a probability that is interpreted and is assigned different value by different people. Complicating decisions in this area are the varying effects that a choice can have on the pregnant person, the fetus/newborn, or the labor and birth process.

The pregnant person should be educated regarding all available choices as to labor and birth options, procedures, settings, and birth attendants. Viewed from an ethics perspective, a goal of beneficence in planning for birth with the patient, accompanied by a scrupulous informed consent process, will assist the clinician in meeting ethical obligations regarding labor and birth choices. While the pregnant person's choices may not be the choice the care provider would make, the labor and birth are the individual's experience, not that of the provider or staff. Autonomy of choice and bodily integrity are basic human rights to be respected and protected by all those involved in healthcare to childbearing individuals. (See Chapter 11, *Risk Assessment during Pregnancy*, for guidance on giving evidence-based information in a nonjudgmental manner that supports the primacy of the pregnant person as decision-maker).

Research in Pregnancy

Participation of pregnant persons in research is controversial (Payne, 2019). Concerns regarding risk to the developing fetus were illuminated by occurrences of fetal damage associated with the use of pharmacologic agents during pregnancy (Vargesson, 2019). The causative link between some pharmaceutical agents and risk to the developing fetus led to a risk-averse approach to research that resulted in automatic exclusion of pregnant persons from being human research subjects (Payne, 2019). This cautionary stance is based on the ethical principles of beneficence and justice (Payne, 2019). However, it is difficult to reconcile this stance with the ethical principle of respect for the autonomy of the pregnant person and also the good that may be derived from research participation. Recognizing the need for this reconciliation, the risk of participating in research during pregnancy has been re-examined. The National Institutes of Health and ACOG now consider complete exclusion from research to be associated with paternalism, which is an affront to the principle of respect for autonomy (Payne, 2019). Further study is required in order to expand the pregnant person's choices regarding research participation.

It should be noted that, differing from clinical treatments and interventions, consent is generally elicited from both parents of the fetus when the pregnant person does have the opportunity to participate in research (Malek, 2017). This requirement is established by institutional review boards to enhance protection of the fetus (Malek, 2017). Though considered ethically sound, this practice may result in the pregnant person's exclusion from research if the fetus's other parent is not willing or available to consent. Further study and consideration are indicated.

Ethics consultation

The goal is the resolution of ethical dilemmas, and ethical conflict involves clinicians, patient, family, or some combination thereof.

The consultant makes recommendations for the amelioration of conflict and the provision of ethical care.

Ethics Consultation

Healthcare **ethics consultation** is the process by which a clinician consults with an expert in bioethics to identify and assess ethical dilemmas and make recommendations on how to move forward within accepted ethical standards (ASBH, 2011). The healthcare ethics consultation process is widely available in both inpatient and outpatient settings but does differ among institutions. Commonly, the process begins when a clinician identifies an ethical dilemma and notifies available institutional representatives who are educated in and knowledgeable about the bioethics of the dilemma (Celie & Prager, 2016; ASBH, 2011). The ethics consultant then gathers information from both the clinician and the medical record to learn the details of the patient's medical status (Fox et al., 2015) and will also gather information regarding the nature of the conflict, the parties involved, and the steps already taken toward resolution. Information may also be sought at meetings with the patient and/or family. Once this information has been secured, the ethics consultant will discuss concerns regarding the patient's values and the clinician's ethical obligations relative to the considered treatment, or the withdrawal or refusal of treatment (Fox et al., 2015). The ethics consultant will ultimately make recommendations for a plan to address and ameliorate the conflict (Celie & Prager, 2016). The clinician should access this valuable resource as a support in the resolution of an ethical conflict in care.

Ethics codes and health equity

ACNM Code of Ethics Explanatory Statement Number 4 (in part): The right to healthcare is a claim that individuals justly make. Justice requires that midwives promote health and the provision of quality, accessible healthcare for all people (ACNM, 2015).

FIGO Statement: Ethical Treatment of Women: Health is a human right, and all women and children deserve access to the highest possible standards of physical, mental, preventive, reproductive, and sexual healthcare (FIGO, 2019).

International Confederation of Midwives Code IIIe: Midwives understand the adverse consequences that ethical and human rights violations have on the health of women and infants and will work to eliminate these violations (ICM, 2014).

Health Equity

The US healthcare system and its institutions, clinicians, and researchers have a documented legacy of racism (Clark, 1998; Prather et al., 2018; Wall, 2018). Racist healthcare treatment has its roots in the racist belief in inferiority of non-White races and subsequent treatment as "less than human" (Clark, 1998, p. 67). The Tuskegee research scandal is one example, and another is the legacy of Dr. J. Marion Sims, a physician who has been lauded as the "father of modern gynecology" but who perfected his techniques by experimenting, without consent, on enslaved Black women (Wall, 2018).

This history of racism and paucity of justice in the distribution of healthcare resources resulted in a lack of healthcare access for people from marginalized groups—including pregnant persons (Prather et al., 2018). The lack of healthcare access is illustrated by the fact that, despite significant biomedical technological advances, the United States has the highest maternal morbidity and mortality rate among higher income countries (Tanne, 2020). Higher morbidity and mortality disproportionately affect people from racial and ethnic minorities, who often receive biased and substandard care (Roeder, 2019). Pregnant persons from marginalized groups or with lower socioeconomic status perceive diminished communication patterns with clinicians, being of lower priority for the provision of care, and a disregard of their choices and values (Janevic et al., 2020).

Ethical principles and ethics codes direct the clinician to embrace social justice, address healthcare disparities, and embed professional values of respect and beneficence. Clinicians must acknowledge that ethics codes mandates are not passive, flowery statements of aspiration. Rather, they are demands for clinicians to meet their ethical obligations by actively working to address health equity for all populations. This may be done in the form of political action and contribution to public policy formation (Farley, 2020). It may also be done by increasing clinician awareness of the historical basis of these inequities and their connection to present-day care, through research and scholarly dissemination (Prather et al., 2018), and via re-organization of care delivery (Janevic, et al., 2020). Individual clinicians have an obligation to self-reflect on their own explicit and implicit biases in order to recognize and remediate the effects of these biases on the care they provide.

Return to the Case Study

The case of Suzanne, a Black cisgender woman barely older than the age of the majority, illustrates patient needs that the clinician has ethical obligations to address. Suzanne has limited financial resources, as evidenced by her low-wage job and inability to access healthcare prior to this pregnancy. Also, Suzanne demonstrates a reluctance to engage with the prenatal office staff, making her vulnerable to Eloise's controlling behavior.

Professional ethics codes mandate that you explore and address healthcare disparities that have affected and may continue to affect Suzanne's well-being during and after this pregnancy. Assign clinicians who are racially concordant with Suzanne if possible, as this may enhance her comfort to ask questions and voice her preferences and reduce the likelihood of bias in clinical encounters. You must ensure that you and all office personnel do not engage, in speech and interventions, in microaggressions that may marginalize and diminish your patient. In addition, Suzanne may need assistance in procuring necessary financial resources for herself and her baby. Arrange to speak with this patient alone, without the presence of Eloise, making every effort to determine what *Suzanne* most desires and values.

The fact that Eloise is paying for Suzanne's healthcare may make Suzanne more vulnerable to coercive control and even psychological abuse, and this should be discussed with Suzanne in the private meeting also. Depending on the outcome of the private meeting, as directed by various ethics codes, arrange for collaboration with healthcare professionals such as social workers and case managers at community organizations to ensure that Suzanne has access to appropriate resources. Follow-up with these concerns at subsequent prenatal office visits is important. A privilege of prenatal care providers is to watch the development of the parental role in the pregnant individual, as well as the growth of the fetus, over the course of pregnancy.

As is consistent with basic ethics principles, patient autonomy must be respected. Suzanne's values and wishes may conflict with Eloise's and Paul's, but you must act consistently within the ethical mandate that recognizes the pregnant person as the decision-maker for pre- and postnatal treatment and interventions. If there is continued conflict between the pregnant person and others involved in the pregnancy, an ethics consultation can assist in facilitating and supporting a respect for Suzanne's autonomy relevant to treatment decisions.

Summary

Advances in technology in pre- and postnatal care have led to an increase in ethical dilemmas that the clinician must be prepared to identify and address. The interconnectedness between a pregnant person and their fetus may necessitate complex treatment decisions. The sheer magnitude of decisions to be made throughout pre- and postnatal care, including recommended testing and monitoring, birth setting, and interventions to which the pregnant person may or may not consent for the newborn, may give rise to ethical dilemmas. Further, the fetus has a parent who is not the pregnant person, and who may have opinions about fetal well-being and participation in treatment decision-making.

The obligations of ethical practice are described and delineated in various ethics codes and embodied in bioethics principles and guidelines. It is incumbent upon clinicians to familiarize themselves with these mandates and resources, and to be able to articulate them, in order to best prepare themselves to achieve excellence in the provision of ethical pre- and postnatal care.

Resources for Healthcare Professionals

American College of Nurse-Midwives. (2015). Code of ethics with explanatory statements. https://www.midwife.org/acnm/files/ACNMLibraryData/UPLOADFILENAME/000000000293/Code-of-Ethics-w-Explanatory-Statements-June-2015.pdf

American College of Obstetricians and Gynecologists. (Reaffirmed 2016). Committee Opinion No. 390: Ethical decision making in obstetrics and gynecology. https://www.acog.org/clinical/clinical-guidance/committee-opinion/articles/2007/12/ethical-decision-making-in-obstetrics-and-gynecology

Resources for the Pre- and Postnatal Family

National Institute of Environmental Health Sciences. Bioethics Resources at the NIH. https://www.niehs.nih.gov/research/resources/bioethics/resources/index.cfm

References

Ali, N. A., Coonrod, D. V., & McCormick, T. R. (2016). Ethical issues in maternal-fetal care emergencies. *Critical Care Clinics, 32,* 137–143. https://doi.org/10.1016/j.ccc.2015.08.007

American College of Nurse-Midwives. (2015). *Code of ethics with explanatory statements.* https://www.midwife.org/acnm/files/ACNMLibraryData/UPLOADFILENAME/000000000293/Code-of-Ethics-w-Explanatory-Statements-June-2015.pdf.

American College of Nurse-Midwives. (2016a). *Planned home birth.* https://www.midwife.org/acnm/files/ACNMLibraryData/UPLOADFILENAME/000000000251/Planned-Home-Birth-Dec-2016.pdf

American College of Nurse-Midwives. (2016b). *Access to comprehensive sexual and reproductive health care services.* https://www.midwife.org/acnm/files/ACNMLibraryData/UPLOADFILENAME/000000000087/Access-to-Comprehensive-Sexual-and-Reproductive-Health-Care-Services-FINAL-04-12-17.pdf

American College of Nurse-Midwives. (2016c). *Shared decision making in midwifery care.* http://midwife.org/ACNM/files/ACNMLibraryData/UPLOADFILENAME/000000000305/Shared-Decision-Making-in-Midwifery-Care-10-13-17.pdf.

American College of Obstetricians and Gynecologists. (2018). *Code of professional ethics of the American College of Obstetricians and Gynecologists.* https://www.acog.org/-/media/project/acog/acogorg/files/pdfs/acog-policies/code-of-professional-ethics-of-the-american-college-of-obstetricians-and-gynecologists.pdf?la=en&hash=CC213370E1EFDCD3E81242D8384BE4AB

American College of Obstetricians and Gynecologists. (Reaffirmed 2020). *Abortion policy.* https://www.acog.org/clinical-information/policy-and-position-statements/statements-of-policy/2020/abortion-policy

American Society for Bioethics and Humanities. (2011). *Core competencies for health care ethics consultation* (2nd ed.). Rittenhouse.

Anthony, D., & Stablein, T. (2016). Privacy in practice: Professional discourse about information control in health care. *Journal of Health Organization and Management, 30*(2), 207–226. https://doi.org/10.1108/JHOM-12-2014-0220

Beauchamp, T. L., & Childress, J. F. (2001). *Principles of biomedical ethics* (5th ed.). Oxford University Press.

Celie, K. B., & Prager, K. (2016). Health care ethics consultation in the United States. *AMA Journal of Ethics, 18*(5), 475–478. https://doi.org/10.1001/journalofethics.2017.18.5.fred1-1605

Chervenak, F. A. & McCullough, L. B. (Eds.). (2021). FIGO *Ethics and Professionalism Guidelines for Obstetrics and Gynecology* (2nd ed). *International Federation of Gynecology and Obstetrics* (FIGO). https://www.figo.org/sites/default/files/2021-11/FIGO-Ethics-Guidelines-onlinePDF.pdf

Clark, P. (1998). A legacy of mistrust: African-Americans, the medical profession, and AIDS. *Linacre Quarterly, 65*(1), Article 8. http://epublications.marquette.edu/lnq/vol65/iss1/8

Dawley, K. (2000). The campaign to eliminate the midwife. *The American Journal of Nursing, 100*(10), 50–56.

Edvardsson, K., Small, R., Lalos, A., Persson, M., & Mogren, I. (2015). Ultrasound's 'window on the womb' brings ethical challenges for balancing maternal and fetal health interests: Obstetricians' experiences in Australia. *BMC Medical Ethics, 16*(31), 1–10. https://doi.org/10.1186/s12910-015-0023-y

Farley, C. L. (2020). Galvanizing global political will in 2020: The year of the nurse and the midwife. *International Journal of Birth and Parent Education, 7*(2), 3–4.

Fishman, M., Paquette, E. T., Gandhi, R., Pendergrast, T. R., Park, M., Flanagan, E., & Ross, L. F. (2020). Surrogate decision making for children: Who should decide? *Journal of Pediatrics, 220*, 221–226. https://doi.org/10.1016/j.jpeds.2019.10.023

Fox, E., Berkowitz, K. A., Chanko, B. L., & Powell, T. (2015). *Ethics consultation: Responding to ethics questions in health care* (2nd ed.). National Center for Ethics in Health Care. Veterans Health Administration. www.ethics.va.gov/ECprimer.pdf. https://doi.org/10.1080/15265161.2015.1134704

Franklin, S. (2013). Conception through a looking glass: The paradox of IVF. *Reproductive Biomedicine Online, 27*, 747–755. https://doi.org/10.1016/j.rbmo.2013.08.010

Halpern, J. (2018). Creating the safety and respect necessary for "shared" decision-making. *Pediatrics, 142*(Suppl 3), S163–S169. http://10.0.6.6/peds.2018-0516G

International Confederation of Midwives. (2014). *International code of midwives.* International Confederation of Midwives. https://www.internationalmidwives.org/about-us/international-confederation-of-midwives

International Federation of Gynecology and Obstetrics. Committee Human Rights Refugees and Violence Against Women. (December 10, 2019). *FIGO statement: Ethical treatment of women.* https://www.figo.org/figo-statement-ethical-treatment-women

Janevic, T., Piverger, N., Afzal, O., & Howell, E. (2020). "Just because you have ears doesn't mean you can hear"—Perception of racial-ethnic discrimination during childbirth. *Ethnicity & Disease, 30*(4), 533–542. https://doi.org/10.18865/ed.30.4.533

Jonsen, A. R. (1993). The birth of bioethics. *Hastings Center Report, 23*(6), S1–S4.

Kidson-Gerber, G., Kerridge, I., Farmer, S., Stewart, C. L., Savoia, H., & Challis, D. (2016). Caring for pregnant women for whom transfusion is not an option. A national review to assist in patient care. *Australian and New Zealand Journal of Obstetrics and Gynaecology, 56*, 127–136. https://doi.org/10.1111/ajo.12420

Lahey, T., DeRenzo, E., Crites, J., Fanning, J., Huberman, B., & Slosar, J. (2020). Building an organizational ethics program on a clinical ethics foundation. *Journal of Clinical Ethics, 31*(3), 259–267. PMID: 32960808

Lee, L. (2017). A bridge back to the future: Public health ethics, bioethics, and environmental ethics. *The American Journal of Bioethics, 17*(9), 5–12. https://doi.org/10.1080/15265161.2017.1353164

Malek, J. (2017). Maternal decision-making during pregnancy: Parental obligations and cultural differences. *Best Practice & Research Clinical Obstetrics and Gynaecology, 43*, 10–20. https://doi.org/10.1016/j.bpobgyn.2017.02.002

Niles, P. M., Stoll, K., Wang, J. J., Black, S., & Vedam, S. (2021). "I fought my entire way": Experiences of declining maternity care services in British Columbia. *PLoS One, 16*(6), e0252645. https://doi.org/10.1371/journal.pone.0252645

Ozar, D. (1999). Profession and professional ethics. In S. G. Post (Ed.), *Encyclopedia of bioethics* (3rd ed.). Macmillan. http://course.sdu.edu.cn/G2S/eWebEditor/uploadfile/20120826203920004.pdf

Payne, P. (2019). Including pregnant women in clinical research: Practical guidance for institutional review boards. *Ethics & Human Research, 41*(6), 35–40. https://doi.org/10.1002/eahr.500036

Prather, C., Fuller, T., Jeffries, W., 4th, Marshall, K., Howell, A., Belyue-Umole, A., & King, W. (2018). Racism, African American women, and their sexual and reproductive health: A review of historical and contemporary evidence and implications for health equity. *Health Equity, 2*(1), 249–259. https://doi.org/10.1089/heq.2017.0045

Rainer, J., Kraenzle Schneider, J., & Lorenz, R. (2018). Ethical dilemmas in nursing: An integrative review. *Journal of Clinical Nursing, 27*, 3446–3461. https://doi.org/10.1111/jocn.14542

Roeder, A. (2019, Winter). America is failing its black mothers. *Harvard Public Health Magazine.* https://www.hsph.harvard.edu/magazine/magazine_article/america-is-failing-its-black-mothers

Salter, E. K. (2017). Conflating capacity and authority: Why we're asking the wrong question in the adolescent decision-making debate. *Hastings Center Report, 47*(1), 32–41. https://doi.org/10.1002/hast.666

Tanne, J. (2020). US lags other rich nations in maternal health care. *BMJ, 371*, m4546. https://doi.org/10.1136/bmj.m4546

Vargesson, N. (2019). The teratogenic effects of thalidomide on limbs. *Journal of Hand Surgery (European Volume), 44*(1), 88–95. https://doi.org/10.1177/1753193418805249

Varkey, B. (2021). Principles of clinical ethics and their application to practice. *Medical Principles and Practice, 30*, 17–28. https://doi.org/10.1159/000509119

Wall, L. (2018). J. Marion Sims and the vesicovaginal fistula: Historical understanding, medical ethics, and modern political sensibilities. *Female Pelvic and Medical Reconstructive Surgery, 24*(2), 66–75. https://doi.org/10.1097/SPV.0000000000000546

White, T. (2019). Driving miss Evers' boys to the historical Tuskegee study of untreated syphilis. *Journal of the National Medical Association, 111*(4), 371–382. https://doi.org/10.1016/j.jnma.2019.01.002

Zielinski, R., Ackerson, K., & Lowe, L. K. (2015). Planned home birth: Benefits, risks, and opportunities. *International Journal of Women's Health, 7*, 361–377. https://doi.org/10.2147/IJWH.S55561

3

Reproductive Tract Structure and Function

LuVerda Sayles Martin

The editors gratefully acknowledge Patricia Caudle, who authored the previous edition of this chapter.

Relevant Terms

Adrenarche—initiation of increased adrenal androgens

Ampulla—wider end of the fallopian tube, the most common site of fertilization

Atresia—degeneration and absorption of immature follicles

Bartholin glands—pea-sized bilateral vulvar glands that secrete fluid to lubricate the vagina

Cervix—lower portion of the uterus

Chadwick's sign—bluish color to the cervix, vagina, and labia due to increased blood flow in pregnancy, can be seen as early as six to eight weeks gestation

Clitoris—erogenous organ with erectile tissue covered by labia minora

Cornua—both sides of the upper outer area of the uterus where the fallopian tubes join the uterus

Ectropion—visible columnar cells at the cervical os

Endocervical canal—passageway within the cervix to the inner uterus

Endometrium—lining of the uterus

Escutcheon—pubic hair

Fimbriae—fingerlike projections that move the egg toward and into the fallopian tube

First polar body—other half of the product of division of the primary oocyte

Fornix (fornices)—spaces around the cervix in the vagina

Fourchette—area immediately below the introitus

Gonadarche—period when ovaries begin to secrete sex hormones

Gonadostat—gonadotropin-releasing hormone pulse generator

Granulosa cells—cells lining an ovarian follicle that become luteal cells after ovulation

Ground substance—mucopolysaccharide between smooth muscle and collagen of the cervix

Hart's line—line of change where skin transitions to smoother, moist skin

Hegar's sign—softening and compressibility of the uterine isthmus

Hymen—membranous ring of tissue at the introitus

Introitus—opening to the vagina

Isthmus—uterine "neck" between cervix and body

Labia majora—two rounded folds of adipose tissue covered with pubic hair

Labia minora—folds of tissue between the labia majora

Lactobacilli—normal bacterial flora of the vagina

Leptin—hormone secreted by fat cells that plays a key role in appetite and metabolism

Meatus—opening of the urethra

Menarche—initiation of menses

Metaplasia—normal replacement of one cell type with another

Mittelschmerz—pain upon ovulation

Myometrium—middle, muscular layer of the uterus

Mucin—glycosylated proteins that form mucus that acts as lubricant and protectant

Nulliparous—a person who has never had a child

Oogenesis—transformation of oogonia into oocytes

Oogonia—primordial female germ cells

Os—opening of the cervix

Parous—person who has had a child

Peritoneum—thin membrane around abdominal organs that covers the bladder, uterus, and rectum

Rectouterine pouch—fold of peritoneum between the uterus and the rectum

Rectovaginal septum—tissue between the rectum and vagina

Rugae—thin ridges of tissue like an accordion that allow for expansion in the vagina

Squamocolumnar junction—where squamous cells and columnar cells meet on the cervix

Skene glands—small bilateral vulvar glands that secrete fluid to lubricate the urethra

Thelarche—breast development

Vasovagal response—bradycardia and syncope

Vesicouterine pouch—fold of peritoneum between the bladder and the uterus

Vesicovaginal septum—tissue between the bladder and the vagina

Vestibule—area inside the labia minora where openings of the urethra and the vagina are found

Zona pellucida—membrane surrounding the plasma membrane of the oocyte

Prenatal and Postnatal Care: A Person-Centered Approach, Third Edition. Edited by Karen Trister Grace, Cindy L. Farley, Noelene K. Jeffers, and Tanya Tringali.
© 2024 John Wiley & Sons Ltd. Published 2024 by John Wiley & Sons Ltd.
Companion website: www.wiley.com/go/grace/prenatal

Anatomy of the Reproductive System

An understanding of the anatomy of the reproductive system is essential in caring for pregnant people. It is important to be able to recognize normal structures and to appreciate that there is a wide variation of normal.

External Genitalia

The vulva is a term designated for the external genitalia. The vulva includes the mons pubis, **labia majora and minora**, **clitoris**, **vestibule**, **hymen**, urinary **meatus**, and Skene and Bartholin glands. Figures 3.1 and 3.2 illustrate the external genitalia and its development from embryonic structures. The external genitals of embryos remain undifferentiated by sex until about the eighth week of gestation.

The mons pubis is the cushion-like area over the pubic bone. In the adult, the mons is covered with curly, coarse pubic hair called the **escutcheon**. The pubic hair distribution is usually triangular but may extend up toward the umbilicus in a diamond shape in people who have higher levels of serum androgens.

The labia majora consist of two rounded folds of adipose tissue covered with pubic hair that extend from the mons to the perineum on either side of the vaginal opening. The **labia minora**, found between the majora, are thinner, pink in color, and hairless (Bickley & Szilagyi, 2020). The labia majora have the same position and general structure as the scrotum and arise from the same tissues during embryonic development.

The labia minora have two folds above where they divide to descend on either side of the vestibule, ending at the **fourchette** just below the **introitus**, or the opening to the vagina. The upper fold forms the prepuce over the clitoris, and the lower fold is the frenulum of the clitoris. The clitoris is an erogenous organ with erectile tissue. Its overall size is 9–11 cm, and it is embryologically homologous to the penis (Pauls, 2015). The clitoris is very sensitive in most people and is a primary source of sexual pleasure.

The vestibule is the area inside the labia minora where the openings to the urethra, vagina, and Skene and Bartholin gland ducts are found. The urethra is just above the vaginal opening and below the pubic arch. The vaginal introitus is rimmed with the hymen or its tags. **Bartholin glands** are located at either side of the lower portion of the introitus. The ducts for these glands open near the hymenal ring at 5 o'clock and 7 o'clock. **Skene glands** and ducts are found near the urethral meatus.

Hart's line is the line of change in the vestibule where keratinized skin meets non-keratinized skin (mucosa). The vulvar skin transitions to smoother, moister skin around the urethral meatus and the introitus.

Below the vulva is the perineal body and anal opening. The perineum is a diamond-shaped area that includes the urogenital triangle and the anal triangle. These structures

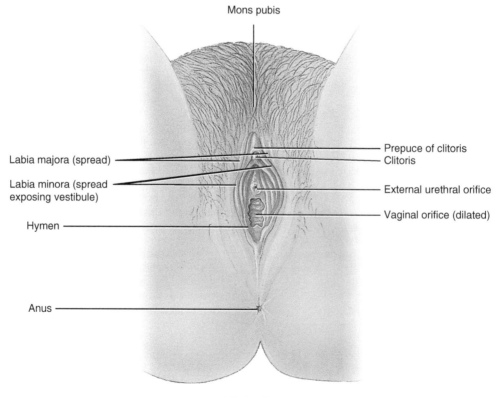

Inferior view

Figure 3.1 External genitalia. Source: Tortora and Derrickson (2017)/with permission of John Wiley & Sons.

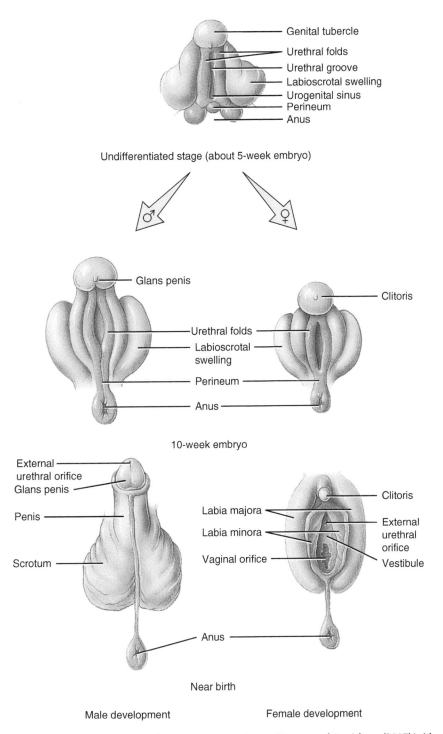

Undifferentiated stage (about 5-week embryo)

10-week embryo

Near birth

Male development   Female development

Figure 3.2   Development of external genitalia from embryonic structures. Source: Tortora and Derrickson (2017)/with permission of John Wiley & Sons.

are examined as part of the external genital examination. Underlying these structures are the superficial muscles of the perineum and anal sphincter. The superficial muscles most often affected by childbirth include the bulbocavernosus muscle, the superficial transverse perineal muscle, and the external and internal anal sphincters.

These structures, with the exception of the internal anal sphincter, converge on the central tendon of the perineum found between the introitus and the anus. The central tendon is part of the perineal body that may tear or be cut by episiotomy during birth (Figure 3.3).

Internal Genitalia

The vagina is a musculomembranous tube that gives access to the **cervix** for coitus and serves as the birth canal. The lower third of the vagina is supported and fixed by the

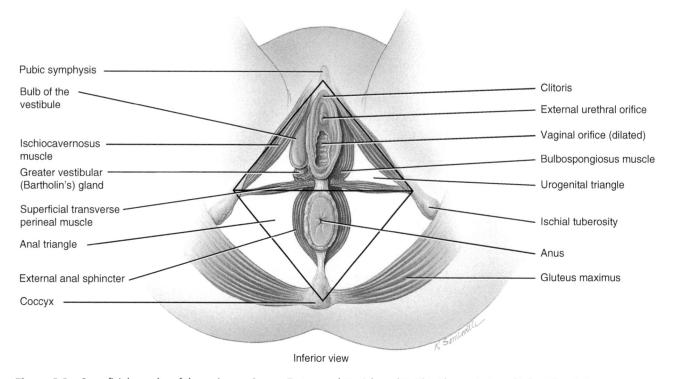

Pubic symphysis
Bulb of the vestibule
Ischiocavernosus muscle
Greater vestibular (Bartholin's) gland
Superficial transverse perineal muscle
Anal triangle
External anal sphincter
Coccyx

Clitoris
External urethral orifice
Vaginal orifice (dilated)
Bulbospongiosus muscle
Urogenital triangle
Ischial tuberosity
Anus
Gluteus maximus

Inferior view

Figure 3.3 Superficial muscles of the perineum. Source: Tortora and Derrickson (2017)/with permission of John Wiley & Sons.

pubococcygeus muscles of the levator ani group. The upper portion of the vagina and the cervix are supported by the cardinal and uterosacral ligaments. This portion of the vagina is capable of incredible expansion to accommodate birth. Vaginal **rugae** allow for elasticity and expansion. Vaginal length varies with genetics, parity, age, and estrogen effect. On average, the length of the vagina is about 9–10 cm (Cunningham et al., 2022). The elastic vagina elongates during intercourse and stretches widely during birth. The spaces around the cervix within the vagina are called the anterior, posterior, and lateral **fornices**.

The rectum supports the middle of the posterior vaginal wall. Some support for the bladder is offered by the anterior vaginal wall (Danhausen et al., 2019). The principal innervations for the vagina are the pudendal nerve and the inferior hypogastric plexus, both of which derive from sacral nerve (S) 2–4. Lymph drainage for the vagina is to the para-aortic nodes.

The vagina is lubricated by an epithelial glycoprotein coat and transudate, cervical mucus from the endocervical columnar epithelium, and by fluids from the Bartholin and Skene glands of the vestibule (Tufts et al., 2019). The milieu of the vagina is acidic and presents a barrier to many bacteria. The pH is normally between 4.0 and 4.5 in people of childbearing age and is maintained by the estrogen effect on the epithelial glycoprotein coat and **lactobacilli** (normal bacterial flora of the vagina). Vaginal secretions increase during pregnancy due to increased vascularity.

The lower portion of the vagina is separated from the urinary bladder by the **vesicovaginal septum** and is separated from the rectum by the **rectovaginal septum,** which is at risk for lacerations and tears during an

operative vaginal birth. The upper vagina, around the cervix, is separated from the rectum via a fold of the **peritoneum** (thin membrane around abdominal organs that covers the uterus, bladder, and rectum) called the **rectouterine pouch** or pouch of Douglas. There is a similar, smaller pouch in front of the cervix and behind the bladder called the **vesicouterine pouch**. During cesarean birth, this area is incised, and the bladder is brought forward (Cunningham et al., 2022).

After ovulation, a secondary oocyte and its corona radiata move from the pelvic cavity into the infundibulum of the uterine tube. The uterus is the site of menstruation, implantation of a fertilized ovum, development of the fetus, and labor.

The cervix is the lower, narrow part of the pear-shaped uterus that protrudes into the vagina (Figure 3.4). About half of the cervix is within the vaginal canal. This part of the cervix has an external **os** followed by a passageway to the uterus called the **endocervical canal**. The canal ends at the internal os, which opens into the uterine cavity. The size and shape of the cervix varies with parity, age, and the amount of estrogen and progesterone available. The cervix of a **nulliparous person** is smaller with a small, circular external os when compared to the cervix of a **parous person**, which is wider with an external os that is slit-like and more open. The length of the cervix plays a role in cervical integrity during pregnancy.

The blood supply to the cervix arrives via the uterine arteries that derive from the internal iliac arteries. The cervical branches of the uterine arteries are located at 3 o'clock and 9 o'clock to the cervical os. Venous blood drains to the hypogastric venous plexus.

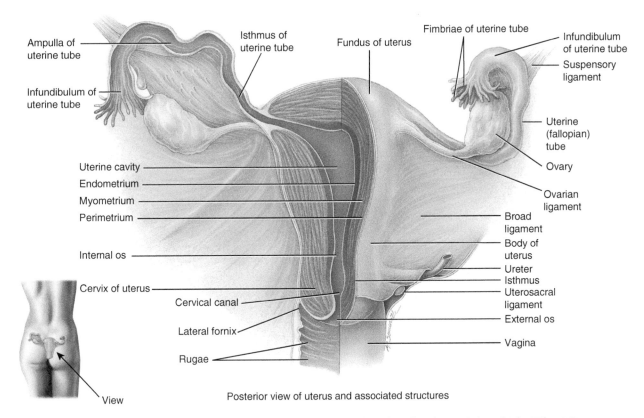

Figure 3.4 The uterus and associated structures. Source: Tortora and Derrickson (2017)/with permission of John Wiley & Sons.

The cardinal and uterosacral ligaments support the cervix and upper vagina. The cardinal ligament attaches to either side of the cervix and extends laterally to attach to connective tissue called the parametrium. The uterosacral ligament attaches to the posterior cervix and extends posteriorly to attach to the fascia of the sacrum. The main nerve supply to the cervix derives from the hypogastric plexus and follows the uterosacral ligament to the posterior cervix. Because there are sensory, sympathetic, and parasympathetic nerve fibers within the endocervical canal, any instrumentation through the cervical os has the potential for causing a **vasovagal response** in some people. Conversely, the external cervix has fewer sensory nerve endings, making small external biopsies less painful for most people.

The structure of the cervix is a complex composition of collagenous connective tissue (smooth muscle and elastic tissue) and **ground substance**, a mucopolysaccharide. There is a much smaller percentage of smooth muscle in the cervix than in the uterine fundus. During pregnancy, the cervix is extraordinarily strong and remains closed as the uterine contents increase in size and volume. Near the end of pregnancy, the cervix softens and becomes distensible, allowing the fetus to be expelled. This dramatic change in the cervix requires enzyme activity, an increase in cervical water content, hormonal changes, and an increase in prostaglandins (Blackburn, 2017). After birth, the dilated cervix will shorten and become firm so that by one week postpartum, the os is dilated to only 1 cm.

Histologically, the cervix has two cell types: the columnar cells that line the endocervical canal and the opening of the cervix, and the squamous epithelium that covers the outside of the cervix. The **squamocolumnar junction** (SCJ), where these two cell layers meet, is where most lower genital tract cancers occur (Danhausen, et al., 2019).

Columnar cells secrete **mucin** (a glycosylated protein that forms mucus that acts as lubricant and protectant) and have a reddened papillary appearance. The squamous epithelium is smooth and pink. At **menarche**, higher levels of estrogen cause glycogenation and other changes in the squamous epithelium. These changes and the increasing acidity in the vagina cause the squamous cells to migrate and cover the columnar cells. **Metaplasia** of the squamous and columnar cells occurs at the SCJ. This makes this area highly susceptible to invasion by human papilloma virus, hyperplasia, and dysplasia. Metaplasia occurs throughout childbearing years. Over time, the SCJ will migrate into the endocervical canal. The SCJ is the most important area for collection of cell samples for cervical cancer screening.

Columnar cells are visible (and called **ectropion**) at the cervical os during adolescence, pregnancy, and while taking oral contraceptive pills due to the higher levels of estrogen during these events. Cervical mucus, produced by columnar cells, changes according to the hormones secreted during the menstrual cycle. During the late follicular phase and ovulation, when estrogen levels are highest, the mucus is clear, stretchy, slick, thin, and abundant. These characteristics of the mucus facilitate sperm passage from the vagina, through the cervix, and into the uterus. Under the influence of progesterone during the luteal phase, the mucus becomes scant, thick, pasty, and opaque. The inhibition of sperm penetration through the thickening of cervical mucus is an important mechanism of progestin-only contraceptives (Regidor, 2018).

Mucus from the columnar cells of the endocervical canal becomes thick and forms a "mucous plug" during pregnancy. This plug helps to prevent the passage of bacteria into the uterus. Increased vascularity and swelling of the cervix during early pregnancy causes a bluish coloring called **Chadwick's sign**.

The uterine cervix is connected to the body of the uterus by the **isthmus**. During early pregnancy, this segment of the uterus softens and becomes compressible, a feature specific to pregnancy known as **Hegar's sign**.

The body or corpus of the uterus (Figure 3.4) is the most dynamic portion of the uterus. The **endometrium** is the innermost lining of the uterus. It responds to ovarian hormones every month, proliferates in preparation for implantation, and then sheds as menses if pregnancy does not occur (Lessey & Young, 2019). This is also where implantation and gestation take place and where the powerful forces of labor are generated. An adult uterus is about 3–4 in (7–10 cm) long before any pregnancies have occurred. After pregnancy and postpartum involution, the range is 4.5–5 in. The weight of the nonpregnant uterus is about 60 g if never pregnant and heavier depending on the number of pregnancies (Cunningham et al., 2022). During pregnancy, the muscles of the uterus hypertrophy and the weight will increase to about 1 kg by 40-week gestation. This hypertrophy does not extend to the cervix, which contains less muscle tissue.

Attached to both sides of the upper, outer portion of the uterus, known as the **cornua**, are the fallopian tubes, round ligaments, and ovarian ligaments. The body of the uterus, unlike the cervix, is mostly muscle tissue. Inside the uterus, the anterior and posterior walls lie close to each other, forming a slit-like space (Cunningham et al., 2022). Within this space of the uterus is the endometrium, the first of three layers in the uterine corpus (Lessey & Young, 2019). The endometrial cyclic response to hormones is explained later in this chapter.

The middle layer of the uterus is the **myometrium**. This layer is composed of smooth muscle united by connective tissue and makes up most of the uterine bulk. The outermost layer is the perimetrium, a thin layer of epithelial cells. The myometrium contains four layers of muscles with blood vessels coursing through each layer. The inner layer of muscle fibers is composed of spirals on the long axis of the uterus. The middle layers of muscle fibers have interlacing fibers that form a figure eight around the abundant blood vessels. When the placenta is expelled after birth, the empty uterus contracts and the muscles of this layer become "living ligatures" that help halt the blood flow. The two outer layers of muscle fibers are smooth muscle in bundles of 10–50 overlapping cells interspersed with connective tissue and ground substance that transmit contractions during labor (Blackburn, 2017). Interestingly, the layers of the myometrium arise from different embryonic locations, so they respond to uterine stimuli in different ways. The result is a rhythmic contractile force that propels the fetus toward the cervical opening regardless of fetal presentation.

Uterine blood supply comes from the internal iliac artery via the ovarian and uterine arteries. These arteries feed the arcuate, radial, basal, and spiral arteries. The spiral arteries of the endometrium change during the menstrual cycle. If pregnancy does not occur during the cycle, the spiral arteries constrict, the endometrial matrix breaks down, and menses occurs. Collateral circulation is enhanced during pregnancy. This arterial system is efficient in supplying nutrients and oxygen to the growing uteroplacental unit and fetus, but if hemorrhage occurs, this interconnected system of vessels makes control of the bleeding difficult.

There are two sets of lymphatics within the uterine body. One set drain into the superficial inguinal nodes and the other set ends in the para-aortic lymph chain (Cunningham et al., 2022). The nerve supply to the uterus is derived mostly from the sympathetic nervous system and partly from the parasympathetic system. The parasympathetic system fibers derive from sacral nerves 2, 3, and 4. The sympathetic system ultimately comes from the aortic plexus just below the sacral promontory. Sensory fibers from the uterus derive from thoracic nerve roots 11 and 12 and carry the pain signals from contractions of labor to the central nervous system. The sensory nerves from the cervix and upper vagina move through the pelvic nerves to sacral nerves 2, 3, and 4. The primary nerve of the lower vagina is the pudendal nerve.

The fallopian tubes (Figure 3.4) extend from the upper sides of the uterus. These oviducts vary from 8 to 14 cm in length. There are three parts: the **fimbriae**, **ampulla**, and the isthmus. The fimbriae open into the abdominal cavity and have fingerlike, ciliated projections, with one longer projection that reaches closer to or touches the ovary, which captures the ovum from the surface of the ovary. The ampulla is the widest section of the uterine tubes. The smooth muscle and ciliated cells within the tubes contract rhythmically all the time. At ovulation, these contractions become stronger and more frequent in order to move the ovum toward the uterine lining. If fertilization occurs, it will typically happen in the ampulla (Blackburn, 2017). The isthmus is the narrowest section of the tubes, connecting the ampulla to the uterine cavity.

The ovaries reside on either side of the uterus and are attached to the ovarian ligament that extends to and attaches to the cornua. Other ligaments help support the ovaries and serve as conduits for vessels and nerves. The top layer of the ovary contains oocytes and developing follicles. The core of the ovary is composed of connective tissue, blood vessels, and smooth muscle. Ovaries vary in size and typically range from 2.5–5 cm long and 1.5–3 cm wide, giving them an almond shape. Ovaries may be palpable during the bimanual examination of the adnexa during pelvic examination (Bickley & Szilagyi, 2020).

Menstrual Cycle Physiology

The menstrual cycle occurs regularly in most people from menarche to menopause with some expected irregularity during the first year after menarche and the years of perimenopause. The cycle is regulated by complex interactions between the hypothalamus, the pituitary gland, the ovaries, and the uterus. This section will highlight the hormonal changes and how these changes affect the ovaries and the uterine lining.

Beginnings

The sex of an embryo is determined at the time of fertilization. The sperm's contribution of an X chromosome combined with the ova-contributed X chromosome produce the basis for a unique human of female sex. Sixteen weeks after fertilization, primordial germ cells called **oogonia** can be detected along the genital ridge in embryos that will develop ovaries (Moore et al., 2019). By seven months of gestation, all of the oogonia have been transformed into primary oocytes and no new oogonia are formed. At birth, the newborn ovaries contain an average of 200,000–400,000 follicles. Each follicle contains a primary oocyte that has already begun the first meiotic division (Moore et al., 2019). At puberty, only

about 10%, or 40,000, of these early follicles will remain due to **atresia**. Of these, only about 400–500 will develop into primary and secondary follicles.

Oogenesis is the sequence of events that transforms the oogonia into an oocyte ready to be fertilized. In early fetal life, oogonia divide via mitosis to form primary oocytes. By birth, the primary oocytes have begun the first meiotic division, but the process is arrested and remains that way until just before ovulation, when the first meiotic division is completed. At this division, a secondary oocyte receives the bulk of the cytoplasm, and the **first polar body** is formed. At ovulation, the secondary oocyte begins its second meiotic division, but the process halts and does not resume unless it is fertilized by a sperm (Moore et al., 2019). The process of oogenesis is depicted in Figure 3.5.

At term, the fetal gonadotropin-releasing hormone pulse generator, or **gonadostat**, is at work. The gonadostat responds to high levels of the pregnant person's estrogen

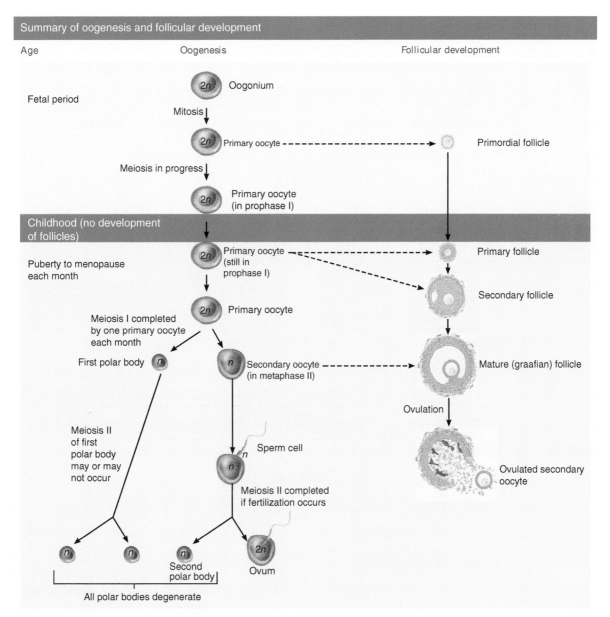

Figure 3.5   Oogenesis. Source: Tortora and Derrickson (2017)/with permission of John Wiley & Sons.

by releasing small amounts of gonadotropin-releasing hormone. After birth, when this estrogen is removed, the gonadotropins, follicle-stimulating hormone (FSH) and luteinizing hormone (LH), are released from the pituitary gland of the newborn and then begin to fall (Tufts et al., 2019). During infancy and childhood, estrogen levels are very low and gonadotropin secretion is restrained in a positive feedback fashion.

Onset of Puberty

When a person with ovaries is 8–12 years old, the gonads begin to produce estrogen and puberty begins with **thelarche** (breast development). Estrogen production begins in response to complex interrelated changes involving the central nervous system, hypothalamus, pituitary, and ovary. The onset of these changes is influenced by factors including genetics, general health, nutrition, geographic location, exposure to light, and

body weight (Silverthorn, 2018; Tufts et al., 2019). It is thought that increasing body fat and the adipose hormone **leptin** facilitate maturation, and both are important to the onset of menses. Reproductive maturation involves the central nervous system and the endocrine system in a sequence of changes that will, ultimately, lead to menarche.

The first in the sequence of events that will lead to reproductive maturation is the release of gonadotropin-releasing hormone from the hypothalamus that will cause the release of FSH and LH from the pituitary. These hormones will induce **gonadarche** and **adrenarche**, and the hormones from the gonads and adrenal glands stimulate the development of secondary sex characteristics such as breast growth, pubic and axillary hair growth, and changes in the vagina (Bickley & Szilagyi, 2020; Tufts et al., 2019). These changes also set the stage for the first ovulation and first ovulatory menstrual period. Figure 3.6 illustrates the sequence for the beginning of hormonal

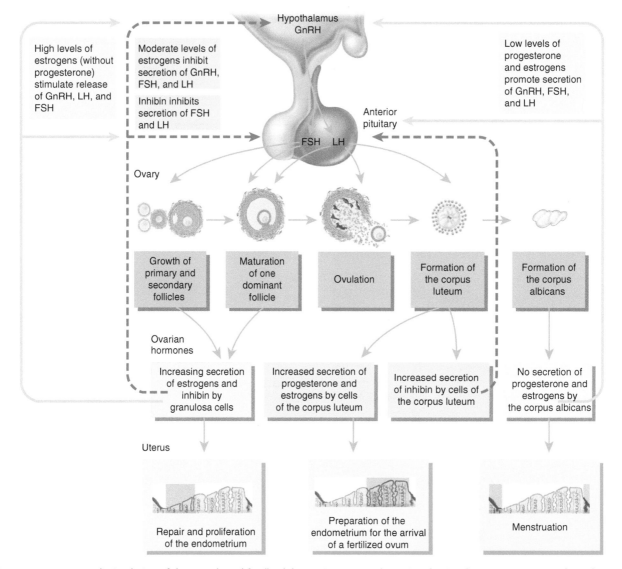

Figure 3.6 Hormonal stimulation of the gonads and feedback loops. GnRH, gonadotropin-releasing hormone. Hormones from the anterior pituitary regulate ovarian function, and hormones from the ovaries regulate the changes in the endometrial lining of the uterus. Source: Tortora and Derrickson (2017)/with permission of John Wiley & Sons.

Table 3.1   Normal Menstrual Cycle Characteristics

Menarche (average age)	
White	12.43 years
Black	~11.5 years
Menstrual cycle length	
First year of menses	32.2 days (range 20–60 days)
Typical menstrual cycle length during the years between menarche and menopause	21–45 days (only 9–15% are 28 days in length)
Flow length	
First year	2–7 days
Typical length	4–6 days (less than 2 or more than 8 considered abnormal)
Flow amount	20–80 mL (second day heaviest)

Source: Adapted from American College of Obstetricians and Gynecologists [ACOG] (2015); Blackburn (2017); and Nelson & Shulman (2018).

stimulation of the ovary and negative and positive feedback loops.

The average age for menarche in the United States varies according to population, race, socioeconomic conditions, and nutrition. Among well-nourished White people, the average age at menarche is 12.43; Black people experience menarche about five or six months earlier (ACOG, 2015). Suggested factors that explain this disparity include structural factors such as disparate exposure to poverty and environmental toxins, as well as interpersonal factors such as experience of racism and discrimination (Shirazi & Rosinger, 2021). Table 3.1 describes the characteristics of the normal menstrual cycle.

Once menarche and ovulatory cycles are established, puberty is complete and the person is physiologically able to reproduce; however, social and cultural norms influence reproductive behaviors and choices once physical reproductive maturity is achieved. Throughout the childbearing years, the hypothalamic–pituitary–ovarian (HPO) axis, and the uterus go through cycles in the production of hormones and changes in the endometrial lining.

The Hypothalamic–Pituitary–Ovarian Axis

Once established, the menstrual cycle continues based on feedback mechanisms between the hypothalamus, pituitary, and the ovary. The hypothalamus is a pearl-sized organ at the base of the brain near the optic chiasm. The cells of the hypothalamus synthesize and secrete many hormones that act on the pituitary and other endocrine glands. The hypothalamus is responsible for regulating thirst, sleep, hunger, libido, and many

endocrine functions (Tufts et al., 2019). The hypothalamus responds to lower serum levels of estrogen near the end of a cycle by secreting an FSH-releasing factor that will travel to the nearby pituitary gland and stimulate the release of FSH. FSH will stimulate the growth of follicles on the ovary, with one follicle becoming dominant for each cycle. Later, when the follicle releases enough estrogen, the hypothalamus will secrete an LH-releasing hormone that will travel to the pituitary and stimulate the release of LH.

The pituitary gland is located in the sella turcica, below the hypothalamus and optic chiasm. It has a stalk connecting it to the hypothalamus and two lobes: anterior and posterior. The anterior lobe synthesizes and secretes FSH, LH, and many other hormones that affect specific target organs. Figure 3.6 depicts the early HPO axis with feedback loops.

The ovaries are the target organs for gonadotropins secreted by the anterior pituitary. They are located on either side of the uterus, suspended by the ovarian ligament. They are covered in follicles, each with the potential for growing and releasing an ovum. Figure 3.7 shows the ovarian surface and the stages of the follicle.

The functioning of the HPO axis is dependent on feedback loop control. The most common form of feedback control is negative feedback. This occurs when rising hormone serum levels cause a decrease in another hormone. The other form of feedback control is positive feedback, where rising levels of one hormone cause a rise in another. These feedback mechanisms help to keep the hormones within normal ranges.

The hormones involved in the menstrual cycle include the gonadotropin-releasing hormones from the hypothalamus, the gonadotropin-stimulating hormones from the pituitary, and the ovarian hormones from the ovary (Table 3.2).

Menstrual Cycle Phases

There are two parts to the menstrual cycle that occur simultaneously. To help clarify what is happening in each part, this section will separate the ovarian cycle and the endometrial cycle.

Ovarian Cycle

There are three phases of the ovarian cycle: follicular phase, ovulation, and luteal phase. The follicular phase begins on the first day of menses and is more variable in length than the luteal phase. It may last from 10 to 21 days (Silverthorn, 2018). The luteal phase is the most predictable in length because of the lifespan of the corpus luteum. It lasts 13–15 days unless a pregnancy occurs and the life of the corpus luteum continues (Nelson & Shulman, 2018).

The follicular phase begins during the last days of the previous cycle when decreasing levels of estrogen and inhibin deliver a negative feedback signal to the hypothalamus and pituitary. This signal stimulates the hypothalamus to release an FSH-releasing factor that

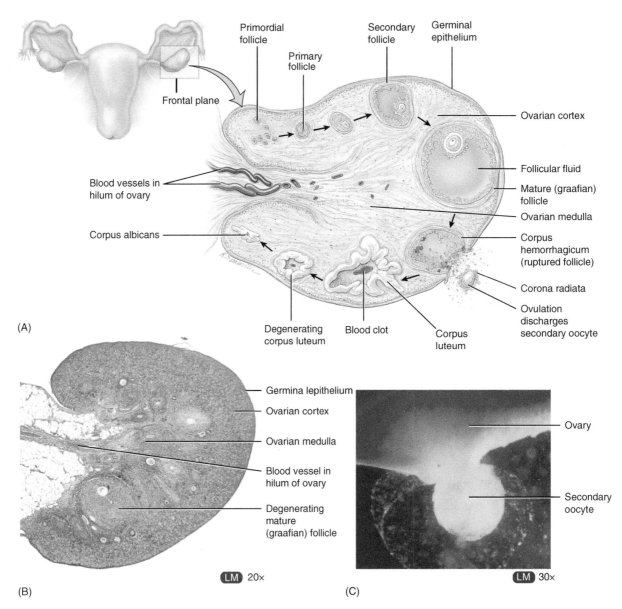

Figure 3.7 Cross section of the ovary during the reproductive years. (A) Frontal section. (B) Hemisection. (C) Ovulation of a secondary oocyte. The ovaries are gonads that produce haploid oocytes. Source: Tortora and Derrickson (2017)/with permission of John Wiley & Sons.

Table 3.2 Hormones of the Menstrual Cycle

Hypothalamus	Follicle-stimulating hormone-releasing factor Gonadotropin-releasing factor Luteinizing hormone-releasing factor
Pituitary	Follicle-stimulating hormone
	Luteinizing hormone
Ovary	Progesterone
	Estrogen
	Testosterone
	Inhibin
	Activin
	Follistatin

Source: Adapted from Tufts et al. (2019).

stimulates the anterior pituitary to release FSH. The primordial follicles on the ovary each contain an oocyte and a layer of **granulosa cells** that will respond to the FSH. It is thought that there is at least a three-month period of stimulation to recruit the dominant follicle for one ovulation (Blackburn, 2017). It is this one primed follicle that responds to FSH first and begins to grow before other follicles on the ovaries that may respond. This follicle takes in more FSH than the others and grows more rapidly. Within this dominant or primary follicle, the oocyte begins to grow and the **zona pellucida** is formed and grows between the oocyte and the granulosa cells (Tufts et al., 2019). Just before ovulation, the corona radiata will form around the zona pellucida. As these changes progress, some of the follicles that had started to respond to FSH but did not fully mature undergo atresia (Nelson & Shulman, 2018).

During the follicular phase, the ovary and the primary follicle secrete both estrogen and progesterone, with estrogen being produced in higher amounts. FSH stimulates the granulosa cells of the dominant follicle to produce much higher levels of estrogen and to upregulate LH receptors within the follicle cells (Tufts et al., 2019). The higher levels of estrogen cause positive feedback stimulation of the hypothalamus and pituitary that result in a rise in LH. Near the end of the follicular phase, the estrogen level will peak, causing LH to surge and reach its highest level about 12–24 hours before ovulation (Blackburn, 2017).

The higher levels of LH are a reliable signal of impending ovulation. LH detection kits are available to help couples determine when ovulation occurs (US Food and Drug Administration [FDA], 2018).

LH has other functions as well. It stimulates ovarian tissue in a way that increases androgen levels and enhances libido (Nelson & Shulman, 2018). It prompts the remaining granulosa cells of the ruptured follicle to become lutein cells so that the corpus luteum is formed. LH is also responsible for stimulating the oocyte to resume meiosis (Silverthorn, 2018).

Ovulation occurs after a surge and peak level of LH, but there are several factors that facilitate the extrusion of the ovum from the follicle. As the follicle and oocyte have grown, the oocyte has shifted to one side of the follicle. When estrogen begins to decrease, the follicle swells and prostaglandins, proteolytic enzymes, and smooth muscle contractions cause the follicular wall to burst open and the ovum is extruded (Blackburn, 2017). The phenomenon of **mittelschmerz** or pain upon ovulation is thought to be due to the rupture of the follicle and the release of the ovum and surrounding fluid that can irritate the abdominal lining.

After ovulation, the remaining cells of the follicle are revascularized and transformed into the corpus luteum by taking up hormones and lutein pigment that gives it a yellow color (Nelson & Shulman, 2018). The corpus luteum continues to secrete estrogen and progesterone, but now progesterone is produced in higher amounts. Progesterone will cause changes in the endometrium and suppress new follicular growth. It will peak between seven and eight days after the rapid increase of LH. This highest level of progesterone corresponds with the time of implantation, if fertilization has occurred. If implantation occurs, the corpus luteum is maintained by the human chorionic gonadotropin (hCG) secreted by the conceptus so that progesterone levels are maintained.

If fertilization has not occurred, the corpus luteum begins involution and estrogen, progesterone, and inhibin levels will fall. Cellular changes during involution will result in a small scar on the ovary called the corpus albicans (Silverthorn, 2018). The decrease in the ovarian hormones causes a negative feedback stimulation of the hypothalamus and pituitary, and the process begins again.

Endometrial Cycle

The endometrial cycle has three phases: proliferative, secretory, and menstrual. These phases correspond with events occurring in the ovarian cycle. Proliferative changes in the endometrial lining occur under the influence of estrogen during the corresponding follicular phase. During this phase, there are both hyperplasia of the endothelial cells and growth of the stroma within the endometrium (Silverthorn, 2018). The endometrial thickness will reach 0.5–5 mm during this phase.

After ovulation, when the corpus luteum begins producing more progesterone, the secretory phase begins. During this phase, the epithelial cells accumulate glycogen, become more tortuous, the spiral arteries coil, and capillary permeability of the stroma increases (Cunningham et al., 2022). If fertilization occurs, the secretory endometrium begins transformation to decidual tissue and will be approximately 5–10 mm deep when implantation begins (Blackburn, 2017).

If fertilization does not occur, then the endometrium degenerates and the menstrual phase begins. The corpus luteum atrophies, estrogen and progesterone production decreases, and prostaglandins are released. Prostaglandins cause vasoconstriction and other changes that lead to ischemia and necrosis of the secretory structures. At the same time, there is the breakdown of proteins within the superficial layer and sloughing. Rupture of capillaries during sloughing leads to bleeding. Bleeding and myometrial contractions help remove the deteriorated endometrium (Tufts et al., 2019).

Menses typically lasts four to six days. The prostaglandins released during menses will cause contractions, ischemia, and pain in some people. These contractions, along with increasing estrogen levels which encourage clot formation, eventually stop the bleeding (Nelson & Shulman, 2018). Figure 3.8 illustrates the endocrine changes, ovarian cycle, and endometrial cycle in one chart.

The menstrual cycle is a complex phenomenon that ensures the continuation of the human race.

Most of the time, all of the components work in harmony, and there is no need to intervene. The journey of embryonic and fetal development that occurs in the uterus is continued in Chapter 4, *Conception, Implantation, and Embryonic and Fetal Development*.

Resources for Clients and Families

Menstruation and the Menstrual Cycle Fact Sheet: https://www.womenshealth.gov/publications/our-publications/fact-sheet/menstruation.html

Resources for Healthcare Providers

Physiology, Female Reproduction: ncbi.nln.nih.gov/books/NBK537132/

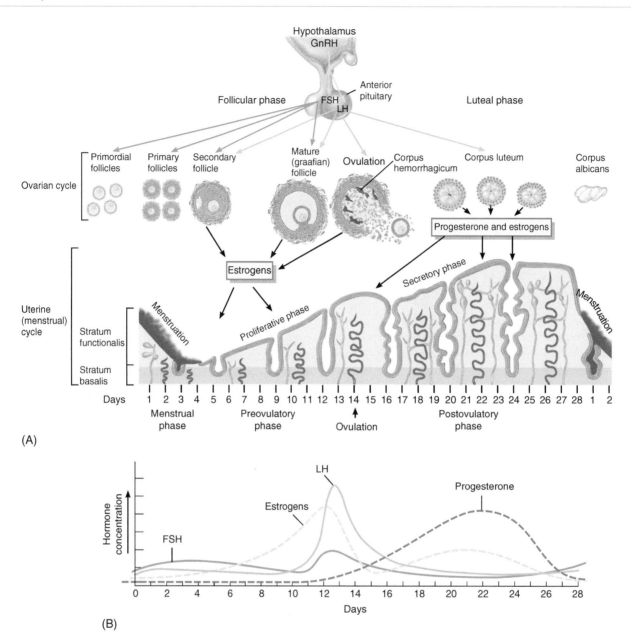

Figure 3.8 Changing hormone levels during the menstrual cycle. (A) Hormonal regulation of changes in the ovary and uterus. (B) Changes in concentration of anterior pituitary and ovarian hormones. Estrogens are the primary ovarian hormones before ovulation; after ovulation, both progesterone and estrogens are secreted by the corpus luteum. Source: Tortora and Derrickson (2017)/with permission of John Wiley & Sons.

References

American College of Obstetricians and Gynecologists (ACOG). (2015). Menstruation in girls and adolescents: Using the menstrual cycle as a vital sign. Committee Opinion No. 651. *Obstetrics and Gynecology, 126*, e143–e146.

Bickley, L., & Szilagyi, P. (2020). *Bates' guide to physical examination and history taking* (13th ed.). Wolters Kluwer/Lippincott Williams & Wilkins.

Blackburn, S. (2017). *Maternal, fetal, & neonatal physiology: A clinical perspective* (5th ed.). Elsevier.

Cunningham, F., Leveno, K., Dashe, J., Hoffman, B., Spong, C., & Casey, B. (2022). *Williams obstetrics* (26th ed.). McGraw-Hill Medical.

Danhausen, K. E., Phillippi, J. C., & McCance, K. L. (2019). Alterations of the female reproductive system. In K. McCance & S. Huether (Eds.), *Pathophysiology: The biologic basis for disease in adults and children* (8th ed., pp. 755–834). Elsevier.

Lessey, B. A., & Young, S. L. (2019). Structure, function, and evaluation of the female reproductive tract. In J. F. Straus & R. L. Barbieri (Eds.), *Reproductive endocrinology* (8th ed., pp. 206–247). Elsevier.

Moore, K., Persaud, T., & Torchia, M. (2019). *Before we are born: Essentials of embryology and birth defects* (10th ed.). Elsevier.

Nelson, A., & Shulman, L. (2018). The menstrual cycle. In R. Hatcher, A. Nelson, J. Trussell, C. Cwiak, P. Cason, M. Policar, A. Aiken, J. Marrazzo, & D. Kowal (Eds.), *Contraceptive Technology* (21st ed., pp. –51). Managing Contraception.

Pauls, R. N. (2015). Anatomy of the clitoris and the female sexual response. *Clinical Anatomy, 28*(3), 376–384. https://doi.org/10.1002/ca.22524

Regidor, P. A. (2018). Clinical relevance in present day hormonal contraception. *Hormone Molecular Biology and Clinical Investigation, 37*(1), 20180030. https://doi.org/10.1515/hmbci-2018-0030

Shirazi, T. N., & Rosinger, A. Y. (2021). Reproductive health disparities in the USA: Self-reported race/ethnicity predicts age of menarche and live birth ratios, but not infertility. *Journal of Racial and Ethnic Health Disparities, 8*(1), 33–46. https://doi.org/10.1007/s40615-020-00752-4

Silverthorn, D. (2018). *Human physiology: an integrated approach* (8th ed.). Pearson.

Tortora, G. J., & Derrickson, B. (2017). *Principles of anatomy & physiology* (13th ed.). Wiley.

Tufts, G., Rodway, G., Huether, S., & Deneris, A. (2019). Structure and function of the reproductive systems. In K. McCance & S. Huether (Eds.), *Pathophysiology: The biologic basis for disease in adults and children* (8th ed., pp. 726–754). Elsevier/Mosby.

US Food and Drug Administration (FDA). (2018). Medical Devices: Ovulation (urine test). Retrieved from https://www.fda.gov/medical-devices/home-use-tests/ovulation-urine-test

4

Conception, Implantation, and Embryonic and Fetal Development

LuVerda Sayles Martin

The editors gratefully acknowledge Patricia Caudle, who authored the previous edition of this chapter.

Relevant Terms

Acrosome reaction—a process that exposes small openings in the head of the sperm that allows it to penetrate the ovum membrane and release its contents

Active transport—movement across a semipermeable membrane against a concentration gradient

Allantois—small appendage of the umbilical vesicle

Angiogenesis—process by which new vessels form from existing vessels

Apoptosis—programmed cell death

Blastocyst—third stage of the conceptus development; postmorula

Capacitation—removal of the glycoprotein coat from the head of the sperm

Chorion—outer membrane that surrounds the embryo/fetus and becomes the fetal part of the placenta

Chorion frondosum—villi at embryonic pole that extend into the decidua; will develop into the placenta

Chorion laeve—smooth chorion that will fuse and disappear

Chorionic villi—projections from the cytotrophoblast to the syncytiotrophoblast that eventually become an arteriocapillary venous network that supplies the embryo

Cleavage—replication process of cells

Cloacal membrane—future site of the anal opening in the embryo

Coelom—cavity that fills with a nutrient lake for molecular exchange between the pregnant person and the embryo

Corona radiata—first layer of the ovum

Cytotrophoblast—inner layer of the trophoblast

Decidual reaction—cellular and vascular changes in the endometrium at implantation

Diploid—contains 46 chromosomes

Ectoderm—outermost layer of the developing embryo

Endoderm—innermost layer of the developing embryo

Extraembryonic somatic mesoderm—layer of mesoderm that will combine with trophoblast to form the chorion

Facilitated diffusion—movement across a semipermeable membrane that needs a transporter but no energy

Gametes—ovum and sperm

Gastrulation—formation of the germ layers of the embryo

Haploid—contains 23 chromosomes

Implantation bleeding—loss of a small amount of blood from the uterine lining during implantation

Lacunae—small spaces or "lakes" within the syncytiotrophoblast

Lanugo—fine, soft hair that covers the fetus

Lipolysis—breakdown of fat molecules

Mesenchymal—cells that can differentiate into many different cell types

Mesoderm—middle layer of the developing embryo

Morula—mulberry-like group of cells, second phase of conceptus cellular development, postzygote

Neurulation—formation of the neural tube

Notochord—rodlike structure that helps organize the nervous system and becomes part of the vertebra and axial skeleton

Oligohydramnios—less than normal amount of amniotic fluid

Oocyte—ovum

Oogonia—primitive ovum

Organogenesis—process by which endoderm, mesoderm, and ectoderm develop into internal organs

Peptide—synthesized from protein

Pinocytosis—carrier molecule is required to engulf molecules and move it across the placental barrier

Placenta accreta—abnormal attachment of the trophoblast to the endometrium

Polyhydramnios—excessive amniotic fluid

Precursors—building blocks or chemicals used to make another chemical

Primitive streak—line of epiblast cells through the middle of the back of the embryo

Pulmonary hypoplasia—poor fetal lung growth

Quickening—fetal movement first felt by the pregnant person

Sacrococcygeal teratoma—cystic tumor with tissue from all three embryonic germ layers

---

Prenatal and Postnatal Care: A Person-Centered Approach, Third Edition. Edited by Karen Trister Grace, Cindy L. Farley, Noelene K. Jeffers, and Tanya Tringali.
© 2024 John Wiley & Sons Ltd. Published 2024 by John Wiley & Sons Ltd.
Companion website: www.wiley.com/go/grace/prenatal

Simple diffusion—movement across a semipermeable membrane from higher to lower concentration

Somites—segmental mass of mesoderm occurring in pairs along the notochord, which develop into vertebrae and muscles

Steroid—hormones that are synthesized from cholesterol

Syncytiotrophoblast—outer layer of the conceptus that sends out fingerlike extensions that take in uterine cells as it invades the endometrium

Teratogen—any substance that can disrupt the development of an embryo

Velamentous insertion—umbilical blood vessels insert into the placenta via the amniotic membrane and are not protected by Wharton's jelly

Vernix caseosa—waxy coating on the fetus that protects the skin

Wharton's jelly—gelatinous connective tissue of the umbilical cord

Zona pellucida—second layer of the ovum

Zygote—first cell created by fusion of ovum and sperm

Introduction

Estrogen produced by the ovarian follicle begins the preparation of the endometrial lining for a potential pregnancy. When the follicle extrudes the ovum, the *corpus luteum* develops and begins to produce more progesterone (literally, progestation). This hormone causes the endometrium to become very receptive to implantation should conception occur. This chapter will outline conception, implantation of the *conceptus* into the receptive uterine lining, and the development of the embryo/fetus and placenta. For purposes of consistency, embryonic and fetal age is based on the estimated time of fertilization unless otherwise stated.

Conception and Implantation

Conception or fertilization occurs in the ampulla of the fallopian tube typically within 24 hours of ovulation. In order for conception to occur, approximately 300–500 sperm must be in the fallopian tube when the ovum arrives. That amount of sperm is needed to produce the enzymes needed for one sperm to fertilize the egg (Blackburn, 2018). During the journey through the cervix and uterus to the fallopian tube, the sperm undergoes **capacitation** so that when it passes through the **corona radiata** (the first layer of the ovum), it can begin the **acrosome reaction** (small openings of the head that release the contents) and bind to the **zona pellucida**, which is the second layer of the ovum. The enzymes that have been released by the other sperm help to remove obstructing cells and allow one sperm to penetrate the zona pellucida and enter the ovum. The entire sperm will be taken into the **oocyte** or ovum. Once the sperm has entered the ovum cytoplasm, a zonal reaction occurs to prevent another sperm from entering. The sperm determines the sex of the embryo by contributing either an X (for female) or a Y (for male) sex chromosome.

Within a few hours, the **haploid** (containing 23 chromosomes) **gametes** (ovum and sperm) will unite within the ovum to form a complete **diploid** (containing 46 chromosomes) cell called the **zygote**, the first cell of a human being. Next, a complex chain of events occurs. All of the information to make a human being is within the zygote. Each cell that develops from this first cell will move and take shape according to the programming of the DNA (deoxyribonucleic acid) from each parent. Cells will change in order to make different tissues, and changing cells will influence each other and migrations of cells form different organs. **Apoptosis** occurs so that cavities are formed and excessive growth does not occur (Beery et al., 2018).

The zygote begins to move toward the uterus and the cell begins the replication process, or **cleavage**. Cleavage divisions come under the control of the zygote at the fourth to eighth stages in human development, and the developing zygote enters the uterine cavity around the fourth day after fertilization (Roberts & Benirschke, 2018). Fluid accumulates in the **morula**, forming a **blastocyst**. The **zona pellucida** is the covering for the blastocyst that works to protect it from the pregnant person's immune system (Blackburn, 2018). About five days after fertilization, a 58-cell blastocyst will shed the zona pellucida and secrete substances that help to make the uterine lining even more receptive to implantation. These substances include human chorionic gonadotropin (hCG).

Spontaneous pregnancy losses that occur during the first two weeks are typically caused by chromosomal abnormalities or by failure of the blastocyst and the **syncytiotrophoblast** to produce enough hCG to maintain the corpus luteum as it produces progesterone. Figure 4.1 depicts the cleavage and travel of the conceptus through the fallopian tube to the uterine implantation site.

Implantation of the blastocyst into the estrogen- and progesterone-primed endometrium begins about 6–10 days after ovulation (Liu, 2018). Most implantations occur on the upper posterior uterine segment closest to the follicle that released the egg. The blastocyst adjusts itself so that the embryonic pole is closest to the endometrial lining (Blackburn, 2018). It will embed entirely into the endometrium where it has adhered itself.

Fertilization usually occurs in the uterine tube.

The embryonic disc appears, and during the second week, it develops the **ectoderm**, **endoderm**, and **mesoderm** layers that will later form all the body systems of the embryo. Structures outside the embryonic disc form the amniotic cavity, the amnion, the umbilical cord beginnings, and the chorionic sac.

The Placenta

Beginnings and Structure

Encircling the blastocyst are trophoblast cells that begin the invasion process by projecting into the uterine lining to reach the pregnant person's blood vessels. These cells will form the placenta. Once adhered to the endometrium, the

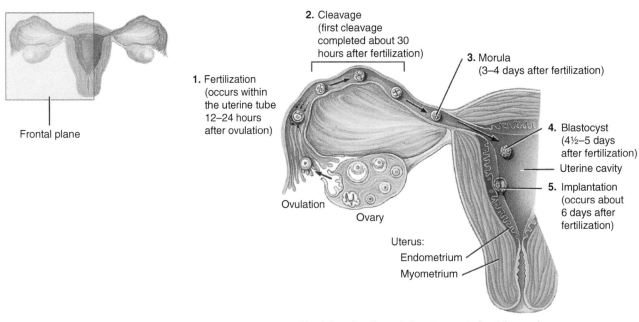

Figure 4.1 Cleavage and travel of the conceptus to the uterus.

trophoblast cells differentiate into two layers. The outer layer is the syncytiotrophoblast, which is a multinuclear protoplasm mass that sends out the fingerlike extensions that take in uterine cells as it invades the endometrium. This layer of the trophoblast secretes both **peptide** and **steroid** hormones important to the maintenance of the pregnancy. The inner layer of the trophoblast has distinct cells and is called the **cytotrophoblast**. These cells secrete peptide hormones needed for the pregnancy.

The syncytiotrophoblast grows and begins to develop small spaces called **lacunae** that will fill with serum from the pregnant person's spiral arteries as the invasion progresses. This fluid will nourish the trophoblast. The pregnant person's arteries become fully dilated and low-resistance, low-pressure continuous flow is established (Cunningham et al., 2022). Communication between the lacunae and uterine vessels begins uteroplacental circulation. The remodeling of the spiral arteries is a critical step in establishing optimal circulation and nourishment for the embryo/fetus. Chronic disorders of pregnancy, such as preeclampsia or intrauterine fetal growth restriction, or both, may result from the incomplete dilation of the spiral arteries at this stage in development (Blackburn, 2018).

The projections from the cytotrophoblast into the syncytiotrophoblast mass become **chorionic villi**. These protrusions develop through three stages to become a functioning arteriocapillary venous network that supplies the embryo. Fetal blood begins to circulate by about 21 days after fertilization within the villi. An exchange via diffusion between the pregnant person's and the embryonic circulations begins, but the blood from each does not combine or meet. More about the cardiovascular development and transfer of nutrients and gases between pregnant person and fetus is presented later in this chapter.

The endometrium is changing under the influence of the progesterone that has been secreted by the corpus luteum. This secretory endometrial lining must be primed for the conceptus to be able to implant. Correct timing is essential. At the midpoint of the secretory phase, the endometrium develops protrusions and chemical changes that enhance the acceptance of the blastocyst (Cunningham et al., 2022).

A **decidual reaction** (cellular and vascular changes in the endometrium at implantation) occurs around the conceptus after it has embedded into the primed endometrium. This reaction provides an area for the conceptus that is protected from the pregnant person's immune system (Moore et al., 2019). If the reaction is abnormal, then **placenta accreta** (abnormal attachment of the trophoblast to the myometrium) or ectopic pregnancy may occur. The *decidua basalis* is directly under the trophoblast and is compressed. The villi at the embryonic pole extend into the decidua basalis and become the **chorion frondosum** that develops into the placenta. The *decidua capsularis* and *decidua vera (or parietalis)* are over the trophoblast. The decidua capsularis will disappear as the embryo develops. The decidua vera fuses with the **chorion laeve** (smooth chorion) and disappears as products of conception fill the uterine cavity.

Implantation bleeding, the loss of a small amount of blood from the uterine lining at implantation, occurs when the invasion of the uterine lining causes an abrupt opening in arterioles or veins. Many pregnant people experience this bleeding, and it is considered physiologic or a normal variant. The appearance of this bleeding occurs at about the same time a menstrual period is anticipated and can be incorrectly interpreted as the last menstrual period. This can affect how the pregnancy is dated, so a careful menstrual history is warranted.

The placenta at term is round and disc-shaped, about 22 cm in diameter, 2–4 cm thick, and weighs about 470 g (Cunningham et al., 2022). The uterine surface is formed by about 20 cotyledons (lobes) attached to the decidua via septa connected to the grooves between the cotyledons. Each lobe contains one main stem villi and its many branches. The fetal side is grayish white and covered by the amniotic membrane.

Chorionic and Amnionic Membranes

At about 14 days post conception, the implanted ovum is visible on the endometrium as a polyp-like protrusion. The embryo, amnion, and yolk sac cavities are within the cytotrophoblast layer. The developing embryo at about 14 days is connected inside the trophoblast via a stalk that will become part of the umbilical cord. The stalk is part of the mesoderm, one of three layers of the developing embryo. The ectoderm is part of the amniotic sac epithelium and the endoderm is opposite the ectoderm, beside the yolk sac (Roberts & Benirschke, 2018). As the embryo grows, it will fold, making the endoderm the innermost portion of the embryo. Eventually, the embryo is surrounded by the amnion and the amniotic fluid (AF).

The yolk sac provides nutrition for the early embryo, and as the embryo folds, the yolk sac is enclosed and becomes the primitive gut (Roberts & Benirschke, 2018). The cytotrophoblast cells encircle the extraembryonic **coelom**, which is a cavity that fills with a nutrient lake for molecular exchange between the pregnant person and the embryo (Ross & Beall, 2018). The coelom disappears by the end of the first trimester, and the AF-filled cavity surrounds the fetus.

One layer of the extraembryonic mesoderm is the **extraembryonic somatic mesoderm**. This layer will combine with the two layers of the trophoblast to form the **chorion** and the chorionic sac. Within the chorion, the embryo, amniotic sac, and umbilical vesicle are attached to the chorion by the connecting stalk that will become the umbilical cord.

The amniotic sac will enclose the embryo and cells from the amniotic membrane will eventually cover the umbilical cord (Roberts & Benirschke, 2018). The amniotic sac lies against but does not normally adhere to the entire chorionic membrane until about 12 weeks. There are no blood vessels in the amnion except in rare instances of a **velamentous insertion** (where blood vessels insert or grow into the amniotic membrane). The amniotic membrane is made up of ectodermal epithelial cells, thin connective tissue, and macrophages.

AF fills the amniotic sac around the embryo. It protects the embryo/fetus from trauma and most bacteria, allows for fetal movement and growth, and facilitates the development of the lungs and limbs (Ross & Beall, 2018). The amount of AF increases steadily between 10 and 30 weeks and then slows. Between 36 and 38 weeks, AF begins to decrease normally. At 41 weeks of gestation, AF begins to decrease more rapidly.

Excessive AF, known as **polyhydramnios**, can occur when the fetus has anencephaly or esophageal atresia, which prevents the swallowing of AF, or when the pregnant person has diabetes. Complications of polyhydramnios include placental abruption, uterine dysfunction, and post-partum hemorrhage.

Oligohydramnios, or below normal AF, can occur when there is an obstruction to fetal urine flow, renal agenesis, or other fetal anomalies; chronic leakage of AF; or rupture of the amniotic membrane. Chronic reduction in AF can cause fetal **pulmonary hypoplasia** or can increase the risk for infection.

Functions of the amniotic fluid

- Protects the embryo/fetus from trauma
- Is a barrier to most bacteria
- Allows for fetal movement and growth
- Facilitates lung and limb development
- Reflects fetal kidney function
- Provides thermoregulation
- Aids in gastrointestinal maturation

The Umbilical Cord

The connecting stalk is the earliest appearance of the umbilical cord. As the embryo folds during the fourth week, the umbilical cord begins to form and the amnion cells near it develop into the covering for the cord (Moore et al., 2019). Once fetoplacental circulation is established, two umbilical arteries within the cord carry deoxygenated blood away from the fetus to the placenta. The placental barrier between the pregnant person and the fetus is thin and allows substances, but not blood, to move back and forth. One umbilical vein within the cord brings oxygen and nutrients back to the fetus from the placenta. These three umbilical vessels are surrounded by **Wharton's jelly**, a gelatinous connective tissue. With a velamentous insertion, this protective coating does not cover the entire umbilical cord.

The umbilical cord is usually between 12 and 35 in (30 and 90 cm) long (Moore et al., 2019). If the umbilical cord is too long, there is danger that it will coil around the fetus, tighten and cut off oxygen and nutrient flow. A true knot in the umbilical cord can be created through fetal movement and is found in about 1 in 100 pregnancies, but only causes problems for 1 in 2000. A longer cord can prolapse with the rupture of amnionic membranes, be occluded by the fetal presenting part, and cause loss of oxygen and nutrients to the fetus. Approximately 1 in 20 umbilical cords are abnormally short (Beall, 2018). The cause of shorter cords is unknown; however, shortened cords may cause decreased fetal movement, placental abruption, or disruption in a part of the cord. A shortened cord can affect fetal descent and expulsion, although there are data that indicate that a vaginal delivery can happen if the cord is as short as 5.125 in (13 cm).

Placental Functions

The placenta and umbilical cord move substances such as nutrients, gases, drugs, and wastes between the pregnant person and the fetus. In addition to the transport of substances, the placenta serves as the organ for gas exchange and waste removal and as an endocrine gland for the fetus. It metabolizes glycogen, cholesterol, and fatty acids for energy and synthesizes and secretes both steroid and peptide hormones (Moore et al., 2019). The placenta can metabolize some drugs via specific enzyme action. In addition, placental cells produce P-glycoprotein, a substance that can pump some drugs away from the fetus (Lassiter & Manns-James, 2017). Shortly after the baby is born, the placenta is expelled from the uterus.

Sociocultural Uses of the Placenta

The American healthcare system has often treated the placenta as biohazardous waste material, although they are sometimes harvested for medical or commercial use. In some cultures, the placenta is used in rituals designed to honor or protect the birthing parent and the baby, such as burying it under a tree. Two alternative trends have emerged with regard to the placenta. The first is lotus birth in which the umbilical cord is not severed at birth and the cord and placenta are kept with the baby until natural separation occurs. The second is placental encapsulation in which the placenta is steamed, dehydrated, ground, and placed into capsules for ingestion in the postpartum period by the birthing parent with reputed effects of enhancing milk supply and preventing depression. Healthcare providers should discuss the pregnant person's preferences for the disposal or use of the placenta in the prenatal period.

Placental Transport

By the third week after fertilization, the embryo has developed a vascular network, and fetal circulation begins and the heart begins to beat around day 21 (Moore et al., 2019). Embryonic circulation is separated from the pregnant person's circulation by a thin membrane often called the placental barrier.

The four main modes of transport for substances across the placental membrane are **simple diffusion** (movement from higher to lower concentration), **facilitated diffusion** (movement that needs a transporter but no energy), **active transport** (movement against a concentration gradient that requires energy), and **pinocytosis** (carrier molecule is required to engulf the molecule and move it across the placental barrier) (Blackburn, 2018; Moore et al., 2019). Most drugs cross the placenta by way of simple diffusion (Lassiter & Manns-James, 2017). Table 4.1 lists the four modes of transport and gives a few examples of substances that are transported via each mode.

Seven factors affect substance transfer across the placenta (Adams et al., 2018):

1. High plasma levels of the specific substance in the pregnant person's circulation can affect transfer. Higher plasma levels will mean that more of the substance is available for transfer to the fetus.
2. Lipid-soluble substances cross the placental barrier better and more rapidly than do water-soluble substances.

Table 4.1 Four Main Transport Mechanisms

Mode of transport	Examples
Simple diffusion	Oxygen, CO_2, carbon monoxide, H_2O, most drugs, steroids, electrolytes, anesthetic gases
Facilitated diffusion	Glucose (facilitated by insulin), cholesterol, triglycerides, phospholipids
Active transport	Amino acids, vitamins, transferrin (carries iron to fetus), iodine, calcium
Pinocytosis	Immunoglobulin G

Source: Adapted from Adams et al. (2018) and Blackburn (2018).

3. The smaller the molecule, the more readily it crosses the placenta. Alcohol, for instance, is a very small molecule and crosses readily. Heparin is a very large molecule and does not cross.
4. Protein binding can make the substance too large to cross.
5. Ionized drugs do not cross as easily as nonionized drugs. An example of this is how nicotine crosses and reaches higher concentrations in the fetus. Nicotine is a weak base and the pregnant person's serum is slightly more acid than fetal serum. Once in the fetus, nicotine becomes ionized in a higher pH environment and will not cross the placenta back to the pregnant person, resulting in higher plasma levels of nicotine in the fetus.
6. If uteroplacental blood flow is compromised, drugs or other substances can stay in the fetus for a long time. This increases the risk for more serious fetal side effects. Diffusion is also affected by the rate of the pregnant person's and fetal blood flow through the villous spaces.
7. The stage of fetal development makes a difference. Before implantation, drug exposure will either destroy the blastocyst or it will not be affected at all. During organ development between weeks 3 and 8, the developing organs may be damaged by teratogenic drugs. This is also the time when the risk for drug-related spontaneous abortion is highest. During the fetal phase, weeks 9–40, drugs will remain for longer in the fetal system due to immature metabolism and excretion processes but are not likely to cause severe malformations. Instead, there may be delayed growth or organ function problems.

Some viruses, bacteria, and protozoa cross the placenta to infect the fetus. Table 4.2 lists the infectious agents that may cross the placental barrier and affect the fetus.

Placental Endocrine Synthesis and Secretion

The placenta uses **precursors** such as cholesterol, estrogen, or protein to synthesize both peptide and steroid hormones. The peptide hormones include, but are not limited to, hCG, human placental lactogen (also called human chorionic somatomammotropin), human chorionic adrenocorticotropin hormone (ACTH), corticotropin-releasing

Table 4.2 Transplacental Infectious Agents

Viruses	Varicella zoster, Coxsackie, parvovirus (B19), cytomegalovirus, rubella, human immunodeficiency virus, polio, zika
Bacteria	*Treponema pallidum* (syphilis), listeriosis, Borrelia (Lyme disease)
Protozoa	Toxoplasmosis

Source: Adapted from Centers for Disease Control and Prevention (2018, October 12), Cunningham et al. (2022), and Moore et al. (2019).

hormone (CRH), relaxin, and inhibin. The steroid hormones include estrogen and progesterone.

The hormone hCG is essential to pregnancy. It is produced by both the syncytiotrophoblast and cytotrophoblast for the first five weeks of pregnancy, thereafter, by the syncytiotrophoblast and fetal kidneys. It is detectible in the pregnant person's serum and urine by seven to nine days after ovulation and is used for pregnancy tests. Plasma levels of hCG double every 31–35 hours until approximately 63–70 days (Liu, 2018). Plasma levels then decline until about 16 weeks and remain stable until birth.

Serum levels of hCG are also used for the diagnosis of various complications in the early weeks of pregnancy. Levels of hCG that are too high may indicate multiple fetuses, fetal hemolytic disease, hydatidiform mole, or Down syndrome. Levels that are too low or that do not double in two days may indicate spontaneous abortion or ectopic pregnancy. hCG is also used in combination with other substances such as estriol and alpha-fetoprotein to screen for other fetal abnormalities.

hCG has many functions including maintenance of the corpus luteum; maintenance of the development of spiral arteries in the myometrium and formation of the syncytiotrophoblast; acting as a luteinizing hormone to stimulate the embryonic/fetal testicle to secrete testosterone; stimulation of the pregnant person's thyroid gland; and promotion of secretion of relaxin (peptide hormone) from the corpus luteum. It may also promote vasodilation and smooth muscle relaxation of the uterus (Moore et al., 2019; Blackburn, 2018). In maintaining the corpus luteum, hCG also prevents menses. Because hCG is synthesized without contribution from the fetus, the pregnant person's serum levels will remain high long after fetal demise, making hCG testing an unreliable method of diagnosing this condition (Blackburn, 2018).

Human placental lactogen is synthesized in the syncytiotrophoblast and can be measured in the pregnant person's serum at about four weeks. Its actions include **lipolysis** (breakdown of fat for energy), increased insulin resistance that facilitates protein synthesis and availability of amino acids and glucose to the fetus, **angiogenesis** (embryo blood vessel formation), and increased synthesis and availability of lipids (Blackburn, 2018). This placental hormone is most involved in maintaining a constant flow of glucose and amino acids to the fetus.

Human chorionic ACTH is important for fetal lung maturation and plays a role in the timing of labor and birth. CRH is produced in the placenta, membranes, and decidua. CRH acts to increase ACTH secretion from the trophoblast, causes smooth muscle relaxation in blood vessels and in the uterus until late in pregnancy, and facilitates immunosuppression in the pregnant person. A rise of CRH from the fetus and the placenta contributes to the genesis of labor.

Relaxin is produced in the corpus luteum, decidua, and the placenta. It acts to quiet the myometrium, facilitate the decidual reaction, remodel collagen, and soften the cervix (Blackburn, 2018). Relaxin also mediates hemodynamic changes of pregnancy and softens ligaments and cartilage in the skeletal system.

Inhibin is another glycoprotein produced by the trophoblast. It acts with sex steroid hormones to decrease the secretion of follicle-stimulating hormone from the pituitary, thereby stopping ovulation during pregnancy.

There are three major estrogens: estrone, estradiol, and estriol. In pregnancy, estriol is the major estrogen. Estriol is synthesized in the placenta from precursors from the pregnant person's and fetal adrenal glands. Dehydroepiandrosterone sulfate (DHEA-S), synthesized from cholesterol in the fetal adrenal glands, is an essential precursor to placental synthesis of estriol (Blackburn, 2018). During pregnancy, estriol production increases about 1000 times that which is seen in nonpregnant people at ovulation (Cunningham et al., 2022). Lower than normal serum levels of estriol are seen when the pregnant person is carrying a fetus with anencephaly or adrenal hypoplasia. Fetal demise can occur because the fetal pituitary is not releasing ACTH or the fetal adrenal glands are not functioning (Blackburn, 2018). Serum and AF estriol levels, along with other substances, are also used to screen for Down syndrome, trisomy 18, and neural tube defects.

Estrogen in pregnancy has many functions. Estrogens induce the proliferation and secretory phase of the endometrium, stimulate phospholipid synthesis, enhance prostaglandin production, and trigger uterine contractions. Estrogens also promote myometrial vasodilation, increase uterine blood flow, prepare the breasts for breastfeeding, affect the pregnant person's renin–angiotensin system, stimulate the liver to produce globulins, and increase fetal lung surfactant production (Blackburn, 2018; Liu, 2018).

Progesterone is secreted by the corpus luteum early in pregnancy and by the placenta after about 8–10 weeks. The precursor for progesterone synthesis is cholesterol. Serum levels of this steroid hormone increase steadily throughout the pregnancy so that by term, 250 mg/day of progesterone is being produced (Liu, 2018). This is about 10 times the amount produced by the corpus luteum during the luteal phase of the menstrual cycle.

Progesterone has a number of essential functions in pregnancy. Progesterone is needed for the preparation of the endometrium for implantation; the maintenance of a quiescent uterus through the relaxation of the smooth muscle; the inhibition of uterine prostaglandin development, thereby delaying cervical softening; the inhibition of the cell-mediated immune system to help prevent the rejection of the conceptus; the reduction of CO_2 sensitivity in the pregnant person's respiratory center; inhibition of prolactin secretion; the relaxation of the pregnant person's smooth muscle in the gastrointestinal and urinary systems; and the elevation of basal body temperature. Additionally, it works to create thicker cervical mucus and a mucous plug that serve as barriers to infectious agents trying to enter the uterus (Blackburn, 2018; Liu, 2018). Unlike estrogen, the fetus is not necessary for the production of progesterone, and serum levels of this hormone will remain high long after fetal demise (Blackburn, 2018). Table 4.3 summarizes the placental hormones and their functions.

The Embryo

Gastrulation (formation of germ layers of the embryo) changes the embryo from a two-layer disc to a three-layer disc. The three layers include the ectoderm, mesoderm, and endoderm. These layers form the basis for all tissues and organs that will develop as the embryo grows. Gastrulation begins with the appearance of the **primitive streak** from the tail through the middle of the back of the embryo to the head (Moore et al., 2019). Cells from the primitive streak and its derivatives will migrate away and form the mesoderm until about the fourth week. Near the tail end of the primitive streak, the **cloacal membrane** develops. This is the future site of the anal opening. Figure 4.2 shows how the primitive streak appears and lengthens.

Table 4.3 Placental Hormones and Their Functions

Human chorionic gonadotropin (hCG)	Maintains the corpus luteum Promotes vasodilation and relaxation of the uterus Stimulates the fetal testicle to secrete testosterone Stimulates the pregnant person's thyroid and secretion of relaxin
Human placental lactogen (hPL)	Lipolysis Increases insulin resistance Angiogenesis Increases synthesis of lipids
Human chorionic adrenocorticotropin (ACTH)	Promotes fetal lung maturation Plays role in timing of labor
Corticotropin-releasing hormone	Acts to increase ACTH secretion from the trophoblast Causes smooth muscle relaxation in blood vessels and uterus Facilitates immunosuppression in the pregnant person Near term, contributes to genesis of labor
Relaxin	Quiets the myometrium Facilitates decidual reaction Remodels collagen Helps soften the cervix Affects cartilage of the pregnant person's skeletal system
Inhibin	Acts with other hormones to decrease release of follicle-stimulating hormone, which stops ovulation
Dehydroepiandrosterone sulfate (DHEA-S)	Essential precursor to placental synthesis of estrogen
Estrogen	Acts to prepare the endometrium for pregnancy Stimulates phospholipid synthesis Enhances prostaglandin production Promotes uterine vasodilation Prepares breasts for lactation Increases fetal lung surfactant production
Progesterone	Essential for preparation of the endometrium for implantation Maintains quiescent uterus Inhibits prostaglandin development Inhibits cell-mediated immune system Reduces CO_2 sensitivity in respiratory center Inhibits prolactin secretion Relaxes smooth muscle Causes increase in basal body temperature Increases cervical mucus and formation of mucous plug

Source: Adapted from Blackburn (2018), Cunningham et al. (2022), and Liu (2018).

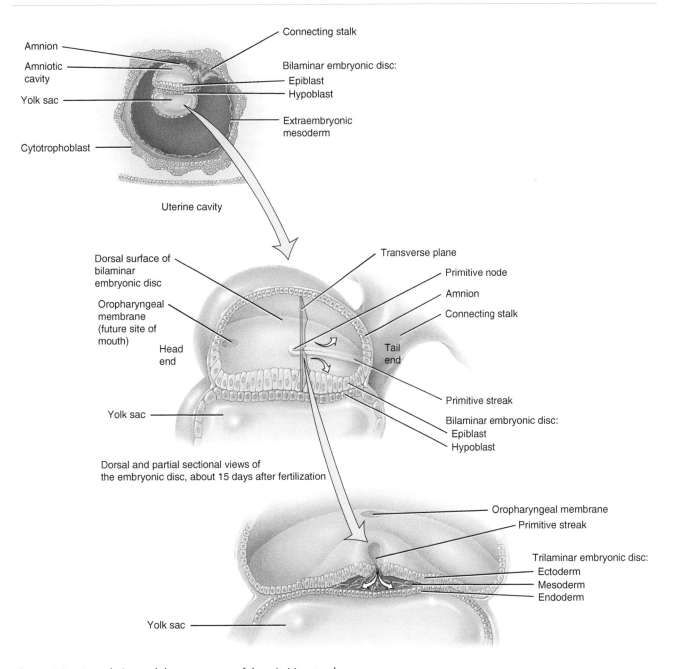

Figure 4.2 Gastrulation and the appearance of the primitive streak.

Parts of the primitive streak that do not degenerate can give rise to a **sacrococcygeal teratoma**, a cystic tumor that contains tissues from all three germ layers (Hamilton, 2019). These tumors can be surgically removed from the neonate without any lasting effect (Table 4.4).

Mesenchymal cells from the primitive node move toward the head and form the notochordal process and canal. The **notochord** is a rodlike structure that helps organize the nervous system and later becomes part of the vertebral column and axial skeleton. As the vertebra develops around the notochord, it will degenerate until only remnants are left in the nucleus pulposus between bony vertebrae. The notochord grows between the ectoderm and the endoderm and stops at the prechordal plate. Before

Table 4.4 Germ Layers and Organogenesis

Ectoderm—central and peripheral nervous systems, muscle, the skin, hair, and nails, mammary glands, pituitary gland, and tooth enamel

Mesoderm—connective tissue, cartilage, bone, striated, and smooth muscle, heart, blood, lymphatic system, kidneys, ovaries, testes, spleen, adrenal glands

Endoderm—lining of the gastrointestinal, urinary, and respiratory tracts, linings of the ear, parts of the pancreas, and thyroid

Source: Adapted from Muhr & Ackerman (2022).

it degenerates, the notochord will cause a thickening of the ectoderm and the formation of the neural plate by the end of week 4. This is where the central nervous system, including the forebrain, begins (Moore et al., 2019). The neural plate and ectoderm also give rise to the retina, iris, optic nerve, and other eye structures. On either side of the notochord, **somites** (a segmental mass of mesoderm occurring in pairs along the notochord) develop, which give rise to the skeleton, muscles, and some of the skin. As somites develop, they can be used to estimate the age of the embryo (Blackburn, 2018). Figure 4.3 shows the notochord process. Near the prechordal plate, layers of ectoderm and endoderm meet and form the oropharyngeal membrane, which will become the mouth.

Gastrulation involves the rearrangement and migration of cells from the epiblast.

Mesenchymal cells migrate to the sides of the primitive streak and fuse with the extraembryonic mesoderm that is part of the amnion and umbilical vesicle. These cells also migrate toward the head and form the cardiogenic mesoderm where the heart will begin development at the end of the third week. The **allantois**, a small appendage of the umbilical vesicle that attaches to the connecting stalk, is involved with blood formation and the development of the urinary bladder. The blood vessels of the allantois become the arteries and vein of the umbilical cord (Moore et al., 2019).

Neurulation is complete at the end of week 4. About day 18, a neural groove and neural folds appear in the neural plate. These early neural folds are the first signs of brain development. Later, the neural folds fuse to form the neural tube that will separate from the surface ectoderm. The edges of the ectoderm will then fuse over the neural tube, becoming the skin of the back. A neural crest forms between the neural tube and the ectoderm (Moore et al., 2019). Neural crest cells migrate and change into spinal ganglia and autonomic nervous system ganglia. These cells also form the ganglia for cranial nerves V, VII, IX, and X; sheaths for peripheral nerves; the pia mater; and arachnoid mater. This is when neural tube defects occur, including anencephaly and meningocele due to failure of primary neurulation, and spina bifida due to failure of secondary neurulation (Shimony, 2018).

The notochordal process develops from the primitive node and later becomes the notochord.

The embryo's first nourishment is from the pregnant person's blood via diffusion through the chorion, extraembryonic coelom, and umbilical vesicle. At the beginning of the third week, blood vessel formation begins in the extraembryonic mesoderm of the umbilical vesicle and connecting stalk (Moore et al., 2019). At the same time, new blood vessels are being formed in the chorion so that by day 21 post-fertilization, the early uteroplacental circulation is functional. At about the same time, the intraembryonic coelom is dividing into the pericardial, pleural, and peritoneal cavities.

Blood formation within the embryo does not begin until week 5. The heart and large vessels develop in the pericardial cavity and the heart begins beating on day 21 or 22 after conception (Moore et al., 2019). The cardiovascular system is the first system in the embryo to function.

Organogenesis

The fourth to eighth week for the embryo is the period of **organogenesis**. All the main organ systems begin to develop during these weeks. This is the time when the embryo is most vulnerable to **teratogens**. As development proceeds, the embryo begins to take on more visual characteristics unique to humans (Table 4.4).

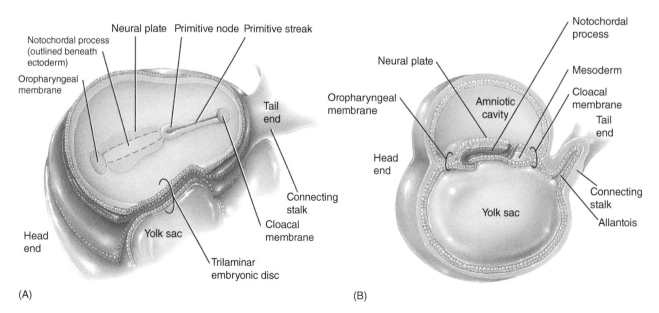

Figure 4.3   Notochord growth. (A) Dorsal and partial sectional views of the trilaminar embryonic disc, about 16 days after fertilization. (B) Sagittal section of the trilaminar embryonic disc, about 16 days after fertilization.

These transformative four weeks begin with the folding of the embryo so that the flat trilaminar disc becomes a curved cylinder (Moore et al., 2019). The curve is toward the connective stalk and umbilical vesicle. Figure 4.4 depicts the folding of the embryo. Once folding is complete, the three layers—ectoderm, mesoderm, and endoderm—begin to divide, migrate, aggregate, and differentiate in precise patterns to form organs.

During the fourth week of development, somites are produced and the neural tube will be open. The pharyngeal arches are visible and the embryo curves more head to tail (Moore et al., 2019). The heart pumps blood even

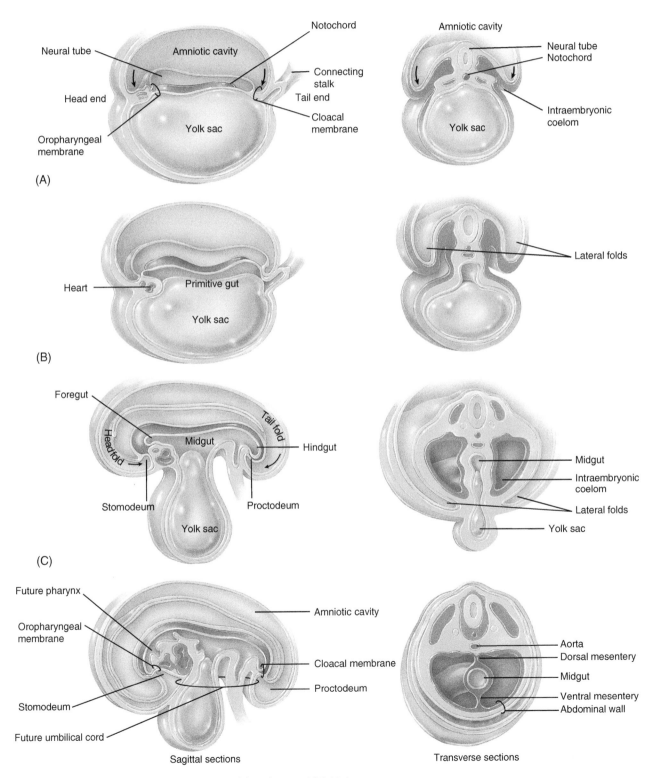

Figure 4.4 Folding of the embryo: (A) 22 days, (B) 24 days, and (C) 28 days.

though chambers are not yet developed. The forebrain causes an elevation of a portion of the head, and there is a tail-like structure opposite the head. Arm buds are seen on either side of the upper embryo.

Embryonic folding converts the two-dimensional trilaminar embryonic disc into a three-dimensional cylinder.

Otic pits are visible where the ears will be, and a thickening on either side of the head marks where the future eye lenses will be. The leg buds become visible at the end of the fourth week.

During week 5, the growth of the head is more rapid than other parts due to the development of the brain and facial features. The embryo is bent in such a way that the face will touch the cardiac prominence. Mesonephric ridges appear that will become the kidneys.

The embryo begins slight movements during week 6 and will reflex to touch. Digital rays, the first stages of fingers and hands, appear. The legs develop about four to five days after the hands. The auricles for the ears begin to be visible. The retinal pigment for the eyes is present. The head is large, and the trunk begins to straighten. The intestines enter the peritoneal cavity near the end of the umbilical cord, and an umbilical hernia occurs to provide room for the intestine (Moore et al., 2019). By the end of week 6, the embryo is about 20 mm in length (Cunningham et al., 2022).

During the seventh week, the limbs develop more rapidly. Digital rays become hand plates and the arms and legs become longer. During this time, the primordial gut and umbilical vesicle shrink to form the omphaloenteric duct (Moore et al., 2019).

During the last week of organogenesis, fingers are webbed, toes are still digital rays, and the scalp veins become visible and form a band around the head. By the end of the eighth week, digits of the hands and feet have grown longer and the webs are gone. Coordinated movements of all four limbs are seen. The femurs are the first bones to begin to ossify. The tail-like structure has disappeared. The head is still larger than the remainder of the body, but its features are human. The neck is visible, eyelids are closing, and auricles, low on the head, are nearing their final shape. Sex identification is not yet possible until 10–12 weeks, but this distinction still cannot be made reliably by ultrasound at this stage.

The Fetus

The end of week 8 and the beginning of week 9 mark the beginning of the fetal period. The fetal period is a time of rapid growth and differentiation of the systems that have been formed during the preceding eight weeks. By convention, the main changes in fetal development are considered to occur every four to five weeks (Moore et al., 2019).

From weeks 9–12, the fetus doubles its crown to rump length. At 9 weeks, the eyes are wide set, the ears low on the head, and the eyelids are fused. The legs are short and thighs are small. The intestines are seen at the end of the umbilical cord until week 10 and by week 11 they will be completely in the peritoneal cavity. Urine formation and micturition begin during this period. The fetus begins to swallow AF that contains the urine. Fetal wastes are passed via fetal blood circulation to the pregnant person through the placental membrane. By the end of week 12, the arm length reaches the proportional length the arms will maintain in relation to the body and leg growth is ongoing.

Separate, uncoordinated limb movements are seen on ultrasound by week 11. By weeks 13–16, the head is smaller in relation to the remainder of the body and the legs are longer. Slow eye movements are seen at 14 weeks and scalp hair has begun to grow. By 16 weeks, fetal ovaries are present and contain ovarian follicles with **oogonia** (primitive ovum). Sixteen weeks is also the time when fetal bones are visible by ultrasound and the eyes are closer together and look forward. At week 14, the fetal crown-rump length has grown to about 7 cm.

Rapid growth occurs between weeks 17 and 20. It is during this time that fetal movements can be felt by the pregnant person (**quickening**). The skin at this stage is covered with **vernix caseosa**, which protects the skin. The skin is also covered with **lanugo**, which helps hold the vernix caseosa to the skin. Eyebrows are visible. The fetal uterus is differentiated and formed, and the testes have started migrating toward the scrotum from the posterior abdominal wall. In the subcutaneous area, brown fat for heat generation begins to be deposited (Moore et al., 2019).

Increased weight gain and a more proportional fetus are seen in weeks 21–25. Rapid eye movements and blink-startle responses become evident between weeks 21 and 23 (Moore et al., 2019). Lung development is nearing completion and surfactant begins to be secreted from the walls of the lungs at 24 weeks. This fluid will help maintain open alveoli and is essential for newborn breathing to begin and continue after birth. Fingernails are seen at 24 weeks (Moore et al., 2019).

Between 26 and 29 weeks, the fetus has the potential to survive if it is born prematurely. The central nervous system has matured enough to direct regular breathing motions and to control body temperature (Moore et al., 2019). The eyelids open and close at 26 weeks and toenails are visible. Brown fat has accumulated and skin wrinkles are smoothed.

Fetal pupils react to light at 30–38 weeks, skin is pink and smooth, and arms and legs become plump. By 35 weeks, the grasp reflex is present and the nervous system is mature enough to function. The abdomen is as wide as the head and the breasts protrude from the chest wall in both sexes. Growth begins to slow, although more brown fat is added during the last weeks before birth (Moore et al., 2019). The fetus at 30 weeks weighs approximately 1800 g, or just under 4 lb. (Cunningham et al., 2022). Fetal growth may be assessed by ultrasound, magnetic resonance imaging (MRI), or fetal monitoring.

Table 4.5   Vulnerable Periods in Embryonic and Fetal Growth and Development

Timing	Physiological events	Potential vulnerabilities
Weeks 1 and 2	Dividing zygote, implantation, bilaminar embryo	Not susceptible to teratogenesis; spontaneous loss may occur, often due to genetic malfunction early in process
Week 3	Neurological system and cardiac system development begins	Anencephaly; neural tube defects; truncus arteriosus, atrial septal defect or ventricular septal defects may occur near the end of this week of development
Week 4	Brain and nervous system, arms, and later in the week, legs; end of week: ears, eyes	Neural tube defects, heart defects, upper, and lower limb defects; low set or deformed ears and deafness; malformed eyes, cataracts, glaucoma
Week 5	Brain and nervous system, heart, arms, legs, ears, eyes, mouth	Same as week 4; add cleft lip
Week 6	Same as week 5; add tooth enamel and hard palate near the end of week 6	Same as week 5; add enamel hyperplasia and staining; cleft palate near end of week 6
Week 7	Same as week 6; add genitalia	Enlargement and degrees of fusion of clitoris/labia may occur at this point
Week 8	Same as week 7; end of this week marks the end of organogenesis	Ears and hearing at risk; eye deformities at week 4; tooth enamel, hard palate, and clitoris/labia still at risk
Week 9	Brain, hard palate, clitoris/labia at risk	Brain development deficiencies major threat; hearing still at risk; other major congenital anomalies become less of a threat; functional defects and minor anomalies still possible
Week 16	Brain	Cognitive impairment; functional defects and minor anomalies continue
Weeks 32–38	Focus on growth and development	Functional and minor anomalies may occur in the central nervous system, ears, eyes, teeth, palate, and external genitalia

Source: Adapted from Moore et al. (2019).

The estimated date of birth is about 266 days after fertilization or 280–283 days after the pregnant person's last normal menstrual period (Moore et al., 2019). It is estimated that about 12% of babies are born after the expected date of birth (EDB) (Moore et al., 2019). The average baby will weigh about 3400 g at birth.

Birth defects have the potential for occurring at many times during embryonic growth and development. Exposure to certain chemicals known as endocrine disruptors has the potential to disrupt normal fetal development. Endocrine disruptors may be naturally occurring or man-made, synthetic chemicals and have been found to lead to adverse pregnancy and birth outcomes (Padmanabhan et al., 2021). Table 4.5 lists vulnerable periods and the defects that can occur.

Summary

There is much more to be learned about the development of a human being from the single-celled zygote. The synthesis of the various cells that grow, produce substances that sustain life, migrate to form organs and tissue, or die away to form hollows and spaces is complex and wondrous. It is easy to see that disruption during any stage can cause a cascade of changes that can lead to birth defects or death. It is important that healthcare professionals respect and support the pregnant person and the embryo/fetus and educate patients and their families to enhance perinatal health.

Resources for Healthcare Providers

For a detailed week-by-week timeline of human development from a cell to a newborn visit: https://embryology.med.unsw.edu.au/embryology/index.php/Human_Development_Movie

Tsiaras, A. (2011). Conception to birth – visualized. https://www.ted.com/talks/alexander_tsiaras_conception_to_birth_visualized?language=en

Khan Academy. (2014). Implantation.https://www.khanacademy.org/test-prep/mcat/cells/embryology/v/implantation

General Embryology: Detailed Animation on Gastrulation (2014).https://www.youtube.com/watch?v=3AOoikTEfeo

Resources for Clients, Their Families, and Healthcare Providers

Fetal Development Timeline: http://www.babycenter.com/0_fetal-development-timeline_10357636.bc

References

Adams, M., Urban, C. & Sutter, R. (2018). Pharmacology: Connections to nursing practice (4th ed.). Pearson.

Beall, M. (2018, June 1). *Umbilical cord complications*. Medscape. https://emedicine.medscape.com/article/262470-overview/article/262470-overview

Beery, T., Workman, M., & Eggert, J. (2018). *Genetics and genomics in nursing and health care* (2nd ed.). F.A. Davis.

Blackburn, S. (2018). *Maternal, fetal, and neonatal physiology: A clinical perspective* (5th ed.). Elsevier.

Centers for Disease Control and Prevention. (2018, October 12). *Zika virus*. https://www.cdc.gov/zika/hc-providers/index.html

Cunningham, F., Leveno, K., Dashe, J., Hoffman, B., Spong, C., & Casey, B. (2022). *Williams obstetrics* (26th ed.). McGraw-Hill Medical.

Hamilton, C. (2019, November 22). *Cystic teratoma*. Medscape. https://emedicine.medscape.com/article/281850-overview

Lassiter, N., & Manns-James, L. (2017). Pregnancy. In M. Brucker & T. King (Eds.), *Pharmacology for women's health* (2nd ed., pp. 1025–1059). Jones & Bartlett.

Liu, J. (2018). Endocrinology of pregnancy. In R. Creasy, C. Lockwood, T. Moore, M. Greene, J. Copel, & P. Silver (Eds.), *Creasy and Resnik's maternal–fetal medicine: Principles and practice* (8th ed., pp. 148–160). Elsevier/Saunders.

Moore, K., Persaud, T., & Torchia, M. (2019). *Before we are born: Essentials of embryology and birth defects* (10th ed.). Elsevier.

Muhr, J. & Ackerman, K. (2022). *Embryology, gastrulation*. National Library of Medicine. https://www.ncbi.nlm.nih.gov/books/NBK554394/#:~:text=Gastrulation%20occurs%20during%20week%203,most%20critical%20steps%20of%20development.

Padmanabhan, V., Song, W., & Puttabyatappa, M. (2021). Praegnatio perturbatio—Impact of endocrine-disrupting chemicals. *Endocrine Reviews, 42*(3), 295–353. https://doi.org/10.1210/endrev/bnaa035

Roberts, D., & Benirschke, K. (2018). Normal early development. In R. Creasy, C. Lockwood, T. Moore, M. Greene, J. Copel, & P. Silver (Eds.), *Creasy and Resnik's maternal–fetal medicine: principles and practice* (8th ed., pp. 39–61). Elsevier/Saunders.

Ross, M., & Beall, M. (2018). Amniotic fluid dynamics. In R. Creasy, C. Lockwood, T. Moore, M. Greene, J. Copel, & P. Silver (Eds.), *Creasy and Resnik's maternal–fetal medicine: Principles and practice* (8th ed., pp. 62–67). Elsevier/Saunders.

Shimony, N. (2018, November 26). *Neural tube defects*. Medscape. http://emedicine.medscape.com/article/1177162-overview

5

Physiologic Alterations during Pregnancy

Ella T. Heitzler

The editors gratefully acknowledge Patricia Caudle, who authored the previous edition of this chapter.

Relevant Terms

Accelerated starvation—ketonemia, ketonuria, and hypoglycemia occur after a period of fasting, and the body starts to break down fat for fuel

Anabolic—construction of molecules for storage

Anagen—active phase of the hair growth cycle

Angiogenesis—growth of new blood vessels

Apoptosis—cell death by the Fas/FasL ligand system, a signaling pathway that plays an important role in the immune system and cancer progression

Bone resorption—osteoclasts break down bone and release calcium

Catabolic—breakdown of molecules for energy

Cytokines—molecule messengers that regulate responses to inflammation

Epulis—localized vascular swelling of gums between teeth

Fas/FasL—cell membrane proteins that can activate cell death

Fibrinolysis—breakup and removal of excess fibrin

Hyperemia—increased blood flow

Hyperplasia—increased number of normal cells in normal tissue

Linea alba—white fibrous structure running from the umbilicus to the symphysis formed by the fusion of the abdominal muscles, visible through the skin of the anterior abdomen

Linea nigra—darkened skin over the linea alba seen in pregnancy

Lipolytic—breakdown of fat

Lordosis—increased inward curve of the lumbar and cervical spine

Melasma—dark discoloration of areas of facial skin

Methylation—the process by which methyl groups are added to a DNA molecule, changing the activity of that DNA segment

Neural tube defects—birth defects of the brain and spinal cord

PCO_2—partial pressure of carbon dioxide in the blood

Pedunculated—attached via a stalk

Pica—a craving for non-food substances

Platelet-derived growth factor—protein that regulates blood vessel formation and growth

Ptyalism—excess salivation

Semiallograft—transplanted tissue that is half-host genetic material; in pregnancy, the fetal-placental unit is half-host genetic material

Telangiectasias—small dilated blood vessels near the skin surface

Telogen—resting phase of the hair growth cycle

Thromboxane—a prostaglandin involved in clotting

Tissue factor—substance that initiates clotting

Trigone—the triangular region of the bladder wall muscle tissue with angles that correspond with ureter and urethra openings

---

Introduction

This chapter outlines physiologic changes and adaptations experienced by the pregnant person as their body accepts, accommodates, and maintains a pregnancy to term. Virtually, every body system is affected by remarkable hormonal, anatomical, physiological, and biochemical changes that occur from fertilization through parturition.

Health equity key points

- The experience of interpersonal and systemic racism may impact blood pressure and/or hypertension during pregnancy.
- Some skin conditions (i.e., melasma and linea nigra) present differently depending on a person's skin tone.

Prenatal and Postnatal Care: A Person-Centered Approach, Third Edition. Edited by Karen Trister Grace, Cindy L. Farley, Noelene K. Jeffers, and Tanya Tringali.
© 2024 John Wiley & Sons Ltd. Published 2024 by John Wiley & Sons Ltd.
Companion website: www.wiley.com/go/grace/prenatal

Hematologic System Adaptations

Pregnancy-related physiologic changes in the hematologic system include increases in blood and plasma volume, and increases in the number of red blood cells (RBCs) and white blood cells (WBCs). These changes lead to increased nutritional requirements for iron and folate. In addition, pregnancy is a hypercoagulable state where changes in specific clotting factors and fibrin and fibrinolytic activities occur.

Blood Changes

Blood is composed of plasma, RBCs and WBCs, platelets, and many smaller molecules with numerous functions. During pregnancy, blood volume increases by approximately 40– 50%, or about 1.2–1.6 L (Blackburn, 2018). The major components, plasma and the RBC mass, increase at different rates and through different mechanisms. The more rapid increase in plasma volume causes hemodilution. This hemodilution lowers the hemoglobin, hematocrit, and RBC count per milliliter. These changes do not affect the mean corpuscular volume or mean corpuscular hemoglobin concentration in a normal pregnancy (Kilpatrick & Kitahara, 2019). Table 5.1 delineates the changes in hematologic laboratory parameters during pregnancy.

Red Blood Cells

The RBC mass will increase by 20–30% by the end of a normal pregnancy (Mastrobattista & Monga, 2019). This increase occurs because of increased production of RBCs in the bone marrow. Progesterone, placental chorionic somatomammotropin, and potentially prolactin have been identified as the hormones of pregnancy that stimulate an increase in erythropoiesis (Mastrobattista & Monga, 2019).

Table 5.1 Changes in Hematologic Laboratory Parameters during Pregnancy

Red blood cells (RBCs)	Increases ~20–30%
RBC indices	Unchanged
Hematocrit	Decreases ~3–5%
Hemoglobin	Decreases 2–10%
White blood cells	Increases 8% (much higher in labor)
Serum ferritin	Decreases 30%
Serum iron	Decreases
Total iron-binding capacity	Increases
Transferrin saturation	Decreases
RBC folate	Decreases
Iron	Decreases
Transferrin	Increases 70%

Source: Adapted from Blackburn (2018) and Kilpatrick and Kitahara (2019).

White Blood Cells

Total WBC count increases during pregnancy, ranging from about 5000 to 12,000 (with values up to 15000 reported) per cubic millimeter (Blackburn, 2018). Most of the increase is in the numbers of neutrophils. Neutrophils function as the first WBC responders in the body's reaction to an infectious or inflammatory process. The WBC count may rise to as high as 30,000 per cubic millimeter during labor and birth without infection. This increase mimics a similar rise in WBCs seen during aerobic exercise.

Plasma

Plasma volume begins to increase as early as six to eight weeks' estimated gestational age (EGA). By about 32-week EGA, plasma volume will have increased to 45% higher than nonpregnant levels (Mastrobattista & Monga, 2019). This increase helps to meet heightened maternal metabolic needs, to circulate blood within the dilated uterine vascular system, to provide nutrients to the growing conceptus, and to protect the pregnant person against the consequences of blood loss during labor and birth. The exact mechanism by which plasma volume expands is uncertain, but the production of nitric oxide, a potent vasodilator synthesized from the endothelium of the blood vessel walls, may lead to vasodilation, causing the renin–angiotensin–aldosterone system (RAAS) to induce sodium and water retention (Mastrobattista & Monga, 2019).

Iron Requirements

An increase in RBC production and a growing fetus and placenta requires increased iron intake and absorption. It is estimated that the pregnant person needs 500 mg of additional iron during pregnancy. This includes 300 mg that is used by the fetus and about 200 mg that is needed for normal daily use and loss (Mastrobattista & Monga, 2019). To meet this need, maternal iron stores are mobilized and increased absorption of dietary iron from the duodenum occurs. Progesterone may mediate a slowed peristalsis in the small intestine and colon, which can enhance iron absorption (Kelly & Savides, 2019).

Many people enter pregnancy with micronutrient deficiencies, particularly iron stores, due to inadequate diets and cyclical menstrual blood loss. The demands of pregnancy will further deplete these stores (Kilpatrick & Kitahara, 2019). Routine iron supplementation in the absence of anemia is not recommended by the US Preventive Service Task Force (USPSTF). However, meta-analysis has shown that prenatal iron supplementation results in lower risk of maternal anemia at term and may result in less risk of having a preterm or low-birth-weight newborn (Peña-Rosas et al., 2015).

The transfer of iron to the fetus occurs via active transport through serum transferrin at the placenta. If the pregnant person's iron stores are low, then the placenta develops more transferrin receptors (Kilpatrick & Kitahara, 2019). This mechanism helps assure iron transfer to the fetus, even when the pregnant person has limited iron, and further depletes their iron stores.

Folate Requirements

Folate is a water-soluble B vitamin that helps tissues grow and function properly. Folate acts as a coenzyme involved in DNA and RNA synthesis and cell division. Specifically, it is required for the process of **methylation** (Scott et al., 1994). Interruption of DNA synthesis or methylation can prevent the proper closure of the neural tube. During pregnancy, folate requirements increase from 400 to 600 µg/d (Kilpatrick & Kitahara, 2019). Studies have demonstrated that adequate folate intake, both before and during early pregnancy, will significantly reduce the occurrence of **neural tube defects** (NTDs).

Changes in Clotting Factors

Blood contains substances to help prevent hemorrhage through clotting and, at the same time, substances that assure that blood stays in liquid form. During pregnancy, factors that promote hemostasis and **fibrinolysis** are enhanced. This adaptation helps control bleeding when there is an increased risk for hemorrhage with implantation and placental development, and again during the third stage of labor when the placenta detaches from the uterine wall. Paradoxically, the prevention of hemorrhage comes with an increased risk for thrombus formation in the uteroplacental and intervillous circulations, and the deep veins of the legs and pelvis.

The changes that occur to enhance hemostasis are many and complex. Not every component of the hemostatic system increases. For instance, the platelet count during pregnancy decreases slightly, but stays within the same normal range as the count for nonpregnant people. This decrease has been attributed to hemodilution, escalated platelet utilization, and increased platelet aggregation in response to increased production of the prostaglandin **thromboxane** A$_2$ (Bowersox, 2021). Platelets are non-nucleated cells synthesized by the bone marrow that play an important role in hemostasis. When there is an injury to a blood vessel, platelets are the first to respond. They work through aggregation, adhesion, and through releasing histamine, serotonin, and **platelet-derived growth factor** (PDGF). Once released, these substances enhance the enlargement of the platelet plug, activate the coagulation cascade, and support the fibrin mesh that develops to further strengthen the plug, and PDGF stimulates smooth muscle blood vessel walls to help healing (Rodger & Silver, 2019).

Progesterone stimulates an increase in **tissue factor** (TF) and plasminogen activator inhibitor type 1 (PAI-1) in the decidua and endometrium (Rodger & Silver, 2019). During pregnancy, fibrinogen doubles, and clotting factors V, VII, VIII, IX, and X and von Willebrand factor all increase. Prothrombin fragments increase and prothrombin time decreases. There is decreased anticoagulation and fibrinolysis; however, bleeding time is about the same. These adaptations serve to control the bleeding that occurs when the placenta detaches. In fact, a fibrin matrix is established in spiral arteries early in pregnancy that will

Table 5.2   Changes in Coagulation Factors in Pregnancy

Platelets	Decreased slightly but within normal prepregnancy limits
Fibrin deposits	Increased
Tissue factor (TF)	Found in amniotic fluid, decidua, placenta, and endometrium
Fibrin–fibrinogen complexes	Increased
Plasminogen-activator inhibitors	Increased
Fibrinogen	Increased
Fibrinolysis	Decreased
Coagulation factors I, VII, VIII, IX, X, and XII	Increased
Coagulation factor XIII	Decreased
von Willebrand factor	Increased
Activated partial thromboplastin time (aPTT)	Decreased slightly
Prothrombin time (PT)	Decreased slightly
Bleeding time	Unchanged
Resistance to activated protein C	Increased
Protein S (coagulation inhibitor)	Decreased
Fibrin degradation products	Increased
D-dimer (marker for fibrinolysis)	Increased

Source: Adapted from Blackburn (2018) and Cunningham et al. (2022).

cause a fibrin mesh to form very quickly over the placenta site. Fibrinolytic activity decreases until about an hour after childbirth. These changes and others are summarized in Table 5.2.

Cardiovascular System Adaptations

The heart and vascular system undergo profound changes beginning as early as five-week gestation. People with healthy hearts seldom report symptoms associated with these changes. There are several signs and symptoms that occur, however, that mimic cardiovascular disease, creating a diagnostic dilemma for the healthcare provider. Up to 4% of pregnant people will have unrecognized cardiovascular disease; this is emerging as a contributor to maternal morbidity and mortality (Mohamad, 2017). Table 5.3 lists the functional cardiovascular signs and symptoms seen in pregnancy.

Anatomical and Functional Cardiac Changes

Ventricular muscle mass increases during the first trimester and left atrial diameter increases as blood volume increases (Mastrobattista & Monga, 2019).

Table 5.3 Signs and Symptoms of A Normal Pregnancy that Mimic Heart Disease

Dyspnea	Progesterone effect on breathing centers and pressure from enlarging uterus leads to increased respiratory rate and metabolic demand
Fatigability	Response to increased metabolic demand
Dependent edema	Venous pressure from gravid uterus, lower colloid osmotic pressure
First heart sound louder	Early closure of mitral valve
Split S_2	Expected at about 30 weeks of gestation
S_3	Heard in up to 90% of pregnant people
Systolic flow murmur	Heard in 95% of pregnant people; begins ~12–20 weeks and disappears about 1 week after birth
Left lateral displacement of the point of maximal impulse	Gravid uterus pressing upward on diaphragm and heart
Mammary souffle	Continuous murmur from mammary vessels, heard best in second intercostal space

Source: Adapted from Blackburn (2018) and Mastrobattista & Monga (2019).

Cardiac output, a measure of functional capacity of the heart, increases by 30–50%, with about half of this increase occurring by eight-week gestation (Blackburn, 2018). The increase in cardiac output comes from increases in both stroke volume and heart rate. Stroke volume causes most of the early rise in cardiac output and then declines as the pregnancy nears term. The pregnant person's heart rate begins to increase at five-week gestation and reaches a maximum increase of about 15–20 beats per minute by 32-week gestation. Increased cardiac output is needed to support the 10-fold increase in uterine blood flow (500–800 mL/min) and the 50% increase in blood flow to the kidneys (Mastrobattista & Monga, 2019). Blood flow is also increased to the breasts and the skin. These adaptations explain the flow murmurs and other changes in signs and symptoms listed in Table 5.3.

Vascular Changes

Collagen throughout the vascular system softens, resulting in increased compliance and decreased vascular resistance beginning around five weeks' gestation (Mastrobattista & Monga, 2019). Vasodilation occurs as a result of the relaxant effects of progesterone and prostaglandin. The low-resistance uteroplacental circulation acts like an arteriovenous connection, thereby contributing to lowered vascular resistance. In addition, there is an increased production of endothelial relaxant factors such as nitric oxide that contribute to lowered vascular resistance. All of these changes contribute to decreased venous resistance that will slow the speed of venous flow and contribute to stasis of the blood, thereby increasing the risk for deep vein thrombosis in pregnancy. These changes also contribute to an increased sensitivity to autonomic blockade, such as that produced by epidural anesthesia, and can result in a sudden drop in blood pressure following epidural administration (Mastrobattista & Monga, 2019).

Blood Pressure Changes

Normally, arterial blood pressure decreases in pregnancy when the arteries relax and peripheral vascular resistance decreases. This decrease in blood pressure begins at about seven-week gestation and persists until around 32-week gestation, when it begins to rise to prepregnancy levels (Mastrobattista & Monga, 2019). Maternal position affects blood pressure measurements. In fact, blood pressure decreases 5–10 mmHg systolic and 10–15 mmHg diastolic when a pregnant person lies on their left side (Mastrobattista & Monga, 2019). Serial blood pressures taken with the pregnant person in a comfortable seated position with their feet on the floor are the best for monitoring for any abnormal changes in blood pressure during pregnancy.

The experience of individual and systemic racism may also impact blood pressure, including during pregnancy, and is implicated in the higher rates of hypertension in people of color. Sims et al. (2012) noted that discrimination was associated with increased prevalence of hypertension in adults aged 35–84 years. Similarly, a meta-analysis by Dolezsar et al. (2014) found perceived racial discrimination was linked with hypertensive status in adults. A similar process may occur during pregnancy.

Supine Hypotensive Syndrome

Supine hypotensive syndrome, defined as at least 15–30 mmHg drop in systolic blood pressure, occurs in up to 15% of pregnant people in the second and third trimesters (Sherman et al., 2016). Lying flat on the back in the supine position after about 30 weeks of gestation can cause the weight of the gravid uterus to compress the inferior vena cava and abdominal aorta, limiting the amount of blood that can return to the heart. This reduction in stroke volume causes a decrease in cardiac output and a decrease in blood pressure (Sherman et al., 2016). Changes in the cardiovascular system can cause a pregnant person to feel faint and can lead to a decrease in fetal heart rate. Rarely, loss of consciousness can occur. People naturally tend to turn to the side when they feel this sensation, and no harm is caused by this temporary state. It can occur during an office visit when a pregnant person is asked to lie on their back for an examination or during labor if they are immobile and supine. Side-lying positions relieve the pressure of the gravid uterus and restore blood flow and blood pressure.

Respiratory System Adaptations

Pregnancy puts less stress on the respiratory system than on the cardiovascular system; however, there are significant adaptations. Although some people may report shortness of breath, respiratory exchange is more efficient during pregnancy. The primary changes occur in lung volume and ventilation as the oxygen demands of pregnancy metabolism and the fetoplacental unit increase. These changes begin early in pregnancy.

Anatomical Changes

Estrogen and the increasing blood volume of pregnancy cause capillary engorgement that leads to swelling and increased mucous production in the nose, sinuses, eustachian tubes, and middle ears. At the same time, progesterone causes a relaxation of veins and increased pooling that further contributes to mucous membrane swelling. The result is increased incidence of pregnancy rhinitis, epistaxis, serous otitis, and congested sinuses (Blackburn, 2018).

The hormone relaxin causes increased pliability of cartilage in the chest, allowing for an increase in chest circumference. As the gravid uterus increases in size, the diaphragm rises about 4 cm, transverse chest diameter expands 2 cm, thoracic circumference expands about 6 cm, and the costal angle widens. There is also an increase in thoracic breathing and more diaphragmatic movement (Blackburn, 2018).

Pulmonary Function Changes

Serum levels of progesterone, a known respiratory stimulant, rise throughout pregnancy. Progesterone is believed to increase ventilation and response to hypercapnia, enhancing sensitivity to carbon dioxide (CO_2) and decreasing the CO_2 threshold (Blackburn, 2018). Progesterone may also impact lung diffusion capacity and substantially lower airway resistance (Blackburn, 2018). The combined effect is mild hyperventilation and mild respiratory alkalosis that occurs as the pregnant person "blows off" CO_2 and decreases the carbon dioxide partial pressure in blood (**PCO_2**). Progesterone has also been implicated in the increase in carbonic anhydrase in RBCs that helps in CO_2 transfer and a decrease in PCO_2 (Whitty & Dombrowski, 2019). Reduced PCO_2 in the pregnant person facilitates the movement of fetal CO_2 waste and enhances the release of oxygen to the fetus via placental exchange pathways (Cunningham et al., 2022).

Table 5.4 lists several pulmonary function parameters that change as adaptation to pregnancy occurs. It is important to note that increased oxygen requirements and adaptations in pulmonary function make respiratory diseases such asthma and pneumonia potentially more serious in pregnancy (Whitty & Dombrowski, 2019).

Renal System Adaptations

The renal and urinary systems undergo dramatic change in response to pregnancy. The kidneys must adjust to increased blood and extracellular fluid volume and

Table 5.4   Changes in Respiratory Parameters in Pregnancy

Total lung capacity	Unchanged or decreased up to 4%
Inspiratory capacity	Increased 5–20% (~300 mL)
Expiratory reserve capacity	Decreased 15–20% (~250 mL)
Residual volume	Decreased by 18%
Tidal volume	Increased by 40–50%
Minute ventilation	Increased by 30–40%
O_2 consumption	Increased by 20% (50% during labor)
Total pulmonary resistance	Reduced
Maternal pH	Mild respiratory alkalosis

Source: Adapted from Cunningham et al. (2022) and Whitty and Dombrowski (2019).

increased wastes. There are changes related to hormonal effects, pressure from the gravid uterus, and from cardiovascular adaptations.

Anatomical Changes

The kidneys grow in volume and length during pregnancy due to an increase in renal vascular and interstitial growth (Mastrobattista & Monga, 2019). The kidneys and ureters dilate when the gravid uterus grows enough to compress the ureters at the pelvic rim and slow urine flow. The right ureter is compressed more than the left due to the right-sided rotation of the uterus, or because of the cushioning provided to the left ureter by the sigmoid colon (Cunningham et al., 2022). Ureter dilation may also be a consequence of progesterone, relaxin, and nitric oxide effects that relax smooth muscle; however, most studies support uterine compression as the most likely cause of these changes (Mastrobattista & Monga, 2019). Dilation of the kidneys and ureters increases the potential for urine stasis and infection. Hydroureter may persist for three to four months after childbirth.

The bladder begins adaptive changes at about 12 weeks of gestation (Cunningham et al., 2022). By then, **hyperemia** and **hyperplasia** of the muscle and connective tissue will cause elevation of the bladder **trigone** and increase the susceptibility to bladder infection. There is reduced bladder capacity and increased incidence of stress incontinence during the third trimester related to pressure on the bladder from the gravid uterus. In addition, pressure from the fetal presenting part may slow blood and lymph drainage, causing the base of the bladder to swell and become more prone to infection.

Renal Function Changes

Renal plasma flow increases 60–80% by mid-pregnancy and then decreases to about 50% above prepregnancy rates by term (Mastrobattista & Monga, 2019). Lateral lying positions increase venous return and renal plasma flow; the left lateral lying position is best for enhancing renal plasma flow. These position changes will lead to increased urine flow and nocturia.

The glomerular filtration rate (GFR) increases significantly within two weeks after conception and is 50% higher than prepregnancy levels by 12-weeks' gestation (Cunningham et al., 2022). This and the weight of the growing uterus on the bladder explain the urinary frequency experienced during the first weeks of pregnancy. The increase in GFR causes increased creatinine clearance and decreased serum creatinine, blood urea nitrogen, and serum osmolarity (Mastrobattista & Monga, 2019).

Renal tubular function also changes in pregnancy. The most impressive tubular function change is the reabsorption of sodium. Sodium retention is promoted by increased levels of estrogen, aldosterone, and deoxycorticosterone, and the increased activity of the RAAS (Mastrobattista & Monga, 2019). Sodium retention is also enhanced by sitting or standing. Interestingly, although sodium is retained during pregnancy, the serum levels of sodium decrease slightly due to hemodilution.

Two other important electrolytes are significantly affected by renal tubular function changes in pregnancy. Potassium is retained, but like sodium, serum levels slightly decrease due to increased plasma volume. Calcium excretion increases while total serum calcium decreases related to a decrease in plasma albumin (Mastrobattista & Monga, 2019). Further discussion of calcium physiology in pregnancy is found in the musculoskeletal section of this chapter.

Glucose excretion increases between 10-fold and 100-fold (Mastrobattista & Monga, 2019), leading to glycosuria in about 17% of normal pregnancies (Cunningham et al., 2022). Increased glycosuria will increase susceptibility to urinary tract infection.

Uric acid excretion increases, and serum uric acid levels decrease between 8- and 24-week gestation. The serum levels begin to rise to near prepregnancy levels by term (Mastrobattista & Monga, 2019). Increased plasma uric acid levels are positively correlated with preeclampsia severity (Ryu et al., 2019), but uric acid level lacks sensitivity and specificity as a diagnostic tool.

About two-thirds of the weight gain in pregnancy is retained fluid related to the changes in renal tubular function. About 6 L of body water is retained in extracellular areas and 2 L is gained in intracellular spaces. Plasma volume increases account for only about one-quarter of the increase in extracellular fluid (Mastrobattista & Monga, 2019). The allocation of fluid is described as about 3.5 L for amniotic fluid, fetus, and placenta, and about 3 L for the pregnant person's blood volume, breasts, and uterus at term (Cunningham et al., 2022). Clinically, edema is associated with retention of more than 1.5 L of interstitial fluid (Blackburn, 2018). Fluid seeps into interstitial spaces of the lower extremities because of increased venous hydrostatic pressure below the uterus when the gravid uterus places pressure on the inferior vena cava and pelvic vessels.

Gastrointestinal System Adaptations

Gastrointestinal (GI) changes related to pregnancy and pregnancy hormones cause discomforts that are experienced in most normal pregnancies. Occasionally, these changes mimic more serious conditions and require careful assessment.

Anatomical Adaptations

The stomach, liver, and intestines are displaced upward and back by the growing uterus. This change will move the appendix as high as the right upper quadrant, causing the pain of appendicitis to be much higher in the abdomen than expected. In most pregnancies, however, the change in location and the compression of the stomach and bowel is well tolerated.

Gastrointestinal Function Changes

The primary cause of changes in GI tract function in pregnancy is progesterone. This hormone relaxes smooth muscle, thereby causing decreased lower esophageal sphincter and intestinal tone. Coupled with restriction by the GI hormone motilin, the result is slowing of peristalsis and increased intestinal transit time. A relaxed lower esophageal sphincter will allow for reflux of stomach contents into the lower esophagus, resulting in heartburn, especially when pressure from the growing uterus is exerted against the stomach. The slowed transit leads to increased absorption of water, vitamin B_{12}, some amino acids, iron, and calcium (Blackburn, 2018; Kelly & Savides, 2019). This also results in dryer, harder stool, an increased incidence of constipation, straining to pass stool, and hemorrhoids.

In the mouth, the gums respond to increased estrogen by becoming hyperemic, friable, and softer. Some pregnant people will develop one or more **epulis**, a localized vascular swelling of the gums. These changes increase the pregnant person's risks for gingivitis and periodontal disease (Blackburn, 2018). There is no evidence that pregnancy increases tooth decay or tooth loss, although this belief is expressed in common folklore (see Chapter 16, *Oral Health*).

Progesterone is an appetite stimulant leading to increased food intake to meet metabolic needs. This may be part of the reason for food cravings, including **pica**, the ingestion of substances such as clay, starch, ice, or other matter with no nutritional value. Iron deficiency may also influence pica (Cunningham et al., 2022).

Ptyalism, or excess salivation, can occur in pregnancy. Often, this is related to a reluctance to swallow saliva due to nausea and vomiting of pregnancy, which is linked to human chorionic gonadotropin (hCG), estrogen, elevated T4, prostaglandin E_2, altered motility related to progesterone, the emotional and psychological state of the pregnant person, and reflux (Kelly & Savides, 2019). However, the exact cause is unknown; the phenomenon of nausea and vomiting has multiple determinants. The nausea likely increases some of the food aversions commonly observed in pregnancy (see Chapter 40, *Hyperemesis Gravidarum*, and Chapter 15, *Common Discomforts of Pregnancy*).

Table 5.5 Liver Function Changes in Pregnancy

Albumin	Decreased
Alkaline phosphatase (ALP)	Increased (also produced in placenta)
Aspartate transaminase (AST)	Slight decrease due to hemodilution
Alanine transaminase (ALT)	Slight decrease due to hemodilution
Bilirubin (conjugated, unconjugated)	Unchanged
Gamma-glutamyl transpeptidase (GGT)	Slight decrease due to hemodilution
Total protein	Decreased

Source: Adapted from Blackburn (2018), Cunningham et al. (2022), and Lee et al. (2019).

Liver and Biliary Changes

Anatomically, the liver is displaced up and back as the uterus grows. The liver does not change in size and hepatic blood flow is unchanged. The production of proteins and enzymes by the liver does change. Plasma proteins, including albumin, decrease in pregnancy, in part, because of hemodilution. Newer studies indicate that the rise in alpha-fetoprotein may cause a drop in serum albumin levels (Lee et al., 2019). The production of fibrinogen and coagulation factors VII, VIII, IX, and X is increased under the influence of estrogen. Progesterone stimulates an increase in cytochrome P450 isoenzymes, a group of enzymes that assist in the metabolism of organic substances and are important in the body's processing of many drugs. Thyroxine-binding and corticosteroid-binding globulins increase as estrogen levels increase (Cunningham et al., 2022; Lee et al., 2019). Serum alkaline phosphatase (ALP) increases due to placental production, while other liver enzymes are slightly decreased or stay the same (Lee et al., 2019). Table 5.5 lists the changes in liver function tests during pregnancy.

The gallbladder may be affected by genetic variations which can lead to differences in biliary bile acid receptors and transporters (Lee et al., 2019). It may also be affected by progesterone-induced slowed peristalsis, causing increased bile volume, bile stasis, and cholesterol saturation. These changes create an environment ripe for gallstone formation.

Metabolic System Adaptations

The pregnant person's metabolism adjusts to ensure that glucose, protein, and fat are metabolized in a way that will meet their energy needs, as well as the needs of the uteroplacental unit and the fetus. To better understand this adaptation, several significant components involved in the process will be described.

Basal Metabolic Rate

By the end of a normal pregnancy, the maternal metabolic rate has increased up to eight times the nonpregnancy rates (Blackburn, 2018). This requires an average of an additional 300 kcal/day, generally starting in the second trimester. While some of this energy is needed for the growth and maintenance of the fetus, placenta, uterus, and breasts, energy is also stored as fat to be used during the last weeks of pregnancy when the fetus is growing more rapidly.

The first two trimesters of pregnancy are dominated by an **anabolic** state (Blackburn, 2018). The pregnant person eats more, moves around less, and stores protein and fat substrates. Weight gain during this half of pregnancy is due to fat storage and the synthesis of protein into growing tissues. During this anabolic state, insulin is also increased and acts like a growth hormone, facilitating the processes of growth.

The third trimester is a more **catabolic** state. **Lipolytic** activity is increased, and pregnancy hormones lead to a relative insulin resistance. Human placental lactogen (hPL), produced by the placenta, has anti-insulin and lipolytic properties that facilitate a change from glucose usage for energy to lipid usage for energy (Blackburn, 2018). This change leads to **accelerated starvation**. When a nonpregnant person is deprived of food, it takes about 14–18 hours before they have used all the glucose-based energy and begin to burn fat. In pregnant persons, fat oxidation begins in about two to three hours (Blackburn, 2018).

Carbohydrate Metabolism

Fasting serum glucose levels are lower in pregnancy than in the nonpregnant state, and after eating, serum glucose and insulin levels are higher for a longer time (postprandial hyperglycemia). Higher levels of insulin cause a suppression of glucagon and maternal insulin resistance increases as the pregnancy advances. Insulin resistance in the maternal skeletal muscle and adipose tissue is mediated by progesterone, estrogen, prolactin, hPL, cortisol, cytokines, and leptin (Cunningham et al., 2022).

Protein Metabolism

Protein is essential to tissue building in pregnancy. The placenta and fetus use amino acids and protein as they grow in mass and develop structure. These substances are also diverted to the liver for gluconeogenesis. Consequently, serum amino acid and serum protein levels are lower in pregnancy (Blackburn, 2018).

Fat Metabolism

Lipids, lipoproteins, and apolipoproteins increase in maternal serum during pregnancy. These increases are due to lipolysis and decreased lipoprotein lipase action in fat tissue. Estradiol effects on the liver also contribute to these changes (Cunningham et al., 2022). Interestingly, these increases are not associated with vascular endothelial dysfunction in healthy pregnant people. Cholesterol, triglycerides, and lipoproteins (VLDL, LDL-C, and HDL-C) increase in late pregnancy (Cunningham et al., 2022; Liu, 2019).

Leptin

Leptin is produced and secreted by maternal fat cells and the placenta. This peptide hormone helps regulate appetite and enhances energy use. It also contributes significantly to fetal growth and development. Serum leptin in pregnancy is two to four times higher than in nonpregnant people (Cunningham et al., 2022). Leptin is increased even further in people with preeclampsia and gestational diabetes. It is well established that leptin levels are increased in people with obesity and the risk of both preeclampsia and gestational diabetes increases with body mass index. Leptin may mediate the relationship between body mass index and these pregnancy complications (Sommer et al., 2015; Taylor et al., 2016).

Insulin

Insulin is a polypeptide hormone synthesized by the beta cells of the islet of Langerhans of the pancreas. It is secreted in response to increased serum glucose, amino acids, free fatty acids, GI hormones, and the parasympathetic nervous system stimulation of the beta cells. Insulin facilitates glucose entry into cells (Brashers & Huether, 2019).

People with normal glucose tolerance will have an increase in insulin during pregnancy in response to estrogen-induced increased hepatic glucose production, and the increased level of serum glucose after a meal. Insulin facilitates movement of glucose into the pregnant person's muscle and fat cells and further suppresses liver production of glucose. Late in pregnancy, insulin sensitivity decreases 50–60%, resistance increases, and approximately three times more insulin is produced. If a person has an elevated BMI or has an abnormal glucose tolerance before pregnancy, their pancreas may not be able to produce the amount of insulin needed to overcome the insulin resistance induced by pregnancy hormones, and gestational diabetes can result (Moore et al., 2019).

Skin Changes

The skin is the body's largest organ. Skin functions as a barrier to infection and ultraviolet radiation; it retains body fluids, regulates body temperature, and produces vitamin D. Skin contains touch and pressure receptors and nociceptors that transmit pain sensation. Skin is part of the integumentary system, which also includes hair, nails, sebaceous glands, and sweat glands. The entire integumentary system is changed during pregnancy. Specifically, there are changes in pigment, vascular supply, and connective tissue of the skin; hair growth; nail structure; and in the sebaceous and sweat gland functions.

Pigmentation Changes

Estrogen and progesterone produced during pregnancy will stimulate the production of melanocyte-stimulating hormone (MSH). The most frequently seen manifestations of increased MSH are hyperpigmentation of the areolae, genital skin, axillae, inner thighs, and the **linea alba**, which becomes the **linea nigra** during pregnancy. Freckles and moles will also darken. These pigment changes can also be seen in people taking oral contraceptives. Pigment changes usually fade after pregnancy or when oral contraceptives are discontinued; however, people with darker skin and hair are more likely to have persistent hyperpigmentation (Blackburn, 2018).

Melasma, or the "mask of pregnancy" occurs as a result of increased MSH in about 70% of pregnant people (Rapini, 2019). This patch of hyperpigmentation is distributed over the forehead, cheeks, and bridge of the nose in a symmetric pattern. About 30% of those affected will have persistent melasma months to years after birth. Exposure to sunlight will exacerbate the hyperpigmentation. Routine use of sunscreen during pregnancy may decrease the degree of discoloration.

Vascular Changes

The hormones of pregnancy cause vasodilation and the proliferation of capillaries in the skin and can result in the development of **telangiectasias** (small, dilated blood vessels near the skin surface) and palmar erythema. Spider angiomas, capillary hemangiomas, varicosities, and palmar erythema are vascular changes which commonly occur during pregnancy. Many integumentary vascular changes regress or completely disappear postpartum (Blackburn, 2018; Rapini, 2019).

Connective Tissue Changes

Estrogen, relaxin, and adrenocorticoids, along with stretching, contribute to *striae gravidarum,* commonly known as stretch marks. The hormones are thought to relax collagen adhesiveness and facilitate the formation of mucopolysaccharide substance that will cause a separation of collagen fibers. Increased cortisol during pregnancy causes the striae to be purplish in color. The usual locations for striae are over the abdomen, breasts, thighs, and buttocks where skin is stretched by the growing fetus, enlarged breast tissue, and weight gain. Striae become prominent by six to seven months of gestation and are most prevalent in people with lighter skin color (Blackburn, 2018). More severe striae occur in teenagers, people with maternal family history of striae, people with obesity or who gain more than 30 lbs in the pregnancy, and people with large babies (Rapini, 2019). Interestingly, there is an increased incidence of pelvic relaxation and prolapse among people who have moderate to severe striae (Norton et al., 2015). Overall, 50–80% of pregnant people have at least a few striae (Rapini, 2019).

Skin tags, called molluscum fibrosum gravidarum, are another connective tissue phenomenon seen in pregnant people. They are small (typically less than 5 mm), soft, **pedunculated** growths that are the same color of the surrounding skin or are hyperpigmented. They appear on the neck, face, axillae, groin, and between and under the breasts (Blackburn, 2018; Rapini, 2019). Skin tags may disappear after birth; however, many persist.

Pruritus

The most commonly reported skin symptom during pregnancy is pruritus, which may be localized or generalized (Blackburn, 2018). Up to 14% of pregnant people report itching (Rapini, 2019). Symptoms commonly occur on the abdomen during later pregnancy and resolve after delivery. Intrahepatic cholestasis of pregnancy (occurs in less than 2% of pregnant people) and pruritic uticarial papules and plaques of pregnancy (PUPPP) are discussed in Chapter 54, *Dermatologic Disorders*.

Secretory Gland Changes

Sebaceous glands secrete more sebum during pregnancy secondary to increased ovarian and placental androgens (Blackburn, 2018). Apocrine sweat glands found in the axillae, scalp, face, abdomen, and genital area have decreased activity during pregnancy, perhaps related to hormonal changes. Eccrine sweat glands that are distributed over the body have an increased activity during pregnancy. This activity increases under the influence of increased thyroid activity, increased maternal metabolic rate, and increased fetal-produced heat. Their main function is to secrete sweat that will evaporate and help dissipate heat (Blackburn, 2018).

Hair and Nail Changes

During pregnancy, estrogen causes an increased number of hairs to remain in the **anagen** phase (growing phase), and a decreased number enter the **telogen** phase (resting phase). When pregnancy hormones are removed after the birth of the placenta, the number of hairs that enter the telogen phase increases, resulting in hair loss (Cunningham et al., 2022). This hair loss is called telogen effluvium and can also occur after surgery, illness, crash dieting, or other stressful life events. Hair loss after giving birth is expected and is easily distinguished from alopecia of other causes. This hair loss will generally resolve by nine months postpartum without treatment (Rapini, 2019).

Nails typically grow faster during pregnancy, but other nail changes are uncommon. However, phenomena such as transverse grooves, increased brittleness, separation of the nail bed at the toe or fingertip, and whitish discoloration have been reported. These changes are benign and disappear during the postpartum period (Blackburn, 2018; Rapini, 2019).

Immune System Adaptations

Pregnancy requires changes in the immune system. In order to accept and maintain a pregnancy to term, some innate, humoral, and cell-mediated immunologic functions must be altered. This section will outline those changes and explain how these alterations may increase risks for infection or provide remission for some autoimmune conditions for the pregnant person.

Fetus as Allograft

The fetus is a **semiallograft** (an allograft is transplanted tissue; "semi" refers to the fact that fetal tissue carries half of the pregnant person's genetic material) that is not rejected by the pregnant person's immune system. Even though half of the genetic material in the fetus is paternal, in most cases, the pregnant person's immune system does not reject the foreign antigens on fetal cells. Several possible theories explaining this phenomenon have been suggested, including that the placenta may be a selective barrier, the immune system may be suppressed, there may be a cytokine shift or an absence of major histocompatibility complex (MHC) class I molecules on the conceptus, and there may be a local immune suppression mediated by **Fas/FasL** (molecules involved with regulation of cell death; Mor & Abrahams, 2019). Additionally, pregnancy protein 13 (PP13), produced solely by the syncytiotrophoblast and released into the pregnant person's circulation during implantation, has been identified as an agent that diverts the immune system so that the placenta will be well established and grow (Than et al., 2014). Furthermore, meta-analysis supports decreased placental production of PP13 as an early predictive sign of preeclampsia development (Wu et al., 2021). The possibility of using serum PP13 testing for predicting preeclampsia is currently under investigation.

The placenta as barrier theory has been discounted; the placenta acts as only a partial barrier to selected substances. In fact, fetal cells can cross into the pregnant person's blood and have been found in circulation and organs years after pregnancy (Boddy et al., 2015). Cell-free fetal DNA also enters the maternal system and laboratory tests can isolate fetal DNA from a maternal venous blood sample and perform a limited number of genetic tests on the DNA (see Chapter 13, *Genetic Counseling, Screening, and Diagnosis*).

Systemic immune suppression does not fully explain how the conceptus is accepted. How could pregnant people have lived to give birth through the millennia if they could not defend themselves against bacteria and viruses? The best argument against this is that people living with human immunodeficiency virus (HIV) infection do not progress into AIDS more rapidly during pregnancy (Mor & Abrahams, 2019).

Another theory has been that pregnancy is anti-inflammatory in nature, which causes abnormal shifts in **cytokines**, the molecular messengers that regulate responses to inflammation. This can contribute to spontaneous pregnancy loss or preeclampsia. Newer information indicates that pregnancy actually occurs in three different phases with regard to maternal immune response: (a) a strong inflammatory response is required for the invasion of the trophoblast and placentation; (b) a quiet anti-inflammatory state follows when the fetus is growing; and (c) a renewed inflammatory response with an increase of immune cells migrating into the uterus to promote contractions, birth, and the rejection of the placenta (Mor & Abrahams, 2019).

Yet another theory is that there is no MHC class I antigen on the trophoblast, so the immune system does not recognize it as foreign antigens. However, the placenta does express human leukocyte antigens (HLA-C, HLA-G, and HLA-E). These are subsets of MHC antigens. So, fetal tissues are capable of initiating a maternal T-cell response (Mor & Abrahams, 2019).

The theory of local immune suppression postulates that immune cells that would recognize the paternal antigens are removed from the pregnant person's system through **apoptosis** (Mor & Abrahams, 2019). In addition, a subset of T lymphocytes called T regulatory cells has been identified as being able to control other T cells that would attack paternal antigens. These are both possible explanations for the survival of the fetal allograft.

It is also important to recognize that several cells of the innate immune system have been identified at the site where the trophoblast implants, including uterine natural killer (uNK) cells, macrophages, and dendritic cells. Basically, this part of the pregnant person's immune system does respond to the conceptus. These noncytotoxic uNK cells, which are specific to pregnancy, contribute to **angiogenesis** and implantation (Mor & Abrahams, 2019). Macrophages clean out dead cells and debris, while dendritic cells help with early implantation. These activities are crucial to placentation and the immune adjustments necessary for a successful pregnancy.

Disorders Related to Immunologic Changes in Pregnancy

During pregnancy, T-helper cells type 1 (Th1) and T-cytotoxic cells (Tc) are suppressed. This has been identified as a reason for remission of autoimmune disorders such as rheumatoid arthritis, multiple sclerosis, and autoimmune thyroiditis during pregnancy (Blackburn, 2018). Suppression of Th1 has also been implicated in the increased susceptibility to viruses, *Candida albicans,* and other organisms. In fact, vulvovaginal candidiasis occurs more often in pregnant people due to increased estrogen and the changes in the cell-mediated immune response. This cell-mediated immune response, along with the changes in the lungs and heart, has also been identified as an explanation for the increase in influenza severity during pregnancy (CDC, 2021). Autoimmune disorders such as uncomplicated systemic lupus erythematosus (SLE) often remain stable during pregnancy due to the increase in type 2 helper cells (Th2) that is normally seen in pregnancy (Blackburn, 2018). Unfortunately, these diseases often flare within six to eight weeks after birth.

There are five inflammatory markers that are increased during pregnancy. These include leukocyte ALP, C-reactive protein, erythrocyte sedimentation rate (due to increased plasma globulins and fibrinogen), complement factors C_3 and C_4, and procalcitonin (Cunningham et al., 2022). This should be taken into consideration when interpreting laboratory measures of these markers during pregnancy.

Some spontaneous abortions are a result of immune system changes in pregnancy. Immunologic factors that have been implicated in spontaneous abortion include infection; increased Th1 activity against the trophoblast; an immune-related failure of the corpus luteum to produce progesterone; HLAs similar to those of the other biological parent; and, in pregnant people with SLE, antiphospholipid antibodies that prevent the development of the placenta (Blackburn, 2018; Cunningham et al., 2022). Recurrent (more than three) spontaneous abortions have been linked with the presence of uNK cells like those found in the periphery rather than the noncytotoxic uNK cells usually found in the decidua (Kuon et al., 2017).

Preterm labor and birth can result from infection that triggers the innate immune system to release inflammatory cytokines, interleukin, and tumor necrosis factors. These cytokines increase the production of prostaglandin that will stimulate contractions. At the same time, enzymes that cause a weakening of the fetal membranes are released and the membranes may rupture prematurely (Cunningham et al., 2022). It is estimated that up to 40% of preterm births occur because of intrauterine infection and inflammatory processes (Cunningham et al., 2022).

Preeclampsia is specific to pregnancy and is a complex chronic disorder that affects many systems. Evidence suggests that preeclampsia has an immunologic component. In fact, preeclampsia has some of the same cellular changes seen in graft rejection including reduced HLA-G on the trophoblast, an increase in Th1 rather than suppression, more immune complexes, increased fibronectin, increased inflammatory cytokines, changes in complement, and the absence of PP13 (Blackburn, 2018; Than et al., 2014).

Unlike the cell-mediated and innate immune systems, the humoral system in pregnancy does not change significantly. However, maternal antibodies can have an effect on the fetus. Humoral immunity occurs when immunoglobulins (Ig) or antibodies are produced by B lymphocytes (plasma cells) in response to a specific antigen. There are five classes of Ig: IgG, IgM, IgE, IgA, and IgD. IgA and IgG are of particular interest during pregnancy. IgA normally protects body surfaces. Its primary benefit in pregnancy is that it is secreted in breast milk and serves to protect the newborn from GI infections (Rote & McCance, 2019; Blackburn, 2018). IgG is also present in breast milk; however, its primary function is enabled by its smaller size and ability to cross the placenta; IgG provides passive immunity to the fetus from infections for which the pregnant person has manufactured specific antibodies (Rote & McCance, 2019).

There are potential problems for the newborn related to IgG crossing the placenta. People with Graves' disease have thyroid-stimulating IgG that may cross the placenta and cause fetal goiter (Cunningham et al., 2022). Similarly, people with myasthenia gravis have antibodies against acetylcholine receptors that may cross the placenta and cause transient muscular weakness in the newborn that will last only a few weeks (Cunningham et al., 2022).

A frequently encountered disorder related to the placental transfer of IgG is rhesus (Rh) incompatibility (Cunningham et al., 2022). This example of isoimmunization has the potential for causing severe hemolytic disease in the fetus. In order to develop IgG antibodies against Rh-positive RBCs, the maternal system must be exposed to the antigen. This means that Rh-positive RBCs must have entered the pregnant person's system, either from an earlier pregnancy or from blood transfusion. Once the IgG to Rh antigen is established, it can cross the placenta to the fetus, recognize fetal Rh-positive RBCs as foreign, mount an attack, and destroy the fetal RBCs. The formation of this antibody occurs only among people with an Rh-negative blood type. The resulting IgG that passes to the fetus is harmful only to the fetus who has inherited Rh-positive RBCs from the other biological parent. The Rh antigen that is most associated with Rh incompatibility and fetal hemolytic disease is D. For this reason, passive immunization has been developed that prevents humoral production of antibodies in people who receive Rh-positive RBCs from the fetus. Other RBC antigen incompatibilities exist including, but not limited to, anti-c, anti-Kell, Kidd, and Duffy (Cunningham et al., 2022). For this reason, RBC antibody titers are drawn from pregnant people during the first prenatal visit (see Chapter 48, *Hematologic and Thromboembolic Disorders*).

ABO incompatibility can also cause newborn hemolytic disease. However, this form of isoimmunization causes a very mild hemolysis and jaundice due to the increased bilirubin release when the RBC is destroyed. Unlike Rh isoimmunization, this incompatibility does not worsen with each pregnancy. The reason ABO incompatibility is less severe is that most of the anti-A and anti-B antibodies from people with O-type blood are IgM-type and are too large to cross the placenta (Blackburn, 2018; Cunningham et al., 2022). If a person has an O-negative blood type and their fetus is A positive, Rh and ABO incompatibility can both occur. However, the pregnant person's natural anti-A antibody will recognize and destroy fetal RBCs that may enter their system before these cells can cause an antibody response against the Rh-positive factor.

Neurological System and Sensory Adaptations

Cognitive impacts during pregnancy, such as problems with memory, attention, and concentration, are likely small and have a questionable impact on daily life (Brown & Schaffir, 2019). However, some evidence indicates more pregnant and early postpartum people self-report difficulty with memory than nonpregnant people (Logan et al., 2014). Furthermore, Hoekzema et al. (2017) found pregnancy led to significant changes in brain structure and gray matter volume that persist at least two years postpartum. Change in sleep patterns is another implicated factor in the cognitive changes of pregnancy reported by some.

During the first trimester, pregnant people tend to sleep longer at night and nap during the day if their schedules allow. This is in response to fatigue related to increased metabolism and the sedative effects of progesterone (Blackburn, 2018). As the pregnancy advances and placental progesterone and estrogen increase, sleep patterns are further altered. Approximately 76% of pregnant people report difficulty falling asleep, staying asleep, frequent nighttime wakening, and poor quality of sleep across all months of gestation (Mindell et al., 2015).

Studies have shown that the rise in the hormones of pregnancy change both rapid eye movement (REM) and nonrapid eye movement (NREM) sleep. Specifically, progesterone seems to enhance NREM, while estrogen and cortisol decrease REM sleep (Blackburn, 2018). An active fetus, increased discomforts of pregnancy, a growing uterus that limits position change, and decreased REM sleep combine to increase sleep disturbances during the last weeks of pregnancy.

Eye changes during pregnancy include corneal edema, decreased corneal sensitivity, decreased intraocular pressure, and transient loss in accommodation (Blackburn, 2018). Corneal edema and decreased sensitivity have been attributed to fluid retention. Decreased intraocular pressure is due to increased aqueous outflow and the effects of progesterone, relaxin, and hCG (Blackburn, 2018). Pregnancy is not an ideal time for a person to be measured for new contact lenses or eyeglasses. The changes in the eyes will resolve after birth.

Estrogen-induced swollen membranes may affect sense of smell, and in some people, sense of hearing (Blackburn, 2018). The diminished sense of smell will affect taste and can lead to food aversions.

Musculoskeletal System Adaptations

The enlarging uterus changes the pregnant person's center of gravity. The spine adjusts by increasing **lordosis**. At the same time, there is increased mobility of the sacroiliac, sacrococcygeal, and pubic joints related to changes in the cartilage brought about by relaxin and progesterone. Changes in the low back and pelvis can cause low-back discomfort, aching, numbness, and tingling in the legs as the pregnancy progresses. Changes in the cervical spine, along with slumping of the shoulders and upper back due to heavier breasts, can stretch the ulnar and median nerves, causing tingling discomfort in the arms and hands.

The growing fetus needs calcium for skeleton and teeth formation and calcification. Calcium demands are greatest in the third trimester of pregnancy. Much of the calcium needed is drawn from the pregnant person's skeleton and enhanced by increased intestinal absorption and decreased urinary excretion of calcium. Changes in calcium concentration require changes in parathyroid hormone, magnesium, phosphate, vitamin D, and calcitonin physiology. Lowered calcium levels in the pregnant person may result in increased bone loss and secondary hyperparathyroidism (Nader, 2019a). Parathyroid hormone acts on bone **resorption**, intestinal absorption, and kidney reabsorption of calcium and phosphate. Parathyroid hormone plasma levels increase steadily as the fetus draws more calcium for bone growth. At the same time, the increased GFR and increased plasma volume in the pregnant person causes a lower serum calcium level.

Vitamin D is either ingested or obtained via synthesis in sun-exposed skin. During pregnancy, the kidney, decidua, and placenta change vitamin D to 1,25-dihydroxyvitamin D_3. This compound further enhances calcium resorption and intestinal absorption of calcium during pregnancy (Cunningham et al., 2022).

Serum calcium levels begin to fall after fertilization regardless of diet (Blackburn, 2018). Calcium levels may be compromised by increased ingestion of phosphate. Too much phosphate will limit calcium absorption in the intestine and increase calcium urinary excretion. Foods high in phosphorus include processed meats, chips, and sodas that are commonly consumed as part of the US diet.

Endocrine System Adaptations

Like other systems, the endocrine glands undergo changes during pregnancy that support fetal growth and pregnancy maintenance. This section is limited to an outline of the changes that occur in the pituitary, thyroid, and adrenal glands, and their hormones. The changes in the parathyroid and the endocrine pancreas have been described earlier in this chapter. Changes in the gonads are explained in Chapter 3, *Reproductive Tract Structure and Function*.

Anatomical Changes

Physiologic pituitary growth occurs in normal pregnancies. In fact, the pituitary will grow to 136% of its original size under the influence of estrogen (Blackburn, 2018; Nader, 2019a). Very rarely, the enlargement will be big enough to increase intracranial pressure or put pressure on the optic chiasm. This may cause headaches or vision changes that will resolve after birth.

The thyroid gland will also increase mildly in size during pregnancy as a result of increased vascularity and some hyperplasia of normal gland cells. Significant enlargement, however, may be a sign of iodine deficiency or other thyroid abnormalities (Nader, 2019b). The adrenal glands do not change in size.

Pituitary Function Changes

The pituitary has two lobes, anterior and posterior, and each lobe secretes hormones activated by the releasing hormones from the hypothalamus. Table 5.6 lists the hormones secreted by the anterior and posterior lobes of the pituitary.

In pregnancy, the most dramatic change in anterior pituitary function is that it secretes 10 times more prolactin (Nader, 2019a). The lactotrophs (cells that secrete prolactin) are stimulated by estrogen and account for most of the cellular growth of the pituitary. Prolactin prepares the breasts for breastfeeding and will maintain breast milk production for the duration of the lactation period (see Chapter 31, *Lactation and Breastfeeding*).

Pituitary growth hormone secretion decreases beginning in the second trimester when placental growth hormone is produced (Nader, 2019a). Thyroid-stimulating hormone (TSH) secretion decreases slightly in the first trimester under the influence of hCG; 10–20% of pregnant people may experience temporary hyperthyroxinemia associated with a larger drop in TSH in the first trimester (Blackburn, 2018). TSH levels then typically return to

Table 5.6 Pituitary Hormones

Anterior pituitary	Target organs
Growth hormone	Bone, muscle, liver
Adrenocorticotropic hormone (ACTH)	Adrenal cortex
Thyroid-stimulating hormone (TSH)	Thyroid gland
Gonadotropic hormones (FSH, LH, and ICSH)	Testis, ovary
Melanocyte-stimulating hormone (MSH)	Anterior pituitary, skin
Prolactin	Mammary glands
Posterior pituitary	Target organs
Antidiuretic hormone (ADH)	Kidney tubules
Oxytocin (OT)	Uterine smooth muscle, mammary glands

Source: Adapted from Brashers and Huether (2019).

normal as the pregnancy progresses. Adrenocorticotropic hormone (ACTH) secretion increases, reaching its highest level during labor (Blackburn, 2018).

Posterior pituitary function also changes. The threshold for release of antidiuretic hormone (ADH) is reset so that the decline in plasma osmolarity can occur. However, the amount of ADH released is not changed (Nader, 2019a). Also, thirst is stimulated by lower levels of osmolarity in pregnant people than in nonpregnant people.

Levels of oxytocin, the second posterior pituitary hormone, rise as pregnancy progresses and play a role in cervical ripening (Blackburn, 2018). Oxytocin levels spike during labor, stimulating, and sustaining uterine contractions. Oxytocin continues to be elevated during lactation and is released when the suckling infant triggers a neural impulse resulting in milk ejection (see Chapter 31, *Lactation and Breastfeeding*).

Oxytocin is also an important facilitator of the bonding process between the parturient and the neonate. Oxytocin is unique to mammals and has central nervous system effects, in addition to effects on the reproductive organs. The importance of oxytocin in regard to social recognition, pair bonding, and other social behaviors has been investigated. Oxytocin release appears to promote feelings of love, gratitude, and security in people (Algoe et al., 2017). Moreover, oxytocin promotes bonding with the newborn and leads to improved mental health and social outcomes (IsHak et al., 2011; Scatliffe et al., 2019).

Thyroid Function Changes

The thyroid gland increases production of thyroid hormones in pregnancy. Increased estrogen causes the liver to produce more thyroxine-binding globulin (TBG) early in pregnancy. As thyroxine (T_4) is bound to TBG, there is a decrease in free T_4 that results in stimulation of the hypothalamus to release thyrotropin-releasing hormone, and in response, the anterior pituitary is stimulated to release TSH (Nader, 2019b). This series of events is an example of a negative-feedback control loop.

At the same time, the thyroid is being stimulated by hCG, which acts like TSH. By 12-week gestation, hCG has reached serum levels that inhibit pituitary production of TSH (Nader, 2019b). Free serum T_4 peaks at around the same time that hCG peaks (Nader, 2019b). Free and total T_3 increase. All these changes in thyroid function lead to an increased basal metabolic rate.

There are significant changes in the thyroid laboratory testing parameters during pregnancy. The third-generation TSH and free T_4 index using the product of T_4 and T_3 resin uptake laboratory tests are commonly utilized to evaluate thyroid function in pregnancy (Nader, 2019b).

Adrenal Function Changes

The adrenal cortex, after stimulation by ACTH, releases glucocorticoids (primarily cortisol), mineralocorticoids (primarily aldosterone), and adrenal androgens and estrogens (Brashers & Huether, 2019). Serum ACTH is lower in early pregnancy but begins to increase as pregnancy progresses. Serum cortisol is increased in pregnancy, and much of it is bound by cortisol-binding globulin that is three times higher during pregnancy. This causes the total cortisol level to rise significantly. Aldosterone levels increase 20-fold during late pregnancy (Nader, 2019a). This increase is necessary because of the antagonistic effects of progesterone including increased sodium excretion (Cunningham et al., 2022). Adrenal testosterone increases in pregnancy due to increased sex hormone-binding globulin produced by the liver (Nader, 2019a).

Corticotropin-releasing hormone (CRH) and ACTH are produced by the placenta and increase significantly during the last weeks of pregnancy (Cunningham et al., 2022). In addition, the fetal adrenal gland secretes high levels of cortisol and dehydroepiandrosterone sulfate (DHEA-S). These substances cause an increase in the production of estriol that will enhance uterine muscle gap junctions and facilitate the development of oxytocin receptors within uterine tissue in preparation for rhythmic, uniform, and coordinated contractions.

Reproductive System Adaptations

See Chapter 3, *Reproductive Tract Structure and Function*, for a description of reproductive system adaptations to pregnancy.

Breast Adaptations

See Chapter 31, *Lactation and Breastfeeding*, for information about the physiology of breast feeding and breast changes during pregnancy.

Summary

Virtually all body systems undergo adaptive changes during pregnancy that are necessary for the well-being of the pregnant person and for fetal growth and development. Understanding the physiology foundational to these changes is imperative for healthcare professionals caring for pregnant people and their babies. Differentiating normal changes from potential or real abnormalities and being able to interpret laboratory findings accurately depend on the knowledge of these miraculous, complex adaptations.

Resources for Clients and Families

Merck Manual (Consumer Version), Physical Changes During Pregnancy: https://www.merckmanuals.com/home/women-s-health-issues/normal-pregnancy/physical-changes-during-pregnancy?query=Physiology%20of%20Pregnancy

Pregnancy Week by Week: https://www.medicinenet.com/stages_of_pregnancy_pictures_slideshow/article.htm

Resources for Healthcare Providers

CDC, COVID-19 Vaccines While Pregnant or Breastfeeding: https://www.cdc.gov/coronavirus/2019-ncov/vaccines/recommendations/pregnancy.html

CDC, Flu & Pregnancy: https://www.cdc.gov/flu/highrisk/pregnant.htm

Merck Manual (Professional Version), Physiology of Pregnancy: https://www.merckmanuals.com/professional/gynecology-and-obstetrics/approach-to-the-pregnant-woman-and-prenatal-care/physiology-of-pregnancy

References

Algoe, S. B., Kurtz, L. E., & Grewen, K. (2017). Oxytocin and social bonds: The role of oxytocin in perceptions of romantic partners' bonding behavior. *Psychological Science*, 28, 1763–1772.

Blackburn, S. (2018). *Maternal, fetal, and neonatal physiology: A clinical perspective* (5th ed.). Elsevier.

Boddy, A. M., Fortunato, A., Wilson Sayres, M., & Aktipis, A. (2015). Fetal microchimerism and maternal health: A review and evolutionary analysis of cooperation and conflict beyond the womb. *BioEssays*, 37(10), 1106–1118.

Bowersox, N. (2021, March 4). *Thrombocytopenia in pregnancy*. Medscape: Drugs & Diseases. https://emedicine.medscape.com/article/272867-overview#a2

Brashers, V., & Huether, S. (2019). Mechanisms of hormonal regulation. In K. McCance, S. Huether, V. Brashers, & N. Rote (Eds.), *Pathophysiology: The biologic basis for disease in adults and children* (8th ed., pp. 644–669). Elsevier/Mosby.

Brown, E., & Schaffir, J. (2019). "Pregnancy brain": A review of cognitive changes in pregnancy and postpartum. *Obstetrical and Gynecological Survey*, 74(3), 178–185.

Centers for Disease Control and Prevention (CDC). (2021, August 26). *Flu vaccine safety and pregnancy: Questions and answers*. https://www.cdc.gov/flu/highrisk/qa_vacpregnant.htm

Cunningham, F. G., Leveno, K. J., Dashe, J. S., Hoffman, B. L., Spong, C. Y., & Casey, B. M. (2022). *Williams obstetrics* (26th ed.). McGraw Hill.

Dolezsar, C. M., McGrath, J. J., Herzig, A. J. M., & Miller, S. B. (2014). Perceived racial discrimination and hypertension: A comprehensive systematic review. *Health Psychology*, 33(1), 20–34.

Hoekzema, E., Barba-Müller, E., Pozzobon, C., Picado, M., Lucco, F., García-García, D., Soliva, J. C., Tobena, A., Desco, M., Crone, E. A., Ballesteros, A., Carmona, S., & Vilarroya, O. (2017). Pregnancy leads to long-lasting changes in human brain structure. *Nature Neuroscience*, 20(2), 287–296. https://doi.org/10.1038/nn.4458

IsHak, W. W., Kahloon, M., & Fakhry, H. (2011). Oxytocin role in enhancing well-being: A literature review. *Journal of Affective Disorders, 130*(1), 1–9.

Kelly, T. F., & Savides, T. J. (2019). Gastrointestinal disease in pregnancy. In R. Resnik, C. J. Lockwood, T. R. Moore, M. F. Greene, & R. M. Silver (Eds.), *Creasy and Resnik's maternal–fetal medicine: Principles and practice* (8th ed., pp. 1158–1172). Elsevier/Saunders.

Kilpatrick, S. J., & Kitahara, S. (2019). Anemia and pregnancy. In R. Resnik, C. J. Lockwood, T. R. Moore, M. F. Greene, & R. M. Silver (Eds.), *Creasy and Resnik's maternal–fetal medicine: Principles and practice* (8th ed., pp. 991–1006). Elsevier/Saunders.

Kuon, R. J., Weber, M., Heger, J., Santillan, I., Vomstein, K., Bar, C., . . . Toth, B. (2017). Uterine natural killer cells in patients with idiopathic recurrent miscarriage. *American Journal of Reproductive Immunology, 78*, e12721. https://doi.org/10.1111/aji.12721

Lee, R. H., Chung, R. T., & Pringle, P. (2019). Diseases of the liver, biliary system and pancreas. In R. Resnik, C. J. Lockwood, T. R. Moore, M. F. Greene, & R. M. Silver (Eds.), *Creasy and Resnik's maternal–fetal medicine: Principles and practice* (8th ed., pp. 1173–1191). Elsevier/Saunders.

Liu, J. H. (2019). Endocrinology of pregnancy. In R. Resnik, C. J. Lockwood, T. R. Moore, M. F. Greene, & R. M. Silver (Eds.), *Creasy and Resnik's maternal–fetal medicine: Principles and practice* (8th ed., pp. 148–160). Elsevier/Saunders.

Logan, D. M., Hill, K. R., Jones, R., Holt-Lunstad, J., & Larson, M. J. (2014). How do memory and attention change with pregnancy and childbirth? A controlled longitudinal examination of neuropsychological functioning in pregnant and postpartum women. *Journal of Clinical and Experimental Neuropsychology, 36*(5), 528–539.

Mastrobattista, J. M., & Monga, M. (2019). Maternal cardiovascular, respiratory, and renal adaptation to pregnancy. In R. Resnik, C. J. Lockwood, T. R. Moore, M. F. Greene, & R. M. Silver (Eds.), *Creasy and Resnik's maternal–fetal medicine: Principles and practice* (8th ed., pp. 141–147). Elsevier.

Mindell, J. A., Cook, R. A., & Nikolovski, J. (2015). Sleep patterns and sleep disturbances across pregnancy. *Sleep Medicine, 16*(4), 483–488.

Mohamad, T. N. (2017, January 10). *Cardiovascular disease and pregnancy.* http://emedicine.medscape.com article/162004-overview

Moore, T. R., Hauguel-DeMouzon, S., & Catalano, P. (2019). Diabetes in pregnancy. In R. Resnik, C. J. Lockwood, T. R. Moore, M. F. Greene, & R. M. Silver (Eds.), *Creasy and Resnik's maternal–fetal medicine: Principles and practice* (8th ed., pp. 1067–1097). Elsevier.

Mor, G., & Abrahams, V. M. (2019). The immunology of pregnancy. In R. Resnik, C. J. Lockwood, T. R. Moore, M. F. Greene, & R. M. Silver (Eds.), *Creasy and Resnik's maternal–fetal medicine: Principles and practice* (8th ed., pp. 127–140). Elsevier.

Nader, S. (2019a). Other endocrine disorders of pregnancy. In R. Resnik, C. J. Lockwood, T. R. Moore, M. F. Greene, & R. M. Silver (Eds.), *Creasy and Resnik's maternal–fetal medicine: Principles and practice* (8th ed., pp. 1135–1157). Elsevier.

Nader, S. (2019b). Thyroid disease and pregnancy. In R. Resnik, C. J. Lockwood, T. R. Moore, M. F. Greene, & R. M. Silver (Eds.), *Creasy and Resnik's maternal–fetal medicine: Principles and practice* (8th ed., pp. 1116–1134). Elsevier.

Norton, P. A., Allen-Brady, K., Wu, J., Egger, M., & Cannon-Albright, L. (2015). Clinical characteristics of women with familial pelvic floor disorders. *International Urogynecology Journal, 26*(3), 401–406.

Peña-Rosas, J. P., De-Regil, L. M., Garcia-Casal, M. N., & Dowswell, T. (2015). Daily oral iron supplementation during pregnancy. *Cochrane Database of Systematic Reviews, 7.* Art. No.: CD004736. https://doi.org/10.1002/14651858.CD004736.pub5

Rapini, R. P. (2019). The skin and pregnancy. In R. Resnik, C. J. Lockwood, T. R. Moore, M. F. Greene, & R. M. Silver (Eds.), *Creasy and Resnik's maternal–fetal medicine: Principles and practice* (8th ed., pp. 1258–1268). Elsevier.

Rodger, M., & Silver, R. M. (2019). Coagulation disorders in pregnancy. In R. Resnik, C. J. Lockwood, T. R. Moore, M. F. Greene, & R. M. Silver (Eds.), *Creasy and Resnik's maternal–fetal medicine: Principles and practice* (8th ed., pp. 949–976). Elsevier.

Rote, N., & McCance, K. (2019). Adaptive immunity. In K. McCance, S. Huether, V. Brashers, & N. Rote (Eds.), *Pathophysiology: The biologic basis for disease in adults and children* (8th ed., pp. 220–254). Elsevier/Mosby.

Ryu, A., Cho, N. J., Kim, Y. S., & Lee, E. Y. (2019). Predictive value of serum uric acid levels for adverse perinatal outcomes in pre-eclampsia. *Medicine, 98*(18), e15462. https://doi.org/10.1097/MD.0000000000015462

Scatliffe, N., Casavant, S., Vittner, D., & Cong, X. (2019). Oxytocin and early parent-infant interactions: A systematic review. *International Journal of Nursing Sciences, 6*, 445–453.

Scott, J. M., Weir, D. G., Molloy, A., McPartlin, J., Daly, L., & Kirke, P. (1994). Folic acid metabolism and mechanisms of neural tube defects. In *Neural tube defects. CIBA foundation symposium* (Vol. 181, pp. 180–191).

Sherman, C., Gauthier, M., & David, M. (2016). Supine hypotensive syndrome of pregnancy. In F. S. Freeman & J. S. Berger (Eds.), *Anesthesiology core review: Part two advanced exam.* McGraw-Hill Medical.

Sims, M., Diez-Roux, A. V., Dudley, A., Gebreab, S., Wyatt, S. B., Bruce, M. A., James, S. A., Robinson, J. C., Williams, D. R., & Taylor, H. A. (2012). Perceived discrimination and hypertension among African Americans in the Jackson heart study. *American Journal of Public Health, 102*(S2), s258–s265.

Sommer, C., Jenum, A. K., Waage, C. W., Morkrid, K., Sletner, L., & Birkeland, K. I. (2015). Ethnic differences in BMI, subcutaneous fat, and serum leptin levels during and after pregnancy and risk of gestational diabetes. *European Journal of Endocrinology, 172*(6), 649–656.

Taylor, B. D., Tang, G., Ness, R. B., Olsen, J., Hougaard, D. M., Skogstrand, K., Roberts, J. M., & Haggerty, C. L. (2016). Mid-pregnancy circulating immune biomarkers in women with preeclampsia and normotensive controls. *Pregnancy Hypertension: An International Journal of Women's Cardiovascular Health, 6*(1), 72–78.

Than, N. G., Balogh, A., Romero, R., Karpati, E., Erez, O., Szilagyi, A., Kovalszky, I., Sammar, M., Gizurarson, S., Matko, J., Zavodszky, P., Papp, Z., & Meiri, H. (2014). Placental protein 13 (PP13)—A placental immunoregulatory galectin protecting pregnancy. *Frontiers in Immunology, 5*, 348. https://doi.org/10.3389/fimmu.2014.00348

Whitty, J., & Dombrowski, M. P. (2019). Respiratory diseases in pregnancy. In R. Resnik, C. J. Lockwood, T. R. Moore, M. F. Greene, & R. M. Silver (Eds.), *Creasy and Resnik's maternal–fetal medicine: Principles and practice* (8th ed., pp. 1043–1066). Elsevier.

Wu, Y., Liu, Y., & Ding, Y. (2021). Predictive performance of placental protein 13 for screening preeclampsia in the first trimester: A systematic review and meta-analysis. *Frontiers in Medicine, 8*, 756383. https://doi.org/10.3389/fmed.2021.756383

6

Physiologic Alterations during the Postnatal Period

Cindy L. Farley and Tanya Tringali

The editors gratefully acknowledge Kaitlin Wilson and Cindy L. Farley, who were coauthors of the previous edition of this chapter.

Relevant Terms

Afterpains—uterine contractions that occur after childbirth and produce pain ranging from mild to labor-like in intensity

Diastasis recti—a midline separation of the rectus abdominus muscles at the linea alba

Genital Hiatus—the distance from the midpoint of the urethral meatus to the posterior margin of the hymen, which is positively associated with symptomatic pelvic organ prolapse

Hyperplasia—enlargement of tissue by an increase in the number of cells

Hypertrophy—enlargement of tissue by the enlargement or growth of cells

Involution—the postpartum process by which the reproductive organs return to a nonpregnant state

Lochia—vaginal discharge resulting from the sloughing of decidual tissue, debris from the products of conception, epithelial cells, red blood cells, white blood cells, and serum

Maternal reset hypothesis—a theory that lactation downregulates the metabolic hyperactivity of pregnancy, thus leading to the many short- and long-term health benefits seen in individuals who lactate

Postpartum—the period after birth beginning at the time of complete expulsion of the placenta and membranes, and continuing until the reproductive structures return to a nonpregnant state; also known as the puerperium or postnatal period

Telogen gravidarum—diffuse hair loss due to postpartum hormonal changes

Uterotonic—substance that induces uterine contractions

Introduction

The **postpartum** period starts with the expulsion of the placenta after the birth of the infant. This event begins a process of **involution** of the reproductive system as it attains a new version of its nonpregnant state. Extensive physiologic changes occur throughout the postpartum body. These changes do not always align with the current time frame of postnatal care. The postpartum period is being reconceptualized to extend at least a year in contrast to the arbitrary six-week time frame (Douthard et al., 2021). It is estimated that over half of preventable maternal mortality and morbidity occurs in the first postpartum year (Davis et al., 2019). A thorough understanding of postpartum physiology can assist the clinician in validating normal changes and recognizing and responding to emerging concerns.

This chapter reviews typical physiologic changes that occur in body systems during the postpartum period. Components of care and psychosocial adaptations of the postpartum individual and family are discussed in Chapter 30, *Components of Postnatal Care*. Breast anatomy, physiology, lactogenesis, and the process of lactation are described in Chapter 31, *Lactation and Breastfeeding*. The return to fertility and postpartum contraceptive options are detailed in Chapter 32, *Contraception in the Postnatal Period*. Complex conditions of postpartum and lactation are covered in Chapter 43, *Common Complications during the Postnatal Period*, and Chapter 44, *Common Lactation and Breastfeeding Problems*.

Prenatal and Postnatal Care: A Person-Centered Approach, Third Edition. Edited by Karen Trister Grace, Cindy L. Farley, Noelene K. Jeffers, and Tanya Tringali.
© 2024 John Wiley & Sons Ltd. Published 2024 by John Wiley & Sons Ltd.
Companion website: www.wiley.com/go/grace/prenatal

Health equity key points

- It is estimated that one-third of maternal deaths occur at the birth and up to one week postpartum and another third occur between one week and one year postpartum.
- In the United States, Black and Native American/Native Alaskan people are three times more likely to die in the postpartum period than White people.
- There is no known physiologic or anatomic basis for racial or ethnic health disparities in postpartum outcomes; these disparities are attributed to the intersection of racism, discrimination, and social determinants of health.
- Postpartum client reports of persistent, severe, or unusual anatomic or physiologic signs or symptoms, particularly of pain and bleeding, deserve prompt and thorough gathering of subjective and objective data before being deemed within normal limits.

Uterus

In a nonpregnant state, the uterus is roughly the size and shape of an inverted pear and weighs only about 100 g. During pregnancy, uterine muscle fibers undergo extensive **hyperplasia** and **hypertrophy**, increasing uterine weight approximately 10-fold to an average weight of about 1000 g (Isley & Katz, 2017). Immediately after the infant is born, the stretched-to-capacity smooth muscle fibers recoil and contract, resulting in a smaller endometrial surface area. This change in the endometrial surface area leads to shearing of the placenta and decidua from the uterine wall (Perlman & Carusi, 2019). The placenta and membranes are usually expelled from the uterus shortly thereafter. After the birth of the placenta, the uterine fundus is located at about the level of or slightly below the umbilicus and remains there for the first two days after birth. The uterus should be firmly contracted and the size of a softball, approximately 17 cm in height, 12 cm in width, and 10 cm thick. In the immediate postpartum period, the uterus tends to be retroverted (Ucci et al., 2021).

It will attain midplane position by the end of the first week and will return to its typical anteverted position at the end of week 2 (Ucci et al., 2021).

The uterus begins this process of involution shortly after birth (Figure 6.1). During pregnancy, there is an increase in blood flow to the uterus with hypertrophy and adaptation of the pelvic vessels. In the puerperium, uterine blood flow decreases, and the vessels revert to their prepregnant state. Involution occurs by a dramatic reduction in the size of the myometrial cells with decreasing quantities of cytoplasm and resorption of the connective tissue (Diniz et al., 2014). The process occurs quickly, with the uterus weighing only 500 g at one week after birth, 300 g at two weeks, and approximately 100 g at four weeks (Paliulyte et al., 2017). Abdominally, the decrease in the size of the uterus is notable by palpation of the uterine fundus and occurs at a rate of about 1 cm a day, as shown in Figure 6.2. The uterine fundus can be difficult to clearly discern in individuals with higher body weights or who have uterine myomas (Ucci et al., 2021). By day 14, the uterus has descended below the rim of the symphysis pubis and is no longer palpable abdominally. Involution may be slowed in people who have had overdistension of the uterus from a multifetal pregnancy or from polyhydramnios.

The uterine contractions that occur after birth are most intense in the first three days postpartum and are commonly called **afterpains**. The contractions are usually more intense in multiparous individuals and can be stimulated with **uterotonic** agents such as oxytocin. Endogenous oxytocin release during infant suckling can also cause afterpains. Uterine contractions are important in maintaining hemostasis in the postpartum period. Failure of the uterus to involute fully is most often related to atony, but it is also seen with retained placental fragments, infection, or lacerations.

After the placenta separates from the endometrium, the uterine muscle fibers contract, effectively ligating the bleeding vessels at the placental site. The compression of these vessels is essential to preventing postpartum

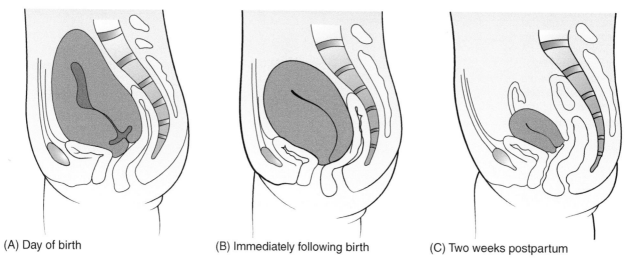

(A) Day of birth   (B) Immediately following birth   (C) Two weeks postpartum

Figure 6.1 Uterine size changes (sagittal view).

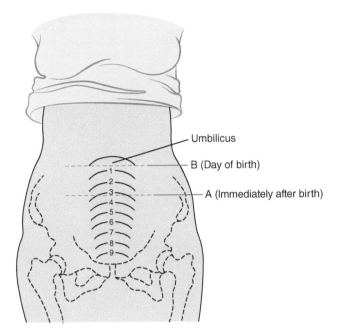

Figure 6.2   Uterine involution (abdominal view).

hemorrhage. After birth, blood loss can range from 150 mL up to 1000 mL and be in the range of normal. Postpartum hemorrhage is defined as a total blood loss of greater than or equal to 1000 mL in either vaginal or cesarean birth, or any amount of blood loss accompanied by signs or symptoms of hypovolemia within 24 hours after the birth (ACOG, 2017). Without the hemostasis provided by the myometrial contraction, profound hemorrhage can occur rapidly. Further blood loss is prevented by the activation of the clotting cascade with placental separation (Osol & Mandala, 2009). This hypercoagulable state remains for the first two weeks to aid in healing of the placental site.

The endometrium is also restored after birth. Excess intracellular proteins as well as intracellular cytoplasm are removed by autolysis with proteolytic enzymes and macrophage degradation. The placental attachment site takes about six weeks to completely exfoliate and regenerate a new endometrial layer.

Lochia

Lochia is vaginal discharge resulting from the sloughing of decidual tissue and includes debris from the products of conception as well as some bacteria, epithelial cells, and red blood cells. Lochia changes in characteristics as the uterus is emptied of necrotic tissue and new endometrium is regenerated at the basal layer adjacent to the myometrium. The average duration of lochial discharge is 24–36 days, although some individuals will have lochia longer than six weeks; this can be a variation of normal (Fletcher et al., 2012). Lochia presents in diverse patterns over time. Lochia rubra begins after the expulsion of the placenta and is composed primarily of blood, along with debris from the placenta, membranes, vernix, lanugo, and decidual tissue. Lochia should not contain large clots; most clots are small and result from pooling of lochia in

the vagina. Lochia rubra is dark red, has a distinctive fleshy odor, and lasts for a few days to a week.

Lochia serosa is a pinkish-brown discharge that lasts for approximately two to three weeks. It consists of blood, wound exudate, erythrocytes, leukocytes, cervical mucus, microorganisms, and decidual tissue and occurs as the uterus begins to regenerate the endometrium and as the placental site is exfoliated and remodeled. This discharge gradually transitions to a pink, yellow, or white color called lochia alba. Lochia alba is primarily leukocytes and decidual cells. It is small to scant in amount and can last up to four weeks.

A transient increase in discharge reverting to lochia rubra can occur between days 7 and 14 postpartum. This corresponds with the sloughing of the eschar tissue that formed at the site of placental detachment. This bleeding episode should be brief and self-limiting and should not be mistaken for the return of menses. Occasionally, an increase in bleeding may be related to the amount and intensity of physical activity in the early postpartum period; increased time spent resting may bring the amount of blood flow back into normal limits.

Cervix

During labor and birth, each contraction of uterine muscle fibers forces the presenting part of the fetus toward and eventually through the cervix and the vagina. Simultaneously, as the muscle fibers shorten with each contraction, the cervix is thinned and drawn over the presenting part, leaving the cervix stretched, edematous, bruised, abraded, and sometimes lacerated. Within hours of birth, healing of the cervix begins. Although the cervix protrudes into the vagina immediately after birth, shortly thereafter, the contracting uterus begins to restore the cervix back into its usual position. As edema resolves, the cervix shortens, thickens, and the epithelium begins to remodel. The cervical os of people who have given birth vaginally or had significant dilation prior to an operative birth does not completely regain its nulliparous appearance; it is usually wider and the cervical os often appears as a transverse slit rather than the more circular os observed in the nulliparous cervix (Figure 6.3).

Vagina

The vaginal muscles and mucosa reach their expansion threshold as the fetus passes through the vagina and over the perineum. After birth, the vagina is often bruised, swollen, abraded, and lacerated. Immediately postpartum, vaginal tone is slack, muscle contractile strength is reduced, and rugae are absent. The vagina begins to heal shortly after birth. By three weeks postpartum, the rugae return but are less prominent than before pregnancy. The vaginal epithelium begins to proliferate at about four weeks after birth. By six weeks postpartum, the vaginal epithelium is usually reconstructed, and vaginal tone is nearly restored. However, like the cervix, the vagina does not completely regain its nulliparous tone or shape and can

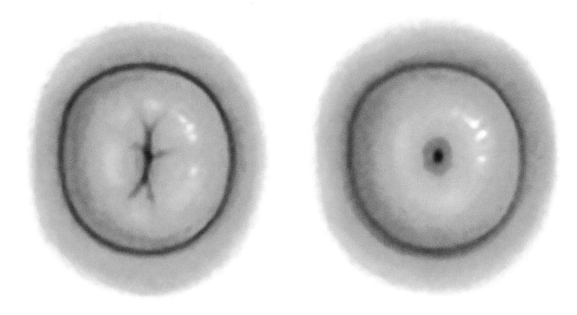

Figure 6.3 Parous and nulliparous cervices.

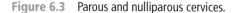

predispose some individuals to later pelvic organ prolapse after childbirth (ACOG & AUGS, 2019). The vaginal microbiome is altered after birth, with a lower abundance of *Lactobacillus* species and greater diversity of other microbiota (Nunn et al., 2021). This change is thought to be related to the decrease in estrogen after birth. The return to a *Lactobacillus* dominant vaginal environment occurs gradually over several months as cyclical hormonal patterns are re-established.

Labia and Perineum

The labia and perineum are often bruised and edematous after birth. Abrasions and small lacerations are common. Lacerations, depending on the severity and the extent of the injury and repair, will vary in healing times from days to weeks. Perineal edema is generally resolved within three to four days. The physiologic reduction in progesterone aids in the rapid return of vulvar tone. Despite proximity to the rectum, healing of the perineal structures after birth is often uncomplicated.

Pelvic Floor

Pelvic floor musculature is changed by both pregnancy and the birth of a baby regardless of the mode of birth, and can include descent of the bladder, uterus, and rectum (Atan et al., 2021). For many, these changes are minor and resolve quickly. However, for others, they can be profound and contribute to pelvic floor dysfunction and pelvic organ prolapse. Changes to the pelvic floor that commonly occur in the postpartum period can be exacerbated by a range of factors including physiologic, hormonal, structural, and genetic, as well as the circumstances of one's labor and birth. During the second stage of labor, the pubococcygeus muscle stretches up to 3.5 times its

original length (Kamel, 2021). This can result in a lengthening of the distance from the midpoint of the urethral meatus to the posterior margin of the hymen, called the **genital hiatus** (Madhu et al., 2018). Excessive stretching or avulsion of the levator ani muscle from its bony insertion greatly increases the risk of developing pelvic organ prolapse (Frawley et al., 2021). Pelvic floor musculature is described in Chapter 3, *Reproductive Structure and Function.*

Rectal Anatomy

Increased blood volume, hormonal changes, and the weight of the gravid uterus during pregnancy contribute to vasocongestion in the rectum. These changes predispose pregnant and postpartum people to internal and external hemorrhoids. Birth can sometimes be traumatic to the nerves that supply the muscles involved in defecation, such as the levator ani and the anal sphincter complex. In some cases, this can contribute to constipation whereas in others, it can lead to fecal incontinence. In many cases, these disorders resolve with time (Palmieri et al., 2021). Lacerations involving the pelvic floor, the anal sphincter complex, and the rectovaginal septum can have long-term sequelae of anal incontinence and urgency, and rectovaginal fistulae that can result in infection, pain, social embarrassment, and isolation.

Additional Physiologic Alterations during the Postpartum Period

In addition to the dramatic changes observed in the reproductive organs during the postpartum period, alterations occur in other organ systems and laboratory values during the postpartum period (Table 6.1). Other significant postpartum physiologic alterations are summarized further.

Table 6.1   Selected Physical Alterations In the Postpartum Period

Physical parameter	Alteration	Return to prepregnant levels
Venous changes	Increased venous diameter and decreased blood flow velocity; there is elevated risk for thrombophlebitis and embolism during this time	Six weeks
Heart rate	Increases in the first hour after birth	Within hours
Cardiac output	Increases significantly in the first hour after birth and remains elevated for the first two days after birth	One week
Blood pressure	Slight increase in both systolic and diastolic values	Two to six months
Coagulation	Increases significantly in the first two days after birth and remains elevated through two weeks	Three to six weeks
Total blood volume	Remains elevated during the first week after birth	One week
Red blood count	Decreases after birth depending on blood loss. May appear falsely low immediately postpartum due to fluid overload in labor	Eight weeks
Total body water	Remains elevated in the first days after birth; diuresis usually begins on about day 2 and continues through day 5 after birth	Five days

Source: Adapted from Blackburn (2016) and San-Frutos et al. (2011).

Weight Loss

An immediate loss of weight occurs with the birth of the baby. Due to the loss of the placenta, amniotic fluid, and blood, expected weight loss right after birth can range from 10 to 15 pounds. Postpartum weight is composed of added uterine and mammary tissues, intracellular and extracellular fluid, and fat. Antidiuretic hormones are triggered after the birth of the placenta, leading to a short period of sodium and water retention. This can make a difference in initial weight loss, particularly if significant amounts of intravenous (IV) fluids were used in labor. Pedal edema can be seen in early postpartum as fluids shift into the interstitial space. As antidiuretic effects of the various hormones lessen, a diuresis begins that effectively eliminates the extra fluid of pregnancy. Postpartum clients commonly report both increased urination and sweating. Many will see an additional loss of four to six pounds in the first week postpartum due to this shift in the fluid compartment. Further weight loss occurs gradually over the next six to nine months.

Hair Loss and Growth

Telogen gravidarum refers to diffuse hair loss that commonly begins between two and four months postpartum and lasts two to five months (Chien Yin et al., 2021). The normal hair growth cycle is interrupted by the sudden withdrawal of pregnancy hormones. This leads to a rapid turnover of hair follicles and excess hair loss as a greater percentage of follicles begin the growth phase. It is a self-limiting physiologic event that can cause distress in some individuals.

Central Nervous System

Structural changes in the brain occur during the early postpartum period. An increase in gray matter volume is found bilaterally and throughout the gyri, the outermost layer of the brain. Greater thickness of these regions is associated with higher parental self-efficacy defined as the cognitive belief in one's capacity to effectively manage parenting-related tasks and overall perceived confidence (Kim et al., 2018). Complex cortico-limbic systems in the brain are engaged in the parental response to infant cues. Cognitive changes in processing systems of the brains of postpartum individuals support empathic responses toward their babies; these changes can persist until at least one year postpartum (Bak et al., 2021).

Endocrine Changes

With the birth of the placenta, there is a rapid clearance of placental steroid hormones. Decreases in estrogen and progesterone are profound. Within 24 hours, estradiol is less than 2% of pregnancy levels; estrogen is almost to prepregnant levels by seven days and progesterone is at nonpregnant levels by 24–48 hours (Blackburn, 2016). Endogenous oxytocin release in the immediate postpartum period facilitates uterine contractions for hemostasis and provides central calming effects that reduce stress and enhance attachment to the newborn. Postpartum prolactin elevations in the first several hours after birth prime the body for milk production and are associated with effects such as decreased anxiety and increased sociability (Buckley, 2015). Thyroid volume, which increased by about 30% during pregnancy, regresses to normal by 12 weeks postpartum (Isley & Katz, 2017). Fasting plasma insulin levels begin to return to normal at 48 hours and are stable by 6 weeks postpartum (Blackburn, 2016).

Immune Response

Pregnancy initiates a subtle immune suppression, particularly in cell-mediated immunity (Singh & Perfect, 2007). This promotes embryonic implantation and protects the growing fetus from a host response. Rapid reversal of these changes along with a rebound effect of heightened inflammatory reactions in the first few months postpartum can lead to an increase in autoimmune disease activity in such conditions as autoimmune thyroiditis, multiple sclerosis, and lupus erythematosus.

Maternal reset hypothesis of lactation and metabolism

Metabolic activity increases significantly during pregnancy. Lactation is integral to the reversal of pregnancy hypermetabolic processes as increased levels of prolactin result in a down regulation of the hypothalamic–pituitary–ovarian axis. This process has been identified as the **maternal reset hypothesis**. This reset of maternal metabolic activity is associated with both short-term and long-term health benefits (Table 6.2). For example, a 39% reduction in breast cancer risk is noted among breastfeeding women (Zhou et al., 2015), as well as a 24% reduction in ovarian cancer risk (Babic et al., 2020). People who have breastfed also have a decreased risk of developing hypertension and type 2 diabetes with longer duration reflecting additional risk reduction. Lactation plays a critical role in resetting metabolism after childbirth, reversing some pregnancy changes, such as the deposits of visceral fat, insulin resistance, and the increase in lipids and triglycerides (Singh et al., 2021).

Table 6.2 Physiologic Benefits of Breastfeeding

Reduction in risk for:
- Breast cancer
- Ovarian cancer
- Hypertension
- Type 2 diabetes
- Hyperlipidemia
- Metabolic syndrome

Source: Adapted from Babic et al. (2020), Singh et al. (2021), and Zhou et al. (2015).

Cardiovascular and Hematological Systems

Increased blood volume is needed to ensure an adequate supply to the uterus and placenta during pregnancy. Once the baby and the placenta are born, the withdrawal of estrogen causes a rapid diuresis for the first 48 hours and a return to normal plasma volume and hematocrit levels. Decreased progesterone leads to removal of excess fluid in the tissues as well as return to normal vascular tone. Cardiac output and blood pressure return to prepregnant levels. Hemoglobin and hematocrit values may be difficult to accurately interpret during the first week postpartum due to the rapid remobilization of fluid into the vascular system as the body begins to diurese.

During pregnancy, there is an increase in coagulation factors and decrease in coagulation inhibitors. This physiologic process occurs to prevent hemorrhage during childbirth. While this measure has a protective function, it creates a hypercoagulable state and increases the risk of developing a venous thromboembolism (VTE). Coagulation factors return to their nonpregnant levels by two weeks postpartum (Patel & Shander, 2020). The highest absolute risk for a pregnancy-related VTE is in the postpartum period. Cardiovascular and hematologic conditions are among the leading causes of maternal mortality and morbidity, including heart disease, stroke, hemorrhage, high blood pressure, and cardiomyopathy (Petersen et al., 2019).

Musculoskeletal System

Pregnancy generates several unique stresses to the musculoskeletal system. It is estimated that about 25% of pregnant people experience some form of temporary alteration in musculoskeletal function during pregnancy (Ferreira et al., 2021). Weight gain puts added stress on ligaments that are softened by circulating hormones, such as relaxin. Weight is distributed anteriorly, favoring a lordotic posture in late pregnancy. The symphysis pubis widens and can lead to pain while walking or during hip abduction. These changes contribute to stride and gait changes (Ferreira et al., 2021). The birth itself is likened to a marathon athletic event and requires the efforts of the smooth muscle of the uterus and the striated muscle of the body to assume various positions and push the baby out. Musculoskeletal aches and pain and joint instability have often been downplayed during pregnancy and birth as it was thought that these symptoms resolve quickly in the postpartum period. However, current thinking suggests a slower return to baseline with some structures permanently altered (Ferreira et al., 2021).

The enlarging gravid uterus forces extensive stretching of the abdominal muscles. This period of protracted abdominal muscle stretching can result in a midline separation of the rectus abdominus muscles at the linea alba, the fibrous connective tissue formed at the midline junction of the right and left rectus abdominis muscles. This separation, known as **diastasis recti (DR)** (Figure 6.4), can readily be seen and palpated at the abdominal midline. DR is often more visible and more easily palpated when the individual is performing movements that contract the abdominal muscles such as an abdominal crunch. Although abdominal exercises may help strengthen these muscles and restore them to a nonpregnant state, some restoration occurs over time and with great variability between individuals (Gustavsson & Eriksson-Crommert, 2020). It is important to note that genetic factors related to the cellular composition of the linea alba may also contribute to DR in some people (Blotta et al., 2018).

Urinary System

The pregnancy-related changes in the renal system are reversed in the postpartum period. The kidneys excrete excess fluids and waste products. With the fall of progesterone levels to a prepregnant state, renal tract dilation resolves. In the early postpartum period, the bladder fills rapidly. This sudden change combined with the transient loss of tone and sensation of fullness puts the postpartum person at risk for bladder overdistention and incomplete emptying. Additional hormonal and mechanical changes during pregnancy, labor, and birth contribute to postpartum anatomical changes such as increased bladder neck mobility, connective tissue weakness, and injury to the levator ani muscle. While these changes often resolve with time, approximately 5–20% of birthing people experience persistent changes that continue into later life (Stroeder et al., 2021). A range of pelvic floor disorders, such as stress urinary incontinence and dyspareunia, can result and impact quality of life.

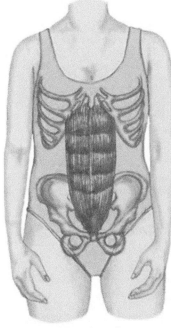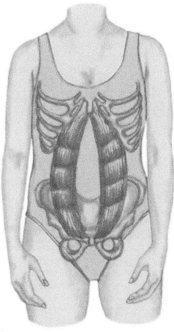

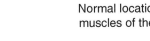

Normal location of rectus muscles of the abdomen   Diastasis recti: separation of the rectus muscles

Figure 6.4   Diastasis recti.

Gastrointestinal Tract

Digestive symptoms common to pregnancy, such as nausea and heartburn, resolve soon after birth. The weight and mechanical impediment of the gravid uterus are lessened after the birth, thus easing these symptoms. Smooth muscle tone returns to normal with reduced progesterone circulation. The first stool is usually passed within two to three days postpartum. Constipation is relieved by increased bowel tone but may persist due to fear of pain with passing stool especially if perineal injuries were sustained or from immobility related to surgical birth. Additionally, some common postpartum medications or supplements can aggravate constipation, such as opioids and iron. Hemorrhoids develop from anatomic clusters of vascular and connective tissue along the anal canal. Pregnancy hormones soften the tissues that support the anal vessels, leading to abnormal downward displacement and venous dilation. The mechanical forces of the gravid uterus regardless of birth route and of pushing during vaginal birth can extrude and exacerbate hemorrhoids in the postpartum period. Anal fissures are linear tears in the anal mucosa, which are most common in the anterior midline and can also develop during pushing (Gardner et al., 2020). As many as one-third of individuals will have hemorrhoids or anal fissures after childbirth.

Summary

Immediately after childbirth, the body begins the journey of returning to its nonpregnant state. While some of the anatomic and physiologic changes that occurred during pregnancy resolve by 6–12 weeks postpartum, other changes persist for longer and some will become part of one's new sense of self and new identity. Healthcare providers can make a positive difference by being attentive to the normal progression of postpartum physiologic adaptations and by supporting people through these profound changes during the postpartum period (Verbiest et al., 2016).

Resources for Clients and Families

March of Dimes. Your body after baby: The first 6 weeks https://www.marchofdimes.org/pregnancy/your-body-after-baby-the-first-6-weeks.aspx

Pregnancy: Physical changes after delivery https://my.clevelandclinic.org/health/articles/9682-pregnancy-physical-changes-after-delivery

Resources for Healthcare Providers

Physiology of the puerperium and lactation https://www.glowm.com/article/heading/vol-15--the-puerperium--physiology-of-the-puerperium-and-lactation/id/415293#.YaVla1NOnVo

Pelvic Guru www.pelvicguru.com

References

American College of Obstetricians and Gynecologists & American Urogynecologic Society (ACOG & AUGS). (2019). Pelvic organ prolapse. *Female Pelvic Medicine & Reconstructive Surgery, 25*(6), 397–408. https://doi.org/10.1097/SPV.0000000000000794

American College of Obstetricians and Gynecologists (ACOG). (2017). Practice bulletin no. 183: Postpartum hemorrhage. *Obstetrics & Gynecology, 130*(4), e168–e186. https://doi.org/10.1097/AOG.0000000000002351. PMID: 28937571

Atan, I. K., Zhang, W., Shek, K. L., & Dietz, H. P. (2021). Does pregnancy affect pelvic floor functional anatomy? A retrospective study. *European Journal of Obstetrics & Gynecology and Reproductive Biology, 259*, 26–31. https://doi.org/10.1016/j.ejogrb.2021.01.047

Babic, A., Sasamoto, N., Rosner, B. A., Tworoger, S. S., Jordan, S. J., Risch, H. A., Harris, H. R., Rossing, M. A., Doherty, J. A., Fortner, R. T., Chang-Claude, J., Goodman, M. T., Thompson, P. J., Moysich, K. B., Ness, R. B., Kjaer, S. K., Jensen, A., Schildkraut, J. M., Titus, L. J., . . . Terry, K. L. (2020). Association between breastfeeding and ovarian cancer risk. *JAMA Oncology, 6*(6), e200421. https://doi.org/10.1001/jamaoncol.2020.0421

Bak, Y., Nah, Y., Han, S., Lee, S., & Shin, N. (2021). Neural correlates of empathy for babies in postpartum women: A longitudinal study. *Human Brain Mapping, 42*, 3295–3304. https://doi.org/10.1002/hbm.25435

Blackburn, S. (2016). *Maternal, fetal, and neonatal physiology: A clinical perspective* (5th ed.). Saunders/Elsevier.

Blotta, R., Costa, S., Trindade, E., Meurer, L., & Maciel-Trindade, M. (2018). Collagen I and III in women with diastasis recti. *Clinics, 73*(5), 1–5. https://doi.org/10.6061/clinics/2018/e319

Buckley, S. J. (2015). *Hormonal physiology of childbearing: Evidence and implications for women, babies, and maternity care.* Childbirth Connection Programs, National Partnership for Women & Families. https://www.nationalpartnership.org/our-work/resources/health-care/maternity/hormonal-physiology-of-childbearing.pdf

Chien Yin, G. O., Siong-See, J. L., & Wang, E. C. E. (2021). Telogen effluvium – A review of the science and current obstacles. *Journal of Dermatological Science, 101*(3), 156–163. https://doi.org/10.1016/j.jdermsci.2021.01.007

Davis, N. L., Smoots, A. N., & Goodman, D. G. (2019). *Pregnancy-related deaths: Data from 14 U.S. Maternal Mortality Review Committees, 2008–2017.* Centers for Disease Control and Prevention, U.S. Department of Health and Human Services. https://www.cdc.gov/reproductivehealth/maternal-mortality/erase-mm/MMR-Data-Brief_2019-h.pdf

Diniz, C. P., Araujo Júnior, E., Lima, M. M., Guazelli, C. A., & Moron, A. F. (2014). Ultrasound and Doppler assessment of uterus during puerperium after normal delivery. *The Journal of Maternal-Fetal & Neonatal Medicine : The Official Journal of the European Association of Perinatal Medicine, the Federation of Asia and Oceania Perinatal Societies, the International Society of Perinatal Obstetricians, 27*(18), 1905–1911. https://doi.org/10.3109/14767058.2014.882895

Douthard, R. A., Martin, I. K., Chapple-McGruder, T., Langer, A., & Chang, S. (2021). U.S. maternal mortality within a global context: Historical trends, current state, and future directions. *Journal of Women's Health, 30*(2). https://doi.org/10.1089/jwh.2020.8863

Ferreira, V., Luamoto, L., & Hsing, W. (2021). Multidisciplinary management of musculoskeletal pain during pregnancy: A review of literature. *The Journal of the International Society of Physical and Rehabilitation Medicine, 4*, 63–69. https://doi.org/10.4103/JISPRM-000099

Fletcher, S., Grotegut, C. A., & James, A. H. (2012). Lochia patterns among normal women: A systematic review. *Journal of Women's Health, 21*(12), 1290–1294. https://doi.org/10.1089/jwh.2012.3668

Frawley, H., Shelly, B., Morin, M., Bernard, S., Bø, K., Digesu, G. A., Dickinson, T., Goonewardene, S., McClurg, D., Rahnama'i, M. S., Schizas, A., Slieker-Ten Hove, M., Takahashi, S., & Voelkl Guevara, J. (2021). An International Continence Society (ICS) report on the terminology for pelvic floor muscle assessment. *Neurourology and Urodynamics, 40*(5), 1217–1260. https://doi.org/10.1002/nau.24658

Gardner, I. H., Siddharthan, R. V., & Tsikitis, V. L. (2020). Benign anorectal disease: Hemorrhoids, fissures, and fistulas. *Annals of Gastroenterology, 33*, 9–18. https://doi.org/10.20524/aog.2019.0438

Gustavsson, C., & Eriksson-Crommert, M. (2020). Physiotherapists' and midwives' views of increased inter recti abdominis distance and its management in women after childbirth. *BMC Women's Health, 20*(1), 1–9. https://doi.org/10.1186/s12905-020-00907-9

Isley, M., & Katz, V. (2017). Postpartum care and long-term health considerations. In S. G. Gabbe, J. R. Niebyl, J. L. Simpson, M. B. Landon, H. L. Galan, E. R. M. Jauniaux, D. A. Driscoll, V. Berghella, & W. A. Grobman (Eds.), *Obstetrics: Normal and problem pregnancies e-book.* ProQuest Ebook Central.

Kamel, R. (2021). Intrapartum ultrasound and levator ani modifications in normal and dystotic labors. In A. Malvasa (Ed.), *Intrapartum ultrasonography for labor management: Labor, delivery and puerperium* (2nd ed.). Springer International.

Kim, P., Dufford, A. J., & Tribble, R. C. (2018). Cortical thickness variation of the maternal brain in the first 6 months postpartum: Associations with parental self-efficacy. *Brain Structure & Function, 223*(7), 3267–3277. https://doi.org/10.1007/s00429-018-1688-z

Madhu, C., Swift, S., Moloney-Geany, S., & Drake, M. J. (2018). How to use the pelvic organ prolapse quantification (POP-Q) system? *Neurourology and Urodynamics, 37*(S6), S39–S43. https://doi.org/10.1002/nau.23740

Nunn, K. L., Witkin, S. S., Schneider, G. M., Boester, A., Nasioudis, D., Minis, E., Gliniewicz, K., & Forney, L. J. (2021). Changes in the vaginal microbiome during the pregnancy to postpartum transition. *Reproductive Sciences, 28*(7), 1996–2005. https://doi.org/10.1007/s43032-020-00438-6

Osol, G., & Mandala, M. (2009). Maternal uterine vascular remodeling during pregnancy. *Physiology, 24*, 58–71. https://doi.org/10.1152/physiol.00033.2008

Paliulyte, V., Drasutiene, G. S., Ramasauskaite, D., Bartkeviciene, D., Zakareviciene, J., & Kurmanavicius, J. (2017). Physiological uterine involution in primiparous and multiparous women: Ultrasound study. *Obstetrics and Gynecology International, 2017*, (6739345), 1–10. https://doi.org/10.1155/2017/6739345

Palmieri, S., De Bastiani, S. S., Degliuomini, R., Ruffolo, A. F., Casiraghi, A., Vergani, P., Gallo, P., Magoga, G., Cicuti, M., Parma, M., Frigerio, M., & Urogynecology-Pelvic Floor Working Group (GLUP) (2022). Prevalence and severity of pelvic floor disorders in pregnant and postpartum women. *International journal of gynaecology and obstetrics: the official organ of the International Federation of Gynaecology and Obstetrics, 158*(2), 346–351. https://doi.org/10.1002/ijgo.14019

Patel, S., & Shander, A. (2020). Physiology and pathology of coagulation in pregnancy. In S. Einav, C. F. Weiniger, & R. Landau (Eds.), *Principles and practice of maternal critical care.* ProQuest Ebook Central.

Perlman, N. C., & Carusi, D. A. (2019). Retained placenta after vaginal delivery: Risk factors and management. *International Journal of Women's Health, 11*, 527. https://doi.org/10.2147/IJWH.S218933

Petersen, E. E., Davis, N. L., Goodman, D., Cox, S., Mayes, N., Johnston, E., . . . Barfield, W. (2019). Vital signs: Pregnancy-related deaths, United States, 2011–2015, and strategies for prevention, 13 states, 2013–2017. *Morbidity and Mortality Weekly Report, 68*(18), 423. https://doi.org/10.15585/mmwr.mm6818e1

San-Frutos, L., Engels, V., Zapardiel, I., Perez-Medina, T., Almagro-Martinez, J., Fernandez, R., & Bajo-Arenas, J. M. (2011). Hemodynamic changes during pregnancy and postpartum: A prospective study using thoracic electrical bioimpedance. *The Journal of Maternal-Fetal & Neonatal Medicine, 24*(11), 1333–1340. https://doi.org/10.3109/14767058.2011.556203

Singh, N., & Perfect, J. R. (2007). Immune reconstitution syndrome and exacerbation of infections after pregnancy. *Clinical Infectious Diseases, 45*(9), 1192–1199. https://doi.org/10.1086/522182

Singh, R. B., Fedacko, J., Pella, D., & Mojto, V. (2021). Lactation and risk of metabolic syndrome. *World Heart Journal, 13*(2), 313–317. https://search.proquest.com/docview/2597848358

Stroeder, R., Radosa, J., Clemens, L., Gerlinger, C., Schmidt, G., Sklavounos, P., Takacs, Z., Meyberg-Solomayer, G., Solomeyer, E. F., & Hamza, A. (2021). Urogynecology in obstetrics: Impact of pregnancy and delivery on pelvic floor disorders, a prospective longitudinal observational pilot study. *Archives of Gynecology and Obstetrics, 304*, 401–408. https://doi.org/10.1007/s00404-021-06022-w

Ucci, M., Mascio, D., Bellussi, F., & Berghella, V. (2021). Ultrasound evaluation of the uterus in the uncomplicated postpartum period: A systematic review. *Journal of Obstetrics & Gynecology MFM, 3*(3), 100318. https://doi.org/10.1016/j.ajogmf.2021.100318

Verbiest, S., Bonzon, E., & Handler, A. (2016). Postpartum health and wellness: A call for quality woman-centered care. *Maternal and Child Health Journal, 20*(1), 1–7. https://doi.org/10.1007/s10995-016-2188-5

Zhou, Y., Chen, J., Li, Q., Huang, W., Lan, H., & Jiang, H. (2015). Association between breastfeeding and breast cancer risk: Evidence from a meta-analysis. *Breastfeeding Medicine, 10*(3), 175–182.

Part II

Preconception, Prenatal Care, and Postnatal Care

7

Preconception and Interconception Care

Cynthia Nypaver

Prenatal and Postnatal Care: A Person-Centered Approach, Third Edition. Edited by Karen Trister Grace, Cindy L. Farley,
Noelene K. Jeffers, and Tanya Tringali.
© 2024 John Wiley & Sons Ltd. Published 2024 by John Wiley & Sons Ltd.
Companion website: www.wiley.com/go/grace/prenatal

Relevant Terms

Chronic disease—diseases of long duration, often characterized by the slow progression of the illness

Developmental Origins of Health and Disease—an upstream approach that addresses how environmental factors experienced in utero impact future health and disease into adulthood

Health indicator—a measurable characteristic that describes the health of a population

Interconception healthcare—a package of healthcare and ancillary services provided to individuals and their families from the time of birth of one child to the conception of the next child

Preconception health—the overall health of people before pregnancy

Preconception healthcare—the preventative biomedical, behavioral, and social interventions aimed at optimizing health before conception to improve perinatal outcomes

Reproductive life plan—a plan for whether, when, and how to have children, including personal goals, priorities, resources, commitments, and cultural values

Screening—examination of asymptomatic people to classify them as likely or unlikely to have the disease that is the object of screening

---

Introduction

Preconception health is the health status of individuals prior to a pregnancy, whether a pregnancy is intended or not. Optimizing preconception health improves perinatal outcomes. **Preconception healthcare** refers to individualized care for the people of reproductive age that aims to reduce maternal and fetal morbidity and mortality should a pregnancy occur. **Interconception healthcare** is care provided between pregnancies and comes under the umbrella term of preconception care; however, this type of care has not been well implemented in practice. Preconception and interconception care aim to increase the probability of a successful conception when pregnancy is desired and to provide contraceptive choices to prevent unintended pregnancy (American Academy of Family Physicians [AAFP], 2023). Preconception care is a continuum of care. Components of preconception healthcare should be addressed with all individuals with reproductive capacity during preventative healthcare visits because more than 40% of pregnancies in the United States are unintended (Guttmacher Institute, 2019). Ideally, individuals will be in optimal health before conception to reduce risks for poor perinatal outcomes. Significant momentum and progress have occurred over the past decade to implement quality and evidence-based preconception healthcare for individuals of reproductive age. It is important to note that many individuals choose not to have children and some are unable to achieve pregnancy. This chapter is written from a preventative, primary care perspective regardless of intent to conceive, linking preconception and contraceptive care if indicated and desired.

Health equity key points

- Many individuals cannot afford preconception or interconception care; they are either uninsured or underinsured.
- Unintended pregnancies remain higher in the United States than in most industrialized countries and is a barrier to seeking preconception or interconception care with noted disparities by race/ethnicity, age, income, and education.
- Increased use of preconception care supports efforts to eliminate health disparities in birth outcomes.
- Chronic stress from the effects of institutional racism leads to increased risk for preterm birth and low birth weight, two of the leading causes of infant mortality.
- Black, Latinx, and Indigenous neighborhoods and those with low incomes are disproportionately exposed to environmental hazardous toxins that contribute to health disparities.
- Transgender men who do not receive equitable reproductive and parenting support as cisgender people are at greater risk for poor health outcomes.

General recommendations for preconception healthcare were first presented by a national working group, the Preconception Care and Health Care (PCHHC) Initiative (Johnson et al., 2006). The PCHHC Initiative consists of a public–private partnership of more than 70 organizations, including professional practice organizations; federal agencies; national and state leaders in maternal–child health; researchers; policymakers; and philanthropists that focus on the improvement of health in people with reproductive capacity and their offspring should they chose to have children. Working groups within the PCHHC Initiative are in the areas of: (a) clinical care; (b) public health; (c) consumer interests; (d) policy and finance; and (e) surveillance and research. Goals of the PCHHC are to: (a) improve reproductive knowledge, attitudes, and beliefs; (b) ensure that all pregnancies that occur are intended and by individuals who are ready to become parents; (c) create health equity in order to eliminate disparities in health outcomes; (d) ensure that all individuals of reproductive age receive evidence-based, quality healthcare to achieve maximal health and minimize risks should they chose to enter into pregnancy; and (e) reduce risk to people who have had prior adverse maternal, fetal, or neonatal outcomes (Johnson et al., 2006; UNC Center for Maternal & Infant Health, 2023).

Over the past decade, the PCHHC Initiative has been instrumental in developing a national strategic plan for preconception health and healthcare, making recommendations for the content of preconception health and healthcare, selecting indicators that will measure the effect of preconception care on preconception health, and developing innovative ways to improve public awareness about the benefits of preconception wellness (Kroelinger et al., 2018). Ten key preconception **health indicators** have been selected and are used as comprehensive evaluation measures of the overall preconception health and practices of the population. The surveillance systems used to collect the data are the Behavioral Risk Factor Surveillance System (BRFSS) and the Pregnancy Risk Assessment Monitoring System (PRAMS). The ten key preconception indicators are listed in Table 7.1.

Challenges to Providing Preconception Care

Although great strides have been made to implement preconception services into routine care for people of reproductive age, there are still significant challenges. A major challenge is that many individuals cannot afford such care; they are either uninsured or underinsured.

While the Affordable Care Act of 2010 expanded coverage for many individuals, 30 million people in the United States are still without health insurance (Sommers, 2020). In addition, many more experience underinsurance, meaning they have coverage, but it is inadequate to protect them against high out-of-pocket costs and delays in obtaining care (Sommers, 2020). Many uninsured individuals have experienced disruptions in coverage, either through gaps or transitions (i.e., losing coverage after

Table 7.1 Ten Key Preconception Risk Indicators (To be Reported in Percentages)

1.	Current smoking (every day or some days)
2.	Depression (prior/current diagnosis)
3.	Diabetes (prior/current diagnosis, excluding gestational diabetes, borderline diabetes, or prediabetes)
4.	Folic acid intake in the month before conception
5.	Heavy alcohol consumption (≥ 8 drinks a week during the three months before conception)
6.	Hypertension (HTN; prior diagnosis of HTN, excluding pregnancy and borderline/pre-HTN)
7.	Normal weight (BMI 18.5–24.6 kg/m^2)
8.	Physical activity (participate in moderate to vigorous physical activity weekly according to recommendations)
9.	Postpartum use of a most or moderate effective method of contraception (someone having a live birth who reports that they or their partner are using a most/moderate effective contraceptive, i.e., intrauterine device, sterilization, implant, or hormonal method)
10.	Unintended pregnancy (someone having a live birth who did not want or plan to conceive prior to pregnancy)

Source: Adapted from Kroelinger et al. (2018).

six-week postpartum; Admon et al., 2021), while others are undocumented immigrants.

Another significant barrier is the healthcare provider's perception of when to provide preconception care. The perception that preconception healthcare is only needed if a person is planning a pregnancy poses a problem since the United States persistently has a high unintended pregnancy rate (AAFP, 2023). While this percentage has decreased over the last decade from greater than half of pregnancies being unintended to around 45%, this rate remains higher than most industrialized countries and disparities exist by race/ethnicity, age, income, and education (Guttmacher Institute, 2019). Individuals with unintended pregnancies are at greater risk for mental and physical health problems.

Other barriers to the provision of preconception healthcare include inadequate training of healthcare providers about integrating preconception healthcare into well visits; lack of clarity about which healthcare provider should be responsible for providing preconception care; individuals being unaware of the importance of preconception care; the absence of supporting policies despite evidence of the health benefits; a fragmented healthcare system; lack of time to incorporate this care into a wellness visit; and inappropriate attitudes toward preconception care at client and provider levels (AAFP, 2023; Goossens et al., 2018). Racial/ethnic minorities and nonbinary gender individuals may avoid care if they experience provider bias or are made to feel marginalized (MacLean, 2021). Avoidance of routine healthcare visits where individuals can receive risk screening and preventative services can lead to poor health outcomes.

Benefits of Preconception Healthcare

Addressing and ameliorating factors that affect pregnancy outcomes before conception has obvious appeal as a preventative strategy since many pathophysiological pathways begin early in pregnancy, sometimes before a person knows they have conceived. Evidence supports a number of interventions that improve pregnancy outcomes and should be initiated in the preconception period (AAFP, 2023; ACOG, 2019a). These include folic acid supplementation, vaccinations, treatment of sexually transmitted infections (STIs), control of **chronic diseases** like diabetes, and **screening** for genetic disorders (American College of Obstetricians and Gynecologists [ACOG], 2019a). Taking folic acid before pregnancy decreases the risk of neural tube defects (NTDs) and perhaps preterm birth (PTB; CDC, 2022; Chiu et al., 2018). Maintaining or achieving healthy weight through diet, exercise, and overall healthy lifestyle improves the health of individuals and their future children. Genetic counseling can provide important information for parents about their risk of having a child with a genetic disorder (see Chapter 13, *Genetic Counseling, Screening, and Diagnosis*). Information on the avoidance of teratogens such as alcohol or medications can prevent such exposures during a pregnancy (ACOG, 2019a).

Increased use of preconception care also supports efforts to eliminate health disparities in birth outcomes. For example, PTB and low birth weight (LBW) disproportionally affect Black infants (Martin et al., 2021). People of color may be particularly vulnerable to chronic stress and its cumulative effects due to traumatic life events and frequent microaggressions surrounding racism, sexism, and classism. Maternal stress activates an increase in the release of cortisol-releasing hormone (CRH), leading to increased risk for preterm labor and birth through neuroendocrine and infection/inflammatory processes (Geronimus et al., 2006; Kim, 2022). Some factors implicated in the etiology of PTB and LBW are amenable to intervention during the preconception period, such as optimizing weight and nutritional status. Additional evidence supports interventions during the postpartum and interconception periods to improve perinatal outcomes in future pregnancies, for example, spacing pregnancies to avoid interpregnancy intervals of six months or less. Individuals should be counseled about risks associated with pregnancies spaced sooner than 18 months (ACOG, 2019a).

The **Developmental Origins of Health and Disease (DOHaD)** framework supports the idea of offering care during the preconception period to improve pregnancy outcomes and to reduce racial and ethnic health disparities (Thiele & Anderson, 2016). This model is an "upstream" approach that addresses how environmental factors experienced by a developing fetus in utero can impact future health and disease as an adult. This approach is particularly applicable to understanding pregnancy outcomes, which are often rooted in exposures and experiences from long before the pregnancy occurs. It also highlights the need for preconception and interconception care, intervening to improve pregnancy outcomes as early as possible in the life course of both parent and child (Thiele & Anderson, 2016).

Evidence Supporting Preconception Healthcare

Elements in preconception care and promotion of healthy behaviors that contribute to the individual's overall health, and also enhance positive perinatal outcomes should a pregnancy occur, include: folic acid supplementation; elimination of alcohol, tobacco products, and harmful drugs; vaccination; management of chronic illnesses like diabetes, hypertension, and thyroid disease; screening for and treating STIs; management of maternal phenylketonuria; weight control; and screening for intimate partner violence (IPV; ACOG, 2019a). Preconception counseling and health promotion by healthcare providers can positively affect a future pregnancy. Preconception counseling with a person who has pregestational diabetes can improve glycemic control prior to pregnancy (Alexopoulos et al., 2019). Smoking cessation programs/strategies should be employed. Unintended pregnancies can be reduced and perinatal outcomes improved in individuals who plan a pregnancy during the preconception period at primary care visits (Henning et al., 2017).

Data supporting the need for preconception health care

- Over 40% of pregnancies in the United States are unplanned[a]
- Potential pregnancy risks among people of reproductive age
  - Alcohol use in past year—66.3%; Heavy drinking (>7 drinks)—5.2%[b]
  - Asthma—approximately 8–10%[c]
  - Obesity—40–42%[d]
  - IPV—41% women; 26% men[e]; Transgender individuals have a two to three times higher risks of physical and sexual IPV compared to cisgender people[f]
  - Daily multivitamin (as proxy for taking daily 0.4 mcg folic acid)—23.6%[g]
  - Hypertension—9.3%[h]
  - Diabetes—4.5% (30% of these are undiagnosed prior to pregnancy)[h]
  - Tobacco use—13.9% aged ≥18 years[i]
  - Illicit drug use in past month—13%[j]
  - Anxiety—19.1%[k]
  - Depression—4.7%[l]
  - Epilepsy—0.64%[m]

Source:
[a] Guttmacher Institute (2019); [b] Boersma et al. (2020); [c] Pate et al. (2021); [d] Hales et al. (2020); [e] CDC (2022b); [f] Peitzmeier et al. (2020); [g] Wong et al. (2019); [h] Azeez et al. (2019); [i] Cornelius et al. (2022); [j] CDC, (2022c); [k] Anxiety & Depression Association of America (2022); [l] Clark, et al., 2020; [m] ACOG, 2020a]

Preconception Care

Preconception care is not a single specialized visit type but rather a continuum of healthcare with every person of reproductive age at every healthcare visit whether or not there is intent to conceive. Primary care providers should routinely ask people with reproductive potential about their reproductive health needs. The One Key Question' Initiative reports that this can be accomplished by simply asking "Would you like to become pregnant in the next year?" (Power to Decide, 2023). This question can lead to dialogue about intentions to avoid or anticipate future pregnancy, including the choice of voluntary childlessness. In addition, healthcare providers must adapt this question to meet the needs of various gender identities and sexual orientations, recognizing that families are created through a variety of means including heterosexual relationships, adoptions, *in vitro* fertilization, surrogacy, and single people desiring parenthood, while some people choose not to have children at all (Mercurio, 2019). The goal is to minimize unintended pregnancies and to optimize health and future perinatal outcomes should pregnancy occur.

The components of preconception healthcare can be grouped into three broad areas: risk assessment and screening; health promotion and counseling; and interventions. Risk assessment and screening is obtained through the health history, physical examination, and laboratory testing. Results from the health history, reproductive health history, physical examination, and laboratory data will provide guidance for the healthcare provider to identify individual **risk factors** that may need counseling or intervention. Several components of health promotion should be addressed with all people of reproductive age including diet, dietary supplements, physical activity, healthy weight, **reproductive life plan** (RLP), and vaccinations. Preconception Health + Health Care Practice Bulletin (2020) and AAFP (2023) provide specific clinical content that should be included in preconception care. A summary of the content for preconception care is provided in Table 7.2. Interventions are tailored individually based upon history, physical, and laboratory findings.

Risk Assessment and Screening

The Preconception Health + Health Care Practice Bulletin (2020) can be used to aid clinicians in performing a complete risk evaluation and appropriate counseling. See *Resources for Healthcare Providers* at the end of this chapter.

Health History

A complete medical, three-generational family, pregnancy, and psychosocial history should be obtained. The areas of nutrition, occupation, environment, and lifestyle habits are of particular importance during the preconception visit. For people who have had a pregnancy complication, the interconception period offers a unique time frame to address risks before a subsequent pregnancy is conceived. Risk assessment should include a careful history of previous pregnancies, including outcomes such as PTB, LBW, and perinatal loss. Information about events, diagnoses, or health behaviors that may have contributed to the outcomes should be obtained. For example, if a person had a previous PTB, the possibility of asymptomatic infections such as periodontal disease or STIs should be considered.

A comprehensive health history is obtained and assessed for factors that may contribute to an unfavorable pregnancy outcome. These factors and their potential contribution to pregnancy complications should be discussed with people during the interconception period. For example, the probable contribution of smoking to LBW or of substance abuse to placental abruption should be communicated in a respectful and caring way with the recognition that some changes are very difficult to make (see Chapter 18, *Substance Use during Pregnancy*). Some people have limited knowledge about pregnancy risks related to chronic medical conditions and the need for optimizing preconception care (Chuang et al., 2010). The long-term implications of pregnancy complications, such as gestational diabetes mellitus (GDM), should be presented to people in the interconception period, with recommendations for possible changes, such as improved diet or weight reduction (Grieger, 2020). Some pregnancy outcomes, such as PTB and LBW, have an increased risk of recurring in subsequent pregnancies, and individuals should be aware of these increased risks. Chronic illnesses and mental illnesses often have exacerbations or a higher prevalence in pregnancy or the postpartum period. Individuals with a prior cesarean birth can be counseled about implications for future vaginal birth versus a repeat cesarean birth. Scoring models to predict vaginal birth after cesarean (VBAC) success may aid in discussion and shared decision-making around a VBAC; however, their accuracy has been called into question (Buckley et al., 2022; Liao et al., 2020; Wyckoff et al., 2020). Predictive scoring models that use race and ethnicity in their calculations are inherently biased contributing to systemic racism that limits the option of VBAC to people of color (Vyas et al., 2019): these should not be used for clinical decision-making in order to provide options with known benefits and to prevent bias and discrimination.

The interconception period is also an excellent time to discuss choices made during the previous pregnancy. For example, topics such as the person's breastfeeding experience should be discussed, assessing problems or successes from previous attempts. Satisfaction with the choice of healthcare provider and site of birth can also be assessed, helping the person to evaluate the various influences on their birth experience and to plan for future births.

Physical Examination

Physical examination should follow the healthcare provider's protocol for a primary care visit assessment.

Table 7.2 Content of Preconception Healthcare for People with Reproductive Capacity

Risk assessment and screening	Health promotion and counseling

• Genetic disorders[a]
• Mental health
• Intimate partner violence
• Infections[a]:
  ○ STIs (gonorrhea and chlamydia)
  ○ Toxoplasmosis
  ○ Cytomegalovirus
  ○ Listeriosis
  ○ Malaria
  ○ Hepatitis B and C
  ○ Tuberculosis
  ○ HSV
  ○ HIV
  ○ Zika virus
• Substance use
  ○ Alcohol
  ○ Tobacco
  ○ Drugs
• Exposures to teratogens
  ○ Medications
  ○ Lead[a]
  ○ Mercury[a]
• Medical conditions[a]
  ○ Asthma
  ○ Diabetes
  ○ Hypertension
  ○ Cardiovascular disease
  ○ Lupus
  ○ Seizure disorder
  ○ Thrombophilia
  ○ Thyroid disease
• Prior perinatal loss[b]
• Prior surgeries[b]
  ○ Uterine, cervical, or vaginal
• Uterine anomalies[a]
• Special populations
  ○ Immigrants/refugees
  ○ Cancer survivors
• People with disabilities
	• Reproductive life plan
	  ○ Short- and long-term reproductive intention
	  ○ Contraceptives including LARCs
	  ○ Timing of conception
	  ○ Preparation for childbirth and parenting
	• Dietary nutrition
	  ○ Calcium (1300 mg/d for teens; 1,000 mg/d ages 19–50)
	  ○ Iodine
	  ○ Essential fatty acids
	  ○ Iron
	  ○ Folic acid
	• Optimal BMI
	  ○ 18.5–24.9 kg/m²
	• Physical activity
	  ○ 150 minutes moderate-intensity weekly
	• Supplements
	  ○ Folic acid (0.4 mg daily)
	  ○ Multivitamin daily
	• Vaccinations
	  ○ Tdap
	  ○ MMR
	  ○ Varicella
	• Influenza
	• COVID-19

Source: Adapted from AAFP (2023); ACOG (2019a); & Preconception Health + Health Care (2023).
Key:
[a] Lab screen recommended.
[b] Screen through history and further work-up as indicated.

It should include a complete physical assessment with determination of body mass index (BMI).

Laboratory Examination

Laboratory testing is similar to the testing performed during pregnancy with a focus on identifying conditions that can be treated before pregnancy. Testing for immunity to rubella, varicella, and hepatitis B is performed so that people who are not immune to these diseases can be vaccinated before becoming pregnant. Testing for syphilis, gonorrhea, and chlamydia are performed so that, if present, the diseases can be treated and eradicated before

pregnancy. Cervical cancer screening is recommended if indicated by current guidelines since treatment for abnormal cytology is ideally performed before pregnancy. Additional screening tests are performed as indicated based on risk factors for the condition.

Mental Health

The US Preventative Services Task Force (USPSTF; 2023) recommends screening (grade B) all adults, including pregnant and postpartum people for depression. This can be done at regular primary care visits for individuals who are not pregnant and during pregnancy and postpartum using a validated tool. Common validated tools used in primary care are the Patient Health Questionnaire (PHQ)-2 or (PHQ)-9. In addition to screening, the healthcare provider must ensure that an adequate referral system is in place for effective diagnosis, treatment, and appropriate follow-up (Siniscalchi et al., 2020). Depression is not the only psychological mood disorder that can affect people of childbearing age. Additional disorders, such as premenstrual dysphoric disorder, post-traumatic stress disorder (PTSD), and anxiety disorders can be detected during primary care and preconception visits.

Psychiatric disorders can complicate pregnancy and adversely affect both mental health and pregnancy outcomes. Mental health disorders increase the risk for miscarriage, GDM, PTB, LBW, hypertensive disorders of pregnancy, vaginal bleeding in pregnancy, and perinatal loss. Preconception depression and anxiety are strong predictors of pregnancy and postpartum depression and anxiety (Montagnoli et al., 2020; Kee et al., 2021). Therefore, interventions such as initiating appropriate medications, making referrals to mental health specialists, and scheduling follow-up care can not only improve current mental status, but also have potential to improve perinatal outcomes associated with depression and anxiety should pregnancy occur.

Bipolar disorder, schizophrenia, and psychosis present additional challenges with teratogenic medications, frequent exacerbations for people who discontinue their medications in pregnancy, and high rates of postpartum exacerbations (Sharma et al., 2020). Factors that contribute to poor perinatal outcomes for people with psychological conditions include higher rates of poverty, smoking, and substance use, which carry risk for PTB, LBW infants, and low Apgar scores (Sharma et al., 2020; Vigod et al., 2020).

It is important to stabilize and provide education for individuals with mental health disorders prior to pregnancy. People should receive counseling on the potential for teratogenic effects of medications, symptom exacerbations, and effects on pregnancy outcomes. Medications should be assessed for safety in pregnancy, and alternative treatments considered. Some individuals may also want to learn about whether their condition has a genetic component and what the risk is for future children. Help in identifying social support and inclusion of friends or family in preconception care is important for these individuals.

Substance Use

Screening for substance use in the preconception period is essential. Asking questions about the use of tobacco, marijuana, prescription opioids, alcohol, and illicit substances provides the opportunity to: (a) counsel individuals about adverse pregnancy outcomes associated with use; (b) offer interventions to promote cessation; (c) refer for intensive counseling services as necessary; and (d) encourage the use of consistent contraception until cessation of the substance use. The Substance Abuse and

Mental Health Services Administration (SAMHSA) provides information about Screening, Brief Intervention, and Referral for Treatment (SBIRT), which is an approach to care that provides early intervention and treatment for substance use disorders (SAMHSA, 2022). See *Resources for Healthcare Providers* at the end of this chapter.

Consuming alcohol (i.e., wine, beer, and liquor) during pregnancy can be harmful to a developing fetus. Alcohol is a known teratogen and is the leading cause of mental disability in children. All people of reproductive age should be screened for alcohol misuse with a validated screening tool (i.e., AUDIT and CAGE; National Institute of Alcohol Abuse and Alcoholism, 2021). Counseling individuals about risks of alcohol is important because alcohol use is legal and common among adults of reproductive age, and exposure with the potential for adverse effects can occur before the person knows they are pregnant, especially if the pregnancy is unintended.

Tobacco addiction is powerful, and the list of detrimental effects on health and pregnancy outcomes is lengthy. Perry et al. (2019) report a moderate increase in risk for fetal gastroschisis if a woman smokes three months before conception, even when she quits during the pregnancy. Other tobacco products and e-cigarettes that contain nicotine are harmful as well. Both active and passive smoking interfere with fertility, regardless of sex (Practice Committee of the American Society of Reproductive Medicine, 2018); therefore, the cessation message may be more effective in a primary care or preconception visit. Helping people quit tobacco use may be the single most useful clinical intervention to improve health over a lifetime. Preconception counseling and behavioral interventions can improve cessation rates. Screening for tobacco use can be done by applying the "5 As":

1. Ask about tobacco use.
2. Advise to quit.
3. Assess willingness to quit.
4. Assist to quit.
5. Arrange follow-up and support (Practice Committee of the American Society of Reproductive Medicine, 2018).

In the preconception period, individuals should be advised of the health risks of tobacco use and its effects on pregnancy. Brief interventions in an office setting can increase and improve efforts to quit tobacco use.

In the United States, during 2019, 10.1 million people aged 12 years and older misused an opioid within the past month and 9.7 million people aged 12 years and older misused a prescription pain reliever within the year (McCance-Katz, 2020). Approximately 5% of pregnant women use at least one addictive substance, the most common being cannabis. Overall, 7% of pregnant women used cannabis and 12.1% of pregnant women used cannabis in the first trimester (National Institute on Drug Abuse, 2020). Polysubstance use is common.

Screening for substance addictions is obtained through a comprehensive history, physical exam, and validated screening tools. A urine drug screen can be obtained with informed consent. Positive findings for opioid use prompts referral to a treatment center that offers medication-assisted treatment with buprenorphine or methadone, behavioral, and psychosocial interventions as well as community recovery support (McCance-Katz, 2020). Individuals with substance use/misuse should never be marginalized, discriminated against, demoralized, or criminalized, but rather offered treatment like any other illness by a healthcare professional. See Chapter 18, *Substance Use during Pregnancy,* for comprehensive information on the topic.

Intimate Partner Violence

Approximately one in three women and about one in four men have experienced IPV during their lifetime (CDC, 2022b). Gender diverse individuals experience IPV at rates estimated to be almost two to three times higher than cisgender individuals, regardless of sex assigned at birth (Peitzmeier et al., 2020). IPV is physical violence, sexual violence, stalking, and/or psychologic aggression by a current or former intimate partner (CDC, 2022b). It is recommended that all people be screened for IPV and reproductive coercion before pregnancy, using either a self-administered, validated questionnaire or a provider interview (ACOG, 2019a). Sabotage of contraceptive methods, pregnancy pressure and controlling the outcome of a pregnancy are forms of reproductive coercion. Many validated screening tools for IPV are available through the Agency for Healthcare Research and Quality (AHRQ; AHRQ, 2015).

Survivors of IPV are at increased risk for unintended pregnancies, depression, anxiety, PTSD, and substance use (CDC, 2022b). A plan for education, support, and referrals for positive screens is an essential element of care. See Chapter 26, *Violence and Trauma in the Perinatal Period,* for more in-depth information.

Genetics

Preconception is the ideal time to screen for genetic conditions. Genetic carrier screening tests are increasingly becoming more affordable and available in the primary care setting. People at risk for having a child with a genetic condition have the opportunity to receive genetic counseling and carefully consider whether they wish to plan a pregnancy or consider alternatives such as adoption, surrogacy, preimplantation testing, or donor sperm or eggs. Preconception counseling provides individuals the opportunity to consider what types of genetic testing, if any, they will perform during pregnancy.

A genetic screening history in the preconception period should mirror genetic screening in prenatal care. Screen for a history of genetic disorders; birth defects; mental disorders; and breast, ovarian, uterine, and colon cancer (ACOG, 2019a). A three-generational medical and ethnic family history is obtained to identify areas of risk for potential offspring and indicate the need for referral for genetic testing. Common autosomal recessive disorders are thalassemia, cystic fibrosis, sickle cell disease, and Tay-Sachs. Couples with a family history of developmental delay, congenital anomalies, or other known or suspected genetic conditions should be referred for genetic counseling. A pregnancy history of three or more consecutive miscarriages prompts testing for potentially contributory genetic conditions such as chromosomal abnormalities or a hereditary thrombophilia (Sak et al., 2019).

Infections

Some infections can impact pregnancy outcomes by directly affecting the fetus or because they are more dangerous during pregnancy. A number of infections are subclinical and screening allows detection and treatment before pregnancy. For example, malaria and syphilis, two conditions that carry high fetal mortality, can be treated preconceptionally to reduce risk for stillbirths (Saito et al., 2020; Tsai et al., 2019). People benefit from information on the risks they have for these infections and the screening recommendations (Table 7.3). Certain infections may be prevented with vaccination; therefore, immunity screening and vaccination are appropriate for varicella, rubella, and hepatitis B. Depending on client history, vaccination might be recommended without first screening for immunity such as with COVID-19, influenza, and human papillomavirus vaccines.

Information on infections to avoid during pregnancy and when trying to conceive is also important. Toxoplasmosis, cytomegalovirus, and listeriosis are infections typically asymptomatic in adults but devastating to the fetus. They can cause cerebral palsy, cognitive impairment, stillbirth, blindness, hearing loss, epilepsy, and other sequelae. Laboratory screening for immunity is not recommended for these infections. Information on how to avoid these infections should be provided and includes frequent and thorough hand washing; cleaning and not sharing eating utensils; safe food handling such as washing fruits and vegetables; thoroughly cooking meats; and not cleaning cat litter boxes unless using gloves and a mask. These precautions are particularly important for people with frequent exposure to young children, such as day care workers (Nypaver et al., 2016).

People living with human immunodeficiency virus (HIV) and acquired immunodeficiency syndrome (AIDS) have specific preconceptional health needs including: discussion about safe sexual practices to avoid transmission; risk factors for and strategies to reduce perinatal transmission; potential effects of antiretroviral (ARV) medications on pregnancy course and outcomes; recommendation not to breastfeed due to increased risk of transmission to the child; and encouragement for partners to receive HIV counseling and screening and if positive, HIV care. People with HIV should achieve viral loads below the limit of detection prior to conception and receive uninterrupted ARV therapy throughout pregnancy. The goal is to achieve optimal health before conception, prevent vertical transmission, and use ARV medications with the safest profiles. Care is best provided by an interdisciplinary team led by an HIV specialist. For those who do not desire pregnancy, all forms of approved

Table 7.3   Screening Recommendations for Infections at a Preconception Visit for People Capable of Pregnancy

Infection	Recommendations with grades[a] for screening	Risk factors
Chlamydia and gonorrhea	Age 24 and younger if sexually active and people with risk factors (B)	• History of or sex partner with an STI • New or multiple sexual partners • Inconsistent condom use • Transactional sex • Incarceration
Hepatitis B (HBV)	People with risk factors (B)	• Born in areas of high prevalence • Household or sexual contact • Injection drug use • HIV or HCV infection • Multiple sex partners • Men who have sex with men • Liver disease • Incarceration • Dialysis
Hepatitis C (HCV)	Adults aged 18–79 years (B)	• Injection drug use
Human immunodeficiency virus (HIV)	Adolescents and adults ages 15–65 years (A) Younger adolescents and older adults with risk factors (A)	• Men who have sex with men • People having sex without condoms or with multiple partners • Injection drug use • Transactional sex • History of or sex partner with an STI
Syphilis	People with risk factors (A)	• Men who have sex with men • Transactional sex • People living with HIV • Incarceration
Latent tuberculosis	People with risk factors (B)	• Contacts of persons with active TB disease • Immigrant from endemic country (most countries in Latin America and the Caribbean, Africa, Asia, Eastern Europe, and Russia) • Live or work where active TB disease is more common such as a homeless shelter, migrant farm camp, prison or jail, or some nursing homes • Injection drug use • People living with HIV or otherwise immunosuppressed • Healthcare workers

Source: Adapted from USPSTF (2023).
[a] Grades for recommendations:
A = high certainty of benefit without harm from this test.
B = high certainty of benefit of this test; moderate certainty test is not harmful.

contraceptives are appropriate; however, some ARV medications may interact with hormonal contraceptives (Thompson et al., 2020).

Transmission of the Zika virus to a developing fetus can be devastating. Zika can cause microcephaly and is associated with other poor outcomes, such as joint and muscle damage. The Zika virus is transmitted by the *Aedes* species mosquito and through sexual intercourse. Signs and symptoms vary in severity and include headache, fever, rash, joint pain, and conjunctivitis, lasting from a few days to a week after exposure. If a woman of reproductive age and their partner present with signs and symptoms or if either party suspects they have been exposed to the Zika virus, both should be tested and counseled to avoid pregnancy with appropriate contraception. Counsel individuals to use condoms and avoid pregnancy for at least three

months. Report positive findings to local or state health departments. There is currently neither a vaccine nor treatment for the Zika virus (CDC, 2022d).

Other infections are of particular concern during pregnancy but do not lend themselves to preconception detection and treatment. Evidence does not support preconception treatment of group B strep, asymptomatic bacteriuria, and parvovirus infections, perhaps because of reinfection potential.

Periodontal infection and disease have been linked to adverse pregnancy outcomes, including PTB, LBW, GDM, and preeclampsia. Information about the risks and appropriate dental hygiene is provided and regular preventative dental care is encouraged (Bobetsis et al., 2020). See Chapter 16, *Oral Health*, for more information on oral health in the perinatal period.

Exposure to Teratogens

Teratogens are substances, like medications, drugs, alcohol, or environmental agents, which can cause a permanent change in fetal growth, structure, or function. Insult to the fetus is agent-dependent, but, in general, the period of organogenesis is the most critical time, often before a person knows they are pregnant. Regularly used prescription and over-the-counter medications and supplements should be reviewed. Teratogenic medications should be discontinued or changed to a medication with a safer pregnancy profile for all people planning a pregnancy. This often is done in collaboration with the other healthcare professionals who originally prescribed the medication. The risks and benefits to the individual and the potential pregnancy and fetus should be balanced when making these decisions. Environmental exposures are not always known; however, they can affect conception and the subsequent pregnancy. History questions should address potential exposures in a person's residence, workplace, and community, including type of work, diet, and use of household agents. Environmental hazards disproportionately affect residents of racial, ethnic, and poor neighborhoods. Researchers have reported that communities that are predominately inhabited by Black, Latinx, and Indigenous people, and people with low incomes are disproportionately located in areas near landfills and industry that emits hazardous toxins, creating environmental injustices or in other words, environmental racism (Ray, 2021; Taylor, 2014). Some toxins of concern in pregnancy can be investigated when history suggests possible environmental exposures. Exposures to chemicals should be investigated individually. The Agency for Toxic Substances and Disease Registry (ATSDR) provides a database that can be searched by agent, providing the clinician with information including data on reproductive effects (ATSDR, 2023). People who use well water should have the water tested for safety. The US Environmental Protection Agency (EPA) offers a plethora of information about private wells, including preventing well water pollution and private well safety publications (U.S. EPA, 2022).

Preconception counseling includes recommendations to avoid common environmental exposures of particular concern in pregnancy such as mercury, lead, and endocrine disrupting compounds (EDCs; ATSDR, 2023; Segal & Giudice, 2019). Mercury is a potent neurotoxin for the developing fetus. People are counseled to avoid consumption of fish known to have higher mercury levels, such as shark, swordfish, king mackerel, marlin, orange roughy, tuna, and tilefish. Seafood and fish with low mercury, like shrimp, salmon, catfish, and pollock can be consumed once or twice weekly (8–12 oz; US Food and Drug Administration [FDA], 2021; Segal & Giudice, 2019).

Lead is another potent neurotoxin. A history of previous lead exposure should prompt more specific questions related to lead exposure and possibly to testing blood lead levels. Houses built before 1978 may contain lead in old paint or the water pipes, therefore people living in these older homes may have lead exposure, particularly if the home is remodeled. People at increased risk for higher lead levels include immigrants from areas without lead regulation, battery factory workers, those who use imported cosmetics, and those who use glazed-pottery cookware. Individuals with lead levels over 20 μg/dL should be referred to a toxicologist for evaluation and possible chelation therapy (Segal & Giudice, 2019).

Exposure to bisphenol (BPA), phthalates, and parabens, referred to as EDCs, is also of concern for a developing fetus, adults, infants, and children. These agents are found in plastics, food, food packaging, and/or personal care items and have been associated with infertility, miscarriage, poor oocyte quality, stillbirth, LBW, PTB, thyroid abnormalities, and early puberty (Segal & Giudice, 2019). The use of insecticides and pesticides should be discouraged as they have been linked with adverse effects such as an increase in NTDs, reduced childhood cognitive development, and an increase in childhood cancers. If a person works in agriculture, they should be instructed to wear gloves and wash hands often (Segal & Giudice, 2019). Chapter 22, *Occupational and Environmental Health in Pregnancy,* provides in-depth information about environmental substance exposure during pregnancy.

Preconception Healthcare for Individuals with Chronic Illnesses

In addition to routine preconception care, people with chronic diseases merit additional consideration since they may be at increased risk of unfavorable pregnancy outcomes, and they may not be aware of those risks (Figure 7.1). In some cases, limited data are available about a particular disease and its associated risks during pregnancy. Preconception counseling should include counseling on any risks to pregnancy and fetal outcomes specific to a diagnosis, as well as risks associated with the physiologic alterations that accompany pregnancy. Generally, an effort should be made to achieve optimum health and chronic disease control before conception. A multidisciplinary approach is often needed in caring for these individuals. Table 7.4 summarizes preconception care recommendations for people with chronic diseases.

Asthma

Asthma is the most common respiratory condition experienced by pregnant people with a prevalence rate in people capable of pregnancy in the United States of approximately 8–10%. Prevalence rates vary by race, according to systemic factors influencing risk, and region of residency, due to environmental factors (Pate et al., 2021). Asthma has been associated with miscarriage, obstetrical hemorrhage, preeclampsia, placental abruption, placenta previa, PTB, LBW, and increased cesarean birth (Bonham et al., 2018). A person planning a pregnancy should be counseled about increased risks during pregnancy. They should be reassured about medication safety and counseled to continue their medications for control and prevention of exacerbations. Explain that

Specific health conditions

Condition	Counsel	Tests	Contraindicated medicaitons§	Contraception†
Asthma*	Women with poor control of their asthma should use contraception until it is well controlled.	See CCGC Asthma Guideline.	No restrictions.	**Safe:** all methods.
Cardiovascular disease*	Pregnancy is a stressor on the cardiovascular system. Discuss potential life-threatening risks especially with pulmonary hypertension. Contraception should be <u>strongly recommended</u> when pregnancy is contraindicated.	Consult with a Cardiac Specialist.	Find an alternate medication for ACE inhibitors and Coumadin beyond 6 weeks gestation.	**Safe:** Copper IUD, sterilization, LNG IUD, ETG implant, DMPA, and POPs. **Avoid:** estrogen-containing methods.
Depression*	Screening prior to pregnancy allows for treatment and control of symptoms that may help prevent negative pregnancy and family outcomes.	Use PHQ-9 or other validated test to monitor.	Paroxetine.	**Safe:** all methods.
Diabetes*	Three-fold increase risk of birth defects, which may be reduced with good glycemic control prior to conception. Women with poor glycemic control should use effective birth control.	Patients should demonstrate good control of blood sugars with HgbA 1c <6.5. Use effective contraception. See CCGC Diabetes Guideline.	ACF Inhibitors, Statins.	**Safe:** all methods (including those with estrogen) are safe for women who are <35 years, non-smokers and no hypertension or vascular disease. **Avoid:** estrogen methods for all other women.
HIV	HIV may be life-threatening to the infant if transmitted. Antiretrovirals can reduce the risk of transmission, but the risk is still about 2%.	Refer to specialist.	Efavirenz (Sustiva®).	**Safe:** all mehods in HIV-infected women who do not have AIDS. Antiretroviral therapy may interfere with hormonal methods. Concomitant use of condoms is strongly recommended.
Hypertension*	Increased maternal and fetal risk during pregnancy, especially pre-eclampsia. Discuss importance of finding alternative to ACE inhibitor prior to pregnancy.	Women with HTN of several years should be assessed for ventricular hypertrophy, retinopathy and renal disease. Consult with a Cardiac Specialist.	ACE Inhibitors.	**Safe:** all methods (including those with estrogen) for women who are <35 years, non-smokers and have controlled hypertension (by way of meds or life style changes). **Avoid:** estrogen methods for all other women.
Obesity*	Use effective contraception until ideal body weight (BMI=18.5– 24.9) is achieved. Offer specific strategies to decrease caloric intake and increase physical activity. For bariatric surgery, avoid pregnancy until weight stabilization and wait 1–2 years after surgery before conceiving.	Screen for diabetes with either a FBS or a 2 hour OGTT with a 75 gram glucose load.	Weight loss medications should not be used during pregnancy.	**Safe:** all methods.
Renal disease	Counsel to achieve optimal control of condition prior to conception. Discuss potential life-threatening risks during pregnancy. Contraception should be <u>strongly recommended</u> to those who do not desire pregnancy.	Consult with Renal Specialist.	Find alternative to ACE Inhibitors if at risk of pregnancy.	**Safe:** Copper IUD and LNG IUD, ETG implant, DMPA, sterilization.
Seizure disorder	Counsel on potential effects of seizures and seizure medications on pregnancy outcomes. Patients should take 4 mg of folic acid per day for at least 1 month prior to conception.	Whenever possbile, monotherapy in the lowest therapeutic dose should be prescribed.	Valproic Acid (Depakote®).	**Safe:** all methods. Certain anticonvulsants decrease levels of steroid hormones and may decrease contraceptive efficacy.
SLE & rheumatoid arthritis	Disease should be in good control prior to pregnancy.	Evaluate for renal function and end-organ disease.	Cyclophosphamide.	**Safe:** Progestin-only methods and IUDs.
Thyroid disease	Proper dosage of thyroid medications prior to conception for normal fetal development. Iodine intake 150 mcg per day.	TSH should be <3.0 prior to pregnancy. Free T4 should be normal.	Redioactive iodine.	**Safe:** all methods.

Other common health conditions		Counsel	Contraception†
Uterine Fibroids, Nulligravidity, Tension Headaches, History of Ectopic Pregnancy, Fibrocystic Breasts or Family History of Breast Cancer, Breastfeeding, and Healthy Women Age >35 years		Reassure patient that these conditions do not generally affect pregnancy. History of ectopic pregnancy: advise to seek care immediately upon conception.	**Safe:** all methods. Progestin-only methods and IUDs may be used immediately post-partum and in breastfeeding women.

*See CCGC guideline
†Contraception column based on ACOG Practice Bulletin No 73, *Use of Hormonal Contraception in Women with Coexisting Medical Conditions, June 2006,* and The World Health organization, *Medical Eligibility Criteria for Contraceptive Use,* 2008 update.
§See Physicians' Desk Reference® (PDR) for comprehensive medications list.
Other Medical Conditions Where Special Counseling Is Recommended
Bipolar Disorder, Migraine Headaches, Phenylketonuria, Schizophrenia.
Contraception key

Barrier Methods: Latex condoms, diaphragm with spermicide, and sponge have a high failure rate with typical use (20–30 pregnancies per 100 women in one year): encourage more effective methods. Condoms are the only contraceptive method that also prevent STIs. When used correctly and consistently, they reduce the risk of infection by 99%. **COC:** Combined Oral Contraceptives (*contains estrogen and progestin*). **DMPA:** Depot Medroxyprogesterone Acetate (*progestin only*). **ETG Implant:** Etonogestrel Implant (*progestin only*).	**LNG IUD:** Levonorgestrel intrauterine device (*progestin only*). **Patch:** Combined contraceptive patch (*contains estrogen and progestin*). **POP:** Progestin only pills (*sometimes referred to as the "mini-pill"*). **Progestin-Only Emergency Contraception:** May be safely used in any woman of reproductive age; there is no medical condition that precludes its use. **Ring:** Combined vaginal ring (*contains estrogen and progestin*).

This guideline is adapted from the AJOG Supplement, December 2008 and CDC Proceedings of the Preconception Heath and Health Care Clinical, Public Health and Consumer Workgroup Meeting, June 2006. The guideline is designed to assist the clinician in preconception and interconception care. It is not intended to replace a clinician's judgment or establish a protocol for all patients. For references and additional copies of the guideline go to www.coloradoguidelines.org or call 720–297–1681. Supported by Grant NO.B04MC11264 from the Maternal and Child Health Bureau (Title V, Social Security Act), Health Resources & Services Administration, Department of Health and Human Services.

Final 12/18/09

Figure 7.1 Preconception occupational/environmental history checklist. Source: McDiarmid & Gehle (2006).

Table 7.4   Summary of Preconception Care for People Capable of Pregnancy, with Selected Chronic Illnesses

Medical condition	Preconception care content
All chronic conditions	• Provide general preconception care • Stabilize condition, optimal health • Recommend contraception appropriate for pregnancy intention and medical condition • Discontinue teratogenic medications if planning a pregnancy or use an effective method of contraception if capable of pregnancy • Discuss potential effect of condition on pregnancy and offspring • Discuss potential effect of pregnancy on long-term health • Recommend optimizing weight and nutrition
Cancer	• Achieve stable remission • Address potential effects on fertility and pregnancy • Address potential recurrence with pregnancy • Consult cancer specialist to review any potential risks to a future pregnancy
Cardiac	• Treat obesity as a disease • Counsel about healthy lifestyle; exercise 30 minutes most days of the week; healthy diet; avoid tobacco products, limit alcohol • Order statin therapy if LDL and/or cholesterol >160 mg/dL (avoid statins in pregnancy)
Chronic hypertension	• Education about increased pregnancy risks for preeclampsia/eclampsia, stroke, cardiac decompensation, renal deterioration, PTB, FGR, placental abruption, fetal demise • Attempt single-agent control of hypertension (<140/90) • ACE inhibitors and ARBs are contraindicated during pregnancy and should be discontinued while attempting conception • Assess baseline renal function, presence of ventricular hypertrophy, and retinopathy
Dermatology	• Strictly avoid conception on isotretinoin (retinoic acid) and for one to two years following etretinate (Tegison)
Diabetes	• Good glycemic control prior to pregnancy (HbA1C <6.5%) • Treatment of diabetic complications • Refer for eye exam to assess for retinopathy
Epilepsy	• Address possibility of increased seizures in pregnancy • Address increased risk for congenital anomalies with seizures, even when no medications, and other adverse pregnancy outcomes associated with seizure disorders • Change anticonvulsant medication, if possible, to one that is not teratogenic
HIV	• Recommend antiretroviral therapy (ARV) before and throughout pregnancy • Encourage use of condoms during intercourse • Counsel regarding prevention of and risk factors for perinatal transmission • Achieve nondetectable viral load before conception • Education about HIV and ARV drugs' effects on pregnancy course • Discussion of risks versus benefits of breastfeeding with HIV • Encourage sexual partner/s to receive counseling and HIV testing—if positive, HIV care
Mental health disorders	• Identify social support • Identify major psychosocial stressors • Refer for counseling or support groups • Consider teratogenicity of medications and possible need to adjust regimen
Obesity	• Screen for diabetes • Screen for CVD and sleep apnea • Strategize ways to maximize health including nutrition, exercise, meditation, and self-care • Delay pregnancy one to two years following bariatric surgery
Phenylalanine hydroxylase deficiency (PAH)	• Dietary and medication control of phenylalanine levels for at least 3 months before conception (<6 mg/dL) • Counsel about reproductive options such as adoption or donor oocyte • Discussion about ability to breastfeed if infant PAH negative
Rheumatoid arthritis	• May prolong time to conception • Risk of postpartum flare • Strictly avoid conception on methotrexate, consider teratogenicity of other medications • Advise partner or sperm donor that leflunomide, sulfasalazine, and cyclophosphamide can reduce fertility

(Continued)

Table 7.4 (*Continued*)

Medical condition	Preconception care content
Sickle cell disease	• Refer for genetic counseling • Baseline renal, pulmonary, cardiac function • Education about risks for exacerbations with pregnancy
Thrombophilia	• Refer for genetic counseling • Obtain thorough history (personal and family) • Assess the need for prophylaxis in pregnancy or postpartum period • Early identification of pregnancy
Thyroid condition	• Control of thyroid hormone levels • Anticipate changes in thyroid medications during pregnancy • Delay pregnancy for at least six months after radioactive iodine therapy

uncontrolled asthma is the greater contributor to poor perinatal outcomes (Bonham et al., 2018).

Cancer Survivors

Survivors of cancer have specific concerns in pregnancy. The most common types of cancer among people capable of pregnancy are breast (most common), thyroid, melanoma, cervical, uterine, and hematologic malignancies. Individuals often want to know whether their cancer treatment will affect fertility. While fertility and pregnancy rates decrease in cancer survivors, especially in cervical cancer survivors, there is no evidence to discourage individuals from having children after surviving most types of cancer (Griffiths et al., 2020). Those who received either radiation therapy or chemotherapy are at risk for PTB, LBW, operative birth, and postpartum hemorrhage (Griffiths et al., 2020). These increased risks should ideally be discussed before a pregnancy to inform decision-making. Some measures can be taken at the time of cancer treatment to preserve fertility, such as cryopreserving oocytes. People may be concerned that the physiologic changes associated with pregnancy such as elevated hormone levels may increase their risk of cancer recurrence. Counseling from a multidisciplinary team should include optimal birth spacing and maternal and birth outcomes. People who wish to become pregnant should discuss their plans with an oncology specialist to determine their risk of cancer recurrence.

Cardiovascular Disease (CVD) and Hypertension

Stroke and heart disease remain a primary cause of death in the United States, and people with reproductive capacity should be screened for and counseled about individual risks for CVD. The International Society of Hypertension provides guidance addressing cholesterol-lowering medications, obesity, risk assessment, and lifestyle issues such as diet and exercise. Statins should be avoided during pregnancy because of their teratogenic potential (Unger et al., 2020).

Blood pressure (BP) should be assessed at every office visit. People with chronic hypertension can experience a worsening of their hypertension during pregnancy and have higher rates of preeclampsia, eclampsia, cardiac decomposition, stroke, renal failure, GDM, postpartum hemorrhage, LBW infants, PTB, and conditions like placental abruption that increases the rate of cesarean births (ACOG, 2019b). These risks should be addressed in preconception counseling. The diagnosis of grade 1 hypertension is made when the BP is 140/90 mmHg or higher on at least two to three occasions, at least one to four weeks apart. The recommended BP goal is below 140/90 mmHg for individuals of reproductive age (Unger et al., 2020). If antihypertensive medication is indicated, initial therapy consists of one of four agents: (a) angiotensin-converting enzyme (ACE) inhibitors; (b) angiotensin receptor blockers (ARBs); (c) thiazide-like diuretics; or (d) calcium-channel blockers (CCBs). However, ACE inhibitors and ARBs are contraindicated during pregnancy and thus should be avoided during the preconception period because of increased risk for miscarriage, fetal growth restriction (FGR), oligohydramnios, intrauterine fetal death, limb defects, and congenital heart defects (Unger et al., 2020).

The preconception period offers an opportunity to decrease the risk for CVD through lifestyle changes. Lifestyle modifications include: 30 minutes of moderate to vigorous aerobic exercise most days of the week: a healthy diet that includes fruits, vegetables, whole grains, low-fat dairy, poultry, fish, and nuts while limiting red meats and high-calorie food or beverages; achieving a normal BMI; avoidance of tobacco products; limiting salt intake; and limiting alcohol intake to <2 drinks per day (Unger et al., 2020). Baseline renal function, presence of ventricular hypertrophy, and retinopathy should be assessed during the preconception period in those with significant cardiovascular conditions, and may require referral to medical specialists.

Diabetes

The prevalence of diagnosed and undiagnosed diabetes in adults aged 18 to 44 years in the United States is estimated to be 4.2% (CDC, 2020a). This estimate does not differentiate between type 1 diabetes, type 2 diabetes, or gestational diabetes; however, the majority of these cases are gestational diabetes (CDC, 2020a). Preconception care for individuals with pregestational diabetes, both type 1 and type 2, has been shown to reduce rates of perinatal mortality and congenital malformation (Alexopoulos et al., 2019). Diabetes during pregnancy is associated with increased risk for miscarriage, still birth, fetal anomalies, preeclampsia, macrosomia, and neonatal hypoglycemia, hyperbilirubinemia, and respiratory distress syndrome, among others (ACOG, 2018a). In addition, a child of a person with diabetes during pregnancy is at increased risk for obesity, hypertension, and diabetes later in life (American Diabetes Association [ADA], 2021). These risks are related not only to hyperglycemia but also to chronic complications and comorbidities of diabetes (ADA, 2021). Preconception care for those with diabetes needs to: (a) incorporate preconception counseling with routine diabetes care starting in adolescence; (b) encourage the use of contraception, especially long-acting reversible contraceptives (LARCs), until euglycemia and ready for pregnancy; (c) provide good glycemic control prior to conception to improve pregnancy outcomes; and (d) offer counseling about the risk and progression of diabetic retinopathy and the importance of receiving regular eye exams during preconception, during each trimester of pregnancy and in the year following birth. Glycemic control is extremely important and the hemoglobin A1C (HbA1C) should be kept as close to normal levels as possible, preferably less than 6.5 (ADA, 2021). It is recommended that individuals with HbA1c levels over 10% avoid pregnancy until blood glucose levels are controlled. Medications must be carefully evaluated for teratogenic potential and changed accordingly. Additional diabetic-specific lab testing (testing after diagnosis of diabetes is made) can include a thyroid-stimulating hormone (TSH) level, creatinine, and urinary albumin-to-creatinine ratio (ADA, 2021). Preconception counseling emphasizes routine physical activity, achievement of a healthy BMI, and the increased fetal risks with poor glycemic control.

Phenylalanine Hydroxylase (PAH) Deficiency

PAH deficiency (formerly known as PKU) is a hereditary disorder that involves a deficiency in PAH, resulting in increased phenylalanine (Phe) levels. High levels of Phe in pregnancy are toxic to the fetal brain and heart increasing the risk for microcephaly, seizures, congenital heart failure and growth delays (ACOG, 2020b). Family planning and preconception counseling about strict diet are paramount in reducing risk of fetotoxicity. It is recommended that Phe levels of <6 mg/dL be achieved at least three months prior to conception and that during pregnancy, these levels be maintained at 2–6 mg/dL (ACOG, 2020b). This can be achieved through dietary restriction and administration of coenzyme tetrahydrobiopterin (BH$_4$). Therefore, people with PAH deficiency should be: (a) managed by practitioners from experienced PAH deficiency centers; (b) referred to a genetic counselor to discuss genetic transmission to a potential fetus; (c) advised about lifelong dietary restrictions; and (d) counseled about reproductive choices like donor egg (ACOG, 2020b).

Systemic Lupus Erythematosus (SLE)

SLE is an autosomal, inflammatory disease that disparately affects Black and Asian women ages 20–30 years. The etiology of SLE is considered multifactorial and can be more common with certain external environmental exposures, such as toxins and hazardous substances discussed in the *Exposure to Teratogens* section of this chapter. This may partially explain why it is more prevalent in some racial and ethnic groups that live in neighborhoods with disproportionate exposure to teratogens (Kinsey et al., 2018). Risks during pregnancy include PTB, FGR, preeclampsia, neonatal lupus, and fetal death (Marder, 2019). Prognosis for perinatal outcomes is best if the person has been in remission for at least six months before conception (Marder, 2019). Any organ can be involved, and it is recommended that those with organ damage be advised to avoid pregnancy. Some SLE medications interact with estrogen; therefore, contraception options may be limited to non-estrogen-containing methods. LARCs may be a good option. For most people, pregnancy is safe if the disease is well controlled. It is essential that people with SLE who are capable of pregnancy receive preconception care and medication adjustment to control the disease. Drugs like hydroxycholoroquine (HCQ) and low dose aspirin to prevent preeclampsia are generally considered safe during pregnancy (Marder, 2019). Immunosuppressive medications are contraindicated during pregnancy and should be discontinued at least three months prior to a conception. Therefore, a highly effective contraceptive should be used if taking immunosuppressive medications in order to avoid an unplanned pregnancy. Referrals to maternal–fetal medicine and a rheumatologist are recommended for coordination of care of people with SLE who are attempting pregnancy (Marder, 2019).

Seizure Disorders

Seizures and the medications used to control them can adversely affect people with childbearing potential and pregnancy outcomes. Ideally, people capable of pregnancy should be counseled frequently about effective contraceptive choices, seizure control, and potential adverse pregnancy outcomes (ACOG, 2020a; Stephen et al., 2019). Estrogen can affect neuronal excitability, leading to increased seizure activity, whereas progesterone exerts an inhibitory effect (ACOG, 2020a; Stephen et al., 2019), resulting in increased seizure activity at specific times during the menstrual cycle, or catamenial epilepsy (ACOG, 2020a). While the first-line treatment for seizure disorders is anticonvulsant medication, progesterone-based hormonal therapy can be used as an adjunct approach to control cycles and provide effective contraception, as well as decrease seizure activity.

Hormonal contraceptives are used less often in people with childbearing potential who have epilepsy than those without epilepsy (Stephen, 2019), therefore contraceptive counseling should be conducted frequently at every visit to avoid unintended pregnancies. Depot medroxyprogesterone acetate (DMPA) has been shown to decrease seizure activity. Levonorgestrel-containing intrauterine devices (IUDs) are another safe and effective option for people with seizure disorders. There is no evidence that combined hormonal contraception (i.e., combined oral contraceptive pills [COCPs], contraceptive patch, or ring) increases epileptic seizures; however, if used in combination with enzyme-inducing antiepileptic drugs such as carbamazepine, felbamate, oxcarbazepine, phenobarbital, phenytoin, primidone, and rufinamide, serum concentration of estrogen is reduced leading to increased risk of contraceptive failure. People who must take an enzyme-inducing antiepileptic drug to control seizures should be counseled to use a non-estrogen-containing method of contraception. The use of COCPs with lamotrigine has been shown to significantly reduce lamotrigine concentrations, increasing the risk of seizures. Therefore, if used together, lamotrigine dose adjustments may be needed. All methods of emergency contraception can be used without restrictions (ACOG, 2020a).

Some antiepileptic drugs have potential for teratogenicity, particularly valproate which increases risk for neurodevelopmental and major congenital malformations. Valproate is also associated with hyperandrogenism, insulin resistance, weight gain, polycystic ovarian syndrome, menstrual disorders, ovulatory failure, and infertility in people with capacity for pregnancy, and should be avoided if possible (Stephen et al., 2019).

For those planning a pregnancy, consultation with a neurologist to optimize antiepileptic drug choice and to decrease teratogenic potential is paramount. Provide education about the possibility of increased seizures in pregnancy and of increased congenital anomalies with seizures, even when no medications are used, and risks of other adverse pregnancy outcomes such as miscarriage, LBW, and developmental disabilities. To minimize these risks, anticonvulsant medication choices should be reviewed for teratogenicity and changed, withdrawn, or reduced when possible. Stabilization before pregnancy is critical because a good predictor of seizure activity during pregnancy is the seizure profile before pregnancy. If a patient is seizure-free 9–12 months before pregnancy, there is a higher likelihood that they will be seizure-free during pregnancy (Vajda et al., 2018).

Thrombophilias

The most common forms of inherited thrombophilias are factor V Leiden mutation, prothrombin G20210A mutation, antithrombin deficiency, protein S deficiency, and protein C deficiency. Any person with a history of a thrombotic event or a family history of a first degree relative who has an inherited thrombophilia should be referred to a medical specialist to undergo individualized risk assessment for therapy. If anticoagulation therapy is indicated, low-molecular weight heparin or unrefractioned heparin is the drug of choice during pregnancy that is initiated early in the first trimester through postpartum. Contraceptives that may be considered for people with a history of inherited thrombophilias include LARCs and barrier methods. Estrogen-containing pills should be avoided (ACOG, 2018b).

Thyroid Disorders

Uncontrolled hyperthyroidism and hypothyroidism are associated with increased maternal and neonatal morbidity. Pregnancy should be delayed for at least six months after completion of treatment with radioactive iodine therapy to minimize potential adverse effects (Lee & Pearce, 2021). Euthyroid status should be achieved before conception. Currently, universal screening for thyroid dysfunction during the preconception period is not recommended in asymptomatic adults (USPSTF, 2021). Preconception counseling should cover risks and control of thyroid levels with medication.

Preconception Health Promotion and Counseling

The purpose of preconception counseling is to improve health behaviors and health status to optimize perinatal outcomes. Adequate counseling covers a wide range of topics and should be addressed with individuals with childbearing potential to promote health. Counseling focuses on education about contraception, diet, immunizations, preparation for pregnancy and childbirth, physical activity, reproductive planning, dietary supplements, and weight. Written material summarizing the essential components of the information should be provided so that the material can be reviewed later. The couple's current healthcare practices should be explored, and recommendations should be within the context of their cultural health beliefs and practices. Listening is as important as speaking when counseling on healthy behaviors (MINT, 2021). Verbally recognize, praise, and reinforce current positive, healthy behaviors. Adequate time should be allotted to provide optimal preconception counseling.

Conception

Many individuals need basic information about the process of conception, including that ovulation is a precursor for conception to occur. Ovulation typically occurs around day 14 of the menstrual cycle; however, the timing varies widely within and between individuals and cannot be determined by simply keeping a calendar, even in those with regular cycles. People can track fertility by monitoring cervical mucous, calendar methods assessing cycle length, basil body temperature monitoring, urinary hormone monitoring, and smartphone-based applications (Simmons & Jennings, 2020). Urinary ovulation prediction tests measure luteinizing hormone (LH), a hormone that typically surges 12–24 hours prior to ovulation. However, the test does not confirm if ovulation actually occurred. Once ovulation occurs, the ovum usually dies within 24 hours if unfertilized. Sperm can live in the vagina, uterus, and fallopian tubes for up to five days. Therefore, there is a fertility window of about six days, and individuals should be counseled that the frequency of intercourse that optimizes conception is about every one to two days during the fertile period (Simmons & Jennings, 2020). If a person less than 35 years old has been trying unsuccessfully to get pregnant for 12 or more months, or if a person who is 35 years or older has not conceived after six months of attempting pregnancy, they should be offered an evaluation for infertility.

Nutrition

A healthy diet provides multiple health benefits not only by reducing risks of medical problems, but also improving perinatal outcomes. Furthermore, the pregnant person's nutritional status is critical for fetal brain development and partly determines the future child's risk for adult-onset diseases like diabetes (Li et al., 2019). Eating is an activity wrapped in emotions, cultural beliefs, and personal preferences. Food choices are made in the context of available resources for purchasing, storing, and cooking. Dietary counseling must take into account the particular beliefs and practices of the individual, as well as the influence of their family and community.

Recommendations for a healthy preconception diet include high-quality carbohydrates such as whole grain products, five to seven daily portions of fresh or frozen fruits and vegetables, and the consumption of a variety of proteins such as lean meats, beans, and low-mercury fish. Ingestion of moderate levels of caffeine (<200 mg/dL) does not appear to increase risks for miscarriage or PTB. Recommended daily allowances (RDAs) for calcium, vitamin D, iron, vitamin A, and vitamin B should be discussed (ACOG, 2019a). Iodine is required for normal thyroid function, and this is typically obtained through dietary salt.

Docosahexaenoic acid (DHA) is an essential omega-3 fatty acid that supports heart health, cognitive function, and mental health. Adequate levels in pregnancy have been associated with decreased risk for FGR, PTB, allergies, and asthma in childhood (Gázquez & Larqué, 2021). Individuals should be counseled to eat 8–12 oz of low-mercury fish weekly.

Dietary Supplements

People in their reproductive years should be asked about taking dietary supplements because some can be harmful during pregnancy, such as herbal or weight loss products and excessive vitamin A intake. The excessive use of vitamin A shortly before and during pregnancy can lead to birth defects (Mousa et al., 2019).

Folic acid supplementation may be the best-known preventative intervention specific to the preconception period. The benefits of supplementation in reducing NTDs and for achieving and maintaining a pregnancy have been well documented (CDC, 2022a; Chiu et al., 2018). People capable of becoming pregnant should be counseled during all primary care and gynecologic visits about dietary folate intake and folic acid supplementation and encouraged to eat a diet containing folate-rich foods. It is recommended that all individuals of reproductive age take 0.4 mg of folic acid daily, one month before conception until 12-week

gestation. Individuals who are at increased risk for NTDs such as those with a prior NTD-affected pregnancy, those with diabetes mellitus, and those who take anticonvulsant medication, should take 4 to 5 mg daily one month prior to conception through the first 12 weeks of pregnancy (Mousa et al., 2019).

All people with reproductive capacity should be screened for dietary calcium intake. If they are not ingesting the RDA through dietary means, then calcium supplements are appropriate. The calcium RDA for adolescents is 1300 mg daily and for adults aged 19–50 years, is 1000 mg daily (National Institute of Health, 2019). Chapter 9, *Nutrition during Pregnancy*, contains more in-depth information on nutrition.

Weight

Maintaining a normal BMI and regular exercise supports ovulatory cycles and decreases risk for miscarriage (Vitner et al., 2019). People of reproductive age with obesity are at greater risk for chronic illnesses and poor perinatal outcomes as well as children with higher risk for future chronic illnesses such as diabetes and CHD. Individuals with elevated or very low BMIs can be offered nutritional consultation as well as provided emotional support and counseling about nutrition and physical activity, ideally with an empowering and nonstigmatizing approach that emphasizes emotional and physical health and well-being (Vitner et al., 2019).

Physical Activity

Regular exercise that incorporates aerobic activity and strength training has many benefits for an individual's health and fertility. Regular exercise is recommended while attempting to conceive. The preconception period is an opportunity to counsel people with reproductive potential on the importance of physical activity. It is recommended that people engage in (a) aerobic activity and (b) strength building exercises. Adults should be advised to engage in at least 150 minutes a week of moderate-intensity or 75–150 minutes of vigorous-intensity aerobic activity weekly, preferable spread throughout the week, and muscle-strengthening activities that involve all major muscle groups on two or more days weekly (US Department of Health and Human Services, 2018).

Preparation for Pregnancy and Childbirth

Some decisions about childbirth are best considered before pregnancy. Several different kinds of healthcare providers offer care during pregnancy and childbirth in the United States, including Certified Nurse-Midwives, Certified Midwives, Certified Professional Midwives, Family Practice Physicians, and Obstetricians. Prenatal care and birth services can be provided in the home, birth centers, and hospitals. Investigating services congruent with a person's preferences and their risk evaluation, and financial issues surrounding these choices, can be done well before pregnancy. Preconception visits with such healthcare providers offer individuals an opportunity to find someone suited to their needs and preferences before conception.

Breastfeeding choices are often not discussed with people until pregnancy, but there are advantages to encouraging this decision earlier. The preconception period offers an opportunity to provide information on the improved health outcomes associated with breastfeeding for both infants and postpartum people. Support from lay and professional educators and social networks increase breastfeeding rates (Westerfield et al., 2018), and the preconception period provides the opportunity to identify such support.

Reproductive Life Plan

The RLP is an individualized plan for reproduction with short- and long-term goals based on personal beliefs and values. The purpose of an RLP is to encourage individual reflection about future intentions regarding pregnancy and then to take appropriate actions to optimize health before an intended pregnancy or to avoid an unwanted pregnancy. The healthcare provider should ask every person with reproductive capacity one question, "Do you plan to get pregnant in the next year?" (Power to Decide, 2023). The answer to this question determines the pathway for management of care. If the person is not planning to get pregnant in the next year, then individualized counseling and management for contraception is recommended. If the answer is yes, then appropriate components of preconception healthcare are pursued based on individualized needs.

Vaccinations

All people of reproductive age should be current with routine vaccinations. Some vaccines are contraindicated in pregnancy, or their safety is undetermined, but immunity to vaccine-preventable diseases can reduce the potential for harm to the developing fetus. In addition, the changes in immune response during pregnancy make many infections more dangerous to the pregnant person, even when not transmitted to the fetus. Treatment for some infections can be problematic in pregnancy due to drug toxicity or teratogenicity. Thus, the preconception period is the best time to recommend these vaccinations, before a fetus can be affected and before the changes in immunity that accompany pregnancy occur.

All recommendations for routine vaccination apply during the preconception period. The CDC's Advisory Committee on Immunization Practices (ACIP) provides general guidance on the principles and logistics of vaccine administration with specific recommendations for pregnancy (CDC, 2023). Table 7.5 provides information on

Table 7.5   Adult Immunizations for People Capable of Pregnancy

Vaccine	Indications and schedule	Pregnancy and other considerations
COVID-19	One to two doses and boosters depending on type of vaccine and per most current recommendations	Recommended before or during pregnancy
Hepatitis A (HAV)	One, two-to-three-dose series, depending on vaccine	Give only if risk factors for HAV
Hepatitis B (HBV)	One, three-dose series	Give only if risk factors for HBV
Haemophilus influenza type b (Hib)	One dose	Give only if risk factors present
Human papillomavirus (HPV)	Two to three doses, depending on age at initial vaccination or condition, through age 45	Not recommended in pregnancy
Influenza inactivated (IIV) or influenza recombinant (RIV4)	One dose annually	Avoid influenza live attenuated (LAIV4; i.e., nasal mist preparations) in pregnancy
Measles, mumps, rubella (MMR)-live attenuated vaccine	One or two doses if nonimmune	Contraindicated in pregnancy
Meningococcal 4-valent conjugate (MenACWY) of polysaccharide (MPSV4)	One to two doses depending on indication	Give only if risk factors present (give to college dorm dwellers)
Meningococcal B (MenB)	Two or three doses depending on vaccine	Give only if risk factors
Pneumococcal 13-valent conjugate (PV13)	One dose	Give only if risk factors
Pneumococcal 23-valent polysaccharide (PPS23)	One to three doses depending on indication	Give only in pregnancy if risk factors present
Tetanus, diphtheria, pertussis (Td/Tdap)	One dose every 10 years; one dose of Tdap every pregnancy (preferably between 27 and 36 weeks gestation)	Substitute Tdap for Td once, then booster every 10 years

Table 7.5 *(Continued)*

Vaccine	Indications and schedule	Pregnancy and other considerations
Varicella (chicken pox)—live attenuated vaccine	Two doses (if born in 1980 or later)	Contraindicated in: pregnancy and presence of immune-compromising conditions
Less common, nonroutine vaccinations	**Indications and schedule**	**Pregnancy and other considerations**
Anthrax—inactivated vaccine	Five doses then yearly (0, 1, 6 month boosters and at 6 months and 12 months after completion of primary series and at 12 month intervals thereafter)	Give only to those with exposure or potential exposure to large amounts of *Bacillus anthracis* bacteria May be given in pregnancy if exposed to *B. anthracis* bacteria
BCG—tuberculosis (TB) vaccine	One dose	• Not routinely given in the US • Give only if TB skin test is negative and individual cannot be separated from TB-positive person • Contraindicated in pregnancy
Rabies—inactivated vaccine	Three doses	Give only to those at high risk for contracting rabies
Small pox vaccine—live vaccinia (pox type-virus related to smallpox)	One dose	• Routine administration in United States stopped in 1992 • Give only if exposed • Immunity wanes in 3–5 years • Contraindicated in pregnancy
Typhoid—2 variations (inactivated and live)	• Inactivated injection—one dose and booster every two years • Live attenuated vaccination- pills—four doses (one pill every other day for one week) and booster in five years	• Live vaccination (pills) contraindicated in pregnancy • Give only if: traveling to typhoid endemic regions, close contact with typhoid carrier, or a lab worker who works with *Samenella typhi* bacteria
Yellow Fever—live attenuated vaccine	One dose	• Give only if travel to yellow fever-endemic regions • Pregnant women should be advised not to travel to yellow fever-endemic regions, if unavoidable, give in pregnancy only if benefit outweighs risks

Source: Adapted from CDC (2023) and Bower et al. (2019).

the CDC recommendations for vaccinations in people capable of pregnancy.

Unique Considerations

There are populations and conditions that require unique consideration for preconception healthcare. These include immigrants, refugees, people with a prior pregnancy loss, and those with disabilities.

Immigrants and Refugees

People who have immigrated or sought refuge from other countries may be at greater risk for country-of-origin endemic infections like malaria, HIV, tuberculosis, and parasites. They may also experience depression, anxiety, or PTSD as a result of violence and trauma experienced in their home countries or during migration, if they lost their homes and/or family members, or simply by being in a foreign land. It is critical that healthcare providers have cultural awareness of the population they care for so that interventions can be uniquely tailored to individual needs.

Refugees are required to have a medical examination typically within one to three months upon arrival in the United States. The purpose of the medical examination is to conduct medical screening, provide health education, follow up on conditions identified in any predeparture exams, and to establish a medical home. The CDC oversees this process and also provides a wealth of information for healthcare providers to assist in determining the best post-arrival screening tests to perform on a variety of populations (CDC, 2022e). The website is provided in the *Resources for Healthcare Providers* section.

Prior Pregnancy Loss

A person with a previous pregnancy loss, defined as a miscarriage, ectopic, stillbirth, or neonatal death, should be carefully evaluated. After a perinatal loss, grief tends to significantly decline by six months for most individuals. Therefore, those who take longer than six months to move through acute feelings of grief and return to activities of daily life should be evaluated for mental health disorders. The loss can trigger psychological distress that may result in major depressive disorder, anxiety, PTSD, or complicated grief (Farren et al., 2020). People may experience disenfranchised grief, which occurs when cultural norms do not recognize the loss of a pregnancy as a significant source of grief for the couple. Thus, grief should be carefully evaluated and openly discussed with every couple who has experienced a pregnancy loss (Farren et al., 2020; Obst et al., 2020).

The preconception period offers an opportunity to discuss what factors may have contributed to the pregnancy loss and to modify the factors that can be changed. The optimum timing of a subsequent pregnancy depends on the health of the individual and the emotional state of the couple. This period is also a good time to evaluate the social support available to the couple. The compassionate prenatal care provider will acknowledge the loss and provide sensitive counseling, recognizing that contemplation of the next pregnancy may bring emotions regarding the prior loss to the surface (Rich, 2018).

Individuals with Disabilities

Nearly 18% of people aged 18–44 years who identify as women in the US report having a disability (Okoro et al., 2018). A greater disparity in health outcomes is reported in individuals who have a disability and who identify as transgender. The intersectionality of having a disability and identifying as transgender compounds the risk for poor outcomes and health disparities. It is important that healthcare providers provide nonjudgmental care to all individuals to break down barriers to care (Disability Rights Education: Defense Fund, 2018). People with the most complex disabilities, such as those that impact self-care and work activities, are less likely to become pregnant than people whose disabilities only affect a single body system. Some people with disabilities have multiple risk factors that can negatively affect pregnancy outcomes. They may receive less routine primary care check-ups and be more likely to smoke, lack social support, and to experience poor mental health, obesity, and asthma (Mitra et al., 2016).

Healthcare should be tailored to address individual needs. The healthcare provider must be able to effectively communicate with the person which may require an interpreter if the person has hearing loss or experiences any other sensory deficit. All healthcare facilities are required to provide accessible medical equipment including wheelchair access (CDC, 2020b). A plethora of resources, including tools and health information about disabilities for healthcare providers is available at the website provided in the *Resources for Healthcare Providers* section of this chapter.

Preconception Care for People Assigned Male at Birth

The health of people assigned male at birth (AMAB) who are planning pregnancy with a partner also matters in the preconception period, not only for their own health and development, but also the impact on reproductive outcomes. The health of sperm plays a critical role in successful conception. In addition to their biological contribution to the pregnancy, AMAB people influence the health of their partners during pregnancy. These influences can be negative (e.g., STIs, tobacco use in the home) or positive (e.g., emotional and financial support). As with all preconception healthcare, the RLP is pivotal in assessing family planning needs (Kotelchuck & Lu, 2017). Preconception care for

AMAB people is focused on: (a) risk assessment and screening; (b) health promotion and counseling; and (c) interventions. A comprehensive history should be taken that includes surgical history, past immunizations, sexual history to identify risks for STIs, occupational/environmental exposures, and a three-generational family history specifically looking for sex-linked and autosomal recessive disorders. Laboratory screening for STIs is indicated if history reveals risk factors. Mental health screening for depression and/or anxiety using a validated tool is also an essential component. One study found that depression in fathers was associated with negative paternal–child and maternal–child relationships as well as poorer childhood emotional and behavioral outcomes (Kotelchuck & Lu, 2017). Tobacco products, heavy alcohol (>2 drinks/day), marijuana, cocaine, and anabolic steroids are associated with abnormal sperm morphology and/or poor sperm quality/quantity (Kotelchuck & Lu, 2017). Medication use is evaluated since some medications can affect sperm quality. The physical exam should include BP, a genital exam, and calculation of BMI. Medical conditions that might impair sperm quality (e.g., diabetes mellitus, obesity, and varicocele) should be addressed with appropriate interventions that will optimize health and fertility before conception. The healthcare provider is well positioned to initiate and facilitate interprofessional collaboration for preconception care of the couple as a whole by providing care for the person who will become pregnant and referral/consultation of the partner or sperm donor with their healthcare provider (Nypaver et al., 2016). Items listed below should be reviewed during an AMAB person's preconception visit.

Components of preconception care for people assigned male at birth

- Develop a RLP.
- Screen for tobacco, heavy drinking, anabolic steroids, marijuana, cocaine, and other illicit drugs and counsel as appropriate.
- Screen and treat for STIs, particularly gonorrhea, chlamydia, and HIV.
- Screen with a three-generational history with particular focus on genetic disorders.
- Screen for immunizations and vaccinate accordingly.
- Screen for depression and anxiety using a validated tool.
- Encourage stress reduction and enhance resilience as it is likely to improve family relationships.
- Counsel about need for normal BMI and that obesity is linked with impaired fertility and damaged sperm.
- Encourage folic acid supplementation as it may protect sperm from DNA damage.
- Encourage regular dental health visits because chronic inflammation, such as with periodontal infections, can damage sperm.
- Counsel to avoid exposure to occupational and environmental toxins that may affect fertility.
- Referral to primary care provider as needed.

Source: Kotelchuck and Lu (2017).

Preconception Care for Gender-Diverse Individuals

Many transgender men with retained reproductive organs may desire pregnancy, yet they often do not receive equitable reproductive support, placing them at risk for poorer health outcomes (MacLean, 2021). Transgender men need individualized care related to transitioning, fertility, contraception, family planning, fertility preserving options, pregnancy, birth, and chest-feeding. The preconception health history should include information about presence or absence of a uterus and ovaries; sexual health; sexual orientation; and pregnancy desires. Unintended pregnancies may occur, especially if there is a belief that testosterone is a contraceptive. The use of testosterone by transgender men can cause amenorrhea, however, ovulation, and pregnancy may still be possible and could lead teratogenic fetal effects should a pregnancy occur. Therefore, any individual who is taking gender affirming hormones and is attempting pregnancy should be advised to discontinue the use of testosterone. Conversely, those who are taking testosterone to transition may experience decreased fertility. Healthcare providers must create a trusting, respectful, and inclusive environment and stay current with language and transsensitivity and clinical care. Additionally, transgender men may be in need of referral to assisted reproductive facilities, especially if their partner is a cisgender female (MacLean, 2021).

Summary

Preconception care has great potential to improve pregnancy outcome and the long-term health of families. Preconception care is likely to have the greatest impact when it is integrated into routine primary care and sexual and reproductive health visits. Interconception care is especially important to provide health-promoting and disease-preventing services as it allows changes in health and lifestyle to begin long before the conception of the next pregnancy. The positive health changes made in preparation for conception pave the way for the physical stamina and emotional resilience needed for the transformative life events of pregnancy and parenting.

Resources for Individuals and Their Families

Association of Maternal & Child Health Programs (AMCHP).Current Initiatives. Available at: https://amchp.org/maternal-infant-health-current-initiatives/

CDC. Before Pregnancy. Planning for pregnancy: Available at: https://www.cdc.gov/preconception/planning.html

Childbirth Connection: Available at: http://www.childbirthconnection.org/planning-pregnancy

March of Dimes: Getting ready for pregnancy: Available at: https://www.marchofdimes.org/find-support/topics/planning-baby/getting-ready-pregnancy-preconception-health

Toxic substances portal. Agency for Toxic Substances and Disease Registry: Available at: https://www.atsdr.cdc.gov

Resources for Healthcare Providers

Agency for Healthcare Research and Quality has research-based tools and other resources to help providers and other make care safer in various healthcare settings. Available at: https://www.ahrq.gov/tools/index.html?search_api_views_fulltext=&field_toolkit_topics=14167&sort_by=title&sort_order=ASC

ATSDR toxic substances portal. Available at: https://www.atsdr.cdc.gov

CDC: Immigrant, Refugee, and Migrant Health information by the CDC, including medical examination for newly arrived refugees. Available at: https://www.cdc.gov/immigrantrefugeehealth/index.html

CDC: CDC information about disability and health information for healthcare providers. Available at: https://www.cdc.gov/ncbddd/disabilityandhealth/hcp.html

Preconception Health + Health Care Practice Bulletin. (2020). Available at: https://beforeandbeyond.org/wp-content/uploads/2021/02/phc-bulletin-0223211.pdf

Power to Decide. Offers training and certification in One Key Question. Available at: https://powertodecide.org/one-key-question

Substance Abuse and Mental Health Services Administration (SAMHSA). Resources for Screening, Brief Intervention, and Referral to Treatment (SBIRT). US Department of Health and Human Services. Available at: https://www.samhsa.gov/sbirt/resources

References

Admon, L. K., Daw, J. R., Winkleman, T. N. A., Kozhimannil, K. B., Zivin, K., Heisler, M., & Dalton, V. K. (2021). Insurance coverage and health care use among low-income women in the US, 2015–2017. *JAMA Network Open*, 4(1), e2034549, 1–4. https://doi.org/10.1001/jamanetworkopen.2020.34549

Agency for Healthcare Research and Quality. (AHRQ). (2015). *Intimate Partner Violence Screening*. https://www.ahrq.gov/ncepcr/tools/healthier-pregnancy/fact-sheets/partner-violence.html

Agency for Toxic Substances and Disease Registry. (2023, April 3). *Agency for toxic substances and disease registry*. https://www.atsdr.cdc.gov

Alexopoulos, A. S., Blair, R., & Peters, A. L. (2019). Management of pre-existing diabetes in pregnancy: A review. *JAMA*, 321(18), 1811–1819. https://doi.org/10.1001/jama.2019.4981

American Academy of Family Physicians (AAFP). (2023, April 5). *Preconception care (position paper)*. https://www.aafp.org/about/policies/all/preconception-care.html

American College of Obstetricians and Gynecologists. (2018a). ACOG practice bulletin no. 190: Gestational diabetes mellitus. *Obstetrics & Gynecology*, 131(2), e49–e64. https://doi.org/10.1097/AOG.0000000000002501

American College of Obstetricians and Gynecologists (ACOG). (2018b). Practice bulletin no. 197: Inherited thrombophilias in pregnancy. *Obstetrics & Gynecology*, 132(1), 249–251. https://doi.org/10.1097/AOG.0000000000002703

American College of Obstetricians and Gynecologists. (2019a). ACOG committee opinion no. 762: Prepregnancy counseling. *Obstetrics & Gynecology*, 133(1), e78–e89. https://doi.org/10.1097/AOG.0000000000003013

American College of Obstetricians and Gynecologists. (2019b). ACOG practice bulletin no. 203. Chronic hypertension in pregnancy. *Obstetrics & Gynecology*, 133(1), e26–e50. https://doi.org/10.1097/AOG.0000000000003020

American College of Obstetricians and Gynecologists. (2020a). Gynecologic management of adolescents and young women with seizure disorders. ACOG committee opinion no. 806. *Obstetrics & Gynecology*, 135(5), e213–e220. https://doi.org/10.1097/AOG.0000000000003837

American College of Obstetricians and Gynecologists (ACOG). (2020b). Management of women with phenylalanine hydroxylase deficiency (phenylketonuria). ACOG committee opinion no. 802. *Obstetrics & Gynecology*, 135(4), e167–e170. https://doi.org/10.1097/AOG.0000000000003768

American Diabetes Association (ADA). (2021). Classification and diagnosis of diabetes: Standards of medical care in diabetes-2021. *Diabetes Care*, 44(Suppl. 1), S1–S232. https://doi.org/10.2337/dc21-S002

Anxiety & Depression Association of American (ADAA). (2022, October 22). *Anxiety disorders: Facts & statistics.* https://adaa.org/understanding-anxiety/facts-statistics

Azeez, O., Kulkarni, A., Kuklina, E. V., Kim, S. Y., & Cox, S. (2019). Hypertension and diabetes in non-pregnant women of reproductive age in the United States. *Preventing Chronic Disease*, 16(E146), 1–9. https://doi.org/10.5888/pcd16.190105

Bobetsis, Y. A., Graziani, F., Gürsay, M., & Madianos, P. N. (2020). Periodontal disease and adverse pregnancy outcomes. *Periodontology 2000*, 83(1), 154–174. https://doi.org/10.1111/prd.12294

Boersma, P., Villarroel, M. A., & Vahratian, A. (2020). *Heavy drinking among U.S. adults, 2018. NCHS data brief no. 374.* National Center for Health Statistics. https://www.cdc.gov/nchs/data/databriefs/db374-h.pdf

Bonham, C. A., Patterson, K. C., & Strek, M. E. (2018). Asthma outcomes and management during pregnancy. *Chest*, 153(2), 515–527. https://doi.org/10.1016/j.chest.2017.08.029

Bower, W.A., Schiffer, J., Atmar, R.L., et al, (2019). Use of Anthrax vaccine in the United States: Recommendations of the Advisory Committee on Immunization Practices, 2019. *MMWR. Recommendations & Reports* 0019, 68(4),1–14. https://doi.org/10.15585/mmwr.rr6804a1.

Buckley, A., Sestito, S., Ogundipe, T., Roig, J., Rosenburg, H. M., Cohen, N., Wang, K., Stoffels, G., Janevic, T., DeBolt, C., Cabrera, C., Cochrane, E., Berkin, J., Bianco, A., & Vieira, L. (2022). Racial and ethnic disparities among women undergoing a trial of labor after cesarean delivery: Performance of a VBAC calculator with and without patient's race/ethnicity. *Reproductive Sciences*, 29, 2030–2038. https://doi.org/10.1007/s43032-022-00959-2

Centers for Disease Control and Prevention. (2020a). *National Diabetes Statistics Report-2020.* Atlanta, GA. Centers for Disease Control and Prevention, U.S. Department of Health and Human Services. 1–30.

Centers for Disease Control and Prevention. (2020b, September 15). *Disability and health promotion: disability and health information for health care providers.* https://www.cdc.gov/ncbddd/disabilityandhealth/hcp.html

Centers for Disease Control and Prevention. (2022a, December 22). *Folic acid.* https://www.cdc.gov/ncbddd/folicacid/index.html

Centers for Disease Control and Prevention. (2022b, October 11). *Violence prevention: preventing intimate partner violence.* https://www.cdc.gov/violenceprevention/intimatepartnerviolence/fastfact.html

Centers for Disease Control and Prevention. (2022c, October 20). *Illicit drug use.* https://www.cdc.gov/nchs/fastats/drug-use-illicit.htm.

Centers for Disease Control and Prevention. (2022d, November 2). *Zika virus.* https://www.cdc.gov/zika/index.html

Centers for Disease Control and Prevention. (2022e, June 16). *Immigrant, refugee, and migrant health.* https://www.cdc.gov/immigrantrefugeehealth/index.html

Centers for Disease Control and Prevention. (2023, February 102). *Immunizations schedules: recommendations for ages 19 years or older, United States, 2023.* https://www.cdc.gov/vaccines/schedules/hcp/imz/adult.html

Chiu, Y. H., Chavarro, J. E., & Souter, I. (2018). Diet and female fertility: doctor, what should I eat? *Fertility and Sterility*, 110(4), 560–569. https://doi.org/10.1016/j.fertnstert.2018.05.027

Chuang, C., Velott, D. L., & Weisman. (2010). Exploring knowledge and attitudes related to pregnancy and preconception health in woman with chronic medical conditions. *Maternal Child Health Journal*, 14(5), 713–719. https://doi.org/1007/s10995-009-0518-6

Clark, T.C., Schiller, J.S., & Boersma, P. (2020). *Early release of selected estimates based on data from the 2019 National Health Interview Survey.* National Center for Health Statistics. https://www.cdc.gov/nchs/data/nhis/earlyrelease/EarlyRelease202009-508.pdf

Cornelius, M. E., Loretan, C. G., Wang, T. W., Jamal, A., & Homa, D. M. (2022). Tobacco product use among adults- United States, 2020. *MMWR Morbidity & Mortality Weekly Report*, 71(11), 397–405. https://doi.org/10.15585/mmwr.mm7111a1

Disability Rights Education & Defense Fund. (2018). *Health disparities at the intersection of disability and gender identify: a framework and literature review.* https://dredf.org/wp-content/uploads/2018/07/Health-Disparities-at-the-Intersection-of-Disability-and-Gender-Identity.pdf.

Farren, J., Jalmbrant, M., Falconieri, N., Mitchell-Jones, N., Bobdiwala, S., Al-Memar, M., Tapp, S., Van Calster, B., Wynants, L., Timmerman, D., & Boone, T. (2020). Postraumatic stress, anxiety, and depression following miscarriage and ectopic pregnancy: a multicenter, prospective, cohort study. *American Journal of Obstetrics & Gynecology*, 222(4), 367.e1–367.e22. https://doi.org/10.1016/j.ajog.2019.10.102

Gázquez, A., & Larqué, E. (2021). Towards an optimized fetal DHA accretion: differences on maternal DHA supplementation using phospholipids vs triglycerides during pregnancy in different models. *Nutrients*, 13(2), 511–533. https://doi.org/10.3390/nu13020511

Geronimus, A. T., Hicken, M., Keene, D., & Bound, J. (2006). "Weathering" and age patterns of allostatic load scores among blacks and whites in the United States. *American Journal of Public Health*, 96(5), 826–833. https://doi.org/10.2105/AJPH.2004.060749

Goossens, J., De Roose, M., Van Hecke, A., & Goemaes, R. (2018). Barriers and facilitators to the provision of preconception care by healthcare providers: A systematic review. *International Journal of Nursing Studies*, 87, 113–130. https://doi.org/10.1016/j.ijnurstu.2018.06.009

Grieger, J. A. (2020). Preconception diet, fertility, and later health in pregnancy. *Fertility, IVF and Reproductive Genetics*, 32(3), 227–332. https://doi.org/10.1097/GCO.0000000000000629

Griffiths, M. J., Winship, A. L., & Hutt, K. J. (2020). Do cancer therapies damage the uterus and compromise fertility? *Human Reproduction Update*, 26(2), 161–173. https://doi.org/10.1093/humupd/dmz041

Guttmacher Institute. (2019). *Fact Sheet: unintended pregnancy in the United States.* https://www.guttmacher.org/sites/default/files/factsheet/fb-unintended-pregnancy-us.pdf

Hales, C.M., Carroll, M.D., Fryar, C.D., & Ogden, C.L. (2020). Prevalence of obesity and severe obesity among adults: United States, 2017–2018. NCHA Data Brief No. 360. National Center for Health Statistics, 2020. https://www.cdc.gov/nchs/data/databriefs/db360-h.pdf

Henning, P. A., Burgess, C. K., Jones, H. E., & Norman, W. V. (2017). The effects of asking a fertility intention question in primary care setting: A systemic review protocol. *Systematic Reviews*, 6(1), 11. https://doi.org/10.1186/s13643-017-0412-z

Johnson, K., Posner, S. F., Bierman, J., Cordero, J. F., Atrash, H. K., Parker, C. S., Boulet, S., & Curtis, M. G. (2006). Select Panel on Preconception. Recommendations to improve preconception health and health care- United States: A report of CDC/ATSDR preconception care work group and the select panel on preconception care. *MMWR Recommendations and Reports*, 55(RR6), 1–23.

Kee, M. Z. L., Ponmudi, S., Phua, D. Y., Rifkin-Graboi, A., Chong, Y. S., Tan, K. H., Chan, J. K. Y., Broekman, B. F. P., Chen, H., & Meaney, M. J. (2021). Preconception origins of perinatal maternal mental health. *Archives of Women's Mental Health*, 24(4), 605–618. https://doi.org/10.1007/s00737-020-01096-y

Kim, S. (2022). Different maternal age patterns of preterm birth: Interplay of race/ethnicity, chronic stress, and marital status. *Research Nursing & Health*, 45, 151–162. https://doi.org/10.1002/nur.22205

Kinsey, D., Paul, C. P., Taylor, D., Caricchio, R., Kulathinal, R. J., & Hayes-Conroy, A. (2018). The whole lupus: Articulating biosocial interplay in systemic lupus erythematosus epidemiology and population disparities. *Health & Place*, *51*, 182–183. https://doi.org/10.1016/j.healthplace.2018.03.007

Kotelchuck, M., & Lu, M. (2017). Father's role in preconception health. *Maternal and Child Health Journal*, *21*(11), 2025–2039. https://doi.org/10.1007/s10995-017-2370-4

Kroelinger, C. D., Okoroh, E. M., Boulet, S. L., Olson, C. K., & Robbins, C. L. (2018). Making the case: The importance of using 10 key preconception indicators in understanding the health of women of reproductive age. *Journal of Women's Health*, *27*(6), 739–743. https://doi.org/10.1089/jwh.2018.7034

Lee, S., & Pearce, E. (2021). Testing, monitoring, and treatment of thyroid dysfunction in pregnancy. *Journal of Clinical Endocrinology & Metabolism*, *106*(3), 883–892. https://doi.org/10.1210/clinem/dgaa945

Li, M., Francis, E., Hinkle, S. N., Ajjarapu, A. S., & Zhang, C. (2019). Preconception and prenatal nutrition and neurodevelopmental disorders: A systematic review and meta-analysis. *Nutrients*, *11*(7), 628. https://doi.org/10.3390/nu11071628

Liao, Q., Luo, J., Zheng, L., Han, Q., Liu, Z., Qi, W., Yang, T., & Yan, J. (2020). Establishment of an antepartum predictive scoring model to identify candidates for vaginal birth after caesarean. *BMC Pregnancy and Childbirth*, *20*(1), 639. https://doi-org.uc.idm.oclc.org/10.1186/s12884-020-03231-0

MacLean, L. R.-D. (2021). Preconception, pregnancy, birthing, and lactation needs of transgender men. *Nursing for Women's Health*, *25*(2), 129–138. https://doi.org/10.1016/j.nwh.2021.01.006

Marder, W. (2019). Update on pregnancy complications in systemic lupus erythematosus. *Current Opinion in Rheumatology*, *31*(6), 650–658. https://doi.org/10.1097/BOR.0000000000000651

Martin, J. A., Hamilton, B. E., Osterman, M. J. K., & Driscoll, A. K. (2021). Births: final data for 2019. *National Vital Statistic Reports*, *70*(2). National Center for Health Statistics.

McCance-Katz, E.F. (2020). *The National Survey on Drug Use and Health: 2019*. Substance Abuse and Mental Health Services Administration. U.S. Department of Health and Human Services. https://www.samhsa.gov/data/sites/default/files/reports/rpt29392/Assistant-Secretary-nsduh2019_presentation/Assistant-Secretary-nsduh2019_presentation.pdf

McDiarmid, M. A., & Gehle, K. (2006). Preconception brief: occupational/environmental exposures. *Maternal and Child Health Journal*, *10*(1), 123–128. https://doi.org/10.1007/s10995-006-0089-8

Mercurio, A. (2019). Integrating sexuality and gender identify into the reproductive life plan. *Journal of Women's Health*, *28*(1), 107–108. https://doi.org/10.1089/jwh.2018.7341

MINT. (2021, November 9). *Understanding motivational interviewing*. https://motivationalinterviewing.org/understanding-motivational-interviewing

Mitra, M., Clements, K. M., Zhang, J., & Smith, L. D. (2016). Disparities in adverse preconception risk factors between women with and without disabilities. *Maternal and Child Health Journal*, *20*(3), 507–515. https://doi.org/10.1007/s10995-015-1848-1

Montagnoli, C., Zanconato, G., Cinelli, G., Tozzi, A. E., Bovo, C., Bortolus, R., & Ruggeri, S. (2020). Maternal mental health and reproductive outcomes: A scoping review of the current literature. *Archives of Gynecology and Obstetrics*, *302*, 801–819. https://doi.org/10.1007/s00404-020-05685-1

Mousa, A., Naqash, A., & Lim, S. (2019). Macronutrient and micronutrient intake during pregnancy: An overview of recent evidence. *Nutrients*, *11*, 443–462. https://doi.org/10.3390/nu11020443

National Institute of Alcohol Abuse and Alcoholism. (November 9, 2021). *Screening tests*. National Institute of Health. https://pubs.niaaa.nih.gov/publications/arh28-2/78-79.htm

National Institute of Health (NIH). (2019, December 6). *Calcium fact sheet for consumers*. Office of Dietary Supplements. https://ods.od.nih.gov/pdf/factsheets/Calcium-Consumer.pdf

National Institute on Drug Abuse. (2020). *Substance use in women research report: substance use while pregnant and breastfeeding*. https://nida.nih.gov/publications/research-reports/substance-use-in-women/substance-use-while-pregnant-breastfeeding.

Nypaver, C. F., Arbour, M., & Niederegger, E. (2016). Preconception care: Improving the health of women and families. *Journal of Midwifery & Women's Health*, *61*(3), 356–364. https://doi.org/10.1111/jmwh.12465

Obst, K. L., Due, C., Oxlad, M., & Middleton, P. (2020). Men's grief following pregnancy loss and neonatal loss: A systematic review and emerging theoretical model. *BMC Pregnancy and Childbirth*, *20*(1), 1–17. https://doi.org/10.1186/s12884-019-2677-9

Okoro, C. A., Hollis, N. D., Cyrus, A. C., & Griffin-Blake, S. (2018). Prevalence of disabilities and health care access by disability status and type among adults—United States, 2016. *MMWR Morbidity and Mortality Weekly Report*, *67*, 882–887. https://doi.org/10.15585/mmwr.mm6732a3

Pate, C. S., Zahran, H. S., Qin, X., Johnson, C., Hummelman, E., & Malilay, J. (2021). Asthma surveillance-United States, 2006–2018. *MMWR Surveillance Summary 2021*, *70*(5), 1–32. https://doi.org/10.15585/mmwr.ss7005a1

Peitzmeier, S. M., Malik, M., Kattari, S. K., Marrow, E., Stephenson, R., Agénor, M., & Reisner, S. L. (2020). Intimate partner violence in transgender populations: Systematic review and meta-analysis of prevalence and correlates. *American Journal of Public Health*, *110*(9), e1–e14. https://doi.org/10.2105/AJPH.2020.305774

Perry, M. F., Mulcahy, H., & DeFranco, E. (2019). Influence of periconception smoking behavior on birth defect risks. *American Journal of Obstetrics and Gynecology*, *220*(6), 588.e1–588.e-7. https://doi.org/10.1016/j.ajog.2019.02.029

Power to Decide. (2023, April 5) *One key question® online*. https://powertodecide.org/one-key-question

Practice Committee of the American Society for Reproductive Medicine. (2018). Smoking and infertility: A committee opinion. *Fertility and Sterility*, *110*(4), 611–618. https://doi.org/10.1016/j.fertnstert.2018.06.016

Preconception Health + Health Care Initiative. (2020). *Women's health practice bulletin* 2020. https://beforeandbeyond.org/wp-content/uploads/2021/02/phc-bulletin-0223211.pdf

Ray, K. (2021). In the name of racial justice: Why bioethics should care about environmental toxins. *Hastings Center Report*, *51*(3), 23–26. https://doi.org/10.1002/hast.1251

Rich, D. (2018). Psychological impact of pregnancy loss: Best practice for obstetric providers. *Clinical Obstetrics and Gynecology*, *61*(3), 628–636. https://doi.org/10.1097/GRF.0000000000000369

Saito, M., Briand, U., Min, A. M., & McGready, R. (2020). Deleterious effects of malaria in pregnancy on the developing fetus: A review on prevention and treatment with antimalarial drugs. *Lancet Child and Adolescent Health*, *4*(10), 761–774. https://doi.org/10.1016/S2352-4642(20)30099-7

Sak, S., Incebiyik, A., Hilali, N. G., Ağacayak, E., Uyanikoğlu, H., Akbas, H., & Sak, M. E. (2019). Cytogenetic screening in couples with habitual abortions. *Journal of Gynecology Obstetrics and Human Reproduction*, *48*(3), 155–158. https://doi.org/10.1016/j.jogoh.2018.10.021

Segal, T. R., & Giudice, L. C. (2019). Before the beginning: Environmental exposures and reproductive and obstetrical outcomes. *Fertility and Sterility*, *112*(4), 613–631. https://doi.org/10.1016/j.fertnstert.2019.08.001

Sharma, V., Sharma, P., & Sharma, S. (2020). Managing bipolar disorder during pregnancy and the postpartum period: A critical review of current practice. *Expert Review of Neurotherapeutics*, *20*(4), 373–383. https://doi.org/10.1080/14737175.2020.1743684

Simmons, R. G., & Jennings, V. (2020). Fertility awareness-based methods of family planning. *Best Practices & Research Clinical Obstetrics and Gynaecology*, *66*, 68–82. https://doi.org/10.1016/j.bpobgyn.2019.12.003

Siniscalchi, K. A., Broome, M. E., Fish, J., Ventimiglia, J., Thompson, J., Roy, P., Pipes, R., & Trivedi, M. (2020). Depression screening and measurement-based care in primary care. *Journal of Primary Care Community Health*, *11*. https://doi.org/10.1177/2150132720931261

Sommers, B. D. (2020). Health insurance coverage: What comes after the ACA? *Health Affairs*, *39*(3), 502–508. https://doi.org/10.1377/hlthaff.2019.01416

Stephen, L. J., Harden, C., Tomson, T., & Brodie, M. J. (2019). Management of epilepsy in women. *The Lancet Neurology*, *18*(5), 481–491. https://doi.org/10.1016/S1474-4422(18)30495-2

Substance Abuse and Mental Health Services Administration (SAMHSA). (2022). *Screening, brief intervention, and referral to treatment (SBIRT)*. U.S. Department of Health and Human Services. https://www.samhsa.gov/sbirt/about

Taylor, P. E. (2014). *Toxic communities: Environmental racism, industrial pollution, and residential morbidity*. New York University Press.

Thiele, D. K., & Anderson, C. M. (2016). Developmental origins of health and disease: A challenge for nurses. *Journal of Pediatric Nursing, 31*(1), 42–46. https://doi.org/10.1016/j.pedn.2015.10.020

Thompson, M. A., Horberg, M. A., Agmu, A. L., Colasanti, J. A., Jain, M. K., Short, W. R., Signh, T., & Aberg, J. A. (2020). Primary care guidance for persons with human immunodeficiency virus- 2020 update by the HIV medicine Association of the Infectious Diseases Society of America. *Clinical Infectious Diseases*, ciaa1391. https://doi.org/10.1093/cid/ciaa1391

Tsai, S., Sun, M. Y., Kuller, J. A., Rhee, E. H., & Dotters-Katz, S. (2019). Syphilis in pregnancy. *Obstetrics and Gynecological Survery, 74*(9), 557–564. https://doi.org/10.1097/OGX.0000000000000713

U.S. Department of Health & Human Services. (2018). *Physical activity guidelines for Americans*. (2nd ed.). https://health.gov/sites/default/files/2019-09/Physical_Activity_Guidelines_2nd_edition.pdf.

U.S. Environmental Protection Agency. (2022). *Private drinking water well*. https://www.epa.gov/privatewells

U.S. Food & Drug Administration. (2021). *Advice about eating fish: for women who are or might become pregnancy, breastfeeding mothers, and young children*. https://www.fda.gov/food/consumers/advice-about-eating-fish

U.S. Preventative Services Task Force. (2023). *A and B recommendations*. https://www.uspreventiveservicestaskforce.org/uspstf/recommendation-topics/uspstf-a-and-b-recommendations

UNC Center for Maternal & Infant Health. (2023). *The national preconception health and health care initiative (PCHHC)*. https://www.mombaby.org/pchhc/

Unger, T., Borghi, C., Charchar, F., Khan, N. A., Poulter, N. R., Prabhakaran, D., Ramirez, A., Schlaich, M., Stergiou, G. S., Tomaszewski, M., Wainford, R. D., Williams, B., & Schutte, A. E. (2020). 2020 International Society of Hypertension global hypertension practice guidelines. *Journal of Hypertension, 38*(6), 982–1004. https://doi.org/10.1161/HYPERTENSIONAHA.120.15026

US Preventative Services Task Force. (2021, November 3). *Thyroid dysfunction: screening*. https://www.uspreventiveservicestaskforce.org/uspstf/recommendation/thyroid-dysfunction-screening

Vajda, F. J. E., O'Brien, T. J., Graham, J. E., Hitchcock, A. A., Lander, C. M., & Eadie, M. J. (2018). Predicting epileptic seizure control during pregnancy. *Epilepsy & Behavior, 78*, 91–95. https://doi.org/10.1016/j.yebeh.2017.10.017

Vigod, S. N., Fung, K., Amartey, A., Bartsch, E., Felemban, R., Saunders, N., Guttman, A., Chiu, M., Barker, L. C., Kurdyak, P., & Brown, H. K. (2020). Maternal schizophrenia and adverse birth outcomes: What mediates the risk? *Social Psychiatry and Psychiatric Epidemiology, 55*(5), 561–570. https://doi.org/10.1007/s00127-019-01814-7

Vitner, D., Harris, K., Maxwell, C., & Farine, D. (2019). Obesity in pregnancy: A comparison of four national guidelines. *The Journal of Maternal-Fetal & Neonatal Medicine, 32*(15), 2580–2590. https://doi.org/10.1080/14767058.2018.1440546

Vyas, D. A., Jones, D. S., Meadows, A. R., Diouf, K., Nour, N. M., & Schantz-Dunn, J. (2019). Challenging the use of race in the vaginal birth after cesarean section calculator. *Women's Health Issues, 29*(3), 201–204.

Westerfield, K. L., Koenig, K., & Oh, R. (2018). Breastfeeding: Common questions and answers. *American Family Physician, 98*(6), 368–373.

Wong, E. C., Rose, C. E., Flores, A. L., & Yeung, L. F. (2019). Trends in multivitamin use among women of reproductive age: United States, 2006–2016. *Journal of Women's Health (Larchmt), 28*(1), 37–45. https://doi.org/10.1089/jwh.2018.7075

Wyckoff, E. T., Cua, G. M., Gibson, D. J., & Egerman, R. S. (2020). Efficacy of the NICHD vaginal birth after caesarean delivery calculator: A single center experience. *Journal of Maternal-Fetal and Neonatal Medicine, 33*(4), 553–557. https://doi.org/10.1080/14767058.2018.1497597

8

Prenatal Care: Goals, Structure, and Components

Emma Clark

The editors gratefully acknowledge Carrie S. Klima, who authored the previous edition of this chapter.

Relevant Terms

Centering Pregnancy—a movement founded in 1993 by Sharon Schindler Rising that changed the prenatal care paradigm by taking pregnant people out of the exam room and placing them into a group setting for assessment, education, and community building.

Children's Bureau—the first federal agency devoted to the welfare of children, signed into law in 1912 by William Howard Taft in response to grassroots efforts led by nurse Lillian Wald. Early agency issues were maternal and infant mortality; its work continues today with child abuse and neglect as leading modern-day concerns.

Community-based organizations—organizations such as Mamatoto Village in Washington, DC, Ancient Song Doula Services in Brooklyn, New York and Birthmark Collective in New Orleans, Louisiana that combat reproductive injustice by expanding access to education and childbirth services for Black women and birthing people, often while also creating employment for birthworkers of color.

Expert Panel on the Content of Prenatal Care—a groundbreaking report published in 1989 that laid out the need to pay attention not only to the birthing person and fetus but also infant and family and emphasized psychosocial and environmental patient and family needs as well as

traditional medical concerns. It included suggestions about visit timing and content that are still being used today.

Feminist movements—social reform efforts advocating for women's rights. First-wave feminism (1880s–1940s) secured the right to vote and hold property for women; second-wave feminism (1960s–1980s) focused on reproductive rights and social equality; third-wave feminism (1990s–present) embraces diversity and intersectionality.

Maternity care desert—areas where there is low or no access to maternity care, no hospitals or birth centers offering pregnancy and birth care, and no perinatal providers.

Maternal morbidity—any short- or long-term health problems that result from being pregnant and giving birth.

Pregnancy-related maternal mortality—the death of a person while pregnant or within one year of the end of pregnancy from any cause related to or aggravated by the pregnancy.

Sheppard–Towner Maternity and Infancy Protection Act—an act of Congress in 1921 that provided federal funds to states for maternity and child healthcare; passed in response to the Children's Bureau finding that 80% of all expecting individuals did not receive any prenatal care at that time.

Introduction

Prenatal care, also referred to as antenatal care, begins "when conception is first considered and continues until labor begins" (Public Health Service Expert Panel on the Content of Prenatal Care, 1989, p. 10). Components of prenatal care include risk identification, prevention and management of pregnancy-related or concurrent diseases, health education, and health promotion (World Health Organization, 2019). While prenatal care has been commonly practiced for more than a century, it has changed little since its initial focus on the detection of preeclampsia/eclampsia. This medical model of pregnancy care was the standard for almost a century before the **Expert Panel on the Content of Prenatal Care**, the first scientific review of prenatal care, was published in 1989.

Prenatal and Postnatal Care: A Person-Centered Approach, Third Edition. Edited by Karen Trister Grace, Cindy L. Farley, Noelene K. Jeffers, and Tanya Tringali.
© 2024 John Wiley & Sons Ltd. Published 2024 by John Wiley & Sons Ltd.
Companion website: www.wiley.com/go/grace/prenatal

Health equity key points

- Early prenatal care legislation and policies, though intended to improve the quality of care, nearly eliminated Black and immigrant traditional midwives, leaving lasting barriers to care for people of color.
- Prenatal care presents an important opportunity to identify and address medical concerns, but mental health and other social issues (e.g., housing) are under-addressed despite their impact on the well-being and health of the pregnant person, the fetus, and the family.
- Racially concordant prenatal care has the potential to begin to address racial disparities in maternal mortality rates, and various models are being implemented nationwide.

A Brief History of Prenatal Care

In 1843, the association between albuminuria and eclampsia was discovered, followed by the conclusion that the presence of proteinuria, edema, and convulsions were related to a common pathology of pregnancy. It was not until the invention of the sphygmomanometer in the late 1800s that blood pressure was included in the triad of symptoms now understood to signify preeclampsia. Concurrently, in Scotland, Dr. John Ballantyne was advocating that obstetrics and midwifery broaden their focus of care from the processes of labor and birth to the antenatal period. He recommended routine prenatal visits and suggested that infections could be transmitted from parent to fetus and that environmental substances, such as heavy metals and nicotine, might adversely affect the fetus. He advocated for the first prenatal beds within hospitals and is commonly referred to as the "father" of prenatal care (Ballantyne, 1923; Dunn, 1993). In the early 1900s, the United States saw similar trends developing in prenatal surveillance for maternal complications, including the routine measurement of blood pressure in pregnancy; however, this practice did not become widespread until 20 years later (Merkatz & Thompson, 1990). In the United States, prenatal care was initially introduced to decrease infant morbidity and mortality and was promoted by social reformers and public health nurses in the early 1900s. An early program in Boston provided self-care information and emotional support by visiting nurses to people enrolled at the Boston Lying-in Hospital. Similar programs began in Baltimore, where the detection of syphilis was emphasized in addition to content on personal hygiene, rest, and diet. In 1917, the Maternity Center Association (MCA) was opened in New York City, providing prenatal care that included a physical exam by a physician, visits with public health nurses at home and at the Center, and an educational emphasis on preparation for labor, birth, and infant care. The MCA reported that the outcomes for almost 9000 pregnant people over a three-year period included a 30% reduction in neonatal death and a 21.5% reduction in maternal mortality. These early attempts at prenatal care were seen by many as a way to address the high rates of **maternal morbidity** and neonatal morbidity and mortality of that time (Merkatz & Thompson, 1990).

As part of this early drive for improved prenatal and childbirth care, **The Children's Bureau** was formed in 1912 to oversee efforts to decrease infant mortality. In 1921, the **Sheppard–Towner Maternity and Infancy Protection Act** was passed, providing funding for pregnancy education, well-baby clinics, and visiting nurse services for pregnant and postpartum clients and their infants as well as midwifery training programs intended to modernize and regulate midwifery practice (Ladd-Taylor, 1988). In 1925, the Children's Bureau published prenatal care standards, which included history, physical exam, and educational content for pregnancy and birth. Little has changed from these standards in the structure and content of prenatal care over the last century. The Sheppard–Towner Act allocated responsibility for prenatal care funding and implementation to individual states, a model still in use (Ladd-Taylor, 1988).

The Sheppard–Towner Act also contained efforts to regulate midwifery and "professionalize" midwifery practice, incorporating modern scientific techniques and eliminating traditional practices. This legislation was driven by racism, sexism, and a conflation of the effects of poverty on childbirth outcomes and how and from whom people accessed prenatal care rather than a full understanding of care being provided and outcomes (Ladd-Taylor, 1988). Tragically, the implementation of the Sheppard–Towner Act caused the near elimination of many immigrant midwives and midwives of color, particularly traditional Black midwives (commonly referred to as "Granny midwives" because they were often older women) working predominately in the southern United States, through denial of permits, intense regulation and surveillance, and reduced demand for services. Meanwhile, individuals such as Mary Breckinridge, who founded the first nurse-midwifery service in rural Kentucky in the 1920s, and Mary Beard, a pioneer in the development of prenatal care, were developing a new cadre of nurse-midwives that combined public health prenatal care with midwifery to decrease maternal and newborn mortality (Dawley, 2003). Notably, many of the same people who were pushing to eliminate traditional Black and other lay midwives were leaders in introducing nurse-midwifery. Given that the now-discredited theory of eugenics played a role in the campaign to eliminate traditional midwives (Dawley, 2003), it is unsurprising that several of them, including Mary Breckenridge, believed in White superiority and wrote about eugenics and the value of segregation. Thus, while the Sheppard–Towner Act contributed greatly to making prenatal care widely available in the United States, it also shaped the racial and ethnic makeup of the midwifery workforce and institutionalization of culturally homogenous practices in ways that continue to have profound consequences on maternal health disparities to this day (Ladd-Taylor, 1988).

With traditional midwives, who had been the maternity care providers for many pregnant people, increasingly unable to practice, childbirth care shifted toward hospitals. Many hospitals, especially in urban areas, developed clinics to care for the large numbers of immigrants who had arrived in the United States in the previous decades. Hospitals were being built in large cities to provide care for the sick and dying; these institutions also allowed opportunities for medical education. The automobile provided mobility and transport to hospitals. Scientific advances, such as anesthesia and twilight sleep, made hospital birth more attractive to many people. Ultimately, this shift from home to hospitals and from midwives to physicians contributed to the medicalization of pregnancy and childbirth that occurred during the twentieth century (Rooks, 1997).

The childbirth education movement arose in response to this growing medicalization of pregnancy and childbirth (see Chapter 27, *Planning for Physiologic Birth*). It began with Grantly Dick-Read and the publication of *Childbirth without Fear* in the 1940s and continued with other methods of prepared childbirth such as Lamaze and the Bradley method. All of these prepared childbirth education models focused on the psychosocial needs of the expecting parent, infant, and family and sought to offer families methods to become active participants in the pregnancy and birth experience. During the second-wave **feminist movement** of the 1960s–1980s, childbirth preparation became more popular and became an adjunct to the traditional prenatal care that was provided mainly by physicians. However, it was heavily geared toward and utilized by middle-class White cisgender women. Low-income, young, unpartnered, LGBTQIA+, and people of color have historically been underserved by childbirth education from a variety of perspectives, including values espoused, information delivery methods, physical or financial access, and time constraints (Morton & Hsu, 2007). Group prenatal care models (discussed further below) can offer a remedy for this by increasing education opportunities within formal prenatal care. **Community-based organizations** such as Mamatoto Village in Washington, DC, Ancient Song Doula Services in New York, and Birthmark Doula Collective in New Orleans have created models that offer in-person and virtual childbirth classes targeted at pregnant people of color.

Innovations in prenatal care have been few since its inception. The discovery of the Rh antigen in 1940 provided insight into a common cause of fetal/infant morbidity and mortality. The immune globulin RhoGAM® was developed in 1963, preventing Rh isoimmunization disease and dramatically reducing morbidity and mortality for infants of Rh-negative individuals (Merkatz & Thompson, 1990). However, underuse of RhoGAM in low-income countries, largely due to lack of prenatal screening, is estimated to result in 114,100 avoidable neonatal deaths a year as well as many disabilities (Bhutani et al., 2013). Obstetric ultrasound for the visualization of the fetus was developed in the 1950s. Though it was developed for use in high-risk pregnancies, the use of ultrasounds was commonplace in hospitals in the United States by the 1970s.

Medications became more commonly prescribed for pregnant people with the introduction of diethylstilbestrol (DES) in the 1940s to prevent miscarriage. It was not until 1971 that the Food and Drug Administration (FDA) determined that DES was contraindicated for the prevention of miscarriage and in fact had long-term consequences such as genital cancers, reproductive tract anomalies, and epididymal cysts in offspring. Another drug with tragic consequences was thalidomide, primarily used in European countries. Thalidomide was touted as a sedative and antiemetic, making pregnant people a potential market for this drug given the common pregnancy discomforts of insomnia, nausea, and vomiting. However, it was quickly recognized as a teratogen, resulting in significant morbidity, mortality, and major limb deformities in affected fetuses. These medications were introduced into practice without long-term studies of their effectiveness and safety for the pregnant person and babies; the tragic outcomes pointed to the need for a more careful approach to the introduction of technologies and therapies during pregnancy (Chalmers, 1986).

This is a cautionary tale, however, since most drugs are not tested on pregnant people and the long-term effects are not known until the drugs have been in widespread use for a period of time. This has made counseling patients on what medications they should or should not continue during pregnancy challenging. The introduction of the COVID-19 vaccine in 2020 brought discussion around how problematic and paternalistic the lack of inclusion of pregnant people in clinical trials can be for developing recommendations and promoting uptake of medications and vaccines in pregnancy (Mena-Tudela et al., 2021).

Current Goals of Prenatal Care

In 1989, "Caring for Our Future: The Content of Prenatal Care" (CPC) was published. This landmark document was the result of a multidisciplinary panel convened by the Department of Health and Human Services to scientifically evaluate the current state of prenatal care. The goals of this Expert Panel group were to "understand, explain and define the content of prenatal care" (Public Health Service Expert Panel on the Content of Prenatal Care, 1989, p. ii). All aspects of care were reviewed, including the prenatal visit schedule and frequency of visits, the evidence for common prenatal care practices, and the health education and psychosocial content of care during pregnancy. The resulting work created objectives for prenatal care, recommendations for maintaining certain care practices; identified practices for which there was little evidence to support their efficacy; and created a broader, more comprehensive view of prenatal care (Public Health Service Expert Panel on the Content of Prenatal Care, 1989).

The Expert Panel also identified the goals of prenatal care for the pregnant person, fetus/infant, and family. For the first time, the goals of prenatal care were expanded to include goals for the infant and family for the first year of life. This expansion of prenatal care challenges prenatal care providers to move beyond simply identifying clients at risk for medical and pregnancy-related conditions to providing effective and timely education to pregnant people and their families as they prepare for the birth of their infant and the nurturing of that infant to maturity.

While the panel identified that prenatal care was a "cornerstone of healthcare delivery in our society" (Public Health Service Expert Panel on the Content of Prenatal Care, 1989), it also identified that prenatal care was often accessed too late to mitigate medical, obstetrical, and psychosocial risk factors that are present in the first trimester of pregnancy. Therefore, preconception care, provided to people as part of comprehensive reproductive and primary care, was promoted to achieve optimal health status of the person at the time of conception. However, preconception care is not often sought, since 45% of all pregnancies in the United States are unintended and many people have difficulty accessing services due to lack of insurance or limited availability of preconception care providers or services in their communities (Finer & Moline, 2016).

Goals of Prenatal Care

Client	Fetus/infant	Family
Increase well-being before, during, and after pregnancy; improve self-image and self-care. Reduce mortality and morbidity, fetal loss, unnecessary interventions. Reduce health risks to subsequent pregnancies and overall health. Promote the development of parenting skills.	Improve health outcomes. Reduce preterm birth, intrauterine growth restriction, congenital, anomalies, and failure to thrive. Promote healthy growth and development. Reduce child abuse and neglect, preventable acute and chronic illness, extended hospital stays after birth.	Promote family development. Reduce unintended pregnancy. Reduce child neglect and family violence.

Source: Public Health Service Expert Panel on the Content of Prenatal Care (1989)/Public Domain/Department of Health and Human Services.

Three basic components of prenatal care were identified: (a) initial and continuing risk assessment; (b) health promotion; and (c) medical and psychosocial interventions and follow-up. The Expert Panel acknowledged that while the focus on medical complications during pregnancy was important, expanding prenatal interventions to address psychosocial concerns such as stress, healthy behaviors, and financial concerns can have a positive effect on pregnancy outcomes and the family after birth. Growing evidence points to the relationship between

psychosocial stressors and medical complications such as hypertension and preterm delivery (Lu et al., 2003; MacKey et al., 2000). These complex problems require interprofessional collaborative approaches to address the medical and psychosocial issues that complicate the pregnancies of people in the United States and across the globe.

Initial and Continuing Risk Assessment

Risk assessment is a dynamic process that begins preconceptionally or at the first prenatal visit and continues throughout pregnancy (Public Health Service Expert Panel on the Content of Prenatal Care, 1989). Risk assessment "enables the prenatal care provider to determine whether the individual, their fetus or infant, or the family are at increased risk of failing to achieve the objectives of prenatal care and should provide a basis for intervention" (Public Health Service Expert Panel on the Content of Prenatal Care, 1989, p. 13; see Chapter 11, *Risk Assessment during Pregnancy*).

Health Promotion

Health promotion includes the education and counseling activities that are intended to assist an individual to attain, maintain, and enhance health; to support healthful behaviors; to increase knowledge about pregnancy, birth, and parenting; and to empower people to take an active role in their care during pregnancy. Individual and group sessions, as well as interpersonal interactions between individuals and their healthcare providers, can enhance health promotion during pregnancy (Enkin et al., 2000; Public Health Service Expert Panel on the Content of Prenatal Care, 1989).

Medical and Psychosocial Interventions and Follow-Up

Medical and psychosocial interventions refer to care strategies planned to cure or ameliorate identified risk factors or conditions diagnosed by the prenatal healthcare team. These interventions can be medically based, such as the treatment of an infection, or can address a psychosocial issue such as intimate partner violence (IPV) identified during pregnancy. Any treatment for an identified prenatal problem should always be evaluated for efficacy, improvement in symptoms, and amelioration of any adverse effects upon maternal and child health (Public Health Service Expert Panel on the Content of Prenatal Care, 1989). This follow-up is a critical aspect of providing prenatal care.

The Expert Panel recognized that the traditional "one-size-fits-all" prenatal care package does not adequately address the needs of all people. For example, the health education needs of nulliparous people are usually different from those of parous people, and people with medical or psychosocial risk factors can have an increased need for surveillance when compared to healthy, low-risk people. Creating individualized, targeted, and appropriate prenatal care and education has the potential to deliver optimal care to the individual and their family in a cost-effective manner. A standard prenatal record was recommended to allow for the smooth transfer of health information across health systems during pregnancy as well as for the collection and analysis of data across populations (Public Health Service Expert Panel on the Content of Prenatal Care, 1989). Electronic health records hold the promise of easier portability of health information from the office to the hospital, as well computer applications that provide decision support for the healthcare provider.

Finally, the panel identified that there was insufficient evidence to support many of the prenatal care practices that were common throughout pregnancy, while other care practices lacked rigorous evaluation. Recognizing that new prenatal care practices will be developed, the panel recommended systematic evaluation of prenatal care practices and policies for efficacy, cost, outcomes, and patient satisfaction (Public Health Service Expert Panel on the Content of Prenatal Care, 1989).

Updates to the "Content of Prenatal Care"

In 2005, an update to the CPC was completed, with a review of relevant literature since the original publication (Gregory et al., 2006). While the structure and overall goals of prenatal care have changed little, advances in genetic testing and prevention of preterm birth (PTB) as well as emerging infectious diseases have added new elements to prenatal care.

Recent decades have witnessed an increase in the knowledge of genetic diseases and options for testing to identify people at risk for these disorders. The identification of risk for genetically transmitted disorders ideally occurs prior to the pregnancy, which then allows for careful pregnancy planning, including the use of reproductive technologies for selected genetic conditions. With the advent of first-trimester screening and sequential screening in the first and second trimesters, adequate counseling for clients and their families regarding their individualized risk is important. Counseling for genetic screening for pregnant people and their families is complex and requires providers to be knowledgeable about risks, screening, testing, and referrals, and to be sensitive to the beliefs and preferences of the individual (see Chapter 13, *Genetic Counseling, Screening, and Diagnosis*).

The prevention of preterm labor and birth has also benefited from improvements to risk assessment. Advances in prematurity prevention require ongoing risk assessment and counseling to assist people in making decisions regarding their pregnancy care (see Chapter 35, *Spontaneous Preterm Birth*).

Emerging infectious diseases have required adaptation to prenatal care, as many infectious diseases increase the risk of maternal and/or neonatal complications or congenital anomalies. One example of significant change in prenatal care practices since the CPC was originally published is in the diagnosis, treatment, and prevention of vertical transmission of human immunodeficiency virus (HIV). Routine screening of all pregnant people for HIV is now recommended, and new treatment modalities and perinatal care practices have been effective in decreasing mother-to-child transmission. Rapid testing is now available, and current recommendations suggest an opt-out approach to testing, with the goal of universal HIV testing for all pregnant people. The 2015–2016 Zika virus epidemic required the development of new guidelines around the prevention of Zika and the clinical management of pregnant people with Zika virus infection (CDC, 2021). Likewise, the COVID-19 pandemic that began in 2020 introduced the need for additional counseling around COVID-19 vaccination during pregnancy and preventing infection during pregnancy (see Chapter 55, *Infectious Diseases*).

Despite these advances, pregnancy-related morbidity and mortality has increased over the last 20 years in the United States, one of only two countries in the world to demonstrate this (Commonwealth Fund, 2020). Causes of increased maternal mortality include preexisting maternal chronic illnesses, hemorrhage, infection, and thromboembolic disease (CDC, 2016). Other contributing factors include a lack of consistent protocols to deal with obstetric emergencies and a lack of consistent data collection measures across states (WHO, 2019). The **pregnancy-related maternal mortality** rate for 2020 was 23.8 deaths per 100,000 live births (Hoyert, 2022). There are huge disparities in pregnancy-related deaths: the maternal death rate for Black individuals (55.3 per 100,000 pregnancies) is 2.9 times the rate for White individuals (19.1) and three times the rate for Hispanic individuals (18.2; Hoyert, 2022). Only small improvements in infant mortality have been made, and Black infants had the highest infant mortality rate (10.5 per 1000 live births), almost twice that of White infants (4.8; March of Dimes, 2022a). Contributing factors for these disparities are complex and multifactorial, including differences in health insurance coverage and access to care as well as structural and systemic racism and discrimination (Artiga et al., 2020). However, prenatal care that is delivered well, recognizes the principles of reproductive justice to begin to account for the social determinants of health, and is tailored to meet the needs of individuals and populations offers an opportunity to address some of these issues.

Structure of Prenatal Care

In 1925, the first published prenatal care guidelines proposed a visit schedule recommending that pregnant people be seen by a physician every month for the first six months, then biweekly until the last month of pregnancy when visits should occur weekly (US Department of Labor: Children's Bureau, 1925). There was no information provided as to how this schedule was determined other than it "was only by intelligent compromise that such a group of physicians agree on what was essential for inclusion in the standards of prenatal care" (US Department of Labor: Children's Bureau, 1925, p. iii). Present-day prenatal care visit practices have changed little in regard to recommendations for when and how frequently people should engage in prenatal care. Despite the urging of the Expert Panel that the number and timing of visits should be reevaluated, prenatal care most often continues to reflect the 1925 guidelines. While the visit schedule has remained virtually unchanged, the recommendations for prenatal care content more often reflect the scientific and technological advances that have evolved to become common and accepted prenatal care practices.

There are many professional, governmental, and public health organizations that contribute to the current-day recommendations for the care of pregnant people and their families during the prenatal period. Professional organizations include the American College of Nurse-Midwives (ACNM), American Congress of Obstetrics and Gynecology (ACOG), the American Academy of Pediatrics (AAP), and the American College of Family Physicians (ACFP). Government agencies include the Agency for Healthcare Research and Quality (AHRQ), the US Preventive Services Task Force (USPSTF), and the Centers for Disease Control and Prevention (CDC). In 1983, the AAP and ACOG published the first guidelines for perinatal care, which summarized goals for prenatal care and provided clinicians with recommendations for care throughout the prenatal, intrapartum, postpartum, and neonatal periods for patients, children, and their families. Regular updates have continued, with the most recent prenatal care guidelines published in 2017.

The Schedule of Prenatal Visits

Evidence suggests that the preconception visit can mitigate selected health, nutritional, and behavioral concerns prior to pregnancy (Beckmann et al., 2014). However, just under half of all pregnancies are unplanned, resulting from contraceptive failures or nonuse of contraception. Thus, the concept of preconception care needs to be introduced to all people capable of pregnancy during primary care. Prenatal care initiated in the first trimester can result in improved health outcomes for the parent and infant (Robbins & Martocci, 2020). AAP/ACOG (2017) recommend that care begin in the first trimester of pregnancy. Healthy People 2030, a set of national objectives to improve health and well-being over the next decade, includes increasing the proportion of pregnant people who receive early and adequate prenatal care as one of its objectives for preventing pregnancy complications and maternal deaths (US Department of Health and Human Services, Office of Disease Prevention and Health Promotion, n.d.). In 2021, 75.6% of pregnant people began prenatal care in the first trimester of pregnancy, an increase from recent years although this varies by age, race, and ethnicity (US Department of Health and Human Services, Office of Disease Prevention and Health Promotion, 2021); medically vulnerable and underserved populations were less likely to begin prenatal care in the first trimester (Robbins & Martocci, 2020).

The Expert Panel and AAP/ACOG recommended that prenatal care should be tailored to meet individual medical, psychosocial, and educational needs. Nulliparous people are expected to have greater educational needs than multiparous people; however, all clients require ongoing risk assessment. The Expert Panel suggested that fewer visits, with more emphasis on education and health promotion, were appropriate for low-risk patients. They postulated that people who received education about pregnancy, healthy behaviors, and symptoms of pregnancy complications would require fewer visits, utilize community resources when appropriate, and be well prepared for birth and parenting (Public Health Service Expert Panel on the Content of Prenatal Care, 1989; see Table 8.1). However, in low- and middle-income countries, evidence emerged that the focused antenatal care model of four goal-oriented visits that was developed in the 1990s was associated with more perinatal deaths than models with more frequent visits. In 2016, the World Health Organization changed its recommendations from four visits to eight *contacts* (a word chosen for connotations of connection; WHO, 2016). In many contexts, contacts may include routine prenatal care visits as well as community outreach programs and lay health worker involvement. However, one study found the pooled prevalence of 8 or more prenatal care contacts in 15 countries was just 13.0% due to inadequate infrastructure, poor levels of education, poverty, and cost of services (Ekholuenetale, 2021). In high-income countries, a reduced number of visits (typically from the standard 12 visits down to 8 visits) reduced costs and was not associated with increased perinatal morbidity, but did decrease patient satisfaction (Dowswell et al., 2015).

Table 8.1 Recommended Prenatal Visit Schedule

	Expert Panel on Content of Prenatal Care (1989)[a]	AAP and ACOG (2017)
	Preconception visit	Preconception visit
First visit	6–8 wk	Prior to 12 wk
Second visit	Within 4 wk	16 wk
Third visit	14–16 wk	20 wk
Fourth visit	24–28 wk	24 wk
Fifth visit	32 wk	28 wk
	32–38 wk (childbirth classes)	
Sixth visit	36 wk	30 wk
Seventh visit	38 wk	32 wk
Eighth visit	40 wk	34 wk
Ninth visit	41 wk	36 wk
Tenth visit		37 wk
Eleventh visit		38 wk
Twelfth visit		39 wk
Thirteenth visit		40 wk

Source: Adapted from Bloch et al. (2009); AAP/ACOG (2017); Public Health Service Expert Panel on the Content of Prenatal Care (1989).
[a] Low-risk, primiparous individuals.

How Much Prenatal Care Is Enough?

What constitutes enough prenatal care? In the late 1960s, data collection regarding the timing of the initiation of prenatal care and the number of prenatal visits began with the addition of this information to the Certificate of Live Birth. Subsequently, there have been several attempts to determine how best to measure the adequacy of prenatal care. Such information can be used to assist researchers and policy makers in the assessment of the sufficiency of prenatal care resources, the effectiveness of prenatal care in addressing morbidities and mortalities, and the identification of areas for research and changes in health policies. The ACOG recommends completing 12–14 visits throughout the pregnancy with a minimum of 9 visits to be considered adequate (AAP/ACOG, 2017; Alexander & Kotelchuck, 1998; Stringer, 1998). The Kessner Index, developed in the 1970s with support from the Institute of Medicine (IOM), considers in what trimester care was initiated, how many prenatal visits were attended, and when the infant was born (Alexander & Kotelchuck, 1998; Institute of Medicine, 2001; Bloch et al., 2009; Stringer, 1998). Care was deemed to be adequate if the number of prenatal visits at birth met or exceeded ACOG recommendations, while inadequate care was defined as less than 50% of the adequate visit criteria. Later, the Adequacy of Prenatal Care Utilization (APNCU) Index was developed by Kotelchuck (1994), proposing separate assessments based on when prenatal care was initiated and how many visits occurred between start of care and giving birth. All of these indices are commonly used in research and evaluation of prenatal care, but they address the quantity, not the quality, of care.

What Happens in Prenatal Care?

The number of prenatal care encounters a person receives only provides a snapshot of the quantity of care. While some evidence suggests that more prenatal care visits may result in improved outcomes for pregnant people and infants, the quality of prenatal care also has an influence on health and psychosocial outcomes. The Expert Panel examined the content of care and developed a framework for organizing prenatal care based on available evidence. Their recommendations for risk assessment included the assessment of maternal blood pressure and laboratory studies. Interventions that resulted in improved maternal and/or infant outcomes included avoidance of substance use, nutritional information, appropriate weight gain in pregnancy, vitamin/mineral supplementation, and breastfeeding support and advice (Public Health Service Expert Panel on the Content of Prenatal Care, 1989). Ideally, the provision of appropriate health promotion content during pregnancy supports changes in maternal behavior. For example, if a pregnant person who smokes is provided with information regarding the dangers of smoking and is given resources to curtail or quit smoking, the expectation is that they will either stop or attempt to stop smoking. However, health behaviors are complex and change is based on more than just knowledge.

Providing all the recommended health information and verifying the person's understanding during prenatal care visits is challenging in the current model of prenatal care due to time constraints in the clinical setting. An early study, which looked at a large population of almost 1000 women, found that only 32% reported receiving all the recommended prenatal advice (Kogan et al., 1994b). Another study with the same population found that people who did not receive all the recommended health advice during pregnancy were at higher risk for delivering a low-birth-weight (LBW) baby (Kogan et al., 1994a). Research continues to evaluate the adequacy of prenatal care and outcomes, with linkages established between inadequate prenatal care and very LBW infants, as well as inadequate maternal weight gain (Xaverius et al., 2016). In today's healthcare environments, pregnant people and their families obtain much of the essential prenatal education through Internet sources of varying accuracy and reliability (Wexler et al., 2020).

Integrating Quality into Prenatal Care

In 2001, the IOM released a landmark report focusing on the changes needed in the US healthcare system to improve safety and quality across all healthcare settings. Their recommendations were intended to serve as a framework to be used by the government, health insurers, healthcare providers, and consumers as they prepared for a 21st century healthcare system. Their recommendations included the following:

- *Safe*—avoiding injuries to patients from the care that is intended to help them
- *Effective*—providing services based on scientific knowledge to all who could benefit and refraining from providing services to those not likely to benefit (avoiding underuse and overuse, respectively)
- *Patient-centered*—providing care that is respectful of and responsive to individual patient preferences, needs, and values and ensuring that patient values guide all clinical decisions
- *Timely*—reducing waits and sometimes harmful delays for both those who receive and those who give care
- *Efficient*—avoiding waste, including waste of equipment, supplies, ideas, and energy
- *Equitable*—providing care that does not vary in quality because of personal characteristics such as gender, ethnicity, geographic location, and socioeconomic status

While the recommendations of the IOM for improving the quality of care are not complex, the ability of the healthcare system to adapt to the needed changes has been poor. Despite evidence about the quantity and the quality of prenatal care, perinatal morbidity and mortality statistics have not significantly improved, and in many sectors, undesirable outcomes have actually increased. For example, approximately 1 in 10 babies (10.1% of live births) in the United States were born preterm in 2020 (March of Dimes, 2022a).

The US Preventative Services Task Force (USPSTF) is an independent panel of experts who make evidence-based recommendations about clinical preventive services. As of February 2022, the USPSTF (n.d.) recommends with a Grade A or B recommendation (high or moderate certainty of benefit) the following directly related to prenatal care:

- Screening for gestational diabetes in asymptomatic pregnant persons at 24 weeks of gestation or after.
- Use of low-dose aspirin (81 mg/day) as preventive medication after 12 weeks of gestation in persons who are at high risk for preeclampsia.
- Screening for asymptomatic bacteriuria using urine culture in pregnant persons.
- Providing interventions during pregnancy and after birth to support breastfeeding.
- Screening for depression in the general adult population, including pregnant and postpartum people. Screening should be implemented with adequate systems in place to ensure accurate diagnosis, effective treatment, and appropriate follow-up.
- All people who are planning or capable of pregnancy take a daily supplement containing 0.4–0.8 mg (400–800 μg) of folic acid.
- Clinicians offer pregnant persons effective behavioral counseling interventions aimed at promoting healthy weight gain and preventing excess gestational weight gain in pregnancy.
- Screening for hepatitis B virus (HBV) infection in pregnant people at their first prenatal visit.
- Screen for HIV infection in all pregnant persons, including those who present in labor or at delivery whose HIV status is unknown.
- Screen for IPV in people of reproductive age and provide or refer people who screen positive to ongoing support services.
- Prophylactic ocular topical medication for all newborns to prevent gonococcal ophthalmia neonatorum.
- Provide or refer pregnant and postpartum persons who are at increased risk of perinatal depression to counseling interventions.
- Screening for preeclampsia in pregnant people with blood pressure measurements throughout pregnancy.
- Rh(D) blood typing and antibody testing for all pregnant people during their first visit for pregnancy-related care; repeated Rh(D) antibody testing for all unsensitized Rh(D)-negative people at 24–28 weeks of gestation, unless the partner or donor is known to be Rh(D)-negative.
- Behavioral counseling for all sexually active adolescents and for adults who are at increased risk for sexually transmitted infections (STIs).
- Early screening for syphilis infection in all pregnant people.
- Ask all pregnant persons about tobacco use, advise them to stop using tobacco, and provide behavioral interventions for cessation to pregnant persons who use tobacco.

Addressing Disparities in Prenatal Care

As discussed above, there are substantial racial and socioeconomic disparities in birth and neonatal outcomes, largely driven by a long history of racism in maternal and newborn healthcare. While access to prenatal care is an important factor in addressing disparities, a recent study found that access to adequate prenatal care alone does not reduce racial disparities in PTB (Thurston et al., 2021); the authors suggest a need to look beyond access to care and focus on quality and responsiveness of service provision as well as interventions that focus on multiple dimensions of health. This recommendation aligns with other research showing that not all racial and ethnic groups receive comparable care. For example, Latinx and Black people are less likely to receive recommended prenatal care content than White people (Artiga et al., 2020; Kogan et al., 1994b; Vonderheid et al., 2003, 2007). Approaches that recognize the principles of reproductive justice may help address some of the social determinants of health (see Chapter 1, *Health Equity*). For example, racially concordant care is being evaluated as an option (see below for further discussion). As noted above, historical developments in prenatal care had profound implications for the racial makeup of the prenatal care workforce, particularly the midwifery workforce.

Another major disparity in prenatal care is the rural/urban divide. In the last decade and a half, a significant number of rural hospitals have closed or discontinued obstetric care due to low birth volumes, low revenue levels due to high rates of Medicaid coverage, and difficulty in attracting and retaining obstetric providers (Center for Medicare and Medicaid Services [CMS], 2019). Fewer than 50% of rural individuals have access to perinatal services, including prenatal care, within a 30-mile drive from their home, and 10% must drive 100 miles or more (CMS, 2019). These conditions are more pronounced in Black and Hispanic communities; low-income individuals are also more affected. Interventions such as expanded use of telehealth services in pregnancy, reimbursement of transportation costs, perinatal regionalization networks that set up care referral system in advance of emergencies when higher level of care is needed, and increasing incentives for providers to practice in areas designated as "**maternity care deserts**" are all aimed at addressing the increased mortality rates seen in rural areas (March of Dimes, 2022b).

Group Prenatal Care: CenteringPregnancy

CenteringPregnancy is a group model of prenatal care that was developed and implemented in 1993 by Sharon Schindler Rising, a nurse-midwife. The ensuing decades have seen a rapid uptake of this group model among prenatal care providers, including midwives, obstetricians, nurse practitioners, and family medicine physicians. CenteringPregnancy builds on the Expert Panel recommendations and combines the essentials of risk assessment, education, and support and bundles prenatal services into a cohesive model of care (Rising, 1998; Rising et al., 2004). In CenteringPregnancy, 8–12 individuals with similar due dates are invited to join a group after their initial prenatal visit. Group members learn self-care skills such as measuring their own weight, blood pressure, and gestational age, and then recording this information in their medical record. This self-assessment is followed by a short individual assessment with their prenatal care provider in the group space and includes assessment of fundal height, fetal position and presentation, fetal heart sounds, and maternal well-being. Concerns and questions are brought to the group for discussion. Healthy snacks and opportunities for socializing among group participants build community and provide peer support for all members.

Group care changes the paradigm of traditional healthcare and builds on the recommendation of the IOM for redesigning healthcare. Groups are patient-centered as the group directs conversations to issues that are important and relevant to their lives and experiences. Groups are efficient for clients, their providers, and health systems. They are planned well in advance so that clients know when all their prenatal appointments will be and health centers can utilize individual exam room space for seeing other patients. Groups are efficient for healthcare providers who need to convey important information only once and other prenatal care services such as social work and lactation support can be bundled into the group setting. Groups always start and end on time, so the time is productive for the client and the prenatal care provider. Group care also provides new opportunities for culturally and/or racially concordant and specific centering care, such as the BElovedBIRTH Black Centering operated by the Alameda (California) Public Health Department. This all Black midwifery-led interprofessional team provides all the benefits of centering as well as improved communication, greater sense of safety and trust, and reduced risk of racial bias/discrimination (Alameda Health System, n.d.).

The potential benefits of CenteringPregnancy continue to be studied with mixed results. A recent systematic review found that CenteringPregnancy had no effect on preterm delivery or birth weight but a reduced rate of postpartum depression at six months compared to standard prenatal obstetric care (Liu et al., 2021). Byerley & Haas (2017) found some benefit to CenteringPregnancy for certain high-risk groups. In the largest randomized controlled trial (RCT) to date, over 1000 women enrolled in group care had a 33% reduction in risk of premature birth when compared to women in individual care (Ickovics et al., 2007). When Black women were evaluated in this study, their risk of premature birth was 41% lower than those enrolled in individual care. Women in groups were more satisfied with their care, initiated breastfeeding more frequently, and felt better prepared for labor, birth, and parenting (Ickovics et al., 2007). Similarly, Gareau et al. (2016), in a large retrospective study of 1262 women in group care, found reductions in relative risk of prematurity (by 36%) and LBW (by 44%) when compared to those in individual care. The authors also estimated that

CenteringPregnancy would result in a savings of over $450,000 per facility based on these reductions. A retrospective analysis found that adolescents enrolled in group care had increased attendance at healthcare visits, lower rates of PTB and LBW babies, and were more satisfied with their care (Grady & Bloom, 2004). When the model was implemented in a large urban public health setting, women in groups were found to have higher rates of attendance at prenatal care visits, improved pregnancy weight gain, and higher satisfaction with care; healthcare providers also believed the model to be effective for patient education and to provide the opportunity for learning and social support (Klima et al., 2009). Group care also has an effect in the postpartum period. Women enrolled in group prenatal care were more likely to be utilizing family planning services in the first year after birth than women enrolled in individual care (Hale et al., 2014).

Making Group Prenatal Care Work

As group care changes how healthcare is delivered, system change is necessary and healthcare providers and support staff require training to become facilitative leaders. Experience suggests that involving key stakeholders within an organization helps create a climate of change that supports CenteringPregnancy. The Centering Healthcare Institute (CHI) is the nonprofit organization that supports healthcare systems and providers to adapt to a new model of group care. Healthcare providers and staff who plan to facilitate group care must attend training sessions to learn group skills and facilitative leadership and to gain practical experience in conducting CenteringPregnancy groups. Health systems must adapt to changes in scheduling systems and work duties and may even adapt physical space to accommodate groups. The CenteringPregnancy model is based on three components, which include Healthcare, Interactive Learning, and Community Building. There are nine defining elements that inform these components and guide health systems and providers to implement and conduct CenteringPregnancy groups. Together, these define the group healthcare experience and reflect the recommendations of the Expert Panel on Prenatal Care as well as the recommendations for healthcare redesign from the IOM (Table 8.2).

Other Alternative Models of Prenatal Care Delivery

While CenteringPregnancy is the most widely available and evaluated alternative model of prenatal care delivery, other innovative models have been developed. Two of these are the JJ Way and HealthConnect One (HC One) Community-Based Doula Program. The JJ Way was created by midwife Jennie Joseph, is currently offered in Florida, and uses a patient-centered, team-based model focused on developing relationships and addressing barriers to care. An initial evaluation found lower rates of preterm and LBW births than the county and state

Table 8.2   Group Care Components and Defining Elements

Component	Defining element
Healthcare	Health assessment occurs in the group space.
	People are involved in self-care activities.
	There is ongoing evaluation.
Interactive learning	Groups are facilitated to be interactive.
	Groups are conducted in a circle.
	Each session has a plan, but emphasis may vary.
	Group size is optimal to promote the process.
Community building	Group members, including facilitators and support people are consistent.
	There is time for socializing and relationship building.

Source: Adapted from Rising and Quimby (2017).

average and eliminated racial disparities in PTB (Novoa, 2020). While the HC One program does not directly provide prenatal care, it provides doulas that accompany pregnant clients to prenatal appointments to provide support and help bridge cultural and structural barriers. Initial evaluation has shown that Black and Hispanic individuals who participated in HC One were less likely to have a cesarean section and more likely to exclusively breastfeed and for longer (AMCHP, 2015). Novoa (2020) notes that what these programs and CenteringPregnancy all have in common is increased access to high-quality preventive care, critical social support through relationship-centered care, and family empowerment.

Components of Prenatal Care Assessment

Prenatal assessment refers to the collection of medical, nutritional, obstetrical, psychosocial, and family histories, as well as physical assessment of the client and fetus. Laboratory studies collected at the initial and subsequent prenatal visits assess selected aspects of maternal and fetal health at the onset of prenatal care, as well as affirmation of ongoing wellness and early detection of pathology. Physical assessment of the client is comprehensive and includes a complete physical exam along with a more targeted exam of the reproductive system at entry into prenatal care. Episodic physical assessment occurs at subsequent prenatal visits and focuses on pregnancy-related changes and overall physical well-being with special attention to potential signs of pregnancy complications. Targeted physical assessments are performed whenever there are signs and symptoms of emerging problems or coexisting disorders. Additionally, the assessment of the fetus is ongoing throughout the pregnancy. Ultrasound screening is commonly performed as indicated to verify viable intrauterine pregnancy, confirm or assign gestational age, assess fetal anatomy, and measure fetal growth and development. Finally, the assessment of past and current psychosocial issues, including mental health status, substance abuse, IPV, and environmental issues such as housing, socioeconomic concerns, and safety, is addressed at entry into care and at each subsequent visit. Risk assessment is integral to each prenatal encounter to evaluate the presence or absence of factors or conditions associated with adverse perinatal outcomes for the pregnant person and or fetus/infant.

While risk assessment is an important component of prenatal care, there is no standardized system that accurately predicts individual risk. The evaluation of risk is confounded due to the complexity of numerous variables, their interactions with each other, and the fact that some conditions may be more highly associated with adverse outcomes than others. Concentrating prenatal resources solely on pregnant people with risk factors may adversely affect those who have been deemed low risk. Pregnant people can experience an adverse outcome without any identifiable risk factors. Some conditions, such as tobacco abuse, are well studied with known sequelae; however, not every pregnant person who smokes experiences these adverse outcomes. Other conditions, such as maternal obesity, may be less well studied or do not have easily implemented interventions to address the identified risks (see Chapter 46, *Obesity in the Perinatal Period*). Risks that involve long-standing habits or lifestyle preferences require a readiness to make behavior change on the part of the individual and persistent effort in creating and maintaining this behavior change (refer to Chapter 11, *Risk Assessment during Pregnancy*).

Health History: Initial Visit

Ideally, the maternal history is obtained at a preconception visit so that health conditions and health behaviors that can adversely affect pregnancy are identified, discussed, and ameliorated. The Expert Panel on Prenatal Care reviewed all components of the health history as well as the scientific evidence for the components of the health history that may impact maternal and fetal pregnancy outcome. With few exceptions, reviewing the health history at the onset of prenatal care is an important activity and is an integral component of evaluating risk status and planning for comprehensive care. The health history not only provides a snapshot of past and current health status but also identifies health behaviors that can negatively impact the pregnancy and can be impacted during the pregnancy. The knowledge of the health history allows healthcare providers to tailor the care in pregnancy to specific health risks and educational opportunities (Table 8.3). In some cases (e.g., prior cesarean section and other previous pregnancy and medical complications), attempts should be made to obtain medical records.

Pregnancy dating is an important activity during the first prenatal visit and the menstrual history is a critical component of this assessment. Ascertaining the last normal menstrual period (LMP) is the first step in determining the gestational age. The reliability of this measure

Table 8.3   Medical and Psychosocial Prenatal History Content

Content	Health information collected
Sociodemographic	Name, age, racial/ethnic group, relationship status, insurance status, emergency contact information
Menstrual history	Menarche, date of last menstrual period (LMP), regularity, frequency, and length of menses, length and character of LMP, bleeding, or spotting since LMP
Past pregnancy history	Gravidity, parity, history of live births, preterm births, miscarriages (circumstances), abortions, stillbirths (circumstances) and living children; history of ectopic pregnancy; pregnancy complications; type of birth (vaginal birth, operative vaginal birth, cesarean section, vaginal birth after cesarean section [VBAC]) and labor/birth complications; history of infertility; and any infertility treatments
Contraceptive history	Previous method use, date of last use
Sexual history	Onset of sexual activity, number of partners, current partner, past/current partner behavior risks, sexual practices, use of safer-sex practices; history of sexually transmitted infections of self and partner, including treatment
Medical/surgical history	Preexisting chronic or episodic maternal medical conditions, especially those that may adversely affect the current pregnancy. These include but are not limited to hypertension, diabetes, thyroid disease, cardiac disease, blood disorders, respiratory illness, and gastrointestinal disorders. Past and current treatments should be obtained. Surgical history includes all relevant surgeries that may impact pregnancy, especially any uterine surgery
Infection history	Common childhood illnesses; communicable diseases
Family/genetic history	Three-generation family pedigree; medical history in first-degree relatives, especially for conditions with familial tendencies such as diabetes; mental, behavioral, and cognitive disorders, atypical physical features or problems, chromosomal anomalies, single gene conditions, consanguinity
Nutrition	Overall dietary history, access to food, vitamin/mineral supplementation, special dietary concerns, vegetarianism, fish intake, exposure to teratogens or infectious agents, history of eating disorders
Smoking	Onset, amount, exposure to second-hand smoke
Alcohol	Onset, amount, duration of use, type of alcohol, family history, dependence. Screening tools are available
Substance use	Type of drug and how it is used; onset, duration, and amount; related behaviors such as sex for drugs or needle-sharing
Social support	Multiple measures, depression, family, relationship
Stress	Multiple measures, acute versus chronic, coping, and support resources, external resources, amenable to interventions, community stressors, financial resources
Intimate partner violence	History, current abuse, type, and severity, resources, children, readiness for intervention, safety plan
Mental health	History or current mental illness, past, and current treatment, medications, safety, potential for self-harm, or harm to others
Teratogen exposure	Environmental, occupational, medication, herbs, home, pets
Occupational	Type of work, heavy lifting, repetitive work tasks, hours per day per week, exposure to chemical or environmental hazards
Activity/exercise	Exercise, type and frequency, resources for increasing activity level, limitations

can be affected by maternal recall, history of irregular menses, recent contraceptive use, lactation, or medication use.

In the early 1880s, German obstetrician Dr. Franz Karl Naegele determined that the mean gestational age of human pregnancy was 280 days or 40 weeks and suggested that the estimated date of birth (EDB) could be established by subtracting 3 months and adding 1 week to the date of the first day of the LMP. Ninety percent of all pregnant people with a known LMP will deliver by the forty-first

week using Naegele's rule. Mean human gestational length has been estimated at ranges between 281 and 287 days with the average being 283 days, somewhat greater than the estimate based on Naegele's rule.

Accurate dating of the pregnancy is critical to the identification of a reliable EDB, accurately interpreting selected prenatal genetic laboratory screening, effectively caring for pregnant people who experience preterm labor or post-term pregnancy, and reducing risks associated with procedures and interventions. Gestational age wheels are commonly used by healthcare providers to calculate the estimated gestational age of the pregnancy; however, slight variations among wheels are common, and the wheels are based on a standard 28-day menstrual cycle. Numerous electronic methods of calculating the gestational age of the pregnancy have supplemented the traditional wheels for calculation of gestational age and due date. Similarly, electronic health records can determine gestational age based on clinical data and can provide consistency across health systems. Ultrasound in early pregnancy is recommended when the LMP is unknown or unreliable (see Chapter 10, *Pregnancy Diagnosis and Gestational Age Assessment*).

The *pregnancy history* will identify any previous pregnancy-related conditions that can impact the current pregnancy. When eliciting the pregnancy history, it is important to explore the circumstances of all pregnancy losses, gestational age at which they occurred, what precipitated the loss, and what, if any, evaluation occurred after the loss, such as genetic testing or autopsy. This information will highlight the potential risk for chromosomal abnormalities, premature labor, or other pregnancy conditions likely to recur. Any operative procedures such as cesarean section are evaluated, along with the indications for the surgery, the stage of labor, and any complications arising from the operative intervention. A history of infertility treatments and assisted reproductive technologies can alert the provider to an increased risk for multifetal pregnancy as well as need for psychosocial and counseling related to increased levels of stress (Velez et al., 2019).

Sexual history provides an opportunity to evaluate risk for STIs and sexual practices that can continue to increase risk for the pregnant person and fetus. The sexual history should be elicited with a nonjudgmental approach using the approach laid out in Chapter 21, *Sexuality*.

The *infection history* will identify preexisting immunity and risks for infection during the pregnancy and the need for immunization during and after pregnancy. Depending on the history of childhood disease and immunization, a pregnant person may have immunity to infections, be at risk for infections, or require targeted education to avoid infectious diseases during the pregnancy. Planning for prenatal and postpartum immunizations will help decrease the risk of selected infectious diseases throughout the lifespan and during future pregnancies.

Family history encompasses the evaluation for medical conditions that can place the pregnant person at a higher risk during pregnancy and may require additional screening and/or evaluation during pregnancy. For example, a client with a first-degree relative with diabetes and one other risk factor like obesity may be at higher risk for diabetes or gestational diabetes and may require early screening (Salmeen, 2016). Genetic histories that are significant for familial or hereditary diseases will alert the provider to the need for additional counseling, testing, or referral to a genetic counselor. Clients are provided with accurate information regarding personalized risk, screening, pregnancy options, benefits and harms of

testing options, and any potential outcomes related to the particular genetic problem. While genetic issues can be complex, all prenatal care providers need skills to discuss basic genetic counseling and testing and to perform a basic three-generation pedigree with genetic history. Numerous resources exist for providers to become more proficient regarding the genetic components of prenatal care, such as the March of Dimes and the International Society of Nurses in Genetics (ISONG; see Chapter 13, *Genetic Counseling, Screening, and Diagnosis*).

Nutritional history provides an assessment of the current diet and nutritional status of a pregnant person, ascertains dietary practices that may impact the pregnancy, and identifies dietary deficiencies that may be amenable to interventions. For example, people who eat a vegan diet may require additional sources of protein, vitamins, and minerals to meet the recommended allowances for pregnancy. People who report consuming foods that can negatively impact pregnancy, such as eating certain fish species, raw meat, or certain cheeses, may be at increased risk for exposure to toxins or infectious diseases and need targeted information to make the necessary dietary changes. Household food insecurity should be assessed, and counseling should reflect realistic access to food sources, cultural and ethnic preferences and practices, and referrals to programs such as the Special Supplemental Nutrition Program for Women, Infants, and Child (WIC; see Chapter 9, *Nutrition during Pregnancy*).

The *psychosocial history* explores life and work concerns and can highlight areas for support, education, and additional resources. Stress from aspects of life such as family, work, or finances and lack of social support can impact pregnancy outcomes. There is also an increasing awareness of the role of intergenerational trauma on stress and its contribution to health disparities. As an intersection between generations, pregnancy, and postpartum can be an optimal time to provide trauma-informed care (Sperlich et al., 2017). It is important to offer opportunities for patients to discuss stress and coping mechanisms, as well as their support systems and broader contextual and community factors that may impact them. This is accomplished through dialogue and open-ended questioning throughout the pregnancy; tools can be used to quantitatively measure stress and coping. The psychosocial history will provide direction for targeted resources that may be needed. It is important for prenatal care providers to become familiar with community resources and agencies that can provide necessary services during pregnancy. The psychosocial history takes place at the initial visit and then is regularly updated at subsequent prenatal visits.

Health History: Subsequent Visits

At each subsequent prenatal visit, the provider continues to assess the client for signs and symptoms associated with common pregnancy problems. Changes in lifestyle, circumstances, exposures, and recent illness are also assessed. Interventions to promote maternal and fetal health discussed at prior visits are evaluated for efficacy. Common pregnancy changes and discomforts are explored. A review of the psychosocial history is completed with periodic assessment of violence, depression, and substance use. Prior to term, symptoms of preterm labor, vaginal bleeding, or leakage of amniotic fluid are often inquired about at each visit.

Physical Assessment

Initial Visit

A general physical examination is conducted on all clients at the first prenatal visit. Since pregnancy affects all body systems, each system is evaluated and the findings recorded. Measuring height and weight on all clients is beneficial, along with calculation of the prepregnant body mass index (BMI). Prepregnancy weight is important as it will guide the recommendations for weight gain during the pregnancy, though this should be done in broader consideration of the client's overall health, well-being, and nutritional needs. Some clients may prefer not to be weighed at all, and this should be respected. Blood pressure, pulse, and respirations are measured on all clients at the initial visit. A pelvic exam to assess for uterine size is especially important in early pregnancy, before 12–14 weeks, and can help in confirming gestational age. Clinical pelvimetry, although commonly done at the initial visit, was studied by the Expert Panel and was found to have poor evidence supporting its efficacy (Public Health Service Expert Panel on the Content of Prenatal Care, 1989). However, it may be useful to assess pelvic adequacy in late pregnancy or during labor. Auscultation of the fetal heart sounds with a handheld Doppler ultrasound device can begin at 10–12 weeks of gestation, although the heart sounds may be heard earlier depending upon maternal habitus and the position of the uterus. The assessment of the location of the fundus can begin when the uterus becomes an abdominal organ sometime after the 12th week of pregnancy. The measurement of fundal height provides information regarding the growing uterus; however, its accuracy is limited by the skill of the clinician, maternal characteristics such as the status of the maternal bladder or abdominal adiposity, and the angle of the examination table. The most common way to measure fundal height is to place a tape measure on the superior border of the symphysis pubis and to bring the tape measure across the contour of the abdomen, in the midline, to the top of the fundus. Using this method, the centimeters should approximately equal (±2 cm) the weeks of gestation after 20 weeks of gestation.

Subsequent Visits

At each subsequent visit, blood pressure and weight are obtained. Weight gain since the last visit and since the onset of pregnancy can inform the client and their provider about the adequacy and pattern of weight gain. Fundal height in centimeters is measured at each visit, along with locating and counting the fetal heart rate. The assessment of client perception of fetal movement usually begins in the second trimester and is determined at each visit. Auscultation of the fetal heart rate using a handheld Doppler ultrasound device can begin as early as 10 weeks and at 16–20 weeks if using a fetoscope. Beginning in the third trimester, Leopold maneuvers are performed. These maneuvers are a series of abdominal examinations that can help the prenatal care provider determine the fetal lie, presentation, position, and engagement of the fetal presenting part into the pelvis. The abdominal exam can also assist the healthcare provider in estimating the fetal weight. Routine cervical examination is not recommended until the 41st week of pregnancy by the Expert Panel but may be appropriate earlier in people at risk for preterm labor (Public Health Service Expert Panel on the Content of Prenatal Care, 1989). The Expert Panel found insufficient evidence to recommend routine urine screening for protein and glucose at each prenatal visit in the absence of symptoms of preeclampsia or infection (Public Health Service Expert Panel on the Content of Prenatal Care, 1989); The ACOG currently states that evidence has not shown a benefit in routine urine screening in the absence of risk factors for urinary tract infections, renal disease, and preeclampsia and in the absence of symptoms of urinary tract infection, hypertension, or unusual edema (ACOG, 2017).

Laboratory Assessment

Routine laboratory screening at the first prenatal visit is important in the diagnosis of anemia, certain infections, and determination of the Rh factor. Subsequent to the Expert Panel, recommendations for additional laboratory studies have been suggested due to new evidence of their association with improved pregnancy outcomes. Numerous organizations and professional organizations contribute to the recommendations for laboratory testing during pregnancy. Not all types of testing are available to all clients due to geographic location, financial resources, insurance coverage, or site of care. Current recommendations for routine laboratory studies and appropriate timing are found in Table 8.4.

Genetic Screening

Prenatal genetic screening has expanded significantly since the Expert Panel reviewed the scientific literature. Some genetic screening is routinely offered to all pregnant people, while other tests are offered to selected groups based on demographic or other risk factors. All discussions regarding genetic testing should be based on the principles of shared decision making with the client and/or their family. Informed consent is necessary to ensure that the pregnant person understands the voluntary nature of genetic testing, the purpose of the test, the limitations of the test, what they will do with the information, and what the implications are for themself, their baby, and future pregnancies. It is important to remember that screening tests are not diagnostic tests. Clients with abnormal screening results are offered confirmation with a

Table 8.4 Recommended Laboratory Studies in Pregnancy

Laboratory study and condition screened for or reason for test	When	Population to be screened	Recommended by whom	Evidence
Hemoglobin or hematocrit, for anemia	Initial, 24–28 wk, and 36 wk in selected populations	All	EPPC	Good
Blood type, Rh factor[a] and antibody testing	Initial	All	EPPC USPHTF ACOG	Good, A, B
Rubella titer	Initial	All	EPPC	Good
Urine dipstick for protein and glucose	Initial	All	EPPC	Good
Purified protein derivative (PPD) skin test or QuantiFERON gold for latent tuberculosis infection	Initial	At risk	EPPC ACOG	Fair
Gonorrhea culture	Initial and 36 wk	Under age 25 and those at risk	EPPC USPHTF ACOG	Good B
Chlamydia[b] culture	Initial and 36 wk	All	EPPC USPSTF	Good B
Rapid plasma reagin (RPR) or venereal disease research laboratory (VDRL) test for syphilis[c]	Initial and 24–28 wk	All	EPPC USPSTF ACOG	Good A
Urine culture for asymptomatic bacteriuria	12–16 wk or first visit	All	USPSTF	Good A
Hepatitis B surface antigen (HBsAg)	Initial	All	EPPC USPSTF ACOG	Good A
HIV (opt out)	Initial	All	EPPC USPSTF ACOG	Good A
Cervical cytology with or without human papillomavirus (HPV) co-testing, for cervical cancer screening	When indicated by age and previous testing	Age 21 and over, every 3–5 yr, depending on age and past screening	ASCCP	Good
Herpes[d] antibodies for evidence of previous infection	Initial	Selected populations	EPPC	Fair, D
Varicella antibodies for evidence of previous infection or immunization	Initial based on history	All	EPPC	Fair
Hemoglobin electrophoresis for hemoglobinopathies (e.g., sickle cell trait, and thalassemia)	Initial	Selected populations	EPPC	Good
Toxoplasmosis antibodies for evidence of previous infection	Initial	Selected populations	EPPC	Good
Urine toxicology for drug screening (offered)	Initial	All	EPPC	Good
Gestational diabetes mellitus screening	24–28 wk	All	USPSTF ACOG	B
Group B streptococcal colonization	35–37 wk	All	ACOG	Good

Recommended by either the Expert Panel on Prenatal Care (EPPC), US Preventative Services Task Force (USPSTF), or ACOG. EPPC labeled evidence as good, fair, and poor, USPSTF rates evidence as A, B, C with A being the highest level of evidence.
[a] The Expert Panel did not include blood type, but it is routinely assessed on all pregnant people in the United States.
[b] Chlamydia is now routinely tested concurrently with gonorrhea. In selected populations, rescreening at 36 wk may be indicated.
[c] Syphilis may be repeated in selected populations at 24–28 wk.
[d] The USPSTF recommends against screening asymptomatic people at any time during pregnancy.

diagnostic test such as chorionic villus testing or amniocentesis (ACOG, 2016; see Chapter 13, *Genetic Counseling, Screening, and Diagnosis*).

Diagnostic Testing

Diagnostic testing in prenatal care was not evaluated by the Expert Panel; however, the use of diagnostic testing has increased significantly over the last decade. Ultrasound is the most commonly used diagnostic test in pregnancy and can provide information about many normal events as well as abnormal processes. First-trimester ultrasound is an accurate way to confirm viability of pregnancy, determine pregnancy location, and estimate gestational age in the absence of a reliable LMP. Ultrasound also plays a role in genetic screening with the evaluation of nuchal translucency and soft markers (see Chapter 12, *Prenatal Ultrasound*). After the first trimester, ultrasound is often used as a screening and diagnostic tool for structural abnormalities at 18–20 weeks of gestation. Diagnostic testing methods of chorionic villi sampling and amniocentesis are used in people at risk for genetic conditions and when screening results are positive.

Preventative Care

Prenatal care is a form of preventative care in many respects. Goals include the prevention of adverse pregnancy outcomes through the identification of risk factors, the treatment of ongoing health issues, and the utilization of health education and preventive health practices to adjust to pregnancy changes and to prepare for a new baby. Most preventative care focuses on maternal care needs but can provide for improved health outcomes for infants as well.

Immunization

Immunizations not only provide immunity for people from vaccine-preventable illnesses but can provide passive immunity for the newborn. While the most opportune time to evaluate for the immunization needs of people is during the preconception period, many vaccines are safe to administer during pregnancy and are recommended to promote optimal maternal health. Live virus vaccines are contraindicated during pregnancy, but can be given in the immediate postpartum period, even if breastfeeding. Current recommendations include that all persons be offered the Tdap vaccine during each pregnancy, ideally between 27 and 36 weeks regardless of prior immunization history, to protect the newborn against pertussis. Immediate postpartum immunization is recommended if Tdap was not administered during pregnancy (CDC, 2017). Pregnant people are recommended to receive the influenza vaccine during or prior to flu season, regardless of trimester of pregnancy. The COVID-19 vaccine, including booster shots, is recommended to all pregnant people; COVID-19 vaccination during pregnancy has been shown to provide antibodies that may protect babies against COVID-19 and to prevent serious sequelae in the pregnant person (CDC, 2022).

The CDC recommends practices that will help to increase immunization acceptance for pregnant people including making a strong recommendation, providing information regarding safety and importance, normalizing immunization practices as a part of standard prenatal care and making it easy to obtain the vaccine in the office setting (CDC, 2017).

Oral Health

Recent evidence suggests that poor oral health may increase the risk of PTB (Perunovic et al., 2016). Encouraging good oral health, including regular brushing and flossing, as well as cleaning and treatment of dental caries, is an important preventative health practice during pregnancy. Clients are encouraged to visit the dentist early in pregnancy. It is safe to receive shielded dental X-rays, have local anesthesia if needed, and use antibiotics that are safe in pregnancy, as needed for dental procedures. Tetracycline and related antibiotics should never be used during pregnancy as they can cause permanent tooth staining in infants exposed during pregnancy. Pregnant people may notice that their gums can bleed more easily during regular tooth brushing, and this observation can prompt questions regarding oral health during regular prenatal visits (see Chapter 16, *Oral Health*).

Mental Health

Mental health issues are an important component of the prenatal care. Maternal stress and anxiety conditions are linked to prematurity and poor infant health outcomes (Staneva et al., 2015). Maternal depression is associated with an increase in premature birth, lower rates of breast/chestfeeding initiation, and neurodevelopmental abnormalities in the newborn (Gentile, 2017; Grigoriadis et al., 2013). Universal screening for depression using a validated instrument for childbearing people is now recommended to be done at least once during the pregnancy and once in the postpartum period. Scores indicating depression should be shared with the person and referrals for mental health services offered for clients with positive scores. Individuals with significant depression may require pharmacological treatment in conjunction with individual or group counseling (see Chapter 47, *Mood and Anxiety Disorders*).

Intimate Partner Violence

IPV "describes physical violence, sexual violence, stalking, and psychological aggression (including coercive acts) by a current or former intimate partner" and affects people of all races and ethnicities and all socioeconomic groups (CDC, 2017). IPV can escalate during pregnancy, making pregnant people more vulnerable to both physical and psychological abuse, or it can decrease, making pregnancy a time of relative safety. It is recommended that all clients be screened for IPV during the first prenatal visit and once each trimester or whenever IPV is suspected based on history or physical examination (CDC, 2017). Many screening tools are available to assist prenatal providers in identifying people who may be experiencing IPV. For example, the following questions may be asked:

- In the last year have you been hit, slapped, kicked, or physically hurt by someone?
- Since you have been pregnant, have you been hit, slapped, kicked, or physically hurt by someone?
- Has anyone ever forced you to have sex with them?
- Are you afraid of your partner or anyone else?

These questions should be asked in private without a partner or other family members present. If the person denies IPV, it is still critical to document findings, express willingness to discuss questions or concerns about IPV, and let them know that you are always available as a resource. A small number of states have mandatory reporting laws, and being familiar with these state laws is important.

If a positive response is elicited, further evaluation is required. The prenatal care provider can provide a safe environment to explore the issue, reassure that this abuse is not their fault, and assess for their current and future safety. IPV is a complex situation and leaving an abusive partner may not be immediately feasible or preferred by the person. Referrals to local resources are critical including counseling and shelters (see Chapter 26, *Violence and Trauma in the Perinatal Period*).

Health Promotion and Education

Perhaps at no other time in a person's life will they have the unique motivation for making health behavior changes as during pregnancy. It is also a time when health behavior changes can have the most impact by improving maternal health, creating a healthier environment for the developing fetus, and setting the stage for maintenance of healthy behaviors after pregnancy. Nutrition and smoking cessation were found to be the two most likely behaviors to improve with counseling (Public Health Service Expert Panel on the Content of Prenatal Care, 1989; see Chapter 24, *Health Education during Pregnancy*).

Nutrition

The US Department of Agriculture (USDA) administers the Women, Infants, and Children (WIC) nutrition program. This program provides supplemental nutrition for pregnant and lactating people, allowing for the addition of healthy foods to meet the needs for increased protein, calcium, fiber, and calories in low-income people.

People who qualify for this program should be directed to enroll in services. For more information on counseling on nutrition in pregnancy (see Chapter 9, *Nutrition during Pregnancy*).

Substance Use

Substance use in pregnancy presents special challenges. Substance use is often underreported. Most illicit drugs have significant effects on the developing fetus and their illegal status also places the person at risk for criminal justice and child protective services involvement. Overall, how substance use affects the individual and their pregnancy will depend on the type of substance or substances used, how long and how frequently they use the substance, and what, if any, comorbidities are present. For example, people who drink alcohol are also more likely to smoke cigarettes. Mental health issues often coexist with substance use and should be assessed during prenatal care.

Use of illicit drugs, particularly opioids, has increased dramatically in recent years; the number of individuals with opioid-related diagnoses documented at delivery increased by 131% from 2010 to 2017 and the number of babies born with neonatal abstinence syndrome increased by 82% in the same period, for all states and demographic groups (Hirai et al., 2021). Pregnant people who use illegal drugs can be incarcerated or face child custody issues after the birth if the infant tests positive for illicit drugs or withdrawal symptoms. Some states require healthcare professionals to test for prenatal drug exposure if they suspect drug use and about half of states require healthcare professionals to report suspected prenatal drug use (Guttmacher Institute, 2022). It is incumbent upon the healthcare provider to know the laws of the state regarding testing and reporting of people who may have a substance use disorder.

Tobacco Use

Experts all agree that there is benefit to counseling pregnant people about the risks of smoking and that smoking cessation programs during pregnancy can decrease the incidence of adverse outcomes (Gregory et al., 2006; Public Health Service Expert Panel on the Content of Prenatal Care, 1989). The adverse effects of smoking in pregnancy are well documented and include an increased risk of ectopic pregnancy, spontaneous abortion, PTB, LBW, placental abruption, and placenta previa. Smoking cessation interventions during prenatal care can be effective as people are often highly motivated to change behaviors that are linked to poorer health outcomes in their infants. Targeted and effective smoking cessation counseling can and should occur during prenatal care. Self-instructional educational programs and toolkits that provide information and support regarding effective counseling techniques are available from ACOG and the CDC.

Alcohol Use

Alcohol use has been associated with a number of adverse pregnancy outcomes. CDC researchers found that one in seven pregnant people reported current drinking estimates that one out of eight people consume some alcohol while pregnant (Gosdin et al., 2022) and every year. People who consume alcohol regularly during pregnancy are at increased risk for spontaneous abortion, placental abruption, and infection. Similarly, the fetus is at an increased risk of LBW, fetal growth restriction, congenital anomalies, PTB, and neonatal depression (CDC, 2016). People should be advised to abstain from alcohol use during pregnancy. Alcohol dependence can develop with regular use, making it difficult for people to stop drinking without assistance from prenatal care providers and mental health specialists. People who report they are unable to stop drinking should be offered a referral to a substance abuse treatment provider or facility.

Substance Use Screening

All people should be screened for substance use in pregnancy (ACNM, 2018). Routine toxicology screening is not recommended during pregnancy. If testing is warranted, the client should be informed, and the provider should understand that, ethically, the client has a right to this information as well as a right to refuse such testing. Coercive or punitive strategies for maternal behaviors deny a client's right to privacy and bodily integrity and are incongruent with a harm-reduction approach to substance use.

Certain substances like heroin are highly addictive and require careful detoxification to prevent maternal and fetal complications. Depending on what substances are used during pregnancy, some infants will require detoxification after birth and require extended hospitalization. Prenatal care provides a unique opportunity to provide services and support to people with substance use disorders. Further information about substance use, screening, and treatment during pregnancy is provided in Chapter 18, *Substance Use during Pregnancy*.

Exercise

Exercise across the lifespan, including pregnancy, is associated with many health benefits and pregnancy can be an ideal time to maintain or initiate physical activity. All people with uncomplicated pregnancies are encouraged to participate in aerobic and strength training exercise before, during, and after pregnancy, aiming for 20–30 minutes of moderate-intensity exercise on most or all of the days of the week (ACOG, 2020). High-contact sports and exercise that has a risk for falling or abdominal trauma should be avoided and sports like scuba diving and skydiving are not recommended. Exercise patterns may change as the pregnancy progresses, and the enlarging abdomen may necessitate alterations in routine exercise regimens. Providers should thoroughly evaluate pregnant people with obstetric or medical complications before making recommendations on exercise in pregnancy (ACOG, 2020). Individuals who have not exercised before pregnancy are encouraged to start with low-intensity, short periods of exercise and gradually increase the period or intensity of exercise as they are able (ACOG, 2020). Adequate hydration during exercise and avoiding exercise in environments with high temperature or humidity are important teaching points regarding prenatal exercise. More detailed information on exercise during pregnancy is provided in Chapter 20, *Physical Activity and Exercise in the Perinatal Period*.

Working and Pregnancy

People throughout the world routinely work during pregnancy. For the majority, there are few risks for adverse health outcomes from continuing work during the pregnancy and there can be benefits of working; however, certain workplaces or occupations may pose risks or may require certain accommodations during pregnancy. There are a wide range of potential exposures to workplace substances and their effects on pregnancy and reproductive outcomes. People who may be exposed to hazardous chemicals, cytotoxic drugs, ionizing radiation, gases, and minerals like lead need to consult their workplace for the evaluation of potential exposures to determine whether it is safe to continue to work in these areas.

The type of work performed, hours worked, and the workplace environment can all contribute to an individual's tolerance of work throughout the pregnancy. While guidelines for occupational tasks have been available since 1981, it was not until 2015 that the National Institute of Occupational Health and Safety (NIOSH) applied their empirically derived guidelines for workplace lifting to pregnant people. These guidelines consider gestational age and the distance an item is being lifted, as well as how frequently the lifting occurs. Lifting any items from the floor is not recommended for any pregnant worker (McDonald et al., 2013). Occupational activities are considered on an individual basis for recommendations regarding continuation, alteration, or discontinuation of that specific job. More detailed information on occupational considerations in pregnancy is provided in Chapter 22, *Occupational and Environmental Health in Pregnancy*.

Some pregnant people will want to stop working prior to the onset of labor due to fatigue and difficulty with the physical demands of advancing gestation. It is common that people can be considered eligible for a pregnancy leave at 38 weeks' gestation. In the United States, paid parental leave benefits vary widely and pregnant people often have short periods of paid leave or no leave at all. The Family Medical Leave Act (FMLA) was enacted in 1993 and provides for unpaid leave of up to 12 weeks due to pregnancy. The Pregnancy Discrimination Act (PDA; 1978) prohibits discrimination based on pregnancy when it comes to any aspect of employment, including hiring, firing, pay, job assignments, promotions, layoff, training, fringe benefits such as leave and health insurance, and any other term or condition of employment. Pregnant people who experience a medical complication related to pregnancy must be treated as any other employee with a short-term disability and must be offered light duty, alternate assignments, or disability leave (Pregnancy Discrimination Act of 1978, 2000).

Health Education throughout Pregnancy

Health education during pregnancy is important for maternal health and psychosocial well-being and helps to prepare for transition to parenthood. The challenge in prenatal care is how to incorporate the necessary health education with ongoing physical and risk assessment, within the prevailing prenatal care system. Health education may not be a priority or may be limited due to the time constraints of prenatal care providers. While pregnant people who attend CenteringPregnancy groups have extensive health education as a major component of prenatal care, those in traditional individual care may need additional resources to meet their ongoing

Table 8.5　Health Education Topics throughout Pregnancy

First trimester	Second trimester	Third trimester
Counseling to promote healthy behaviors and avoidance of teratogens	Counseling to promote healthy behaviors and avoidance of teratogens	Counseling to promote healthy behaviors and avoidance of teratogens
Nutritional information, recommended weight gain, referrals for WIC if appropriate	Nutritional information, healthy weight goals	Nutritional information, healthy weight goals
Safety such as seatbelts, work safety, food safety, safer sex	Physiologic and emotional changes in changes in pregnancy	Physiologic and emotional changes in pregnancy
Physiologic and emotional changes in early pregnancy	Common pregnancy discomforts and recommendations	Common pregnancy discomforts and recommendations
Common pregnancy discomforts and recommendations	Fetal growth and development, anticipated fetal movement	Fetal growth and development, anticipated fetal movement
Exercise	Common screening and diagnostic tests, such as genetic screening, ultrasound	Common screening and diagnostic tests, such as group B strep screening
Prenatal care content and frequency of visit	Danger signs to report and how to contact provider	Danger signs to report and how to contact provider
Common screening and diagnostic tests, such as genetic screening	Signs and symptoms of preterm labor	Signs and symptoms of preterm labor
Danger signs to report and how to contact provider	Breastfeeding promotion	Breastfeeding promotion, preparation, class
Explanations of philosophy of care of the prenatal providers, scope of practice, and place of birth	Birth preparation, available educational opportunities	Labor and birth preparation, childbirth education class, visit to birth place, birth plan
Community resources for pregnant and parenting families		Preparation for baby, car seat, infant feeding, newborn care
		Preparation for parenting, roles, support, pediatric care and provider, parenting class, sibling adjustment
		Signs and symptoms of labor, when to notify provider, when and how to arrive at place of birth
		Postpartum changes, postpartum depression, activity, plan of care during postpartum period
		Contraceptive plans
		Post-term pregnancy expectations

Source: Adapted from AAP/ACOG (2017), Merkatz and Thompson (1990), Public Health Service Expert Panel on the Content of Prenatal Care (1989).

educational needs. In order to obtain in-depth and comprehensive health education, it may be necessary for pregnant individuals to attend classes outside of their regularly scheduled visits or to seek outside resources, such as books and online resources. Prenatal care providers should be familiar with common consumer resources for their clients (see *Resources for Clients and Their Families*). The Expert Panel recommended health promotion content be provided based on the needs of pregnant people throughout the pregnancy. Early pregnancy concerns will be different from those at the end of pregnancy. Anticipatory guidance is critical so that clients will know what to expect at each stage of pregnancy. This will help them to identify common changes and discomforts and alert them to danger signs that may indicate the need for evaluation. Preparation for labor, birth, and early parenting is important to help promote a successful transition to parenthood and ensure that pregnant people have appropriate resources and information (Table 8.5; see Chapter 24, *Health Education during Pregnancy*).

Summary

Prenatal care has the potential to affect the health of the pregnant person, their infant, and the family in a positive way. Current trends in healthcare emphasize the importance of evidence-based care to achieve improved health outcomes. Pregnancy and childbirth care represent one of the largest expenditures of healthcare dollars for both public and private insurers, yet despite this significant expenditure, the United States ranks well below other industrialized and some lower-income countries in maternal and newborn health outcomes. The current system of maternity care is procedure intensive, and that overuse is contributing to excessive harm and costs. Significant racial disparities exist in maternal and infant outcomes, as do rural/urban and socioeconomic disparities. Many childbearing people lack choice in their healthcare provider, place of birth, and childbirth experience due to institutional policies, reimbursement issues, and provider availability and preferences. Prenatal care providers have a unique opportunity to change how pregnant people and their families experience pregnancy and birth. Transforming Maternity Care is a group of over 100 experts in maternity healthcare and health policy brought together to create a blueprint for achieving a safer, cost-effective, and person-centered prenatal care system (Cook Carter et al., 2010). These changes may not be easy but are necessary to improve the health of families and communities. Prenatal care is over 100 years old with many traditional aspects that remain important today, but it is time to integrate current evidence into best care practices.

2020 Vision for a high-quality, high-value maternity care system

1. Each person is engaged as a partner in their own care and education during pregnancy; they receive affirmation and practical support for their role as the natural leader of their care team to the extent that they so desire and is encouraged to provide input to shape their own care.
2. Each person's preferences are known, respected, and matched with individually tailored care that meets their needs and reflects their choices during pregnancy, delivered by a care team whose composition is also customized based on their needs and preferences.
3. Each person has access to complete, accurate, up-to-date, high-quality information, decision support, and education to help ensure that they feel emotionally and psychologically prepared to make decisions during their pregnancy, and confident about their birth care options and choices well in advance of the onset of labor.
4. Education and care during pregnancy are designed and delivered to be empowering to people, emphasizing a climate of confidence.
5. Education and care during pregnancy include support for breastfeeding; most people make decisions about infant feeding well before they give birth.
6. Each pregnant person receives personalized coaching and has access to high-quality resources for comprehensive health promotion, disease prevention, and improved nutrition and exercise for optimal wellness during their pregnancy.
7. Care during pregnancy is available when needed and can be accessed in a time and place that is convenient and accessible for each person, and balanced with concerns for value and efficiency.
8. Care during pregnancy acknowledges the social context in which pregnancy occurs for each person and includes opportunities for social networking and access to adequate professional and peer support during pregnancy.

Source: Adapted from Cook Carter et al. (2010).

Resources for Clients and Their Families

American Pregnancy Association: http://www.american-pregnancy.org/
Childbirth Connection for Women: https://nationalpartnership.org/childbirthconnection/
March of Dimes: http://www.marchofdimes.com
Occupational Safety and Health Administration (OSHA): http://www.osha.gov

Resources for Healthcare Providers

Agency for Healthcare Research and Quality (AHRQ): http://www.ahrq.gov
American Academy of Pediatrics (AAP): http://www.aap.org/en-us/Pages/Default.aspx
American College of Family Physicians (ACFP): http://www.aafp.org/online/en/home.html
American College of Nurse-Midwives (ACNM): https://midwife.org/
American Congress of Obstetricians and Gynecologists (ACOG): http://www.acog.org
Centering Healthcare Institute: https://www.centering-healthcare.org/index.php
Centers for Disease Control and Prevention: http://www.cdc.gov/
Childbirth Connection: https://nationalpartnership.org/childbirthconnection/
United States Department of Agriculture (USDA) Supplemental Nutrition Program for Women, Infants, and Children (WIC) Nutrition Program: http://www.fns.usda.gov/wic
US Preventive Services Task Force (USPSTF): http://www.ahrq.gov/clinic/uspstfix.htm

References

Alameda Health System. (n.d.). *BElovedBIRTH Black Centering*. https://www.alamedahealthsystem.org/family-birthing-center/black-centering

Alexander, G. R., & Kotelchuck, M. (1998). Quantifying the adequacy of prenatal care: A comparison of indices. *Public Health Reports*, *111*, 408.

American Academy of Pediatrics and the American College of Obstetricians and Gynecologists. (2017). *Guidelines for perinatal care* (8th ed.). https://www.acog.org/clinical-information/physician-faqs/-/media/3a22e153b67446a6b31fb051e469187c.ashx.

American College of Nurse-Midwives. (2018). Position statement: Substance use disorders in pregnancy. *American College of Nurse-Midwives*. http://www.midwife.org/acnm/files/acnmlibrarydata/uploadfilename/000000000052/PS-Substance-Use-Disorders-in-Pregnancy-FINAL-20-Nov-18.pdf

American College of Obstetricians and Gynecologist (ACOG). (2020). Physical activity and exercise during pregnancy and the postpartum period: ACOG committee opinion, number 804. *Obstetrics and Gynecology*, *135*(4), e178–e188.

American College of Obstetricians and Gynecologists (ACOG). (2016). Practice bulletin no. 162: Prenatal diagnostic testing for genetic disorders. *Obstetrics and Gynecology*, *127*(5), e108–e122.

Artiga, S., Pham, O., Orgera, K., & Ranji, U. (2020). *Racial disparities in maternal and infant health: An overview*. Kaiser Family Foundation. https://www.kff.org/report-section/racial-disparities-in-maternal-and-infant-health-an-overview-issue-brief

Association of Maternal and Child Health Programs. (2015, December). *Innovation station: The HealthConnect One community-based doula program*. https://amchp.org/wp-content/uploads/2021/05/HealthConnect.pdf.

Ballantyne, J. W. (1923). An address on the new midwifery: Preventive and reparative obstetrics. *BMJ (Online)*, *1*(3250), 617–621.

Beckmann, M. M., Widmer, T., & Bolton, E. (2014). Does preconception care work? *Australian and New Zealand Journal of Obstetrics and Gynaecology*, *54*(6), 510–514.

Bhutani, V. K., Zipursky, A., Blencowe, H., Khanna, R., Sgro, M., Ebbesen, F., Bell, J., Mori, R., Slusher, T. M., Fahmy, N., Paul, V. K., Du, L., Okolo, A. A., de Almeida, M.-F., Olusanya, B. O., Kumar, P., Cousens, S., & Lawn, J. E. (2013). Neonatal hyperbilirubinemia and Rhesus disease of the newborn: Incidence and impairment estimates for 2010 at regional and global levels. *Pediatric Research*, *74*(S1), 86–100. https://www.nature.com/articles/pr2013208

Bloch, J., Dawley, K., & Suplee, P. (2009). Application of the Kessner and Kotelchuck prenatal care adequacy indices in a pre-term birth population. *Public Health Nursing*, *26*(5), 449.

Byerley, B. M., & Haas, D. M. (2017). A systematic overview of the literature regarding group prenatal care for high-risk pregnant women. *BMC Pregnancy and Childbirth*, *17*, 329.

Center for Medicare and Medicaid Services. (2019). *Issue brief: Improving access to maternal health care in rural communities*. https://www.cms.gov/About-CMS/Agency-Information/OMH/equity-initiatives/rural-health/09032019-Maternal-Health-Care-in-Rural-Communities.pdf.

Centers for Disease Control and Prevention (CDC). (2016). *Fetal alcohol spectrum disorders*. https://www.cdc.gov/ncbddd/fasd/index.html.

Centers for Disease Control and Prevention (CDC). (2017). *Injury center: Violence prevention*. https://www.cdc.gov/violenceprevention/intimatepartnerviolence

Centers for Disease Control and Prevention (CDC). (2021). *Zika and pregnancy: Prenatal care*. https://www.cdc.gov/pregnancy/zika/testing-follow-up/prenatal-care.html

Centers for Disease Control and Prevention (CDC). (February18, 2022). *COVID-19 vaccines while pregnant or breastfeeding*. https://www.cdc.gov/coronavirus/2019-ncov/vaccines/recommendations/pregnancy.html#:~:text=COVID%2D19%20vaccination%20is%20recommended,it's%20time%20to%20get%20one.

Chalmers, I. (1986). Minimizing harm and maximizing benefit during innovation in health care: Controlled or uncontrolled experimentation? *Birth (Berkeley, Calif.)*, *13*(3), 155–164.

Commonwealth Fund. (2020). *Maternal mortality in the United States: A primer*. https://www.commonwealthfund.org/publications/issue-brief-report/2020/dec/maternal-mortality-united-states-primer.

Cook Carter, M., Corry, M., Delbanco, S., Foster, T. C.-S., Friedland, R., Gabel, R., Gipson, T., Jolivet, R. R., Main, E., Sakala, C., Simkin, P., & Simpson, K. R. (2010). 2020 Vision for a high-quality, high-value maternity care system. *Women's Health Issues*, *20*(1), S7–S17. https://www.whijournal.com/article/S1049-3867(09)00139-X/fulltext

Dawley, K. (2003). Origins of nurse-midwifery in the United States and its expansion in the 1940s. *Journal of Midwifery & Women's Health*, *48*(2), 86–95.

Dowswell, T., Carroli, G., Duley, L., Gates, S., Gülmezoglu, A. M., Khan-Neelofur, D., & Piaggio, G. (2015). Alternative versus standard packages of antenatal care for low-risk pregnancy. *Cochrane Database of Systematic Reviews*, *7*, CD000934. https://www.cochranelibrary.com/cdsr/doi/10.1002/14651858.CD000934.pub3/full

Dunn, P. M. (1993). Dr John Ballantyne (1861–1923): Perinatologist extraordinary of Edinburgh. *Archives of Disease in Childhood*, *68*(1 Spec No, 66–67.

Ekholuenetale, M. (2021). Prevalence of eight or more antenatal care contacts: Findings from multi-country nationally representative data. *Global Pediatric Health*, *8*, 2333794–2333794X211045822

Enkin, M., Keirse, M., Neilson, J., Crowther, C., Duley, L., Hodnett, E., & Hofmeyr, J. (2000). *A guide to effective care in pregnancy and childbirth* (3rd ed.). Oxford University Press.

Finer, L., & Moline, R. (2016). Declines in unintended pregnancy in the United States, 2008–2011. *New England Journal of Medicine*, *324*(9), 843–852.

Gareau, S., Lòpez-De Fede, A., Loudermilk, B. L., Cummings, T. H., Hardin, J. W., Picklesimer, A. H., Crouch, E., & Covington-Kolb, S. (2016). Group prenatal care results in medicaid savings with better outcomes: A propensity score analysis of CenteringPregnancy participation in South Carolina. *Maternal and Child Health Journal*, *20*(7), 1384–1393. https://doi.org/10.1007/s10995-016-1935-y

Gentile, S. (2017). Untreated depression during pregnancy: Short- and long-term effects in offspring. A symptomatic review. *Neuroscience*, *342*(7), 154–166.

Gosdin, L. K., Deputy, N. P., Kim, S. Y., Dang, E. P., & Denny, C. H. (2022). Alcohol consumption and binge drinking during pregnancy among adults aged 18–49 years – United States, 2018–2020. *MMWR Morbidity and Mortality Weekly Report 2022*, *71*(1), 10–13.

Grady, M. A., & Bloom, K. C. (2004). Pregnancy outcomes of adolescents enrolled in a CenteringPregnancy program. *Journal of Midwifery and Women's Health*, *49*(5), 412–420.

Gregory, K. D., Johnson, C. T., Johnson, T. R., & Entman, S. S. (2006). The content of prenatal care. Update 2005. *Women's Health Issues*, *16*(4), 198–215.

Grigoriadis, S., Vonderhorten, E., Mamisashvili, L., & Ross, L. (2013). The impact of maternal depression during pregnancy on perinatal outcomes: A systematic review and meta-analysis. *Journal of Clinical Psychiatry*, *74*(4), e321–e341.

Guttmacher Institute. (February 1 2022). *Substance use during pregnancy*. https://www.guttmacher.org/state-policy/explore/substance-use-during-pregnancy.

Hale, N., Billlings, D., & Covington-Kolb, S. (2014). The impact of CenteringPregnancy group prenatal care on postpartum family planning. *American Journal of Obstetrics and Gynecology*, *210*, 50.e11–50.e7.

Hirai, A., Ko, J. Y., Owens, P. L., Stocks, C., & Patrick, S. W. (2021). Neonatal abstinence syndrome and maternal opioid-related diagnoses in the US, 2010–2017. *JAMA: The Journal of the American Medical Association*, *325*(2), 146–155. https://doi.org/10.1001/jama.2020.24991

Hoyert, D. (2022). *Maternal mortality rates in the United States, 2020*. National Center for Health Statistics. https://doi.org/10.15620/cdc:113967

Ickovics, J. R., Kershaw, T. S., Westdahl, C., Magriples, U., Massey, Z., Reynolds, H., & Rising, S. S. (2007). Group prenatal care and perinatal outcomes – A randomized controlled trial. *Obstetrics and Gynecology (New York. 1953)*, *110*(2), 330–339. https://doi.org/10.1097/01.AOG.0000275284.24298.23

Institute of Medicine. (2001). *Crossing the quality chasm*. National Academy Press.

Klima, C., Norr, K., Vonderheid, S., & Handler, A. (2009). Introduction of CenteringPregnancy in a public health clinic. *Journal of Midwifery & Women's Health*, *54*(1), 27–34.

Kogan, M. D., Alexander, G. R., Kotelchuck, M., & Nagey, D. A. (1994a). Relation of the content of prenatal care to the risk of low birth weight. Maternal reports of health behavior advice and initial prenatal care procedures. *JAMA: The Journal of the American Medical Association*, *271*(17), 1340–1345.

Kogan, M. D., Alexander, G. R., Kotelchuck, M., Nagey, D. A., & Jack, B. W. (1994b). Comparing mothers' reports on the content of prenatal care received with recommended national guidelines for care. *Public Health Reports*, *109*(5), 637–646.

Kotelchuck, M. (1994). The Adequacy of Prenatal Care Utilization Index: Its US distribution and association with low birthweight. *American Journal of Public Health*, *84*(9), 1486–1489. https://doi.org/10.2105/AJPH.84.9.1486

Ladd-Taylor, M. (1988). "Grannies" and "spinsters": Midwife education under the Sheppard-Towner Act. *Journal of Social History*, *22*(2), 255–275. http://www.jstor.org/stable/3788221

Liu, Y., Wang, Y., Wu, Y., Chen, X., & Bai, J. (2021). Effectiveness of the CenteringPregnancy program on maternal and birth outcomes: A systematic review and meta-analysis. *International Journal of Nursing Studies*, *120*, 103981.

Lu, M. C., Tache, V., Alexander, G. R., Kotelchuck, M., & Halfon, N. (2003). Preventing low birth weight: Is prenatal care the answer? *The Journal of Maternal-fetal and Neonatal Medicine*, *13*(6), 362–380.

MacDonald, L. A., Waters, T. R., Napolitano, P. G., Goddard, D. E., Ryan, M. A., Nielsen, P., & Hudock, S. D. (2013). Clinical guidelines for occupational lifting in pregnancy: Evidence summary and provisional recommendations. *American Journal of Obstetrics and Gynecology*, *209*(2), 80–88.

MacKey, M. C., Williams, C. A., & Tiller, C. M. (2000). Stress, preterm labour and birth outcomes. *Journal of Advanced Nursing*, *32*(3), 666–674.

March of Dimes. (2022b). *Nowhere to go: Maternity care deserts across the United States 2022 reports*. https://www.marchofdimes.org/sites/default/files/2022-10/2022_Maternity_Care_Report.pdf

March of Dimes (MOD). (2022a). *Peristats*. http://www.marchofdimes.org/peristats/Peristats.aspx.

Mena-Tudela, D., Aguilar-Camprubí, L., Quifer-Rada, P., Paricio-Talayero, J. M., & Padró-Arocas, A. (2021). The COVID-19 vaccine in women: Decisions, data and gender gap. *Nursing Inquiry, 28*(3). https://doi.org/10.1111/nin.12416

Merkatz, I., & Thompson, J. E. (Eds.) (1990). *New perspectives on prenatal care*. Elsevier.

Morton, C., & Hsu, C. (2007). Contemporary dilemmas in American childbirth education: Findings from a comparative ethnographic study. *The Journal of Perinatal Education, 16*(4), 25–37. https://doi.org/10.1624/105812407X245614

Novoa, C. (2020). *Ensuring healthy births through prenatal support: Innovations from three models*. https://www.americanprogress.org/article/ensuring-healthy-births-prenatal-support.

Perunovic, N. D., Rakic, M. M., Nikolic, L. I., Jankovic, S. M., Aleksic, Z. M., Plecas, D. V., & Cakic, S. S. (2016). The association between periodontal inflammation and labor triggers (elevated cytokine levels) in preterm birth: A cross-sectional study. *Journal of Periodontology, 87*(3), 248–256.

Pregnancy Discrimination Act of 1978. Pub. L. 95-555, 92 Stat. 2076 (codified as amended at 42 U. S. C. §2000e(k) (2000) https://www.eeoc.gov/statutes/pregnancy-discrimination-act-1978

Public Health Service Expert Panel on the Content of Prenatal Care. (1989). *Caring for our future, the content of prenatal care: A report of the Public Health Service Expert Panel on the Content of Prenatal Care*. Department of Health and Human Services.

Rising, S. S. (1998). Centering pregnancy. An interdisciplinary model of empowerment. *Journal of Nurse-Midwifery, 43*(1), 46–54.

Rising, S. S., Kennedy, H. P., & Klima, C. S. (2004). Redesigning prenatal care through CenteringPregnancy. *Journal of Midwifery and Women's Health, 49*(5), 398–404.

Rising, S. S., & Quimby, C. (2017). *The CenteringPregnancy model*. Springer Publishing Co.

Robbins, C., & Martocci, S. (2020). Timing of prenatal care initiation in the Health Resources and Services Administration Health Center Program in 2017. *Annals of Internal Medicine, 173*(11 Suppl), S29–S36. https://doi.org/10.7326/M19-3248

Rooks, J. (1997). *Midwifery and childbirth in America*. Temple University Press.

Salmeen, K. (2016). Gestational diabetes mellitus testing: Making sense of the controversy. *Journal of Midwifery and Women's Health, 61*(2), 209–219.

Sperlich, M., Seng, J., Rowe, H., Fisher, J., Cuthbert, C., & Taylor, J. (2017). A cycles-breaking framework to disrupt intergenerational patterns of maltreatment and vulnerability during the childbearing year. *Journal of Obstetric, Gynecologic, and Neonatal Nursing, 46*(3), 378–389. https://doi.org/10.1016/j.jogn.2016.11.017

Staneva, A., Bogossian, F., Pritchard, M., & Wittkowski, A. (2015). The effects of maternal depression, anxiety, and perceived stress during pregnancy on preterm birth: A systematic review. *Women and Birth, 28*(3), 179–193.

Stringer, M. (1998). Issues in determining and measuring adequacy of prenatal care. *Journal of Perinatology: Official Journal of the California Perinatal Association, 18*(1), 68.

Thurston, H., Fields, B. E., & White, J. (2021). Does increasing access to prenatal care reduce racial disparities in birth outcomes? *Journal of Pediatric Nursing, 59*, 96–102.

US Department of Health and Human Services, Office of Disease Prevention and Health Promotion. (n.d.) *Healthy People 2030 pregnancy and childbirth objectives*. https://health.gov/healthypeople/objectives-and-data/browse-objectives/pregnancy-and-childbirth

US Department of Health and Human Services, Office of Disease Prevention and Health Promotion. (2021). Increase the proportion of pregnant women who receive early and adequate prenatal care — MICH-08. https://health.gov/healthypeople/objectives-and-data/browse-objectives/pregnancy-and-childbirth/increase-proportion-pregnant-women-who-receive-early-and-adequate-prenatal-care-mich-08

US Department of Labor: Children's Bureau. (1925). Standards of prenatal care. U.S. Government; Report No.: 153.

US Preventative Service Task Force (USPSTF). (n.d.) *Recommendations*. https://www.uspreventiveservicestaskforce.org/uspstf/index.php/topic_search_results?topic_status=P&gender%5B%5D=14&searchterm

Velez, M., Hamel, C., Hutton, B., Gaudet, L., Walker, M., Thuku, M., Cobey, K. D., Pratt, M., Skidmore, B., & Smith, G. N. (2019). Care plans for women pregnant using assisted reproductive technologies: A systematic review. *Reproductive Health, 16*(1), 9–19. https://doi.org/10.1186/s12978-019-0667-z

Vonderheid, S. C., Montgomery, K. S., & Norr, K. F. (2003). Ethnicity and prenatal health promotion content. *Western Journal of Nursing Research, 25*(4), 388–404.

Vonderheid, S. C., Norr, K. F., & Handler, A. S. (2007). Prenatal health promotion content and health behaviors. *Western Journal of Nursing Research, 29*(3), 258–276.

Wexler, A., Davoudi, A., Weissenbacher, D., Choi, R., O'Connor, K., Cummings, H., & Gonzalez-Hernandez, G. (2020). Pregnancy and health in the age of the Internet: A content analysis of online "birth club" forums. *PLoS One, 15*(4), e0230947. https://doi.org/10.1371/journal.pone.0230947

World Health Organization. (2016). *WHO recommendations on antenatal care for a positive pregnancy experience. Executive summary*. World Health Organization. https://www.who.int/publications/i/item/9789241549912

World Health Organization (WHO). (2019). *Maternal mortality*. https://www.who.int/news-room/fact-sheets/detail/maternal-mortality.

Xaverius, P., Aman, C., Holtz, L., & Yarberm, L. (2016). Risk factors associated with very low birth weight infants in a large urban. *Maternal Child Health Journal, 20*(3), 623–629.

9

Nutrition during Pregnancy

Rhea Williams

The editors gratefully acknowledge Robin G. Jordan, who was author of the previous edition of this chapter.

Relevant Terms

Adequate intake—reference value set for nutrient levels when sufficient scientific evidence is not available

Basal metabolic rate—the number of calories burned as the body performs basic life-sustaining functions

Body mass index—a measure of weight in kilograms divided by height in meters squared. BMI categories include underweight, healthy weight, overweight, and obese. During pregnancy, only the prepregnant BMI is relevant to weight gain guidelines

Dietary reference intake—standardized nutrient level for populations used to set nutritional goals

Fiber—nondigestible carbohydrates and lignin that are found in plants; beneficial to gastrointestinal function

Food-borne illness—illness resulting from the consumption of food contaminated with pathogenic bacteria (e.g., *Escherichia coli*), viruses (e.g., norovirus), or parasites (e.g., *Toxoplasma gondii*)

Food insecurity—the limited or uncertain availability of nutritionally adequate and safe foods

Food deserts—neighborhoods or communities with little access to fresh fruits and vegetables and other wholesome foods, generally in impoverished areas lacking large grocery stores and farmer's markets

Fortification—the addition of one or more essential nutrients to a food item, regardless of whether it is normally contained in the food

Glycemic index—a numeric indicator of how quickly a particular food causes glucose levels to rise after eating and how quickly the carbohydrates convert to glucose in the body

Macronutrients—dietary components that provide energy; macronutrients are proteins, fats, and carbohydrates

Micronutrients—dietary nutrients required in small quantities that orchestrate a range of physiologic functions

Monounsaturated fats—have one double bond; plant sources of an unsaturated fatty acid (UFA) include nuts and vegetable oils such as canola, olive, safflower, and sunflower oils

Omega-3 fatty acids—essential fatty acids obtained only in the diet, such as eicosapentaenoic acid (EPA) and docosahexaenoic acid (DHA) found primarily in fish and shellfish; also called n-3 fatty acids

Omega-6 fatty acids—essential fatty acids found only in the diet, such as linoleic acid; primary sources are liquid vegetable oils such as soybean, corn, and safflower oil; also called n-6 fatty acids

Ovo-lacto vegetarians—those persons following a diet that does not include meat, poultry, or fish/seafood but does contain eggs and dairy foods

Polyunsaturated fats—hydrocarbon chain has two or more carbon–carbon double bonds; found mostly in nuts, seeds, fish, seed oils, and can reduce LDL cholesterol

Portion size—the amount of a particular food chosen to be eaten at one sitting; this differs from serving size

Recommended daily allowance—levels of nutrient intake advised by experts based on sufficient scientific evidence

Saturated fats—have no double bond and are generally solid at room temperature; typically found in animal products such as meat and milk, and coconut and palm oils

Serving size—a standardized specific amount for the five food groups set by the US Department of Agriculture (USDA)

Trans fats—are minimally found in natural foods; most are created in an industrial process that adds hydrogen to liquid vegetable oils to make them more solid. Found in mass produced baked goods, snack foods and margarine, trans fats are linked with heart disease, inflammation processes, and insulin resistance

Vegan—those persons following a diet that does not include meat, poultry or fish/seafood, dairy, eggs, or honey

Vegetarians—those following a diet that generally does not include meat, poultry, or fish/seafood

---

Prenatal and Postnatal Care: A Person-Centered Approach, Third Edition. Edited by Karen Trister Grace, Cindy L. Farley, Noelene K. Jeffers, and Tanya Tringali.
Companion website: www.wiley.com/go/grace/prenatal

Introduction

Nutrition plays a major role in maternal and child health. Nutrient needs typically increase more during pregnancy than during any other stage of an adult person's life. An increase in select nutrients is required during the prenatal period for the fetal development and growth of maternal tissue that supports human gestation. Healthy eating behaviors during pregnancy enable optimal gestational nutrition and weight gain, both of which are linked to positive birth outcomes and the reduction of perinatal complications. The association between maternal nutrition and birth outcome is complex and is influenced by many biological, socioeconomic, and cultural factors, which vary widely in different populations.

There is a growing understanding of the significant influence that prenatal nutrition has on health status throughout life. Understanding the relationship between maternal nutrition and birth outcomes provides a basis for developing nutritional interventions that will improve birth outcomes and long-term quality of life and reduce mortality, morbidity, and healthcare costs. Providers of prenatal care must appreciate the complex relationship between maternal nutritional status and health outcomes to provide comprehensive and effective dietary guidance to pregnant individuals. This chapter provides foundational information on nutritional needs during pregnancy; impact of nutrition on maternal, child, and adult health; assessment of nutritional status; and nutritional counseling and modification strategies.

Health equity key points

- Melanin absorbs the ultraviolet rays that start the DNA synthesis of vitamin D. The more pigmented skin a person has, the higher the likelihood they will need vitamin D supplementation.
- Poverty, access to nutritional services and programs, living in rural areas or **food deserts**, living with food insecurity, lower education, and racism in healthcare are all social determinants that contribute to nutritionally associated health inequities.

Prenatal Nutrition and Health Outcomes

Maternal nutrition plays a crucial role in influencing fetal development and birth outcomes. Poor pregnancy nutrition is linked with adverse conditions, such as fetal growth restriction (FGR), preterm birth (PTB), low birth weight, preeclampsia, gestational diabetes mellitus (GDM), and certain congenital anomalies (Berti et al., 2016). Some of these adverse outcomes have lifelong consequences for growth, development, and quality of life in offspring.

Nutrition during the first trimester of pregnancy is especially important as it can affect fertility, placental development, and significantly influence pregnancy outcome (Tsakiridis et al., 2020). The placenta is the interface between the maternal and fetal circulations; optimal placental functioning is critical for effective fetal nutrition and oxygenation and, consequently, fetal growth. In turn, placental ability to supply nutrients to the fetus depends on placental size, morphology, blood supply, and transport ability. During normal pregnancy, the placenta undergoes physiologic changes to maximize efficiency for the progressively increasing fetal demand for nutrients. Changes in these factors caused by undernutrition or overnutrition, especially in early pregnancy, can significantly alter nutrient availability to the fetus for the entire pregnancy. Animal studies indicate that low nutrient intake during placental development suppresses cell proliferation and vascular development (Nusken et al., 2016), explaining the higher incidence of FGR in those with insufficient weight gain during pregnancy.

Fetal Origins of Disease

Prenatal nutrition not only affects fetal growth and development but also has a significant influence on adult health. Evidence from both epidemiological studies in humans and experimental studies in animals indicates that prenatal maternal nutrition has long-lasting consequences and predisposes the offspring to the development of several chronic diseases. Links are well established between low birth weight and increased risk of heart disease, diabetes, hypertension, and stroke in adulthood (Langley-Evans, 2015; Lagisz et al., 2014). In addition, infants born with FGR are at risk for physical and mental impairments in childhood and as adults (Salam et al., 2014).

Increasing evidence implicates maternal obesity as a major determinant of offspring health during childhood and later adult life (Godfrey et al., 2017). Individuals with prepregnancy obesity have a higher risk of giving birth preterm. Those children born preterm to mothers with prepregnancy obesity have a higher risk of poorer neurocognitive function compared to preterm infants born to mothers entering pregnancy at a normal weight (Jensen et al., 2017). Evidence suggests causal implications of prepregnancy obesity for immune disorders, cardiovascular disease, and infectious-disease-related conditions in offspring (Godfrey et al., 2017; Wilson & Messaoudi, 2015), possibly due to higher levels of inflammatory processes in individuals with obesity (Hrolfsdottir et al., 2016).

Understanding Food Units and Recommendations

Nutrition experts have produced a set of standards that define the amounts of energy, nutrients, and other dietary components that best support health based on scientific evidence. These recommendations are called **dietary reference intake** (DRI), the general term for a set of reference values used for planning and assessing nutrient intake for healthy people. DRIs reflect the collaborative efforts of scientists in the United States and Canada and take into account the amount of nutrients needed to promote health and to prevent chronic diseases.

Table 9.1 Food Groups and Subgroups

Food group	Subgroup and examples
Vegetables	Dark-green vegetables: all fresh, frozen, and canned dark-green leafy vegetables and broccoli, cooked or raw: for example, broccoli; spinach; romaine; collard, turnip, and mustard greens Red and orange vegetables: all fresh, frozen, and canned red and orange vegetables, cooked or raw: for example, tomatoes, red peppers, carrots, sweet potatoes, winter squash, and pumpkin Beans and peas: all cooked and canned beans and peas: for example, kidney beans, lentils, chickpeas, and pinto beans; does not include green beans or green peas (see additional comment under protein foods group) Starchy vegetables: all fresh, frozen, and canned starchy vegetables: for example, white potatoes, corn, and green peas Other vegetables: all fresh, frozen, and canned other vegetables, cooked or raw: for example, iceberg lettuce, green beans, and onions
Fruits	All fresh, frozen, canned, and dried fruits and fruit juices: for example, oranges and orange juice, apples and apple juice, bananas, grapes, melons, berries, and raisins
Grains	Whole grains: All whole grain products and whole grains used as ingredients, for example, whole-wheat bread, whole grain cereals and crackers, oatmeal, and brown rice Refined grains: All enriched refined grain products and enriched refined grains used as ingredients, for example, white breads, enriched grain cereals and crackers, enriched pasta, and white rice
Dairy products	All milks, including lactose-free and lactose-reduced products and fortified soy beverages, yogurts, frozen yogurts, dairy desserts, and cheeses. Most choices should be fat-free or low-fat. Cream, sour cream, and cream cheese are not included due to their low calcium content
Proteins	All meat, poultry, seafood, eggs, nuts, seeds, and processed soy products. Meat and poultry should be lean or low-fat. Beans and peas are considered part of this group, as well as the vegetable group, but should be counted in one group only

Source: US Department of Agriculture and US Department of Health and Human Services (2020).

There are two sets of values used as DRIs that help set nutritional goals for individuals. The **recommended daily allowance** (RDA) is the foundation of the DRI. The RDA refers to the average daily intake that is sufficient to meet the nutrient **requirements** of nearly all healthy individuals in each age and gender group. RDAs are based on scientific evidence with an emphasis on human experiments. The **adequate intake** (AI) values were established whenever scientific evidence was insufficient to generate an RDA, using scientific findings as much as possible. Some nutrients have an RDA and others have an AI. Both the RDA and AI are nutrient reference values set by experts to promote optimal health during various life stages.

The US Department of Agriculture (USDA) has established food guides based on DRIs to help individuals build healthy diets. The USDA Food Guide is a plan that builds a diet recommending specific daily amounts of food from each of the five major food groups (Table 9.1). An understanding of this foundational content enables healthcare providers to make accurate dietary assessments and recommendations during pregnancy.

Food Servings

The amount of food eaten is an important contributing factor to achieving or maintaining a healthy weight. This is a modifiable factor that can present many opportunities for therapeutic person-based education for persons who are underweight or overweight. Many people are not aware of what constitutes a serving of a particular food item. The **serving size** of a given food is the amount recommended by the USDA. The USDA specifies food measures based

on weight in ounces or amounts in cups of food rather than a visual estimate. Fruits, vegetables, and milk are measured in one-cup servings, and whole grains, meats, and beans are measured in 1-oz servings. People often confuse the "serving" recommendation to mean "portions" with no regard to size. For example, 6–11 daily servings of whole grains are recommended during pregnancy. The USDA indicates that one serving equals 1 oz, which translates into one slice of bread or cup of rice or pasta.

The USDA food guides provide guidance on food selections and serving and **portion sizes** that will provide adequate amounts of nutrients for a healthy pregnancy diet (Table 9.2).

Nutritional Needs in Pregnancy

The need for most nutrients increases during pregnancy to meet physiologic pregnancy demands. The pregnant person's **basal metabolic rate** (BMR) is elevated to support maternal pregnancy changes, fetal growth needs increase during pregnancy, and the body stores fat to prepare for lactation. Increased high-quality nutrient intake is needed to account for these physiologic activities.

Fluid Intake

Fluid requirements increase during pregnancy to approximately 3 L/day, approximately 8–12 8-oz glasses per day, primarily due to the increase in blood volume, production of amniotic fluid, and increase in BMR. Adequate fluid intake also prevents urinary tract infection and constipation. Fluid needs are even higher in warm weather and during exercise. Pregnant people should be encouraged to

Table 9.2 Serving Size Guidelines and Pregnancy Needs

Food	Amount per day	Food group serving size	Comments
Grains	6 oz; 1 oz is a serving	✓ 1 slice of bread ✓ 1 cup of dry cereal ✓ ½ cup of cooked rice, pasta, or cereal	✓ >3 oz/day should be whole grain ✓ Choose low-sugar cereals.
Vegetables	2–3 cups	✓ Most vegetables = ½ cup ✓ 1 cup greens like lettuce or spinach	✓ Select various color vegetables.
Fruits	2 cups	✓ 1 cup fresh fruit or 100% fruit juice ✓ ½ cup dried fruit ✓ A single piece of fruit	✓ Choose whole fruit instead of juice more often.
Dairy	3–4 cups	✓ 1.5 oz natural cheese ✓ 2.0 oz processed cheese ✓ 1 cup milk ✓ 1 cup yogurt ✓ 1 cup fortified soymilk	✓ Choose low-fat or skim milk and yogurt.
Proteins	5–6 oz	✓ ¼ cup beans ✓ 1 oz meat, poultry, seafood, shellfish ✓ 1 egg ✓ 1 tbsp peanut or other nut butters	✓ Eat seafood twice per week. ✓ Select lean meats and poultry.
Other calories such as oils	6 tsp	✓ 1 tsp vegetable oil ✓ 1½ tsp mayonnaise ✓ 2 tsp French dressing	✓ Use vegetable oils rather than solid fats like butter or lard.

drink fluids regularly throughout the day, as well as respond to sensations of thirst.

High consumption of sugary drinks during pregnancy has been associated with an increased risk of GDM as it contributes to a proinflammatory state within the body (Nicolì et al., 2021), PTB (Gete et al., 2020), and obesity in children (Phelan et al., 2011). Animal and human studies suggest that high sugar consumption during pregnancy is a risk factor for ADHD in offspring (Choi et al., 2015; Yu et al., 2016). Consumption of high-sugar drinks, such as sodas, some sports drinks, fruit drinks, and flavored water, should be discouraged during pregnancy, and the rationale behind these recommendations should be explained. Fruit juices, while containing some **micronutrients**, are a more nutritious drink but contain high amounts of natural sugars and should be limited. The ready availability of pre-packaged and high-sugar fluids contributes to reduced water consumption. Increasing water intake and reducing high-sugar fluid intake is encouraged.

Macronutrients

Total Energy

Caloric recommendation in pregnancy is currently based on the level of daily activity, pregnancy trimester, and the person's prepregnancy **body mass index (BMI).** During the first trimester, there is no increased energy cost associated with a singleton pregnancy in a person who has a normal BMI. Weight gain during the first trimester should be minimal, ranging from 0 to 4 lb. It is not uncommon for a person to lose or not gain any weight because extreme nausea, vomiting, or fatigue prevents them from eating their normal diet, while others may gain weight because of increased hunger, fluid retention, or reduced physical activity. In most cases, pregnant people need to increase caloric intake by 340 kcal/day (example: two eggs and one slice of bread) during the second trimester and 450 kcal/day (example: tuna salad sandwich) during the third trimester for a singleton pregnancy. People with a BMI in the underweight range should increase their caloric intake in the first trimester by approximately 150 kcal/day (example: apple with 2 tbsp of peanut butter).

Carbohydrates

Carbohydrates are the primary source of fuel for fetal growth and development and maternal neurologic support. Glucose is the primary monosaccharide in the carbohydrate family used for fuel. Carbohydrates are found

---

Benefits of adequate water consumption in pregnancy

- Promotes adequate blood volume to carry fetal nutrients.
- Aids digestion.
- Regulates body temperature.
- Decreases constipation, swelling, headache, risk of urinary tract infection, heartburn, and cramping.
- Prevents dehydration.

Strategies to promote adequate water consumption:

- Flavor water with lemon or lime.
- Set a timer to drink water.
- Drink small amounts every hour excluding the last two hours before bedtime.
- Bring a water bottle to work and keep it filled and nearby.
- Fill a large pitcher with daily water amount to drink during the day.

in two different forms: simple and complex. Simple carbohydrates are digested quickly and are transformed into glucose to be used as energy. Simple carbohydrates are found naturally in foods such as fruits, milk, and milk products. They are also found in processed and refined foods such as candy, table sugar, syrups, and soft drinks. Simple carbohydrates increase serum glucose levels quickly because they are easily broken down into its simplest usable form. This can present a problem among pregnant individuals with impaired glucose metabolism, preexisting diabetes, history of GDM, or risk factors for GDM. When the body quickly processes glucose into its energy form, the rise and fall in blood glucose levels occurs rapidly. Symptoms of hyperglycemia can include hunger, thirst, blurred vision, nausea, and vomiting, while symptoms of hypoglycemia can include sweating, headache, dizziness, and syncope. Additionally, refined sugars increase the inflammatory signaling in the body, which can contribute to inflammatory-related diseases such as diabetes.

Complex carbohydrates, also known as starches, are found in some cereals, whole grain foods, vegetables like broccoli and corn, and legumes. Complex carbohydrates take longer to digest, are important sources of dietary **fiber**, and promote satiety for longer periods. Complex carbohydrates take longer to break down into glucose and tend to maintain blood glucose levels more evenly over time.

The recommended RDA carbohydrate intake for pregnant people is 175 g/day divided over meals and snacks throughout the day. Most US individuals eat enough carbohydrates to meet normal pregnancy requirements. Pregnant people should be advised that low-carbohydrate diets are not healthy during pregnancy though people with GDM benefit from a mild restriction on carbohydrates. As with other nutrients, the quality of the carbohydrate food source should be evaluated. The majority of carbohydrate intake should come from complex carbohydrates and naturally occurring sugars, rather than processed or refined sugars, to improve blood glucose control. Complex carbohydrates are low on the **glycemic index** (GI) and glycemic load. Additionally, complex carbohydrates have lower inflammatory responses within the body and are supportive of a balanced gut microbiome.

Fats

Fats are sources of vitamins and concentrated calories and contribute to cell development. Fats are essential components of a healthy prenatal diet. While an RDA or AI has not been established for fats as a group, the recommendation is for fats to make up 20–35% of the total daily caloric intake (IOM, 2020). An evaluation of the type of fats frequently consumed by the pregnant person should be done during the nutritional intake history. **Monounsaturated fats** (olive, canola, and peanut oils) and **polyunsaturated fats** (flaxseed and corn oils) should predominate in the diet, while **saturated** (coconut oil and lard) and **trans fats** (packaged baked goods and chip snacks) should be limited.

Omega-3 Fatty Acids

Fatty acid intake during pregnancy is essential for fetal brain and eye development and the child's subsequent neurodevelopment. The three main **omega-3 fatty acids** are alpha-linolenic acid (ALA), eicosapentaenoic acid (EPA), and docosahexaenoic acid (DHA). DHA is important for the structure, growth, and development of the fetal central nervous system and the retina. DHA forms a major part of fetal neural tissue that maintains optimal neurotransmitter function. The fetus and nursing newborn acquires DHA from the pregnant or nursing person. DHA accrues rapidly in the brain during the third trimester and the first six weeks of life. DHA naturally occurs in human milk, and omega-3 supplementation during pregnancy and lactation increases levels of DHA in breast milk and nursing infants.

Omega-3 fatty acids must be ingested in the diet; they are not made in the body. ALA comes from plants and is found in vegetable, flaxseed, walnut, canola, and soybean oils. ALA is the most common omega-3 fatty acid found in a standard American diet and is used to form the more functionally essential omega-3 fatty acids, EPA, and DHA. Although most people easily ingest the recommended amount of ALA, it is not well converted to EPA and DHA. Therefore, preformed EPA and DHA are required for optimal health in most people, especially during periods of rapid growth and development such as pregnancy and in the first year of life. EPA and DHA are known as the long-chain or marine omega-3 fatty acids since they are mainly found in fish and fish oils. EPA and DHA have significant health benefits; however, both are especially low in the typical American diet.

Recommendations for Omega-3 Intake in Pregnancy

RDAs or DRIs have not been set for DHA and EPA and daily intake recommendations for omega-3 fatty acids vary among expert groups:

- 200 mg/day minimum—The European Perinatal Lipid Intake (Perlip) Group
- 300 mg/ DHA—The National Institute of Health (NIH)
- 200–500 mg/day of EPA plus DHA—The World Health Organization (WHO)
- 500 mg/day of DHA plus EPA—The Academy of Nutrition and Dietetics

Higher intakes (up to 1 g/day of DHA and 2.7 g/day total long-chain polyunsaturated fatty acid [LC-PUFA]) have been shown in randomized trials to have no significant adverse effects in pregnancy (Makrides et al., 2006). It is reasonable to advise an intake of 300–500 mg of DHA per day through supplementation or from eating fatty fish such as wild caught salmon, see Figure 9.1. Pregnant individuals living with low resources in the United States are especially vulnerable to inadequate omega-3 intake. A recent study found that this population had a mean omega-3 intake of only 89 mg daily, highlighting the need for particular focus in nutrition information and support

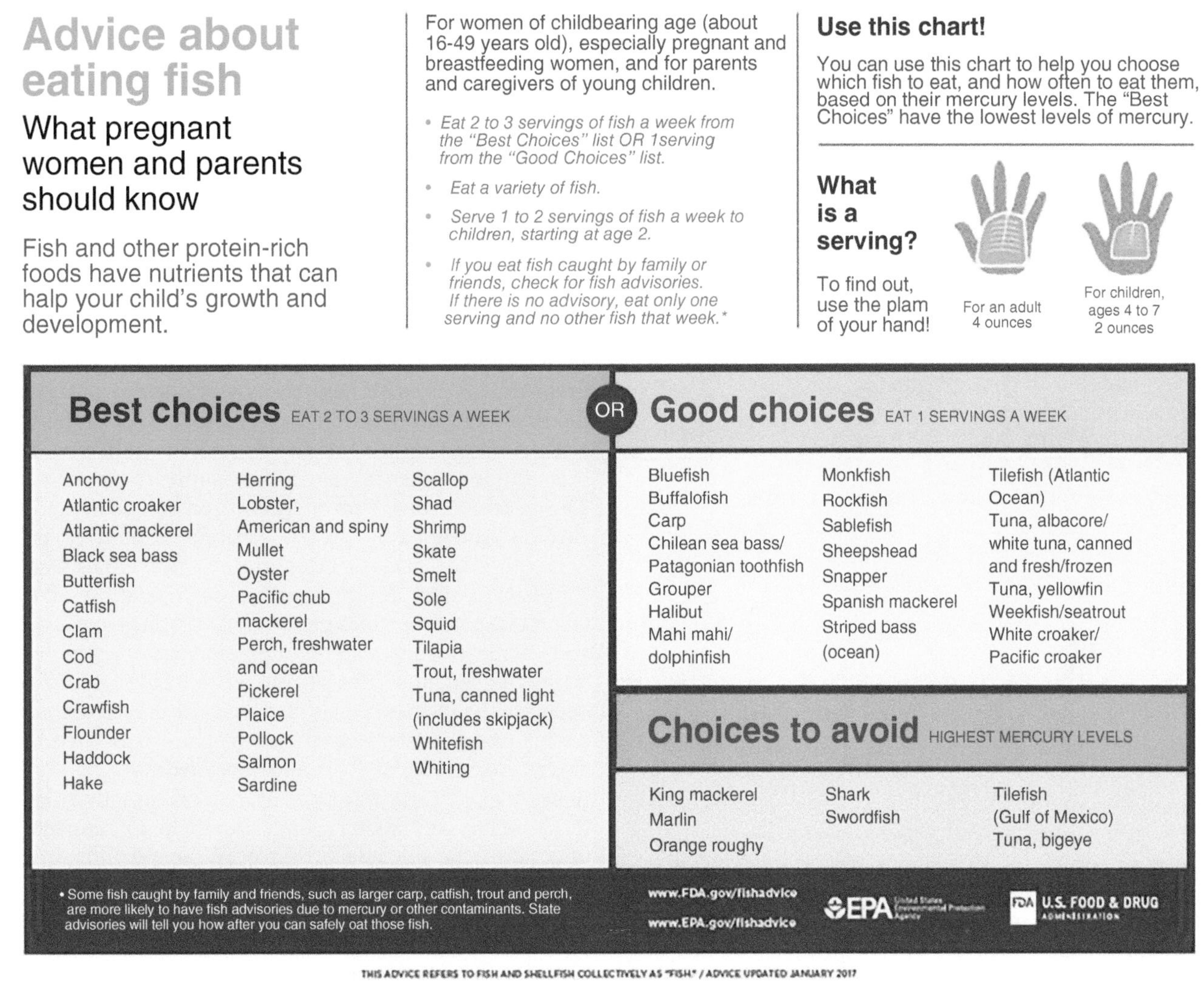

Advice about eating fish

What pregnant women and parents should know

Fish and other protein-rich foods have nutrients that can halp your child's growth and development.

For women of childbearing age (about 16-49 years old), especially pregnant and breastfeeding women, and for parents and caregivers of young children.

- *Eat 2 to 3 servings of fish a week from the "Best Choices" list OR 1serving from the "Good Choices" list.*
- *Eat a variety of fish.*
- *Serve 1 to 2 servings of fish a week to children, starting at age 2.*
- *If you eat fish caught by family or friends, check for fish advisories. If there is no advisory, eat only one serving and no other fish that week.**

Use this chart!

You can use this chart to help you choose which fish to eat, and how often to eat them, based on their mercury levels. The "Best Choices" have the lowest levels of mercury.

What is a serving?

To find out, use the plam of your hand!

For an adult 4 ounces

For children, ages 4 to 7 2 ounces

Best choices EAT 2 TO 3 SERVINGS A WEEK   **OR**   **Good choices** EAT 1 SERVINGS A WEEK

Best choices			Good choices		
Anchovy	Herring	Scallop	Bluefish	Monkfish	Tilefish (Atlantic
Atlantic croaker	Lobster,	Shad	Buffalofish	Rockfish	Ocean)
Atlantic mackerel	American and spiny	Shrimp	Carp	Sablefish	Tuna, albacore/
Black sea bass	Mullet	Skate	Chilean sea bass/	Sheepshead	white tuna, canned
Butterfish	Oyster	Smelt	Patagonian toothfish	Snapper	and fresh/frozen
Catfish	Pacific chub	Sole	Grouper	Spanish mackerel	Tuna, yellowfin
Clam	mackerel	Squid	Halibut	Striped bass	Weekfish/seatrout
Cod	Perch, freshwater	Tilapia	Mahi mahi/	(ocean)	White croaker/
Crab	and ocean	Trout, freshwater	dolphinfish		Pacific croaker
Crawfish	Pickerel	Tuna, canned light			
Flounder	Plaice	(includes skipjack)			
Haddock	Pollock	Whitefish			
Hake	Salmon	Whiting			
	Sardine				

Choices to avoid HIGHEST MERCURY LEVELS

King mackerel	Shark	Tilefish
Marlin	Swordfish	(Gulf of Mexico)
Orange roughy		Tuna, bigeye

• Some fish caught by family and friends, such as larger carp, catfish, trout and perch, are more likely to have fish advisories due to mercury or other contaminants. State advisories will tell you how after you can safely oat those fish.

www.FDA.gov/fishadvice
www.EPA.gov/fishadvice

EPA United States Environmental Protection Agency

FDA U.S. FOOD & DRUG ADMINISTRATION

THIS ADVICE REFERS TO FISH AND SHELLFISH COLLECTIVELY AS "FISH" / ADVICE UPDATED JANUARY 2017

Figure 9.1   Environmental Protection Agency (2022)/Public Domain/US Environment Protection Agency.

(Nordgren et al., 2017). It is helpful to counsel pregnant people on optimal supplementation methods; fat-soluble vitamin supplementation should be done in conjunction with a meal containing healthy fats.

Protein

Protein intake is essential to pregnancy because it forms the structural basis for the new cells and tissues in the pregnant person and fetus. Nitrogen is the primary element in protein that differentiates it from fats and carbohydrates. Protein sources include meat, fish, poultry eggs, dairy products, tofu and other soy products, legumes, nuts, and seeds. The RDA for protein intake during pregnancy and lactation is approximately 71 g/day for most pregnant people. The average protein intake for US women ages 20–44 is 78.5 g/day; thus, protein needs are easily met by most individuals (Murphy et al., 2021). Pregnant people who choose to eat no meat or animal protein and those living with **food insecurity** may experience protein deficiency.

When evaluating a diet for protein intake, the overall quality of the diet should be considered. Protein sources

with higher saturated fat intake are associated with alterations in gut microbiota that are likely to impair glucose metabolism (Ponzo et al., 2019). A person may have an adequate protein intake, but if their overall caloric intake is low, some of the amino acids from protein are used for energy rather than for building blocks. The quality of the protein should also be evaluated. Low-fat protein sources and food preparation methods should predominate in the prenatal diet. High-protein prenatal diets (above the RDA) are generally not recommended as these can lead to stress on the renal system from protein metabolism.

Micronutrients

Iron

Iron needs increase in pregnancy to support the increased maternal red blood cell mass and to build fetal iron stores needed for the first several months of life. In the first trimester, requirements are reduced because menstruation has ceased, the demands of the fetus are still small, and the expansion of the red cell mass during pregnancy is not yet significant. The need for additional iron begins early in the second trimester and reaches a

Table 9.3   Select Daily Macronutrient and Micronutrient Dietary Reference Intakes in Pregnancy

	Calcium (mg)	Vitamin D (mg)	Iron (mg)	Folate (mcg)	DHA and EPA (mg)	Carbohydrate (g)	Fiber (g)	Protein (g)
14–18 years old pregnant	1300	600	27	400	200–300	175	28	71
19–50 years old pregnant	1000	600	27	400	200–300	175	28	71

Source: Adapted from IOM National Academies Dietary Reference and Intake Tables (2020).

peak toward the end of the third trimester. Iron deficiency anemia during pregnancy increases risk for adverse birth outcomes, including low birth weight and perinatal mortality, and may increase the risk of PTB. See Chapter 48, *Hematologic and Thromboembolic Disorders*, for more on iron deficiency anemia. The RDA during pregnancy is 27 mg/day, which is the amount of iron commonly found in most prenatal vitamin formulations (Table 9.3).

Iron Absorption

Iron absorption refers to the amount of dietary iron that the body obtains and uses from food. Healthy adults absorb only about 10–15% of dietary iron, but individual absorption is influenced by the body's needs and conditions (Abbaspour et al., 2014). Iron absorption increases when body stores are low. When iron stores are high, absorption decreases to help protect against the toxic effects of iron overload. A person's body absorbs iron more efficiently during pregnancy, offering a protective effect against anemia.

Iron absorption is also influenced by the type of dietary iron consumed. Dietary iron has two forms: heme iron and nonheme iron. Heme is found in meat, poultry, and fish. Nonheme iron is found in eggs and plant-based foods, such as legumes, vegetables, fruit, grains, nuts, and iron-fortified grain products. Iron utilization from heme iron provides for a higher bioavailability of iron than nonheme sources or from ferrous sulfate iron supplementation (Moustarah & Mohiuddin, 2021). Absorption of heme iron from meat proteins is efficient and is not significantly affected by other food consumed at the same time. In contrast, nonheme iron in plant foods is not absorbed as efficiently and is significantly influenced by other food components ingested at the same meal. Meat proteins and vitamin C will improve the absorption of nonheme iron. Tannins, as found in tea, calcium, and some substances found in legumes and whole grains, can decrease the absorption of nonheme iron (National Institutes of Health [NIH], 2022a). Foods that enhance nonheme iron absorption should be encouraged, such as such as vitamin C-rich fruits and vegetables, especially when only vegetarian nonheme sources of iron are consumed. Individuals following **vegan** diets may consider temporarily consuming animal protein during pregnancy if this does not conflict with their values.

Iron Supplementation

Pregnant people with hematocrit levels less than 33% in the first and third trimesters or less than 32% in the second trimester should be supplemented with oral iron preparations and encouraged to consume iron-rich foods. The gastrointestinal side effects of iron supplementation, such as constipation, painful passage of hard or tarry black stool, and nausea, often prompt individuals to stop supplementation. Intermittent supplementation of one tablet one to three times per week can reduce side effects and increase acceptance of supplementation, while still improving anemia (Pena-Rosas et al., 2015a), and can decrease the incidence of high hemoglobin concentration during mid and late pregnancy, which are associated with an increased risk of PTB and low birth weight (Pena-Rosas et al., 2015b). Additionally, increasing activity level, fluid intake, and dietary fiber can help to reduce the uncomfortable side effects of iron. When recommending supplementation with iron, it is important not to take it in conjunction with calcium, caffeinated products, or high-fiber foods, which can inhibit iron absorption. Dietary sources of vitamin C can enhance iron absorption.

Folate

Folate, or folic acid, is a water-soluble form of vitamin B_9 found in foods such as leafy green vegetables, bananas, lentils, and fortified cereal products. It is well established that adequate folate intake before conception and during the first month after conception reduces the risk of neural tube defects (NTDs), including anencephaly and spina bifida. Supplementation of grain products with folic acid was initiated in 1998 by a mandate from the FDA in response to evidence regarding NTD prevention. The **fortification** program has been effective in reducing the incidence of all NTDs by 70% (Blencowe et al., 2010). Additionally, folic acid taken in the early weeks of pregnancy can reduce the risk of cardiovascular anomalies, perhaps by as much as 40% (Feng et al., 2015). Low levels of folate in early pregnancy are associated with lower placental weight and birth weight, and increased incidence of preeclampsia (Bergen et al., 2012). Expert groups advocate that people with capacity for pregnancy take folic acid supplements; however, most do not consume folic acid supplements regularly. During pregnancy, a person should consume 400 mcg of folate prior to and during pregnancy. Most prenatal vitamin formulations have at least 400 mcg of folic acid.

Calcium

The growing fetus requires adequate calcium for skeletal growth and development. Fetal calcium concentrations exceed maternal levels, indicating active transport of calcium across the placenta (Kovacs, 2014). The high fetal demand for calcium during pregnancy is facilitated by a maternal increase in calcium absorption ability during pregnancy. The RDA for elemental calcium is 1000 mg/day in pregnant and lactating people 19–50 years of age and 1300 mg for those 14–18 years old (IOM, 2020).

Many people who are capable of pregnancy in the United States do not consume the DRI for calcium. People at risk for lower calcium intake include adolescents, those who are lactose intolerant, who are following a vegetarian or vegan diet, and who have low income. **Vegetarians** might absorb less calcium than omnivores because they consume more plant products containing oxalic and phytic acids, which can block calcium absorption. People who begin pregnancy with adequate daily intake may not need additional calcium, but individuals with suboptimal intakes (<500 mg) require additional amounts to meet both maternal and fetal bone needs.

Rich natural sources of well-absorbed calcium include broccoli, kale, cabbage, milk, yogurt, and cheese. Thirty percent of the calcium levels in those foods are absorbed into the body. Calcium content varies slightly by fat content; the more fat, the less calcium the food contains. Calcium-fortified foods, such as orange juice and cereals, are also excellent sources. Calcium citrate may be the better supplementation choice because it does not depend on optimal stomach acid conditions for absorption like calcium carbonate. Additionally, if supplementing, doses more than 500 mg should be taken in split doses and separate from iron to maximize absorption (National Institutes of Health [NIH], 2020).

Vitamin D

Vitamin D, a fat-soluble molecule acquired through exposure to sunlight or diet, has been identified as a steroid hormone precursor that modulates the long-term programming of human health. Vitamin D helps the body use calcium and maximizes fetal bone growth. Supplementation with vitamin D can improve birth outcomes, such as reducing risk of PTB, LBW, and preeclampsia (Perez-Lopez et al., 2015; Sablok et al., 2015; Wei, 2014). There is a wide divergence of recommendations for prenatal vitamin D intake. The commonly followed guidelines issues by the NIH (2022b) and Institute of Medicine (IOM; 2020) recommend 600 IU daily during pregnancy. The Endocrine Society supports a daily intake of 4000-IU vitamin D_3 to achieve a circulating 25-hydroxyvitamin D of 40–60 ng/mL (100–150 nmol) during pregnancy (Curtis et al., 2018). This higher recommendation considers both observational and randomized controlled trial data. Research is ongoing in this area to reach consensus on recommendations. It is especially important to ensure adequate vitamin D intake during the winter months. Individuals with dark pigmented skin may need additional supplementation or exposure to sunlight compared to those with lighter pigmentation since sunlight helps the body synthesize vitamin D. Prenatal vitamin formulations typically contain between 400 and 600 IU vitamin D.

Weight Gain in Pregnancy

Once pregnancy is confirmed, monitoring gestational weight gain is incorporated as part of the prenatal care regimen. At the first prenatal visit, prepregnancy BMI is calculated using previously measured weights and heights or self-reported prepregnancy weight to establish the appropriate weight gain range. The weight gain range serves as the person's weight gain goal.

The total amount of weight gained in normal-term pregnancies varies considerably. As pregnancy progresses, weight is distributed across the fetus, placenta, amniotic fluid, uterus, mammary glands, blood, and adipose tissue compartments. Normal fetal growth is relatively uniform until the mid-second trimester. At term, there is much greater variation in fetal weight.

Average pregnancy weight gain distribution

- 6–8 lb baby
- 1.5 lb placenta
- 2 lb amniotic fluid
- 2 lb uterus growth
- 2 lb breast growth
- 8 lb added and body fluids
- 7 lb added muscle and fat stores

Source: Rasmussen and Yaktine (2009).

As more individuals of childbearing age have become heavier, recommendations have been reexamined to achieve a balance between the risks due to overweight or obese status and fetal growth needs. The IOM issues pregnancy weight gain recommendations based on prepregnancy weight (Table 9.4). People who gain weight within the IOM guidelines are more likely to have better maternal and infant outcomes (ACOG, 2013). The pattern of gestational weight gain, like total gestational weight gain, is also highly variable, even among those with good pregnancy outcomes.

Weight gain higher than IOM recommendations is linked with the same prenatal, intrapartum, and postpartum complications as prepregnancy obesity, such as preeclampsia and macrosomia. Excess weight gain during pregnancy and failure to lose weight after pregnancy are important and identifiable predictors of long-term obesity and weight-related complications later in life. While it is a standard of care to provide weight gain guidance, caution is advised when approaching the conversation. The use of motivational interviewing (MI) and therapeutic communication techniques is recommended. Conversations about weight can be very stigmatizing and

Table 9.4 IOM Recommendations for Total and Rate of Weight Gain during Pregnancy by Prepregnancy BMI

Prepregnancy BMI category	Recommended total weight gain (lb) range	Recommended weekly weight gain range, second and third trimesters (lb/week)[a]
Underweight: BMI <18.5	28–40	1–1.3
Normal weight: BMI 18.5–24.9	25–35	0.8–1
Overweight: BMI 25–29.9	15–25	0.5–0.7
Obese: BMI ≥30	11–20	0.4–0.6

Source: Rasmussen and Yaktine (2009)/The National Academies Press.

[a] Calculations assume 1.1–4.4 lb weight gain in the first trimester.

interrupt the patient–provider relationship. If weight-based counseling is provided, it is ideal to counsel periconceptually and at the first prenatal visit on their recommended weight gain range, based on IOM recommendations. The same caution is advised when monitoring weight during pregnancy. It should be approached with care as it can create a barrier between the provider and the pregnant person if weight is addressed disproportionate to dietary quality, or if the approach is stigmatizing or biased.

Overweight and Obesity in Pregnancy

Approximately 39% of women aged 20–39 in the United States are in the obese category by BMI (Hales et al., 2020). Overweight or obesity status prior to pregnancy is linked with increased risks for pregnancy complications such as GDM and preeclampsia (Dow & Szymanski, 2020), NTDs, omphalocele, and cardiac anomalies (Marchi et al., 2015). Obesity doubles the risk of stillbirth and neonatal death (Yao et al., 2014), and this can increase as high as threefold when BMI reaches 40 and over (Aune et al., 2014).

There is ongoing debate regarding the optimal amount of weight that people with severe obesity should gain during pregnancy. Some have advocated for no weight gain or even weight loss for people with obesity during pregnancy, which is associated with a higher risk of SGA (Devlieger et al., 2020), but can result in risk reduction of other perinatal complications such as operative birth and preeclampsia (Liang et al., 2018). Currently, weight gain recommendations below the IOM guidelines cannot be routinely recommended.

To avoid feeling shamed or stigmatized, clients should be able to measure their own weights in a private area or may wish to face away from the scale and not be told what their weight. Clients have a right to decline to be weighed; indeed, some providers avoid weighing altogether if it is a trigger for their clients. Issues related to obesity in pregnancy are covered in detail in Chapter 46, *Obesity in the Perinatal Period*.

Underweight in Pregnancy

The percentage of women who started their pregnancy underweight in the United States is approximately 4% (Centers for Disease Control and Prevention [CDC], 2016). People who begin their pregnancy underweight as defined by a BMI of less than 18.5 have a greater risk of PTB, even if only mildly underweight (Bhuyar & Dharmale, 2018), suggesting that a small variation in maternal weight is sufficient to increase the risk. Underweight individuals also have an increased risk of neonatal complications, infant low birth weight, and FGR (Gennette et al., 2017).

Screening for additional risk factors such as smoking, drug and alcohol use, and eating disorders should be done since these are often coexisting comorbidities in those who are underweight and malnourished. Additional factors that may promote inadequate weight gain include prolonged nausea and vomiting, conditions such as hyperemesis gravidarum, food aversions, lactose intolerance, cultural food practices, minimal resources such as poverty, poor prepregnancy diet, and excessive physical activity.

Strategies to improve weight gain begin with the development of a nutrition plan. A daily prenatal vitamin should be offered during pregnancy to help support nutrient needs of the pregnant person and growing fetus. The optimal weight gain for those who start pregnancy underweight is between 28 and 40 lb. A goal of 1–2 lb/week is appropriate.

Advice for achieving a healthy weight gain in pregnancy

- Eat breakfast.
- Eat fiber-rich foods such as oats, beans, peas, lentils, grains, seeds, fruits, and vegetables, as well as whole grain bread and pastas, and brown rice.
- Eat low-fat proteins such as fish (low in mercury) and lean meats.
- Eat at least five portions of various fruits and vegetables daily.
- Limit fried food, drinks, and desserts high in added sugars (such as cakes, pastries, and sodas).
- Limit foods high in empty calories (such as most fast foods and chips).
- Monitor portion size of meals and snacks.
- Make activities such as walking, cycling, swimming, aerobics, and gardening part of daily life.
- Minimize sedentary activities, such as sitting for long periods watching television, at a computer, or playing video games.
- Practice mindful eating. Remove distractions such as television, phone usage, and work while eating.

Pre- and Postnatal Flavor Learning

Recent research has suggested that flavor preferences start in utero based on what the pregnant person consumes. Through the maternal diet, the fetus is exposed to biochemicals in amniotic fluid that create taste and odor sensations. Infants and children have been found to be more accepting of a variety of foods when a variety of foods were consumed during pregnancy. This flavor learning carries over into the feeding method. Exclusively bottle-fed newborns are exposed solely to the flavor of formula and do not benefit from the ever-changing flavor profiles of breast milk. These prenatal and early life flavor exposures can modulate children's flavor preferences with the potential to improve lifelong health (Esposito et al., 2009; Mennella, 2014). Teaching about pre- and postnatal flavor learning can empower pregnant and breastfeeding people to influence their child's future nutritional health by eating a wide variety of healthy food.

Food Safety During Pregnancy

What is safe to eat and what should not be consumed during pregnancy can be an area of confusion. Pregnant individuals are at an increased risk for getting select **food-borne illnesses** because of the hormonal changes that occur during pregnancy. While such changes are necessary for the survival of the fetus, they also suppress the mother's immune system, thereby increasing the chance of infection from certain food-borne pathogens. All pregnant individuals should be provided with information on food safety and foods to avoid. Table 9.5 contains a list of select foods and beverages that should be avoided during pregnancy.

Food-Borne Infections

Certain organisms can cross the placenta and cause fetal infection. Infection can result in miscarriage, stillbirth, PTB, fetal infection, and neonatal illness. Examples of pathogens of special concern during pregnancy are

Table 9.5   Foods and Beverages to Avoid During Pregnancy

Food to avoid	Rationale	Do not consume
Alcohol	Alcohol is a known teratogen that may result in negative behavioral or neurological consequences in the offspring	Alcohol in any form
Raw fish	Raw or undercooked fish and shellfish are more likely to contain parasites and bacteria than foods made from cooked fish	Sushi; sashimi; raw or undercooked oysters, clams, and mussels; scallops; ceviche
Raw eggs	Raw eggs can contain salmonella and other food-borne illness-causing bacteria	Cookie dough, fresh eggnog, Hollandaise sauce, Béarnaise sauce, homemade mayonnaise and ice cream, mousse, meringue, tiramisu made with uncooked eggs
Raw milk	Some cheeses are made with unpasteurized milk. These cheeses are typically produced and sold locally. Potential pathogens are *Listeria* and *Escherichia coli*. Review labels and look for, "Made with pasteurized milk"	Raw milk such as goat's milk cheeses like chevre; queso fresco, Brie, Camembert; soft, blue-veined cheeses, such as Danish blue, gorgonzola, and Roquefort
Raw sprouts	Bacteria can get into the sprout seeds through cracks in the shell before the sprouts are grown. Once this occurs, these bacteria are nearly impossible to wash out	Alfalfa, clover, radish sprouts in salads or on sandwiches
Unpasteurized juice	Unpasteurized juices may contain harmful bacteria such as *E. coli*. Unpasteurized juices must have a warning on the label	Unpasteurized apple cider, health-food store juices, juice bar juices
Smoked meats and seafood refrigerated pate, meat spreads from a meat counter	Possible source of *Listeria*	Refrigerated smoked seafood like whitefish, salmon, and mackerel; meat, fish, and vegetable pate. Foods that do not need storage refrigeration, like canned tuna or salmon, are okay to eat. Refrigerate after opening
Unheated lunch meats, hot dogs, store-made protein salads	Possible source of *Listeria;* to eat safely, lunch meats and hot dogs should be reheated until steaming hot	Store-made salads such as ham salad, chicken salad, egg salad, tuna salad, or seafood salad
Excessive caffeine	Possible increased risk of miscarriage	>200 mg caffeine: about two 8-oz cups of coffee

Source: US Department of Agriculture (2017).

Listeria monocytogenes, Toxoplasma gondii, Brucella species, *Salmonella* species, and *Campylobacter jejuni.*

Listeriosis is a form of infection that may result when foods containing the bacteria *L. monocytogenes* are consumed, which is widely found in soil, groundwater, plants, and animals. *L. monocytogenes* is often carried by humans and animals and can survive unfavorable conditions, including refrigeration temperatures, food preservatives, and conditions with little or no oxygen. It is easily destroyed by cooking. Once in the bloodstream, *Listeria* bacteria can travel to any site, but seem to prefer the central nervous system and the placenta. The fetus is unusually vulnerable to listeriosis, and infection can cause early pregnancy loss, stillbirth, or infection of the neonate and significant health problems. There is an estimated 14-fold increase in the incidence of listeriosis among pregnant adults compared to nonpregnant adults; approximately one-third of all cases occur in pregnancy (Pouillot et al., 2012).

Listeriosis is more common in the third trimester, and signs and symptoms are easily missed. A nonspecific flu-like illness with symptoms such as fever, chills, headache, muscle aches, and backaches is the most common presentation. Foods typically associated with listeriosis have a long shelf life and are eaten without further cooking. Outbreaks have involved foods such as coleslaw, Mexican-style soft cheeses, milk, pate, pork tongue, hot dogs, processed meats, and deli salads. Safe food handling should be encouraged to avoid infection from *L. monocytogenes* (Madjunkov et al., 2017).

Safe food handling

- Wash hands frequently during food preparation.
- Wash fruits and vegetables before eating or preparation.
- Wash kitchen surfaces, cutting boards, and utensils before and after food preparation, especially after contact with raw meat or poultry.
- Separate raw meat, poultry, and seafood from other foods.
- Cook food to proper temperatures.
- Refrigerate foods quickly to prevent harmful bacteria from proliferating.
- Refrigerate all perishable foods at or below 40 °F.
- Reheat leftover foods to 165 °F before eating.

Source: Adapted from US Department of Agriculture (2017).

Toxoplasmosis, the infection caused by the parasite *T. gondii,* can be passed to humans by water, dust, soil, or through eating contaminated foods. It is estimated that 1.5 million people in the United States become infected with *T. gondii* each year (CDC, 2018). Most individuals do not experience symptoms and will develop a protective resistance to the parasite. However, if a person not previously exposed to *T. gondii* first acquires the parasite a few months before or during pregnancy, they may pass the organism to the fetus. This could result in stillbirth, fetal death, or neonatal health problems such as eye or brain damage. Symptoms in the baby may not be visible at birth but can appear months or even years later.

Toxoplasmosis most often results from eating raw or undercooked meat, especially pork, and wild game meat, eating unwashed fruits and vegetables, cleaning a cat litter box, or handling contaminated soil. To avoid infection from *T. gondii*, it is important that safe food-handling procedures are practiced. Meats should be cooked to the appropriate internal temperature with a three-minute rest time, as this kills *T. gondii* (CDC, 2018).

Prevention of food-borne toxoplasmosis

- Cook food to safe temperatures. A food thermometer should be used to measure the internal temperature of cooked meat. Do not sample meat until it is cooked. USDA recommends the following for meat preparation.
- Whole cuts of meat (excluding poultry): cook to at least 145 °F (63 °C) as measured with a food thermometer placed in the thickest part of the meat, then allow the meat to rest for three minutes before carving or consuming.
- Ground meat (excluding poultry): cook to at least 160 °F (71 °C); ground meats do not require a rest time.
- Poultry (whole cuts and ground): cook to at least 165 °F (74 °C), and for whole poultry allow the meat to rest for three minutes before carving or consuming.
- Freeze meat for several days at subzero (0 °F) temperatures before cooking to greatly reduce chance of infection.
- Peel or wash fruits and vegetables thoroughly before eating.
- Wash cutting boards, dishes, counters, utensils, and hands with hot soapy water after contact with raw meat, poultry, seafood, or unwashed fruits or vegetables.

Source: CDC Toxoplasmosis Prevention and Control (2018).

Prevention of environmentally acquired toxoplasmosis

- Avoid drinking untreated drinking water.
- Wear gloves when gardening and during any contact with soil or sand because it might be contaminated with cat feces that contain *Toxoplasma*, and wash hands with soap and warm water afterward.
- Teach children the importance of washing hands to prevent infection.
- Keep outdoor sandboxes covered to prevent introduction of cat feces.
- Feed cats only canned or dried commercial food or well-cooked table food, not raw or undercooked meats.
- Change the litter box daily if you live with a cat, especially one that goes outdoors. The *Toxoplasma* parasite does not become infectious until one to five days after it is shed in a cat's feces.
- During pregnancy:
  - Avoid changing cat litter if possible. If no one else can perform the task, wear disposable gloves and wash hands with soap and warm water afterward.
  - Keep cats indoors if possible.
  - Do not adopt or handle stray cats, especially kittens.

Campylobacteriosis is an infection caused by consuming food or water that contains the bacteria *C. jejuni or Campylobacter coli*. It is a very common cause of diarrhea accompanied by fever in the United States. These organisms are found in the intestinal tracts of animals, especially chickens, and in untreated water. People are infected most often by consuming raw unpasteurized milk and raw milk products, raw or undercooked poultry or meat, and raw shellfish (CDC, 2011). Maternal campylobacteriosis infection can be transmitted to the fetus through the placenta. While *Campylobacter* infections are usually self-limited and rarely cause mortality, consequences of fetal infection include abortion, stillbirth, or PTB. Maternal symptoms usually appear within two to five days after eating the contaminated food and include fever, stomach cramps, muscle pain, diarrhea, nausea, and vomiting. The diagnosis is established by stool culture and infection is treated with erythromycin. To avoid campylobacteriosis, pregnant people are advised to practice safe food-handling procedures, to consume only pasteurized milk and milk products, and to thoroughly cook meat, poultry, and shellfish (CDC, 2011).

Alcohol, Caffeine, and Artificial Sweeteners

Alcohol is a teratogen, and no safe level of alcohol consumption during pregnancy has been established. All pregnant people should be counseled to abstain from drinking alcoholic beverages. Some individuals are concerned about alcohol intake in early gestation before they knew they were pregnant. During conception and for about two weeks thereafter, most cells of the conceptus are not yet committed to a specific developmental sequence. One damaged cell can be replaced by another, and normal development will usually ensue, although the embryo will not survive if too many cells are damaged or killed. This is known as the "all or none" period where the fetus is generally not susceptible to teratogens (Cragan et al., 2006). Those who ingested alcohol in the first few weeks of pregnancy should be offered reassurance regarding this early exposure.

Excessive caffeine intake during pregnancy is associated with an increased risk of spontaneous miscarriage and low birth weight (James, 2021). Caffeine intake less than 200 mg/day is encouraged (March of Dimes [MOD], 2020). Average caffeine content of brewed coffee is 188 mg for 16 oz, with a range of 143–300 mg, although caffeine content can vary widely among different type of beans used within one brand. Carbonated sodas contain caffeine amounts between 18 and 48 mg/12-oz can, whereas energy drinks have higher caffeine content of 33–75 mg/8.4 oz (McCusker et al., 2006). Encourage awareness regarding the different caffeine contents of various coffee and cola drinks and encourage a reasonable intake.

Few studies have investigated whether regular intakes of foods containing artificial sweeteners are safe during pregnancy. Moderate intake of non-nutritive sweeteners (NNSs) that are classified by the FDA as "generally recognized as safe" within acceptable daily intakes is considered safe in pregnancy. NNSs that are generally recognized as safe include aspartame, sucralose, neotame, and stevia. Sucralose may not cross the fetal placental barrier, while saccharine can cross the placental barrier and reach the fetus (Halasa et al., 2021). NNS that crosses the placenta may have long-term metabolic effects throughout childhood (Halasa et al., 2021). Careful consideration should be made when counseling about NNS intake during pregnancy. Recent evidence links prenatal NNS exposure with higher birth weight and higher rates of childhood obesity (Azad et al., 2016), and high prenatal NNS intake with PTB (Petherick et al., 2014).

Factors Influencing Nutritional Intake

Resource Availability

There are significant differences in food choices in different socioeconomic classes that lead to both under- and overnutrition. Class differences in diet are of particular concern with respect to health inequalities. Individuals with nutritional deficits are often found in low socioeconomic populations and commonly involve multiple nutrients. Food insecurity and food deserts are associated with risk of excessive weight gain during pregnancy and pregnancy complications such as GDM (Laraia et al., 2010).

Food Insecurity and Social Determinants

Social determinants of health have a direct impact on nutritional quality. Poverty, access to nutritional services and programs, living in rural areas or food deserts, lower education, and racism in healthcare are all social determinants that contribute to nutritionally associated health inequities (Healthcare Value Hub, 2020).

Healthy People 2030 (HP2030) has identified food insecurity as a primary factor in the economic stability domain under the social determinants of health. HP2030 seeks to reduce the food insecurity rate to 6% from 10.5% of households (US Department of Health and Human Services, n.d.), due to risks associated with food insecurity such as obesity and chronic disease. It affects one in eight adults and approximately 11% of households in the United States (Healthcare Value Hub, 2020). Lower socioeconomic status, lower levels of education, living in rural areas, Black race, and family structures were all associated with an increased likelihood of food insecurity and poor diet quality (Demétrio et al., 2020; Parker et al., 2020). Race is a risk factor for food insecurity due to longstanding effects of systemic racism. Black pregnant people are more likely to experience food insecurity in pregnancy compared to non-Black pregnant people, and individuals entering pregnancy with existing food insecurity have increased odds of excessive or inadequate weight gain during pregnancy (Demétrio et al., 2020). Individuals with very low food security have reduced food diversity and decreased dietary intake (Healthcare Value Hub, 2020). Individuals with food insecurity will likely choose to consume empty calories or skip meals because of the lack of access to high-quality nutrient dense foods. Access to nutritionally dense foods is very important during the prenatal period because of the direct correlation with birth outcomes (Grieger & Clifton, 2015).

Culture and Family

Traditions, beliefs, and values are among the main factors that influence food preference, mode of food preparation, and nutritional status. The shaping of food choices takes place in the home, which typically reflects cultural preferences and norms. Diverse cultural components of behavior have significant impacts on patterns of eating irrespective of socioeconomic status. Many cultures have food beliefs, customs, or proscriptions specific to pregnancy that are considered important to maternal–fetal, physical, emotional, and spiritual health. Some food beliefs may have an influence on dietary choices, but can often be incorporated into a healthy diet. Foods from all cultures can enable a healthy pregnancy diet, and nutritional advice should be provided within the context of the person's cultural preferences (see Chapter 19, *Culture and Community*).

Completing a Nutritional Assessment

A dietary assessment informs the healthcare provider about the pregnant person's daily nourishment and provides a foundation for prenatal nutritional counseling. At the initial prenatal visit, the person's attitudes toward weight gain, physical activity, and nutrition during pregnancy should be assessed and individualized advice provided based on this assessment. Simple dietary assessments, such as 24-hour diet recalls and food records and checklists, can be used to evaluate diet and nutrient intakes throughout pregnancy. A complete nutritional assessment includes relevant history, relevant physical examination, and laboratory testing. An assessment of nutritional status begins with taking an accurate history of factors that can influence eating behaviors and nutrition. Much of this information is obtained during routine questioning at the first prenatal visit (Table 9.6). Risk factors for inadequate nutrition during pregnancy include adolescence, smoking or other substance use, brief interconception period, multiple gestation, high or low BMI, restrictive diet patterns, bariatric surgery, and social issues such as homelessness, poverty, or domestic violence.

After the general history is taken, a more specific history regarding diet is obtained in order to make a complete evaluation and relevant plan for pregnancy nutrition (Table 9.7). It is important to consider using closed- and open-ended questions when evaluating dietary quality. While closed-ended questions provide valuable quick information, open-ended questions provide in depth insight into factors that influence dietary choices. Starting the Conversation (STC) is a validated, efficient eight-item screening tool designed for assessment and counseling in busy clinical settings to identify dietary patterns and readiness to make changes (Paxton et al., 2011). This tool has been adapted for using with pregnant individuals to offer guidance for healthy choices (Widen & Siega-Riz, 2010; Figure 9.2). Depending on the person's responses to the questions and readiness to change, appropriate advice for dietary improvement and guidance with goal setting can

Table 9.6 Factors that Influence Nutritional Status

Relevant medical history	✓ Preexisting conditions such as diabetes or cardiovascular disease ✓ Bariatric surgery or gastrointestinal disorders that can contribute to gut dysbiosis ✓ Anemia or other nutritional deficiencies ✓ Past or current eating disorder ✓ Food allergies or intolerances
Psychosocial and personal history	✓ Tobacco, alcohol, or substance use ✓ Current exercise and activity patterns ✓ Economic status and resources ✓ Living situation and family structure ✓ Family or intimate partner violence ✓ Support systems ✓ Prior history of depression and current emotional health ✓ Feelings about pregnancy ✓ Educational level ✓ Cognitive level ✓ Ethnic/cultural group and food preferences and prohibitions ✓ Language proficiency
Past and current pregnancies	✓ Gravidity and parity ✓ History of preterm birth or low-birth-weight infant ✓ Gestational diabetes ✓ Interconception interval ✓ Breastfeeding history ✓ Weight gain pattern in prior pregnancy ✓ Reports of nausea and vomiting, heartburn, and constipation ✓ Hyperemesis gravidarum

be provided. To facilitate the counseling session, responses are organized into three columns. The left column indicates the healthiest dietary habits, the center column indicates less healthy habits, and the right column indicates the least healthy practices. Responses in the left column are scored 0, and responses in the center column and right column are scored 1 and 2, respectively. Total scores range from 0 to 14, with higher scores reflecting poor diet habits and lower scores healthy diet habits.

The physical exam to assess nutritional status includes parameters evaluated at the first prenatal visit. The determination of weight and BMI status is done first. The remainder of the exam includes skin, hair, nails, mucosa, heart, thyroid, and screens for signs of nutritional deficiencies (Table 9.8).

Using Nutrition Resources

Smartphone applications and web resources provide additional mechanisms to monitor dietary intake and quality. The instant feedback and tailored approach provided with Internet-based technologies can improve nutritional self-efficacy and knowledge. Specific and personalized dietary information delivered through a multimedia method can improve dietary behaviors (Livingstone et al., 2016).

Table 9.7   Components of a Detailed Nutritional Health History

Topic	Questions
Food resources	Do you or your family run out of food before there is money to buy more? If so, please share what do you do until you are able to purchase food.
Food assistance programs	Does your family receive food stamps? Utilize community food pantries? Are they enrolled in the WIC program?
Food preparation and cooking resources	Who purchases and prepares the family food? Do you have a working refrigerator, stove, oven, and freezer?
Eating away from home	How often do you or your family eat away from home? What types of foods? Fast food?
Usual eating pattern	What are the typical patterns of eating meals and snacks? Describe a typical day when you are in your home and when you are out for the day? Please include the estimated time of day you typically consume each meal or snack. Do you skip meals? If so, would you mind sharing why?
Cultural/ethnic/religious food practices	What types of foods do you eat, and how are they prepared? Do you have specific cultural food beliefs or traditions related to pregnancy?
Dietary supplements	Do you take vitamin supplements and herbal preparation? If so, what types? How often, and in what doses?
Dieting practices	Have you dieted frequently in the past, gained and lost weight? What diet methods were used? Do you have any concerns about your weight? Would you like to discuss them further?
Activity level	What are your current daily activity levels? Regular exercise habits?
Detailed diet history	This can be done with screening tools (like STC; see Figure 9.1) and/or a one- to three-day food diary to be brought at the next visit. If asking for a food diary, be sure to have the patient include a day at home and a day outside of the house.

MyPlate, for example, is an illustrative and interactive tool provided by the USDA that helps people analyze their personal dietary habits and provides daily recommendations for healthy eating during pregnancy based on individual BMI, physical activity level, and gestational age (see *Resources for Clients and Their Families*). People can enter food data themselves and evaluate areas of adequacy and those areas that need improvement. This self-assessment can help empower individuals to evaluate nutritional choices and make changes during pregnancy as needed and monitor their progress. The tool provides an individualized estimate of nutrients needed by food groups and the daily amount recommended in cups or ounces for each food group. This type of information may be more practically usable than the general advice given by many clinicians of simply encouraging an additional 300 cal/day. People can see how their food choices compare to what they need during pregnancy and can develop printable daily menu plans specific to pregnancy needs. Additionally, MyPlate uses a visual plate icon to estimate the relative portion sizes of the food groups people should eat at a meal they have planned, thus enhancing the knowledge of appropriate servings and portion size. A checklist is provided to aid in meeting their daily nutritional goals (Figure 9.3).

Some people do not have fluency in or access to computer-based technologies to use these platforms; these individuals rely on the clinician to provide resources. Resources like the USDA Food Tracker can be used in an office setting to enter a person's information and provide resources to print and take home. Additionally, packets of printed materials on pregnancy nutritional needs and strategies for healthy eating and weight control can be created at this website.

The Women, Infants, and Children's (WIC) program is a supplemental food and nutrition program for pregnant and postpartum people and children under five years old. Through the WIC program, financial assistance in purchasing food, counseling and information on healthy eating, breastfeeding support and information, and referrals to healthcare and other community resources, such as food kitchens and food pantries, are available. All prenatal care providers should be familiar with program services provided and should facilitate enrollment for eligible people. Those who need more comprehensive dietary guidance, such as those with diabetes and obesity, and who follow restrictive diets, benefit from referral to a dietitian who can help them meet pregnancy nutritional needs.

Counseling for Optimal Prenatal Nutrition

Detailed and personalized advice on weight gain and food selection can assist in the attainment of pregnancy weight and nutrition goals. Weight should not be the primary focus as it can be stigmatizing. It is important to focus on the quality of food, identifying what the person wants to learn and what their goals are when approaching a therapeutic nutrition education session. A lack of advice and support from healthcare professionals can lead individuals to seek information for themselves,

Starting the conversation on healt y eating for pregnant women

ARE YOU READY TO WORK ON HEALTHY EATING DURING YOUR PREGNANCY?
___ I'm ready to make some changes and I would like help
___ I'm not sure if I'm ready to change the way I eat but I would like to start the conversation
___ I'm not ready to change the way I eat at this time

HOW WELL DO YOU EAT?	TIPS TO HELP YOU EAT WELL
How many times a week do you eat food that is fried or high in fat? ☐ Less than 1 ☐ 1-3 ☐ 4 or more	**Eat less fast food.** • If you eat fast food, order grilled chicken, a salad or plain burger.
How many servings of fruit and vegetables do you eat each day? ☐ 5 or more ☐ 3-4 ☐ 2 or less	**Aim for 5 or more servings of fruits and vegetables a day.** • Add a fruit and a vegetable to each meal. • Raw fruits and vegetables are easy snacks.
How many regular sodas, juice or glasses of sweetened beverages do you drink each day? ☐ Less than 1 ☐ 1-2 ☐ 3 or more	**Beverage calories add up.** • Drink water throughout the day. • If you drink milk, switch from whole or 2% to 1% or skim. • Limit soda and other sweet drinks to one or less per day.
How many times a week do you eat beans (like pinto or black beans), chicken or fish? ☐ 3 or more ☐ 1-2 ☐ Less than 1	**Eat more beans, chicken and fish.** • Beans are a great substitute for meat. • Eat up to 12 oz. of low-mercury fish weekly like canned light tuna, salmon or pollock. • Eat baked, broiled, or grilled chicken and fish. • Avoid high mercury fish like shark, swordfish, king mackerel and tilefish.
How many times a week do you eat regular (not low-fat) snack chips or crackers? ☐ 1 or less ☐ 2-3 ☐ 4 or more	**Hold the chips.** • Try popcorn, but limit oil, butter or salt. • Try nuts such as almonds or walnuts, but limit your serving to 2 Tablespoons.
How many times a week do you eat desserts and other sweets? ☐ 1 or less ☐ 2-3 ☐ 4 or more	**Be smart with your sweet tooth.** • Eat smaller amounts of dessert. • Try desserts with less fat and calories like fruit, sherbet or angel food cake.
How much butter, lard and animal fat (visible fat in red meat, chicken skin) do you eat? ☐ Very little ☐ Some ☐ A lot	**Cut back on animal fats.** • Use a small amount of plant-based oils and trans-fat free margarines. • Season foods with spices and fresh herbs.

0 x (____) +   1 x (____) +   2 x (____) = Total Score _____

IF YOU FEEL THIS WAY	TRY THESE THINGS
Healthy food costs too much.	**Eating well can save you money.** • Eat less meat and more beans. • Eat canned or frozen fruits and vegetables. • Eat at home instead of going out.
Healthy food doesn't taste as good as junk food.	**Don't give up your favorite foods—just eat smaller amounts.** • Try new foods and recipes.
I eat when I'm bored, tired, angry or depressed.	**Find something else to distract you.** • Work on a hobby, call a friend, go for a walk. • Keep only healthy snacks around.
It's hard to be healthy when I eat out.	**Avoid all-you-can-eat places and restaurants that don't offer healthy options** • Order grilled or low-fat sandwiches and salads instead of fried foods. • Ask for low-fat dressing on the side. • Ask for half portions, share with a friend, or bring leftovers home.
I eat too much at social events.	**You can still eat healthy at social events.** • Eat a healthy snack before you go. • Choose a few things to eat. • Bring healthy dishes to potlucks.
I eat too much when I'm cooking or cleaning.	**Don't just eat because it is there.** • Chew gum or a toothpick. • Ask someone else to put away leftovers while you wash dishes.
I tend to skip regular meals, but snack in front of the TV and throughout the day.	**Make time for regular meals.** • Sit down at the table and eat healthy meals with friends, family and/or co-workers. • Pack lunch and snacks to take to work or for travel.

Making a Plan

What goal(s) can you set for yourself now?
Before my next visit, I am going to:
___ Eat fried foods less often
___ Aim to eat 5 or more fruits and vegetables per day
___ Eat smaller portions
___ Instead of regular sodas, juice and sugar sweetened beverages, drink water or skim milk
___ Keep healthy snacks around
___ Other _____

Figure 9.2   Starting the Conversation with pregnant women. Used with permission from Wiley.

Table 9.8   Clinical Signs of Nutritional Status

Body area	Signs of adequate nutrition	Signs of inadequate nutrition
Weight	Normal for height, body build	Overweight or underweight
Hair	Shiny, firm, not easily plucked	Stringy, brittle, sparse
Skin	Smooth, good color	Rough, dry, scaly, petechiae, pale, bruised
Oral membranes	Reddish/pink	Mucosa swollen, boggy tissue
Gums	Pink, no swelling or bleeding	Spongy, bleeds easily, inflamed, gums receding
Teeth	No cavities, no pain	Black caries, absent teeth, worn surfaces, malpositioned teeth
Eyes	Bright, clear, no sores, moist	Pale conjunctiva, dryness, redness
Nails	Firm, pink	Brittle, ridged, spoon-shaped

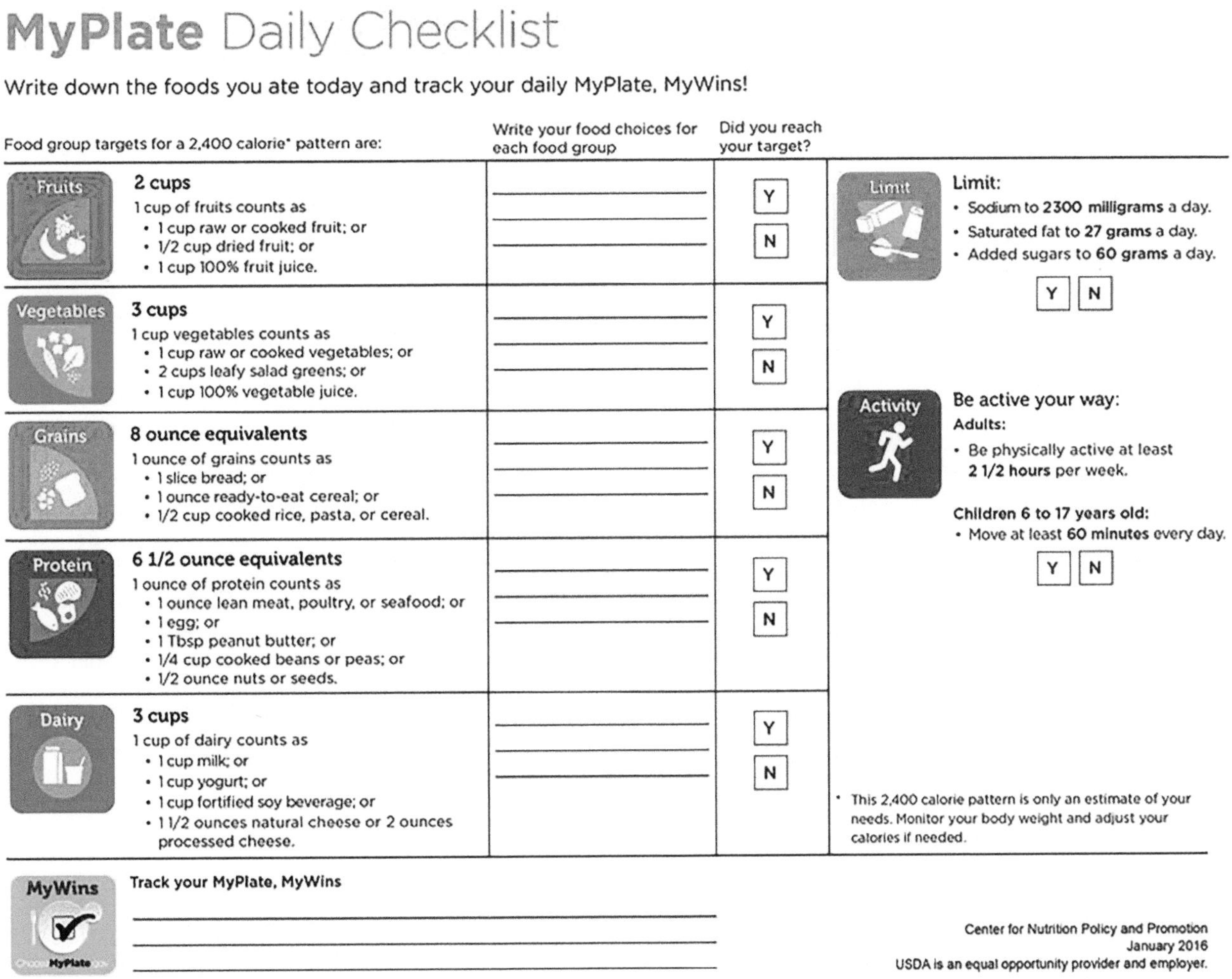

MyPlate Daily Checklist

Write down the foods you ate today and track your daily MyPlate, MyWins!

Food group targets for a 2,400 calorie* pattern are:

		Write your food choices for each food group	Did you reach your target?

Fruits — **2 cups**
1 cup of fruits counts as
- 1 cup raw or cooked fruit; or
- 1/2 cup dried fruit; or
- 1 cup 100% fruit juice.

Y / N

Vegetables — **3 cups**
1 cup vegetables counts as
- 1 cup raw or cooked vegetables; or
- 2 cups leafy salad greens; or
- 1 cup 100% vegetable juice.

Y / N

Grains — **8 ounce equivalents**
1 ounce of grains counts as
- 1 slice bread; or
- 1 ounce ready-to-eat cereal; or
- 1/2 cup cooked rice, pasta, or cereal.

Y / N

Protein — **6 1/2 ounce equivalents**
1 ounce of protein counts as
- 1 ounce lean meat, poultry, or seafood; or
- 1 egg; or
- 1 Tbsp peanut butter; or
- 1/4 cup cooked beans or peas; or
- 1/2 ounce nuts or seeds.

Y / N

Dairy — **3 cups**
1 cup of dairy counts as
- 1 cup milk; or
- 1 cup yogurt; or
- 1 cup fortified soy beverage; or
- 1 1/2 ounces natural cheese or 2 ounces processed cheese.

Y / N

Limit:
- Sodium to **2300 milligrams** a day.
- Saturated fat to **27 grams** a day.
- Added sugars to **60 grams** a day.

Y / N

Activity — **Be active your way:**
Adults:
- Be physically active at least **2 1/2 hours** per week.

Children 6 to 17 years old:
- Move at least **60 minutes** every day.

Y / N

* This 2,400 calorie pattern is only an estimate of your needs. Monitor your body weight and adjust your calories if needed.

MyWins — Track your MyPlate, MyWins

Center for Nutrition Policy and Promotion
January 2016
USDA is an equal opportunity provider and employer.

Figure 9.3   USDA MyPlate Pregnancy Food Plan Checklist for women needing 2400 daily calories. US Department of Agriculture (2021)/ US Department of Agriculture.

sometimes from unreliable web sources (Kennedy et al., 2017). There is much conflicting advice on what constitutes an optimal diet in pregnancy. Health professionals are a trusted source of nutrition and weight management advice, and therefore, it is very important that the advice offered is consistent and evidence-based and able to counter any conflicting advice received from family, friends, and the media. Advice provided during prenatal care regarding weight gain, diet, and exercise is brief and is generally not related to weight management during pregnancy (Brown & Avery, 2012). Interventions focused on a person's personal diet are the most effective and are associated with reductions in maternal gestational weight gain and improved perinatal outcomes (Thangaratinam et al., 2012). Providing a pregnant person with specific dietary information, guidance, and support throughout the course of prenatal care can help them achieve pregnancy weight gain goals. Additionally, the provider should not unilaterally set goals for the pregnant person, but rather work alongside the person setting both short- and long-term dietary goals utilizing principles of shared decision-making.

Strategies to promote optimal pregnancy nutrition

- Utilize motivational interviewing.
- Provide positive feedback on healthful dietary practices.
- Share findings on dietary areas of adequacy/excess/deficiency.
- Share specific nutrient information on how much is taken in now and what is needed daily.
- Provide information on how specific nutrients are useful to fetal and maternal health.
- Provide specific suggestions for change with examples.
- Assess diet and weight gain at each visit, unless the individual finds this triggering and requests that weight not be discussed or monitored.

After subjective and objective dietary quality data points are obtained, MI can be used to facilitate behavior change to optimize pregnancy outcomes. MI is a method of communication with a client that is centered around the person, not the practitioner, and incorporates active listening and providing information and advice to empower a person to change particular behaviors. MI values autonomy and personal choice. There are four fundamental actions for MI that include (a) engaging, (b) focusing, (c) evoking, and (d) planning. The first action, engaging, establishes the mutually beneficial trusting relationship between the pregnant person and practitioner via active listening, positive reinforcement of strengths while respecting personal decision-making. Focusing is the process of beginning the language focused on behavior change. Evoking helps the person establish their motivation for behavior change without judgment. It is important to consider that people may not be ready to make a behavior change. Finally, the planning action establishes the process of the client-selected behavior change that is supported by the practitioner. MI has been shown to have a positive impact on pregnancy-related behavior changes for improved birth outcomes (Rasouli et al., 2018).

Special Issues in Prenatal Nutrition

Adolescent Pregnancy

Adolescence represents the second major growth phase in an individual's life. The additional energy and nutrient demands of pregnancy place adolescents at nutritional risk. Pregnant teens are more likely to have a background of poverty, be a member of an ethnic minority, and engage in smoking, alcohol, and substance use, placing them at further risk for poor pregnancy outcomes. It is important to note that the link between teenage pregnancy and ethnic minority groups is secondary to the impact of systemic racism and bias. The racial makeup of a person is not inherently the risk; rather, it is how the marginalized racial group is treated in the United States. Adolescents may not have adequate knowledge of nutrition, and their present-focused orientation may inhibit them from linking current behaviors, such as eating poorly, to later outcomes. Poor dietary habits are common among adolescents, and many enter pregnancy with suboptimal iron status, unhealthy weight, and low intake of several key nutrients. Teens are more likely than adults to consume energy-dense, micronutrient-poor diets and to experience adverse pregnancy outcomes such as LBW (Karataşlı et al., 2019).

Assessment

In addition to the routine history and physical examination, the evaluation of a pregnant teen's nutritional status includes the number of years since onset of menarche. Teens who conceive within two years of the onset of menarche are at highest risk for poor pregnancy outcomes due to their own physiologic immaturity. The greater the amount of uncompleted growth at conception, the greater the energy and nutrient needs above those normally required during pregnancy.

Pregnancy Nutritional Needs

Adolescence is a critical time of life to accumulate bone for peak bone mass; thus, ensuring adequate calcium intake during pregnancy is important to later health. The DRI is 1300 mg calcium/day for those 18 years of age or younger who are pregnant and those who are lactating. Many pregnant adolescents consume diets that provide less than recommended intakes of key nutrients. Low calcium intakes are well documented in adolescents. Improving maternal calcium intake and vitamin D status during pregnancy has a positive effect on fetal skeletal development in pregnant adolescents (Young et al., 2012). During pregnancy, intestinal calcium absorption doubles to meet fetal demand for calcium, but if maternal intake of calcium is insufficient to meet the combined needs of the pregnant person and fetus, the maternal skeleton will undergo resorption during the third trimester. Teen pregnancy can be associated with osteoporosis later in life (Cho et al., 2012).

Pregnant teens have a high prevalence of anemia. Concern is especially warranted because the iron requirements for adolescents are relatively high due to growth spurts, sexual maturation, and menstrual losses. Pregnancy places an additional burden on iron stores, predisposing the pregnant teen to anemia. Supplementation with iron and folic acid significantly reduces anemia and improves outcomes in this population (Salam et al., 2016).

Counseling

Pregnancy can motivate many pregnant adolescents to improve their diets to have a healthy baby. Pregnancy provides a window of opportunity for educating young people about the importance of healthy eating. Adolescents tend to retain more weight postpartum, which can have a lifelong effect on their BMI (Danilack et al., 2018; Groth et al., 2013; Joseph et al., 2008). Prenatal nutrition and activity counseling to promote optimal weight gain can reduce postpartum weight retention and improve long-term health. Developing strategies for working with pregnant adolescents can increase healthy habits and improve outcomes.

Strategies for dietary change in pregnant adolescents

- Establish a positive, supportive relationship.
- Assess the teen's perspective of their diet.
- Determine the teen's willingness to learn.
- Use specific foods rather than nutrients in teaching.
- Use images of food on handouts to display optimal food choices.
- Follow up on diet and physical activity at each visit.
- Provide verbal positive feedback for improvements.
- Include relevant family members in planning.
- Consider introducing smartphone tracking if desired.

To facilitate dietary change, healthcare providers should work within the context of the pregnant adolescent's current eating habits. For example, adolescents often eat fast food and other convenience foods. While these may not be the best options, pregnant adolescents can be assisted to choose healthier foods such as salads and milk instead of French fries and soft drinks when eating at fast-food restaurants. Frequent meals and snacking are another common characteristic of adolescent eating behaviors. Working within this habit, pregnant adolescents can be encouraged to carry healthy snacks such as fruits, cheese sticks, nuts, or granola bars.

Concrete and practical strategies can help adolescents track nutritional goals. For example, a smartphone app or a wipe-away board that lists the daily servings of all food groups can be used to mark off the servings consumed throughout the day. Adolescents tend to think concretely and can relate to specific foods better than vague nutrients of which they may have little knowledge. Providing literature that has food pictures can help by illustrating easily understood healthy food choices.

Most pregnant adolescents live with their immediate or extended family. These relationships can greatly influence not only what the pregnant adolescent eats but also when and under what circumstances. An evaluation of the family food dynamics and meals is important to enable the healthcare provider to work within the family norms for improving adolescent nutrition. Pregnant adolescents with limited resources should be encouraged to utilize the WIC program to supplement current food sources.

Vegetarian and Vegan Diets in Pregnancy

Approximately 5% of the US adult population follows a **vegetarian** diet and 3% report themselves as **vegan** (Reinhart, 2018). Vegetarian diets are defined as dietary patterns that exclude or rarely include animal flesh such as meat, poultry, and fish/seafood. Individuals that further restrict animal protein sources and refrain from eating dairy, eggs, and honey are considered vegan. Vegetarians who avoid flesh yet do eat animal products, such as cheese, milk, and eggs, are considered **ovo-lacto vegetarians**. All vegetarian diets emphasize foods of plant origin, particularly vegetables, legumes, and fruits. Vegetarian diets are associated with health advantages, including lower blood cholesterol levels, lower risk of heart disease, lower risk of hypertension and type 2 diabetes, and lower levels of obesity and various cancers (Marsh et al., 2012; Yokoyama et al., 2014). Vegetarian diets tend to be lower in saturated fat and cholesterol and have higher levels of dietary fiber, magnesium, potassium, vitamins C and E, flavonoids, and other phytochemicals (Ghosh et al., 2016). However, individuals following vegan and vegetarian diets may have lower intakes of vitamin B_{12}, calcium, vitamin D, and omega-3 fatty acids (Pistollato et al., 2015).

The American Dietetic Association considers a vegetarian diet compatible with all life stages, including pregnancy and lactation (Melina et al., 2016). When vegan and vegetarian diets are the result of a free choice and are not linked with limited access to food or with poverty, pregnancy outcomes are similar to those reported in the omnivorous population (Piccoli et al., 2015).

AI of iron, folate protein, B_{12}, vitamin D, calcium, and omega-3 fatty acids should be considered when planning vegetarian diets (Haider et al., 2018; Piccoli et al., 2015; Table 9.9). A reliable source of vitamin B12, such as many prenatal vitamins or fortified nondairy milk or cereal, should be included.

People choose a vegetarian diet for many reasons, including religious beliefs, ethical concerns about animal rights, health, and environmental issues. Perhaps because of this awareness, those following a vegetarian diet tend to be well informed about a balanced diet. A thorough diet history and accurate diet counseling in addition to consultation with a dietician will help to optimize pregnancy outcomes.

Protein

Pregnant vegetarians and vegans consume lower levels of protein and higher levels of carbohydrates than pregnant nonvegetarians. Protein needs in pregnancy can be met from plant sources with adequate planning. Dried beans and other legumes, soy products like tofu, and nut butters are good protein sources toward meeting the 71 g daily protein recommendation in pregnancy. Cheeses, dairy proteins, and eggs are excellent sources for those following ovo-lacto vegetarian diets.

Table 9.9 Vegetarian and Vegan Diet Nutrient Sources

Whole grains, breads, cereals
Nine or more servings
Serving = 1 slice of bread, 1/2 bun or bagel
½ cup cooked cereal, rice, or pasta
3/4–1 cup ready-to-eat cereal

Vegetables
Four or more servings
Serving = ½ cup cooked or 1 cup raw vegetables
Choose several dark-green vegetables daily
Choose at least one yellow or orange vegetable daily

Fruits
Four or more servings
Serving = ½ cup cooked, 1 cup raw fruits
1 piece of fruit, ¾ cup fruit juice, ¼ cup dried fruit

Legumes, soy products, nondairy milks
Five to six servings
Serving = ½ cup cooked beans, tofu, tahini, or tempeh
8-oz fortified soymilk or other nondairy milk
3-oz plant-based protein source

Nuts, seeds, wheat germ
One to two servings
Serving = 2 tbsp nuts or seeds
2 tbsp nut butter, 2 tbsp wheat germ

Source: Adapted from: National Academies Dietary Reference and Intake Tables (2017).

B Vitamins

B vitamin deficiency is of particular concern for vegetarians. Individuals on vegetarian diets have lower serum B_{12} levels than those whose diets include animal protein (Piccoli et al., 2015). Many foods are fortified with vitamin B_{12} including meat substitute products, soy milks, tofu, cereals, and nutritional yeasts. Four servings daily of B_{12} fortified foods are recommended during pregnancy.

Iron

Iron needs may be greater for those on a vegetarian or vegan diet because of less efficient absorption of iron from plant sources. It can be difficult for any pregnant person to meet increased iron needs through diet alone. Therefore, iron supplements or prenatal vitamins containing iron are often required regardless of diet. Vegetarians or vegans should include iron-rich plant foods daily, in addition to taking their prescribed vitamins or supplements. Iron supplements should not be taken at the same time as tea, coffee, or calcium supplements. Dairy products decrease iron absorption and should not be taken with supplements. Iron sources include whole and enriched grains, legumes, nuts, seeds, dark-green vegetables, dried fruit, beans, lentils, and blackstrap molasses. Including vitamin C-rich foods at meals can increase absorption of iron from these sources.

Calcium

Calcium needs must be met from sources other than dairy for people following a vegan diet. Adequate calcium intake for vegetarians and vegans is 1200–1500 mg/day,

higher than for omnivores due to lower calcium absorption in many plant-based calcium sources. Many vegetables contain calcium but may have low bioavailability (e.g., spinach). Other greens with high calcium bioavailability, such as kale, broccoli, cabbage, and bok choy, should be encouraged. Other excellent sources of calcium include tofu and soybeans, dark-green leafy vegetables, beans, figs, sunflower seeds, tahini, almond butter, calcium-fortified nondairy milk, and calcium-fortified cereals and juices. If these foods are included in the diet every day, pregnancy calcium needs are easily met.

Vitamin D

Inadequate vitamin D may be a concern for those following vegetarian and vegan diets. Apart from foods such as eggs and salmon with bones, few foods naturally contain vitamin D. Fortified foods include soy milk and some breakfast cereals. Vitamin D is also included in most prenatal vitamin supplements; additional supplementation may be recommended.

Omega-3 Fatty Acids

DHA and EPA, essential for fetal brain and nervous system development, pose challenges for pregnant vegetarians since they are found primarily in fatty fish. It is important to include adequate amounts of short-chain fatty acids such as ALA found predominantly in chia seeds, flaxseeds, and walnuts. ALA is endogenously converted to long-chain omega-3 fatty acids, though in small amounts. Minimal amounts of dietary **omega-6 fatty acids**, found in vegetable oils and margarines, are essential to optimize conversion to DHA and EPA. Eggs from chickens fed a DHA-rich diet, and foods fortified with microalgae-derived DHA are additional food sources. Supplements made from marine fish may be acceptable for some following vegetarian diets.

Pregnancy after Bariatric Surgery

Bariatric surgery has become more common and often improves fertility in childbearing-aged people struggling with obesity. The knowledge of the unique nutritional needs of this population is important for prenatal care providers. Bariatric surgery reduces the risk of GDM, preeclampsia and macrosomia, yet can increase risk of FGR (Chilelli et al., 2014).

Bariatric surgery itself causes macro- and micronutrient deficiencies, and pregnancy can exacerbate these deficiencies. Both malabsorption procedures such as the Roux-en-Y gastric bypass (RYGB) and restrictive procedures such as lap-band can cause significant nutritional deficiencies, especially in those with nausea and vomiting of pregnancy. A physically smaller stomach space is created during bariatric surgery, necessitating small portions. The most common nutritional deficiencies in pregnant people postbariatric surgery are vitamin B, folate, and iron (Shankar et al., 2010). All pregnant individuals with a history of any type of bariatric surgery should be screened for various nutritional deficits at the first prenatal visit and then once per trimester (Carreau et al., 2017).

Dumping syndrome is a condition in which glucose passes quickly into small intestine, causing hypoglycemia and hyperinsulinemia, and producing symptoms such as palpitations, fatigue, irritability, and sweating. Recommendations to eat complex carbohydrates rather than simple carbohydrates can help avoid this condition. Screening for GDM with the oral glucose tolerance testing using glucose solution should be avoided; fasting and postprandial blood glucose level monitoring can be used instead (Carreau et al., 2017). The evaluation of fetal growth is of particular concern for this population. A multidisciplinary approach to care involving the bariatric surgeon and a nutritionist can be used to provide care during pregnancy following bariatric surgery.

It is important to recognize the disordered eating that led to the excessive weight that necessitated bariatric surgery. For many people who have had bariatric surgery, food was familiar comfort, and excessive eating was a coping mechanism needed to deal with a past trauma. Often, this trauma was childhood sexual abuse and/or physical abuse (Richardson et al., 2014). Trauma-informed care is particularly important; see Chapter 26, *Violence and Trauma in the Perinatal Period*, for more on trauma-informed care.

Eating Disorders

Approximately 5–10% of people with the capacity for pregnancy struggle with an eating disorder (Sebastiani et al., 2020). Eating disorders are thought to arise from the interplay of genetics, biology, and psychosociocultural factors. Eating disorders are classified as anorexia nervosa, bulimia, or eating disorders not otherwise specified (EDNOS) such as binge eating.

Condition	Symptom criteria
Anorexia nervosa	Intense fear of weight gain and of becoming fat Unwillingness to maintain normal body weight Body image disturbances Amenorrhea for a minimum of three months
Bulimia nervosa	Recurrent uncontrolled binge eating two times per week for at least three months Use of measures to prevent weight gain such as laxatives, enemas, diuretics, self-induced vomiting, excessive exercise Body image disturbances

EDNOS is a diagnosis of exclusion; it involves those who exhibit some symptoms but do not fit the criteria of anorexia or bulimia. Some examples include binge eating and those individuals with a normal weight but who purge after eating, chew and spit out food rather than swallowing to prevent weight gain, psychiatric impairment related to diet pills and diuretics, or obsessive preoccupation with cosmetic surgery to deal with shape and weight issues (Reiter & Graves, 2010).

There is a correlation between the severity of eating disorders and the incidence of pregnancy-associated morbidities and epigenetic remodeling in the neonate. In one study, women with eating disorders had a greater likelihood of anemia, pregnancy loss, and cesarean section (Sebastiani et al., 2020). Infants born to women with eating disorders have an increased risk of growth restriction, very premature birth, small for gestational age, low birth weight, low Apgar score, and perinatal death (Sebastiani et al., 2020).

It is not uncommon for eating disorders to go unrecognized in pregnancy; early detection can minimize complications. Individuals with eating disorders may present with the following signs and symptoms: severe anxiety, body dissatisfaction, food obsession, negative affectivity, exercise obsession, and depressive symptoms (Reiter & Graves, 2010; Stice et al., 2011). A lack of weight gain over two consecutive visits, unexplained electrolyte disorders, and/or dental erosion can be cues to prompt further history and evaluation for eating disorders (Harris, 2010).

All pregnant people should be asked about a history of eating disorders at the initial prenatal visit. Specific areas of inquiry include reproductive history, history of amenorrhea lasting longer than three months, eating habits, exercise history, history of frequent weight loss and gain, and prior history of eating disorders. Screening tools designed to detect eating disorders, such as SCOFF, can be used to identify those who need further assessment.

SCOFF tool to screen for eating disorders

S—Do you make yourself *sick* because you are uncomfortably full?
C—Do you worry about loss of *control* over your eating?
O—Have you recently lost *one* stone (14 lb) in three months?
F—Do you believe you are *fat* although others say you are thin?
F—Would you say *food* predominates your life?

One point is given for each "yes" answered and a score of 2 or more indicates the presence of an eating disorder is likely (Harris, 2010).

Pregnancy can be a strong motivator to change eating habits as up to 70% of individuals have improved symptoms during pregnancy (Harris, 2010). Successful strategies to assist those with eating disorders include care from the same healthcare provider throughout the entire pregnancy whenever possible. This will provide some consistency and allow for a trusting relationship to develop. An increased prenatal visit schedule will allow for small goal setting using MI techniques and increase the likelihood of success. Discussing appropriate food portions and

Table 9.10 Pica Evaluation and Management

Pica substance	Potential signs and symptoms	Potential problems	Management
Dirt, clay, paint chips	Fatigue Muscle weakness Constipation Sensitive or broken teeth Abdominal bloating Nausea and vomiting	Elevated blood lead levels Anemia Parasitic infection	Consider tests for anemia, lead levels, hypokalemia Examine teeth Monitor for inadequate weight gain
Ice	Sensitive or broken teeth	Anemia Inadequate weight gain	Test for anemia Examine teeth
Starch	Excessive weight gain Abdominal bloating		Test for anemia Monitor for excessive weight gain Consider monitoring for elevated blood glucose levels
Baking soda	Fatigue Muscle weakness Abdominal bloating	Rhabdomyolysis Cardiomyopathy	Test for anemia Consider metabolic panel Suggest alternative methods to relieve heartburn Medical referral if symptomatic

Source: Adapted from Childress and Myles (2013).

necessary nutrients and vitamins may increase the likelihood of appropriate weight gain. Potential obstacles may arise from reintroduction of food and the physiologic changes of pregnancy affecting the gastrointestinal system. Pregnant individuals identified with an eating disorder also benefit from referral to a nutritionist and a mental healthcare provider (Paslakis & de Zwaan, 2019).

Pica

Pica is derived from the Latin word for magpie, a bird known for its unusual and indiscriminate eating habits. It is defined as the compulsive and purposeful intake of non-nutritive substances that the consumer does not define as food for greater than a one-month duration (Al Nasser et al., 2022). People who practice pica ingest products such as ice (pagophagia—70% of pica practices), dirt/clay (geophagia—18% of pica practices), corn starch (amylophagia), soap (4% of pica practices), gravel, charcoal, ash, paper, chalk, cloth, baby powder, coffee grounds, eggshells, and nail polish (Lopez et al., 2007; Mills, 2007; Young, 2010).

The etiology of pica is poorly understood. Pica can be viewed in a variety of ways: as an eating disorder, in response to a nutritional deficiency (zinc, iron, calcium), as a response to psychological distress, or as a cultural practice. Pica may be initiated by individuals who enjoy the taste, texture, and smell of the substance ingested. Cultural values and traditions can strongly influence the practice and acceptance of pica. Pica may also be a psychological and behavioral response to stress, but no clear etiology has been established (Al Nasser et al., 2022; Mills, 2007).

Complications vary based on the type of pica practices. Pica is associated with iron deficiency anemia, though it is unclear whether iron deficiency anemia is a result of pica or may be a predisposing factor to pica (Johnson, 2017). Signs, symptoms, and management of pica depend on the substance being consumed (Table 9.10). It should be noted that pica practices vary in their potential for harm. Depending on the substance ingested, pica can lead to heavy metal poisonings, dental and gastrointestinal tract damage, and nutrient deficiencies (Al Nasser et al., 2022). A referral to nutritional services for detailed evaluation and assessment can be useful in reducing pica practices.

Pica is a condition that often goes unreported and undiagnosed, primarily because of embarrassment and guilt. A nonjudgmental, understanding, and culturally supportive environment can facilitate reporting of pica. The person should be told that the information shared will be confidential and that they will not be judged. The substance and amount consumed should be identified and counseling regarding potential effects, and nutritional management for all individuals practicing pica provided. The goal is to change potentially harmful eating behaviors and support the person in making the change.

Summary

Pregnancy is a critical time in human development, and outcomes can be strongly influenced by prenatal nutrition. Facilitating early prenatal care appointments allows for the best opportunity to assess nutritional habits and status and to recommend dietary modifications, thus improving both perinatal outcomes and the person's long-term health. It is imperative for prenatal care providers to have the knowledge and resources to be able to provide relevant information on prenatal diet choices and influences on pregnancy and fetal health. It is also critical to prioritize adequate time during prenatal care visits to evaluate and address nutrition throughout pregnancy.

Promoting positive eating habits and lifestyle choices can influence family health for years to come.

Resources for Clients and Their Families

USDA interactive website for pregnant people on healthy eating during pregnancy called MyPlate: https://www.myplate.gov/myplate-plan

International Food Information Council, Healthy Eating during Pregnancy Brochure: https://foodinsight.org/healthy-eating-during-pregnancy

CDC website with consumer information on food safety during pregnancy: http://www.cdc.gov/pregnancy/infections.html

EPA and FDA joint website providing information and handouts on fish safety in pregnancy: https://www.fda.gov/Food/ResourcesForYou/Consumers/ucm393070.htm

EPA website for local fish advisories: https://fishadvisoryonline.epa.gov/General.aspx

Glycemic index and glycemic load for 100+ foods: https://www.health.harvard.edu/diseases-and-conditions/glycemic-index-and-glycemic-load-for-100-foods

Resources for Healthcare Providers

Motivational Interviewing: www.motivationalinterviewing.org

EPA and FDA handout on fish consumption during pregnancy: https://www.fda.gov/food/consumers/advice-about-eating-fish

USDA Interactive Dietary Reference Intake and Estimated Energy Requirement: https://www.nal.usda.gov/fnic/interactiveDRI

Information on the supplemental food and nutrition program, WIC: http://www.fns.usda.gov/wic

References

Abbaspour, N., Hurrell, R., & Kelishadi, R. (2014). Review on iron and its importance for human health. *Journal of Research in Medical Sciences: The Official Journal of Isfahan University of Medical Sciences*, 19(2), 164. PMCID: PMC3999603

Al Nasser Y, Muco E, Alsaad AJ. Pica. [Updated 2021 Jul 29]. In: StatPearls [Internet]. StatPearls Publishing. https://www.ncbi.nlm.nih.gov/books/NBK532242

American College of Obstetricians and Gynecologists. (2013). ACOG Committee opinion no. 548: Weight gain during pregnancy. *Obstetrics and Gynecology*, 121(1), 210–212. https://doi.org/10.1097/01.aog.0000425668.87506.4c

Aune, D., Saugstad, O. D., Henriksen, T., & Tonstad, S. (2014). Maternal body mass index and the risk of fetal death, stillbirth, and infant death: A systematic review and meta-analysis. *JAMA*, 3JJ(15), 1536–1546.

Azad, M. B., Sharma, A. K., de Souza, R. J., Dolinsky, V. W., Becker, A. B., Mandhane, P. J., Turvey, S. E., Subbarao, P., Lefebvre, D. L., & Sears, M. R. the Canadian Healthy Infant Longitudinal Development Study Investigators. (2016). Association between artificially sweetened beverage consumption during pregnancy and infant body mass index. *JAMA Pediatrics*, 170(7), 662–670. https://doi.org/10.1001/jamapediatrics.2016.0301

Bergen, N. E., Jaddoe, V. W. V., Timmermans, S., Hofman, A., Lindemans, J., Russcher, H., Raat, H., Steegers-Theunissen, R. P. M., & Steegers, E. A. P. (2012). Homocysteine and folate concentrations in early pregnancy and the risk of adverse pregnancy outcomes: The generation R study. *BJOG: An International Journal of Obstetrics & Gynaecology*, 119(6), 739–751.

Berti, C., Cetin, I., Agostoni, C., Desoye, G., Devlieger, R., Emmett, P. M., Ensenauer, R., Hauner, H., Herrera, E., Hoesli, I., Krauss-Etschmann, S., Olsen, S. F., Schaefer-Graf, U., Schiessl, B., Symonds, M. E., & Koletzko, B. (2016). Pregnancy and infants' outcome: Nutritional and metabolic implications. *Critical Reviews in Food Science and Nutrition*, 56(1), 82–91.

Bhuyar, S., & Dharmale, N. (2018). Effect of maternal body mass index on pregnancy outcomes. *International Journal of Reproduction, Contraception, Obstetrics and Gynecology*, 7(12), 4949–4956.

Blencowe, H., Cousens, S., Modell, B., & Lawn, J. (2010). Folic acid to reduce neonatal mortality for neural tube defects. *International Journal of Epidemiology*, 39(Suppl. 1), i110–i121.

Brown, A., & Avery, A. (2012). Healthy weight management during pregnancy: What advice and information is being provided. *Journal of Human Nutrition and Dietetics*, 25(4), 378–387.

Carreau, A. M., Nadeau, M., Marceau, S., Marceau, P., & Weisnagel, S. J. (2017). Pregnancy after bariatric surgery: Balancing risks and benefits. *Canadian Journal of Diabetes*, 41(4), 432–438.

Centers for Disease Control and Prevention (CDC). (2011). Vital signs: Incidence and trends of infection with pathogens transmitted commonly through food—Foodborne diseases active surveillance network, 10 US sites, 1996-2010. *MMWR Morbidity and Mortality Weekly Report*, 60(22), 749–755.

Centers for Disease Control and Prevention (CDC). (2016). Prepregnancy body mass index by maternal characteristics and state: Data from the birth certificate, 2014. *National Vital Statistics, Report*, 65(6). https://www.cdc.gov/nchs/data/nvsr/nvsr65nvsr65_06.pdf.

Centers for Disease Control and Prevention (CDC). (2018, September 27). *Toxoplasmosis - Prevention & Control*. https://www.cdc.gov/parasites/toxoplasmosis/prevent.html

Childress, K. M. S., & Myles, T. (2013). Baking soda pica associated with rhabdomyolysis and cardiomyopathy in pregnancy. *Obstetrics & Gynecology*, 122(2, PART 2), 495–497.

Chilelli, N. C., Burlina, S., Dalfra, M. G., & Lapolla, A. (2014). A focus on the impact of bariatric surgery on pregnancy outcome: Effectiveness, safety and clinical management. *Journal of Obesity and Weight Loss Therapy*, 4(210), 2.

Cho, G., Shin, J., Yi, K., Park, H., Kim, T., Hur, J., & Kim, S. (2012). Adolescent pregnancy is associated with osteoporosis in postmenopausal women. *Menopause*, 19(4), 456–460.

Choi, C. S., Kim, P., Park, J. H., Gonzales, E. L. T., Kim, K. C., Cho, K. S., Son, J. S., Kim, K.-H., Kim, Y.-S., Kim, E. S., Park, S. H., Yoon, J. H., Choi, S.-M., Lee, H., Oh, W. S., Choi, S.-Y., Kim, N.-J., Choi, J.-P., Park, S. Y., . . . Shin, C. Y. (2015). High sucrose consumption during pregnancy induced ADHD-like behavioral phenotypes in mice offspring. *The Journal of Nutritional Biochemistry*, 26(12), 1520–1526.

Cragan, J. D., Friedman, J. M., Holmes, L. B., Uhl, K., Green, N. S., & Riley, L. (2006). Ensuring the safe and effective use of medications during pregnancy: Planning and prevention through preconception care. *Maternal and Child Health Journal*, 10(Suppl. 1), 129–135.

Curtis, E. M., Moon, R. J., Harvey, N. C., & Cooper, C. (2018). Maternal vitamin D supplementation during pregnancy. *British Medical Bulletin*, 126(1), 57–77. https://doi.org/10.1093/bmb/ldy010

Danilack, V. A., Brousseau, E. C., & Phipps, M. G. (2018). The effect of gestational weight gain on persistent increase in body mass index in adolescents: A longitudinal study. *Journal of Women's Health*, 27(12), 1456–1458.

Demétrio, F., Teles, C. A. D. S., Santos, D. B. D., & Pereira, M. (2020). Food insecurity in pregnant women is associated with social determinants and nutritional outcomes: A systematic review and meta-analysis. *Ciência & Saúde Coletiva*, 25, 2663–2676.

Devlieger, R., Ameye, L., Nuyts, T., Goemaes, R., & Bogaerts, A. (2020). Reappraisal of gestational weight gain recommendations in obese pregnant women: A population-based study of 337,590 births. *Obesity Facts*, 13(4), 333–348.

Dow, M. L., & Szymanski, L. M. (2020). Effects of overweight and obesity in pregnancy on health of the offspring. *Endocrinology and Metabolism Clinics of North America*, 49(2), 251–263.

Environmental Protection Agency. (2022). *EPA-FDA Advice about Eating Fish and Shellfish*. EPA. https://www.epa.gov/fish-tech/epa-fda-advice-about-eating-fish-and-shellfish

Esposito, L., Fisher, J. O., Mennella, J. A., Hoelsher, D. M., & Huang, T. T. (2009). Developmental perspectives on nutrition and obesity from gestation to adolescence. *Preventing Chronic Disease, 6*(3), 1–11.

Feng, Y., Wang, S., Chen, R., Tong, X., Wu, Z., & Mo, X. (2015). Maternal folic acid supplementation and the risk of congenital heart defects in offspring: A meta-analysis of epidemiological observational studies. *Scientific Reports, 5,* 8506.

Gennette, S., Varlamov, A., & Eason, R. (2017). Pregnancy outcomes in underweight versus ideal weight women at time of delivery [33F]. *Obstetrics & Gynecology, 129,* 69S–70S.

Gete, D., Waller, M., & Mishra, G. (2020). Effects of maternal diets on preterm birth and low birth weight: A systematic review. *British Journal of Nutrition, 123*(4), 446–461. https://doi.org/10.1017/S0007114519002897

Ghosh, S., Shukla, R., Mujalde, V. S., Chaturvedi, V., & Barolia, D. K. (2016). Maternal vegetarian diet in pregnancy, a predisposition to hypospadias? *International Journal of Research in Medical Sciences, 5*(1), 344–345.

Godfrey, K. M., Reynolds, R. M., Prescott, S. L., Nyirenda, M., Jad-doe, V. W., Eriksson, J. G., & Broekman, B. F. (2017). Influence of maternal obesity on the long-term health of offspring. *The Lancet Diabetes & Endocrinology, 5*(1), 53–64.

Grieger, J. A., & Clifton, V. L. (2015). A review of the impact of dietary intakes in human pregnancy on infant birthweight. *Nutrients, 7*(1), 153–178. https://doi.org/10.3390/NU7010153

Groth, S. W., Holland, M. L., Kitzman, H., & Meng, Y. (2013). Gestational weight gain of pregnant African American adolescents affects body mass index 18 years later. *Journal of Obstetric, Gynecologic, & Neonatal Nursing, 42*(5), 541–550.

Haider, L. M., Schwingshackl, L., Hoffmann, G., & Ekmekcioglu, C. (2018). The effect of vegetarian diets on iron status in adults: A systematic review and meta-analysis. *Critical Reviews in Food Science and Nutrition, 58*(8), 1359–1374.

Halasa, B. C., Sylvetsky, A. C., Conway, E. M., Shouppe, E. L., Walter, M. F., Walter, P. J., Cai, H., Hui, L., & Rother, K. I. (2021). Non-nutritive sweeteners in human amniotic fluid and cord blood: Evidence of transplacental fetal exposure. *American Journal of Perinatology.* Epub ahead of print

Hales, C. M., Carroll, M. D., Fryar, C. D., & Ogden, C. L. (2020). *Prevalence of obesity and Severe Obesity Among Adults: United States, 2017-2018. NCHS Data Brief, no 360.* National Center for Health Statistics.

Harris, A. A. (2010). Practical advice for caring for women with eating disorders during the prenatal period. *Journal of Midwifery and Women's Health, 55*(6), 579–586.

Healthcare Value Hub. (2020). *Social determinants of health: Food insecurity in the United States.* Altarum Healthcare Value Hub. https://www.healthcarevaluehub.org/advocate-resources/publications/social-determinants-health-food-insecurity-united-states

Hrolfsdottir, L., Schalkwijk, C. G., Birgisdottir, B. E., Gunnarsdottir, I., Maslova, E., Granstrom, C., Strom, M., Olsen, S., & Halldorsson, T. I. (2016). Maternal diet, gestational weight gain, and inflammatory markers during pregnancy. *Obesity, 24*(10), 2133–2139.

Institute of Medicine. (IOM). (2020). *Dietary reference intakes tables and application.* National Academies. https://www.ncbi.nlm.nih.gov/books/NBK222881/

James, J. E. (2021). Maternal caffeine consumption and pregnancy outcomes: A narrative review with implications for advice to mothers and mothers-to-be. *BMJ Evidence-Based Medicine, 26*(3), 114–115. https://doi.org/10.1136/bmjebm-2020-111432

Jensen, E. T., van der Burg, J. W., O'Shea, T. M., Joseph, R. M., Allred, E. N., Heeren, T., Leviton, A., & Kuban, K. C. K. on behalf of the Extremely Low Gestational Age Newborns Study Investigators(2017). The relationship of maternal prepregnancy body mass index and pregnancy weight gain to neurocognitive function at age 10 years among children born extremely preterm. *The Journal of Pediatrics, 187,* 50–57.

Johnson, D. (2017). PICA during pregnancy. *International Journal of Childbirth Education, 32*(1), 45–47.

Joseph, N. P., Hunkali, K. B., Wilson, B., Morgan, E., Cross, M., & Freund, K. M. (2008). Pre-pregnancy body mass index among pregnant adolescents: Gestational weight gain and long-term postpartum weight retention. *Journal of Pediatric and Adolescent Gynecology, 21*(4), 195–200.

Karataşlı, V., Kanmaz, A. G., İnan, A. H., Budak, A., & Beyan, E. (2019). Maternal and neonatal outcomes of adolescent pregnancy. *Journal of Gynecology Obstetrics and Human Reproduction, 48*(5), 347–350.

Kennedy, R. A. K., Mullaney, L., Reynolds, C. M. E., Cawley, S., McCartney, D. M. A., & Turner, M. J. (2017). Preferences of women for web-based nutritional information in pregnancy. *Public Health, 143,* 71–77.

Kovacs, C. S. (2014). Osteoporosis presenting in pregnancy, puerperium, and lactation. *Current Opinion in Endocrinology, Diabetes and Obesity, 21*(6), 468–475.

Lagisz, M., Blair, H., Kenyon, P., Uller, T., Raubenheimer, D., & Nakagawa, S. (2014). Transgenerational effects of caloric restriction on appetite: A meta-analysis. *Obesity Reviews, 15*(4), 294–309.

Langley-Evans, S. C. (2015). Nutrition in early life and the programming of adult disease: A review. *Journal of Human Nutrition and Dietetics, 28*(s1), 1–14.

Laraia, B. A., Siega-Riz, A. M., & Gundersen, C. (2010). Household food insecurity is associated with self-reported pregravid weight status, gestational weight gain, and pregnancy complications. *Journal of the American Dietetic Association, 110*(5), 692–701.

Liang, Y., Gong, Y., Zhang, X., Yang, D., Zhao, D., Quan, L., Zhou, R., Bao, W., & Cheng, G. (2018). Dietary protein intake, meat consumption, and dairy consumption in the year preceding pregnancy and during pregnancy and their associations with the risk of gestational diabetes mellitus: A prospective cohort study in Southwest China. *Frontiers in Endocrinology, 9,* 596. https://doi.org/10.3389/fendo.2018.00596

Livingstone, K. M., Celis-Morales, C., Navas-Carretero, S., San-Cristobal, R., Macready, A. L., Fallaize, R., Forster, H., Woolhead, C., O'Donovan, C. B., Marsaux, C. F. M., Kolossa, S., Tsirigoti, L., Lambrinou, C. P., Moschonis, G., Godlewska, M., Surwiłło, A., Drevon, C. A., Manios, Y., Traczyk, I., ... Kolossa, S. (2016). Effect of an internet-based, personalized nutrition randomized trial on dietary changes associated with the Mediterranean diet: The Food4Me Study. *The American Journal of Clinical Nutrition, 104*(2), 288–297.

Lopez, L. B., De Portela, M. L., & Soler, C. R. (2007). Nutrient intake in women with pagophagia and other forms of pica during the pregnancy. *Nutricion Hospitalaria, 22*(6), 641–647.

Madjunkov, M., Chaudhry, S., & Ito, S. (2017). Listeriosis during pregnancy. *Archives of Gynecology and Obstetrics, 296,* 143–152.

Makrides, M., Duley, L., & Olsen, S. F. (2006). Marine oil, and other prostaglandin precursor, supplementation for pregnancy uncomplicated by pre-eclampsia or intrauterine growth restriction. *Cochrane Database of Systematic Reviews, 3,* CD003402.

March of Dimes (MOD). (2020). *Caffeine in pregnancy.* https://www.marchofdimes.org/pregnancy/caffeine-in-pregnancy.aspx

Marchi, J., Berg, M., Dencker, A., Olander, E. K., & Begley, C. (2015). Risks associated with obesity in pregnancy, for the mother and baby: A systematic review of reviews. *Obesity Reviews, 16*(8), 621–638.

Marsh, K., Zeuschner, C., & Saunders, A. (2012). Health implications of a vegetarian diet: A review. *American Journal of Lifestyle Medicine, 6*(3), 250–267.

McCusker, R. R., Goldberger, B. A., & Cone, E. J. (2006). Caffeine content of energy drinks, carbonated sodas, and other beverages. *Journal of Analytical Toxicology, 30,* 112–114.

Melina, V., Craig, W., & Levin, S. (2016). Position of the academy of nutrition and dietetics: Vegetarian diets. *Journal of the Academy of Nutrition and Dietetics, 116*(12), 1970–1980.

Mennella, J. A. (2014). Ontogeny of taste preferences: Basic biology and implications for health. *The American Journal of Clinical Nutrition, 99*(3), 704S–711S.

Mills, M. E. (2007). Craving more than food: The implications of pica in pregnancy. *Nursing for Women's Health, 11*(3), 266–273.

Moustarah, F., & Mohiuddin, S. S. (2021). *Dietary iron.* In *StatPearls.* StatPearls Publishing. PMID: 31082013

Murphy, M. M., Higgins, K. A., Bi, X., & Barraj, L. M. (2021). Adequacy and Sources of Protein Intake among Pregnant Women in the United States, NHANES 2003–2012. *Nutrients*, 13(3), 795. https://doi.org/10.3390/nu13030795

National Institutes of Health (NIH). (2022a). *Dietary Supplement Fact Sheet—Iron*. Office of Dietary Supplements National Institutes of Health. https://ods.od.nih.gov/factsheets/Iron-HealthProfessional/#h3

National Institutes of Health (NIH). (2022b). *Dietary Supplement Fact Sheet—Vitamin D*. Office of Dietary Supplements National Institutes of Health. https://ods.od.nih.gov/factsheets/VitaminD-HealthProfessional

National Institutes of Health (NIH). (2020). *Calcium-Fact Sheet for Health Professionals*. Office of Dietary Supplements National Institutes of Health. https://ods.od.nih.gov/factsheets/Calcium-HealthProfessional/

Nicolì, F., Prete, A., Citro, F., Bertolotto, A., Aragona, M., de Gennaro, G., Del Prato, S., & Bianchi, C. (2021). Use of non-nutritive-sweetened soft drink and risk of gestational diabetes. *Diabetes Research and Clinical Practice*, 178, 108943. https://doi.org/10.1016/j.diabres.2021.108943

Nordgren, T. M., Lyden, E., Anderson-Berry, A., & Hanson, C. (2017). Omega-3 fatty acid intake of pregnant women and women of child-bearing age in the United States: Potential for deficiency? *Nutrients*, 9(3), 197.

Nusken, E., Gellhaus, A., Kuhnel, E., Swoboda, I., Wohlfarth, M., Vohlen, C., Schneider, H., Dotsch, J., & Nusken, K.-D. (2016). Increased rat placental fatty acid, but decreased amino acid and glucose transporters potentially modify intrauterine programming. *Journal of Cellular Biochemistry*, 117, 1594–1603.

Parker, H., Tovar, A., McCurdy, K., & Vadiveloo, M. (2020). Socio-economic and racial prenatal diet quality disparities in a national US sample. *Public Health Nutrition*, 23(5), 894–903. https://doi.org/10.1017/S1368980019003240

Paslakis, G., & de Zwaan, M. (2019). Clinical management of females seeking fertility treatment and of pregnant females with eating disorders. *European Eating Disorders Review*, 27(3), 215–223. https://doi.org/10.1002/erv.2667

Paxton, A. E., Strycker, L. A., Toobert, D. J., Ammerman, A. S., & Glasgow, R. E. (2011). Starting the conversation: Performance of a brief dietary assessment and intervention tool for health professionals. *American Journal of Preventive Medicine*, 40(1), 67–71.

Pena-Rosas, J. P., De-Regil, L. M., Garcia-Casal, M. N., & Dowswell, T. (2015b). Daily oral iron supplementation during pregnancy. *The Cochrane Database of Systematic Reviews*, 7. https://doi.org//10.1002/14651858.CD004736.pub5

Pena-Rosas, J. P., De-Regil, L. M., Gomez Malave, H., Flores-Urrutia, M. C., & Dowswell, T. (2015a). Intermittent oral iron supplementation during pregnancy. *The Cochrane Database of Systematic Reviews*, 10, CD009997. https://doi.org/10.1002/14651858.CD009997.pub2

Perez-Lopez, F. R., Pasupuleti, V., Mezones-Holguin, E., Benites-Zapata, V. A., Thota, P., Deshpande, A., & Hernandez, A. V. (2015). Effect of vitamin D supplementation during pregnancy on maternal and neonatal outcomes: A systematic review and meta-analysis of randomized controlled trials. *Fertility and Sterility*, 103(5), 1278–1288.

Petherick, E. S., Goran, M. I., & Wright, J. (2014). Relationship between artificially sweetened and sugar-sweetened cola beverage consumption during pregnancy and preterm delivery in a multi-ethnic cohort: Analysis of the born in Bradford cohort study. *European Journal of Clinical Nutrition*, 68(3), 404–407.

Phelan, S., Hart, C., Phipps, M., Abrams, B., Schaffner, A., Adams, A., & Wing, R. (2011). Maternal behaviors during pregnancy impact off-spring obesity risk. *Experimental Diabetes Research*, 2011, 985139.

Piccoli, G. B., Clari, R., Vigotti, F. N., Leone, F., Attini, R., Cabiddu, G., Mauro, G., Castelluccia, N., Colombi, N., Capizzi, I., Pani, A., Todros, T., & Avagnina, P. (2015). Vegan-vegetarian diets in pregnancy: Danger or panacea? A systematic narrative review. *BJOG: an international journal of obstetrics and gynaecology*, 122(5), 623–633. https://doi.org/10.1111/1471-0528.13280

Pistollato, F., Cano, S. S., Elio, I., Vergara, M. M., Giampieri, E., & Battino, M. (2015). Plant-based and plant-rich diet patterns during gestation: Beneficial effects and possible shortcomings. *Advances in Nutrition: An International Review Journal*, 6(5), 581–591.

Ponzo, V., Fedele, D., Goitre, I., Leone, F., Lezo, A., Monzeglio, C., Finocchiaro, C., Ghigo, E., & Bo, S. (2019). Diet-gut microbiota interactions and gestational diabetes mellitus (GDM). *Nutrients*, 11(2), 330. https://doi.org/10.3390/nu11020330

Pouillot, R., Hoelzer, K., Jackson, K. A., Henao, O. L., & Silk, B. J. (2012). Relative risk of listeriosis in Foodborne Diseases Active Surveillance Network (FoodNet) sites according to age, pregnancy, and ethnicity. *Clinical Infectious Diseases*, 54(Suppl. 5), S405–S410.

Rasmussen, K. M., & Yaktine, A. L. Committee to Reexamine IOM Pregnancy Weight Guidelines, Institute of Medicine, National Research Council (2009). *Weight gain during pregnancy: Reexamining the guidelines*. The National Academies Press.

Rasouli, M., Mousavi, S. A., Khosravi, A., Keramat, A., Fooladi, E., & Atashsokhan, G. (2018). The impact of motivational interviewing on behavior stages of nulliparous pregnant women preparing for childbirth: A randomized clinical trial. *Journal of Psychosomatic Obstetrics and Gynecology*, 39(3), 237–245.

Reinhart, R. J. (2018). *Snapshot: Few Americans vegetarian or vegan*. Gallup. https://news.gallup.com/poll/238328/snapshot-few-americans-vegetarian-vegan.aspx

Reiter, C. S., & Graves, L. (2010). Nutrition therapy for eating disorders. *Nutrition in Clinical Practice*, 25(2), 122–136.

Richardson, A. S., Dietz, W. H., & Gordon-Larsen, P. (2014). The association between childhood sexual and physical abuse with incident adult severe obesity across 13 years of the National Longitudinal Study of Adolescent Health. *Pediatric Obesity*, 9(5), 351–361.

Sablok, A., Batra, A., Thariani, K., Batra, A., Bharti, R., Aggarwal, A. R., Kabi, B. C., & Chellani, H. (2015). Supplementation of vitamin D in pregnancy and its correlation with feto-maternal outcome. *Clinical Endocrinology*, 83(4), 536–541. https://doi.org/10.1111/cen.12751

Salam, R. A., Das, J. K., & Bhutta, Z. A. (2014). Impact of intrauterine growth restriction on long-term health. *Current Opinion in Clinical Nutrition & Metabolic Care*, 17(3), 249–254.

Salam, R. A., Hooda, M., Das, J. K., Arshad, A., Lassi, Z., Middleton, P., & Bhutta, Z. (2016). Interventions to improve adolescent nutrition: A systematic review and meta-analysis. *Journal of Adolescent Health*, 59(4), S29–S39.

Sebastiani, G., Andreu-Fernández, V., Herranz Barbero, A., Aldecoa-Bilbao, V., Miracle, X., Meler Barrabes, E., Balada Ibañez, A., Astals-Vizcaino, M., Ferrero-Martínez, S., Gómez-Roig, M. D., & García-Algar, O. (2020). Eating disorders during gestation: Implications for mother's health, fetal outcomes, and epigenetic changes. *Frontiers in Pediatrics*, 8, 587. https://doi.org/10.3389/fped.2020.00587

Shankar, P., Boylan, M., & Sriram, K. (2010). Micronutrient deficiencies after bariatric surgery. *Nutrition*, 26(11), 1031–1037.

Stice, E., Marti, C. N., & Durant, S. (2011). Risk factors for onset of eating disorders: Evidence of multiple risk pathways from an 8-year prospective study. *Behaviour Research and Therapy*, 49, 622–627.

Thangaratinam, S., Rogozinska, E., Jolly, K., Glinkowski, S., Rose-boom, T., Tomlinson, J. W., Kunz, R., Mol, B. W., & Khan, K. S. (2012). Effects of interventions in pregnancy on maternal weight and obstetric outcomes: Meta-analysis of randomised evidence. *BMJ: British Medical Journal*, 344, e2088. https://www.bmj.com/content/bmj/344/bmj.e2088.full.pdf

Tsakiridis, I., Kasapidou, E., Dagklis, T., Leonida, I., Leonida, C., Bakaloudi, D., & Chourdakis, M. (2020). Nutrition in pregnancy: A comparative review of major guidelines. *Obstetrical & Gynecological Survey*, 75(11), 692–702. https://doi.org/10.1097/OGX.0000000000000836

US Department of Agriculture. (2021). *Your MyPlate Plan - 2400 calories, ages 14+ years*. https://www.myplate.gov/myplate-plan/results/2400-calories-ages-14-plus

US Department of Agriculture and US Department of Health and Human Services. (2020, December). *Dietary Guidelines for Americans, 2020-2025. 9th Edition*. https://www.dietaryguidelines.gov

US Department of Health and Human Services. (n.d.). *Objectives and data: Healthy People 2030*. https://health.gov/healthypeople/objectives-and-data

USDA. (2017). *Food safety*. https://www.fns.usda.gov/ofs/food-safety

Wei, S. Q. (2014). Vitamin D and pregnancy outcomes. *Current Opinion in Obstetrics and Gynecology, 26*(6), 438–447.

Widen, E., & Siega-Riz, A. M. (2010). Prenatal nutrition: A practical guide for assessment and counseling. *Journal of Midwifery & Women's Health, 55*(6), 540–549.

Wilson, R. M., & Messaoudi, I. (2015). The impact of maternal obesity during pregnancy on offspring immunity. *Molecular and Cellular Endocrinology, 418*, 134–142.

Yao, R., Ananth, C. V., Park, B. Y., Pereira, L., Plante, L. A., & Perinatal Research Consortium. (2014). Obesity and the risk of stillbirth: A population-based cohort study. *American Journal of Obstetrics and Gynecology, 210*(5), 457–e1.

Yokoyama, Y., Nishimura, K., Barnard, N. D., Takegami, M., Wata-nabe, M., Sekikawa, A., & Miyamoto, Y. (2014). Vegetarian diets and blood pressure: A meta-analysis. *JAMA Internal Medicine, 174*(4), 577–587.

Young, B. E., McNanley, T. J., Cooper, E. M., McIntyre, A. W., Witter, F., Harris, Z. L., & O'Brien, K. O. (2012). Maternal vitamin D status and calcium intake interact to affect fetal skeletal growth in utero in pregnant adolescents. *The American Journal of Clinical Nutrition, 95*(5), 1103–1112.

Young, S. L. (2010). Pica in pregnancy: New ideas about an old condition. *Annual Review of Nutrition, 30*, 403–422.

Yu, C. J., Du, J. C., Chiou, H. C., Feng, C. C., Chung, M. Y., Yang, W., Chen, Y. S., Chien, L. C., Hwang, B., & Chen, M. L. (2016). Sugar-sweetened beverage consumption is adversely associated with childhood attention deficit/hyperactivity disorder. *International Journal of Environmental Research and Public Health, 13*(7), 678. https://doi.org/10.3390/ijerph13070678

10

Pregnancy Diagnosis and Gestational Age Assessment

Joyce D. Cappiello and Janet L. Engstrom

Relevant Terms

Amenorrhea—the absence of menstruation; suggestive of pregnancy in a person of reproductive age who has a history of regular menstrual cycles

Basal body temperature—temperature upon awakening, before rising, engaging in any activity, or consuming any food or beverage

Chadwick's sign—bluish discoloration of the vagina

Dickinson's sign—softening of the uterus in the area of implantation; creates a sensation of inconsistency in the uterus during a bimanual exam, described as a feeling of "furrows and grooves"

Endocrine pregnancy test—biochemical measurement of the pregnancy-related hormone human chorionic gonadotropin (hCG), sometimes called "beta-hCG" because the test targets the beta subunit of the hormone

Estimated date of birth, also known as estimated date of delivery or estimated due date, and previously called the estimated date of confinement—approximate date of expected birth, calculated as 280 days from the first day of the last menstrual period, or 266 days from the date of conception

Fetal heart activity, fetal heart sounds or fetal heart tones—fetal heart activity can be observed using real-time ultrasound; fetal heart sounds or tones can be heard by using a handheld Doppler ultrasound unit or auscultated using a fetoscope

Fetoscope—modified stethoscope used to auscultate fetal heart sounds; the stethoscope has a headpiece that is placed against the examiner's frontal bones to facilitate the transfer of the faint sounds of the fetal heartbeat

Fundal height measurements—distance between the uppermost border of the symphysis pubis and the uppermost border of the uterine fundus in the midline of the pregnant person's abdomen, measured in centimeters; used to assess fetal growth and determine whether the size of the uterus is appropriate for the gestational age of the pregnancy

Gestational age—estimated duration of a pregnancy in weeks counted from the first day of the last menstrual period

Gestational weeks—number of weeks since the first day of the last menstrual period, also known as menstrual weeks

Goodell's sign—softening of the uterine cervix

Hegar's sign—softening and compressibility of the lower uterine segment

Jacquemin's sign—bluish or violet discoloration of the vaginal mucosa near the urethra

Ladin's sign—a small spot of softening in the anterior center of the lower uterine segment

Leopold's maneuvers—a series of maneuvers used to systematically palpate the fetus through the pregnant person's abdomen to assess fetal size, position, and presentation

McDonald's sign—ability to move the uterus and cervix toward each other during a bimanual exam due to softening of the lower uterine segment

Positive sign of pregnancy—findings directly attributable to the fetus that can be detected by a healthcare provider; considered "absolute" proof of pregnancy

Presumptive sign of pregnancy—physiologic and anatomic changes experienced or noticed by a person capable of becoming pregnant, suggestive of pregnancy but not diagnostic

Probable sign of pregnancy—physiologic and anatomic changes that can be observed or palpated by a healthcare provider, suggestive of pregnancy but not diagnostic

Postconceptional weeks—terminology used by embryologists (but not in clinical practice) to describe the age of the embryo or fetus; the calculation is based on the date of conception: postconceptional weeks are two weeks less than the number of gestational weeks

Pseudocyesis—a condition in which a person thinks that they are pregnant and may have pregnancy-related symptoms, but there is not a pregnancy present

Quickening—perception of the first fetal movement by the pregnant person, also known as "feeling life"

Prenatal and Postnatal Care: A Person-Centered Approach, Third Edition. Edited by Karen Trister Grace, Cindy L. Farley, Noelene K. Jeffers, and Tanya Tringali.
© 2024 John Wiley & Sons Ltd. Published 2024 by John Wiley & Sons Ltd.
Companion website: www.wiley.com/go/grace/prenatal

Introduction

The diagnosis of pregnancy is an important life event, and the decisions that accompany the confirmation of a pregnancy have ramifications for the person's physical, psychosocial, and economic well-being. Although the health and well-being of the pregnant person and the developing fetus are the primary concern when a pregnancy is identified, the diagnosis also raises important moral, ethical, legal, psychosocial, and personal questions that must be carefully considered and addressed by the pregnant person in a relatively short period of time.

The diagnosis of pregnancy also begins a process of determining the **gestational age** of the pregnancy and estimating the approximate date of birth, procedures known as gestational aging or "dating" the pregnancy. Many of the clinical signs used to diagnose pregnancy are also used to determine the gestational age of the pregnancy and estimate the date of birth, so the diagnosis and dating of a pregnancy are closely related activities. Knowledge of the gestational age of a pregnancy is essential to almost every aspect of prenatal care, so accurate estimation of the gestational age is an important component of prenatal care and is initiated at the time of pregnancy diagnosis and reevaluated throughout the pregnancy. Knowledge of the **estimated date of birth** (EDB) is also important and helps the pregnant person, their significant others, and healthcare providers plan for the impending birth. The EDB is also known as the estimated date of delivery or estimated due date (EDD), but the term "estimated date of birth" is the preferred terminology for person-centered care.

This chapter presents the clinical, biochemical, and biophysical methods of diagnosing pregnancy, establishing the gestational age, and calculating the EDB. Also described are the health, psychosocial, and economic considerations that must be addressed at the time of pregnancy diagnosis. The appropriate counseling that should accompany pregnancy testing and the diagnosis of pregnancy is also reviewed.

Health equity key points

- The rhetoric of choice regarding a pregnancy diagnosis as experienced by people of color and those in poverty is overshadowed by the harsh realities of racism and economic scarcity. The rhetoric of choice has been further confounded by the overturning of the 1973 Roe vs. Wade decision and recent legislative changes in some states that do not allow pregnant individuals to make their own pregnancy-related decisions and have made some pregnancy options illegal. Although these legislative changes impact all pregnant people in those states, historically, these changes have the most negative impact on people of color and those with the fewest economic resources.
- The reproductive justice movement goes beyond the issue of choice and incorporates social inequities, such as poverty, welfare reform, economic injustice and the well-being of people into a framework for decision-making around pregnancy.

Benefits of Early Pregnancy Diagnosis and Gestational Age Assessment

Pregnancy raises a number of health issues and decisions, so early diagnosis of a pregnancy is ideal. Early pregnancy diagnosis is important for individuals who decide to terminate the pregnancy because early termination is associated with lower morbidity and mortality for the pregnant person and allows more options in pregnancy termination methods, depending on the state where the person resides. For people who decide to continue the pregnancy, early diagnosis facilitates early entry to prenatal care and provides the opportunity to advise the pregnant person to avoid potential teratogens and avoid or minimize potentially harmful exposures such as alcohol, tobacco, and illicit drugs. For individuals with preexisting medical conditions such as diabetes, seizure disorders, and hypertension, early pregnancy diagnosis facilitates management of these conditions and allows the selection of medications most compatible with pregnancy.

Early pregnancy diagnosis also facilitates the accurate assessment of gestational age. The calculation of the gestational age and EDB begin at the time of pregnancy diagnosis, and both are reevaluated throughout the pregnancy because knowledge of the gestational age is essential to many aspects of routine prenatal care. For example, the timing and interpretation of many screening and diagnostic procedures depend on knowledge of the gestational age. Most notable is the need for accurate dating of the pregnancy to determine when to perform blood and ultrasound testing for genetic screening as well as for more invasive testing such as chorionic villi sampling and genetic amniocentesis. Knowledge of the gestational age is also required to know when to perform procedures such as screening for diabetes or administering Rh immune globulin.

The appropriate diagnosis and treatment of pregnancy complications, such as preterm labor and postterm pregnancy, also depend on an accurate assessment of the gestational age. In the case of preterm labor, decisions about whether to use medications such as tocolytics and antenatal steroids or to transport the pregnant person to a regional perinatal center depend on knowledge of the gestational age. Knowledge of the gestational age is also essential to the identification of pregnancy problems that cause the uterus to be abnormally large or small, such as fetal growth restriction, fetal macrosomia, amniotic fluid volume disorders, multiple gestation, and hydatidiform mole. Knowledge of the gestational age is also essential to the correct timing of procedures, such as the induction of labor and scheduled cesarean birth. If healthcare providers do not have an accurate assessment of gestational age in these situations, they may overlook important pregnancy complications and fail to intervene when indicated, or they may intervene inappropriately.

Knowledge of the gestational age is also essential to providing relevant and timely health education throughout pregnancy. The need for information varies through the various stages of pregnancy. Early in pregnancy, teaching focuses on the avoidance of teratogens, nutrition, a healthy lifestyle, and the warning signs and symptoms of early pregnancy complications such as miscarriage and ectopic pregnancy. Later in pregnancy, teaching focuses on the preparation for labor and birth, selection of an infant feeding method, and preparation for infant care and parenting. Additional education that should be provided later in pregnancy includes information about the recognition of complications associated with more advanced pregnancy such as preterm labor, preterm rupture of the membranes, and preeclampsia.

In summary, early pregnancy diagnosis with concurrent and ongoing assessment of gestational age is a cornerstone of prenatal care and provides the timeline for clinical assessments, interventions, counseling, and education. Early pregnancy diagnosis also provides the opportunity for pregnant individuals to appreciate the experience of early pregnancy and make health and lifestyle changes to optimize pregnancy outcomes. Early pregnancy diagnosis is more important than ever in states that limit or no longer allow individuals to make their own pregnancy-related decisions. In these states, healthcare professionals must provide careful and thorough advisement and planning to protect the health, safety, and freedom of all pregnant individuals.

Pregnancy Diagnosis

The diagnosis of pregnancy has changed dramatically in recent decades with the introduction of readily available sensitive and specific home and laboratory pregnancy tests and easy access to real-time ultrasonography. Although modern biochemical pregnancy tests and biophysical methods of identifying a pregnancy have greatly advanced pregnancy care, assessment of the clinical signs and symptoms of pregnancy remain an important component of prenatal care. In fact, the diagnosis of pregnancy usually begins with a person's recognition of subjective symptoms associated with pregnancy, such as the absence of menstrual bleeding at the anticipated time or a cluster of symptoms such as nausea, vomiting, and fatigue.

Although no single subjective symptom or cluster of symptoms is absolutely diagnostic of pregnancy, documentation of clinical signs and symptoms augments the information gleaned from biochemical pregnancy tests and biophysical assessments such as ultrasound. Reports of pregnancy-related symptoms provide the opportunity to teach the person about the normal physiological changes that occur during pregnancy and how to mitigate unpleasant symptoms. Listening carefully to a person's reports of pregnancy-related symptoms also provides the opportunity to determine whether the symptoms are within the range of normal or indicative of a pregnancy complication or other health problem.

Knowledge of the signs and symptoms of pregnancy also enables healthcare providers to consider the possibility of pregnancy when individuals capable of becoming pregnant seek care for symptoms that they attribute to other health problems. For example, people occasionally seek care for a symptom such as **amenorrhea** or nausea, thinking that the symptom is related to a normal physiologic event such as menopause, a serious health problem such as cancer, a physical change such as weight loss, or a stressful life event. Healthcare providers must be vigilant in their differential diagnosis to exclude pregnancy as a cause of the symptoms in any person capable of becoming pregnant, even at the extreme ends of the reproductive years and in individuals who have previously undergone tubal sterilization. Indeed, for many of the symptoms described in this chapter, pregnancy should be at the top of the list of differential diagnoses in any person potentially capable of becoming pregnant.

Historically, the signs and symptoms of pregnancy have been organized into three categories: presumptive, probable, and positive. Presumptive signs are those noted by the pregnant individual and are considered subjective symptoms of pregnancy. Probable signs are those that can be observed or palpated by the healthcare provider and are considered objective signs of pregnancy. Positive signs of pregnancy are those that can be directly attributed to the fetus such as seeing the embryo on ultrasound or hearing the fetal heartbeat. The positive signs of pregnancy are the only signs that are considered absolute proof of pregnancy. These presumptive, probable, and positive signs of pregnancy are summarized in Table 10.1 and described in the following paragraphs.

Presumptive Signs of Pregnancy

The presumptive signs of pregnancy are symptoms and findings that are experienced or noticed by the individual. These subjective symptoms are the least accurate method of diagnosing pregnancy because they can be caused by many conditions other than pregnancy.

Amenorrhea

Amenorrhea, or the absence of menstruation, is strongly suggestive of pregnancy in a person with a history of regular menstrual cycles. However, amenorrhea is less predictive of pregnancy in individuals with preexisting amenorrhea, irregular menstrual cycles, or people who are lactating or perimenopausal. Additionally, some pregnant people experience bleeding early in pregnancy that can be mistaken for menses and delay the diagnosis of pregnancy.

Breast Changes

There are several breast changes that occur during pregnancy. Enlargement of the breasts is one of the earliest symptoms of pregnancy, occurring as early as the fourth week after the last menstrual period (LMP). Tenderness, throbbing, stretching, tingling, and fullness of the breasts are also common in the early weeks of pregnancy. Other changes include enlargement and increased pigmentation of the nipples and areola with increased protuberance of the Montgomery glands. Secretion of colostrum or milk occurs in some individuals, and is more likely to occur in

Table 10.1   Signs and Symptoms of Pregnancy

Category	Defining characteristic of the category	Sign or symptom
Presumptive signs	Physiological and anatomical changes that are experienced or noticed by the pregnant person Subjective sensations or assessments noted by the pregnant person Suggestive but not diagnostic of pregnancy	Amenorrhea Breast changes Vaginal changes Skin changes Nausea and vomiting Urinary frequency Fatigue Fetal movement
Probable signs	Physiological and anatomical changes that can be observed or palpated by a healthcare provider Objective findings on clinical exam by a healthcare provider Suggestive but not diagnostic of pregnancy	Enlargement of the abdomen Vaginal changes Cervical changes Uterine changes Palpation and ballottement of the fetus Basal body temperature elevation Endocrine pregnancy tests
Positive signs	Findings directly attributable to the fetus that can be detected by the healthcare provider Considered absolute proof of pregnancy Diagnostic of pregnancy	Detection of the embryo or fetus by ultrasound or X-ray Identification of fetal heart activity by a healthcare provider Detection of fetal movement by a healthcare provider

the second half of pregnancy and in people who have previously been pregnant and given birth.

Vaginal Changes

Pregnancy is often associated with an increase in the normal vaginal discharge, a symptom known as leukorrhea. The increased discharge is odorless and not irritating, and is not indicative of any inflammatory or infectious process.

Skin Changes

Skin changes that may be noted during pregnancy include increased pigmentation in areas such as the nipple, areola, axilla, genitals, and in the line down the center of the abdomen and around the umbilicus, an area known as the *linea nigra*. Many pregnant people also experience changes in pigmentation on the face, known as chloasma. Other skin changes include the appearance of striae, most often on the abdomen and breasts, but they may also appear on the buttocks and thighs. Changes in the vasculature of the skin include vascular spiders and palmar erythema and tend to appear later in pregnancy.

Subjective Sensations

There are many subjective sensations associated with pregnancy including nausea and vomiting, urinary frequency, and fatigue. The prevalence of these symptoms varies widely, which limits their usefulness in pregnancy diagnosis. When these subjective symptoms occur, they tend to be the most pronounced in the early weeks of pregnancy.

Another subjective sensation is fetal movement. Although long considered a hallmark of pregnancy, a person's perception of fetal movement is classified as a subjective sensation and is therefore considered a **presumptive sign of pregnancy**. The first perception of fetal movement, also known as "**quickening**," is a pivotal event in the pregnancy and an important milestone in parental role development and attachment to the fetus (Bloom, 1995; Lerum & LoBiondo-Wood, 1989). Historically, quickening was thought to reflect the moment when the fetus "came to life," and the pregnant person's perception of fetal movement is still often termed "feeling life" (Engstrom, 1985b). In the era before biochemical and biophysical methods of diagnosing pregnancy were widely available, quickening was often a person's only method of verifying the existence of a pregnancy. Although quickening remains an important and notable pregnancy event, its role in the diagnosis of pregnancy has lessened with the advent of modern chemical and biophysical tests. Quickening usually occurs between 14 and 22 weeks of gestation, but has been reported earlier and later in gestation (Engstrom, 1985b; O'Dowd & O'Dowd, 1985). Quickening is usually noted at about 16–17 weeks of gestation in people who have previously given birth and at about 18–19 weeks in people who have not previously given birth (Gillieson et al., 1984; O'Dowd & O'Dowd, 1985).

Probable Signs of Pregnancy

The probable signs of pregnancy are physiological and anatomical changes that can be detected by the healthcare provider. Although the probable signs of pregnancy are more objective, observable, and verifiable than the subjective sensations reported by individuals, the probable signs of pregnancy are still not absolute signs of pregnancy. Thus, even in the presence of several clinically detectable signs, the pregnancy must still be verified by another method.

Enlargement of the Abdomen

Enlargement of the abdomen is one of the classic signs of pregnancy. However, the uterus is usually not palpable through the pregnant person's abdomen until about 12 weeks of gestation. Although the pattern of abdominal enlargement during pregnancy is generally predictable, there is variation among different individuals. Additionally, the ability to accurately assess the size of the uterus through the abdomen may be hindered by the amount of adipose tissue and the strength of the abdominal musculature, as well as by the skill of the examiner. Another limitation of using abdominal enlargement as a sign of pregnancy is that any abdominal mass can be misidentified as the uterus and, periodically, a person will experience enlargement of the abdomen due to a cancerous or noncancerous tumor and mistakenly assume that the enlargement is due to pregnancy. Individuals can also experience abdominal enlargement and think they are pregnant despite the absence of any documentation of a pregnancy. In such cases, the person may simply be mistaken, and incorrectly assumed that pregnancy was the cause of their abdominal enlargement. In other cases, abdominal enlargement may be related to a strong desire for a pregnancy, which can be associated with the development of pregnancy-related symptoms in the absence of a pregnancy, a condition known as **pseudocyesis** (Gaskin, 2012).

Vaginal Changes

Changes in the color of the vaginal mucosa are often noticed during early pregnancy and usually begin in the anterior, lower portion of the vagina, close to the vaginal opening. The change begins in the area of a venous plexus and is described as a bluish or purplish spot known as **Jacquemin's sign** (Figure 10.1). Over time, the dusky blue or violet color spreads from the lower anterior vaginal wall to the entire vaginal mucosa. The bluish color of the vaginal mucosa is known as **Chadwick's sign** and occurs as early as six weeks of gestation.

Cervical Changes

Cervical changes noted during pregnancy include changes in cervical color and consistency. Similar to the vagina, the cervix becomes bluish purple or violet color in appearance. The softening of the cervix is remarkable and is known as **Goodell's sign**. A classic description of cervical consistency is that the nonpregnant cervix is as firm as the tip of the nose, whereas the pregnant cervix is as soft as the cheek or lips. The softening of the cervix begins on the lateral sides at 3 o'clock and 9 o'clock. These areas of softening are described by examiners as grooves

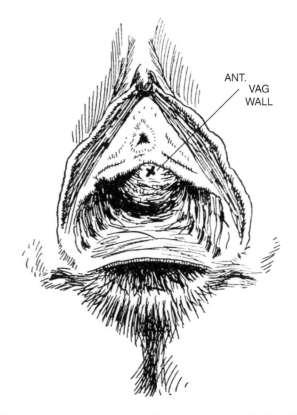

Figure 10.1 Jacquemin's sign of pregnancy. Source: McDonald (1908)/American Journal of Obstetrics and Diseases of Women and Children.

along the sides of the cervix. These grooves appear early but eventually disappear as the remainder of the cervix softens.

Uterine Changes

The uterus undergoes several changes during pregnancy. One of the first changes noted is the softening of the lower uterine segment. The softening is known as **Ladin's sign** and begins as a single soft spot in the center of the anterior aspect of the lower uterine segment (Munsick, 1986). The softening spreads throughout the lower uterine segment and is called **Hegar's sign** (Spreet, 1955). The softening of the lower uterine segment is readily detectable upon bimanual pelvic examination and is so pronounced that the lower segment can easily be compressed, giving the impression that there is no lower uterine segment whatsoever—just a cervix and the corpus of the uterus (McDonald, 1908). The softening and compressibility of the lower uterine segment is illustrated in Figure 10.2.

The softening of the lower segment also makes this area of the uterus more flexible and acts like a hinge, enabling the examiner to bend the uterus so that the fundus and the cervix move toward each other, a finding known as **McDonald's sign** (Figure 10.3).

Other areas of the uterus also demonstrate softening during pregnancy. The first area of uterine softening

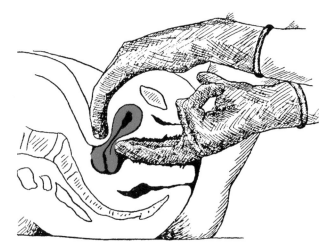

Figure 10.2 Hegar's sign of pregnancy. Source: McDonald (1908)/American Journal of Obstetrics and Diseases of Women and Children.

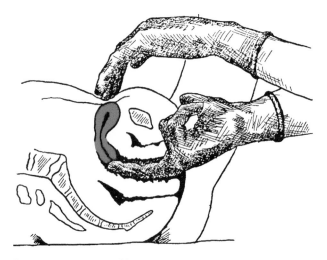

Figure 10.3 McDonald's sign of pregnancy. Source: McDonald (1908)/American Journal of Obstetrics and Diseases of Women and Children.

occurs in the area where the conceptus implanted. This area of softening is surrounded by areas of the firmness and is described by examiners as a sensation of "furrows and grooves" and is known as **Dickinson's sign**. Although present in most pregnant people, these changes are subtle and may not be noticed by a novice examiner.

The uterus also demonstrates changes in size and shape. The nonpregnant uterus is described as shaped like a flattened pear, with the narrowest diameter in the sagittal (anterior–posterior) plane. The first change in the shape and size of the uterus occurs at the site of implantation; the uterus enlarges asymmetrically in that area. Shortly thereafter, the uterus increases in the anterior–posterior diameter becoming pear shaped by four to five weeks of gestation. The uterus continues to enlarge and become rounder through the first trimester of pregnancy, acquiring the shape and size of a juice orange by 6 weeks of gestation, a navel orange by 8 weeks, and a grapefruit by 12 weeks (Fox, 1985; Margulies & Miller, 2001).

Uterine size and shape on bimanual examination	
4–5 weeks	Pear
6 weeks	Juice orange
8 weeks	Navel orange
12 weeks	Grapefruit

The uterus can be palpated by the examiner through the pregnant person's abdomen at approximately 12 weeks of gestation, when the uterine fundus is located immediately above the symphysis pubis. Subsequently, the uterine fundus is located approximately halfway between the symphysis pubis and umbilicus at 16 weeks of gestation, at the umbilicus at about 20 weeks, about halfway between the umbilicus and the xiphisternum at 28 weeks, and at the xiphisternum at 36 weeks (Andersen et al., 1981; Engstrom, 1988). However, there is wide variation among pregnant people in when the uterine fundus reaches these landmarks due to anatomic differences among individuals, the adiposity and muscularity of the abdomen, and the size of the uterus (Andersen et al., 1981; Engstrom, 1988; Jimenez et al., 1983).

Location of the uterine fundus during pregnancy	
12 weeks	At the symphysis pubis
16 weeks	About halfway between the symphysis pubis and umbilicus
20 weeks	At the umbilicus
28 weeks	About halfway between the umbilicus and the xiphisternum
36 weeks	At the xiphisternum

Contractions of the uterus, known as Braxton-Hicks contractions, can often be detected early in pregnancy. These contractions are painless and are usually not perceptible by the pregnant person until later in pregnancy. The contractions can be palpated early in pregnancy by the healthcare provider and are often stimulated by a bimanual or abdominal examination. However, these contractions are subtle and may not be detected by a novice examiner.

Palpation and Ballottement of the Fetus

The palpation of the fetus by a healthcare provider is another **probable sign of pregnancy**. Even before fetal parts can be palpated, the examiner can "bounce" the fetus between the examiner's hands, a finding known as ballottement. Later, individual fetal parts such as the head, buttocks, back, and extremities are palpable. Although the palpation of the fetus is useful in identifying fetal position and presentation, and in estimating fetal weight later in pregnancy, these signs have limited value in pregnancy diagnosis since they occur later in pregnancy and are only detectable once the fetus is large enough to be palpated.

Basal Body Temperature

The **basal body temperature** (BBT) can be useful in identifying a pregnancy. The BBT is the person's oral temperature taken upon first awaking in the morning, before any activity, or any oral intake of food or beverages. The temperature is ideally obtained at approximately the same time each day, after a full night of undisturbed rest. The BBT is influenced by the presence of progesterone, which has a thermogenic effect on body temperature, causing it to increase. Normally, BBTs are lower (below 98 °F/36.6 °C) during the follicular phase (first half or approximately the first 14 days) of the menstrual cycle when serum progesterone levels are consistently low. Around the time of ovulation, temperatures begin to increase as progesterone is beginning to be produced by the luteinized follicle. Progesterone is produced in large amounts by the corpus luteum after ovulation, and body temperature remains elevated throughout most of the luteal phase (second half or last 14 days of the cycle). In the presence of a pregnancy, the temperature remains elevated throughout the remainder of the pregnancy. The amount of temperature increase associated with ovulation and pregnancy varies but is usually about 0.4–0.8 °F, and postovulatory temperatures are usually above 98 °F/36.6 °C.

Endocrine Pregnancy Tests

Modern **endocrine pregnancy tests** measure the hormone human chorionic gonadotropin (hCG). The tests are often called "beta-hCG" because the tests target the beta subunit of the hormone. The tests can be performed on urine or serum and are classified as qualitative, semiquantitative, and quantitative. Qualitative tests simply detect the presence of hCG, and the results are reported as positive or negative, with positive indicating the presence of

enough of the hormone to be associated with a pregnancy. There are also semiquantitative or multilevel pregnancy tests that measure hCG in categories of units (IU/L; Cole, 2012). Semiquantitative tests are used to follow urine hCG levels in special circumstances such as after the termination of a molar pregnancy, after medication abortion, and after embryo transfer using assisted reproductive technology (Hoppenot et al., 2016; Raymond et al., 2017; Shochet et al., 2017). Quantitative pregnancy tests measure the precise level of hCG in the serum and report the findings in units (IU/L). Serum pregnancy tests are used to diagnose pregnancy and to monitor pregnancy progress in selected pregnancy complications such as suspected ectopic pregnancy or threatened abortion (Table 10.2).

There are two additional categories of urine pregnancy tests: point-of-care tests used in healthcare settings and over-the-counter pregnancy tests used for home testing. Although promotional materials for both point-of-care and over-the-counter tests claim high sensitivity and specificity and indicate that pregnancy can be detected several days before the missed menstrual period, the accuracy of both types of products varies widely (Cervinski et al., 2009; Cole, 2012). When the tests are positive, there is a high probability that the person is pregnant. False positive tests are uncommon but can occur in someone who has recently been pregnant and in individuals with certain cancers and other medical conditions. In contrast, false negative rates can be high in early pregnancy (Cole, 2012). The tests are most likely to be inaccurate when the level of hCG is the lowest during the first two to three weeks after conception (Cervinski et al., 2009; Cole, 2012; Greene et al., 2013). Many commonly used point-of-care pregnancy tests fail to detect pregnancy at the time of the missed menstrual period; the false negative rate at the time of missed menses is 33–60%, depending on the brand of test used (Cervinski et al., 2009; Cole, 2012). Thus, when a person has a negative test around the time of the missed menstrual period, it is reasonable to perform another

Table 10.2   Types of Endocrine Pregnancy Tests

Type of test	Type of specimen	Characteristics of the test
Qualitative	Urine	Used to diagnose pregnancy Reported as positive or negative Available over-the-counter and in healthcare settings
Semiquantitative or multilevel	Urine	Used to follow hCG levels after using assisted reproductive technology, medication abortion, and termination of a molar pregnancy Reported in categories of units of hCG (<25, 25–99, 100–499, 500–1999, 2000–9999, or ≥10,000 mIU/mL) Available in some healthcare settings
Quantitative	Serum	Used to diagnose pregnancy Reported in units (IU/L) Used to follow hCG levels when pregnancy complications are suspected Available in healthcare settings

pregnancy test four to seven days later. Four days is selected as the minimum interval between tests because the level of hCG increases exponentially in early pregnancy, nearly doubling every other day. Thus, by four to seven days, the levels should be substantially increased, and the test should be positive if a viable pregnancy is present.

Positive Signs of Pregnancy

The positive signs of pregnancy are signs that are directly attributed to the fetus and can be detected by the examiner. The positive signs of pregnancy are considered absolute signs of pregnancy. There are three positive signs of pregnancy: identification of **fetal heart activity**, detection of the embryo or fetus by ultrasound or X-ray, and detection of fetal movement by the examiner.

Identification of Fetal Heart Activity

Fetal heart activity can be visualized using real-time ultrasound or by hearing **fetal heart sounds** using Doppler ultrasound or auscultation. In most settings in the United States, fetal heart sounds are assessed during the prenatal period using a handheld Doppler ultrasound unit. Early in pregnancy, the best place to listen for fetal heart sounds is in the suprapubic area slightly above the pubic bone in the center of the pregnant person's abdomen. The fetal heart rate is faster than the normal adult heart rate and is typically heard at a rate of 110–160 beats per minute. When using a handheld Doppler ultrasound device, fetal heart sounds should be heard by 12 weeks of gestation and are often heard as early as 10 weeks. Real-time ultrasound can be used to identify fetal heart activity as early as six weeks of gestation (Richards, 2021).

Historically, fetal heart sounds, also called fetal heart "tones," were auscultated using a modified stethoscope known as a **fetoscope**. The fetoscope has a headpiece added to a stethoscope that provides additional stimulation of the examiner's frontal head bones to facilitate the conduction of the sounds, thereby enabling the healthcare provider to hear the faint sounds of early fetal heart activity (Figure 10.4) Although the fetoscope is primarily of historic interest in the United States, it is still used to assess fetal heart activity in some settings, especially in low-resource settings or when avoidance of technology is desired. Fetal heart sounds are not usually heard with a fetoscope until 15–22 weeks of gestation (Engstrom, 1985b). Later in pregnancy, fetal heart sounds can be auscultated with a standard stethoscope.

Detection of the Embryo or Fetus by Ultrasound or X-Ray

Observation of the embryo or fetus by ultrasound or X-ray is a definitive sign of pregnancy. X-ray is rarely used during pregnancy, but ultrasonography is widely used and can detect the gestational sac as early as four to five weeks

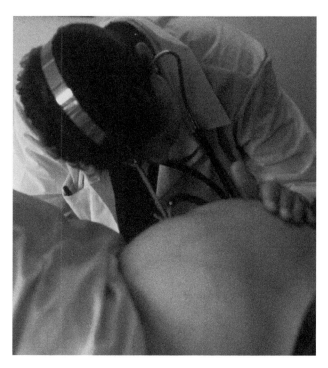

Figure 10.4   Auscultation of fetal heart sounds with a fetoscope. Source: Courtesy of Virginia Michels, MSN, CNM.

of gestation (Richards, 2021). The embryo can be observed by six weeks of gestation on ultrasound, and embryonic heart activity can also be observed at that time (Richards, 2021).

Detection of Fetal Movement by the Examiner

The third **positive sign of pregnancy** is the detection of fetal movement by the examiner. The fetus is usually not palpable by a healthcare provider until the second half of pregnancy. The detection of fetal movement usually occurs during the routine prenatal examination of the pregnant abdomen. The abdomen is systematically palpated using a series of procedures known as **Leopold's maneuvers** (McFarlin et al., 1985; Sharma, 2009). Leopold's maneuvers are described below and depicted in Figure 10.5. All palpation is performed gently using a circular motion with the flat portion of the fingers rather than the tips. To relax the pregnant person's abdominal musculature during the exam, the head of the exam table is raised slightly, and the person's legs are flexed and bent at the knees. In addition to confirming the presence of a fetus, Leopold's maneuvers are also used to identify fetal size, position, and presentation. Including the pregnant person in the palpation of the fetus can also facilitate parental–fetal attachment (Nishikawa & Sakakibara, 2013).

Gestational Age Assessment

Once the presence of a pregnancy is confirmed, the gestational age of the pregnancy should be determined. Knowledge of the gestational age is such an important

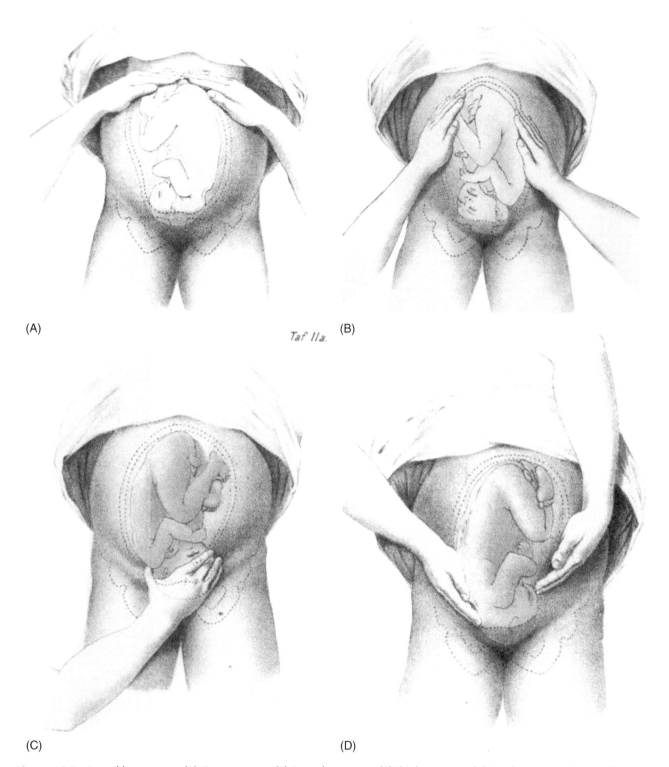

(A)

Taf IIa.

(B)

(C)

(D)

Figure 10.5   Leopold maneuvers. (A) First maneuver; (B) Second maneuver; (C) Third maneuver; (D) Fourth maneuver. Source: Sharma (2009)/Springer Nature.

component of prenatal care that gestational age assessment begins at the time of pregnancy diagnosis. At each prenatal visit, the clinician verifies the gestational age and compares the size of the uterus to the calculated gestational age to determine whether uterine size and fetal growth are consistent with the gestational age. The dates of other events such as quickening, hearing the fetal heart sounds for the first time, and when the uterine fundus reaches the level of the umbilicus are also compared to the estimated gestational age to determine whether the timing of these events is consistent with the estimated gestational age.

Leopold maneuvers

First maneuver	Facing the head of the examination table, systematically palpate the uterine fundus to determine which fetal parts are present. The buttocks feel irregular and soft, whereas the head is round and hard. The absence of any part in the area may indicate a transverse lie.
Second maneuver	Facing the head of the examination table, systematically palpate each side of the uterus. Place one hand on each side of the uterus, near the fundus. The examiner's left hand should be placed on the right side of the uterus and the right hand on the left side of the uterus. Hold the left hand stable while palpating with the right hand. Move the hands systematically from the fundus to the symphysis to cover all the areas. Then, repeat the procedure holding the right hand still while palpating with the left hand along the right side of the uterus. The fetal back is usually along one side of the uterus and the "small parts" (arms and legs) are along the other side. The back feels smooth and firm. The fetal extremities are small and very irregular.
Third maneuver	Facing the head of the examination table, the examiner separates the thumb and fingers of the right hand to form a large "C." Palpate the lateral borders of the uterus immediately above the symphysis pubis to determine whether the head or buttocks are in the area. The absence of any part in the area may indicate a transverse lie.
Fourth maneuver	Face the foot of the examination table and place both hands along the lateral uterine borders immediately above the symphysis pubis. Gently glide the hands along the fetal presenting part into the pelvis to identify the presenting part and its relationship to the pelvis.

Source: Adapted from McFarlin et al. (1985) and Sharma (2009).

Terminology Used to Describe Gestational Age

In clinical practice, gestational age is usually calculated by using the date of first day of the LMP. The first day of the LMP is used regardless of the time of day menstruation started or the amount of menstrual flow. When calculated from the first day of the LMP, the duration of human pregnancy is 280 days or 40 weeks. The first day of the LMP is used to determine the number of **gestational weeks** for a pregnancy. Although *gestational weeks* is the current preferred terminology, the terms *gestational age, menstrual weeks*, and *menstrual age* are also used. The first day of the LMP is considered the start of Week 1. Many prenatal care providers record the number of days in the current week in addition to the number of weeks. For example, a note in a person's health record who is currently 35 weeks plus an additional 6 days of pregnancy may be recorded using any of the following notations: 35 weeks 6 days, 35 6/7 weeks, or 35.[6] The number of gestational weeks is never rounded up to the next week.

Although the phrase "gestational weeks" is the accepted terminology in clinical practice, embryonic development is described in **postconceptional weeks**, beginning with the date of conception. When postconceptional weeks are used, the duration of pregnancy is 266 days or 38 weeks. Although useful in understanding embryonic development, the terminology of postconceptional weeks is not used in the clinical setting because of the potential confusion with the standard use of gestational weeks. The terminology *gestational weeks* or *gestational age* is always used when communicating in the clinical setting.

Pregnancy is also sometimes described in months and trimesters. The relationship between gestational weeks, lunar months, and trimesters is depicted in Table 10.3. The terminology surrounding the use of months is fraught with confusion and can easily lead to miscommunication. When months are used to describe pregnancy, the months are lunar months, each consisting of 28 days. Thus, a normal pregnancy is 10 lunar months. Lunar months are shorter than calendar months, so 10 lunar months translates to about 91/3 calendar months. For these reasons, prenatal care providers should avoid using the terminology of months whenever possible.

Pregnancy is also described in trimesters. Surprisingly, the method of dividing the pregnancy into trimesters has varied over time and has included schemes that divided the pregnancy into unequal trimesters. The current recommended approach divides gestation into three more equally spaced trimesters. The first trimester begins on the first day of the LMP, and that day is identified as Week 1—Day 0 (Week 1 0/7). The first trimester lasts through the end of the 13th week (13 weeks 6 days or 13 6/7 weeks). The second trimester begins at the start of the 14th week (14 weeks 0 days or 14 0/7 weeks) and continues through the end of the 27th week (27 weeks 6 days or 27 6/7 weeks). The third trimester extends from the first day of the 28th week (28 weeks 0 days or 28 0/7 weeks) through the end of the pregnancy (ACOG, 2017).

Current trimester terminology		
Trimester	Begins	Ends
First	First day of the last menstrual period is the first day of Week 1 (1 0/7 weeks)	13 6/7 weeks
Second	Week 14 (14 0/7 weeks)	27 6/7 weeks
Third	Week 28 (28 0/7 weeks)	Time of Birth

Because the terminology surrounding trimesters is varied and each trimester spans a long time period that includes important events and milestones, the terminology *trimesters* should only be used in the broadest sense, such as when discussing how to focus health education or the period of pregnancy when selected pregnancy discomforts and complications are most likely to occur. For example, ectopic pregnancy usually occurs in the first trimester of pregnancy, whereas preeclampsia is most likely to become symptomatic in the third trimester.

Table 10.3   Timing of Events in Gestation

Trimester	Lunar month	Week of gestation	Event
First	1	1	First day of the last menstrual period (LMP). Follicular phase of the menstrual cycle begins.
		2	Follicular phase of the menstrual cycle continues. Ovulation occurs. Fertilization of the oocyte (conception) occurs on approximately day 14 of a perfect menstrual cycle.
		3	Basal body temperature increases. Conceptus is transported through the fallopian tube and into the uterus. Preliminary attachment of the conceptus to the endometrium occurs.
		4	Conceptus is implanted in the endometrium. Urine and serum endocrine pregnancy tests (hCG) may be positive. Gestational sac observed on ultrasound at 4–5 weeks. Breast tenderness and fullness may occur.
	2	5	
		6	Embryo is observed on ultrasound. Fetal heart activity is observed on real-time ultrasound. The uterus becomes more rounded and is approximately the size of a juice orange. Jacquemin's, Chadwick's, Goodell's, Ladin's, Hegar's, McDonald's, and Dickinson's signs may appear between 6 and 12 weeks.
		7	
		8	The uterus is the size of a navel orange.
	3	9	
		10	Fetal heart sounds are usually heard with Doppler ultrasound at 10–12 weeks.
		11	
		12	The uterus is the size of a grapefruit. The uterus is palpable at the symphysis pubis.
		13	
Second	4	14	Quickening usually occurs between 14 and 22 weeks.
		15	Fetal heart sounds are usually first auscultated with a fetoscope between 15 and 22 weeks.
		16	The uterus is about halfway between the symphysis pubis and the umbilicus.

(Continued)

Table 10.3 (*Continued*)

Trimester	Lunar month	Week of gestation	Event
	5	17	
		18	
		19	
		20	The uterus is at about the level of the umbilicus. Fundal height measurements (in centimeters) are approximately equal to the number of gestational weeks from 20 to 36 weeks (±3 cm).
	6	21	
		22	
		23	
		24	
	7	25	
		26	
		27	
Third		28	The uterus is about halfway between the umbilicus and the xiphisternum.
	8	29	
		30	
		31	
		32	
	9	33	
		34	
		35	
		36	The uterus is at the xiphisternum.
	10	37	
		38	
		39	
		40	

Source: Adapted from Baskett and Nagele (2000), Hunter (2009), and Loytved and Fleming (2016).

Devices Used to Calculate the Gestational Age

Gestational age should be calculated at the time of pregnancy diagnosis and verified at each healthcare encounter thereafter. Verifying the gestational age at each visit during pregnancy assures that the prenatal care provider has an accurate assessment of the gestational age at that encounter and prevents the problem of carrying forward a calculation error from a previous visit. Although this precaution may seem trivial, an error of even a few days in estimating the gestational age can result in serious health consequences for the pregnant person and the fetus.

There are several electronic calculators that can be used to assist with the calculation of gestational weeks and the EDB. These devices are available online and as applications for mobile devices such as cellular phones and electronic tablets. The electronic calculators are uniformly accurate and are the preferred method for calculating gestational weeks and the EDB (Smout et al., 2012).

Gestational weeks can also be calculated using a manual calculator, commonly known as a "wheel" because of its circular design and rotating wheels. There are a number of small, handheld, manual, cardboard, or plastic devices available, and they are often given to healthcare providers as a promotional item advertising maternity care products. Although handy in low-resource settings, the accuracy of these devices varies widely. There are significant differences between the gestational age and EDB calculations made with various devices, as well as differences between healthcare providers when using the same device (McParland & Johnson, 1993; Ross, 2003; Smout et al., 2012). The devices also yield different results from electronic calculators, with differences as large as five days reported (Ross, 2003). Thus, the use of manual calculators should be avoided except in low-resource settings where there is no access to an electronic calculator. In those settings, all healthcare providers should use the same brand of device and verify that they all obtain the same result when using the device. Before selecting a manual calculator, the device should be validated with an electronic calculator to assure its accuracy.

Methods of Estimating the Gestational Age

There are several methods of estimating gestational age, including the date of the LMP, the date of conception, the date of a single act of coitus or insemination, the date of a sustained increase in BBT, **fundal height measurements**, and ultrasound. The timing of these events and the timing of the appearance of many of the clinical signs of pregnancy described previously in this chapter are summarized in Table 10.3.

Last Menstrual Period

The date of the first day of the LMP is the most commonly used method of estimating gestational age and the EDB. When this date is known and the person has regular menstrual cycles, the estimation of gestational weeks and the EDB is usually accurate. Some individuals are unable to accurately recall the date of the LMP, and even when a person presents with an accurate LMP, the estimation of the gestational weeks may be inaccurate if the person has irregular cycles, cycles longer or shorter than 28 days, a recent pregnancy, is lactating, or has recently used hormonal contraception.

The standard calculation of the EDB is based on an average pregnancy interval of 280 days and assumes that ovulation and fertilization take place on day 14 of the cycle. The EDB can be calculated using the following procedure, named Naegele's rule (Baskett & Nagele, 2000; Hunter, 2009; Loytved & Fleming, 2016):

Naegele's rule for calculating the EDB

Naegele's rule	Example
1. Use the first day of the LMP.	8-10-2024
2. Subtract 3 from the number of months.	5-10-2024
3. Add 7 to the number of days	5-17-2024
4. Adjust the year if the birth will occur in the next year.	5-17-2025

Naegele's rule is easy to apply and does not require the use of any devices or calculators. However, the calculation provides only one date, the EDB. The calculation does not assist healthcare providers during pregnancy with calculating the gestational weeks, information that is needed at each prenatal visit. Thus, gestational weeks must be calculated using a gestational calculator. Additionally, Naegele's calculation does not account for differences in the number of days in the various months throughout the year. Depending on the particular months included in the pregnancy, the difference between the

calculation made by Naegele's rule and the calculation of the EDB using 280 days from the LMP can be different by as many as 3 days (McParland & Johnson, 1993; Ross, 2003). For these reasons, Naegele's rule is not used as the only method of estimating the EDB in most settings. However, Naegele's rule is easy to use and may be the only method available in low-resource settings. Calculations made using Naegele's rule should be verified with a validated electronic or manual gestational calculator when possible. However, it is important to emphasize that all EDBs are an approximate date of birth, and the actual date of birth varies in different individuals and is influenced by many factors (Lawson, 2021). For these reasons, many pregnancy care providers are providing an estimated range of dates when the birth is most likely to happen rather than a single estimated date.

Because the LMP is essential in calculating gestational weeks, a thorough menstrual history is an essential component of pregnancy diagnosis and the initial prenatal visit. For individuals who initially respond that they do not recall the exact date of the LMP, many can be assisted to recall the date by viewing a calendar or thinking about events at the time of the LMP. The regularity of cycles as well as the normality of the LMP should also be documented. It is also important to determine whether the individual has recently used hormonal contraception, had a recent gestation or lactation, or any other factor that may influence the regularity of menstrual cycles or delay ovulation.

The primary limitation of using the LMP is error in recall over time (Lynch & Zhang, 2007; Wegienka & Baird, 2005). Even when individuals are certain of the date of the LMP, the actual date of ovulation and conception may be unknown. The time between the first day of the LMP and ovulation varies widely, even in individuals who have cycles of the same length, and even in the same person from month to month (Lynch & Zhang, 2007). The calculated gestational age based on the LMP is a relatively good estimate in a person with regular cycles who is certain of the date of the LMP, but that estimate will always be limited by the variability in the timing of ovulation. Research has suggested that when the LMP is used to calculate the EDB, the prediction is one to three days earlier than sonographic estimates of gestational age, resulting in more pregnancies being classified as postterm when the LMP is used (Hoffman et al., 2008; Nakling et al., 2005; Savitz et al., 2002; Taipale & Hiilesmaa, 2001). For these reasons, some experts have recommended using ultrasound estimates of gestational age rather than the LMP when the ultrasound estimate is obtained between 6 and 20 weeks of gestation and is performed by a skilled sonographer (Gardosi, 1997; Nakling et al., 2005; Richards, 2021; Taipale & Hiilesmaa, 2001). However, a joint statement by the American College of Obstetricians and Gynecologists, the American Institute of Ultrasound in Medicine, and the Society for Maternal-Fetal Medicine recommends using the date of the LMP unless the difference between the LMP and ultrasound estimated gestational weeks exceeds a certain number of days for each period of gestation. These recommendations are summarized in Table 10.4 (ACOG, 2017).

Table 10.4 Accuracy of Ultrasound Assessments of Gestational Age and Recommendations for when to Adjust Gestational Age

Structures measured for gestational age assessment	Weeks of gestation	Accuracy of gestational age assessments	Redate pregnancy if LMP and ultrasound estimates of gestational age differ by
CRL	6 0/7 to 8 6/7 wk	±5 d	More than 5 days
	9 0/7 to −13 6/7 wk	±7 d	More than 7 days
BPD, HC, AC, and FL	14 0/7 to 15 6/7 wk	±7 d	More than 7 days
	16 0/7 to −21 6/7 wk	±10 d	More than 10 days
	22 0/7 to 27 6/7 wk	±14 d	More than 14 days
	28 0/7 wk until birth	±21 d	More than 21 days

Source: ACOG (2017) and Richards (2021).
CRL = Crown-rump length, BPD = Biparietal diameter, HC = Head circumference, AC = Abdominal circumference, FL = Femur length.

Known Date of Conception

The gestational age of a pregnancy can be most accurately calculated when assisted reproductive technology procedures, such *in vitro* fertilization, are used to achieve pregnancy. In these cases, the date of conception is certain and can be used to accurately calculate gestational age. The calculation is performed by adding 38 weeks (266 days) to the date of conception.

Occasionally, a person will report a single act of unprotected coitus that led to the pregnancy. However, even when the person knows the precise date of coitus or insemination, the actual date of conception is unknown because sperm can reside in the cervix, uterus, and fallopian tubes for up to six days before fertilizing the egg (Wilcox et al., 2000). Thus, estimates made using a single act of coitus or insemination are likely to be accurate within one week.

Change in Basal Body Temperature

Occasionally, a person can provide BBTs from the cycle in which conception occurred. Although neither the day of ovulation nor the day of conception can be pinpointed from a BBT graph, the change in temperature associated with ovulation can provide an excellent estimate of the date of conception and is likely to be accurate within one week.

Fundal Height Measurements

Fundal height measurements, also known as symphysis-fundus measurements, are a measure of the distance between the uppermost border of the symphysis pubis and the uppermost border of the uterine fundus in the midline of the pregnant person's abdomen. The measurements are a routine part of the prenatal exam and can be useful in determining whether uterine size is appropriate for the number of gestational weeks. Abnormally large or small fundal height measurements can indicate that the estimated gestational age may be incorrect or that a pregnancy complication such as fetal growth restriction, macrosomia, amniotic fluid abnormality, or multifetal

gestation may be present (Grantz et al., 2021; Morse et al., 2009; Roex et al., 2012).

Fundal height measurements are recorded in centimeters, and the measurements are approximately equal to the number of gestational weeks between 20 and 36 weeks of gestation. However, many factors influence these measurements, so differences of up to 2–3 cm between the measurements and the number of gestational weeks are considered acceptable. The pattern of measurements is also important, with sudden increases or decreases in the measurements suggesting potential complications. Although fundal height measurements are used to corroborate pregnancy dating, the measurements are not accurate enough to be used as the only method of estimating gestational age except in very-low-resource settings where ultrasound is not available (Self et al., 2022; White et al., 2012).

Many different methods of measuring the fundal height have been reported in the literature, and the different measurement techniques yield significantly different measurements, so it is important that the measurements be consistently performed using the same measurement technique (Engstrom, 1985a; Engstrom & Sittler, 1993). Additionally, there can be significant differences in the measurements obtained by different healthcare providers, so it is important that all healthcare providers within a clinical setting agree upon how the measurement should be obtained and consistently use the same measurement technique (Engstrom et al., 1993b). Some prenatal care providers have difficulty identifying the uterine fundus accurately, so all providers should have the opportunity to learn how to obtain the measurements and verify that their measurements are the same as those obtained by other healthcare providers (Engstrom et al., 1993a, 1993b). The recommended fundal height measurement procedure is described below and depicted in Figure 10.6.

Provider bias in obtaining fundal height measurements is also an important problem. When healthcare providers can see the numeric centimeter markings on the tape measure, they are more likely to record the number as

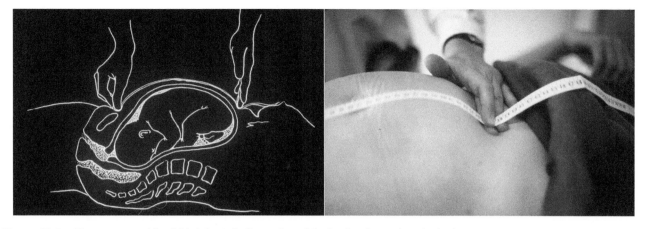

Figure 10.6   Measurement of fundal height. Left: Illustration of the landmarks used to obtain the measurement. Source: Engstrom and Sittler (1993)/with permission of Elsevier. Right: Photograph of the placement of the tape measure and the technique of holding the tape measure at the uterine fundus. Source: Courtesy of Virginia Michels.

Fundal height measurement procedure

- Ask the pregnant person if they need to use the restroom before beginning the prenatal exam.
- Place the person in a supine position with the head of the exam table flat and the person's legs extended.
- Lower the person's clothing so that the pubic area is exposed and use a drape or sheet to discreetly cover the area.
- Place the tape measure in the midline of the pregnant person's abdomen with the numeric centimeter markings on the tape measure facing the abdomen, so the clinician cannot see the markings.
- Identify the uppermost border of the symphysis pubis and place the zero mark of the tape measure on that point.
- Identify the uppermost border of the uterine fundus and bring the tape measure to that point.
- The tape measure should be in contact with the skin of the abdomen throughout the length of the measurement.
- Mark the fundal height on the tape measure by tearing, folding, or holding the tape measure at that point.
- Turn the tape measure over, read the measurement, and record the measurement in the person's prenatal health record.

---

being closer to the number of gestational weeks (Engstrom et al., 1994; Jelks et al., 2007). Thus, the measurements should be obtained with the numeric centimeter markings facing away from the examiner, toward the pregnant person's abdomen.

The pregnant person's position during fundal height measurement also significantly influences the measurements, so it is important to consistently use the same position for all measurements (Engstrom et al., 1993c). The measurements are closest to the actual number of gestational weeks when the pregnant person is in the supine position with the head of the table flat and the person's legs extended (Engstrom & Sittler, 1993). However, the supine position should be avoided for extended periods of time during pregnancy, so a pregnant

person should only be placed in this position for the time that the measurement requires, and then, the head of the exam table should be elevated and the person's legs should be bent at the knees. Bladder fullness is known to increase the fundal height measurement, so patients should be asked if they need to use the restroom before the fundal height is measured (Engstrom et al., 1989).

Fundal height measurements can be plotted on a fundal height growth curve to graphically depict uterine growth during pregnancy. However, the limits of normal on the published curves vary widely, so the fundal height growth curves should be used with caution and tested in the clinical setting before adopting their routine use (Engstrom & Work, 1992).

Ultrasound

Ultrasound is widely used to estimate gestational age, and the technology can provide a very accurate assessment of the gestational age early in pregnancy (American College of Obstetricians and Gynecologists [ACOG], 2017). The earliest structure visible is the gestational sac, which can be identified as early as four to five weeks of gestation (Richards, 2021). Although measurements of the gestational sac can be used to estimate gestational age, the estimates are not as accurate as when other fetal parameters are measured, so gestational sac measurements should not be used as the only method of estimating gestational age (Richards, 2021). Measurements of the embryo and fetus such as crown-rump length, biparietal diameter, head circumference, femur length, and abdominal circumference are the most accurate predictors of gestational age when the measurements are obtained during the first half of pregnancy (ACOG, 2017).

During the first trimester of pregnancy, the crown-rump length of the embryo provides a very accurate estimate of the gestational age. The crown-rump length can be used to accurately estimate gestational age within 5 days from 6 to 8 weeks of gestation, and within 7 days from 9 to 13 weeks. By 14 weeks of gestation, the crown-rump length becomes less accurate, so other fetal parameters, such as the fetal biparietal diameter, head circumference, abdominal circumference, and femur length, are used to estimate gestational age (ACOG, 2021). Gestational age assessments made using these fetal measurements can accurately estimate gestational age within 7 days from 14 to 15 weeks, and within 10 days from 16 through 21 weeks of gestation (ACOG, 2017).

In the second half of pregnancy, the amount of error in the sonographic estimation of gestational age increases rapidly because fetal growth becomes more variable. The error in gestational age assessment increases to 14 days from 22 to 27 weeks of gestation. After 27 weeks, the error in gestational age estimates is large, with errors as large as 21 days. Thus, the timing of ultrasound examinations for gestational aging is extremely important, and when verification of gestational age is needed, it should be obtained during the first half of pregnancy, ideally in the first trimester but before 22 weeks of gestation (ACOG, 2017).

Counseling for Pregnancy Diagnosis

Conduct all counseling about the results of a pregnancy test in a neutral manner, with no assumption that a positive or negative test is the desired result. For example, avoid statements such as "Congratulations, your test is positive" or, "Good news, your test is negative," when reporting pregnancy results. Instead, deliver the results accurately, clearly, in a simple manner, and avoid value statements, such as, a "good" or "bad" result. Similarly, conduct all discussions about reproductive options in a nondirective and noncoercive manner. Equally important is the confidential nature of any discussion related to pregnancy testing. There are some exceptions to confidentiality, such as reporting suspected neglect and abuse or if the person is unable to consent due to age or disability. Healthcare providers must know state reporting regulations and advise the individual of any exceptions to confidentiality.

Urine pregnancy test results are reported as positive or negative, with positive indicating the presence of a pregnancy and negative indicating that the individual is not pregnant or the pregnancy is too early to be detected. Although the language of positive and negative test results is obvious to healthcare professionals, the meaning of positive and negative tests is not clear to many patients. Additionally, individuals may be so anxious about the test results that they may not completely understand the terminology. When reporting the pregnancy test results, it is best practice to clarify the meaning of a positive and a negative test. For example, a healthcare provider might say, "Your pregnancy test is positive; that means that you are pregnant," or "Your test is negative; that means that you are not pregnant or that the pregnancy is so early that the test may not yet detect the pregnancy."

Many individuals who visit a healthcare facility for pregnancy testing have already performed a home pregnancy test and have an idea of whether they are pregnant or not. These individuals often seek healthcare because they are looking for the confirmation of the result or are

hoping the home test result is incorrect. Research indicates that most individuals decide about their pregnancy within one day of receiving pregnancy test results, suggesting that most individuals already suspect they are pregnant and have some sense of how they feel about the pregnancy prior to taking a test (Branum & Ahrens, 2017; Brauer et al., 2019).

Deliver the pregnancy test results promptly; the individual should not be required to sit through counseling or education sessions before receiving the results. After stating the test results, it is beneficial to allow the person a moment to process the information and to collect their thoughts. Although healthcare providers are often tempted to manage the situation by providing information and referrals, it is helpful to engage in active listening by giving the individual time to reflect on how they feel about the pregnancy test result. Nonverbal clues may provide a sense of how the individual feels about the result. If the individual's feelings are not evident, healthcare providers can elicit their feelings by asking, "How are you feeling about this?" or "Is this what you were expecting?" or "You seem upset/sad/shocked/happy." Additional areas to explore include the individual's support system and how they might respond to the news of the pregnancy. Neutral comments such as "Tell me more about what is concerning you" or "Many individuals have mixed feelings about a pregnancy" can often open the conversation and elicit concerns.

Counseling after a Negative Pregnancy Test

If a pregnancy test is negative and the individual is disappointed, further assessment is warranted. If they desire a pregnancy, this is an ideal time to discuss preconception care. If there is a concern of infertility, recognize the individual's disappointment and obtain a detailed gynecological, reproductive, and health history. Provide counseling to optimize the probability of conceiving and referrals to fertility specialists provided when indicated.

If an individual is relieved by a negative test result, this is a teachable moment for contraceptive counseling. Following a negative test, people are often highly motivated to use an effective method of birth control and learn about emergency contraception. Both prescription and nonprescription emergency contraceptive products are available. Advise individuals that these products are often kept "behind the counter" even though they are available without a prescription. A negative pregnancy test also provides an opportunity for an individual to think about preconception health and reproductive planning.

The term pregnancy intention has historically been used to describe pregnancy planning and decision-making. Dichotomous terms of planned and unplanned, intended or unintended pregnancy, are helpful for researchers and academics but do not capture decision-making nuances. Many groups, especially groups of people of color, have challenged the traditional language of researchers to consider reproductive rights and decision-making with a human rights framework. The reproductive justice framework expands pregnancy decision-making to include social issues such as economic justice, education, housing, immigration, environmental, political, and other social and cultural contexts (Price, 2020). Since this chapter is citing research that uses the terms of intended or unintended, such terminology is used for consistency.

Counseling after a Positive Pregnancy Test

If the individual is pleased with the positive pregnancy results, they should be congratulated and referred or scheduled for early pregnancy care. Essential information to provide at the time of pregnancy diagnosis includes the importance of avoiding alcohol, drugs, unnecessary medications, and potential teratogens. Also important is information about the signs and symptoms of early pregnancy complications such as ectopic pregnancy and miscarriage. If they are not already taking a supplement, all people should be advised to immediately start taking a folic acid supplement of 0.4 mg/day (400 pg/day). If the individual's financial resources are limited, give information about state Medicaid programs for prenatal care as well as the Women, Infants, and Children (WIC) nutrition program.

Options Counseling for Unintended Pregnancy

In the United States, 49% of all pregnancies are categorized as unintended (consisting of pregnancies that are mistimed or unwanted). With progress historically slow in meeting the Healthy People National Public Health Goal of reducing unintended pregnancy, many individuals will experience unintended pregnancy (Office of Disease Prevention and Health Promotion, n.d.). For the first time in four decades, there has been a decline in abortion rates among all demographic groups; however, the decline varies widely by groups (Jones & Jerman, 2017). The decline in abortion rates and unintended pregnancy is thought to be due to expanded access to contraception, especially long-acting methods (Nash & Dreweke, 2019; Jones & Jerman, 2017). People with limited financial resources and people and individuals of color continue to face barriers to reliable contraception (Dickman et al., 2021).

Healthcare providers should expect to encounter people with unintended pregnancies in a wide variety of clinical settings and should be prepared to provide sensitive and nonjudgmental counseling. An individual with a newly diagnosed pregnancy may need support in deciding whether to continue or terminate the pregnancy. If deciding to terminate an early pregnancy, the individual may have the option of medication or procedural (aspiration/surgical) abortion, depending on the state in which they live (Guttmacher Institute, 2023). If continuing the pregnancy, the individual will have to decide whether to parent the child or plan for adoption.

The issue of providing comprehensive reproductive healthcare for an individual with an unintended pregnancy raises personal and professional ethical conflicts for some healthcare providers. To effectively facilitate the decision-making process for individuals facing unintended pregnancy, it is helpful for healthcare providers to examine their personal beliefs and biases that may interfere with providing person-centered care. Value clarification enables healthcare providers to resolve these conflicts in a way that ensures patient safety and preserves the integrity of the provider (Guiahi et al., 2021). Resources for value clarification are provided at the end of this chapter.

Midwifery and nursing organizations have historically articulated ethical guidelines for the advanced practice nurse and midwife (see section: Professional Ethics and Standards for Reproductive Options Counseling). Healthcare providers should remember that they are not personally responsible for ethical consequences of the decisions made by the people they serve who are exercising their right to autonomy in decision-making about their own bodies and health (Beal & Cappiello, 2008; Cappiello et al., 2011). The exercise of professional right of conscience is generally discussed in the content of refusal to participate in specific healthcare services, such as provision of contraception, sterilization, emergency contraception, and abortion care. Harris (2012), however, suggests that the professional right of conscience rules and legislation fail to protect providers who choose to provide reproductive health services. That is, if acting from a moral perspective, healthcare providers should be free from harassment and stigma for the conscious provision of reproductive health services. Facilitating evidenced-based, person-centered early pregnancy decision-making and care can be defined as the conscientious provision of reproductive healthcare. For more discussion, see Chapter 2, *Ethics in Perinatal Care*.

Healthcare providers can assist individuals experiencing ambivalence or uncertainty about pregnancy by helping them identify life circumstances that affect the decision to parent a child at this point in their lives. Several interconnected social factors motivate the decision to continue or terminate a pregnancy. Individuals who feel that they cannot continue a pregnancy often report resource limitations. Financial constraints, lack of partner support, responsibility to others, wanting to limit childbearing as they feel too young, want to space children, or do not want more children are common reasons (Chae et al., 2017). These factors can be explored in the discussion of pregnancy options. Ask the individual to identify their support systems. Many people want to involve a partner, a friend, or a family member in their decision. If a partner or support person is in the waiting room, ask the individual if they want the person involved in this discussion.

It is important to discuss a timetable for decision-making about the pregnancy. The assessment of the gestational age of the pregnancy is essential to determine whether the person is close to the legal time limit for pregnancy termination. Approximately 4% of abortions occur after 15 weeks and 1% after 21 weeks (Guttmacher Institute, 2019). The majority of pregnancies are diagnosed in the first trimester when there is more time available to decide what is suited to their personal situation. The Roe vs. Wade Supreme Court decision of 1973 that permits abortion up to 24 weeks was overturned on June 24, 2022. Several states have passed laws to drastically reduce the legal limit of abortion to six weeks pregnancy (White et al., 2021) or eliminate abortion at any stage of pregnancy (see Center for Reproductive Rights, 2022; Guttmacher Institute, 2022, Kaiser Family Foundation, 2022 for up-to-date state policies). The ramifications of the Supreme Court decision are evolving as this book goes to press. The limitations on a previously guaranteed constitutional right will exacerbate existing disparities in access to reproductive healthcare. Immigration status, race, ethnicity, disability, geographic location, gender identity, and economic status are existing barriers to healthcare that will intensify under the new restrictions. This new era demands that clinicians engage in advocacy to eliminate barriers to reproductive health needs for all people.

The healthcare provider must assess if the individual has accurate and adequate information to make an informed decision, and whether they understand the information and have the capacity to decide. The possibility that the individual's decision is being coerced or manipulated by someone else must also be explored. Healthcare providers should provide any additional information and service required and, if needed, arrange for counseling appointments. Healthcare providers must know what local referral resources are available to provide referrals for care in a seamless manner. It is important to have printed information for counseling services, adoption agencies, abortion services, and prenatal care providers. Many patients need support beyond simply providing local agencies' names and contact information. With the increase of state restrictions on abortion access, care coordination may take the form of assessing the need for travel to another state, lodging with 24-hour waiting periods, financial aid, childcare, and other needs (Guttmacher Institute, 2023; Nash, 2021; Simmonds & Likis, 2011). In some areas, abortion doulas are available to provide individuals with support at the time of abortion (Chor et al., 2018).

When referring an individual for counseling and services, it is important to be aware that some clinics have a history of unethical practices in pregnancy counseling.

Professional ethics and standards for reproductive options counseling

- The American College of Nurse-Midwives' (ACNM) Code of Ethics emphasizes conflict resolution, respect for human and reproductive rights, and midwives' respect for their own dignity. Midwives follow guidelines in Standard VIII of the Standards for the Practice of Midwifery to incorporate new procedures into their practice, including abortion (ACNM, 2013) and has position statements on Midwives as Abortion Providers (2019) and Access to Comprehensive Sexual and Reproductive Healthcare Services (2016).

- The American Nurses' Association Position Statement on nursing and sexual and reproductive health (SRH) affirms that (a) Everyone has the right to privacy and the right to make decisions about SRH based on full information and without coercion, (b) Nurses are obligated to share with their patients in an unbiased manner all relevant information about SRH choices that are available and to support that patient regardless of the decisions that patient makes, (c) Abortion is a reproductive health alternative that nurses and other providers can discuss when counseling patients, (d) SRH care should be widely available, accessible, and affordable for all, and (e) Nurses have the right to refuse to participate in SRH care based on ethical grounds, as long as patient safety is assured, and alternative sources of care have been arranged (2022).

- The National Association of Nurse Practitioners in Women's Health (NPWH) mission includes "protecting and promoting a woman's right to make her own choices regarding her health and well-being within the context of her lived experience and her personal, religious, cultural, and family beliefs." (2022). NPWH guidelines for practice and education identify the Women's Health Nurse Practitioner entry-level practice competencies which include: provide nondirective pregnancy options counseling to include parenting, abortion, and adoption, with indicated referrals; and provide medication abortion within state abortion and scope of practice regulations (NPWH, 2020).

- The Association of Women's Health, Obstetric and Neonatal Nurses (AWHONN) promulgates care that is provided in a nonjudgmental and nondiscriminatory manner and that is sensitive to patient diversity and patient preferences whenever possible. AWHONN supports and promotes a woman's right to evidence-based, accurate, and complete information and access to the full range of reproductive healthcare services (AWHONN, 2022).

- The National Organization of Nurse Practitioner Faculties (NONPF) articulates the obligation for nurse practitioners to develop strategies to prevent one's own personal biases from interfering with delivery of quality care and preserves the patient's control over decision-making by negotiating a mutually acceptable plan of care (NONPF, 2017).

- The American Academy of Physicians Assistants (AAPA) promotes patient autonomy women's right to access the full range of reproductive healthcare services, including fertility treatments, contraception, sterilization, and abortion. Physician assistants have an ethical obligation to provide balanced and unbiased clinical information about reproductive healthcare (AAPA, 2013).

- Professional nursing organizations that denounced the Supreme Court decision on Dobbs v. Jackson Women's Health Organization: American Nurses Association; American Academy of Nursing; American College of Nurse-Midwives; Association of Women's Health, Obstetric and Neonatal Nurses; Nurse Practitioners Women's Health. (Joint Statement from the Reproductive Healthcare Nursing Organizations on the US Supreme Court Ruling on *Dobbs v. Jackson Women's Health Organization,* 2022). Source: https://cdn.ymaws.com/npwh.org/resource/resmgr/Joint_Maternal_Health_Statem.pdf.

For example, clinics known as *crisis pregnancy centers* are nonprofit organizations ostensibly established to provide supportive services to pregnant or parenting people. The centers offer free pregnancy testing and ultrasound screening but do not provide a full range of reproductive options. Typically, these centers do not support an individual's autonomy to explore other options beyond parenting or adoption and have been known to provide false, misleading, and coercive health information to pregnant patients (Bryant & Swartz, 2018).

Generally, healthcare issues are considered confidential, but some states require parental notification or parental consent for a teenager deciding about a pregnancy. In the case of abortion, many states with parental notification or parental consent laws have judicial bypass arrangements for teenagers that are unable to involve their parents. Healthcare providers must be aware of the state policies regarding these matters. Resources to find those regulations are provided at the end of the chapter.

When counseling an individual with an unintended pregnancy, the healthcare provider also explores whether they are at risk for intimate partner violence (IPV). Approximately one in five women is abused during pregnancy by a close partner and 40% of women experience sexual violence in their lifetime (Chisholm et al., 2017). One of the leading causes of maternal mortality is homicide (Wallace et al., 2021). Effects on the pregnancy may include miscarriage, placental abruption, pelvic fracture, fetal injury, still birth, preterm delivery, low birth weight, and poor pregnancy weight gain. Reproductive coercion (RC) is a term that connects sexual and reproductive violence with unintended pregnancy. RC includes pregnancy coercion and can occur in relationships where physical or sexual IPV is present or absent (Fay & Yee, 2018; Grace & Anderson, 2018; Holliday et al., 2017).

For example, RC might include tampering with birth control pills or poking a hole in a condom or lying about having a vasectomy. The ACOG recommends screening for RC at annual examinations, new patient visits, at diagnosis of pregnancy, and if continuing the pregnancy, in each trimester and postpartum (ACOG, 2013). RC rates vary by race and ethnicity with higher prevalence among groups that also experience other health disparities (Basile et al., 2021). In their most current bulletin on IPV and pregnancy, ACOG recommends the use of a framing statement such as "We've started talking to all of our patients about safe and healthy relationships because it can have such a large impact on your health" (2013). Inform the person that everything that is said is confidential unless what is said is of such nature that you are bound by state law to report. For instance, if the person states that they plan to cause immediate harm to someone or a minor discusses events that meet the definition of statutory rape, the healthcare provider is bound to report to the appropriate protection agency. After the framing and confidentiality statements, proceed with more specific questions. See Chapter 26, *Violence and Trauma in the Perinatal Period,* for more on IPV.

Suggested steps in pregnancy options counseling

1.	Explore how the person is feeling about the positive test result.
2.	Assess for any immediate health concerns.
3.	Provide nonjudgmental, nondirective counseling using specific counseling techniques.
4.	Address issues of ambivalence.
5.	Explore current life circumstances.
6.	Screen for IPV and RC.
7	Help the individual to identify support systems.
8.	Assure that the informed-consent process includes accurate, evidenced-based information about the options of parenting, adoption, and abortion.
9.	Assess that the individual is capable of understanding the information and that their decision-making is not coerced.
10.	If the individual is not ready to make a decision, discuss a timetable for decision-making after estimating gestational age by LMP/clinical exam and/or ultrasound.
11.	Support the individual in their decision-making.
12.	Provide resources, referrals, and care coordination to quality providers.

Providing Evidence-Based Information about Pregnancy Options

To provide accurate information and support to an individual newly diagnosed as pregnant, the healthcare provider must be knowledgeable about all reproductive options. The options available in the United States include continuing the pregnancy and parenting, continuing the pregnancy, planning an adoption, and, in some states, terminating the pregnancy. Pregnancy care is described throughout the majority of this textbook. However, many healthcare providers have limited knowledge of pregnancy termination procedures and adoption services. If a person indicates that they want to continue the pregnancy, consider asking these additional questions (Open Adoption and Family Services, n.d.):

- How do you feel about parenting at this time?
- What supports do you feel that you need to make your vision of parenting a reality?
- If the choice to parent does not feel right, what do you know about adoption?

Adoption Counseling

Present adoption information in as much detail as possible, including the options of open, closed, familial, and state adoption as well as foster care. Appropriate language to use in discussions about adoption is summarized in the textbox. Most adoption agencies provide some degree of openness in the adoption process. Open adoption can range from simply sharing information between the birth parent and the adoptive family prior to placement to arrangements in which birth parents choose the adoptive family and maintain ongoing contact once the child is born. Birth parents work with agencies that support them in creating adoption plans and agreements that are non-coercive, and fully explain rights and the range of options available. Some individuals are interested in familial adoptions, in which a member of their family assumes the legal rights of the child. It is important to refer individuals to agencies that can help them navigate the legal and emotional nuances.

Positive language for discussing adoption	
Preferred language	Negative language that should *not* be used
Planning an adoption for your child	Giving your child away
Choosing an adoptive family for your child	Putting your child up for adoption
Birth mother, birth father, birth parent	Real or natural parents
Deciding to parent the child	Keeping the child

Source: Adapted from Open Adoption and Family Services (n.d.).

Pregnancy Termination Counseling

Options for early pregnancy termination include medication and procedural (aspiration/surgical) abortion. Medication abortion has been available since 2000 in the United States with updated indications in 2016. In 2016, the FDA approved the "evidence-based dosage" of mifepristone 200 mg. orally followed by 800 mcg (4 pills) of misoprostol self-administered buccally at home. The National Abortion Federation Clinical Practice Guidelines (2022) discuss sublingual and vaginal route protocols in addition to buccal administration. Misoprostol is not administered orally as the efficacy is slightly reduced. The miscarriage-like bleeding event lasts four to six hours after taking misoprostol, followed by one to three weeks of spotting or bleeding. A follow-up visit (in person or virtual) is scheduled 7–14 days later to confirm the success of the medication abortion. Efficacy rates for medication abortion (mifepristone and misoprostol) were 99.6% effective in a study of pregnancies up to 64 days compared to 99.8% for procedural abortion (Abbas et al., 2015; Danco, 2016; Ireland et al., 2015; US Food & Drug Administration [USFDA], 2016). Many people value the privacy of medication abortion and perceive it as a less invasive, more "miscarriage-like" event. Note that mifepristone and misoprostol are considered a safe and effective option for miscarriage management (Chu et al., 2020). Unlike most medications, mifepristone has historically not been dispensed through pharmacies although a recent ruling allows pharmacy dispensing (Kaiser Family Foundation, 2022; USFDA, 2023). During the pandemic, the telehealth restriction under the Risk Evaluation and Mitigation System (REMS) was lifted, meaning that mifepristone could be mailed rather than limited to in-person supervision by a healthcare provider. In December 2021, the FDA made permanent the telehealth provision of mifepristone through mail order pharmacies. In other parts of the globe where mifepristone is unavailable, misoprostol alone abortions are common.

Although the risk profile of mifepristone is very low, in the past 19 years, 20 deaths of women having a medication abortion have been reported to the FDA (Aultman et al., 2021). One death was due to an ectopic pregnancy; screening for early ectopic pregnancies is very important. There have been nine cases of sepsis reported. A cluster of cases were reported in the early 2000s with *Clostridium sordellii*, an organism also reported in miscarriage, childbirth, aspiration, and other nonpregnancy-related events. One death was related to hemorrhage; access to follow-up care is essential. Four deaths were related to drug toxicity/overdose, three cases were possible homicides, one was suicide, and one was unknown.

Vacuum aspiration procedures have a high success rate at 99% and are usually completed within minutes. The procedures can be performed up to 14–15 weeks of gestation in an outpatient setting with sedation if desired. Infection and perforation are extremely rare, occurring in less than 1% of procedures (Cameron, 2018). Vacuum aspiration procedures usually require only one visit, and for individuals who must travel long distances to find an abortion provider, this may be an advantage.

Abortions performed later in pregnancy may use a dilation and evacuation (D & E) procedure. Complication rates are somewhat higher for procedures provided between 14 and 24 weeks than for the first-trimester procedures. General anesthesia, sometimes used in abortion procedures at any gestation, carries risks. Less than 1% of all abortions are provided after 20 weeks of gestation (Guttmacher Institute, 2019). The most common indications for later procedures are severe fetal abnormalities or severe medical complications of the pregnant person. Rarely are induction or instillation techniques used.

Healthcare providers need to be familiar with the current evidence related to abortion care. Many individuals have misunderstandings about the safety of abortion and its impact on their long-term health. For example, information in the lay press has inaccurately linked abortion to breast cancer and mental health problems. Research has failed to substantiate a relationship between abortion and breast cancer (ACOG, 2021; Tong et al., 2020) or depression and mental illness (National Academies of Sciences, Engineering, and Medicine, 2018; Rocca et al., 2020). Similarly, the lay press has carried inaccurate statements about the fetus's ability to experience pain during abortions under 20 weeks' gestation (Brugger, 2012, Royal College Obstetricians Gynaecologists [RCOG], 2010).

Some healthcare providers will perform medication abortion and aspiration abortion procedures as a component of their practice. Nurse practitioners and midwives interested in expanding their practice to include medication or aspiration procedures must know their state-based scope of practice regulations specific to the provision of abortion services (Taylor et al., 2018). Additionally, midwives and nurse practitioners must follow the guidelines of their professional organizations on how to add skills such as medication and procedural abortion services to their practice.

Healthcare providers should be aware of the increase of self-managed abortions in the United States, through ordering of medications from the internet. A study by Aiken (2018) found that individuals chose to induce an abortion outside the context of professional healthcare networks due to barriers of access to safe and legal abortion. Such barriers included cost, long travel distances, lack of transportation, difficulty finding a clinic, waiting periods, and ultrasound requirements. Some people, though, with access in their state preferred the privacy of a self-managed medication abortion. Altman et al. (2019) found that implicit bias, judgment, and power dynamics experienced by people of color in other aspects of reproductive care, such as pregnancy and birth, informed their opinions of healthcare systems and providers. Given the structural racism in society and in healthcare, self-managed abortion may provide a sense of safety and autonomy not experienced in the current health delivery system. The World Health Organization 2022 Abortion Care Guidelines state that it is possible for people to manage the medication abortion process on their own, and that this should not automatically be considered a "last resort" option or the result of a nonfunctioning health system, but rather recognized as a potentially empowering approach that some people may prefer (WHO, 2022).

Those who choose self-managed abortions are not likely to interface with healthcare providers unless they experience complications (Bixby Center for Global Reproductive Health, n.d.). However, when providers do interface with patients self-managing an abortion, it is important to remember that patients may face legal risks for terminating their pregnancy depending on state law. According to current legal analysis, no state laws mandate reporting of self-managed abortion to law enforcement or vital statistics (Harris & Grossman, 2020). Clinicians are only required to report the abortions they provide, although policies could change. It is important to avoid the criminalization of a person who self-managed their abortion (Verma et al., 2022). Patients may be reluctant to share information with a healthcare provider. If the provider has sufficient history to appropriately care for a patient about their reason for visit, further questioning is not necessary and may protect an individual from legal prosecution. Incomplete self-managed abortion and spontaneous miscarriage present with similar symptoms, and the management is the same. A health history that has appropriate detail to care for the patient might not need to solicit detail about the cause of the pregnancy loss (Harris & Grossman, 2020). Some patients who cannot access safe abortion medications may resort to less effective or dangerous methods, such as drinking toxic fluids or inflicting direct injury to the cervix, uterus, or vagina (Moseson et al., 2020). The reality of increasing abortion restrictions means providers may care for people who have resorted to desperate measures. Overall, the emerging data on self-managed abortion suggests that it is safe and effective even when only misoprostol is available (Conti & Cahill, 2019; Johnson et al., 2023; WHO, 2022).

It is imperative for healthcare providers to understand the laws in their state, to provide nonjudgmental care to those in need of healthcare services, and to lobby legislators for laws that ensure pregnant individuals can make their own pregnancy-related decisions.

Summary

Pregnancy diagnosis and gestational age assessment are essential components of prenatal care. Early and accurate pregnancy diagnosis facilitates subsequent healthcare services and an individual's personal health behaviors. Pregnancy diagnosis should be accompanied by unbiased, nondirective, and noncoercive counseling about pregnancy options. Early pregnancy diagnosis also allows the opportunity to accurately assess the gestational age, essential to all aspects of prenatal care. Although endocrine pregnancy tests and ultrasonography play increasingly important roles in pregnancy diagnosis and gestational aging, clinical methods of assessing the signs of pregnancy and gestational age remain an important part of prenatal care and augment assessments made by biochemical and biophysical methods.

Resources for Clients and Their Families

Adoption information: www.openadopt.org
Patient information on self-managed abortion Plan C: https://www.plancpills.org
Pregnancy Options Workbook: http://www.pregnancyoptions.info/pregnant.htm

Resources for Healthcare Providers

Abortion care toolkit for nurse-midwives, nurse practitioners and physician assistants: *Abortion Provider Toolkit (2018)*. UCSF Bixby Center for Global Reproductive Health. https://aptoolkit.org/understanding-abortion-care
Adoption information: www.openadopt.org
Guttmacher Institute (2023). State laws and policies: An overview of abortion laws. https://www.guttmacher.org/state-policy/explore/overview-abortion-laws
Options Counseling (2021). Reproductive Health Access Project https://www.reproductiveaccess.org/resource/options-counseling
Society of Family Planning Interim Clinical Recommendations: Self-managed abortion. (2022). https://www.societyfp.org/society-of-family-planning-interim-clinical-recommendations-self-managed-abortion/

Values Clarification Workshop Curriculum (2013). Reproductive Health Access Project. http://www.reproductiveaccess.org/integrating_reprohealth/values_clar.htm

References

Abbas, D., Chong, E., & Raymond, E. (2015). Outpatient medical abortion is safe and effective through 70 days gestation. *Contraception, 92*(3), 197–199.

Aiken, A., Broussard, K., Johnson, D., & Padron, E. (2018). Motivations and experiences of people seeking medication abortion online in the United States. *Perspectives on Sexual & Reproductive Health, 50*(4), 157–163. https://doi.org/10.1363/psrh.12073

Altman, M., Oseguera, T., McLemore, M., Kantrowitz-Gordon, I., Franck, L., & Lyndon, A. (2019). Information and power: Women of color's experiences interacting with health care providers in pregnancy and birth. *Social Science &Medicine, 238*, 112491. https://doi.org/10.1016/j.socscimed.2019.112491

American Academy of Physicians Assistants. (2013). *Guidelines for the ethical conduct of the physician assistant profession.* https://www.aapa.org/wp-content/uploads/2017/02/16-EthicalConduct.pdf

American College of Nurse-Midwives (ACNM). (2013). *Code of ethics.* https://www.midwife.org/acnm/files/ACNMLibraryData/UPLOAD-FILENAME/000000000048/Code-of-Ethics.pdf

American College of Nurse-Midwives (ACNM). (2016). *Access to comprehensive sexual and reproductive health care services.* https://www.midwife.org/acnm/files/ACNMLibraryData/UPLOADFILE-NAME/000000000087/Access-to-Comprehensive-Sexual-and-Reproductive-Health-Care-Services-FINAL-04-12-17.pdf

American College of Nurse-Midwives (ACNM). (2019). *Position Statement: Midwives as abortion providers.* https://www.midwife.org/acnm/files/acnmlibrarydata/uploadfilename/000000000314/PS-Midwives-as-Abortion-Providers-FINAL-August-2019.pdf?mc_cid=b4924e8c2d&mc_eid=UNIQID

American College of Obstetricians & Gynecologists (ACOG). (2013). Committee opinion no. 554: Reproductive and sexual coercion. *Obstetrics and Gynecology, 121*, 411–415. https://doi.org/10.1097/01.AOG.0000426427.79586.3b

American College of Obstetricians & Gynecologists (ACOG). (2009, reaffirmed 2021). Committee opinion no. 434. Induced abortion and breast cancer risk. *Obstetrics and Gynecology, 113*, 1417–1418. https://www.acog.org/clinical/clinical-guidance/committee-opinion/articles/2009/06/induced-abortion-and-breast-cancer-risk

American College of Obstetricians and Gynecologists (ACOG). (2017). Methods for estimating the due date, committee opinion no. 700. *Obstetrics & Gynecology, 129*, e150–e154.

American Nurses Association; American Academy of Nursing; American College of Nurse-Midwives; Association of Women's Health, Obstetric and Neonatal Nurses; Nurse Practitioners Women's Health. (2022). Joint Statement from the Reproductive Healthcare Nursing Organizations on the US Supreme Court Ruling on *Dobbs v. Jackson Women's Health Organization*, 2022. https://cdn.ymaws.com/npwh.org/resource/resmgr/Joint_Maternal_Health_Statem.pdf

Andersen, H. F., Johnson, T. R., Barclay, M. L., & Flora, J. D. (1981). Gestational age assessment. I. Analysis of individual clinical observations. *American Journal of Obstetrics and Gynecology, 139*, 173–177.

Association of Women's Health, Obstetric and Neonatal Nurses. (2022). AWHONN position statement. AWHONN strengthens position statement on health care decision making for reproductive care. *Journal of Obstetric, Gynecologic, & Neonatal Nursing, 51*(5), e6. https://www.jognn.org/article/S0884-2175(22)00286-6/fulltext

Aultman, K., Cirucci, C. A., Harrison, D. J., Beran, B. D., Lockwood, M. D., & Seiler, S. (2021). Deaths and severe adverse events after the use of mifepristone as an abortifacient from September 2000 to February 2019. *Issues in Law & Medicine, 36*(1), 3–26.

Basile, K. C., Smith, S. G., Liu, Y., Miller, E., & Kresnow, M. J. (2021). Prevalence of intimate partner reproductive coercion in the United States: Racial and ethnic differences. *Journal of Interpersonal Violence, 36*(21–22), NP12324-NP12341. https://doi.org.unh.idm.oclc.org/10.1177/0886260519888205

Baskett, T. F., & Nagele, F. (2000). Naegele's rule: A reappraisal. *British Journal of Obstetrics and Gynaecology, 107*, 1433–1435.

Beal, M. W., & Cappiello, J. D. (2008). Professional right of conscience. *Journal of Midwifery and Women's Health, 53*, 406–412. https://doi.org/10.1016/j.jmwh.2008.05.009

Bixby Center for Global Reproductive Health. (n.d.). *Self-managed abortions: What health care workers need to know.* https://bixbycenter.ucsf.edu/sites/bixbycenter.ucsf.edu/files/Self-managed%20abortion-what%20healthcare%20workers%20need%20to%20know.pdf

Bloom, K. C. (1995). The development of attachment behaviors in pregnant adolescents. *Nursing Research, 44*, 284–289.

Branum, A. M., & Ahrens, K. A. (2017). Trends in timing of pregnancy awareness among US women. *Maternal and Child Health Journal, 21*(4), 715–726. https://doi.org/10.1007/s10995-016-2155-1

Brauer, M., van Ditzhuijzen, J., Boeije, H., & van Nijnatten, C. (2019). Understanding decision-making and decision difficulty in women with an unintended pregnancy in the Netherlands. *Qualitative Health Research, 29*(8), 1084–1095. https://doi.org/10.1177/1049732318810435

Brugger, E. C. (2012). The problem of fetal pain and abortion: Toward an ethical consensus for appropriate behavior. *Kennedy Institute of Ethics Journal, 22*(3), 263–287.

Bryant, A., & Swartz, J. (2018). Why crisis pregnancy centers are legal but unethical. *AMA Journal of Ethics., 20*(3), 269–277. https://doi.org/10.1001/journalofethics.2018.20.3.pfor1-1803

Cameron, S. (2018). Recent advances in improving the effectiveness and reducing the complications of abortion. *F1000Research, 7*(F1000 Faculty Rev), 1881. https://doi.org/10.12688/f1000research.15441.1

Cappiello, J., Beal, M., & Hudson-Gallogly, K. (2011). Applying ethical practice competencies in the prevention and management of unintended pregnancy. *Journal of Obstetric, Gynecologic, and Neonatal Nursing, 40*(6), 808–816. https://doi.org/10.1111/j.1552-6909.2011.01307.x

Center for Reproductive Rights. (2022). *After ROE fell: Abortion laws by state.* https://reproductiverights.org/maps/abortion-laws-by-state

Cervinski, M. A., Lockwood, C. M., Ferguson, A. M., Odem, R. R., Stenman, U. H., Alfthan, H., Grenache, D. G., & Gronowski, A. M. (2009). Qualitative point-of-care and over-the-counter urine hCG devices differentially detect the hCG variants of early pregnancy. *Clinica Chimica Acta, 406*, 81–85.

Chae, S., Desai, S., Crowell, M., & Sedgh, G. (2017). Reasons why women have induced abortions: A synthesis of findings from 14 countries. *Contraception, 96*(4), 233–241. https://doi.org/10.1016/j.contraception.2017.06.014

Chisholm, C., Bullock, L., & Ferguson, J., II (2017). Intimate partner violence and pregnancy: Epidemiology and impact. *American Journal of Obstetrics and Gynecology, 217*(2), 141–144. https://doi.org/10.1016/j.ajog.2017.05.042

Chor, J., Lyman, P., Ruth, J., Patel, A., & Gilliam, M. (2018). Integrating doulas into first-trimester abortion care: Physician, clinic staff, and doula experiences. *Journal Midwifery & Women's Health, 63*(1), 53–57. https://doi.org/10.1111/jmwh.12676

Chu, J. J., Devall, A. J., Beeson, L. E., Hardy, P., Cheed, V., Sun, Y., Roberts, T. E., Ogwulu, C. O., Williams, E., Jones, L. L., La Fontaine Papadopoulos, J. H., Bender-Atik, R., Brewin, J., Hinshaw, K., Choudhary, M., Ahmed, A., Naftalin, J., Nunes, N., Oliver, A., & Izzat, F. (2020). Mifepristone and misoprostol versus misoprostol alone for the management of missed miscarriage (MifeMiso): a randomised, double-blind, placebo-controlled trial. *Lancet, 396*(10253), 770–778. https://doi-org.unh.idm.oclc.org/10.1016/S0140-6736(20)31788-8

Cole, L. A. (2012). The hCG assay or pregnancy test. *Clinical Chemistry and Laboratory Medicine, 50*, 617–630.

Conti, J., & Cahill, E. P. (2019). Self-managed abortion. *Current Opinion in Obstetrics & Gynecology, 31*(6), 435–440. https://doi-org.unh.idm.oclc.org/10.1097/GCO.0000000000000585

Danco. (2016). *Mifepristone prescribing information.* https://www.earlyoptionpill.com/for-health-professionals/prescribing-mifeprex

Dickman, S. L., White, K., & Grossman, D. (2021). Affordability and access to abortion care in the United States. *JAMA*

Internal Medicine, 181(9), 1157–1158. https://doi.org/10.1001/jamainternmed.2021.3502

Engstrom, J. L. (1985a). *Fundal height and abdominal girth measurements during pregnancy* (Doctoral dissertation). University of Illinois at Chicago, Chicago, IL.

Engstrom, J. L. (1985b). Quickening and auscultation of fetal heart tones as estimators of the gestational interval: A review. *Journal of Nurse-Midwifery, 30,* 25–32.

Engstrom, J. L. (1988). Measurement of fundal height. *Journal of Obstetric, Gynecologic, and Neonatal Nursing, 17,* 172–178.

Engstrom, J. L., McFarlin, B. L., & Sampson, M. B. (1993a). Fundal height measurement. Part 4—Accuracy of clinicians' identification of the uterine fundus during pregnancy. *Journal of Nurse-Midwifery, 38,* 318–323.

Engstrom, J. L., McFarlin, B. L., & Sittler, C. P. (1993b). Fundal height measurement. Part 2—Intra- and interexaminer reliability of three measurement techniques. *Journal of Nurse-Midwifery, 38,* 17–22.

Engstrom, J. L., Ostrenga, K. G., Plass, R. V., & Work, B. A. (1989). The effect of maternal bladder volume on fundal height measurements. *British Journal of Obstetrics and Gynaecology, 96,* 987–991.

Engstrom, J. L., Piscioneri, L. A., Low, L. K., McShane, H., & McFarlin, B. (1993c). Fundal height measurement. Part 3—The effect of maternal position on fundal height measurements. *Journal of Nurse-Midwifery, 38,* 23–27.

Engstrom, J. L., & Sittler, C. P. (1993). Fundal height measurement. Part 1—Techniques for measuring fundal height. *Journal of Nurse-Midwifery, 38,* 5–16.

Engstrom, J. L., Sittler, C. P., & Swift, K. E. (1994). Fundal height measurement. Part 5—The effect of clinician bias on fundal height measurements. *Journal of Nurse-Midwifery, 39,* 130–141.

Engstrom, J. L., & Work, B. A. (1992). Prenatal prediction of small-and large-for-gestational age neonates using fundal height growth curves. *Journal of Obstetric Gynecologic & Neonatal Nursing, 21,* 486–495.

Fay, K., & Yee, L. (2018). Reproductive coercion and women's health. *Journal of Midwifery & Women's Health, 63*(5), 518–525. https://doi.org/10.1111/jmwh.12885

Fox, G. N. (1985). Teaching first trimester uterine sizing. *Journal of Family Practice, 21,* 400–401.

Gardosi, J. (1997). Dating of pregnancy: Time to forget the last menstrual period. *Ultrasound in Obstetrics and Gynecology, 9,* 367–368.

Gaskin, I. M. (2012). Has pseudocyesis become an outmoded diagnosis? *Birth, 39,* 77–79.

Gillieson, M., Dunlap, H., Nair, R., & Pilon, M. (1984). Placental site, parity, and date of quickening. *Obstetrics & Gynecology, 64,* 44–45.

Grace, K. T., & Anderson, J. C. (2018). Reproductive coercion: A systematic review. *Trauma, Violence, & Abuse, 19*(4), 371–390. https://doi.org/10.1177/1524838016663935

Grantz, K. L., Ortega-Villa, A. M., Pugh, S. J., Bever, A., Grobman, W., Newman, R. B., Owen, J., Wing, D. A., & Albert, P. S. (2021). Combination of fundal height and ultrasound to predict small for gestational age at birth. *American Journal of Perinatology.* https://doi.org/10.1055/s-0041-1728837

Greene, D. N., Schmidt, R. L., Kamer, S. M., Grenache, D. G., Hoke, C., & Lorey, T. S. (2013). Limitations in qualitative point of care hCG tests for detecting early pregnancy. *Clinica Chimica Acta, 415,* 317–321.

Guiahi, M., Wilson, C., Claymore, E., Simonson, K., & Steinhauer, J. (2021). Influence of a values clarification workshop on residents training at Catholic Hospital programs. *Contraception, 3,* 1–6. https://doi.org/10.1016/j.conx.2021.100054

Guttmacher Institute. (2019). *Induced abortion in the United States.* https://www.guttmacher.org/fact-sheet/induced-abortion-united-states

Guttmacher Institute. (2023). *State laws and policies: An overview of abortion laws.* https://www.guttmacher.org/state-policy/explore/overview-abortion-laws

Harris, L. H. (2012). Recognizing conscience in abortion provision. *The New England Journal of Medicine, 367*(11), 981–983. https://doi.org/10.1056/NEJMp1206253

Harris, L. H., & Grossman, D. (2020). Complications of unsafe and self-managed abortion. *The New England Journal of Medicine,* 382(11), 1029–1040. https://doi-org.unh.idm.oclc.org/10.1056/NEJMra1908412

Hoffman, C. S., Messer, L. C., Mendola, P., Savitz, D. A., Herring, A. H., & Hartmann, K. E. (2008). Comparison of gestational age at birth based on last menstrual period and ultrasound during the first trimester. *Paediatric and Perinatal Epidemiology, 22,* 587–596.

Holliday, C. N., McCauley, H. L., Silverman, J. G., Ricci, E., Decker, M. R., Tancredi, D. J., Burke, J. G., Documét, P., Borrero, S., & Miller, E. (2017). Racial/ethnic differences in women's experiences of reproductive coercion, intimate partner violence, and unintended pregnancy. *Journal of Women's Health, 26*(8), 828–835. https://doi-org.unh.idm.oclc.org/10.1089/jwh.2016.5996

Hoppenot, C., Zimmerman, L., Arlandson, M., Lurain, J. R., & Patel, A. (2016). Follow-up after molar pregnancy evacuation: Feasibility of using semi-quantitative urine pregnancy tests. *Journal of Reproductive Medicine, 61,* 192–196.

Hunter, L. A. (2009). Issues in pregnancy dating: Revisiting the evidence. *Journal of Midwifery & Women's Health, 54,* 1184–1190.

Ireland, L. D., Gatter, M., & Chen, A. Y. (2015). Medical compared with surgical abortion for effective pregnancy termination in the first trimester. *Obstetrics & Gynecology, 126*(1), 22–28. https://doi.org/10.1097/AOG.0000000000000910

Jelks, A., Cifuentes, R., & Ross, M. G. (2007). Clinician bias in fundal height measurement. *Obstetrics and Gynecology, 110,* 892–889.

Jimenez, J. M., Tyson, J. E., & Reisch, J. S. (1983). Clinical measures of gestational age in normal pregnancies. *Obstetrics and Gynecology, 61,* 438–443.

Johnson, D. M., Michels, G. M., Gomperts, R., & Aiken, A. R. A. (2023). Safety and effectiveness of self-managed abortion using misoprostol alone acquired from an online telemedicine service in the United States. *Perspectives on Sexual & Reproductive Health, 55*(1), 4–11. https://doi-org.unh.idm.oclc.org/10.1363/psrh.12219

Jones, R., & Jerman, J. (2017). Population group abortion rates and lifetime incidence of abortion: United States 2008–2014. *American Journal Public Health, 107,* 19-4-1909. https://doi.org/10.2105/AJPH.2017.304042

Kaiser Family Foundation. (2022). *Women's Health Policy. Interactive: How state policies shape access to abortion coverage.* https://www.kff.org/womens-health-policy/issue-brief/interactive-how-state-policies-shape-access-to-abortion-coverage

Lawson, G. W. (2021). Naegele's rule and the length of pregnancy—A review. *Australian and New Zealand Journal of Obstetrics and Gynaecology, 61,* 177–182.

Lerum, C. W., & LoBiondo-Wood, G. (1989). The relationship of maternal age, quickening, and physical symptoms of pregnancy to the development of maternal-fetal attachment. *Birth, 16,* 13–17.

Loytved, A. A. L., & Fleming, V. (2016). Naegele's rule revisited. *Sexual & Reproductive Healthcare, 8,* 100–101.

Lynch, C. D., & Zhang, J. (2007). The research implications of the selection of a gestational age estimation method. *Paediatric and Perinatal Epidemiology, 21*(Suppl. 2), 86–96.

Margulies, R., & Miller, L. (2001). Fruit size as a model for teaching first trimester uterine sizing in bimanual examination. *Obstetrics and Gynecology, 98,* 341–344.

McDonald, E. (1908). The diagnosis of early pregnancy. *American Journal of Obstetrics and Diseases of Women and Children, 57,* 323–346.

McFarlin, B. L., Engstrom, J. L., Sampson, M. B., & Cattledge, F. (1985). The concurrent validity of Leopold's maneuvers in determining fetal presentation and position. *Journal of Nurse-Midwifery, 30,* 280–284.

McParland, P., & Johnson, H. (1993). Time to reinvent the wheel. *British Journal of Obstetrics and Gynaecology, 100,* 1061–1062.

Morse, K., Williams, A., & Gardosi, J. (2009). Fetal growth screening by fundal height measurement. *Best Practice & Research Clinical Obstetrics and Gynaecology, 23,* 809–818.

Moseson, H., Herold, S., Filippa, S., Barr-Walker, J., Baum, S. E., & Gerdts, C. (2020). Self-managed abortion: A systematic scoping review. *Best Practice & Research Clinical Obstetrics & Gynaecology, 63,* 87–110. https://escholarship.org/content/qt1mj5832t/qt1mj5832t.pdf

Munsick, R. A. (1986). Correct use of Hegar's sign [letter]. *American Journal of Obstetrics and Gynecology, 154,* 691–692.

Nakling, J., Buhaug, H., & Backe, B. (2005). The biologic error in gestational length related to the use of the first day of the last menstrual period as a proxy for the start of pregnancy. *Early Human Development, 81*, 833–839.

Nash, E. (2021). *For the first time ever, U.S. states enacted more than 100 abortion restrictions in a single year.* Guttmacher Institute. https://www.guttmacher.org/article/2021/10/first-time-ever-us-states-enacted-more-100-abortion-restrictions-single-year

Nash, E., & Dreweke, J. (2019). The U.S. abortion rate continues to drop: Once again, state abortion restrictions are not the main driver. *Guttmacher Policy Review, 22*, 41–48. https://www.guttmacher.org/sites/default/files/article_files/gpr2204119.pdf

National Abortion Federation. (2022). *Clinical policy guidelines for abortion care.* https://prochoice.org/providers/quality-standards

National Academies of Sciences, Engineering, and Medicine. (2018). *The safety and quality of abortion care in the United States.* The National Academies Press. https://doi.org/10.17226/24950

National Association of Nurse Practitioners in Women's Health (NPWH). (2020). *The women's health nurse practitioner: Guidelines for practice and education* (8th ed.), p. 14. https://npwh.org/store/download.aspx?id=3EFB421A-26DF-4BE7-AA8D-A7D08F3FFF70

National Association of Nurse Practitioners in Women's Health (NPWH). (2022). *Reproductive rights policy summary.* https://cdn.ymaws.com/npwh.org/resource/resmgr/positionstatement/npwh_reproductive_rights_pol.pdf

National Organization of Nurse Practitioner Faculties (NONPF). (2017). *Nurse practitioner core competencies content.* https://cdn.ymaws.com/http://www.nonpf.org/resource/resmgr/competencies/2017_NPCoreComps_with_Curric.pdf

Nishikawa, M., & Sakakibara, H. (2013). Effect of nursing intervention program using abdominal palpation of Leopold's maneuvers on maternal-fetal attachment. *Reproductive Health, 10*, 12.

O'Dowd, M. J., & O'Dowd, T. M. (1985). Quickening—A re-evaluation. *British Journal of Obstetrics and Gynaecology, 92*, 1037–1039.

Office of Disease Prevention and Health Promotion. (n.d.). *Reduce the proportion of unintended pregnancies — FP-01.* Healthy People 2030. https://health.gov/healthypeople/objectives-and-data/browse-objectives/family-planning/reduce-proportion-unintended-pregnancies-fp-01/data

Open Adoption and Family Services. (n.d.). *OA&FS statement regarding Supreme Court decision to overturn Roe v. Wade.* https://www.openadopt.org

Price, K. (2020). What is reproductive justice? How women of color activists are redefining the pro-choice paradigm. *Meridians, 19*(S1), 340–362. https://doi.org/10.1215/15366936-8566034

Raymond, E. G., Shochet, T., Blum, J., Sheldon, W. R., Platias, I., Bracken, H., Dabash, R., Weaver, M. A., Ngoc, N. T. N., Blumenthal, P. D., & Winikoff, B. (2017). Serial multilevel urine pregnancy testing to assess medical abortion outcome: A meta-analysis. *Contraception, 95*, 442–448.

Richards, D. S. (2021). Obstetric ultrasound: Imaging, dating, growth, and anomaly. In M. B. Landon, H. L. Galan, E. R. M. Jauniaux, D. A. Driscoll, V. Berghella, W. A. Grobman, S. J. Kilpatrick, & A. G. Cahill (Eds.), *Gabbe's obstetrics: Normal and problem pregnancies* (8th ed., pp. 156–179). Elsevier.

Rocca, C., Samari, G., Foster, D., Gould, H., & Kimport, K. (2020). Emotions and decision rightness over five years following an abortion: An examination of decision difficulty and abortion stigma. *Social Science & Medicine, 248*, 112782. https://doi.org/10.1016/j.socscimed.2019.112704

Roex, A., Nikpoor, P., Eerd, E. V., Hodyl, N., & Dekker, G. (2012). Serial plotting on customized fundal height charts results in doubling of antenatal detection of small for gestational age fetuses in nulliparous women. *The Australian and New Zealand Journal of Obstetrics and Gynaecology, 52*, 78–82.

Ross, M. G. (2003). Circle of time: Errors in the use of the pregnancy wheel. *Journal of Maternal-Fetal & Neonatal Medicine, 14*, 370–372.

Royal College of Obstetricians and Gynecologists. (2010). *Fetal awareness: Review of research and recommendations for practice.* www.rcog.org.uk/globalassets/documents/guidelines/rcogfetalawareness-wpr0610.pdf

Savitz, D. A., Terry, J. W., Dole, N., Thorp, J. M., Siega-Riz, A. M., & Herring, A. H. (2002). Comparison of pregnancy dating by last menstrual period, ultrasound scanning, and their combination. *American Journal of Obstetrics and Gynecology, 187*, 1660–1666.

Self, A., Daher, L., Schlussel, M., Roberts, N., Ioannou, C., & Papageorghiou, A. T. (2022). Second and third trimester estimation of gestational age using ultrasound or maternal symphysis-fundal height measurements: A systematic review. *British Journal of Obstetrics & Gynaecology.* https://doi.org/10.1111/1471-0528.17123

Sharma, J. B. (2009). Evaluation of Sharma's modified Leopold's maneuvers: A new method for fetal palpation in late pregnancy. *Archives of Gynecology and Obstetrics, 279*, 481–487.

Shochet, T., Comstock, I. A., Ngoc, N. T. N., Westphal, L. M., Sheldon, W. R., Loc, L. T., & Blumenthal, P. D. (2017). Results of a pilot study in the U. S. and Vietnam to assess the utility and acceptability of multi-level pregnancy test (MLPT) for home monitoring of hCG trends after assisted reproduction. *BMC Women's Health, 17*(1), 67.

Simmonds, K., & Likis, F. (2011). Caring for women with unintended pregnancies. *Journal of Obstetric, Gynecologic, and Neonatal Nursing, 40*, 794–807. https://doi.org/10.1111/j.1552-6909.2011.01293.x

Smout, E. M., Seed, P. T., & Shennan, A. H. (2012). The use and accuracy of manual and electronic gestational age calculators. *The Australian and New Zealand Journal of Obstetrics and Gynaecology, 52*, 440–444.

Spreet, H. (1955). Alfred Hegar: Hegar's sign and dilators. *Obstetrics and Gynecology, 6*, 679–683.

Taipale, P., & Hiilesmaa, V. (2001). Predicting delivery date by ultrasound and last menstrual period in early gestation. *Obstetrics and Gynecology, 97*, 189–194.

Taylor, D., Safriet, B., Kruse, B., Dempsey, G., & Summers, L. (2018). *AP toolkit.* UCSF Bixby Center for Global Reproductive Health. https://aptoolkit.org/understanding-abortion-care

Tong, H., Wu, Y., Yan, Y., Dong, Y., Guan, X., Liu, Y., & Lu, Z. (2020). No association between abortion and risk of breast cancer among nulliparous women: Evidence from a meta-analysis. *Medicine, 99*(19), e20251. https://doi.org/10.1097/MD.0000000000020251

U.S. Food & Drug Administration. (2023). *Information about Mifepristone for medical termination of pregnancy through ten weeks gestation.* https://www.fda.gov/drugs/postmarket-drug-safety-information-patients-and-providers/information-about-mifepristone-medical-termination-pregnancy-through-ten-weeks-gestation

US Food & Drug Administration. (2016). *Mifeprex (mifepristone) Information.* https://www.fda.gov/drugs/postmarket-drug-safety-information-patients-and-providers/mifeprex-mifepristone-information

Verma, N., Goyal, V., Grossman, D., Perritt, J., & Shih, G. (2022). *Society of Family Planning interim clinical recommendations: Self-managed abortion.* https://www.societyfp.org/society-of-family-planning-interim-clinical-recommendations-self-managed-abortion

Wallace, M., Gillispie-Bell, V., Cruz, K., Davis, K., & Vilda, D. (2021). Homicide during pregnancy and the postpartum period in the United States, 2018–2019. *Obstetrics & Gynecology, 138*(5), 762–769. https://doi.org/10.1097/aog.0000000000004567

Wegienka, G., & Baird, D. D. (2005). A comparison of recalled date of last menstrual period with prospectively recorded dates. *Journal of Women's Health, 14*, 248–252.

White, K., Vizcarra, E., Palomares, L., Dane'el, A., Beasley, A., Ogburn, T., Potter, J., & Dickman, S. (2021). Initial impacts of Texas' Senate Bill 8 on abortions in Texas and at out-of-state facilities. *Research Brief.* https://sites.utexas.edu/txpep/files/2021/10/initial-impacts-SB8-TxPEP-brief.pdf

White, L. J., Lee, S. J., Stepniewska, K., Simpson, J. A., Dwell, S. L. M., Arunjerdja, R., Singhasivanon, P., White, N. J., & Nosten, & McGready, R. (2012). Estimation of gestational age from fundal height: A solution for resource-poor settings. *Journal of the Royal Society, Interface, 9*, 503–510.

Wilcox, A. J., Dunson, D., & Baird, D. D. (2000). The timing of the "fertile window" in the menstrual cycle: Day specific estimates from a prospective study. *British Medical Journal, 321*, 1259–1262.

World Health Organization. (2022). *Abortion care guidelines.* https://www.who.int/publications/i/item/9789240039483

11

Risk Assessment during Pregnancy

Robin G. Jordan

Relevant Terms

Absolute risk—the probability that an event will occur

Allostatic load—the wear and tear consequences of chronic exposure to elevated neuroendocrine responses to frequent and repeated stress; higher allostatic load can result in accelerated disease processes

Attributable risk—the incidence of adverse events resulting from exposure to the risk factor

Iatrogenic risk—risk inadvertently introduced by healthcare provider action or medical intervention

Negative predictive value—the true negatives among all those with negative screens; reflects the probability that a negative test indicates actually not having the underlying condition being tested

Positive predictive value—the true positives among all those with positive screens; reflects the probability that a positive test indicates actually having the underlying condition being tested

Relative risk—estimate of the probability of an adverse event in one group compared to another group

Risk factor—any attribute, characteristic, or exposure of an individual that increases the likelihood of developing a disease or injury

Salutogenesis—the study of the origins of health that include a person's sense of self-determination, self-efficacy, and resilience that lead toward human wellness and flourishing

Sensitivity—proportion of positive screens among those known to have the condition being screened

Specificity—proportion of negative screens among those known not to have the condition being screened

Soft markers—slight deviations from normal findings on ultrasound that may or may not indicate increased risk for defect or anomaly

Weathering—adverse physical consequences of chronic stress, advances the aging process

Introduction

The word *risk* denotes a danger or hazard, the possibility of harm. In healthcare, the word *risk* is used to indicate the likelihood that a particular adverse health event will occur. Risk assessment is the systematic clinical process of identifying and analyzing conditions that could result in adverse perinatal outcomes. Risk assessment is done to determine if intervention is available to potentially improve the health outcome for the pregnant person and/or fetus with the risk factor. For risks that cannot be modified, plans are made to ameliorate or respond to potential adverse effects.

The assessment of risk status is done at each encounter and guides healthcare provider management and client behaviors and decisions regarding care in various birth settings. In situations of known risk during pregnancy or birth, successful planning or intervention can improve the likelihood of positive outcomes. Misapplication of the risk assessment can introduce problems that diminish optimal perinatal outcomes, which is contrary to the goal of risk assessment. Over the past few decades, the pregnancy and childbirth processes have been greatly transformed by two cultural shifts: the pathologization of the pregnant body and the use of medical technology in an attempt to preempt childbearing risk, with broad and significant effects on pregnant people. The appropriate application of the risk assessment process and the interpretation and management of risk during prenatal care requires an understanding of childbearing physiology, the benefits and limitations of the risk assessment process, and an appropriate appraisal of theoretical, perceived, and actual risk. Healthcare providers must also skillfully communicate appropriate evaluations of risk without inducing undue fear.

This chapter will focus on the risk assessment process, limitations, and potential problems of risk assessment, and appropriate risk management and communication of childbearing risk to pregnant clients and their families.

Health equity key points

- Risk calculations incorporating race and ethnicity are inherently biased and can limit important childbirth options.
- Childbirth care for Black pregnant people is paradoxically overmedicalized and medically neglected, imparting risks due to systemic racism.

Prenatal and Postnatal Care: A Person-Centered Approach, Third Edition. Edited by Karen Trister Grace, Cindy L. Farley, Noelene K. Jeffers, and Tanya Tringali.
© 2024 John Wiley & Sons Ltd. Published 2024 by John Wiley & Sons Ltd.
Companion website: www.wiley.com/go/grace/prenatal

Process and Purpose of Risk Assessment

Risk assessment is ideally started prior to conception during routine health screening visits (see Chapter 7, *Preconception and Interconception Care*). Many pregnancies are unplanned, and the process is initiated at the first prenatal visit. Risk assessment is primarily accomplished via history, physical exam, and laboratory studies. Subjective and objective data assessment of the medical, psychosocial, nutritional, genetic, occupational, social, and environmental factors is evaluated in an ongoing process throughout prenatal care. Data are gathered at each prenatal visit to evaluate changes in risk status. Risk status can change to a higher risk or a lower risk during prenatal care.

Benefits of Risk Assessment

Ideally, risk assessment directs each pregnant individual to the best place for birth and the most appropriate healthcare provider and allocates appropriate resources to foster optimal maternal and infant outcomes (Jordan & Murphy, 2009). Pregnant people identified at increased risk for adverse outcome can be directed to facilities with the availability of appropriate specialty care. Those considered lower risk can explore options regarding the place of birth and birth attendants.

The identification of **risk factors** can start the process of offering or recommending interventions to improve health-promoting behaviors. Lifestyle issues, such as diet, exercise, smoking, and other substance use, can be addressed and remediated with education, support, and motivational strategies to change behavior, thus reducing perinatal risk. The knowledge of the presence of risk factors can alert healthcare providers to recommend specific measures to evaluate and monitor risk such as laboratory screening or diagnostic testing and fetal surveillance techniques. Risk information also allows the provider and client to be aware of and watchful for the development of associated conditions or symptoms in an effort to prevent adverse outcomes.

Limitations of Risk Assessment

Poor Predictive Value

The validity of many risk-scoring tools is undetermined, and the benefit of prenatal risk-scoring systems remains undocumented (Davey et al., 2015). Many risk assessment tools are poor predictors of actual outcome. For example, one study showed no evidence of efficacy for current methods used to predict preeclampsia in pregnant women (Henderson et al., 2017). It is common for individuals with risk factors to have a normal pregnancy and birth course. Conversely, those with no risk factors can develop complications.

Risk-scoring tools to predict select conditions have improved over the last decade. For example, some improved screening methods to predict preterm birth (PTB) have shown an increase in their **positive predictive value**. However, these tools are better at identifying those who are *not* at risk for PTB and have limited data to support their routine use (Berghella & Saccone, 2019; Esplin et al., 2017; van Baaren et al., 2014). Although many factors have been shown to increase risk for PTB, the majority of cases of PTB occur in those without any identifiable risk factor (Vogel et al., 2018).

Lack of Precision

Definitions of risk factors vary considerably, and many are neither quantifiable nor modifiable. While factors may be associated with increased risk for a particular event, the relationship of these factors in causing or contributing to the event may be tenuous or spurious. For example, it is well established that unmarried women have higher rates of PTB and low-birth-weight infants than married women (Barr & Marugg, 2019). This is an association, not causation, and a factor that is not amenable to change by provider intervention.

The high numbers of "risk factors" included in standard risk assessment forms result in large numbers of clients being labeled "at risk." However, many of these so-called risk factors are statistically *associated* with adverse outcomes, with no evidence of actual causation. Placing clients in risk categories based on methods with poor predictive value for actual occurrence of adverse event can lead to erroneous decisions by healthcare providers and pregnant individuals (Jordan & Murphy, 2009). Importantly, prenatal risk assessment processes lack the means to determine the effect of risk accumulation, or the existence of multiple factors and their effect on each other.

Using race as a variable in risk-scoring tools can result in healthcare decisions with potential to disadvantage non-White clients. For example, a commonly used scoring tool to predict the risk of vaginal birth after cesarean (VBAC) incorporates race as a variable in its calculation and predicts a higher risk for those who are Black or Hispanic. The tool also found correlations with increased VBAC risk and type of insurance and marital status; however, those variables are not used in the risk calculations (Grobman et al., 2007). The health benefits of a successful VBAC are well established, yet Black and Hispanic patients continue to have higher rates of cesarean section compared to White clients. Making healthcare decisions based on race can limit VBAC as an option for Black and Hispanic patients and exacerbate health outcome disparities (Vyas et al., 2020).

Nonmodifiable Risk Factors

Some risk factors are not amenable to modification, such as socioeconomic status or age. It is still important, however, to identify these nonmodifiable risk factors so that appropriate screening tools may be offered when available. For example, a 40-year-old pregnant person is at higher risk for certain fetal anomalies. While age cannot be changed, screening or diagnostic testing can be offered to determine if the outcome associated with increased age (anomaly) has occurred. This is then followed up with appropriate counseling and options moving forward, depending on the test results.

Race and ethnicity are often mentioned as nonmodifiable risk factors. While race and ethnicity are associated with disparities in many health outcomes, it is important to note that race or ethnicity itself is not the root cause. Factors such as discrimination, stigma, stress, and structural bias moderate and mediate the relationship between race/ethnicity and poor health outcomes. Developing concepts of **allostatic load**, stress biomarkers, **weathering**, and other areas of emerging research continue to add to the understanding of racial and ethnic health disparities.

Disadvantages of Risk Assessment and Risk Management

It is clear that the identification of risk factors during the course of prenatal care is important to maternal and fetal health and to help guide care decisions. The disadvantages and potential problems of inappropriate risk assessment and risk management in childbearing care are not as readily recognized. There has been a broad shift in maternity care over the past several decades toward a focus on potential risk and risk management. Many more pregnant individuals are labeled "at risk" than in the past. This has fundamentally altered not only the way in which pregnancy is perceived by patients and providers but also how pregnancy and birth are experienced.

Unnecessary Interventions

The effect of the evaluation of risk and the use of subsequent interventions can have a profound influence on a person's sense of self, body, and the course of pregnancy, labor, birth, and early postpartum. The proliferation of prenatal testing in pregnancy surveillance has led prenatal care to serve as a platform for testing as a technologic imperative: "we have the technology; therefore, we must use it" (Topçu & Brown, 2019). The use of prenatal ultrasound offers an example.

Consider the common situation of a pregnant cisgender woman in the last month of pregnancy who has been told by her prenatal care provider that she has a "large baby." Ultrasound for the evaluation of estimated fetal weight at 38 weeks indicates that the fetus is over 8 lb. The client is encouraged to consider labor induction for "impending macrosomia" soon to avoid potential intrapartum problems attributed to macrosomia at term. Induction of labor prior to the physiological preparation necessary for labor to ensue is associated with an increase in cesarean births (Banner & D'Souza, 2021) and with limited mobility that can contribute to labor dysfunction (Ondeck, 2014). Healthcare provider and ultrasound estimates of fetal weight are prone to clinically significant error with accuracy decreasing as fetal weight increases (Dimassi et al., 2015; Sekar et al., 2016). A California study found that 29% of clients were told they "had a big baby" during the last weeks of gestation; however, the average weight of the babies studied was 7 pounds, 8 oz

(Sakala et al., 2018). Despite these uncertainties, the provider's advice to proceed with induction prompts the woman to agree to labor induction with known **iatrogenic risks** to reduce the possibility of a poorly qualified risk.

Additionally, institutional culture and provider preference can have a significant effect on the increased use of pregnancy and birth technology, separate from any evidence-based indication for use. Hospital personnel holding a heightened fear of vaginal birth and with an overall perception of cesarean section safety, have significantly higher incidence of cesarean section in term, singleton, vertex, nulliparous pregnancies than personnel in hospitals with a culture of supporting vaginal birth (White-VanGompel et al., 2019). It is difficult for clients to challenge or question respected healthcare providers' information and course of action, and many feel disempowered to speak up about their desires for their birth experience and to engage in discussion regarding information and decisions presented by medical personnel (Happel-Parkins & Azim, 2016).

Normalization of Technology and Illusion of Risk Control

The use of medical technology during pregnancy and childbirth has expanded, and its routine use has become an expectation of the public and clinicians. Technologic strategies to preempt adverse events give both clients and clinicians a sense of certainty and control over the unknown that is often unfounded. Prenatal ultrasound serves to illustrate these concepts. Multiple ultrasound examinations are perceived by provider and recipient as an essential component of routine pregnancy care. A study examining ultrasound use in a low-risk pregnant population found a mean of 4.2 ultrasounds per pregnancy (Harris et al., 2015). The most recent *Listening to Mothers III* survey found that 70% had three or more ultrasounds and 23% had six or more (Childbirth Connections, 2013). If the fetus can be "seen," pregnant clients and their providers feel relieved and reassured despite the low positive predictive value of an ultrasound to detect many abnormalities (Thomas et al., 2017). Additionally, it is not uncommon for ultrasound to visualize **soft markers** or findings of undetermined significance, which generate further ultrasound and diagnostic evaluations. These uncertain ultrasound findings of possible abnormality introduce another risk: an increase in maternal stress and anxiety, which can persist into the postpartum period, influencing attachment to the fetus/newborn, even if these soft marker findings are ultimately determined to be of no significance (Gross et al., 2021; Viaux-Savelon et al., 2012).

Salutogenesis and Potential for Health

Salutogenesis is the study of the origins of health and encompasses the capacity for wellness and human flourishing rather than simply surviving. The concept includes social and physical determinants of health and allows for care that considers how to create, enhance, and improve health and well-being (Downe et al., 2020). Salutogenesis moves beyond the narrow goal of a safe birth and includes the potential for positive life transformations through the experience of pregnancy, birth, and parenting. However, the focus of contemporary childbearing research and practice is pathology, illness, and disease detection and treatment, despite the fact that the majority of women can give birth safely without medical intervention or treatment (Downe et al., 2020). This approach to childbirth assumes a mechanistic view of the body with a set of narrow data as the sole measures of success. A birth may be documented as "normal"; however, if the client felt violated, ignored, or coerced, it may have been experienced by the individual as trauma, yet this adverse experience and its health implications likely remain unaddressed.

Risk assessment is a significant and embedded component of pathology-focused childbearing care and, thus, is limited in scope for discovering a person's potential for health and wellness. Prenatal risk assessment tools generally lack evaluation of salutogenic factors such as self-determination (the belief that one has the ability and right to make one's own decisions), self-efficacy (the confidence that one has the ability to exert control over one's situation/environment), and resilience (ability to bounce back after a negative situation and remain hopeful). By limiting the evaluation of risk to a set of physiologic factors, problems, and deficits, opportunities to foster enduring positive health benefits are missed.

Salutogenesis underpins a holistic philosophy of care that views the physical, emotional, spiritual, and social aspects of health as equally important to the person, with each component vital to the other. Providing care that incorporates these elements of salutogenesis has potential to transform the way childbearing care is provided and promote a higher level of overall health of childbearing individuals and their families. The midwifery approach to childbearing focuses on pregnancy and birth as a normal physiologic process with potential for human growth and empowerment: salutogenesis provides a compatible and promising path to care that serves as a catalyst for long-term well-being of families (Muggleton & Davis, 2022).

The Label of High Risk

Prenatal care providers should be aware that classifying a person as "high risk" can produce negative psychological effects. When individuals are labeled "high risk" during pregnancy, they can experience increased anxiety, negative self-perception (Lee et al., 2012), increased stress, and loss of control (Holness, 2018). Those with nonmodifiable risk factors, such as age, who are told they are "high risk," experience increased feelings of guilt, even though no high-risk condition has been detected and nothing can be done about the factor that placed them in that risk category (Isaacs & Andipatin, 2020). Healthcare providers are influenced by the very label that they assign and can adopt an assumption of abnormality and birth as a potential emergency when caring for clients labeled "high risk" (Naylor-Smith et al., 2018). Interventions with iatrogenic risk are applied, thus shaping clinical care and heightening the sense of risk and danger.

Misapplication of Risk Assessment and Risk Management

American healthcare culture is risk averse, based on the belief that risk can be identified, prevented, managed, and controlled. If an adverse event occurs, legal redress is directed at the party perceived as incorrectly managing risk. Risk aversion and obstetrical interests have led to exaggerated perceptions of pregnancy risk and the ability of technology and intervention to reduce risk (Jordan & Murphy, 2009). A reconceptualization of childbearing as potentially pathologic and requiring routine intervention and invasive surveillance to maintain "safety" has occurred over the past several decades with the rise of technology use in healthcare. Universal applications of medical intervention once reserved for individual indications are now standard obstetrical care as a preemptive strategy to prevent adverse outcomes, regardless of a person's actual risk status. Despite this increased use of medical interventions during childbearing care, maternal and infant outcomes have not appreciably improved in the last decade, and outcomes such as maternal mortality and low-birth-weight infants have increased or remained stable, with Black, Hispanic, and Native American people experiencing an extraordinarily high burden of adverse outcomes (Heck et al., 2021; Hoyert, 2022). Population health trends, such as the increasing rates of obesity, are often cited as the reason for the need for increasing technology use however, but this may be considered patient-blaming and used as justification for a provider preference to intervene (Cole et al., 2019).

Nocebo (Latin for "I shall harm") effects are the inadequately recognized opposite of placebo (Latin for "I shall please") effects. Nocebo is defined as the perception of negative effects from an inert or sham treatment, whereas placebo is the perception of positive effects from an inert or sham treatment. It is argued that nocebo effects are common in contemporary childbearing care practices (Hotelling, 2013; Symon et al., 2015). Prenatal visits become an opportunity to be reminded of pregnancy risks. Consider communication such as, "Let us get another ultrasound just in case," or "I think your baby is getting large," or "We do not want you going past your due date." This unrecognized negative effect can create a climate of doubt rather than instilling confidence in pregnant individuals regarding their abilities to labor and birth. The cumulative effect of persistent focus on potential perinatal problems regardless of actual risk can undermine confidence in the ability to maintain health throughout pregnancy and to give birth (Hotelling, 2013; Symon et al., 2015). See Chapter 27, *Planning for Physiologic Birth*, for further information about childbearing confidence.

A variety of factors contribute to healthcare providers treating pregnancy with medical intervention regardless of risk, indication, or evidence. Obstetric care is an area of high liability, and healthcare provider litigation fears are a real concern. Defensive medical practice is a phenomenon influencing the healthcare decisions of obstetricians and, therefore, influencing the pregnancy and birth experience and outcomes. A majority of obstetricians have engaged in defensive care practices, such as prescribing medication or ordering ultrasound without indication (Asher et al., 2013). Obstetricians report that the fear of litigation and defensive medicine practices contributes to increased use of childbirth interventions such as cesarean section (Cheng et al., 2014; Frakes & Gruber, 2020). This "risk to the healthcare provider" is a distinct factor in obstetrical decision making (Williams et al., 2021).

Healthcare provider lifestyle issues can create incentives for the misapplication of risk evaluations and management decisions. Healthcare providers attending to labor and birth have lives characterized by unpredictability, less control over personal time, heavy workload, and long hours. The process of labor for a given individual is unknown: when it will start, how long it will be, when it will end, and how the process will unfold. These factors create challenges in other aspects of life. Provider incentives to control patient scheduling and workload and to maximize daytime births to allow for more personal time (Barber et al., 2011; Nijagal et al., 2015), as well as surgical financial incentives (Alexander, 2017; Foo et al., 2017) have been linked to increasing use of practices such as elective labor induction and cesarean section.

Some of the following examples used to illustrate the potential problems of misapplication of risk evaluation and management sections are related to labor and birth; however, many decisions related to labor and birth are discussed and determined during prenatal care. Therefore, an understanding of the association between prenatal application of risk assessment, risk management, childbearing experiences, and outcomes is vital.

Introduction of Actual Risk

Surgical cesarean section, once reserved for situations of fetal and or maternal risk, has increased in the United States by approximately 60% from 1996 to 2009 (Martin et al., 2014), and currently stands at a rate of 31.8% of all births (Osterman et al., 2022). One in three births occur via cesarean section. This dramatic rise in cesarean birth has not resulted in improved health outcomes. In fact, the overuse of cesarean has been linked with secondary poor outcomes such as placenta accreta, placenta previa, emergency cesarean hysterectomy, maternal morbidity and mortality, and a higher rate of uterine rupture in subsequent pregnancies (Al-Zirki et al., 2016; De Mucio et al., 2019). Recent research suggests a link between adverse cesarean section and adverse childhood psychological outcomes such as disordered sensory perception conditions and poorer mother–infant relationships (Chen & Tan, 2019). VBAC is the safer option for most people, rather than a repeat cesarean section. However, when obstetricians discuss the benefits and risks of VBAC, the common focus is on the risks of VBAC with less emphasis on information regarding the risk of a repeat cesarean (Munro et al., 2017). In an effort to eliminate the perceived risk of vaginal birth, the use of a

major surgical procedure without true indication has caused an increase in real and measurable risk to the client and fetus.

Increase in Financial, Physical, and Emotional Costs

The routine use of nonindicated and nonevidence-based interventions incurs financial costs to society and is an acute burden to the current healthcare system already under financial strain. For example, operative birth requires expensive operating room facilities and personnel, and longer hospital stays. There is a physical cost to parturients with the routine use of nonevidence-based interventions. This can be illustrated by the routine use of continuous electronic fetal monitoring in all laboring individuals. This practice results in immobility, adding to physical discomfort, prolonging labor (Alfirevic et al., 2017), changing critical hemodynamics that lead to indeterminate or abnormal fetal heart rate patterns, causing additional interventions, and an increase in operative birth (Paterno et al., 2016). The physical cost of cesarean section is readily apparent in longer recovery time and increased risk of future childbearing complications.

Emotional costs of attempts to preemptively manage perceived pregnancy and birth risks can be difficult to quantify and easier to set aside as less important. However, childbirth is not only a physical event, it is also a major emotional and transformative event in a person's life. Prenatal and birth technology has led to a transfer of authoritative birth knowledge from women themselves to medical professionals (Davis-Floyd, 2001). Reliance on technology can diminish a sense of personal and experiential knowledge of one's own pregnancy health, instead creating a reliance on external measures. Individuals may wait to obtain results of tests to "prove" all is well before announcing the pregnancy and envisioning the baby, creating a delay in the prenatal attachment process (Lawson & Turriff-Janasson, 2006). Survey research indicates that as many as 67% of women report an abnormal test result during pregnancy, the majority relating to an ultrasound scan eventually found to be normal; more than half of these women report being acutely worried and one-quarter are still concerned five weeks later (Peterson et al., 2009).

There is a compelling argument that risk assessment has become a way of controlling childbirth choices. Clients rely on the expertise of health professionals to help them make pregnancy-related decisions and have great trust in this expertise as well as in medical technical measures to provide security and protection from risk during childbearing (Regan et al., 2013). This can create a climate of intimidation and reluctance to question authoritatively provided information. Pregnant individuals can feel that they possess little power to challenge medical authority during the vulnerable course of pregnancy and childbirth.

Birth Fear

Fear of childbirth, or *tocophobia* (or tokophobia), is a phenomenon that has increased since 2000 (O'Connell et al., 2017). It is believed to be the most common driver of maternal request for elective cesarean section without medical indication (Otorepec, 2022). Commonly reported fears about normal pregnancy include such issues as going past the due date, pain, the labor process, fear of the unknown, and loss of control (Demsar et al., 2018; O'Donovan & O'Donovan, 2018). Multiparous clients with a prior traumatic birth experience are at risk for significant secondary tocophobia (Donel, 2019). Social media, the medical community, and family and friends are predominant sources of childbirth information and also the sources of significant misinformation, instilling childbirth fear. A simple internet search of "childbirth" results in scores of posts recounting childbirth horror stories.

Negative information or misinformation about childbirth through healthcare provider discussions, conversations with others, or through experience can lead individuals to catastrophize the event of childbirth before it occurs (Greathouse, 2014). Escalating interventions and cesarean birth rates are seen as proof that birth is dangerous and frightening. While some anxiety about birth is normal and serves a useful purpose as a prompt to seek safety and security, excessive fear of birth can lead to the expectation of birth interventions (Fenwick et al., 2015; Preis et al., 2018), physical labor dysfunction, and increased perception of pain, (Deng et.al, 2021) and a personal sense of failure (Nilsson & Lundgren, 2007). Elevated fear of childbirth has a strong association with maternal request for an elective cesarean birth (Kanellopoulos & Gourounti, 2022; O'Donovan & O'Donovan, 2018).

Perspective of Risk and Risk Assessment

Antepartum care is an opportunity for healthcare providers to perform wholistic appraisals of pregnancy risk and to help individuals develop an appropriate sense of confidence regarding their health and their childbearing abilities. The underlying belief that childbirth is a normal physiologic human function forms the foundation for applying evidence-based care practices to pregnancy. Childbearing is not without risk; however, the translation of theoretical and actual risks into a meaningful probability is essential in order to explain risk assessment to pregnant individuals and their families in a realistic way.

Risk assessment in pregnancy includes both primary and secondary preventions. For example, primary prevention of gestational diabetes involves helping people develop healthy eating and activity patterns before becoming pregnant. Secondary prevention involves screening healthy asymptomatic pregnant individuals for evidence of abnormal glucose tolerance to detect those who have gestational diabetes. Screening tests and evaluations should be accurate, and accuracy is evaluated by **sensitivity**, **specificity**, and **predictive value** of the screening test (Figure 11.1), which is dependent on the prevalence of the condition in the population being screened. When screening large numbers of asymptomatic individuals in a population that has a low prevalence of the condition, the number of false positive screens will increase as more and more healthy people are screened. For example, a 5% false positive rate in 10,000 healthy people will create 500

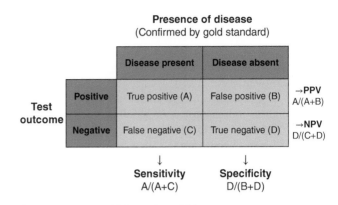

Figure 11.1 Sensitivity and specificity.

false positive diagnoses. Therefore, it is important to consider the consequences of false positive screen results on healthy people, such as the introduction of additional risk from added stress and invasive procedures.

Explaining Risk to Clients

Healthcare providers discuss risk or risk factors with pregnant clients frequently in the course of prenatal care, and the different ways risk can be expressed and communicated should be understood. In general, risk can be expressed in several ways using the same underlying data. **Absolute risk** is the probability or chance that an event will occur. **Relative risk** is an estimate of the probability of an adverse event in one group (for example, with prior cesarean birth) relative to another (no prior cesarean birth). **Attributable risk** refers to how many additional adverse outcomes can be ascribed to the risk factor.

Healthcare providers' communication regarding risk of an event has a strong influence on how risk is perceived by clients. The following example illustrates how a realistic understanding of the risk of an adverse event depends on provider presentation. Consider the following statements when counseling an individual pregnant for the second time interested in having a vaginal birth after having a cesarean birth (VBAC):

- "Your risk of uterine rupture during labor and birth is 0.2%." (absolute risk of adverse event)
- "Your risk of uterine rupture during labor and birth is 37 times higher than a person who has had no previous cesarean section." (relative risk)
- "VBAC creates 1.9 additional uterine ruptures for every 1000 cesarean births." (attributable risk)

Each of these statements is based on exactly the same underlying data, but each conveys a different perspective. A client who is counseled about an adverse event that is 37 times more likely to happen if a particular course of action is taken will most likely interpret the risk as much higher than the person who is counseled that they have a 2 in 1000 risk of the same adverse event. Additionally, a client who is advised only of the risks of VBAC and not the risks of cesarean birth may view their risk level differently and, thus, may view their choices differently. And importantly, the risk of the adverse event not occurring should be stated as well. For the prior example, it would be:

- "Your risk of *not* experiencing a uterine rupture during labor and birth is 99.8%." (absolute risk of positive outcome)

People who receive the labels of "positive" or "abnormal" test results perceive themselves to be at much higher risk than those who received "negative" or "normal" interpretive results, even when the actual risk numbers are the same. In a study examining risk communication, women who were told their risk of 5/1000 meant "abnormal test result" showed greater interest in further diagnostic testing compared with women who were told the risk of 5/1000 meant "normal test result" (Zikmund-Fisher et al., 2007). A significant concern is the variation in interpretation of the meaning of judgment terms such as "low risk" or "high risk." To one person, a low risk is equated with a risk of 1%, whereas to a second person, a low risk might be 10%. When communicating about pregnancy risks, it is best to not apply interpretive labels such as "abnormal" or "high risk" to testing results that can increase the perception of risk and can further affect intentions to act on that risk. Using numerical risk when available will help individuals make better-informed decisions rather than decisions based on their perceptions as to whether their risk had increased or decreased.

Research indicates that people misinterpret risk when it is stated as a probability with the numerator of 1 (Sirota et al., 2018). For example, some may perceive the risk of 1/250 as greater than 1/25 simply because they see only the larger number. Converting risk probabilities to use standard denominators can facilitate communication and understanding of risk. The Paling Palette is a tool that efficiently and effectively communicates risk in an understandable manner using a denominator of 1000 and includes the probability of both adverse events occurring and adverse events not occurring (Figure 11.2). For example, when talking with a person regarding their chances for successful VBAC and their risk of uterine rupture, all risks should be presented numerically with a denominator of 1000. The discussion should include the probability that no adverse effect will occur. This balanced presentation of risk can lead to a more realistic appraisal and understanding of potential problems (Table 11.1).

Research suggests that healthcare providers differ in the extent to which they communicate known risk factors to clients. While most people expressed desire to know about specific risk so they could plan and prepare, providers were concerned about alienation of clients, perceptions of blame, and risk estimate uncertainty as reasons to withhold some risk information (Tesfalul et al., 2021). This discrepancy in risk communication can have implications for client perinatal health.

Potential Problems of Risk Miscommunication

Informed Compliance

The principles of informed choice may not be applied when healthcare providers consider tests to be routine or necessary. *Informed compliance* is a term that means rather than making a choice, the client takes the action directed by the provider. Information about a particular course of action can be provided in a way that affects the perception of risk. Power imbalances in the client–provider relationship can foster a climate where the person providing the information influences client's actions. This can be illustrated with the common clinical scenario of a pregnant person at the first prenatal care visit. They are provided literature about maternal serum genetic screening, informed that this is done between 10 and 13 weeks of gestation, and instructed to let the clinician know if they have questions. This presentation can foster the belief that all pregnant people should have this test, and that it would be deviant to decline it. Some individuals may follow along without a full understanding of the genetic screening test and its implications. In this example, the healthcare provider most likely believes the acts of talking about and giving written information regarding the serum quad screen implies an informed client who could then give informed consent to have the test. When clients lack full information on the benefits, risks, limitations and implications of tests and procedures, and the freedom to decline without sanction, it is not possible for them to have the opportunity to make an informed choice.

Illusion of Choice

Information about risk can also be framed by the clinician toward offering a superior choice over another to avoid provider-perceived health outcome risks. The practice can lead to an *illusion of choice*.

This concept is illustrated by the situation of a pregnant person at 39 weeks of gestation assessed by the healthcare provider as having a big baby. The choice of labor induction is offered at 39 weeks with the advice that it can reduce the risk of potential problems related to suspicion of macrosomia. The discussion focuses on possible fetal risks without quantification of those risks. Importantly, equal information of the risks of labor induction, the relative plasticity of the pelvis in late pregnancy, the inaccuracy of estimating fetal weight in late pregnancy, and the capacity of the fetal head to mold during labor is not presented, and therefore, this client does not have a complete picture of the various risks. The client may feel that they are being offered a decision that avoids a potential threat. In reality, the potential for harm by waiting for natural labor may be quite remote, while a decision to induce labor brings new and undisclosed yet quantifiable risks with potential for maternal and fetal harm.

Informed Consent

Pregnancy is a unique time in life when an individual seeks expert healthcare information and opinion, even though they are not experiencing illness. It is the responsibility of prenatal healthcare providers to provide pregnant people with complete information in an understandable format.

Pregnant clients need to understand all aspects of care offerings so that they can make the best decision for themselves. Discussions on childbearing risk should culminate in a mutually agreeable decision about how to proceed

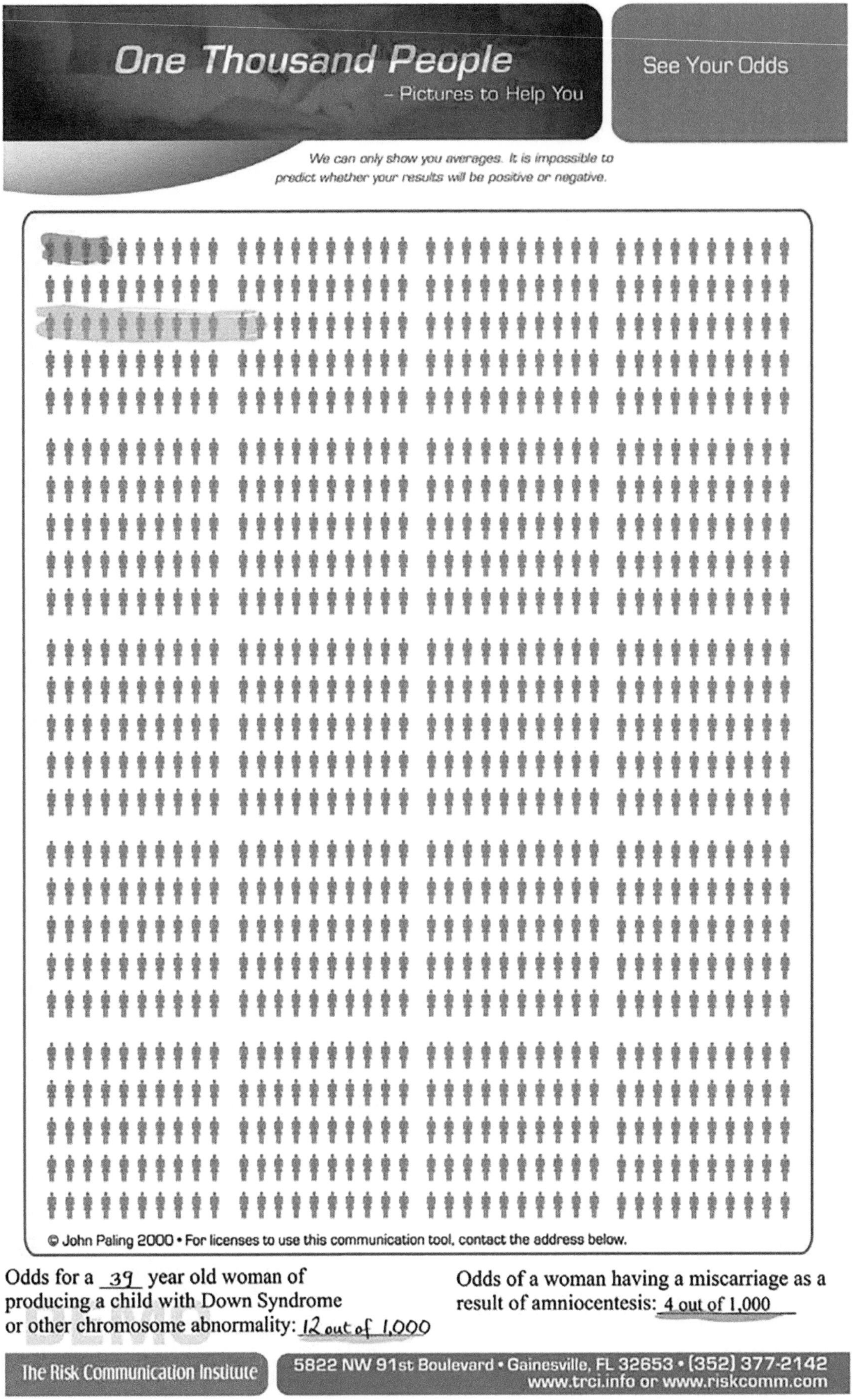

Figure 11.2   The Paling Palette Risk Communication Tool Paling Palettes©. Reproduced from J. Paling 2008/with permission of J. Paling.

Table 11.1   Principles of Communicating Risk

1. *Provide numeric likelihoods of risks and benefits.* Describing risk with words only can inflate or minimize risk and does not provide enough detail to make an informed decision.
2. *Provide absolute risks, not just relative risks.* Risk perception can be significantly influenced with relative risk.
3. *Keep denominators constant for comparisons.* A single denominator should be chosen for comparisons, preferably 1 in 1000.
4. *Explain the risk numbers by using visual aids.* These give context and increase understanding for the largest number of patients.
5. *Make the differences between baseline and treatment risks and benefits clear.* Use pictographs to show baseline risks in one color and the risks due to treatment in a different color.
6. *Reduce the amount of information to what is essential when possible.* Clinicians are often motivated to provide people with as much information as possible. However, with excess information, they may not know where to focus their attention and what information should be most important in their decisions.
7. *Provide both positive and negative frames.* People are unduly influenced by whether a treatment is described in positive or negative terms. When possible, describe the risks and benefits using both frames.
8. *Limit using interpretive labels to convey risk information.* Avoid using phrases like "You have a high risk for a certain condition."
9. *Test communications prior to use.* It is critical to test educational materials prior to use to determine understandability and to ensure that bias is eliminated in the materials.

Source: Adapted from Fagerlin and Peters (2011).

with the risk information presented. Informed consent is not a signature on a document; it is a process of communication and exchange between a client and healthcare provider to foster the ability to make the best decision about their own healthcare. Applying informed consent principles to commonly used technology such as nonindicated ultrasound, genetic screening, and elective induction allows the depth of information for an informed decision and permits informed refusal without sanction.

Knowledge for informed consent

- The known or presumptive diagnosis requiring treatment
- The nature and purpose of proposed treatments
- Whether these are time-sensitive decisions
- The benefits and risks associated with proposed treatment and without treatment
- Potential complications and side effects
- Likelihood of treatment success for this patient
- Reasonable alternatives available
- Benefits and risk associated with alternatives

Informed consent not only ensures client protection against unwanted or unnecessary medical treatment but also promotes active involvement in care and planning for the major life event of childbearing. The informed consent process requires adequate time for skillful communication, seeking understanding of the person's perspective, verifying their understanding of the information provided, and respecting their choices. Written material, smartphone apps, and other electronic resources are useful adjuncts to promote the understanding of conditions, testing, and risk during prenatal care. Clients prefer information to be provided during a face-to-face discussion, and written material should supplement, not replace, these important discussions (Willis et al., 2015).

The inherent inequalities in male–female power and in professional status between the client and the healthcare provider have a great influence on what happens to clients during prenatal care (Darilek, 2018). This is especially true for Black pregnant clients, who experience greater power imbalance and significant levels of medical neglect and unnecessary intervention during pregnancy and childbirth (Campbell, 2021). Equalizing the power balance between client and healthcare provider within the context of a caring relationship promotes open dialogue. When clients are able to form trusting relationships with their healthcare providers, they are more likely to have confidence to ask questions and to make choices about their care, rather than simply being "compliant" (Ward, 2018).

Fostering the transition of authoritative childbirth knowledge from the healthcare provider to the pregnant person should be a prenatal care goal. Each prenatal encounter should leave the individual feeling heard and valued. Validating and affirming experiential knowledge of pregnancy can empower people to rely less on outsiders' opinions of their pregnancy needs and support their autonomous care decisions.

Summary

While childbirth is not without risk, the "risk" of having a healthy vaginal birth is far greater than that of an adverse or operative event. Communicating this most likely outcome can help instill confidence and promote a balanced perspective of childbirth in pregnant individuals. The risk assessment process guides healthcare providers by delineating consultation and referral patterns. Evaluations of pregnancy risk are ongoing throughout prenatal care and can improve perinatal outcomes in some situations. However, the translation of theoretical and potential risks into reasonable, evidence-based, person-centered care practices requires a broad understanding of what risk assessment can and cannot do. Transforming risk assessment into universal applications of prenatal surveillance and risk management strategies regardless of actual risk lacks evidence of improved outcomes and introduces new potential for harmful consequences. An awareness of the pitfalls of risk-based pregnancy evaluation and management can assist the healthcare provider in avoiding inappropriate distortion of pregnancy risk and its harmful consequences.

Resources for Healthcare Providers

The Risk Communication Institute: For healthcare professional and consumers, offering information and visual aids to help communicate risk: http://www.risk comm.com

The Risk Communication Institute. (2008). The Paling Palettes. https://riskcomm.com/palettes.php?p=3

References

Alexander, D. (2017). *Does physician pay affect procedure choice and patient health? Evidence from medicaid c-section use.* Working Paper 2017-07. https://www.econstor.eu/bitstream/10419/200597/1/888171676.pdf

Alfirevic, Z., Devane, D., Gyte, G. M., & Cuthbert, A. (2017). Continuous cardiotocography (CTG) as a form of electronic fetal monitoring (EFM) for fetal assessment during labour. *The Cochrane Library*, 2, CD006066.

Al-Zirqi, I., Stray-Pedersen, B., Forsen, L., Daltveit, A. K., & Vangen, S. (2016). Uterine rupture: Trends over 40 years. *BJOG: An International Journal of Obstetrics & Gynaecology*, 123(5), 780–787.

Asher, E., Dvir, S., Seidman, D. S., Greenberg-Dotan, S., Kedem, A., Sheizaf, B., & Reuveni, H. (2013). Defensive medicine among obstetricians and gynecologists in tertiary hospitals. *PLoS One*, 8(3), e57108. https://doi.org/10.1371/journal.pone.0057108

Banner, H., & D'Souza, R. (2021). Towards an evidence-based approach to optimize the success of labor induction. *Best & Research: Clinical Obstetrics &Gynecology*, 77, 129–143. https://doi.org/10.1016/j.bpobgyn.2021.08.006

Barber, E., Eisenberg, D., & Grubman, W. (2011). Type of attending obstetrician call schedule and changes in labor management and outcome. *Obstetrics & Gynecology*, 118(6), 1371–1376.

Barr, J. J., & Marugg, L. (2019). Impact of marriage on birth outcomes: Pregnancy risk assessment monitoring system, 2012–2014. *The Linacre Quarterly*, 86(2–3), 225–230. https://doi.org/10.1177/0024363919843019

Berghella, V., & Saccone, G. (2019). Fetal fibronectin testing for reducing the risk of preterm birth. *Cochrane Database of Systematic Reviews*, 7. https://doi.org/10.1002/14651858

Campbell, C. (2021). Medical violence, obstetric racism, and the limits of informed consent for black women. *Michigan Journal of Race & Law*, 47. https://doi.org/10.36643/mjrl.26.sp.medica

Chen, H., & Tan, D. (2019). Cesarean section or natural childbirth? Cesarean birth may damage your health. *Frontiers in Psychology*, 10, 351. https://doi.org/10.3389/fpsyg.2019.00351

Cheng, Y. W., Snowden, J. M., Handler, S. J., Tager, I. B., Hubbard, A. E., & Caughey, A. B. (2014). Litigation in obstetrics: Does defensive medicine contribute to increases in caesarean delivery? *The Journal of Maternal-Fetal & Neonatal Medicine*, 27(16), 1668–1675.

Childbirth Connections. (2013). *Listening to mothers III: Pregnancy and birth.* https://www.nationalpartnership.org/our-work/resources/health-care/maternity/listening-to-mothers-iii-pregnancy-and-birth-2013.pdf

Cole, L., LeCouteur, A., Feo, R., & Dahlen, H. (2019). "Trying to give birth naturally was out of the question": Accounting for intervention in childbirth. *Women and Birth*, 32(1), e95–e101. https://doi.org/10.1016/jwombi.2018.04.101

Darilek, U. (2018). A woman's right to dignified, respectful healthcare during childbirth: A review of the literature on obstetric mistreatment. *Issues in Mental Health Nursing*, 39(6), 538–541. https://doi.org/10.1080/01612840.2017.1368752

Davey, M. A., Watson, L., Rayner, J. A., & Rowlands, S. (2015). Risk-scoring systems for predicting preterm birth with the aim of reducing associated adverse outcomes. *Cochrane Database of Systematic Reviews*, 10. https://doi.org/10.1002/14651858

Davis-Floyd, R. (2001). The technocratic, humanistic, and holistic paradigms of childbirth. *International Journal of Gynecology & Obstetrics*, 75(Suppl. 1), S5–S23.

De Mucio, B., Serruya, S., Aleman, A., Castellano, G., & Sosa, C. G. (2019). A systematic review and meta-analysis of cesarean delivery and other uterine surgery as risk factors for placenta accreta. *International Journal of Gynecology & Obstetrics*, 147(3), 281–291. https://doi.org/10.1002/ijgo.12948

Demsar, K., Svetina, M., Verdenik, I., Tul, N., Blickstein, I., & Globevnik Velikonja, V. (2018). Tokophobia (fear of childbirth): Prevalence and risk factors. *Journal of Perinatal Medicine*, 46(2), 151–154. https://doi.org/10.1515/jpm-2016-0282

Deng, Y., Lin, Y., Yang, L., Liang, Q., Fu, B., Li, H., Zhang, H., & Liu, Y. (2021). A comparison of maternal fear of childbirth, labor pain intensity and intrapartum analgesic consumption between primiparas and multiparas: A cross-sectional study. *International Journal of Nursing Sciences*, 8(4), 380–387. https://doi.org/10.1016/j.ijnss.2021.09.003

Dimassi, K., Douik, P., Ajroudi, M., Triki, A., & Gara, M. F. (2015). Ultrasound fetal weight estimation: How accurate are we now under emergency conditions? *Ultrasound in Medicine & Biology*, 41(10), 2562–2566.

Donel, J. (2019). Tocophobia: Overwhelming fear of pregnancy and childbirth. *International Journal of Reproduction, Contraception, Obstetrics and Gynecology*, 8(11), 4641–4646. https://doi.org/10.18203/2320-1770

Downe, S., Calleja-Aguis, J., Balaam, M. C., & Frith, L. (2020). Understanding childbirth as a complex salutogenic phenomena: The EU COST birth action collection. *PLoS One*, 15(8), e0236722. https://doi.org/10.1371/journal.pone.0236722

Esplin, M. S., Elovitz, M. A., Iams, J. D., Parker, C. B., Wapner, R. J., Grobman, W. A., Simhan, H. N., Wing, D. A., Haas, D. M., Silver, R. M., Hoffman, M. K., Peaceman, A. M., Caritis, S. N., Parry, S., Wadhwa, P., Foroud, T., Mercer, B. M., Hunter, S. M., Saade, G. R., & Reddy, U. M. (2017). Predictive accuracy of serial transvaginal cervical length and quantitative vaginal fetal fibronectin levels for spontaneous preterm birth among nulliparous women. *JAMA*, 317(10), 1047–1056. https://doi.org/10.1001/jama.2017.1373

Fagerlin, A., & Peters, E. (2011). Quantitative information. In B. Fischoff, N. T. Brewer, & J. S. Downs (Eds.), *Communicating risks and benefits: An evidence-based user's guide* (pp. 53–64). US Department of Health and Human Services, Food & Drug Administration. https://www.fda.gov/files/about%20fda/published/Communicating-Risk-and-Benefits-An-Evidence-Based-User%27s-Guide-%28Printer-Friendly%29.pdf

Fenwick, J., Toohill, J., Creedy, D. K., Smith, J., & Gamble, J. (2015). Sources, responses and moderators of childbirth fear in Australian women: A qualitative investigation. *Midwifery*, 31(1), 239–246.

Foo, P. K., Lee, R. S., & Fong, K. (2017). Physician prices, hospital prices, and treatment choice in labor and delivery. *American Journal of Health Economics*, 3(3), 422–453.

Frakes, M., & Gruber, J. (2020). Defensive medicine and obstetric practices: Evidence from the military health system. *Journal of Empirical Legal Studies*, 17(1), 4–37.

Greathouse, K. (2014). *The "Nightmare" of childbirth: The prevalence and predominant predictor variables for tokophobia in American women of childbearing age* [Unpublished doctoral dissertation]. The Chicago School of Professional Psychology.

Grobman, W. A., Lai, Y., Landon, M. B., Spong, C. Y., Leveno, K. J., Rouse, D. J., Varner, M. W., Atef, H. M., Caritis, S. N., Harper, M., Wapner, R. J., Sorokin, Y., Miodovnik, M., Carpenter, M., O'Sullivan, M. J., Sibai, B. M., Langer, O., Thorp, J. M., Ramin, S. M., & Mercer, B. M. (2007). Development of a nomogram for prediction of vaginal birth after cesarean delivery. *Obstetrics & Gynecology*, 109, 806–812. https://doi.org/10.1097/01.AOG.0000259312.36053.02

Gross, M. S., Ju, H., Osborne, L. M., Jelin, E. B., Sekar, P., & Jelin, A. C. (2021). Indeterminate prenatal ultrasounds and maternal anxiety: A prospective cohort study. *Maternal and Child Health Journal*, 25(5), 802–812. https://doi.org/10.1007/s10995-020-03042-x

Happel-Parkins, A., & Azim, K. A. (2016). At pains to consent: A narrative inquiry into women's attempts of natural childbirth. *Women and Birth*, 29(4), 310–320. https://doi.org/10.1016/j.wombi.2015.11.004

Harris, J. M., Franck, L., Green, B., Wilson, S., & Michie, S. (2015). The relationship between frequency of obstetric ultrasound scans and birthplace preference-a case control study. *Midwifery*, *31*(1), 31–36.

Heck, J. L., Jones, E. J., Bohn, D., McCage, S., Parker, J. G., Parker, M., Pierce, S. L., & Campbell, J. (2021). Maternal mortality among American Indian/Alaska native women: A scoping review. *Journal of Women's Health*, *30*(2), 220–229. https://doi.org/10.1089/jwh.2020.8890

Henderson, J. T., Thompson, J. H., Burda, B. U., Cantor, A., Beil, T., & Whitlock, E. P. (2017). *Screening for preeclampsia: A systematic evidence review for the US preventive services task force.* Agency for Healthcare Research and Quality. https://pubmed.ncbi.nlm.nih.gov/28813128

Holness, N. (2018). High-risk pregnancy. *Nursing Clinics*, *53*(2), 241–251.

Hotelling, B. A. (2013). The nocebo effect in childbirth classes. *The Journal of Perinatal Education*, *22*(2), 120.

Hoyert, D. L. (2022). *Maternal mortality rates in the United States, 2020.* NCHS Health E-Stats. https://doi.org/10.15620/cdc:113967

Isaacs, N. Z., & Andipatin, M. G. (2020). A systematic review regarding women's emotional and psychological experiences of high-risk pregnancies. *BMC Psychology*, *8*(1), 1–11. https://doi.org/10.1186/s40359-020-00410-8

Jordan, R., & Murphy, P. (2009). Risk assessment and risk distortion: Finding the balance. *Journal of Midwifery & Women's Health*, *54*(3), 191–200.

Kanellopoulos, D., & Gourounti, K. (2022). Tocophobia and women's desire for a caesarean section: A systematic review. *Maedica*, *17*(1). https://doi.org/10.26574/maedica.2022.17.1.186

Lawson, K. L., & Turriff-Janasson, I. S. (2006). Maternal serum screening and psychosocial attachments to pregnancy. *Journal of Psychosomatic Research*, *60*, 371–378.

Lee, S., Ayers, S., & Holden, D. (2012). Risk perception of women during high-risk pregnancy: A systematic review. *Health, Risk & Society*, *14*(6), 511–531.

Martin, J. A., Hamilton, B. E., & Osterman, M. J. (2014). *Birth in the United States: 2013.* National Center for Health Statistics. https://www.cdc.gov/nchs/data/databriefs/db175.htm

Muggleton, S., & Davis, D. (2022). Applying salutogenesis in midwifery practice. In M. M. Mittlemark, G. F. Bauer, L. Vandrager, J. M. Pelican, S. Sagy, M. Eriksson, B. Lindstrom, & C. M. Magistretti (Eds.), *The handbook of salutogenesis* (pp. 459–464). Springer. https://doi.org/10.1007/978-3-030-79515-3_42

Munro, S., Kornelsen, J., Corbett, K., Wilcox, E., Bansback, N., & Janssen, P. (2017). Do women have a choice? Care providers' and decision makers' perspectives on barriers to access of health services for birth after a previous cesarean. *Birth*, *44*(2), 153–160.

Naylor-Smith, J., Taylor, B., Shaw, K., Hewison, A., & Kenyon, S. (2018). 'I didn't think you were allowed that, they didn't mention that.' A qualitative study exploring women's perceptions of home birth. *BMC Pregnancy and Childbirth*, *18*(1), 1–11. https://doi.org/10.1186/s12884-018-1733-1

Nijagal, M. A., Kuppermann, M., Nakagawa, S., & Cheng, Y. (2015). Two practice models in one labor and delivery unit: Association with cesarean delivery rates. *American Journal of Obstetrics and Gynecology*, *212*(4), 491–e1. https://doi.org/10.1016/j.ajog.2014.11.014

Nilsson, C., & Lundgren, I. (2007). Women's lived experience of fear of birth. *Midwifery*, *25*(2), 1–9.

O'Connell, M. A., Leahy-Warren, P., Khashan, A. S., Kenny, L. C., & O'Neill, S. M. (2017). Worldwide prevalence of tocophobia in pregnant women: Systematic review and meta-analysis. *Acta Obstetricia et Gynecologica Scandinavica*, *96*(8), 907–920. https://doi.org/10.1111/aogs.13138

O'Donovan, C., & O'Donovan, J. (2018). Why do women request an elective cesarean delivery for non-medical reasons? A systematic review of the qualitative literature. *Birth*, *45*(2), 109–119. https://doi.org/10.1111/birt.12319

Ondeck, M. (2014). Healthy birth practice# 2: Walk, move around, and change positions throughout labor. *The Journal of Perinatal Education*, *23*(4), 188.

Osterman, M. J., Hamilton, B. E., Martin, J. A., Driscoll, A. K., & Valenzuela, C. P. (2022). Births: Final data for 2020. *National Vital Statistics Report*, *70*(17), 1–50. https://doi.org/10.15620/cdc:112078

Otorepec, I. R. (2022). Tocophobia. *The Journal of Sexual Medicine*, *19*(5), S226.

Paterno, M. T., McElroy, K., & Regan, M. (2016). Electronic fetal monitoring and cesarean birth: A scoping review. *Birth*, *43*(4), 277–284. https://doi.org/10.1111/birt.12247

Peterson, J., Paulitsch, M., Guethlin, C., Gensichen, J., & Albrecht, J. (2009). A survey on worries of pregnant women—Testing the German version of the Cambridge worry scale. *BMC Public Health*, *9*, 490.

Preis, H., Gozlan, M., Dan, U., & Benyamini, Y. (2018). A quantitative investigation into women's basic beliefs about birth and planned birth choices. *Midwifery*, *63*, 46–51. https://doi.org/10.1016/j.midw.2018.05.002

Regan, M., McElroy, K. G., & Moore, K. (2013). Choice? Factors that influence women's decision making for childbirth. *The Journal of Perinatal Education*, *22*(3), 171. https://doi.org/10.1891/1058-1243.22.3.171

Sakala, C., Declercq, E. R., Turon, J. M., & Corry, M. P. (2018). *Listening to mothers in California: A population-based survey of Women's childbearing experiences, full survey report.* National Partnership for Women & Families. https://www.chcf.org/wp-content/uploads/2018/09/ListeningMothersCAFullSurveyReport2018.pdf

Sekar, R., Khatun, M., Barrett, H. L., & Duncombe, G. (2016). A prospective pilot study in assessing the accuracy of ultrasound estimated fetal weight prior to delivery. *Australian and New Zealand Journal of Obstetrics and Gynaecology*, *56*(1), 49–53.

Sirota, M., Juanchich, M., & Bonnefon, J.-F. (2018). "1-in-X" bias: "1-in-X" format causes overestimation of health-related risks. *Journal of Experimental Psychology: Applied*, *24*(4), 431–439. https://doi.org/10.1037/xap0000190

Symon, A., Williams, B., Adelasoye, Q. A., & Cheyne, H. (2015). Nocebo and the potential harm of 'high risk' labelling: A scoping review. *Journal of Advanced Nursing*, *71*(7), 1518–1529.

Tesfalul, M. A., Feuer, S. K., Castillo, E., Coleman-Phox, K., O'Leary, A., & Kuppermann, M. (2021). Patient and provider perspectives on preterm birth risk assessment and communication. *Patient Education and Counseling*, *104*(11), 2814–2823. https://doi.org/10.1016/j.pec.2021.03.038

Thomas, G. M., Roberts, J., & Griffiths, F. E. (2017). Ultrasound as a technology of reassurance? How pregnant women and health care professionals articulate ultrasound reassurance and its limitations. *Sociology of Health & Illness*, *39*(6), 893–907.

Topçu, S., & Brown, P. (2019). The impact of technology on pregnancy and childbirth: Creating and managing obstetrical risk in different cultural and socio-economic contexts. *Health, Risk & Society*, *21*(3–4), 89–99. https://doi.org/10.1080/13698575.2019.1649922

van Baaren, G. J., Vis, J. Y., Wilms, F. F., Oudijk, M. A., Kwee, A., Porath, M. M., Scheepers, H. C. J., Spaanderman, M. E. A., Bloemenkamp, K. W. M., Haak, M. C., Bolte, A. C., Bax, C. J., Cornette, J. M. J., Duvekot, J. J., Bijvanck, B. W. A. N., van Eyck, J., Franssen, M. T. M., Sollie, K. M., Vandenbussche, F. P. H. A., . . . Moi, B. W. J. (2014). Predictive value of cervical length measurement and fibronectin testing in threatened preterm labor. *Obstetrics & Gynecology*, *123*(6), 1185–1192.

Viaux-Savelon, S., Dommergues, M., Rosenblum, O., Bodeau, N., Aidane, E., Philippon, O., Mazet, P., Vibert-Guigue, C., Vauthier-Brouzes, D., Feldman, R., & Cohen, D. (2012). Prenatal ultrasound screening: False positive soft markers may alter maternal representations and mother-infant interaction. *PLoS One*, *7*(1), e30935.

Vogel, J. P., Chawanpaiboon, S., Moller, A. B., Watananirun, K., Bonet, M., & Lumbiganon, P. (2018). The global epidemiology of preterm birth. *Best Practice & Research. Clinical Obstetrics & Gynaecology*, *52*, 3–12. https://doi.org/10.1016/j.bpobgyn.2018.04.003

Vyas, D. A., Eisenstein, L. G., & Jones, D. S. (2020). Hidden in plain sight—Reconsidering the use of race correction in clinical algorithms. *New England Journal of Medicine*, *383*(9), 874–882.

Ward, P. (2018). Trust and communication in a doctor-patient relationship: A literature review. *Journal of Health Communication, 3*(3), 36.

White-VanGompel, E., Perez, S., Datta, A., Wang, C., Cape, V., & Main, E. (2019). Cesarean overuse and the culture of care. *Health Services Research, 54*(2), 417–424. https://doi.org/10.1111/1475-6773.13123

Williams, P. L., Williams, J. P., & Williams, B. R. (2021). The fine line of defensive medicine. *Journal of Forensic and Legal Medicine, 80*, 102170. https://doi.org/10.1016/j.jflm.2021.102170

Willis, A. M., Smith, S. K., Meiser, B., Muller, C., Lewis, S., & Halliday, J. (2015). How do prospective parents prefer to receive information about prenatal screening and diagnostic testing? *Prenatal Diagnosis, 35*(1), 100–102.

Zikmund-Fisher, B. J., Fagerlin, A., Keeton, K., & Ubel, P. A. (2007). Does labeling prenatal screening test results as negative or positive affect a woman's responses? *American Journal of Obstetrics and Gynecology, 197*, 528e1–528e6.

12

Prenatal Ultrasound

Jenna Shaw-Battista

The editors gratefully acknowledge Cynthia Parke and Robin G. Jordan, who authored the previous edition of this chapter.

Relevant Terms

Amniotic fluid index (AFI)—sum of the deepest amniotic fluid pocket in each abdominal quadrant

Amniotic fluid volume (AFV)—assessment of amniotic fluid amount in the uterus, utilized in scoring of the biophysical profile (BPP) and defined as adequate if one pocket of at least 2 cm fluid is present

Anechoic—tissues that do not produce a returning echo and appear dark on ultrasound images, e.g., amniotic fluid and blood

Artifacts—misleading or incorrect information appearing on the visual display

As low as reasonably achievable (ALARA)—guiding principle to keep ultrasound exposure as low as possible while still acquiring the information needed for diagnostic images

American Registry for Diagnostic Medical Sonography (ARDMS)—national certification body for sonographers

Biometry—the direct ultrasound measurement of the fetal parts

Cavitation—generation, growth, and vibration of air bubbles within tissues caused by ultrasound

Chemical pregnancy—colloquial term meaning a conception that produces measurable levels of β-hCG but does not develop far enough to be seen on ultrasound

Doppler effect—change in the frequency of wave lengths as the source of the waves and observer move toward or away from each other

Echogenicity—term used to describe the ability of body tissues and structures to create an echo in which an ultrasound signal is bounced back and returns.

Enhancement artifact—can occur with fluid-filled structures, is seen as increased echogenicity (whiteness) posterior to fluid-filled structures.

Frequency—number of vibrations produced per unit of time

Hertz (Hz)—measurement unit for the frequency of sound waves

Hyperechogenic—ultrasound waves producing a greater number of returning echoes

Hypoechogenic—ultrasound waves producing lower levels of returning echoes

Likelihood ratio—ratio of sensitivity to specificity for a given diagnostic test that reflects reliability; used in the evaluation of soft markers for fetal anomalies detected on prenatal ultrasound

Limited ultrasound—performed when a focused maternal/fetal ultrasound assessment is indicated for a clinical situation

Nuchal translucency (NT)—an abnormal collection of fluid in the posterior cervical area of the fetus may be detectable in a specialized ultrasound done in conjunction with maternal serum draw at 10–13 weeks to determine potential risk for major congenital anomalies; one of the noninvasive genetic screening and testing strategies available

Piezoelectric crystals—material housed within the ultrasound transducer that generates the ultrasound by converting electrical impulse energy into sound waves which are directed into the body, and then detects the returning sound echoes and converts them back into electrical energy for visual representation in ultrasound images

Point-of-care (POC) ultrasound—a type of limited ultrasound performed during a patient encounter to obtain immediate clinical information and enhance care; is often performed by a nonsonographer and not interpreted further, e.g., fetal presentation assessment

Pregnancy of unknown viability—a term given to an intrauterine pregnancy in a situation where there are not enough criteria to confidently categorize an intrauterine pregnancy as either viable or nonviable

Reverberation artifact—production of false echoes when ultrasound bounces between two interfaces with high acoustic impedance or resistance

Shadowing artifact—characterized by a signal void behind structures that strongly absorb or reflect ultrasonic waves can cause image distortion

Single deepest pocket—also known as the *maximum vertical pocket*, the measurement of the deepest pocket of amniotic

---

Prenatal and Postnatal Care: A Person-Centered Approach, Third Edition. Edited by Karen Trister Grace, Cindy L. Farley, Noelene K. Jeffers, and Tanya Tringali.
© 2024 John Wiley & Sons Ltd. Published 2024 by John Wiley & Sons Ltd.
Companion website: www.wiley.com/go/grace/prenatal

fluid observed within the uterus that is at least 2 cm deep by 1 cm wide and free of umbilical cord and fetal parts

Soft markers—minor sonographic findings associated with increased risk for fetal aneuploidy particularly if multiple markers are identified

Sonographer—a skilled medical imaging professional within the allied health sector who operates an ultrasound machine to perform diagnostic medical sonographic examinations.

Registered Diagnostic Medical Sonographer—the credential Registered Diagnostic Medical Sonographer is used by those who have passed the national certification exam provided by ARDMS

Specialized ultrasound—a targeted anatomic examination to assess specific maternal/fetal structures

Standard ultrasound—examination performed to visualize a list of specific maternal/fetal structures and functions which were identified by expert groups and vary by pregnancy trimester

Introduction

Advances in ultrasound research, equipment, and software have increased the application of ultrasound imaging as a diagnostic tool in all areas of healthcare, including sexual and reproductive healthcare. The benefits of this noninvasive diagnostic tool include the safe ability to recognize normal and diagnose abnormal conditions with near immediate interpretation, and increased safety of invasive procedures when ultrasound is used for guidance.

This chapter reviews the use of ultrasound during the antepartum period. Whether ordering or performing ultrasound, healthcare providers must understand the limitations of ultrasound in the particular context and setting in which it is being used. These topics will be addressed in this chapter along with the mechanism and use of this assessment tool, the experience of undergoing ultrasound, the importance of accurate education regarding the type and purpose of the exam, and implications of findings. This chapter also covers the basic physics, types of scans, safety data, and indications for ultrasound during pregnancy. General considerations for both normal and abnormal ultrasound findings will be covered. Detailed content needed to perform ultrasound exams is beyond the scope of this text, as are diagnostic and management plans for varied conditions identified on ultrasound exam. Like any diagnostic modality, results must be viewed within the context of a complete assessment of the pregnant person and fetus. The training, certification, and experience of those performing ultrasound are also important considerations.

The Physics and Mechanics of Ultrasound

Ultrasound is the use of timed, high-frequency sound waves to produce a visual image. Medical ultrasound imaging uses frequencies of 3–15 MHz (mega**Hertz**), with 3–5 MHz commonly used in prenatal ultrasound. Ultrasound vibrations move at different speeds through different mediums and travel faster through firmer travel faster through firmer substances or structures which are rigid and dense. **Frequency** of sound waves, or the number of vibrations per unit of time, is the energy that is transformed into a visual image. Higher frequencies have a greater number of vibrations, shorter sound waves, and better image resolution, but also less tissue penetration or depth of viewing.

Ultrasound equipment includes a probe that contains a transducer. Probes are marketed in three different shapes: linear, sector, and array. The probe shape helps determines the way sound waves are distributed. The abdominal and transvaginal probes used in sexual and reproductive healthcare are curvilinear, and the images produced are fan shaped. Ultrasound providers must understand probe type and frequency selection for clinical situations encountered. Additionally, all probes have an indicator notch or ridge used to establish the orientation of the objects being scanned when operating the probe. Proper orientation is an important component of obtaining clinically relevant data and communicating with other healthcare team members.

Housed within the probe is a transducer that contains **piezoelectric crystals** that convert electrical energy into the mechanical energy of sound waves. Sound waves pass

Health equity key points

- The application of ultrasound technology to prenatal care shaped clinical guidelines and accelerated shifting cultural perceptions about the fetus, while presenting new ethical challenges related to the priorities, autonomy, and bodily integrity of the pregnant person.
- Contemporary guidelines for perinatal care and fetal imaging recommend that ultrasound for genetic screening purposes should be offered to all pregnant people regardless of age, though insurance coverage is not yet aligned with these recommendations.
- Inequities in the ability to access routine and specialized ultrasound imaging differentially burden individuals living in

rural areas and disenfranchised communities, and persons of color.
- Politicians seeking to prevent pregnancy terminations have mandated viewing of prenatal ultrasounds by people seeking abortions, which disproportionately affects communities with barriers to imaging, and is not supported by research evidence or endorsed by sexual and reproductive healthcare organizations.
- Research is underway on the optimal number, timing, and indications for pregnancy ultrasound, which will inform ongoing public health efforts to address perinatal inequities in imaging as well as abortion access and pregnancy outcomes.

into the body and come in contact with tissues, which cause echoes to bounce or reflect back to the crystals. The crystals convert the echoes into electrical energy that is displayed as an image on the monitor display screen. The material on the cover of a probe and the gel used during the examination enable the sound waves to be effectively transmitted into the body and read as echoes.

There are two main types of display modes used in ultrasound examinations. A-mode (amplitude mode) is the simplest type of ultrasound, which consists of a one-dimensional fixed beam. B-mode (brightness mode) is the mode typically used during pregnancy, also known as two-dimensional (2D) ultrasound. In B-mode, each returning echo provides a brightness-regulated display, which produces a cross-sectional view of objects in real time. As the transducer is held steady, the sound waves slice through the tissue and echoes return to create an image, many times a second.

The use of M-mode (motion mode) and Doppler mode imaging modalities enhance scanning and imaging ability for sexual and reproductive health indications. M-mode displays motion of an object and is widely used in echocardiography. Doppler mode uses detectable changes in high-frequency sound waves, based on the **Doppler effect**, to create clear digital images in real time. In Doppler ultrasound, the transducer is held still but the object is moving, such as with blood flow. Color flow Doppler superimposes color on the returning echo to allow better visualization and assess blood flow dynamics. An additional ultrasound enhancement is three-dimensional (3D) imaging, which is essentially a systematic series of conventional 2D image slices on which the machine software is moving the transducer automatically. The software also utilizes artificial lighting and other enhancements to create realistic images. Though images are enhanced, 3D technology does not provide more clinically useful information than 2D imaging and is not required for standard sexual and reproductive health ultrasound examinations.

Echogenicity is an important aspect of ultrasound images and refers to the number of echoes transmitted by a transducer which are bounced back by internal body tissues and structures, thereby contributing to the quality of the image produced. The strength of the returning echo is dependent on the density of the tissue being scanned. The denser the tissue, the greater the reflection, and the brighter the appearance on the monitor image. High levels of returning echoes are termed **hyperechogenic** and appear as white areas of images produced by echoes from dense or rigid tissue such as bone. Low levels of returning echoes are termed **hypoechogenic,** are produced by less dense tissues such as muscle, and are displayed within an image as shades of gray. **Anechoic** structures produce no echo return and will appear black in images, such as amniotic fluid, or fluid within cavities like the fetal stomach or bladder.

As transmitted ultrasound travels through the body, it becomes weaker (attenuated) because the sound waves are reflected, scattered, and absorbed, which is of limited clinical significance. Absorption is the conversion of the sound energy into heat, which will always occur to some degree but increases when higher ultrasound frequency is used. The safety of ultrasound with regard to heat generation will be discussed later.

Ultrasound waves may also be refracted or bent and cause **artifacts** that produce imaging errors. The identification of refraction artifacts is essential for sonogram providers. Artifacts may distort the size, position, and shape of the studied structures or even mimic structures that are not actually present. The most common artifacts are **reverberation**, **shadowing**, and **enhancement** which providers of ultrasound must take steps to prevent, correctly identify, and accurately interpret (Chudleigh et al., 2017).

Types of Scans

Ultrasound is increasingly used as an assessment and diagnostic tool in sexual and reproductive healthcare. As with any clinical tool, it should be used by trained individuals according to best practice guidelines and incorporated into a comprehensive patient assessment. The American Institute of Ultrasound in Medicine (AIUM), the American College of Radiology (ACR), the American College of Obstetricians and Gynecologists (ACOG), and the Society of Radiologists in Ultrasound (SRU) have jointly defined three types of obstetric ultrasound exams: limited or point of care (POC), standard, and specialized (American Institute of Ultrasound in Medicine [AIUM], 2018a).

Limited ultrasound is performed during any trimester when a focused ultrasound assessment is indicated on the basis of the clinical situation. A limited examination is performed when a specific question requires investigation. Examples include determination of fetal presentation, amniotic fluid measurement, and verification of fetal cardiac activity. Limited exams have these benefits: they provide immediate information thus preventing delay in treatment; improve continuity of care thus enhancing the patient care experience; and improve effectiveness and safety of procedures such as intrauterine device (IUD) insertion and external cephalic version.

POC ultrasound is a type of limited ultrasound often done at the bedside and interpreted directly by the healthcare provider. As limited ultrasound examinations are narrowed in scope, they do not replace a standard examination (Menihan & Kopel, 2014). Examples of POC ultrasound include scans performed only for localization of the placenta or determination of presenting part at term and during labor.

Standard ultrasound is the routine examination of maternal and fetal structures. Expert groups have developed lists of components examined during a standard exam during each trimester of pregnancy. A standard obstetric ultrasound in the first trimester includes evaluation of the presence, size, location, and number of gestational sac(s) and the presence of a yolk sac and embryo/fetus. When an embryo/fetus is detected, it should be measured to verify pregnancy dating and cardiac activity recorded. Maternal reproductive structures are identified. A standard ultrasound in the second or third trimester includes an evaluation of fetal presentation, **amniotic fluid volume**, cardiac activity, placental position, fetal **biometry**, and fetal number, plus an anatomic survey. Placental appearance and location with proximity to the cervical os, and umbilical cord assessments are also included. This scan is generally performed by a **sonographer** and interpreted by a radiologist or other physician.

Specialized ultrasounds are ordered to follow up on suspected complications of pregnancy and are targeted to provide further diagnostic information. A detailed anatomic examination is performed when a fetal anomaly is suspected based on history, biochemical abnormalities, or the results of either the limited or standard scan. Specialized examinations also include fetal Doppler ultrasound, a biophysical profile (BPP), and a fetal echocardiogram and repeat scans to evaluate known or suspected problems such as fetal growth restriction. Evaluation of **nuchal translucency (NT)** and cervical length (CL) measurement are other examples of specialized ultrasound examinations.

There can be overlapping of the definition of types of scans. Two exams may be considered as standard and/or specialized as they are recommended in some practice areas routinely. An example is the ultrasound used in the first-trimester genetic screening evaluating NT along with maternal serum measurements for genetic risk screening. This exam may be considered specialized in that specific education, training, and credentialing is recommended for those performing NT measurements. In the same way, CL measurement may be classified as included in the standard first-trimester exam, or it can be considered a specialized exam or performed as a limited exam in maternity triage.

Use of Prenatal Ultrasound

Prenatal application of ultrasound technology varies by gestational and clinical presentation, as well as healthcare provider training and sociodemographic factors associated with pregnancy imaging access and utilization. Common indications for prenatal ultrasound include documentation of fetal viability, gestational age, and fetal number, placental location and condition, detection of fetal anomalies, and evaluation of fetal growth and amniotic fluid. Ultrasound examinations are performed either intravaginally or abdominally depending on gestational age and indication for the exam. A written or electronic request for an obstetric ultrasound is made by the ordering healthcare provider who will not perform an ultrasound exam themselves. Included in the request should be the indication for the exam, pertinent history and or differential diagnoses, and any pertinent maternal or fetal clinical signs and symptoms.

First-Trimester Ultrasound

First-trimester ultrasound usually begins with a transabdominal scan and may proceed to include a transvaginal scan as well. The transvaginal approach is the preferred method before 10 weeks of gestation due to its superior

Table 12.1 Indications for First-trimester Ultrasound

Confirmation of pregnancy location
Confirmation of fetal viability with cardiac motion
Confirmation of fetal number and evaluation of membrane characteristics (i.e., monochorionic and diamniotic)
Estimation of gestational age
Evaluation of vaginal bleeding, pain, and uterine mass
Evaluation of suspected complications such as gestational trophoblastic disease or ectopic pregnancy
Measurement of nuchal translucency to screen for fetal aneuploidy
Assessment for certain fetal anomalies such as anencephaly
Adjunct to procedures such as:
  Embryo transfer
  Chorionic villi sampling
  Intrauterine device removal
  External cephalic version

Source: Adapted from AIUM (2021) and AIUM (2018a).

image quality. The transvaginal probe will be in closer proximity to the uterus and fallopian tubes and uses higher frequencies (7–9 MHz). Clinical indications for first-trimester ultrasound are noted in Table 12.1.

Evaluation of suspected spontaneous or missed abortion is a common situation in which ultrasound is used in the first trimester. Verification of both viable and intrauterine pregnancy in the presence of an elevated beta human chorionic gonadotropin (β-hCG) is essential, particularly when vaginal bleeding and/or abdominal or pelvic pain is present. A β-hCG of 1000–2000 IU/L has been historically referred to as the *discriminatory zone* and cited as the threshold above which a pregnancy should be visualized by transvaginal ultrasound. However, isolated case reports exist of normal pregnancies following abnormal β-hCG absolute values. Providers should cautiously interpret lab values and correlate with ultrasound findings before determining a plan of care. Table 12.2 lists the pregnancy findings, expected timing, and markers of viable and nonviable pregnancies. While a known last menstrual period (LMP) is helpful for dating, its accuracy can vary depending on the length and regularity of cycles and other factors. See Chapter 10, *Pregnancy Diagnosis and Gestational Age Assessment*, for guidelines on when to adjust the estimated due date based on ultrasound results. Follow-up scans are done at a minimum interval of five to seven days regardless of any known β-hCG values, with serial imaging as the definitive means to establish a viable or nonviable pregnancy.

Before viability can be demonstrated, the diagnostic term, **pregnancy of unknown viability (PUV)**, is used. The expected developmental landmarks are the gestational sac present at 5 weeks gestation, a yolk sac visible at 5.5 weeks, fetal pole by 6–6.5 weeks, and cardiac activity typically by 5 weeks and expected in embryos at 7 weeks or >7 mm in crown rump length (CRL). Until cardiac activity is demonstrated in an intrauterine pregnancy, the viability of the pregnancy cannot be confirmed. Differential diagnoses for the finding of PUV include gestational age <5 weeks of gestation; anembryonic or **chemical pregnancy;** embryonic demise; delayed,

Table 12.2   Characteristics of Early Pregnancy Viability and Failure

Characteristic	Timing	Description
Gestational sac	5 weeks' gestation	Normally located in the endometrium, with smooth, round, regular appearance; Demonstrates a hyperechoic ring; Sac growth >0.6 mm/day If >20 mm, yolk sac should be seen If ≥25 mm, embryo should be seen
Yolk Sac	5.5 weeks' gestation	Normal size <6.0 mm; Located within the chorioamniotic space; Round or spherical shape; Bright echogenic rim
Embryo with cardiac motion	5.5–7 weeks' gestation	Cardiac motion should be seen in embryos with CRL >7 mm Fetal heart rate normally above 85 beats per minute
Ultrasound findings diagnostic of nonviable pregnancy	5–8 weeks gestation	CRL ≥7 mm and no cardiac activity Mean sac diameter ≥25 mm and no visible embryo Absence of embryo with heartbeat ≥2 weeks after a scan that showed gestational sac without a yolk sac Absence of embryo with heartbeat ≥11 days after scan that showed gestational sac with a yolk sac

Source: Adapted from Chudleigh et al. (2017) and Doubilet et al. (2013).

Table 12.3   Components of the First-trimester Standard Exam

ACOG	AIUM
Evaluate maternal structures: uterus, adnexa, cervix, and cul-de-sac	Evaluate uterus (including cervix and cul-de-sac) and adnexa for presence of gestational sac
Confirm presence of gestational sac and yolk sac, measure both	Evaluate gestational sac for yolk sac and embryo and measure CRL if present
Confirm presence of embryo ± cardiac activity, measure CRL	Evaluate for presence or absence of fetal cardiac activity
Confirm fetal number	Document fetal number. If multiple gestation, document amnionicity and chorionicity
Evaluate for early detection of severe fetal anomalies	Assess appropriate embryonic and fetal anatomy, including the nuchal region

Source: Adapted from ACOG (2016) and AIUM (2018a, 2018b).

incomplete, threatened, or inevitable abortion; molar pregnancy; and ectopic pregnancy.

The components identified in a first trimester ultrasound exam are listed in Table 12.3. In addition to pregnancy viability, pregnancy location is also a critically important component of an early pregnancy ultrasound. This is most urgent in the presence of bleeding or pain, or a β-hCG level that is abnormal for gestational age and/or not rising as expected. The diagnostic term **pregnancy of unknown location (PUL)** is used until an intrauterine pregnancy is seen. Thorough evaluation of the adnexa in an early pregnancy is an essential part of the ultrasound exam even when an intrauterine pregnancy is confirmed. Rare heterotopic pregnancy must be ruled out, which is the rare circumstance that both intrauterine and ectopic pregnancies occur simultaneously. Caution should be

used in making the presumptive diagnosis of an intrauterine gestational sac in the absence of a definite embryo or yolk sac since without these findings, an intrauterine fluid collection could represent a pseudogestational sac associated with an ectopic pregnancy. A pseudogestational sac may appear thin without a rim of thick chorionic tissue, and the intrauterine fluid collection may have a small "beak" or teardrop appearance that connects with or points toward the uterine cavity line. Follow-up ultrasound with or without serial evaluation of maternal serum β-hCG levels is appropriate in cases of PUL to avoid missed ectopic pregnancy requiring life-saving treatment and to prevent inappropriate intervention in a potentially viable early pregnancy (AIUM, 2018a).

Early ultrasonography for pregnancy dating should be routinely offered to ensure intrauterine pregnancy and prevent induction of labor for prolonged pregnancy, particularly for pregnant persons with a history of irregular cycles or bleeding, uncertain timing of LMP, or if there is a discrepancy in uterine size compared with gestational age. A first-trimester ultrasound between 6 and 13 6/7 weeks of gestation measures the CRL with an accuracy of ±5–7 days and can be performed during a prenatal intake appointment at the POC (ACOG, 2022).

Second-Trimester Ultrasound

There are multiple indications for a second-trimester ultrasound (Table 12.4), though no benefit has been clearly established for routine fetal anatomy scans in the general population. It is recommended that a genetic screening ultrasound to detect fetal anomalies be offered with informed consent to all pregnant people in the second-trimester (ACOG, 2016), though the overall detection rate for fetal anomalies with second-trimester ultrasound is reported to be between 19% and 89% and varies greatly by type of anomaly, examiner skill, maternal habitus, and ultrasound equipment (Bardi et al., 2019; Rydberg & Tunon, 2017). In the absence of specific

Table 12.4   Indications for Second-trimester Ultrasound

Estimate gestational age: size-date discrepancy, interval fetal growth, fetal number
Evaluate fetal number
Pelvic/abdominal pain or bleeding
Assessment of amniotic fluid or for premature rupture of membranes
Placental localization or follow-up, evaluation of placenta abruption
Measurement of cervical length
Confirm fetal viability
Fetal anatomic scan; follow-up to abnormal biochemical markers; increased risk for fetal aneuploidy; evaluation for fetal anomalies
Evaluate maternal pelvic mass or uterine anomaly
Adjunct to procedure: amniocentesis, cerclage placement, external cephalic version
Confirm presenting part
Evaluate fetal well-being

Source: Adapted from: AIUM (2021), AIUM (2018a), and Chudleigh et al. (2017).

indications, the optimal time for an optional single ultrasound examination is at 18–22 weeks of gestation, which allows for a survey of fetal anatomy and an accurate estimation of gestational age in most cases.

In addition to fetal anatomy components of standard second-trimester ultrasounds (Table 12.5), sonographers should assess preterm birth risk with CL measured by transvaginal ultrasound in the second-trimester. This recommendation is not uniformly implemented across geographical regions or socioeconomic status. Studies demonstrate that pregnant persons who are indigenous experience significant barriers to pregnancy ultrasound exams in Canada (Adams, Yao, et al., 2022), while Black and Latina parturients are more likely to experience late or no standard second-trimester transvaginal ultrasound CL measurement compared to White counterparts in the United States (Haviland et al., 2016), which are examples of the many ways structural inequalities and racism impact perinatal care and outcomes, and have prevented health equity to date.

Pregnancy Dating in the Second Trimester

Pregnancy dating by ultrasound is best accomplished in the first trimester of pregnancy when the margin of error is smallest. A second-trimester ultrasound exam at 18–20 weeks of gestation with measurements of the head circumference,

Table 12.5   Fetal Anatomical Components and Measurements of a Standard Second-trimester Ultrasound Examination

Head and neck	Measurement of biparietal diameter and head circumference of fetal skull Lateral cerebral ventricles—the two largest of the four ventricles in the brain Choroid plexus (multi-lobed vascular structure in the pia mater that is part of the blood–brain barrier) Midline falx—the dura mater fold that dips inward between cerebral hemispheres Cavum septi pellucidi (CSP)—membrane separating the horns of the right and left lateral ventricles, filled with cerebral spinal fluid Cerebellum—located under cerebral hemispheres, controls motor function. Cistern magna—one of the three key openings in the subarachnoid space in the meninges surrounding the brain Upper lip to r/o clefting defects Facial profile and eye orbits Nuchal fold
Chest	Heart: Measure fetal heart rate, four-chamber view, right and left ventricular outflow tract Diaphragm: Intact
Abdomen	Measurement of abdominal circumference Stomach: Presence, size, location Kidneys Urinary bladder Umbilical cord: Cord vessel number, and integrity of fetal abdominal wall at insertion site
Spine	Examine full length: Cervical, thoracic, lumbar, sacral areas Examine skin and hair over spine
Extremities	Count 12 long bones Hands: Count fingers in open hand when possible, observe for movement Legs: Measure femur length, confirm presence of three long bones in each limb Feet: determine presence and shape of two and carrying angle to the tibia, assess and count toes, observe for movement
Genitalia	Presence or absence of penis, scrotum, descended testicles, or visualization of vulva, clitoris, labia, uterus, ovaries
Placenta	Assess localization and measure position relative to internal cervical os if proximate

Source: Adapted from ACOG (2020), AIUM (2018a), and AIUM (2021).

Table 12.6   Measurement of Amniotic Fluid

	Single deepest pocket	Amniotic fluid index
Oligohydramnios	<2 × 1 cm	<5 cm
Normal	>2 and <8 cm	AFI >5 and <24 cm
Polyhydramnios	>8 cm	>24 cm

biparietal diameter, abdominal circumference, and femur length has an accuracy of ±7–10 days (ACOG, 2022). See Chapter 10, *Pregnancy Diagnosis and Gestational Age Assessment,* for a further discussion of the role of ultrasound in establishing gestational age in pregnancy.

Amniotic Fluid Evaluation

Observation of the amniotic fluid level is an important second-trimester scan component. Amniotic fluid can be measured in a second-trimester exam either by using the **single deepest vertical pocket** (also known as the **maximum vertical pocket**) or with an **amniotic fluid index** (AFI). The AFI is obtained by dividing the gravid abdomen into four quadrants using the umbilicus and linea nigra if present, identifying and measuring the deepest pocket in each quadrant, and adding those four sums together for a cumulative result. Fluid pockets should each measure at least 2 × 1 cm to be included in the total AFI. Normal parameter for the **single deepest pocket** is at least 2 cm. The use of the single deepest pocket method results in fewer obstetric interventions without a significant difference in perinatal outcomes (Kehl et al., 2016; Nabhan & Abdelmoula, 2008). Table 12.6 provides standard descriptive measurements for amniotic fluid amounts.

Placental Localization

Placental localization is a key component of the second-trimester standard ultrasound exam. The exam and report should include the measurement of the distance between the lower placental edge and the cervical os. Normal placental location is 2 cm or more from the internal os.

Placental position early in pregnancy does not correlate well with location at the time of childbirth. In pregnancy less than 16 weeks of gestation, placenta previa is overdiagnosed (AIUM, 2018a). Previa and low-lying placentas must be confirmed by transvaginal ultrasound in the second trimester, and follow-up examinations will help to determine the evolving relationship between placenta and internal cervical os, placental edge thickness and architecture, and CL with implications for type and timing of delivery. The characteristics of these ultrasound features may help differentiate between pregnant persons who are at highest risk for developing symptoms and need closer monitoring versus asymptomatic expectant patients who can safely continue their pregnancies to term and anticipate a normal vaginal delivery (Vintzileos et al., 2015). After 16 weeks of gestation, ultrasound has a high negative

predictive value for placenta previa. Transvaginal scanning provides more accurate information and can be performed safely in the second trimester even in the presence of a true placenta previa. Abnormal placental implantation, such as placenta accreta or vasa previa, is evaluated whenever previa is found, especially if the maternal history includes cesarean birth.

Third-Trimester Ultrasound

Ultrasounds done in the third trimester are typically for follow-up or continued surveillance of findings from a previous ultrasound or when clinical findings indicate need for further investigation. Some of these conditions include bleeding, abdominal pain, fetal growth restriction, multiple gestation, and placental abnormalities. Ultrasound in the third trimester is also used for people with high-risk conditions as part of fetal surveillance methods, as with the BPP or assessment of amniotic fluid (Table 12.4). POC ultrasound is often used in the third trimester to gain specific and limited information, such as presenting part close to term or at the onset of labor. Similar to second-trimester fetal anatomy scans, there is no indication to perform routine third-trimester ultrasound in low-risk pregnancies, doing so has not improved perinatal outcomes studied to date. The balance of risks and benefits of routine ultrasound in advanced pregnancy may change with research on the latest noninvasive prenatal screening options and introduction of new technologies in the future. Presently, ultrasounds without specific indication performed in the third trimester may increase the likelihood of labor induction and lack demonstrable clinical benefit to parent or child (Bricker et al., 2015; Henrichs et al., 2019).

Soft Markers

Some ultrasound findings are considered variations of normal yet can indicate an increased risk for fetal aneuploidy particularly when multiple markers are present. **Soft markers** are typically identified on a standard second-trimester ultrasound, but may also be identified in the first trimester. Soft markers were first identified in the 1980s, and their use in pregnancy management has evolved. The most commonly studied soft markers of aneuploidy include a thickened nuchal fold, limb shortening, mild fetal pyelectasis, echogenic bowel, echogenic intracardiac focus, and choroid plexus cyst (Table 12.7). These soft markers are further evaluated utilizing a **likelihood ratio (LR)**. The LR is an assessment of how likely it is that the patient actually has the condition being tested compared to those who do not have the condition. A positive LR in the low range is generally considered to be nonsignificant especially if the soft marker is found in isolation. Individual soft markers vary in their degree of association with fetal aneuploidy and, thus, in their individual LR (Liu et al., 2021). The LR increases when more than one marker is identified. Other risk factors such as advanced maternal age, prior genetic history, and maternal serum screening results are considered in the overall risk

Table 12.7 Common Soft Marker Ultrasound Findings

Soft marker	Associations	Comments
Echogenic intracardiac focus	Fetal aneuploidy	Lower risk in isolation Seen as small bright spot
Mild renal pelvic dilation	Congenital hydronephrosis Fetal aneuploidy	Lower risk in isolation Neonatal follow-up to rule out congenital hydronephrosis
Single umbilical artery	Renal and cardiac anomalies	Lower risk in isolation Warrants detailed ultrasound evaluation of fetal kidneys and heart
Echogenic bowel	Fetal aneuploidy Cystic fibrosis Congenital infection Structural bowel defects	Higher risk in isolation Graded I, II, and III Grades II and III require further investigation
Thickened nuchal fold	Fetal aneuploidy Single gene disorders (Noonan's syndrome, skeletal dysplasia) Congenital heart disease	Higher risk in isolation Expert ultrasound review recommended Fetal karyotyping recommended
Mild cerebral ventriculomegaly	Abnormal neurodevelopment Congenital infection	Higher risk in isolation Expert ultrasound review recommended Fetal karyotyping recommended Neonatal follow-up recommended
Shortened humerus or femur	Fetal aneuploidy	Higher risk in isolation
Choroid plexus cysts	Fetal aneuploidy	Lower risk in isolation
Enlarged cistern magna	Trisomy 18 Dandy-Walker syndrome	Lower risk in isolation

Source: Adapted from Liu et al. (2021) and Society for Maternal-Fetal Medicine (2021).

evaluation. Caution must be used in interpretation since many soft markers are nonspecific and transient, especially when they are isolated findings.

The presence of one or more soft markers can indicate increased risk but is not diagnostic of fetal anomalies. Specialized ultrasound for the evaluation of soft markers coupled with maternal serum screenings can decrease the need for amniocentesis and fetal karyotyping particularly in pregnant persons with risk factors for aneuploidies.

Contemporary guidelines for perinatal care and fetal imaging recommend that ultrasound for genetic screening purposes should be *offered* to all pregnant people though health insurance may not cover all options (ACOG, 2016, 2022) and access inequities exist for disenfranchised communities. After receiving information on the benefits and limitations of the procedure, pregnant people who decline ultrasound screening should have their decision viewed through the lens of patient autonomy with documentation of the informed consent process and stated reasons for declining. This will improve patient care and coordination and may help guard against wrongful birth litigation.

Prenatal ultrasound examinations should always be presented as a choice rather than mandatory procedures. Education about the purposes, benefits, and limitations of ultrasound is not always provided to patients prior to scans as it should be (Vuorenlehto et al., 2021). Many

people approach the second-trimester ultrasound as a routine procedure that allows them to see the baby and confirm that all is well, rather than one that can reveal fetal anomalies (Skelton et al., 2022). Appropriate anticipatory guidance is, therefore, indicated to correct any misunderstandings and provide accurate information about what ultrasound exams do and do not assess, and the limits of the tool's diagnostic, much less prognostic, capability.

Research has demonstrated that the routine use of early ultrasound can improve early detection of multiple gestation and reduce the incidence of post-term pregnancy with improved accuracy of pregnancy dating, but routine scans in the second half of low-risk pregnancies do not improve perinatal outcomes overall (Bricker et al., 2015; Henrichs et al., 2019; Whitworth et al., 2015). Despite the lack of supportive evidence for routine scans as normal pregnancies progress, studies have shown that prenatal care providers and pregnant people may perceive prenatal care is inadequate if ultrasounds are not performed (Thomas et al., 2017), which necessitates appropriate health education for both patients and healthcare providers and shared clinical decision-making particularly since there are significant socioeconomic and geographical barriers to imaging during pregnancy for low-income persons and those living rurally (Adams, Yao et al., 2022; Adams, Burbridge, Chatterson, Babyn et al., 2022; Peterman et al., 2022). Simultaneously, ultrasound is a tool that may be overused in contemporary prenatal care for communities with many resources, and though used to provide reassurance, it has a limited ability to provide such reassurance, which must be disclosed during informed consent discussions beforehand.

Interpreting and Communicating Results

Prenatal healthcare providers often have the responsibility to review ultrasound results and reports and communicate them to parturients. Parameters for fetal biometry are evaluated utilizing a software system within the ultrasound machine. Biometric parameters are printed within the report and typically include basic interpretation by a radiologist, along with the listing and description of normal and abnormal findings. Reports are typically provided to the ordering provider who is responsible for communicating results to the patient, although this may have already been done at the time of imagining depending on the type of sonographer and clinical scenario. For example, a patient with an abnormal fetal anatomy scan may be informed of results if there is a radiologist or maternal-fetal medicine physician onsite to interpret findings when imaging is conducted. In other settings, sonologists take images and measurements to send for interpretation by supervising providers after the visit is over, who then communicate results to ordering clinicians if not also the patient directly. Effective communication is a critical component of diagnostic imaging. Systems are needed to ensure that ultrasound results are conveyed in a timely fashion to those responsible for treatment decisions. Effective methods of communication should promote timely and high-quality patient care and support the ordering healthcare provider in this endeavor while minimizing the risk of communication errors (AIUM, 2020). Pregnant persons should be informed of the process by which ultrasound results will be communicated prior to the exam. If prenatal ultrasound results are within normal limits, this is communicated to the pregnant person, and questions regarding the findings or experience of the ultrasound exam are reviewed. If discrepancies or abnormalities are noted among findings, such as in pregnancy dating or interval fetal growth, further information is collected which may include present and prior pregnancy history, additional data and documentation from the sonographer, and information on the interpretation provided by the reading physician. A plan for appropriate follow-up should be made and assistance given for scheduling, further counseling, and/or referral.

Abnormal results must be promptly shared with the pregnant person, preferably face to face by their prenatal care provider. A communication policy within a prenatal care practice and knowledge of the communication policy for the sonography service are both important components of optimizing care in difficult clinical situations. It may be the policy of the sonography service to not communicate with the patient directly concerning findings such as uncertain pregnancy viability and abnormal-

ities during the examination. Pregnant persons can experience significant anxiety and suffering while waiting for ultrasound reports and may be motivated to seek attention and answers from their provider. Sonographer training on how best to communicate bad news, policies of immediate notification of the healthcare provider, and an immediate patient visit with prompt communication regarding findings are effective strategies to facilitate supportive care (Tomlin et al., 2020). In a study of expectant parents who were informed of lethal findings on fetal ultrasound, the reported best interactions with care providers were with those perceived to be supportive and aligned in their interactions and goals with that of their patients' preferences and priorities (Denney-Koelsch et al., 2015).

The Experience of Prenatal Ultrasound

Most pregnant people view ultrasound as a positive experience (Øyen & Aune, 2016) and parental bonding can be accelerated in the short term after visualizing the fetus during an ultrasound (Jong-Pleij et al., 2013). For expectant fathers and partners, the ultrasound can be a confirmation of the pregnancy and can assist them in adjusting to becoming a parent (Skelton et al., 2022). Ultrasound is typically highly desired by the pregnant person because they want to see the baby and obtain reassurance of fetal health, and often to discover fetal sex (Øyen & Aune, 2016; Thomas et al., 2017).

In contrast, people seeking to terminate pregnancy may not wish to view the fetus during ultrasound exams and should not be compelled to do so. Mandatory ultrasound viewing may alter pregnant persons' perceptions of the fetus and decision about abortion in a coercive imposition of politics into the exam room, but actual effects appear to be minimal in studies of people already certain about the decision, contrary to the intentions of antiabortion lawmakers (Kimport et al., 2018; Kimport & Weitz, 2015; Upadhyay et al., 2017). The introduction of mandatory ultrasound viewing disproportionately affected Black women in Wisconsin, when it joined nine other states requiring it in 2013 (Upadhyay et al., 2017). Mandatory ultrasounds do not improve the safety of medication abortion in the first trimester, and professional organizations do not endorse mandated ultrasound exams without clinical indication or mandated viewing for any pregnant person (ACOG, 2022; Upadhyay et al., 2017).

Most people report transvaginal ultrasound feels similar to a vaginal exam with minimal discomfort during the procedure (Deed et al., 2014) that may include sensations of cold (from the transducer gel) and pressure. Anecdotal reports regarding patient maltreatment during ultrasound examination include stories of bruising, residual soreness, and transient cramping after abdominal ultrasound; however, this phenomenon has not been studied. Disrespectful care to childbearing individuals occurs often enough that it has been described as a global epidemic (Miller & Lalonde, 2015). Providers should seek feedback from clients on their ultrasound experiences and follow-up with due diligence and due process when complaints are reported.

The experience of receiving an ultrasound begins with education from the healthcare provider on the indication for the exam, what information can be gained, limits to that information, and any risks to the procedure. The pregnant person's expectations and understanding of the purpose of the ultrasound examination should be explored. Research indicates that expectant parents are often unaware of the possibility of adverse ultrasound findings, including soft markers for anomalies that may be detected (Øyen & Aune, 2016). Studies have found that women who received false-positive findings of a soft marker on ultrasound have higher rates of postpartum depression and anxiety, and deficits in knowledge with potential implications for parent–infant interactions (de Souza et al., 2022; Viaux-Savelon et al., 2012). These data reveal that screening ultrasounds are not entirely benign procedures and highlight the importance of informed consent, which requires a balanced discussion about what the sonographer will be looking for, can and cannot see, and what findings may indicate about risk versus definitive diagnosis of fetal anomalies, to ensure the full understanding of the choice to undergo or decline ultrasound examination.

The possibility of a misdiagnosis and the concept of a screening versus diagnostic test and thus possible limitations of the exam also should be reviewed. It is a common belief that a "normal" ultrasound report is a statement of 100% health for their baby. While a number of fetal anomalies can be recognized by ultrasound, approximately half of defects remain undetected (Rydberg & Tunon, 2017). Some patients can feel pressured to have an ultrasound they do not want, as it has become a routine and expected procedure regardless of risk status (Øyen & Aune, 2016). It should be noted that for people with uncomplicated pregnancies, an ultrasound is not a necessary aspect of prenatal care or one which has been demonstrated to optimize perinatal outcomes, unless there is a specific indication for imaging (Bricker et al., 2015; Henrichs et al., 2019). The pregnant person's concerns need to be voiced and their autonomy respected, and it is always their right to accept or decline sonography whether it is medically indicated or not. It may be hard to convey the absence of clinical rationale for routine or repeated ultrasound exams to expectant parents, as they are likely excited to view their developing fetus and aware of pregnant peers receiving multiple ultrasounds in other care settings.

The widespread use of ultrasound in prenatal care has increased possibilities to monitor and diagnose fetal conditions and risks prioritizing fetal considerations over the health interests and priorities of the pregnant person. Research has elucidated obstetricians' views on prenatal ultrasound and their reports that imaging creates an early sense of the fetus as a distinct patient with increased attention paid to the fetus as gestational age advances, and in situations where parental and fetal health interests seem to conflict or are uncertain (Edvardsson et al., 2015; Moncrieff et al., 2021). These recent research findings are aligned with sentinel anthropological research on the impact of ultrasound technology, when it was a new innovation, which first allowed the fetus to be viewed as a separate entity from its parent. This capability accelerated a dramatic shift away from historical cultural perspectives of the fetus and pregnant person as one interconnected being until the newborn was ascribed personhood at birth or at a later survival date or an event such as religious ceremony (Davis-Floyd, 2003; Davis-Floyd & Sargent, 1997).

Research identifies additional financial considerations in the experience of prenatal ultrasound related to time and travel in addition to the cost of the procedure. There are significant barriers to ultrasound assessments for low-income pregnant persons and those in rural locations (Adams, Burbridge, Chatterson, Babyn, et al., 2022; Adams, Yao, et al., 2022; Peterman et al., 2022), given consolidated services and prenatal ultrasound cost of $150–$1500 depending on patient share and whether the provider is in-network. Informed consent must include the knowledge of insurance coverage to ensure accurate expectations of ultrasound exams and health plan benefits.

Patient Education

Anticipatory guidance and health education are necessary when ordering exam to help ensure informed consent and the best possible experience of prenatal ultrasound. Patient education best begins with a review of the pregnant person's knowledge base regarding ultrasound, with education provided from this foundation, and misconceptions identified and explained. Important teaching points should be adapted to meet the needs of the individual and their family. When an ultrasound exam is ordered for further evaluation of abnormal signs and symptoms, gentle preparation about the potential for bad news is best initiated by the ordering provider. A plan for follow-up regardless of exam findings can reduce patient anxiety.

Prenatal ultrasound teaching points

- Purpose of the examination and its limitations
- How and where the examination will be done
- Exploration of financial considerations for the exam
- Preparation for the exam: two-piece, loose clothing, potential need to fill the bladder
- Who will perform the ultrasound and if that person can provide information on results during the examination or not
- Qualifications of the sonographer for a specialized exam
- Anticipated and potential results, with an explanation of potential further plan of care
- Acknowledgment that ultrasound does not detect all abnormal fetal conditions; thus, a normal ultrasound report is not a guarantee of fetal/neonatal health status
- Method and anticipated time of communicating results
- Choices for genetic screening ultrasound with or without other forms of prenatal assessment for fetal anomalies
- Right to view the screen and to have a chaperone present during exam

Safety

With over 50 years of use of ultrasound in pregnancy care and considerable research, ultrasound is considered a safe procedure with no reliable evidence of human harm or damage from physical effect of diagnostic ultrasound. However, experts acknowledge that there is a limit to what is known about long-term effects of ultrasound. Theoretical concerns of possible harm from are twofold: mechanical and thermal effects. Mechanical vibrations are propagated through tissue, creating a potential impact from physical forces generated by the ultrasound waves, such as radiation, streaming, free radicals, and cavitation (Abramowicz, 2013; Sande et al., 2021). **Cavitation** refers to the potential for ultrasound to mechanically create or disturb gas bubbles which may then expand or collapse, affecting nearby tissue in unknown ways. Cavitation is more likely with low frequencies, long pulses, and high negative pressures, which are all avoided in prenatal ultrasound exams.

The second main ultrasound concern is regarding thermal energy generated with sound waves. Tissue is exposed to ultrasound waves, which produce heat. A low risk of thermal or mechanical effect is seen with a thermal index (TI) or mechanical index (MI) value of less than 1. As a safeguard, if an ultrasound machine is capable of producing output levels of greater than 1, then either the TI or MI must be displayed on the screen and monitored by the operator. If an ultrasound machine does not have such a display screen, the equipment has its own inner safeguard and will not operate if the safe TI or MI are exceeded. The recognition of potential harm is expressed in guidelines issued by expert groups mandating use of the lowest possible ultrasonic exposure setting to gain the necessary diagnostic information under the "**as low as reasonably achievable**" or **ALARA principle**. This is accomplished in practice by using the lowest power, least amount of time, use of power or color Doppler only when medically necessary, not using pulsed Doppler unless medically necessary (this imaging creates the most energy), and keeping TI less than or equal to 1.

Although most studies have not shown adverse clinical outcomes from ultrasound exposure, a current concern is that modern machines have substantially higher output potential than machines used when most of the safety studies were performed. In 1992, the US Food and Drug Administration (FDA) increased the upper limit for permissible output of ultrasound machines almost eightfold (94–720 mW/cm² in obstetric ultrasound) (Menihan & Kopel, 2014). Additionally, the output display standard was created by the AIUM and the National Electrical Manufacturers Association as a safety measure when performing prenatal ultrasound examination with increasingly powerful machines. Thus, the responsibility of ensuring safety during an ultrasound examination was placed on the user. However, studies have shown that clinicians performing obstetric ultrasound are largely unaware of the output display standard and do not routinely monitor or adjust this in practice (Sheiner & Abramowicz, 2008).

Current research results on long-term effects of ultrasound reflect routine care practices 15–25 years ago. Prenatal ultrasound has increased in intensity, use, and exposure, with many people receiving multiple scans in one pregnancy (You et al., 2010). While animal studies have documented neurobehavioral deficits and physiologic brain changes related to ultrasound, no independent, peer-reviewed human research has confirmed a cause-and-effect relationship with prenatal ultrasound exposure. Epidemiologic studies and professional organizations support the safety of diagnostic ultrasound use during pregnancy. While considered generally safe, recent FDA statements regarding the use of prenatal diagnostic ultrasound, as well as ongoing attention in the scientific literature, continue to stress its conservative use for indicated purposes (ACNM, 2018; ACOG, 2021; AIUM, 2018a; USFDA, 2020).

Overuse of Ultrasound

The use of ultrasound has significantly increased over time as the indications for use have evolved into an expected and routine part of maternity care. A study examining ultrasound use in a low-risk pregnant population found a mean of 4.2 ultrasounds per pregnancy (Harris et al., 2015), while the most recent *Listening to Mothers III* survey found the proportion of pregnant persons who had five or more ultrasounds increased from 23% in 2005 to 34% in 2012 (Declercq et al., 2013). Childbearing families often wait with anticipation for an ultrasound examination to reveal fetal sex. The healthcare provider can feel caught between the pregnant person's expectations or desires for ultrasound and actual medical indications for ultrasound imaging, with marketing and financial considerations among other conflicting factors, which could result in an ethical dilemma. Adequate information regarding the medical indications for ultrasound and a trusting provider–patient relationship can help inform expectations about appropriate prenatal application of ultrasound technology and avoidance of nonmedical scans done for entertainment and bonding purposes.

Recreational Prenatal Ultrasound

Commercial enterprise has developed around the recreational application of prenatal ultrasound. "Keepsake" ultrasound pictures and videos are offered in shopping malls, private homes, professional studios, and even popup shops in hotel rooms (Roberts et al., 2015). These images are marketed as early baby pictures for the family photo albums, to share with family and friends, post on social media, and promote bonding with the fetus. The FDA, along with a number of professional obstetric and sonographic organizations, have issued warnings against use of ultrasound for nonmedical purposes (USFDA, 2014, 2020). The implementation and/or maintenance of technical safeguards, operator training, qualifications, expertise, standards for infection control, and competency are not ensured. As a result, fetal energy exposure may not be appropriately monitored, and operators of the equipment may not be adequately trained to recognize fetal and placental abnormalities that may adversely affect fetal and maternal outcomes. Some exposure times can exceed one hour as video is captured, violating the principles of ALARA (AIUM, 2018a; USFDA, 2020).

Other potential harms include false-positive diagnoses, leading to unnecessary investigations and anxiety; false reassurance to the expectant parent that everything is "normal," and physical harm if unsafe levels of abdominal pressure and fetal maneuvering are used to obtain a suitable commercial product. In addition, the FDA cautions that those who subject patients to ultrasound exposure using a diagnostic ultrasound device without a healthcare provider's order may be in the violation of state or local laws or regulations regarding the use of a prescription medical device. These recommendations have been endorsed nationally and internationally by government agencies and professional medical and sonographic organizations (AIUM, 2018a; USFDA, 2014).

Who Performs Prenatal Ultrasounds

Standards and systematic training with prenatal ultrasound certification are recommended to ensure that the screening and diagnostic tool is used correctly. Additionally, it is important for the healthcare provider ordering exams to know the credentials of ultrasound providers they utilize for their patients. Lack of proper training in the performance or interpretation of ultrasound increases the risk of a missed or incorrect diagnosis and potential incorrect management as a result.

Standard and specialized exams should be performed by experienced sonographers who have completed training and are registered, carrying the initials **Registered Diagnostic Medical Sonographer** (RDMS) after national certification through the **American Registry for Diagnostic Medical Sonography** (ARDMS). Additional certifications are recommended for specific procedures such as NT and CL measurements, which are available through the Fetal Medicine Foundation (FMF) and the Perinatal Quality Foundation (PQF) for healthcare providers performing or reading these measurements.

Adding Ultrasound to Scope of Practice

A range of healthcare providers are eligible to expand their scope of practice to include POC ultrasound, and national certification in prenatal ultrasound is available to certified midwives and nurse-midwives, women's health nurse practitioners, and physician's assistants (AIUM, 2018a). Clinical guidelines for prenatal ultrasound are provided by national organizations including American College of Nurse-Midwives (ACNM), ACOG, Association of Women's Health and Neonatal Nurses (AWHONN), and Society for Maternal-Fetal Medicine (SMFM), and include documentation of didactic and clinical education with supervised skill performance. Courses in limited prenatal sonography

are available from a number of programs throughout the United States. The ACNM and the American Registry for Diagnostic Medical Sonography have established a national certification exam specifically for certified nurse-midwives and certified midwives in the United States. The scope of professional practice defined by the state professional body regulations and healthcare institutions outline additional parameters for who may perform prenatal ultrasound examinations with sufficient and verified training in specific settings.

Adding ultrasound to American Midwifery Certification Board-certified midwife or nurse-midwife practice

1. Study the 2018 ACNM Position Statement "Ultrasound in Midwifery Practice."
2. Investigate the Nurse Practice Act for your state of practice, the hospital or group policy, and practice guidelines.
3. Complete necessary didactic and clinical training and experience.
4. Document a check-off of skills demonstrating competency.

Summary

Prenatal ultrasound is a helpful skill for clinicians who work with pregnant persons, and POC limited obstetrical ultrasound can help to address disparities in access to standard imaging, as well as perinatal outcomes, for socioeconomically disenfranchised and rural communities, and pregnant persons of color. Perinatal healthcare providers can develop ultrasound exam skills through postgraduate education programs as specified by their professional organizations, regulation by their state practice acts, employers' policies and procedures, and requirements for ARDMS certification if applicable. First-trimester ultrasound is recommended for accurate pregnancy dating as well as confirming fetal viability, number, and location. This type of limited obstetrical scan is commonly provided during routine early prenatal care, with a more detailed and formal ultrasound assessment of fetal anatomy in the second trimester. The fetal anatomy ultrasound performed at approximately 20 weeks of gestation is a common experience in contemporary prenatal care, though research does not support any improvement in outcomes in normal pregnancy for healthy persons. Similarly, existing data do not support routine ultrasound in the third trimester.

Research is ongoing to identify the optimal number and timing of prenatal scans based on the preexisting risk and current health status of the pregnant person, and results from any pregnancy genetic or carrier screening performed. Additionally, new methods of prenatal imaging are being explored, for example, telerobotic prenatal ultrasound screening with potential to expand access to underserved communities, and possible utility in cases where infectious disease is present (Adams, Burbridge, Chatterson, McKinney, et al., 2022). This research should be accompanied by careful consideration of impact on perceptions of the fetus and parenthood, the experience of undergoing prenatal imaging, and effectiveness and cost comparison with other perinatal care practices.

Resources for Clients and their Families

- United States Food and Drug Administration
  - Ultrasound Imaging https://www.fda.gov/radiation-emitting-products/medical-imaging/ultrasound-imaging

Resources for Healthcare Providers

- American College of Nurse-Midwives
  Information about adding sonography to clinical midwifery practice: http://www.midwife.org/Midwife-Sonography-Certification
- American College of Obstetricians and Gynecologists
  - Clinical guidelines for obstetricians
  - ACOG Ultrasound FAQs for patients: https://www.acog.org/womens-health/faqs/ultrasound-exams#:~:text=It%20allows%20your%20obstetrician%2Dgynecologist,to%20help%20guide%20these%20procedures
- American Institute for Ultrasound in Medicine
  Guidelines for training, performance and documentation of ultrasounds https://www.aium.org/resources/guidelines.aspx
- American Registry for Diagnostic Medical Sonography (ARDMS)
  - Training and certification as sonographer
  - Ob/Gyn certification: https://www.ardms.org/get-certified/rdms/obstetrics-gynecology
  - Midwife Sonography certificate: https://www.ardms.org/get-certified/midwifery
- Association of Women's Health and Neonatal Nurses (AWHONN)
  - Guidelines: Ultrasound examinations performed by nurses in obstetric, gynecologic and reproductive medicine settings: Clinical competencies and education guide, 4th Edition: https://my.awhonn.org/productdetails?id=a1B2E000008LOXfUAO

References

Abramowicz, J. S. (2013). Benefits and risks of ultrasound in pregnancy. *Seminars in Perinatology, 37*(5), 295–300. https://doi.org/10.1053/j.semperi.2013.06.004

Adams, S., Burbridge, B., Chatterson, L., McKinney, V., Babyn, P., & Mendez, I. (2022). Telerobotic ultrasound to provide obstetrical ultrasound services remotely during the COVID-19 pandemic. *Journal of Telemedicine Telecare, 28*(8), 568–576.

Adams, S., Yao, S., Mondal, P., Lim, H., Mendez, I., & Babyn, P. (2022). Sociodemographic and geographic disparities in obstetrical ultrasound imaging utilization: A population-based study. *Academic Radiology, 29*(5), 650–662.

Adams, S. J., Burbridge, B., Chatterson, L., Babyn, P., & Mendez, I. (2022). A telerobotic ultrasound clinic model of ultrasound service delivery to improve access to imaging in rural and remote communities. *Journal of the American College of Radiology, 19*(1 Pt B), 162–171.

American College of Nurse-Midwives (ACNM). (2018). *Ultrasound in midwifery practice.* http://www.midwife.org/acnm/files/acnmlibrarydata/uploadfilename/000000000318/Ultrasound-in-Midwifery-Practice-FINAL-11-24-18.pdf

American College of Obstetricians and Gynecologists (ACOG). (2016). Practice bulletin number 175. Ultrasound in pregnancy. *Obstetrics & Gynecology, 128*, e241–e256.

American College of Obstetricians and Gynecologists (ACOG). (2020). Committee opinion number 815. Increasing access to abortion. *Obstetrics & Gynecology, 136*, e107–e115.

American College of Obstetricians and Gynecologists (ACOG). (2021). Committee opinion number 723. Guidelines for diagnostic imaging during pregnancy and lactation. *Obstetrics & Gynecology, 130*, e210–e216.

American College of Obstetricians and Gynecologists (ACOG). (2022). Committee opinion number 700. Method for estimating the due date. *Obstetrics & Gynecology, 129*, e150–e154.

American Institute of Ultrasound in Medicine (AIUM). (2018a). AIUM-ACR-ACOG-SMFM-SRU practice parameter for the performance of standard diagnostic obstetric ultrasound examinations. *Journal of Ultrasound Medicine, 37*, E13–E24. https://doi.org/10.1002/jum.14831

American Institute of Ultrasound in Medicine (AIUM). (2018b). *Training guidelines for advanced clinical providers in women's health performing and interpreting limited obstetric ultrasound.* https://www.aium.org/officialStatements/70

American Institute of Ultrasound in Medicine (AIUM). (2020). AIUM practice parameter for documentation of an ultrasound examination. *Journal of Ultrasound Medicine, 39*, E1–E4.

American Institute of Ultrasound in Medicine (AIUM). (2021). Practice parameter for the performance of detailed diagnostic obstetric ultrasound examinations between 12 weeks 0 days and 13 weeks 6 days. *Journal of Ultrasound Medicine, 40*, E1–E16. https://doi.org/10.1002/jum.15477

Bardi, F., Smith, E., Kuilman, M., Snijders, R. J. M., & Bilardo, C. M. (2019). Early detection of structural anomalies in a primary care setting in the Netherlands. *Fetal Diagnosis & Therapy, 46*, 12–19. https://doi.org/10.1159/000490723

Bricker, L., Medley, N., & Pratt, J. J. (2015). Routine ultrasound in late pregnancy (after 24 weeks' gestation). *The Cochrane Database of Systematic Reviews, 6*, CD001451. https://doi.org/10.1002/14651858.CD001451.pub4

Chudleigh, T., Smith, A., & Cumming, S. (2017). *Obstetric & gynaecological ultrasound how, why and when.* Elsevier Health Sciences.

Davis-Floyd, R., & Sargent, C. F. (1997). *Childbirth and authoritative knowledge: Cross-cultural perspectives.* University of California Press.

Davis-Floyd, R. E. (2003). *Birth as an American rite of passage* (2nd ed.). University of California Press.

de Souza, V., Parlato-Oliveira, E., Anchieta, L. M., Machado, A., & Savelon, S. V. (2022). The effects of prenatal diagnosis on the interaction of the mother-infant dyad: A longitudinal study of prenatal care in the first year of life. *Frontiers in Psychology, 13*, 804724. https://doi.org/10.3389/fpsyg.2022.804724

Declercq, E.R., Sakala, C., Corry, M.P., Applebaum, S. & Herrlich, A. (2013). *Listening to MothersSM III: Pregnancy and birth.* Childbirth Connection https://www.nationalpartnership.org/our-work/resources/health-care/maternity/listening-to-mothers-iii-pregnancy-and-birth-2013.pdf

Deed, K., Childs, J., & Thoirs, K. (2014). What are the perceptions of women towards transvaginal sonographic examinations? *Sonography, 1*(2), 33–38.

Denney-Koelsch, E. M., Côté-Arsenault, D., & Lemcke-Berno, E. (2015). Parents' experiences with ultrasound during pregnancy with a lethal fetal diagnosis. *Global Qualitative Nursing Research, 2*, 2333393615587888.

Doubilet, P. M., Benson, C. B., Bourne, T., Blaivas, M., Society of Radiologists in Ultrasound Multispecialty Panel on Early First Trimester

Diagnosis of Miscarriage and Exclusion of a Viable Intrauterine Pregnancy, Barnhart, K. T., Benacerraf, B. R., Brown, D. L., Filly, R. A., Fox, J. C., Goldstein, S. R., Kendall, J. L., Lyons, E. A., Porter, M. B., Pretorius, D. H., & Timor-Tritsch, I. E. (2013). Diagnostic criteria for nonviable pregnancy early in the first trimester. *The New England Journal of Medicine*, 369(15), 1443–1451. https://doi.org/10.1056/NEJMra1302417

Edvardsson, K., Small, R., Lalos, A., Persson, M., & Mogren, I. (2015). Ultrasound's 'window on the womb' brings ethical challenges for balancing maternal and fetal health interests: Obstetricians' experiences in Australia. *BMC Medical Ethics*, 16(1), 1–10.

Harris, J. M., Franck, L., Green, B., Wilson, S., & Michie, S. (2015). The relationship between frequency of obstetric ultrasound scans and birthplace preference—A case control study. *Midwifery*, 31(1), 31–36.

Haviland, M. J., Shainker, S. A., Hacker, M. R., & Burris, H. H. (2016). Racial and ethnic disparities in universal cervical length screening with transvaginal ultrasound. *The Journal of Maternal-Fetal & Neonatal Medicine*, 29(24), 4078–4081.

Henrichs, J., Verfaille, V., Jellema, P., Viester, L., Pajkrt, E., Wilschut, J., van der Horst, H. E., Franx, A., de Jonge, A., & IRIS study group. (2019). Effectiveness of routine third trimester ultrasonography to reduce adverse perinatal outcomes in low risk pregnancy (the IRIS study): Nationwide, pragmatic, multicentre, stepped wedge cluster randomised trial. *BMJ (Clinical Research Ed.)*, 367, l5517.

Jong-Pleij, E. A. P., Ribbert, L. S. M., Pistorius, L. R., Tromp, E., Mulder, E. J. H., & Bilardo, C. M. (2013). Three-dimensional ultrasound and maternal bonding, a third trimester study and a review. *Prenatal Diagnosis*, 33(1), 81–88.

Kehl, S., Schelkle, A., Thomas, A., Puhl, A., Meqdad, K., Tuschy, B., Berlit, S., Weiss, C., Bayer, C., Heimrich, J., Dammer, U., Raabe, E., Winkler, M., Faschingbauer, F., Beckmann, M. W., & Sütterlin, M. (2016). Single deepest vertical pocket or amniotic fluid index as evaluation test for predicting adverse pregnancy outcome (SAFE trial): A multicentre, open-label, randomized controlled trial. *Ultrasound in Obstetrics & Gynecology*, 47(6), 674–679. https://doi.org/10.1002/uog.14924

Kimport, K., Johns, N., & Upadhyay, U. (2018). Coercing women's behavior: How a mandatory viewing law changes patients' preabortion ultrasound viewing practices. *Journal of Health Politics, Policy & Law*, 43(6), 941–960.

Kimport, K., & Weitz, T. A. (2015). Constructing the meaning of ultrasound viewing in abortion care. *Sociology of Health and Illness*, 37(6), 856–869.

Liu, Y., Jing, X., Xing, L., Liu, S., Liu, J., Cheng, J., Deng, C., Bai, T., Xia, T., Wei, X., Luo, Y., Zhou, Q., Zhu, Q., & Liu, H. (2021). Noninvasive prenatal screening based on second-trimester ultrasonographic soft markers in low-risk pregnant women. *Frontiers in Genetics*, 12, 793894. https://doi.org/10.3389/fgene.2021.793894

Menihan, C. A., & Kopel, E. (2014). *Point-of-care assessment in pregnancy and women's health: Electronic fetal monitoring and sonography*. Lippincott Williams & Wilkins.

Miller, S., & Lalonde, A. (2015). The global epidemic of abuse and disrespect during childbirth: History, evidence, interventions, and FIGO's mother–baby friendly birthing facilities initiative. *International Journal of Gynecology & Obstetrics*, 131, S49–S52.

Moncrieff, G., Finlayson, K., Cordey, S., McCrimmon, R., Harris, C., Barreix, M., Tunçalp, Ö., & Downe, S. (2021). First and second trimester ultrasound in pregnancy: A systematic review and metasynthesis of the views and experiences of pregnant women, partners, and health workers. *PLoS One*, 16(12), e0261096. https://doi.org/10.1371/journal.pone.0261096

Nabhan, A. F., & Abdelmoula, Y. A. (2008). Amniotic fluid index versus single deepest vertical pocket as a screening test for preventing adverse pregnancy outcome. *Cochrane Database of Systematic Review 2008*, 3, CD006593.

Øyen, L., & Aune, I. (2016). Viewing the unborn child-pregnant women's expectations, attitudes and experiences regarding fetal ultrasound examination. *Sexual & Reproductive Healthcare*, 7, 8–13.

Peterman, N. J., Yeo, E., Kaptur, B., Smith, E. J., Christensen, A., Huang, E., & Rasheed, M. (2022). Analysis of rural disparities in ultrasound access. *Cureus*, 14(5), e25425.

Roberts, J., Griffiths, F. E., Verran, A., & Ayre, C. (2015). Why do women seek ultrasound scans from commercial providers during pregnancy? *Sociology of Health & Illness*, 37(4), 594–609.

Rydberg, C., & Tunon, K. (2017). Detection of fetal abnormalities by second-trimester ultrasound screening in a non-selected population. *Acta Obstetricia et Gynecologica Scandinavica*, 96(2), 176–182.

Sande, R., Jenderka, K. V., Moran, C. M., Marques, S., Jimenez Diaz, J. F., Ter Haar, G., Marsal, K., Lees, C., Abramowicz, J. S., Salvesen, K. Å., Miloro, P., Dall'Asta, A., Brezinka, C., & Kollmann, C. (2021). Safety aspects of perinatal ultrasound. *European Journal of Ultrasound*, 42(6), 580–598. https://doi.org/10.1055/a-1538-6295

Sheiner, E., & Abramowicz, J. S. (2008). Clinical end users worldwide show poor knowledge regarding safety issues of ultrasound during pregnancy. *Journal of Ultrasound in Medicine*, 27(4), 499–501. https://doi.org/10.7863/jum.2008.27.4.499

Skelton, E., Webb, R., Malamateniou, C., Rutherford, M., & Ayers, S. (2022). The impact of antenatal imaging on parent experience and prenatal attachment: A systematic review. *Journal of Reproductive and Infant Psychology*. https://doi.org/10.1080/02646838.2022.2088710

Society for Maternal-Fetal Medicine. (2021). SMFM consult series #57: Evaluation and management of isolated soft ultrasound markers for aneuploidy in the second trimester. *American Journal of Obstetrics & Gynecology*, 225(4), B2–B15.

Thomas, G. M., Roberts, J., & Griffiths, F. E. (2017). Ultrasound as a technology of reassurance? How pregnant women and health care professionals articulate ultrasound reassurance and its limitations. *Sociology of Health & Illness*, 39(6), 893–907.

Tomlin, L., Parsons, M., Kumar, P. V., Arezina, J., Harrison, R., & Johnson, J. (2020). Learning how to deliver bad and challenging news: Exploring the experience of trainee sonographers—A qualitative study. *Ultrasound*, 28(1), 30–37. https://doi.org/10.1177/1742271X19876087

United States (US) Food and Drug Administration (FDA). (2020, September 28). *Ultrasound imaging*. https://www.fda.gov/radiation-emitting-products/medical-imaging/ultrasound-imaging

Upadhyay, U. D., Kimport, K., Belusa, E., Johns, N. E., Laube, D. W., & Roberts, S. (2017). Evaluating the impact of a mandatory preabortion ultrasound viewing law: A mixed methods study. *PLoS One*, 12(7), e0178871.

US FDA. (2014, December 16) *Avoid fetal "keepsake" images, heartbeat monitors*. https://www.fda.gov/consumers/consumer-updates/avoid-fetal-keepsake-images-heartbeat-monitors

Viaux-Savelon, S., Dommergues, M., Rosenblum, O., Bodeau, N., Aidane, E., Philippon, O., & Cohen, D. (2012). Prenatal ultrasound screening: False positive soft markers may alter maternal representations and mother-infant interaction. *PLoS One*, 7(1), e30935.

Vintzileos, A. M., Ananth, C. V., & Smulian, J. C. (2015). Using ultrasound in the clinical management of placental implantation abnormalities. *American Journal of Obstetrics and Gynecology*, 213(4), S70–S77.

Vuorenlehto, L., Hinnelä, K., Äyräs, O., Ulander, V. M., Louhiala, P., & Kaijomaa, M. (2021). Women's experiences of counselling in cases of a screen-positive prenatal screening result. *PLoS One*, 16(3), e0247164. https://doi.org/10.1371/journal.pone.0247164

Whitworth, M., Bricker, L., & Mullan, C. (2015). Ultrasound for fetal assessment in early pregnancy. *The Cochrane Database of Systematic Reviews*, 2015(7), CD007058. https://doi.org/10.1002/14651858.CD007058.pub3

You, J. J., Alter, D. A., Stukel, T. A., McDonald, S. D., Laupacis, A., Liu, Y., & Ray, J. G. (2010). Proliferation of prenatal ultrasonography. *Canadian Medical Association Journal*, 182(2), 143–151.

13

Genetic Counseling, Screening, and Diagnosis

Aishwarya Arjunan and Susan Hancock

The editors gratefully acknowledge Robin G. Jordan, who was the author of the previous edition of this chapter.

Relevant Terms

Alpha-fetoprotein (AFP)—plasma protein produced by the fetus and measured in maternal serum as a marker for risk of neural tube defects

Aneuploidy—one or more missing or extra chromosomes leading to an unbalanced number of chromosomes within a cell; the second most common cause of chromosomal abnormalities

Autosomal dominant disorder—a condition or disease caused by an individual having a mutation on one copy of a particular gene

Autosomal recessive disorder—a condition or disease caused by an individual having mutations on each copy (i.e., two mutations) of a particular gene. Generally, the mutations are inherited from the parents and/or donors.

Cell-free DNA—extracellular DNA that is present in the blood because of cell degradation. Cell-free DNA originating from the placenta enables noninvasive prenatal screening (NIPS) to screen for fetal chromosome differences.

Confined placental mosaicism—a mosaic abnormality in the placental tissue but not in the fetus; can increase risk for pregnancy complications and loss

Consanguinity—the characteristic of being descended from the same ancestor as another person

Detection rate—percentage of those actually affected and called "screen positive" by the test/screen, often used synonymously with sensitivity

False negative rate—the percentage of individuals *with* a particular disease, condition or mutation that *are not* detected by a screening test (false negative rate = 1 − sensitivity)

False positive rate—the percentage of individuals *without* a particular disease, condition, or mutation who *are* identified as having a condition, disease or mutation by a screening test (false positive rate = 1 − specificity)

Fetal fraction—the amount of cell-free DNA in the maternal blood that is of placental origin, the basis of noninvasive prenatal screening

Karyotype—the chromosomal makeup of an individual, typically made up of 46 chromosomes arranged in 23 pairs

Monogenic—disease or conditions caused by mutations in a single gene

Mosaicism—a condition in which cells within the same person have a different genetic makeup, caused by an error in cell division or a gene mutation in the gamete or embryo: some cells will have the mutation, some will not; can result in a minor difference (a person's eyes are different colors) or more significant syndromes

Negative predictive value (NPV)—the chance that an individual with a negative screening result is truly negative and does not have a specific disease, mutation or condition. NPV is determined by sensitivity, specificity, and prevalence of the condition

Neural tube defects—birth defect of the spinal cord, spine, or brain; categorized as either **open**, where the brain and/or spinal cord are exposed through an opening in the skull or vertebrae, or **closed,** where the defect is covered by skin

No call—when cell-free DNA testing results are not reported, indeterminate, or unable to be interpreted; can indicate a higher risk for aneuploidy in some individuals

Nuchal translucency—ultrasound measurement of the fetal neck; used in the screening for Down syndrome and other conditions

Positive predictive value (PPV)—percentage of individuals with a positive screening test that actually have the disease, mutation, or condition; PPV is determined by sensitivity, specificity, and prevalence of the condition

Prenatal diagnosis—making a certain diagnosis of a genetic condition or birth defect prior to birth

Prenatal genetic screening—evaluations that identify fetuses at risk for genetic conditions or birth defects prior to birth

Residual risk—the remaining risk of having a particular disease, condition, or mutation following a negative screening result

Sensitivity—ability of a screening test to correctly identify individuals who have the disease or condition. The higher the test sensitivity, the more likely it is to correctly identify those who DO have the disease or condition

Specificity—ability of a screening test to correctly identify individuals who do not have the disease or condition. The higher the test specificity, the more likely it is to

---

Prenatal and Postnatal Care: A Person-Centered Approach, Third Edition. Edited by Karen Trister Grace, Cindy L. Farley, Noelene K. Jeffers, and Tanya Tringali.
© 2024 John Wiley & Sons Ltd. Published 2024 by John Wiley & Sons Ltd.
Companion website: www.wiley.com/go/grace/prenatal

correctly identify those who do NOT have the disease or condition

Spina bifida occulta—the mildest form of neural tube defects, a gap in between one or more vertebrae

Trisomy 13—an extra copy of chromosome 13 is present in each cell; also known as Patau syndrome

Trisomy 18—an extra copy of chromosome 18 is present in each cell; also known as Edwards syndrome

Trisomy 21—an extra copy of chromosome 21 is present in each cell; also known as Down syndrome

X-linked—a condition or disease caused by a mutation on one or both copies of a gene located on the X chromosome(s)

Introduction

Over the past four decades, there have been major advances in the science of genetics and the application of this knowledge to **prenatal screening** and testing during pregnancy. The option of screening for and diagnosing genetic disorders and birth defects during pregnancy has become an integral part of prenatal care. Genetic screening ideally begins in preconception with a comprehensive family history discussion and the consideration of laboratory tests such as carrier screening. Additional screening is typically discussed and offered at the first prenatal visit and later in pregnancy screening is offered for certain fetal conditions such as **neural tube defects** (NTDs) and trisomies 13, 18, and 21. The baseline risk of some types of birth defects is approximately 3% of all births, with higher risk for those with selected risk factors, such as family history or increased maternal age. Birth defects are the leading cause of infant death in the United States. Genetic screening and testing allow pregnant individuals and families to know their risk of a genetic disorder or birth defect and to make decisions regarding pregnancy that are best for them. According to the American College of Obstetricians and Gynecologists (ACOG), *prenatal genetic testing should be based on individual values and preferences with pretest counseling to facilitate informed decision-making. Counseling should be performed in a clear, objective, and nondirective fashion, allowing patients sufficient time to understand and make informed decisions regarding testing* (American College of Obstetricians and Gynecologists [ACOG], 2017b).

This chapter reviews genetic screening using the personal health and multigenerational family history as well as the genetic screening procedures offered to all pregnant patients. Indications for targeted genetic screening and diagnostic tests for those with specific risk factors are reviewed as well as the indications for referral for genetic counseling. Finally, the essential components of genetic counseling are described, including the ethical and social issues as well as strategies for counseling families about their options for genetic testing.

Family History and Risk Evaluation

A multigenerational family history should be obtained at the first prenatal visit if not completed during the preconception period. This can be done using a checklist filled out by the patient or by verbal questioning about whether there is a family history of disorders, conditions, or health problems. Another method of evaluating the family history often used by genetic counselors is the pedigree.

Health equity key points

- Provide genetic testing education materials that reflect gender, race, and ethnic diversity.
- People in rural areas, with limited financial resources, or without insurance may have decreased access to genetic screening and testing.
- Using race/ethnicity to determine the type of screening a patient is offered increases healthcare disparities and results in suboptimal care.
- Patients with high body mass index (BMI) are more likely to experience noninvasive prenatal screening test failure, leading to more unnecessary invasive procedures and potential for anxiety; appropriate pretest counseling should be provided, and testing options that are valid in people with higher BMIs should be developed.
- Genetic testing can imply ableism bias; include value of and preparation for a child with a genetic condition in counseling.

A pedigree is a visual diagram to evaluate genetic relationships and assess the risk to individuals of developing certain diseases or conditions. This visual form of documenting family health history offers a more comprehensive method of capturing significant health patterns than can be achieved with a narrative description. A pedigree captures at least three generations and includes self-reported ethnicity, age, age of death if deceased, relevant health history, illness, and age of onset of the condition for each individual and any information about known genetic mutations or variants. The ideal pedigree tool is tailored for use in the prenatal care setting. The most useful family history includes medical, developmental, and pregnancy outcome information on first-, second-, and third-degree relatives (Table 13.1). Online resources are available to create a pedigree, generate a personal genetic screening risk assessment, and engage the pregnant patient, their

Table 13.1 Degree of Relationship and Shared Genes

First-degree relatives	Second-degree relatives	Third-degree relatives
50% shared genes	25% shared genes	12.5% shared genes
Children Siblings Parents	Aunts and uncles Nieces and nephews Half siblings Grandparents	Cousins Great-grandparents

partner, and/or family members as active participants in the process. The use of an electronic genetic screening system can also expedite the sometimes lengthy intake, risk assessment, and decision-making process (see *Resources for Pregnant People, Their Families, and Healthcare Providers*).

Genetic Screening Tests

All pregnant individuals are offered a number of genetic testing and screening procedures. Most of the screening tests are noninvasive and provide an estimated risk or risk score for certain birth defects or genetic disorders. When screening the fetus for chromosomal aneuploidies where risk is associated with age, pregnant individuals with a risk above a certain cutoff are considered "screen positive" and are at an increased risk of carrying an affected fetus. Those with a risk score below the cutoff are considered "screen negative" and are not at an increased risk of carrying an affected fetus. **Prenatal genetic screening** choices are best discussed as early as possible in pregnancy, ideally at the first prenatal visit, so that first-trimester screening options and personal decisions for pregnancy are available.

Maternal serum screening tests are blood tests measuring serum markers found in the pregnant individual associated with selected birth defects and genetic disorders. The screening tests typically measure three to five serum markers. Based on the results of the tests, the patient's risk of having an affected infant is calculated using an algorithm that factors in the amounts of serum markers and information about the patient, including age, weight, race, and gestational age at the time of the screening, all of which can influence test results. The raw value of the maternal serum markers is converted to a multiple of the median (MoM) that is similar to a standard deviation and allows for the comparison of results between patients as well as laboratories. The result is often noted as "screen positive/screen negative" or "abnormal/normal," with the patient's specific numeric risk provided.

It is imperative that the correct information is used for the calculation to provide the most accurate risk assessment. For example, using a gestational age that is incorrectly calculated by as little as one week can change the risk assessment. Thus, whenever there is an abnormal test result for the estimated gestational age, dating parameters should be reviewed. An ultrasound may be needed to confirm gestational age if one has not already been done. If there is a discrepancy in gestational age estimated by ultrasound and the last menstrual period of more than 5 days in the first trimester and 10 days in the second trimester, then the test result must be reinterpreted using the gestational age from the ultrasound (Delaney & Roggensack, 2017).[1]

Screening for Neural Tube Defects

Neural tube defects (NTDs) are a complex group of disorders ranging in severity from **spina bifida occulta** to anencephaly and are one of the most common congenital malformations worldwide. NTDs are caused by a combination of multiple genes and multiple environmental factors and develop in the first four weeks of pregnancy, often before an individual may even know that they are pregnant. The incidence of NTD is approximately 6.5 per 10,000 live births in the United States (Williams et al., 2015). It is well established that adequate folic acid is preventative for NTD, and all childbearing-aged and pregnant people are advised to consume 400-mcg folic acid daily. The introduction of folic acid fortification to cereal and grains sold in the United States has reduced the incidence of NTDs by approximately 28–35% (Williams et al., 2015). In the United States, NTD prevalence is highest among Hispanic populations, with non-Hispanic White and non-Hispanic Black populations having lower incidences (Egbe et al., 2015; Williams et al., 2015). It is important to hold in mind that associations between race and/or ethnicity and incidence of a multifactorial condition (such as NTD) typically does not indicate a singular genetic propensity within that population to develop said condition, but rather serves as a proxy for myriad social, demographic, environmental, and systemic pressures that cannot be easily measured in terms of their impact to risk and health.

Although the history of an NTD in an immediate family member increases the chance of having an infant with an NTD, the vast majority of people who have a fetus with an open NTD have a negative family history. Known risk factors account for fewer than 50% of NTD cases (Agopian et al., 2013).

Risk factors for NTD

- Family history of NTD
- Diabetes
- Obesity
- Opioid use
- Maternal hyperthermia in early gestation
- Medications
  - Antiseizure medications
  - Sulfonamide antibiotics
  - Pain medications (nonsteroidal anti-inflammatory drugs [NSAIDs] and opioids)
- Ethnicity

Source: CDC (2022).

Screening for NTD is offered to all pregnant patients presenting for prenatal care prior to 23 completed weeks of gestation (Table 13.2). Screening may be performed via level II ultrasound or maternal serum **alpha-fetoprotein (AFP),** a protein made in the fetal liver that can be measured in maternal serum and amniotic fluid. The optimal time for NTD screening is at 16–18 weeks of gestation, but

---

1 Note that this guidance is specific to risk assessment for aneuploidy and NTDs via maternal serum markers and is different from guidance on changing EDBs.

Table 13.2 Prenatal Genetic Screening Options

Test	Conditions screened	Components	Ideal or required timing	Sensitivity for Down syndrome	Benefits and limitations
First-trimester Screen	Trisomy 13 Trisomy 18 Trisomy 21	NT plus PAPP-A hCG	Blood test at 10–13 weeks gestation NT at 11–14 weeks gestation	Detection 82–87% False positive 5%	Benefits: Allows for earlier diagnosis Safer and earlier termination choices Limitations: Does not screen for NTD Requires availability of certified technician
Triple screen	NTD Trisomy 18 Trisomy 21	AFP hCG uE3	16–18 weeks gestation	Detection 69% False positive 5%	Limitations: Lower sensitivity for Down syndrome compared to other tests Later gestation termination risks
Quad screen	NTD Trisomy 18 Trisomy 21	AFP hCG uE3 DIA	15–22 weeks gestation	Detection 81% False positive 5%	Benefits: Widely available Screens for NTD Later gestation termination risks
Penta screen	NTD Trisomy 18 Trisomy 21	AFP hCG uE3 DIA h-hCG	15–22 weeks gestation	Detection 83% False positive 5%	Limitations: Later diagnosis Later gestation termination risks Not widely available
Integrated screen	NTD Trisomy 13 Trisomy 18 Trisomy 21	NT plus PAPP-A AFP hCG uE3 DIA	Blood test #1 at 10–13 weeks gestation NT at 11–14 weeks gestation Blood test #2 at 15–22 weeks gestation Risk assigned after all tests results reported	Detection 96% False positive 5%	Benefits: High DS detection rate Screens for NTD Limitations: Later diagnosis Later gestation termination risks Increased patient anxiety with waiting time between tests
Serum-integrated screen	NTD Trisomy 18 Trisomy 21	PAPP-A AFP hCG uE3 DIA	Blood test #1 at 10–13 weeks gestation Blood test #2 at 15–22 weeks gestation Risk assigned after both tests results reported	Detection 88% False positive 5%	Benefits: Improved detection over quad screen Limitations: NT not done Later diagnosis Later gestation termination risks
Sequential screen	NTD Trisomy 13 Trisomy 18 Trisomy 21	NT plus PAPP-A AFP hCG uE3 DIA	Blood test #1 at 10–13 weeks gestation NT at 11–14 weeks gestation Blood test #2 at 15–22 weeks gestation Risks assigned in both first and second trimester	Detection 95% False positive 5%	Benefits: Allows for earlier diagnosis for some Limitations: Two risk assessments may be confusing to patients
NIPS screen	Trisomy 13 Trisomy 18 Trisomy 21 Optional: additional panels including sex chromosome aneuploidy, microdeletion syndromes, rare aneuploidies, and copy number variants	Cell-free placental DNA in maternal serum	9–10 weeks through term	Detection >99% False positive <0.5%	Benefits: Highest detection and lowest false positive rate for DS Limitations: No-calls occur and necessitate screen positive follow-up. Some additional panel options not recommended by ACOG

Source: Adapted from ACOG (2020), Quest Diagnostics (2022), and Taylor-Phillips et al. (2016).
NT, nuchal translucency by ultrasound; AFP, alpha-fetoprotein; hCG, human chorionic gonadotropin; uE3, unconjugated estriol; DIA, dimeric inhibin A; h-hCG, hyperglycosylated human chorionic gonadotropin.

it can be done between 15 and 22^6/$_7$ weeks of gestation. Fetuses with an opening in the skull or spine leak extra AFP into the amniotic fluid. In addition to NTD, fetuses with other openings such as the ventral wall defect gastroschisis can also be identified with serum AFP screening. Level II ultrasound has a higher sensitivity for NTD detection than AFP alone, and is an accepted substitute or adjunct to serum AFP screening (ACOG, 2017c).

Screening for Aneuploidy

Prenatal detection of fetal **aneuploidy,** which increases with maternal age, is one of the major goals of prenatal genetic screening. Two of the most commonly encountered aneuploidies are **trisomy 18** and **trisomy 21**.

Trisomy 21, also known as Down syndrome, is the most common chromosome anomaly found in newborns and is the leading genetic cause of intellectual disability. Down syndrome occurs in approximately 1 in 700 live births (National Down Syndrome Society, 2022). The features of Down syndrome can include variable intellectual disability, hypotonia, distinctive facial features, heart defects, gastrointestinal anomalies, vision and hearing problems, thyroid problems, increased incidence of leukemia and Alzheimer features, and spine instability. Children with Down syndrome typically reach their developmental milestones later than children without Down syndrome.

A major risk factor for Down syndrome is increased maternal age. Although older individuals are at higher risk, the majority of children with Down syndrome are born to people younger than age 35 since the majority of pregnancies occur in this age group. Therefore, all pregnant patients presenting for prenatal care prior to 22 weeks of gestation are offered Down syndrome screening.

Trisomy 18, also known as Edwards syndrome, is a chromosomal disorder affecting many parts of the body and characterized by severe intellectual disabilities, congenital heart disease, renal malformations, low set ears, and clenched fists. The estimated incidence of trisomy 18 is 1 per 2500 pregnancies. An unknown number of cases spontaneously abort during the first trimester, and at least half of the pregnancies carried to term result in an intrauterine fetal demise. Given this, the birth incidence of trisomy 18 is much lower at 1/6000–1/8000. It has been noted that 90–95% of liveborns with trisomy 18 die within the first year (Cereda & Carey, 2012).

Trisomy 13, also known as Patau syndrome, is a very rare condition occurring in approximately 1 per 16,000 live births (National Library of Medicine, 2021). The disorder is characterized by multiple organ system defects, physical abnormalities, and severe neurological deficits, and many affected babies do not survive longer than weeks or months.

Whereas NTD risk assessment based on maternal serum analytes considers AFP measurement alone, aneuploidy risk assessments based on serum analytes include marker combinations of AFP, human chorionic gonadotropin (hCG), unconjugated estriol (uE3), pregnancy-associated plasma protein-A (PAPP-A), dimeric inhibin

A (DIA), and/or hyperglycosylated human chorionic gonadotropin (h-hCG). There are several methods of aneuploidy risk screening available in the first and second trimesters (Table 13.2).

First-Trimester Screening

First-trimester screening is performed between 11 and 13 6/7 weeks of gestation and includes **nuchal translucency** (NT) measurement by ultrasound and maternal serum measurement of free or total β-hCG and PAPP-A. An increase in NT is an independent risk factor for aneuploidy and certain cardiac and genetic defects, with risk increasing with the size of translucency. Patients who screen positive are given the option of having a diagnostic test such as an amniocentesis or chorionic villus sampling (CVS) to determine if the fetus is affected.

First-trimester screening offers several potential advantages over second-trimester screening. When test results are negative, anxiety can be reduced earlier in pregnancy. If results are positive, early screening allows the option of first-trimester **prenatal diagnosis** by CVS, which can be performed between 10 and 12 weeks of gestation. First-trimester screening also affords greater privacy and less health risk if they choose to terminate the pregnancy. Another advantage of first-trimester screening is that the **detection rate** is superior to second-trimester screening, thus reducing the need for invasive testing and associated risk. For those who undertake first-trimester screening for Down syndrome, second-trimester AFP screening and ultrasound examination are offered to screen for open NTDs.

Second-Trimester Screening

Maternal multiple marker serum (MMS) screening may be offered in the second trimester to detect trisomy 18, trisomy 21, and NTDs. The tests are commonly known by the number of markers or analytes measured, with detection rates increasing with the number of markers (Table 13.2). The quad screen measures four markers and detects approximately 80% of fetuses with Down syndrome (ACOG, 2020). The quad screen also measures AFP and, therefore, screens for NTD, with a detection rate of 80–90%, depending on the nature of the defect (Driscoll & Gross, 2009). The penta screen includes measurement of a fifth analyte, h-hCG, which increases the Down syndrome detection rate by 2% over the quad screen (Quest Diagnostics, 2022). However, limited performance data are available, and it is not widely used (ACOG, 2020). It is important to note that of all patients who have a positive serum screening test, only a small number are actually carrying a fetus with an NTD or chromosomal abnormality.

Maternal serum screening results can be affected by factors such as multiple gestation, maternal weight, and inaccurate pregnancy dating. If pregnancy dating is well established and serum screening indicates a high level of AFP, this is considered a marker for an increased risk of NTD. If the AFP is low and hCG and inhibin A levels are high, this indicates a higher risk of Down syndrome. Genetic counseling and additional testing such as a targeted ultrasound and amniocentesis for diagnosis are offered with a positive screen.

Integrated and Sequential Screening

Integrated screening combines both first-trimester NT measurement and first-trimester serum testing along with second-trimester quad screen (Table 13.2). NT is measured by ultrasound between 11 and 13 6/7 weeks of gestation. A risk score is then reported in the second trimester based on the combined serum and NT measurement results. This test provides the highest **sensitivity** with the lowest **false positive rate** of the maternal serum marker screen choices, limiting the number of invasive amniocenteses done for positive results. The availability of technicians trained in NT measurement can limit access to this test for those in rural and underserved areas. Since the integrated screen measures AFP, it also screens for NTD. Variations of integrated screening protocols are also available. Serum-integrated screen is the same as the integrated screen except the NT measurement is not done. Although the serum-integrated screen has a lower detection rate than the integrated screen, it may be preferred when NT measurement is not available.

Sequential integrated screening is a method in which NT and the same first- and second-trimester serum screens are done, but the patient is informed of the first-trimester screening results when they come in instead of waiting for the second-trimester screening results to issue a risk score. If the first-trimester screen is positive, either **cell-free DNA** (cfDNA) serum testing (discussed below) for further risk analysis or CVS for diagnosis is offered. When the first-trimester results are negative, the second-trimester serum screen is completed, and markers from tests are combined to provide a final risk estimate. Thus, the sequential integrated screen enables earlier diagnosis for pregnant individuals with a first-trimester elevated risk while maintaining a high detection rate.

Noninvasive Prenatal Screening

Noninvasive prenatal screening (NIPS) relies on the presence of cfDNA from the placenta circulating in the pregnant person's bloodstream. Most of the cfDNA in a patient's sample is maternal in origin; however, a small proportion of the cfDNA originates from the placenta. Many laboratories measure this proportion and report it as a percentage known as the **fetal fraction.** The laboratory analyzes the cfDNA in the maternal serum sample and reports risk of trisomy 13, 18, and 21. Some cfDNA laboratories also offer additional screening for sex chromosome abnormalities, such as monosomy X (Turner syndrome). Other options available include screening for rare aneuploidies, specified microdeletion syndromes, such as DiGeorge syndrome, or missing or extra portions of chromosomes of a certain size, such as 5–7 Mb or larger. Blood may be drawn for NIPS beginning as early as 9–10 weeks of gestation with results typically available within 7–10 days. NIPS has a reported 99% **specificity** and sensitivity for Down syndrome, with slightly lower rates for trisomies 13 and 18 (ACOG, 2020). Prenatal screening using cfDNA has far superior **positive predictive values (PPV)** than serum marker measurements and ultrasound, and positive NIPS test results for Down syndrome are likely to be true positives. In a large study directly comparing NIPS versus traditional screening methods for Down syndrome in a general prenatal population, NIPS provided an 80.9% PPV, whereas first-trimester screening was much lower at 5.4% PPV (Norton et al., 2015). Even with these very high PPVs, NIPS is a screening test, and it is important that those who test positive are offered diagnostic testing.

In a small number of cases, the fetal fraction is too low to be measured or results are indeterminate and are labeled a **no-call** result. No-call results are more common in pregnant patients with elevated BMI and those carrying a fetus with aneuploidy (Skrzypek & Hui, 2017). Patients with no-call results are offered additional genetic counseling, ultrasound, and diagnostic procedures due to the potential increased risk of an affected fetus. A redraw for NIPS after no-call result may occur but is not encouraged, as many redraws result in recurrent no-calls and delays in diagnosis (ACOG, 2020).

NIPS has several benefits. The high sensitivity of the screening significantly reduces the number of invasive diagnostic procedures performed and associated risk to the pregnant person and fetus. Screening and diagnostic testing can be performed sooner than conventional methods, allowing pregnant individuals more options for pregnancy planning. However, NIPS does not assess the risk of fetal anomalies such as NTDs or ventral wall defects. Those who elect to have NIPS are also offered maternal serum AFP screening and/or ultrasound evaluation for NTD risk assessment.

Despite a high sensitivity in detecting aneuploidy, NIPS is not diagnostic and does not replace CVS or amniocentesis. Management decisions, including pregnancy termination, should never be based on NIPS results alone. Patients who screen positive are offered CVS or amniocentesis for diagnosis. It should also be clearly communicated that a negative NIPS result does not guarantee an unaffected fetus.

Recommendations for the use of NIPS in the general prenatal population have become uniform in recent years. The current recommendations from the ACOG, The Society for Maternal-Fetal Medicine (SMFM), and The American College of Medical Genetics and Genomics (ACMG) state that all pregnant individuals should be offered prenatal screening for aneuploidy regardless of maternal age at the time of childbirth or risk for chromosomal abnormality. As of 2020, the ACOG in conjunction with the SMFM included NIPS as one of the several screening options available to all pregnant patients and, together with ACMG, they further state that it is the most sensitive and specific screening option available for common fetal aneuploidies (ACOG 2020; Gregg et al., 2016)

Genetic Screening by Ultrasound

Ultrasonography can be diagnostic for fetal structural defects, such as heart defects or open NTDs. If a serum screening indicates a higher risk for NTD or Down syndrome, a more comprehensive ultrasound is performed to more thoroughly examine fetal anatomy, and additional testing may be offered.

Although ultrasound is not diagnostic for fetal chromosome anomalies and has limited utility in genetic screening, recent advances in ultrasound technology have improved the ability of ultrasound in detecting "soft" markers indicating an increased risk for fetal aneuploidy. Ultrasound soft markers, such as short femur, short humerus, choroid plexus cysts, or increased NT, and structural anomalies such as ventricular septal defects suggest an increased risk of aneuploidy. (See Chapter 12, *Prenatal Ultrasound,* for more detailed information.) However, ultrasound also detects findings that have undetermined significance, which generate uncertainty over fetal health and increase family anxiety and stress (Kowalcek, 2017; Larsson et al., 2009; Viaux-Savelon et al., 2012). In many cases of soft marker findings or findings of unknown significance, no actual problem is found. Many soft markers do not require additional follow-up if aneuploidy screening is negative (ACOG, 2020).

A fetal anomaly ultrasound between 16 and 20 weeks of gestation has been integrated into routine prenatal care practices. This detailed scan systematically examines fetal anatomy for major structural anomalies. Healthcare providers need to be cognizant that this standard ultrasound is a type of genetic screening. Indeed, in professional and consumer literature, it is termed the *fetal anomaly scan.* When offering the fetal anomaly scan, the same approach should be used as with other genetic screening methods. Simply saying "We are going to get an ultrasound to check on the baby, see if everything is okay" is not informed consent, nor is it full disclosure. Pregnant people in the United States have come to expect ultrasound as part of prenatal care and generally see this as a pleasant opportunity to see the baby and discover the fetal sex and often do not realize that this is a form of genetic screening (Ahman et al., 2010; Van der Zalm & Byrne, 2006). In comparison to uptake rates of serum screening for genetic conditions, the uptake rates of the second-trimester ultrasound are extremely high, close to 100%. This may be a reflection of preference for less invasive screening or may reflect patients' limited understanding and knowledge about prenatal genetic screening and the role of ultrasound compared to the significant impact a positive screening result may have on their lives (Skirton & Barr, 2010).

When unexpected abnormalities are found on an ultrasound, patients may feel frightened, unprepared, and uninformed (Ahman et al., 2010). They may experience heightened anxiety and distress (Kaasen et al., 2010), and normal attachment behaviors can be negatively impacted (Viaux-Savelon et al., 2012). Offering a routine anomaly scan ultrasound should be appropriately framed within the context of genetic screening and information provided to patients on the conditions being screened for, detection rate, false positive rate, and any risks and benefits. As with all screening tests, patients have the right to accept or decline testing without sanction.

Carrier Screening

Carrier screening allows individuals and couples to find out if they are carriers of select genetic conditions that are typically inherited in an **autosomal recessive** or **X-linked** fashion. According to a joint statement from multiple leading genetics organizations, *the goal of preconception and prenatal carrier screening is to provide couples with information to optimize pregnancy outcomes based on their personal values and preferences* (Edwards et al., 2015).

Sex chromosomes (X and Y) determine the chromosomal sex of the fetus but do not determine gender, which is a social construct. Typically, XX is associated with female sex, and XY with male sex. Intersex, also known as differences of sexual development (DSD) or sex trait variations, describes sex characteristics that are different than the two most common presentations. These are understudied and may result from differences in chromosomes, genes, and/or hormones. The vast majority of conditions included in carrier screening panels are autosomal recessive. Most individuals that are carriers for an autosomal recessive condition do not know that they are a carrier because there often is not a known family history. A child is at risk for an autosomal recessive condition if both biological parents or donors are carriers for the same condition. If the parents and/or donors are carriers of the same genetic condition, there is a 25% chance of having a child with the condition, a 50% chance a child will be a carrier, and a 25% chance the child will not have the condition nor be a carrier (see Figure 13.1). While carrier screening is ideally done in the preconception period, the vast majority of individuals are screened at their first prenatal appointment. Typically, the pregnant individual or egg donor is offered carrier screening first, and if they screen positive, the partner or sperm donor is screened to determine their carrier status. If both parents (or parent and donor) are found to be carriers of the same disease, prenatal diagnostic testing is offered to determine if the fetus is affected. If carrier screening is done during the preconception period, individuals have expanded reproductive health choices such as preimplantation genetic diagnosis, use of an egg or sperm donor, adoption, or choosing not to have children.

While the majority of conditions on carrier screening panels are autosomal recessive conditions, some conditions inherited in an X-linked fashion can also be included, for example, fragile X syndrome. With X-linked conditions, a child is at risk if the pregnant person or egg donor is a carrier of the X-linked condition. Additionally, an offspring with XY chromosomes has a 50% chance of inheriting the mutation and manifesting the disease, whereas an offspring with XX chromosomes has a 50% chance of inheriting the mutation and may be at risk for symptoms

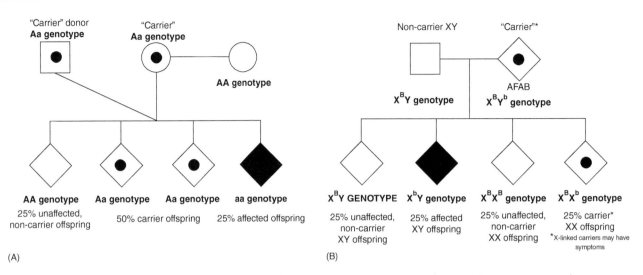

Figure 13.1 Carrier inheritance (A) autosomal recessive inheritance pattern: same-sex couple conceiving using a sperm donor (B) X-linked inheritance pattern: nonbinary individual AFAB (assigned female at birth) who is a manifesting carrier. Arjunan et al. (2022)/MDPI/Public Domain.

related to the disease but generally not to the same extent or severity as an XY offspring (see Figure 13.1).

Common conditions or diseases included on carrier screening panels include **monogenic** disorders such as cystic fibrosis (CF), fragile X syndrome, sickle cell disease, alpha- and beta-thalassemia, spinal muscular atrophy, and Tay–Sachs disease (Table 13.3). Couples with **consanguinity** are at higher risk for offspring with **autosomal recessive disorders** and can benefit from carrier screening. If a pregnant patient or their partner has a family history indicating genetic risk for a specific disease, screening for that disease and genetic counseling should be offered.

Carrier screening can have significant impacts beyond a single pregnancy. When a person tests positive, their relatives may carry the same gene mutation. The individual is encouraged to share the risk information with relatives and inform them of carrier screening availability; however, doing so is their choice. Additionally, they should be informed that positive genetic results could impact future life and health insurance coverage and costs (ACOG, 2017b).

Expanded Carrier Screening

At the onset of carrier screening, individuals were offered screening for one or a handful of conditions depending on their self-reported ethnicity or family history. As the knowledge of genetics has grown along with technological advances, we now have the ability to screen individuals for mutations in hundreds of genes simultaneously. The process of screening for many genes at the same time is known as expanded carrier screening (ECS).

Currently, the ACOG and the ACMG recommend that all individuals planning a pregnancy, regardless of self-reported ethnicity, be offered screening at minimum for CF, spinal muscular atrophy, and the hemoglobinopathies. There are also certain genetic conditions that have a higher prevalence in individuals of defined ancestral background (Table 13.3). However, anyone can be a carrier for these conditions even if they are not within the high-risk population. The United States, and indeed the world, is multiethnic and multiracial with much intermixing of groups, and genetic disorders continue to expand to outside traditionally affected ethnic groups. Additionally, studies have shown that self-reported ethnicity is an imperfect indicator of genetic ancestry (Kaseniit et al. 2020). Thus, there has been a trend in preconception and prenatal practice of moving away from ethnicity-based carrier screening to more panethnic screening such as ECS where all individuals are offered screening for the same large panel of conditions regardless of their self-reported ethnicity. Ethnicity-based screening, panethnic screening, and ECS are all acceptable screening strategies (ACOG, 2017a). However, since a standard ECS panel has not been defined, prenatal care providers are advised to develop their own standard approach to expanded screening. ACOG (2017a) recommends that genes included on expanded carrier panels should meet the following criteria:

- has a carrier frequency of 1/100 or greater
- causes physical or cognitive impairment requiring medical or surgical intervention
- can be diagnosed prenatally and the information used to optimize pregnancy, labor, childbirth, and newborn care
- does not have onset in adulthood.

In 2021, the ACMG took the ACOG recommendations a few steps further by stating that all pregnant patients and those planning a pregnancy should be offered screening for an expanded panel of 97 autosomal recessive genes and 16 X-linked genes regardless of self-reported ethnicity (Gregg et al., 2021). The ACMG developed this recommended panel of 113 genes by including those genes that have a severe or moderate phenotype, a carrier frequency

Table 13.3   Example of Conditions, Carrier Frequencies, and Condition Characteristics*

Condition	Ethnicity and carrier frequency	Condition characteristics
Thalassemia	Southeast Asian (Cambodian, Hmong, Thai, Laotian, Vietnamese) 1/4 to 1/60 carrier African American 1/15 to 1/50 carrier Mediterranean (Greek, Italian) 1/20 to 1/50 carrier	• Alpha-thalassemia disease can range from mild to a severe anemia that causes stillbirth. • Person pregnant with an affected baby may develop serious health problems during the pregnancy. • Beta-thalassemia disease causes severe anemia and poor growth beginning in infancy/early childhood. • Lifespan is often shortened. • Hemoglobin E/beta-thalassemia disease is a variable condition that causes moderate to severe anemia. • Usually cannot be cured but can be managed.
Sickle cell disease	African ancestry 1/8–10 carrier	• Blood disorders beginning in infancy/early childhood; cause anemia, bone pain, and frequent serious infections. • Lifespan may be shortened. • Treatment may include frequent hospital stays, medications, and blood transfusions. • Carriers are at higher risk for asymptomatic bacteriuria in pregnancy; urine culture & sensitivity each trimester recommended. • Severity varies. Some live without serious illness. • Usually cannot be cured but can be managed.
Fragile X syndrome	People with XX chromosomes 1/151 carrier People with XY chromosomes 1/468 affected	• X-linked condition. • Mild to severe intellectual disabilities. • Behavioral, developmental, learning delays, and disorders such as autism, ADHD. • People with XY chromosomes usually have a more severe presentation. • Characteristic physical features: ○ Long narrow face ○ Prominent jaw and forehead ○ Protuberant ears ○ Unusually flexible fingers
Cystic fibrosis	European/White 1/29 carrier	• Body produces thick mucus in the lungs and in the gastrointestinal system. • Can lead to severe infections, difficulty absorbing food, poor growth. • Lifespan may be shortened to 30–40 years. • Treatment includes pancreatic enzymes, respiratory treatments, lung transplant may ultimately be necessary.
Tay–Sachs disease	Ashkenazi Jewish 1/30 carrier French Canadian 1/15 to 1/30 carrier Louisiana Cajun 1/27 carrier	• Brain and nervous system disease. • Progressive muscle weakness, mental deterioration, and blindness. • Death occurs by about 3–5 years of age. • No treatment or cure.
Canavan disease	Ashkenazi Jewish 1/55 carrier General population 1/300	• Brain and nervous system disease. • Progressive loss of myelin causing muscle weakness, mental deterioration, and seizures. • Death usually occurs by 10 years of age. • No treatment or cure.
Familial dysautonomia	Ashkenazi Jewish 1/27 carrier	• Disease of the nervous system begins in infancy. • Can lead to pain insensitivity, unstable blood pressure and/or temperature, problems with speech and movement, difficulty swallowing. • The average lifespan is 30 years. • No cure, treatment focuses on symptom relief.
Spinal muscular atrophy	European/White 1/47 carrier Asian 1/59 carrier Ashkenazi Jewish 1/67 carrier	• Severe neuromuscular disease. • Rapid progressive muscle weakness and paralysis. • The average lifespan is 2 years. • Death is caused by respiratory failure.

Source: Adapted from American Society of Hematology (2022), Cystic Fibrosis Foundation (2017), Familial Dysautonomia Foundation (n.d.), National Tay-Sachs & Allied Diseases Association (2021), and CDC (2016).*not an inclusive list.

of at least ≥1/200 for autosomal recessive conditions and a 1/40,000 disease prevalence for X-linked conditions.

Diagnostic Prenatal Genetic Testing

Amniocentesis and CVS are the two most commonly performed diagnostic procedures. Percutaneous umbilical blood sampling (PUBS) can be indicated in certain circumstances. The advantage of diagnostic testing is that fetal **karyotype** can be accurately determined and the developing fetus can be tested to determine if they might be affected with a genetic condition identified via carrier screening. Newer technologies also allow for an even more in-depth analysis of the fetal genetic makeup via microarray analysis and whole exome sequencing (WES). In practice, diagnostic genetic testing is routinely offered to all pregnant people who will be age 35 or older at the time of birth, as the incidence of aneuploidy increases with maternal age. However, professional societies such as ACOG and ACMG currently recommend that all pregnant individuals, regardless of age or *a priori* risk, be offered the option of prenatal diagnostic testing, affording all patients the opportunity to choose a testing strategy that is best aligned with their individual goals and values (ACOG, 2016; Gregg et al., 2016). The superior accuracy and increased use of NIPS has significantly reduced the number of invasive diagnostic tests performed (Warsof et al., 2015).

Diagnostic Procedures

Amniocentesis

Amniocentesis was the first prenatal diagnostic procedure to examine fetal chromosomes and involves withdrawing a small amount of amniotic fluid from the amniotic sac. Within the fluid, there are skin and other cells from the fetus. These cells contain the fetal chromosomes that can then be analyzed for structural and numerical chromosomal abnormalities. The procedure involves cleaning the patient's abdomen with an antiseptic wash, and under ultrasound guidance, a needle is inserted and a small amount of amniotic fluid, about 20 mL, is removed. The amniotic fluid is centrifuged, and the cells are prepared for genetic analysis. A small portion of the fluid is used to measure the level of AFP to screen for open NTDs. Amniocentesis is typically performed between 15 and 20 weeks of gestation when the amnion and chorion are fused. Complications are rare and include chorioamnionitis and transient amniotic fluid leakage or spotting. Procedure-related pregnancy loss rates are low, from approximately 1 in 370 to 1 in 900 pregnancies (ACOG, 2016).

Chorionic Villus Sampling

CVS can diagnose Down syndrome, **confined placental mosaicism**, and other chromosomal abnormalities, but does not detect NTD. It is performed in the first trimester of pregnancy between 10 and 12 6/7 weeks of gestation and involves removing a small sample of the placenta. There are several approaches to obtaining the sample. The

location of the placenta determines which method is used. The transcervical approach involves inserting a small catheter through the cervix using ultrasound guidance. A catheter is directed to the placenta and gentle suction is applied to remove a small amount of chorionic villi (about 20–25 mg). The transabdominal approach is similar in technique to amniocentesis in that a needle is inserted through the abdomen, under ultrasound guidance, but the needle is directed to the placenta rather than the amniotic fluid. Suction is applied and a small amount of placental tissue is removed. Lidocaine may be used with the transabdominal approach.

CVS allows for earlier diagnosis and either advanced preparation for a child with a genetic condition or safer pregnancy termination options. Privacy is also enhanced since it can be done before the pregnancy is visually noticeable. CVS pregnancy loss rates have lowered over time, as clinicians have gained experience and loss rates of 1 in 455 are reported (ACOG, 2016).

Percutaneous Umbilical Blood Sampling

PUBS, also called cordocentesis, is a less commonly performed diagnostic test in which a needle is inserted under ultrasound guidance into the umbilical cord and a small amount of blood is withdrawn. Procedure-related risks are significant and include fetal bleeding, umbilical cord hematoma, maternal–fetal hemorrhage, and fetal bradycardia. However, in certain circumstances, such as the evaluation of hydrops or the need to obtain a specimen of fetal blood, it has a place in the armament of available diagnostic procedures.

Diagnostic Evaluations

Karyotype

Karyotype analysis can be performed on the prenatal sample collected via any of the above prenatal diagnostic procedures. This is a microscopic evaluation of the chromosomal makeup of the fetus, and it allows for the diagnosis of large changes to the chromosomal structure including aneuploidy or large segments of chromosome material that are deleted, duplicated, and/or rearranged. This is the oldest method of analyzing fetal chromosomes. Karyotype is unable to discern small submicroscopic differences of the chromosomes, many of which are pathogenic.

Chromosomal Microarray Analysis

Chromosomal microarray analysis (CMA) is a genetic test on fetal cells obtained by CVS or amniocentesis, PUBS, or direct tissue sampling that analyzes small amounts of genetic material that traditional karyotyping cannot detect. CMA is sensitive for many disorders and can identify potential intellectual disabilities and congenital abnormalities and aid in determining etiologies of stillbirth (Dugoff et al., 2016). It is often used postnatally in cases of fetal structural anomalies and unexplained fetal demise. The American Society for Maternal Fetal Medicine recommends that CMA counseling and testing be offered to those who undergo invasive diagnostic testing to augment karyotyping (Dugoff et al., 2016). CMA testing poses a unique challenge for patients and providers in that a patient can receive a normal karyotype result from the amniocentesis and abnormal CMA results. It is not uncommon for the significance of some abnormal CMA results to be unknown, thereby introducing uncertainty and making already difficult decisions even more challenging (Werner-Lin et al., 2016).

Prenatal Whole Exome Sequencing

As with the above prenatal genetic evaluations, WES can be performed on a fetal sample collected by any of the previously described procedures. This analysis provides the most comprehensive genetic evaluation of the fetus of any of those described in this chapter; WES involves sequencing of the coding regions of DNA and can detect mutations as small as a single base abnormality, which can identify single-gene diseases, for example, CF, not diagnosable via karyotype or microarray analysis. As with CMA, WES can lead to findings that are of uncertain significance based on current knowledge. WES is currently the least employed of the diagnostic evaluations described; however, it is becoming more commonly recommended in cases of fetal anomalies (Jelin & Vora, 2018; Pratt et al., 2020).

Psychosocial Considerations in Genetic Testing

Psychosocial considerations are central to all interactions with patients and their families. It is important to take the time to understand the patient's expectations and goals. Developing and building rapport with the patient will help establish a working alliance and fully informed decision-making. Family history is one important tool a healthcare provider can utilize to assess and address psychosocial issues (Uhlmann et al., 2011; Weil, 2000). Learning about the patient's family history allows one to understand both existing and absent relationships and level of connectedness in a family. Nuances in how the individual responds to questions can also help elucidate information about the patient's social support system and their concerns for the appointment. Gaining an understanding of the patient's priorities, preferences, and support system will all be crucial in recognizing the type of care that they may need from their provider.

As genetic technology has evolved, so have the testing options available to individuals during their pregnancies. Individuals are also learning and accessing information from a variety of sources, such as friends and family, online support groups, discussion forums, and advocacy groups. In a highly technological information age, pressures and expectations about lifestyle behavior choices in pregnancy, including genetic testing, are hard to escape. Information about new procreative technologies and appropriate behavior is available in popular magazines, reality television shows, and books for pregnant people and those considering pregnancy. In this context, the domain of pregnancy-related responsibilities seems infinitely expandable.

A study done by Gregg and colleagues (1993, p. 69) suggests that:

> When the participants made choices about prenatal testing and other procreative technologies, they experienced subtle and overt outside pressures on their choices and behaviors. They faced advice and comments from strangers, acquaintances, coworkers, family members and health providers. Women felt they had choices, but they were burdened with their own and other people's expectations that they make the "right" choices. *Women in the study experienced feelings of guilt and ambivalence both before and after they made prenatal screening and testing choices.* The women in the study discovered that their prenatal choices were double-edged swords. Though they welcomed the freedom to make prenatal choices, they discovered that these choices were accompanied by social and internal pressures and feelings of ambivalence and guilt.

In order to make the best decision, an individual considering genetic testing must simultaneously weigh and compare several areas of risk: (a) the chance of giving birth to an unaffected versus affected child; (b) the risk of having an abnormal test result; and (c) the risk that the test may cause harm. Numerous hypothetical tradeoffs and considerations of possible scenarios depending on choices made are required in the process of making a decision.

How risks are perceived individually can differ from the way that they are perceived in relationship to each other. Scenarios are created on how the pregnant person and their partner might think, feel, act, and respond to the news of a baby with a problem and then weighed against each other. This personal risk assessment is made even more complex because of the value-laden nature of the potential outcomes being weighed. Additionally, the process of making a decision about prenatal testing can include some discussion with the patient's partner or family members. The negotiation about testing choices is likely to involve not only two potentially different perceptions of risk but also two somewhat different sets of values, attitudes, and prior experiences. It is important to recognize and remember that there is no prescriptive process when it comes to psychosocial counseling. Each patient experiences their pregnancy differently. Provider goals may be similar for each patient, but the best execution and accomplishment of those goals are different depending on the patient's needs. See Chapter 11, *Risk Assessment during Pregnancy*, for further discussion of risk perception.

Genetic testing is a serious undertaking for pregnant individuals and their families. Prenatal healthcare providers must be aware of the ways in which prenatal testing can change a person's experience of pregnancy. For example, some patients who undergo serum screening with full understanding of the implications of information gained from testing suspend emotional attachment to their fetus pending the results of the testing (Lawson & Turriff-Jonasson, 2006; Rowe et al., 2009). In other studies, patients receiving screening results indicating a higher risk for a fetus with Down syndrome describe the waiting time until definitive diagnosis as a time when they repress the pregnancy (Baillie et al., 2000; Georgsson et al., 2006; Susanne et al., 2006). They avoid thinking about the baby and deny their pregnancy in different ways, such as expressing no feelings of happiness about the pregnancy, not informing family or friends about the pregnancy, not preparing baby supplies, or not thinking about baby names. This "timeout" lasted even beyond when the normal result from the invasive test was received. Even after a reassuring diagnostic test, some people exhibit higher levels of anxiety and worry about the health of their fetus, indicating that false positive results can have a lasting effect on pregnant people (Allison et al., 2011; Green et al., 2004; Sapp et al., 2010). Prenatal healthcare providers need to be aware of the ways in which prenatal testing changes experiences of pregnancy.

While the above may imply that prenatal testing infuses an unnecessary level of anxiety into the prenatal experience, some studies have indicated that patients find value in having complete information in advance. Hurford et al. (2013) evaluated mothers of children with Down syndrome that were diagnosed prenatally. The vast majority indicated an increase in anxiety due to diagnosis; however, they indicated *"the benefit of knowing and having time to process the prenatal diagnosis overshadowed the negative consequence of increased stress and anxiety during the pregnancy."* (p. 593)

Considerations for Genetic Testing

Genetic counseling is more than providing a pregnant person with information. It is a form of communication that facilitates decisions on a course of action that are made solely by the pregnant person. This counseling takes time, and it is imperative that adequate time be allocated during prenatal care visits to cover genetic testing choices and their implications. The addition of NIPS, CMA, and carrier screening choices has added another layer of complexity to the already-wide array of genetic screening choices to consider. A small study noted that many individuals receiving positive results from genetic screening report a lack of understanding of the implications of the testing and also confuse it with other genetic screening options (Rothwell et al., 2017). Particular attention to ensuring patients' understanding of the expanded genetic screening choices is an important component of prenatal genetic pretest counseling. Inviting the pregnant person to bring their partner to prenatal care visits when genetic testing choices are discussed can facilitate informed discussions and test understanding, but can also add divergent opinions and social pressures to decision-making.

Pretest Counseling

Pretest counseling is perhaps the most important component of preconception and prenatal genetic testing and screening. The purpose of pretest counseling is to provide full and balanced information on genetic screening options to allow pregnant patients to make their best personal choice. Supporting patient autonomy and facilitating patient decision-making is important when talking to people about their screening and testing options (Eunpu, 1997). It is important to provide counseling in a manner that empowers patients to make decisions that are best for them and their families through information about their risks and options, in a culturally respectful, confidential manner. When making decisions about genetic risk and testing choices, pregnant individuals and their families need to know the following to make an informed choice (Hodgson & Gaff, 2013):

- the condition(s) for which the test is directed
- the parental or fetal numerical risk for the condition
- the test to detect the condition
- when and how the test is performed
- risks and benefits of the test
- that an assessment of probability is not a diagnosis
- the meaning of the test results
- the probability of false positive and **false negative** results
- that a negative test does not guarantee a good outcome
- implications of a positive test result, including psychological effects
- choosing no testing is an equal option
- that the pregnant person and their partner will be faced with decisions if the results are positive
- how common the abnormalities are and possible consequences for the child and the family
- options after diagnosis
- resources for additional information.

These points of discussion cover the principles of informed consent. It is especially important to explain false positives when discussing genetic screening options. For example, the quad screen has a false positive rate of 5%. This means that 1 out of 20 pregnant patients who have the test will have a positive screen yet have a baby without the condition. Some of these individuals with positive screens will undergo invasive diagnostic testing in order to determine whether the pregnancy is affected or not.

Another consideration to discuss is the question, "What would you do in the event of positive results?" Some people would agree to invasive testing, and others would not want to introduce added risk. Informed consent requires taking the time needed to adequately educate about the implications of genetic screening. However, it is important to recognize that intended responses to a hypothetical situation can change when individuals are faced with real results. Providers should discuss all options available to the individual, regardless of their stated intent.

Consider this scenario. A pregnant patient wants to have the first-trimester screening or quad screen but tells you they would never agree to invasive testing. This is a potential dilemma for them and illustrates why understanding the patient's goals is important and can help facilitate decision-making. Some questions to consider in this situation:

- What information is the patient hoping to learn from the screening?
- Are there other noninvasive evaluations that the patient would be interested in pursuing?

- What resources or information would be helpful for the patient if they were to receive a positive result?
- Would the patient worry during the entire pregnancy about something being wrong with the baby?
- Would they use the information to prepare for a potential confirmatory diagnosis at birth?

Since most patients with positive quad screen results ultimately are found to have an unaffected fetus, it is important to set expectations for the patient. These points are essential to bring up in discussions of genetic testing options to encourage pregnant individuals to fully consider the possible results in making their testing decisions. Discussions on prenatal genetic testing can be complex and providing written material to supplement the discussions will allow patients time to integrate the information with their own needs and values.

Posttest Counseling

Results should be provided in a timely manner to allow for optimal reproductive choice as indicated. When an aneuploidy screen result is negative, it is recommended that the patient's risk for Down syndrome be provided in numerical form (Cartier et al., 2012). For example, a 33-year-old pregnant individual at 13 weeks of gestation with a negative NIPS result would have a < 1 in 10,000 chance of having a child with Down syndrome (National Society of Genetic Counselors, n.d.). Reassurance is offered and any questions or concerns addressed. All pregnant patients are also advised that a negative screening test carries **residual risk** and does not guarantee the birth of an unaffected baby.

For individuals who screen positive, it is important to reiterate that a positive screening result does not mean a positive diagnosis. Counseling includes a discussion of individual risk score indicated by the result, such as "1 in 100 chance of being affected" and supported with a visual tool such as the Paling Palette to aid in comprehension (see Chapter 11, *Risk Assessment during Pregnancy*, for a Paling Palette example). Framing risk in the negative, such as "99/100 chance of not being affected," should accompany the positive risk statement to present a comprehensive risk picture. Risks can be communicated in both fractions and percentages to aid in comprehension. More specific information about the condition is relevant to posttest counseling. Diagnostic testing options following a positive screen are presented, with a clear equal option to decline further testing. At this point, it is appropriate to remind the patient that if they choose diagnostic testing and results are positive, they have the option of terminating, depending on state law and gestational age, or continuing the pregnancy and either parenting or placing the child for adoption. It is also important to make patients aware of resources supporting either decision, including advocacy and support groups. Historically, face-to-face conversations were often viewed as the preferred mode of delivery of positive results to a patient; however, with the expansion of telehealth as a result of

COVID-19 pandemic restrictions, providers have had to become skilled at delivering such results remotely. Interprofessional care is typically introduced at this juncture with genetic counselors and maternal–fetal medicine or obstetrical referral.

When providing results of carrier screening, it is important to recognize that there is a broad range of clinical presentations, or phenotypes, for many genetic disorders, and genetic testing cannot predict all outcomes. For example, prenatal CF carrier testing can identify when both partners in a couple or donor are carriers. When these CF mutations are identified, prenatal diagnosis can be performed to determine whether a fetus has inherited a CF gene mutation from each parent and/or donor. Knowing that a fetus has inherited two CF mutations, however, does not predict the severity of CF in the baby, which is dependent on the particular combination of mutations and is not always known. For couples and individuals in this situation, the ethical dilemma may involve the decision to continue or to end a pregnancy without having knowledge of the severity of the disorder.

Disclosing a prenatal diagnosis to expectant parents is challenging no matter how much experience one has. Skotko et al. (2009) highlight how best to deliver a prenatal diagnosis of Down syndrome, which can be extrapolated to other prenatal diagnoses. They found that patients prefer to receive the diagnosis (Carroll et al., 2018):

- From a provider knowledgeable about the condition and able to sensitively deliver the diagnosis
- As soon as possible, after diagnostic testing
- With their partner
- At a preestablished time, in person or by phone
- With accurate information about the condition
- With opportunities to reach out to other parents of children with the diagnosis
- Avoiding words like "unfortunately" or "I have bad news"
- Using words like "I have unexpected news"
- With opportunities to resume discussion later, after the impact of the immediate news

Continuing with the example of Down syndrome, it is estimated that 67% of prenatal Down syndrome diagnoses are terminated (Natoli et al., 2012). Due to this, some providers may expect their clients to choose this option. Be careful not to *assume* anything and be ready to support the individual's decision, even if it differs from what you would choose. Adoption of an affected child is another option that should be discussed. A survey of families waiting to adopt children with Down syndrome revealed that few families learned of this option from healthcare providers, even though many were eager to do so. Primary motivators for adopting these children were positive experiences with people with Down syndrome in the past as well as the perception of having sufficient resources to care for a child with special needs (Lindh et al., 2007).

The Role of Professional Genetic Counselors

Genetic counselors are healthcare professionals with specialized graduate degrees and experience in the areas of medical genetics and counseling. They combine their in-depth knowledge of genetic tests and genetic technology with their psychosocial counseling skills to promote patient autonomy and facilitate the decision-making process to ensure that patients are receiving the appropriate follow-up. Genetic counselors work in both clinical, research, and industry areas of healthcare.

Prenatal genetic counselors are those that specialize in preconception and prenatal care. They may be involved in pre- and posttest patient counseling or may primarily focus on the posttest process. Individuals who screen positive on universally offered prenatal screening tests or who have certain risk factors are often referred to a genetic counselor for a more in-depth discussion. The role of a genetic counselor in the prenatal clinic has evolved not only because of the expansion and availability of genomic testing but also due to the increased numbers of genetic counselors in practice. Some experts advocate for a professional genetic counselor to be a part of the prenatal healthcare team to provide pretest and posttest counseling to all pregnant people (Minkoff & Berkowitz, 2014). However, it is important to note that initial genetic counseling can be provided by any prenatal care provider. A professional genetic counselor is most necessary for positive test results.

Consider referral to a genetic counselor

- Screen positive on serum marker screening
- Fetal abnormalities detected on prenatal ultrasound
- Screen positive on NIPS
- Screen positive on carrier screening
- Personal or family history of a known or suspected genetic disorder, birth defect, or chromosome abnormality
- Family history of intellectual disability of unknown etiology
- Those with a medical condition known or suspected to affect fetal development
- Those who are considering invasive prenatal diagnostic testing
- Those who pursue invasive prenatal diagnostic testing (for review of results)
- Teratogenic exposure

The Role of Consent in Genetic Testing

It is important to recognize that the concepts of "consent," "informed consent," "informed refusal," and "shared decision-making" differ, and all are important components of genetic counseling. Simple consent to or refusal of a procedure or test applies to decisions that are of low risk and cases in which there are limited options (Whitney et al., 2003). When decisions involve significant risk and/or uncertainty and where there are available options to consider, shared decision-making is most appropriate

(Whitney et al., 2003). This is often the case with genetic testing decisions.

Despite the ethical responsibility to provide informed consent, many patients are offered testing without being informed of the side effects, complications, and implications of positive test results, or that the tests were optional (Dahl et al., 2011; Press, 2000; Sheinis et al., 2017). Informed compliance, where patients are given an explanation of testing procedure with limited or no additional information, while not an ethical practice, can be a common prenatal care practice (Ackmann, 2005; van den Berg et al., 2005). The ACOG published in 2017 clear guidelines for providers, emphasizing the necessity of pre- and posttest counseling as it relates to genetic testing. (ACOG, 2017b).

In a commonly accepted definition, informed consent is a process consisting of five components: (a) competence to understand and decide; (b) disclosure of risks and benefits; (c) understanding of information and plans; (d) autonomy in choosing testing or no testing; and (e) consent or authorizing the choice (Beauchamp & Childress, 2001). A meta-analysis of 78 studies of prenatal screening found an overwhelming inadequacy in achievement of informed consent, with healthcare providers consistently failing to meet criteria 2–5 (Seavilleklein, 2009). It is a primary responsibility of the prenatal healthcare provider to obtain informed consent or refusal, not simply consent or informed compliance. It is each person's individual choice to accept or decline any testing options. Pregnant people deserve to have a full understanding of what will happen to them and their fetus before proceeding with any type of testing or treatment.

The power of technology to identify the genetic traits of embryos and fetuses is rapidly increasing. New genetic testing options will continue to bring additional ethical challenges to healthcare providers and to pregnant people and families. The ability to appropriately manage resolution of ethical dilemmas and conflicts that may result from genetic screening and diagnosis is an essential skill for prenatal care providers (see Chapter 2, *Ethics in Perinatal Care*).

Prenatal Genetic Counseling and the Healthcare Provider

Prenatal diagnosis and counseling can be an emotional issue for both patient and provider. Providers are likely to have an opinion about whether testing is valuable or not, in which situation it is more valuable, what patients should do with the results of their tests, and when certain tests should be ordered. The challenge for healthcare providers is to be objective and provide counseling on all testing choices that supports patient autonomy. To do this, healthcare providers must remain current in their knowledge of genetic testing and closely examine personal biases. Abortion is one of the many choices involved in genetic counseling and testing, and this topic may evoke strong feelings. It is each pregnant person's own choice to have or not have prenatal genetic screening and testing and what to do with that information. It is the responsibility of the healthcare provider to give appropriate, nonjudgmental, and complete information that fully enables pregnant patients to make these decisions, and that provides respect and support to them in their right to make decisions that will affect their lives.

Addressing Health Disparities and Bias in Reproductive Genetics Care

Perinatal genetic screening and counseling and providers who work in this area are not immune to systemic issues of bias and discrimination and must be aware of personal biases in order to promote more equitable practice and help individuals achieve optimal health. Gender bias is especially common in reproductive healthcare, including in genetic counseling. Sample pedigrees generally only show examples of inheritance for a male/female pairing; patient education materials can be presented in more gender-inclusive fashion. Carrier screening historically used race and self-reported ethnicity to determine what tests individuals would be offered. This is biased toward those of European ancestry because genomic databases predominantly contain genomic profiles from individuals of European ancestry (Landry et al., 2018). While professional guidelines have started to move away from recommending race and self-reported ethnicity to dictate the type of testing offered, it is uncertain how providers have changed their practice. Rural communities are often underserved by perinatal healthcare and are disproportionately affected by site closures and staffing shortages, all of which contributes to health disparities (Centers for Medicare & Medicaid Services [CMMS], 2019). These challenges can also decrease access to genetic testing options both before and during pregnancy. Limited financial resources and lack of health insurance or reliance on public insurance can also limit access due to the cost of some genetic screening and testing options. Patients with high BMI are more likely to experience a test failure or no-call results if they opt for the NIPS test, leading to additional tests and potential for invasive procedures and anxiety in this population. High BMI is more prevalent in certain racial and ethnic groups (Muzzey et al., 2020) creating greater disparity for those with intersecting identities of high BMI and race. Increased risk with advancing age and genetic tests previously reserved for individuals who become pregnant at age 35 and beyond, has contributed to an over-pathologizing of pregnancy for those over age 35. And finally, concerns regarding the implications of genetic testing on the disability community have existed for decades (Steinbach et al., 2016). Some argue that the very concept of genetic testing implies a hierarchy of desirability with children, with those affected by genetic conditions deemed undesirable. Studies of healthcare providers reveal significant bias against disabled people and negative beliefs about their potential quality of life (Iezzoni et al., 2021).

These examples of health inequities, though not exhaustive, must be actively considered and intentional action must be taken to diminish the disparities experienced by patients. As prenatal care and genetic screening continue to evolve, it is certain that additional health disparities will occur if the impact of new care approaches is not carefully and proactively considered. Being aware of and addressing existing and potential inequities will help ensure excellent care for all patients.

Summary

Offering pregnant individuals genetic testing choices is standard care and allows patients and families control over aspects of their reproductive and family lives. The goal of screening is to identify early disease or risk in order to implement preventive therapy and to provide patients with information relevant to reproductive decisions. Prenatal genetic tests offer increasingly comprehensive identification of genetic conditions and susceptibilities. It is essential that these testing options be offered with a nondirective approach and complete information, so pregnant patients have a full understanding of testing ramifications. For those choosing to undergo prenatal testing, most will get results confirming an unaffected fetus. Some will learn their baby has a defect or developmental condition, and in some cases, testing will yield results that are indeterminate. Prenatal genetic testing offers more information about the unborn fetus, yet raises additional questions about what to do with the information. Prenatal healthcare providers must be aware of the implications for care and emotional impact of prenatal genetic testing. The skills to provide true informed consent as well as navigate the ethical dilemmas that may arise are essential. Genetic testing technologies are expanding rapidly and will continue to give pregnant people more reproductive choices while potentially creating ethical challenges. Lifelong learning in this area is a commitment to excellence in care for childbearing individuals and families.

Resources for Pregnant People, Their Families, and Healthcare Providers

Disability Language Style Guide is provided by the National Center on Disability and Journalism. This resource offers helpful guidance on the appropriate use of words describing disability and the associated communities. https://ncdj.org/style-guide

Down Syndrome Diagnosis Network (DSDN) has resources for both patients and professionals in view of a prenatal diagnosis or screen positive for Down syndrome: https://www.dsdiagnosisnetwork.org

Genetics Home Reference by the National Institutes of Health (NIH) offers information on all genetic conditions with guidelines and resources for professionals: http://ghr.nlm.nih.gov

Genetic Support Foundation has information for consumers and professionals: https://geneticsupportfoundation.org/pregnancy-genetics

Lettercase: The National Center for Prenatal and Postnatal Resources is a nationally recognized source of current and balanced information for both patients and providers. Booklets are available for Down syndrome, Turner syndrome, and several other chromosomal abnormalities when diagnosed or suspected prenatally. www.lettercase.org

National Genetics Education and Family Support Center provides information and resources surrounding genetics and genetic testing. https://nationalfamilycenter.org

National Institutes of Health (NIH) website is devoted to genetic research and educating professionals about genetics: http://www.genome.gov/Education

National Society for Genetic Counselors website has a resource section for professionals: http://www.nsgc.org

Norton and Elaine Sarnoff Center for Jewish Genetics provides education resources related to hereditary cancers and genetic disorders more common among persons of Jewish descent. https://www.jewishgenetics.org/

Perinatal Quality Foundation has a NIPS/Cell Free DNA Screening Predictive Value online calculator to determine PPV or NPV based on NIPS results: https://www.perinatalquality.org/vendors/nsgc/nipt

Pregnancy and Health Profile (PHP) has free prenatal genetic screening risk assessment and clinical decision-making tool for providers and patients: https://www.hrsa.gov/advisorycommittees/mchbadvisory/heritabledisorders/meetings/twentyeighth/prenatalfamilyhistoryscott.pdf

References

Ackmann, E. A. (2005). Prenatal testing gone awry: The birth of a conflict of ethics and liability. *Indiana Health Law Review*, *2*, 199–224.

Agopian, A., Tinker, S., Lupo, P., Canfield, M., & Mitchell, L. (2013). Proportion of neural tube defects attributable to known risk factors. *Birth Defects Research Part A: Clinical and Molecular Teratology*, *97*(1), 42–46.

Åhman, A., Runestam, K., & Sarkadi, A. (2010). Did I really want to know this? Pregnant women's reaction to detection of a soft marker during ultrasound screening. *Patient Education and Counseling*, *81*(1), 87–93.

Allison, S. J., Stafford, J., & Anumba, D. O. (2011). The effect of stress and anxiety associated with maternal prenatal diagnosis on feto-maternal attachment. *BMC Women's Health*, *11*(1), 33.

American College of Obstetricians and Gynecologists (ACOG). (2016). Prenatal diagnostic testing for genetic diseases. ACOG practice bulleting no. 162. *Obstetrics & Gynecology*, *127*(5), e108–e122.

American College of Obstetricians and Gynecologists (ACOG). (2017a). Carrier screening for genetic conditions. Committee opinion no. 691. American. *Obstetrics & Gynecology*, *129*(3), e41–e55.

American College of Obstetricians and Gynecologists (ACOG). (2017b). Counseling about genetic testing and communication of test results. ACOG Committee opinion no. 693. *Obstetrics & Gynecology*, *129*(4), 771–772.

American College of Obstetricians and Gynecologists (ACOG). (2017c). Neural tube defects. ACOG practice bulletin no. 187. *Obstetrics & Gynecology*, *130*(6), e279–e290.

American College of Obstetricians and Gynecologists (ACOG). (2020). Practice bulletin 226: Screening for fetal chromosomal abnormalities. *Obstetrics and Gynecology*, *136*(4), e48–e69.

American Society of Hematology. (2022). *Sickle cell trait*. http://www.hematology.org/Patients/Anemia/Sickle-Cell-Trait.aspx

Arjunan, A., Darnes, D. R., Sagaser, K. G., & Svenson, A. B. (2022). Addressing reproductive healthcare disparities through equitable carrier screening: Medical racism and genetic discrimination in United States' history highlights the needs for change in obstetrical genetics care. *Societies*, *12*(2), 33. https://doi.org/10.3390/soc12020033

Baillie, C., Smith, J., Hewison, J., & Mason, G. (2000). Ultrasound screening for chromosomal abnormality: Women's reactions to false positive results. *British Journal of Health Psychology*, *5*(4), 377–394.

Beauchamp, T. L., & Childress, J. F. (2001). *Principles of biomedical ethics* (5th ed.). Oxford University Press.

Carroll, C., Carroll, C., Goloff, N., & Pitt, M. B. (2018). When bad news isn't necessarily bad: Recognizing provider bias when sharing unexpected news. *Pediatrics*, *142*(1), e20180503. https://doi.org/10.1542/peds.2018-0503

Cartier, L., Murphy-Kaulbeck, L., Wilson, R. D., Audibert, F., Brock, J. A., Carroll, J., Cartier, L., Gagnon, A., Johnson, J.-A., Langlois, S., Murphy-Kaulbeck, L., Okun, N., & Pastuck, M. (2012). Counselling considerations for prenatal genetic screening. *Journal of Obstetrics and Gynaecology Canada*, *34*(5), 489–493.

Centers for Disease Control and Prevention (CDC). (2016). *Key findings: Prevalence of Fragile X premutation prevalence of CGG expansions of the FMR1 gene in a US population-based sample*. https://www.cdc.gov/ncbddd/fxs/features/fxs-prevalence-keyfindings.html

Centers for Disease Control and Prevention (CDC). (2022). *5 Ways to lower the risk of having a pregnancy affected by a neural tube defect*. https://www.cdc.gov/ncbddd/birthdefects/5-ways-to-lower-the-risk.html

Centers for Medicare & Medicaid Services. (2019). *Improving access to maternal health care in rural communities: Issue brief*. https://www.cms.gov/About-CMS/Agency-Information/OMH/equity-initiatives/rural-health/rural-maternal-health

Cereda, A., & Carey, J. C. (2012). The trisomy 18 syndrome. *Orphanet Journal of Rare Diseases*, *7*(1), 81.

Cystic Fibrosis Foundation. (2017). *About cystic fibrosis*. https://www.cff.org/What-is-CF/CF-Genetics

Dahl, K., Hvidman, L., Jorgensen, F. S., Henriques, C., Olesen, F., Kjaergaard, H., & Kesmodel, U. S. (2011). First-trimester down syndrome screening: Pregnant women's knowledge. *Ultrasound in Obstetrics and Gynecology*, *38*, 145–151.

Delaney, M., & Roggensack, A. (2017). No. 214—Guidelines for the management of pregnancy at 41+ 0 to 42+ 0 weeks. *Journal of Obstetrics and Gynaecology Canada*, *39*(8), e164–e174.

Quest Diagnostics. (2022). *Penta screen*. https://testdirectory.questdiagnostics.com/test/test-guides/TS_Penta_Screen/penta-screen?p=td

Driscoll, D., & Gross, S. (2009). Screening for fetal aneuploidy and neural tube defects. *Genetics in Medicine*, *11*(11), 818–821.

Dugoff, L., Norton, M., Kueller, J., & Society for Maternal-Fetal Medicine (SMFM). (2016). The use of chromosomal microarray for prenatal diagnosis. *American Journal of Obstetrics and Gynecology*, *215*(4), B2–B9.

Edwards, J. G., Feldman, G., Goldberg, J., Gregg, A. R., Norton, M. E., Rose, N. C., Schneider, A., Stoll, K., Wapner, R., & Watson, M. S. (2015). Expanded carrier screening in reproductive medicine-points to consider: A joint statement of the American College of Medical Genetics and Genomics, American College of Obstetricians and Gynecologists, National Society of Genetic Counselors, Perinatal Quality Foundation, and Society for Maternal-Fetal Medicine. *Obstetrics & Gynecology*, *125*(3), 653–662. https://doi.org/10.1097/AOG.0000000000000666

Egbe, A., Lee, S., Ho, D., & Uppu, S. (2015). Effect of race on the prevalence of congenital malformations among newborns in the United States. *Ethnicity & Disease*, *25*(2), 226–231.

Eunpu, D. L. (1997). Systemically-based psychotherapeutic techniques in genetic counseling. *Journal of Genetic Counseling*, *6*(1), 1–20. https://doi.org/10.1023/A:1025630917735

Familial Dysautonomia Foundation, Inc. (n.d.). *FD fact sheet*. https://familialdysautonomia.org/about-fd

Georgsson, S., Ohman, S., Saltvedt, U., Waldenstrom, C., Grunewald, S., & Olin-Lauritzen, S. (2006). Pregnant women's responses to information about an increased risk of carrying a baby with down syndrome. *Birth*, *33*(1), 664–673.

Green, J. M., Hewison, J., Bekker, H. L., Bryant, L. D., & Cuckle, H. S. (2004). Psychological aspects of genetic screening of pregnant women and newborns: A systematic review. *Health Technology Assessment*, 8(33), 1–109.

Gregg, A. R., Aarabi, M., Klugman, S., Leach, N. T., Bashford, M. T., Goldwaser, T., Chen, E., Sparks, T. N., Reddi, H. V., Rajkovic, A., Dungan, J. S., Professional Practice, A. C. M. G., & Committee, G. (2021). Screening for autosomal recessive and X-linked conditions during pregnancy and preconception: A practice resource of the American College of Medical Genetics and Genomics (ACMG). *Genetics in Medicine: Official Journal of the American College of Medical Genetics*, 23(10), 1793–1806. https://doi.org/10.1038/s41436-021-01203-z

Gregg, A. R., Skotko, B. G., Benkendorf, J. L., Monaghan, K. G., Bajaj, K., Best, R. G., Klugman, S., & Watson, M. S. (2016). Noninvasive prenatal screening for fetal aneuploidy, 2016 update: A position statement of the American College of Medical Genetics and Genomics. *Genetics in Medicine*, 18(10), 1056–1065.

Gregg, R. (1993). "Choice" as a double-edged sword: Information, guilt and mother-blaming in a high-tech age. *Women & Health*, 20(3), 53–73.

Hodgson, J., & Gaff, C. (2013). Enhancing family communication about genetics: Ethical and professional dilemmas. *Journal of Genetic Counseling*, 22(1), 16–21.

Hurford, E., Hawkins, A., Hudgins, L., & Taylor, J. (2013). The decision to continue a pregnancy affected by Down syndrome: Timing of decision and satisfaction of receiving a prenatal diagnosis. *Journal of Genetic Counseling*, 22(5), 587–593. https://doi.org/10.1007/s10897-013-9590-6

Iezzoni, L. I., Rao, S. R., Ressalam, J., Bolcic-Jankovic, D., Agaronnik, N. D., Donelan, K., Lagu, T., & Campbell, E. G. (2021). Physicians' perceptions of people with disability and their health care. *Health Affairs*, 40(2), 297–306. https://doi.org/10.1377/hlthaff.2020.01452

Jelin, A. C., & Vora, N. (2018). Whole exome sequencing: Applications in prenatal genetics. *Obstetrics and Gynecology Clinics of North America*, 45(1), 69–81.

Kaasen, A., Helbig, A., Malt, U. F., Naes, T., Skari, H., & Haugen, G. (2010). Acute maternal social dysfunction, health perception and psychological distress after ultrasonographic detection of a fetal structural anomaly. *BJOG: An International Journal of Obstetrics and Gynaecology*, 117(9), 1127–1138.

Kaseniit, K. E., Haque, I. S., Goldberg, J. D., Shulman, L. P., & Muzzey, D. (2020). Genetic ancestry analysis on >93,000 individuals undergoing expanded carrier screening reveals limitations of ethnicity-based medical guidelines. *Genetics in Medicine*, 22(10), 1694–1702. https://doi.org/10.1038/s41436-020-0869-3

Kowalcek, I. (2017). Anxiety associated with prenatal diagnosis. *Journal of Gynecology and Obstetrics Bulletins*, 1(2), 1–2.

Landry, L. G., Ali, N., Williams, D. R., Rehm, H. L., & Bonham, V. L. (2018). Lack of diversity in genomic databases is a barrier to translating precision medicine research into practice. *Health Affairs*, 37(5), 780–785. https://doi.org/10.1377/hlthaff.2017.1595

Larsson, A., Svalenius, E., Marsal, K., & Dykes, A. (2009). Parental level of anxiety, sense of coherence and state of mind when choroid plexus cysts have been identified at a routine ultrasound examination in the second trimester of pregnancy: A case control study. *Journal of Psychosomatic Obstetrics and Gynaecology*, 30, 95–100.

Lawson, K. L., & Turriff-Jonasson, S. I. (2006). Maternal serum screening and psychosocial attachment to pregnancy. *Journal of Psychosomatic Research*, 60(4), 371–378.

Lindh, H. L., Steele, R., Page-Steiner, J., & Donnenfeld, A. E. (2007). Characteristics and perspectives of families waiting to adopt a child with down syndrome. *Genetics in Medicine*, 9(4), 235–240.

Minkoff, H., & Berkowitz, R. (2014). The case for universal prenatal genetic counseling. *Obstetrics & Gynecology*, 123(6), 1335–1338.

Muzzey, D., Goldberg, J. D., & Haverty, C. (2020). Noninvasive prenatal screening for patients with high body mass index: Evaluating the impact of a customized whole genome sequencing workflow on sensitivity and residual risk. *Prenatal Diagnosis*, 40(3), 333–341. https://doi.org/10.1002/pd.5603

National Down Syndrome Society. (2022). *Facts about Down syndrome*. http://www.ndss.org/about-down-syndrome/down-syndrome-facts

National Library of Medicine. (2021). *Trisomy 13*. MedlinePlus. https://medlineplus.gov/genetics/condition/trisomy-13

National Society of Genetic Counselors. (n.d.). *NIPT/Cell free DNA screening predictive value calculator*. Retrieved August 26, 2022 from https://www.perinatalquality.org/vendors/nsgc/nipt

National Tay-Sachs & Allied Diseases Association. (2021). *Tay-Sachs disease*. https://www.ntsad.org/index.php/the-diseases/tay-sachs

Natoli, J. L., Ackerman, D. L., McDermott, S., & Edwards, J. G. (2012). Prenatal diagnosis of down syndrome: A systematic review of termination rates (1995–2011). *Prenatal Diagnosis*, 32(2), 142–153. https://doi.org/10.1002/pd.2910

Norton, M. E., Jacobsson, B., Swamy, G. K., Laurent, L. C., Ranzini, A. C., Brar, H., Tomlinson, M. W., Pereira, L., Spitz, J. L., Hollemon, D., Cuckle, H., Musci, T. J., & Wapner, R. J. (2015). Cell-free DNA analysis for noninvasive examination of trisomy. *New England Journal of Medicine*, 372(17), 1589–1597. https://doi.org/10.1056/NEJMoa1407349

Pratt, M., Garritty, C., Thuku, M., Esmaeilisaraji, L., Hamel, C., Hartley, T., Millar, K., Skidmore, B., Dougan, S., & Armour, C. M. (2020). Application of exome sequencing for prenatal diagnosis: A rapid scoping review. *Genetics in Medicine*, 22(12), 1925–1934. https://doi.org/10.1038/s41436-020-0918-y

Press, N. (2000). Assessing the expressive character of prenatal testing: The choices made or the choices made available. In E. Parens & A. Asch (Eds.), *Prenatal testing and disability rights* (pp. 214–233). Georgetown University Press.

Rothwell, E., Johnson, E., Mathiesen, A., Golden, K., Metcalf, A., Rose, N. C., & Botkin, J. R. (2017). Experiences among women with positive prenatal expanded carrier screening results. *Journal of Genetic Counseling*, 26(4), 690–696.

Rowe, H., Fisher, J., & Quinlivan, J. (2009). Women who are well informed about prenatal genetic screening delay emotional attachment to their fetus. *Journal of Psychosomatic Obstetrics and Gynecology*, 30(1), 34–41.

Sapp, J. C., Hull, S. C., Duffe, S., Zornetzer, S., Sutton, E., Marteau, T. M., & Biesecker, B. B. (2010). Ambivalence toward undergoing invasive prenatal testing: An exploration of its origins. *Prenatal Diagnosis*, 30, 77–82.

Seavilleklein, V. (2009). Challenging the rhetoric of choice in prenatal screening. *Bioethics*, 23, 68–77.

Sheinis, M., Bensimon, K., & Selk, A. (2017). Patients' knowledge of prenatal screening for trisomy 21. *Journal of Genetic Counseling*, 27(1), 95–103.

Skirton, H., & Barr, O. (2010). Antenatal screening and informed choice: A cross-sectional survey of parents and professionals. *Midwifery*, 26(6), 596–602.

Skotko, B. G., Kishnani, P. S., Capone, G. T., & Down Syndrome Diagnosis Study Group. (2009). Prenatal diagnosis of down syndrome: How best to deliver the news. *American Journal of Medical Genetics. Part A*, 149A(11), 2361–2367.

Skrzypek, H., & Hui, L. (2017). Noninvasive prenatal testing for fetal aneuploidy and single gene disorders. *Best Practice & Research Clinical Obstetrics and Gynaecology*, 42, 26–38.

Steinbach, R. J., Allyse, M., Michie, M., Liu, E. Y., & Cho, M. K. (2016). "This lifetime commitment": Public conceptions of disability and noninvasive prenatal genetic screening. *American Journal of Medical Genetics Part A*, 170A(2), 363–374. https://doi.org/10.1002/ajmg.a.37459

Susanne, G. O., Sissel, S., Ulla, W., Charlotta, G., & Sonja, O. L. (2006). Pregnant women's responses to information about an increased risk of carrying a baby with Down syndrome. *Birth (Berkeley, California)*, 33(1), 64–73.

Taylor-Phillips, S., Freeman, K., Geppert, J., Agbebiyi, A., Uthman, O. A., Madan, J., Clarke, A., Quenby, S., & Clarke, A. (2016). Accuracy of non-invasive prenatal testing using cell-free DNA for detection of down, Edwards and Patau syndromes: A systematic review and meta-analysis. *BMJ Open*, 6(1), e010002.

Uhlmann, W., Schuette, J. & Yashar, B. (2011). *A guide to genetic counseling* (2nd ed.). Wiley-Blackwell.

van den Berg, M., Timmermans, D. R., Ten Kate, L. P., van Vugt, J. M., & van der Wal, G. (2005). Are pregnant women making informed choices about prenatal screening? *Genetics in Medicine, 7*(5), 332–338.

Van der Zalm, J. E., & Byrne, P. J. (2006). Seeing baby: Women's experience prenatal ultrasound examination and unexpected fetal diagnosis. *Journal of Perinatology, 26*(7), 403–408.

Viaux-Savelon, S., Dommergues, M., Rosenblum, O., Bodeau, N., Aidane, E., Philippon, O., Mazet, P., Vibert-Guigue, C., Vauthier-Brouzes, D., Feldman, R., & Cohen, D. (2012). Prenatal ultrasound screening: False positive soft markers may alter maternal representations and mother-infant interaction. *PLoS One, 7*(1), e30935.

Warsof, S. L., Larion, S., & Abuhamad, A. Z. (2015). Overview of the impact of noninvasive prenatal testing on diagnostic procedures. *Prenatal Diagnosis, 35*(10), 972–979.

Weil, J. (2000). *Psychosocial genetic counseling.* Oxford University Press.

Werner-Lin, A., McCoyd, J. L., & Bernhardt, B. A. (2016). Balancing genetics (science) and counseling (art) in prenatal chromosomal microarray testing. *Journal of Genetic Counseling, 25*(5), 855–867.

Whitney, S. N., McGuire, A. L., & McCullough, L. B. (2003). A typology of shared decision making, informed consent, and simple consent. *Annals of Internal Medicine, 140*(1), 54–59.

Williams, J., Mai, C. T., Mulinare, J., Isenburg, J., Flood, T. J., Ethen, M., Frohnert, B., & Kirby, R. S. (2015). Updated estimates of neural tube defects prevented by mandatory folic acid fortification—United States, 1995–2011. *MMWR Morbidity Mortality Weekly Reports, 64*(1), 1–5.

14

Assessment of Fetal Well-Being

Jenifer Fahey

Relevant Terms

Acidemia—increased concentration of hydrogen ions in blood (increased acidity of blood); normal, term newborn umbilical cord arterial blood pH is 7.27 ± 0.07

Acidosis—increased concentration of hydrogen ions in tissue, increased acidity of tissue.

Asphyxia—combination of hypoxia and metabolic acidosis due to profound and/or prolonged lack of oxygen. Asphyxia is associated with a risk of brain damage.

Auscultated acceleration test (AAT)—a simple evaluation of fetal health in which the examiner listens for fetal heart rate accelerations with a fetoscope, Doptone, or other device

Fetal heart rate (FHR) accelerations—an abrupt increase in FHR that usually occurs in conjunction with fetal movement, typically determined visually on an electronic fetal monitor heart tracing

Fetal heart rate baseline—the baseline FHR is the predominant heart rate during a 10-minute segment rounded to the nearest 5 beats per minute (bpm); normal range of FHR is 110–160 bpm

Fetal heart rate variability—fluctuations in the baseline FHR that are irregular in frequency and amplitude; the degree of variability is an indicator of fetal oxygenation

Fetal growth restriction (FGR)—a fetus that does not grow to its genetically determined potential, often clinically defined as a fetus whose estimated fetal weight (EFW) is below a certain percentile (e.g., <10th or <5th percentile)

Hypoxemia—decreased oxygen content of blood; normal, term fetal scalp blood PO_2 is 21.8 ± 2.6 (mmHg)

Hypoxia—decreased oxygen content in tissue

Iatrogenic—an illness or disorder caused inadvertently by a medical provider or by medical treatment or diagnostic procedures

Iatrogenic prematurity—the induced or operative birth of a fetus prior to reaching term gestation

Negative predictive value—likelihood that if a test is negative, the condition is truly absent in that individual; the nonstress test (NST) has good negative predictive value for fetal acidemia

Oligohydramnios—less than normal amniotic fluid volume (AFV); variously defined as an AFV of ≤200–500 mL, diagnosed with ultrasound by a largest vertical pocket (LVP) of ≤2 cm or an amniotic fluid index (AFI) of ≤5 cm

Polyhydramnios—greater than normal amniotic fluid volume; commonly defined as an amniotic fluid volume of >2100 mL—diagnosed with ultrasound by an AFI of ≥25 cm at any gestational age, or a single measurement of any LVP >8 cm

Positive predictive value—likelihood that if a test is positive, the condition is truly present in that individual; the NST has poor positive predictive value for fetal acidemia

Sensitivity—ability of a test to identify that a condition or disease is present, for example, the ability of the NST to identify the presence of fetal academia; the NST has poor sensitivity for fetal acidemia

Specificity—ability of a test to identify that a condition or disease is absent, for example, the ability of the NST to determine that acidemia is not present; the NST has excellent specificity for acidemia

---

Introduction

One of the primary responsibilities of prenatal care providers is to monitor fetal well-being to determine if intervention is necessary to prevent fetal neurologic impairment or demise. There are multiple techniques and technologies available to assist in this task—from time-honored measures such as measurement of fundal growth and fetal movement counts (FMCs) to the newer,

technologically based tests such as ultrasound assessment of fetal breathing movements and Doppler velocimetry. Collectively referred to as "antenatal fetal testing" or "antenatal fetal surveillance," the monitoring conducted using these technologies is aimed at identifying fetuses with signs of compromised oxygenation that may benefit from intervention. These tests can also be used to monitor the status of the fetus with compromised oxygenation to detect signs of worsening status and help

Prenatal and Postnatal Care: A Person-Centered Approach, Third Edition. Edited by Karen Trister Grace, Cindy L. Farley, Noelene K. Jeffers, and Tanya Tringali.
© 2024 John Wiley & Sons Ltd. Published 2024 by John Wiley & Sons Ltd.
Companion website: www.wiley.com/go/grace/prenatal

optimize the timing of intervention. This makes it possible to prolong pregnancy in order to minimize the risks from prematurity, while also allowing for intervention early enough to prevent fetal death or complications from fetal **asphyxia**.

Prenatal care providers will conduct some of these tests, while others may be performed by specialists or subspecialists such as perinatologists. In these cases, the primary prenatal care provider is responsible for ensuring that, when necessary, individuals in their care are appropriately referred for testing and assessment. Often, it is also the responsibility of the primary prenatal care provider to interpret the results of those tests and to make an appropriate management plan based on the findings. In all cases, the prenatal care provider must be able to educate the pregnant person regarding the indications for testing, testing procedures, test results, and the management plan based on those results. This chapter focuses on those assessment techniques that evaluate fetal circulation and oxygenation starting at approximately 24 weeks estimated gestational age (EGA) but prior to the onset of labor.

These tests of fetal well-being include the following:

- FMCs
- Nonstress test (NST)
- Contraction stress test (CST)
- Biophysical profile (BPP)
- Amniotic fluid volume (AFV) or amniotic fluid index (AFI)
- Doppler flow studies.

This chapter includes a description of each test, indications for testing, testing procedures, interpretation of test results, and general management principles. Screening for genetic anomalies and fetal growth assessment are addressed in Chapters 13 and 34. The topic of intrapartum fetal heart rate (FHR) monitoring is outside the scope of this text.

> **Health equity key points**
>
> - Black pregnant individuals are at increased risk for fetal death. Racism and bias at the individual and population level are key determinants of this increased risk.
> - Standardized, evidence-based guidelines for the initiation and periodicity of fetal assessment as well as for the management of patient concerns regarding fetal well-being, such as reports of decreased fetal movement, is one way in which healthcare systems can work to reduce the impacts of bias in the arena of fetal surveillance.
> - Fetuses that are small for gestational age (SGA) may be so for normal, constitutional reasons that differ across populations or for pathologic reasons that may warrant intervention.
> - Instructions (both spoken and written) regarding fetal well-being that are in the correct language and at the appropriate reading and health literacy level are necessary to promote equitable access to appropriate antenatal fetal assessment and intervention.

Physiologic Principles

Many cases of fetal neurologic damage and demise result from conditions that lead to fetal **hypoxia** and **acidemia**. The causes of fetal hypoxia may be acute (e.g., placental abruption following trauma) or chronic (e.g., decreased unteroplacental flow due to maternal hypertension) and can be categorized as preplacental/maternal, uteroplacental, and postplacental/fetal, as outlined in Table 14.1. Often etiological factors will overlap/interact. When the fetus experiences hypoxia, irrespective of the cause, it will respond with compensatory mechanisms that are protective and adaptive and allow the fetus to withstand periods of decreased oxygenation without central nervous system damage. These mechanisms include the following:

Table 14.1 Causes of Fetal Hypoxia

Type	Description	Causes or associated conditions
Preplacental/ maternal hypoxia	The fetus is hypoxic due to maternal hypoxia	- Hypoxic environment such as high-altitude - Preexisting maternal cardiovascular disease such as cyanotic heart disease, heart failure and pulmonary hypertension - Chronic pulmonary disease such as poorly controlled asthma, tuberculosis, or cystic fibrosis - Maternal hematologic disorders such as severe anemia, sickle-cell disease, or thalassemia
Uteroplacental hypoxia	Fetus becomes hypoxic due to abnormalities of the placenta	- Abnormal placentation early in gestation - Placental vascular disease later in pregnancy
Postplacental/ fetal hypoxia	The fetus becomes hypoxic due to fetal conditions or abnormal uterine artery circulation	- Progressive fetal cardiac failure such as complete congenital heart block, complex congenital heart malformations - Genetic anomalies - Mechanical compression, rupture, or thrombotic occlusion of the uterine artery

Source: Adapted from Hutter and Jaeggi (2010) and Kingdom and Kaufmann (1997).

- Redirection of blood flow to preferentially perfuse vital organs including the heart, adrenal glands, and brain
- Decreased perfusion to kidneys, gastrointestinal tract, and lower extremities
- Decreased fetal movement
- Slowing of the FHR.

These compensatory mechanisms produce signs that can be used by clinicians to identify and evaluate fetal hypoxia. Decreased amniotic fluid production resulting from decreased fetal urine production due to compromised kidney perfusion and a loss of accelerations on the FHR tracing believed to be related to the compensatory decrease in fetal movement are examples of clinical signs of compromised fetal oxygenation. Chronic and/or profound hypoxia can also produce clinical signs including **fetal growth restriction** (FGR) and resistance in venous circulation detectable via Doppler ultrasonography.

The antenatal fetal tests described in this chapter are not able to predict or assist in the management of acute hypoxic events leading to fetal neurological damage or demise such as placental abruption, cord accidents, or maternal cardiovascular events. Similarly, they are of no or limited usefulness in the case of nonhypoxic etiologies of fetal neurologic damage or demise such as preterm rupture of membranes, chorioamnionitis, or genetic anomalies.

Indications

Antenatal fetal testing in a low-risk population has been demonstrated to have low **sensitivity** and **specificity** as well as poor **positive predictive value** for fetal compromise. Current evidence does *not* support the routine use of antepartum fetal testing in uncomplicated pregnancies prior to 41 weeks' EGA (ACOG, 2021; Grivell et al., 2010). There is evidence from observational studies, however, that in populations at increased risk of fetal asphyxia, antenatal surveillance may help improve outcomes (Kontopoulos & Vintzileos, 2004). One of the tasks for prenatal care providers is, therefore, to identify those pregnant persons who may benefit from antenatal fetal testing and to either conduct this assessment or to refer them to receive this assessment.

Table 14.1 lists some of the conditions that are associated with an increased risk of asphyxia and fetal death. Increased fetal surveillance is recommended for pregnant persons with one or more of these conditions. FGR has emerged as the single most significant risk factor for intrauterine fetal demise (IUFD; Flenady et al., 2011; Gardosi et al., 2005; Manning, 2009). Therefore, timely recognition of fetal growth disorders is critical so that an appropriate surveillance and management plan can be put in place (see Chapter 34, *Amniotic Fluid and Fetal Growth Disorders*). Additional factors associated with IUFD include extremes of maternal age, grand multiparity, Black race (which, as discussed below, is now understood to be related to the health impacts of racism), prenatal smoking, use of assisted reproductive technologies, fetal anomalies, and male fetal sex (a consistent finding, the

pathophysiology of which is still being elucidated; Flenady et al., 2011; Signore et al., 2009). However, increased antenatal fetal surveillance for these indications has not been proven to improve outcomes (O'Neill & Thorp, 2012).

There is insufficient evidence to make specific recommendations regarding what type of antenatal fetal testing is best, when this surveillance is started, or how often it is repeated. The decision to initiate testing must consider the prognosis for neonatal survival, which is impacted by multiple factors including maternal condition and gestational age. The risks to the neonate related to **iatrogenic prematurity** must be weighed against the risks of continuation of pregnancy, a task that is made particularly difficult due to the low positive predictive value of available antenatal fetal tests. A fetal surveillance plan must, therefore, be determined based on the clinical picture and individual risk factors and will often require consultation with a specialist or subspecialist.

Black pregnant people are more likely to experience a fetal demise. The Centers for Disease Control and Prevention (CDC) analyzed 2015–2017 US fetal death report data and found that non-Hispanic Black (Black) pregnant individuals had more than twice the fetal mortality rate compared with non-Hispanic White (White) and Hispanic individuals (Pruitt et al., 2020). Disparities in outcomes by race often persist even after researchers control for socioeconomic and health factors (Wang et al., 2020). While the mechanisms that result in this increased risk related to race are complex and still being elucidated, there is now an understanding that the impact of both racism and bias at the individual and systems level are key determinants. Research has demonstrated that provider bias decreases the probability that the concerns of Black individuals will be addressed with treatment and referrals (Bailey et al., 2017; FitzGerald & Hurst, 2017). The implementation of standardized, evidence-based guidelines for initiation and periodicity of fetal assessment and for management of patient concerns regarding fetal well-being, such as reports of decreased fetal movement, are ways in which healthcare systems can work to reduce the impacts of bias in the arena of fetal surveillance.

Interprofessional Care

Some of the conditions listed in Table 14.2 are conditions that may require a team approach to care. Primary prenatal care providers ensure that pregnant patients are appropriately screened for these conditions with a thorough history, appropriate lab work and diagnostic tests, and monitoring of fetal and maternal health status throughout pregnancy. When a complex pregnancy condition develops, the healthcare provider must decide whether independent management of the patient is still appropriate or whether consultation, collaborative management, or transfer of care is indicated. This decision will be influenced by the practice site, the personnel and facility resources, and by the clinical situation.

Table 14.2 Conditions Associated with An Increased Risk of Fetal Death

Maternal medical conditions
Pregestational diabetes mellitus
Hypertensive disorders
Thyroid disorders (poorly controlled)
Renal disease
Cardiac disease (cyanotic)
Systemic lupus erythematosus (SLE)
Hemoglobinopathies
Antiphospholipid syndrome
Obesity
Pregnancy-related conditions
Fetal growth restriction
Decreased fetal movement
Placental abruption
Hypertensive disorders of pregnancy
Gestational diabetes that is poorly controlled and/or requiring medication
Post-term pregnancy
Oligohydramnios
Multiple gestation with growth discrepancy
Isoimmunization
Previous IUFD
Intrahepatic cholestasis of pregnancy

Source: Adapted from Signore et al. (2009), American College of Obstetricians & Gynecologists (2021), and Gardosi et al. (2013).

Fetal Assessment Methods

Monitoring of Fetal Movement

Decreased movement is a known fetal response to hypoxia and has been demonstrated to be associated with an increased risk of fetal death (O'Sullivan et al., 2009; Sinha et al., 2007). The fetus experiencing hypoxia will preferentially perfuse vital organs such as the adrenal glands, heart, and brain. This is accomplished, in part, through a decrease or cessation of fetal movement that reduces the overall fetal demand for oxygen. Research has repeatedly found that perception of decreased fetal movement by the pregnant person is associated with an increased risk of poor perinatal outcomes including stillbirth (Heazell & Frøen, 2008). In theory, therefore, if a pregnant person detects a decrease in activity, this can trigger additional assessments and interventions in time to avoid fetal injury or death.

Fetal movement monitoring is an attractive fetal assessment modality because it is easily taught to patients and can be conducted at home without the need for healthcare personnel or expensive equipment. There are two approaches to patient monitoring of fetal movement— qualitative and quantitative. In a qualitative approach, pregnant patients are asked to report a subjective decrease in fetal movement, while in a quantitative approach, patients are asked to count fetal movements and report if the number of movements does not meet a specific threshold. Quantitative assessments of fetal movement are referred to as FMC. Current evidence suggests that a pregnant person's perception of a decrease in fetal movement may be more effective than formal FMC as a screening tool for detecting the compromised fetus (Sterpu et al., 2020).

Studies investigating the effectiveness of FMC in reducing the incidence of IUFD have produced mixed results. Some observational studies have shown a significant decrease in IUFD rate in pregnant individuals who conducted regular FMCs and reported decreased fetal movement to their healthcare providers (Moore & Piacquadio, 1989; Neldam, 1980; Tveit et al., 2009). However, other larger studies examining the effectiveness of FMC interventions in reducing fetal deaths have shown no effect (Grant et al., 1989; Mangesi et al., 2015; Norman et al., 2018). A meta-analysis of five randomized control trials representing more than 450,000 fetuses showed no difference in perinatal outcomes, including perinatal death, between groups who received counseling to conduct FMC and those who did not (Bellussi et al., 2020). Currently, there are insufficient data, therefore, to recommend for or against routine FMC for any pregnant individual, even those considered at high risk for fetal demise.

Experts who support the use of FMC suggest that the failure of FMC to consistently improve outcomes may be related to the fact that fetal death is a rare event and sample sizes, even pooled ones, are simply too small to detect differences between groups. Additionally, false negative results during additional testing and unclear or nonexistent protocols for the management of decreased fetal movement resulting in delays in intervention may further dilute the potential impact of maternal reporting of decreased fetal movement on perinatal outcomes. Further complicating the observed relationship between the perception of decreased fetal movement and fetal outcomes is that a pregnant individual who may have a qualitative decrease in fetal movement that accurately reflects compromised oxygenation may not report this decrease if they also conduct an FMC, and it does not meet the quantitative criteria for reporting (false negative for FMC). Part of the difficulty in maximizing the potential effectiveness of FMC is the wide range of normal fetal activity patterns as well as the fact that the maternal perception of fetal movement can be highly variable among individuals and even in the same person. Studies correlating perceived fetal movement with sonographic evidence of fetal movements demonstrate that pregnant persons feel only a fraction of the total number of fetal movements and that there is a wide variation from individual to individual in the percentage of fetal movements perceived (Brown et al., 2016; Hijazi & East, 2009). The factors that affect the perception of fetal movement are summarized in the following textbox.

> ### Factors influencing the perception of fetal movement
>
> - Fetal position
> - Amniotic fluid volume
> - Placental location
> - Maternal position
> - Maternal attention to fetal movement
> - Certain medications
> - Alcohol
> - Smoking

A pregnant person asked to conduct formal FMCs must receive clear instructions on the procedures used for counting. There are several techniques for conducting FMCs, of which the Cardiff "count to ten" technique is probably the most popular. Instructions for the most used FMC methods are included below:

1. *Cardiff "count to ten"*—The pregnant person starts counting at the same time each day and records how long it takes for them to count 10 movements. If they do not feel 10 movements in 12 hours or if it takes progressively longer to get to 10 movements (e.g., usually it takes 5 hours and suddenly it is taking more than 5 hours), they should report decreased fetal movement to the healthcare provider (Pearson & Weaver, 1976).
2. *Liston*—This method is similar to Cardiff, but 10 movements should be felt in 6 hours (Liston et al., 1982).
3. *Moore*—This method is similar to Cardiff and Liston, but 10 movements should be felt in 2 hours (Moore & Piacquadio, 1989).
4. *Sadovsky*—The pregnant person counts how many movements they have in a specific period (at the same time every day) and reports to their healthcare provider if the number of movements is decreased (Sadovsky & Yaffe, 1973).

Currently, in addition to insufficient evidence to support FMC, there is also insufficient evidence to support one FMC method over another. However, there is agreement that if providers are going to recommend FMC, it is best for an individual to only use one method and conduct the counts around the same time of day. Conducting FMC in the early evening in a semireclined position may help improve the perception of fetal movement. In addition to instructions on how to conduct FMC, patients should receive clear directions on how to proceed if they perceive decreased fetal movement. In individuals at an increased risk for fetal demise, FMCs are conducted in addition to and *not* in place of additional fetal surveillance. In other words, FMC should not be the sole method of antenatal fetal surveillance in pregnancies at increased risk of fetal demise.

All pregnant clients are counseled to be aware of fetal movement in the third trimester and encouraged to report significant changes and/or decreases in fetal movement. Approximately 40% of pregnant individuals become concerned about decreased fetal movement at least once during a pregnancy (Saastad et al., 2012). Pregnant clients are advised that additional evaluation will be needed if they report a decrease in fetal movement; however, most episodes of decreased fetal movement are transient and further evaluation will reveal a normal, well-oxygenated fetus. To avoid unnecessary maternal anxiety, it is important that prenatal care providers educate all pregnant clients on fetal behaviors and movement patterns. This education includes information on the following:

1. Maternal awareness of fetal movement (quickening) is not expected to begin until sometime between 16- and 20-week gestation, and primigravidas experience fetal movement a little later than multigravidas.
2. By 26–28 weeks of gestation, pregnant individuals should feel distinct fetal movement several times a day.
3. The fetus has a circadian rhythm that becomes evident in the second trimester and, therefore, will be more active during some portions of the day than others.
4. Short periods (20–40 minutes) of reduced fetal activity can be normal but should not exceed 90 minutes.
5. There are normal variations in the quality of fetal movement with progressive gestational age. In other words, the movement of the 28-week fetus will feel different from the movement at 38 weeks, but the amount of movement should be similar.
6. Despite the commonly held belief that eating or drinking will stimulate fetal movement, low glucose levels have not been associated with a decrease in fetal movement (Velazquez & Rayburn, 2002).
7. Substances such as smoking (Coppens et al., 2001), alcohol, and some medications such as benzodiazepines and opioids can produce a transient reduction in fetal movement (Olesen & Svare, 2004).
8. During labor, it may be difficult to perceive fetal movement, particularly during contractions. A healthy fetus remains active in labor and fetal movement may be detectable between contractions.
9. A complete cessation of fetal movement is never normal and should be reported immediately.

Care of a Pregnant Individual Reporting Decreased Fetal Movement

All patients who report decreased fetal movement should be evaluated. Ideally, cessation of fetal movement is assessed as soon as possible. History and physical are the first components of evaluation.

> ### History and physical for a report of decreased fetal movement
>
> **History:**
>
> Onset of decreased movement
> Previous episodes of decreased movement
> Associated factors such as bleeding and rupture of membranes
> Maternal activities that day
> Recent smoking, alcohol, and substance use

Medication history
Presence of conditions such as hypertension, FGR, and diabetes
Previous history of adverse perinatal outcome

Physical:

Weight and blood pressure
Fundal height measurement and comparison
Fetal heart rate auscultation

A pregnant person who reports decreased fetal movement can receive additional assessment such as an NST and/or BPP. The ideal timing for this follow-up testing is unknown, but most studies that reported a decreased incidence of fetal death conducted additional testing within 1–12 hours of the report of the decrease in fetal movement. Fetal anomalies may be ruled out prior to intervening for decreased fetal movement. The algorithm in Figure 14.1 outlines the steps in the management of decreased fetal movement.

Nonstress Test

An NST is a method of antenatal fetal surveillance that utilizes the visual record of FHR that is produced by an electronic fetal monitor (EFM) to assess fetal oxygenation status. It is used to help guide management by detecting FHR patterns that may indicate hypoxemia and warrant intervention as well as those that signal adequate fetal oxygenation and, thus, do not require intervention. Selected terms related to FHR monitoring used in this section are defined at the beginning of the chapter. For a more detailed discussion of this terminology and FHR pattern interpretations, healthcare providers can refer to the report from the 2008 National Institute of Child Health and Human Development Research Planning Workshop (Macones et al., 2008).

As gestational age advances and the fetal nervous system develops and matures, the parasympathetic system gains increased influence over FHR modulation. This neurological maturation results in certain FHR tracing characteristics, which include a decrease in the average **FHR baseline** and an appearance of **FHR variability** and **FHR accelerations**.

Fetal heart rate accelerations definition

The National Institute of Child Health and Human Development (NICHD) defines the normal amplitude and duration of accelerations as 15 beats per minute (bpm) above baseline lasting at least 15 seconds in a fetus of 32 or more weeks of gestational age and 10 bpm above baseline lasting 10 seconds or more in a fetus at less than 32 weeks of gestational age (Macones et al., 2008). Accelerations lasting 2 minutes or more, but less than 10 minutes, are considered prolonged accelerations. An increase in FHR above baseline that lasts 10 minutes or more is considered a change in baseline.

Key points on fetal movement

- Decreased fetal movement is associated with an increased risk of fetal death.
- There are two broad categories of fetal movement monitoring: (a) general maternal awareness of fetal movement patterns in which a pregnant person is informed that by 26–28 weeks of gestation they should feel fetal movement multiple times a day, and that a cessation of fetal movement is never normal; and (b) formal FMC in which a pregnant person is instructed on a particular method of counting in which a specific number of fetal movements are expected during a specific time period. FMCs are conducted using the same technique at least once a day usually at the same time of the day.
- There is insufficient evidence to support a strategy of *routine* FMCs in pregnancy even for pregnant individuals at high risk of fetal demise.
- The benefits of FMC in those with an increased risk for fetal **hypoxemia** may outweigh the inconvenience, limited evidence, and risks associated with FMC.
- Pregnant individuals who are going to conduct FMC are instructed in one clear, consistent method for FMC and given explicit instructions for when and how to notify a healthcare provider and how to seek additional evaluation if they do not experience the targeted number of movements.
- All pregnant individuals are advised on the normal parameters of fetal movement and asked to be aware of their baby's patterns of movement.
- All pregnant persons are advised to immediately report a complete cessation of fetal movement, a marked decrease in the usual pattern of fetal movement, or a progressive decrease in fetal movement that has occurred over the course of a couple of days.
- Ideally, all patients who report decreased fetal movement (whether qualitatively or quantitatively decreased) should receive prompt evaluation of fetal well-being.

While the presence of gestational-age-appropriate accelerations is a sign of adequate fetal oxygenation, the lack of accelerations is not a good predictor of fetal hypoxia. However, studies have shown that a loss of FHR accelerations and variability often precede fetal demise due to progressive hypoxia (Cetrulo & Schifrin, 1976; Kodama et al., 2009; Low et al., 2001; Pillai & James, 1990). These findings have provided hope that antenatal FHR monitoring will allow the identification of fetuses at risk for demise due to progressive hypoxia with enough time to intervene to prevent fetal death and provides the theoretical underpinnings for the fetal NST.

During a fetal NST, the FHR is monitored for 20 minutes, and then, the recorded visual output (i.e., "tracing" or "strip") is evaluated for the presence of gestational-age-appropriate FHR accelerations and categorized as reactive or nonreactive.

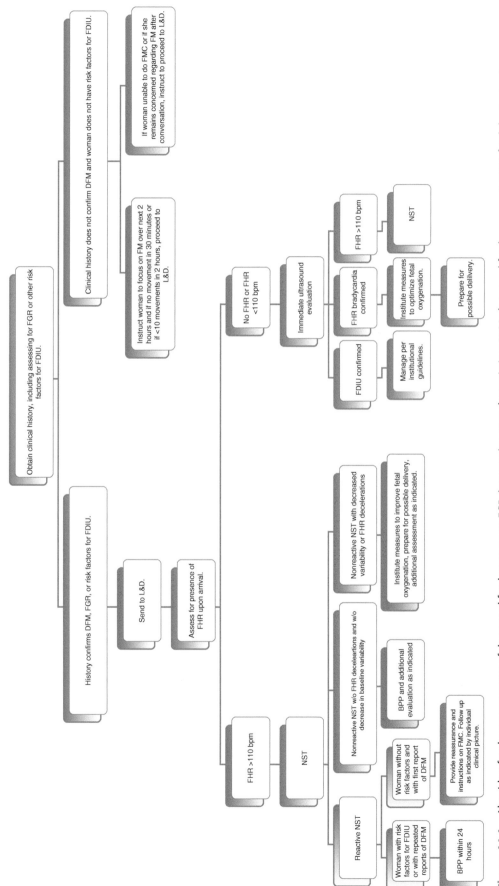

Figure 14.1 Algorithm for the management of decreased fetal movement. FGR, intrauterine growth restriction; DFM, decreased fetal movement; FDIU, fetal demise in utero; FHR, fetal heart rate; NST, nonstress test. Adapted from Liston et al. (2007) and Franks and Nightingale (2014).

Reactivity is defined using the following parameters:

Two accelerations of ≥ 15 bpm above baseline lasting ≥ 15 seconds in a fetus at ≥ 32-week EGA

or

Two accelerations of ≥ 10 bpm above baseline lasting ≥ 10 seconds in a fetus at < 32 weeks' EGA

An example of a reactive NST is provided in Figure 14.2. A reactive NST indicates a well-oxygenated fetus at the moment of testing. If the strip does not meet the criteria for reactivity in the initial 20 minutes of monitoring, the testing can be extended for an additional 20 minutes. If in that additional time the strip still does not meet gestational-age-appropriate criteria for reactivity, then the NST is considered nonreactive. A nonreactive strip is considered an abnormal finding in any fetus >30 weeks' gestational age, and further evaluation is warranted. Similarly, loss of FHR reactivity in a fetus that previously had exhibited FHR accelerations is a finding that warrants further evaluation regardless of gestational age.

A reactive NST is a sensitive predictor of a fetus that is adequately oxygenated at the time of testing and, in the absence of intervening factors, typically is not repeated for a week because the risk of fetal death in the seven days following a reactive NST is very small (2.3–7 per 1000; Manning, 2009). It must be kept in mind, however, that this is due in great part to the fact that fetal demise at >28 weeks' EGA is already a relatively rare event occurring at a rate of approximately 3 deaths per 1000 live births (Gregory et al., 2022). There are pregnant persons, including those who have diabetes or preeclampsia, who are at increased risk for accelerated compromise of fetal oxygenation and for whom more frequent fetal testing may be indicated. The decision for frequency of fetal testing is, therefore, based on a comprehensive and evolving clinical picture and not on past reactive NSTs, irrespective of how recent that testing may have been.

While a reactive NST correlates highly with a well-oxygenated fetus, a nonreactive NST has very poor positive predictive value for **hypoxemia** and **acidosis**. Studies indicate that the NST has low sensitivity (50–62%) for predicting fetal hypoxemia—especially in low-risk populations (Khooshideh et al., 2009; Ocak et al., 1992). Intervention for a nonreactive NST must, therefore, be undertaken with caution, especially if the fetus is premature because intervention based solely on a nonreactive NST can lead to an increase in the rate of labor induction, cesarean section, and iatrogenic prematurity without a decrease in perinatal morbidity and mortality. To avoid unnecessary interventions, therefore, additional testing is often warranted to determine whether a nonreactive strip is due to compromised fetal oxygenation or to another, nonhypoxic cause of nonreactivity such as a fetal sleep cycle, maternal sedation, or maternal smoking.

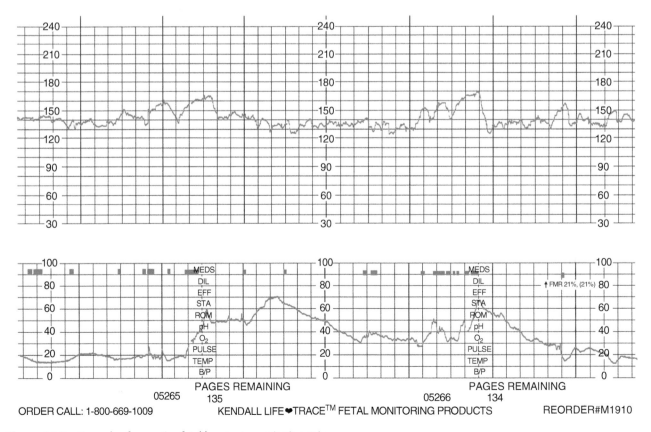

Figure 14.2 Example of a reactive fetal heart rate monitoring strip.

These additional testing modalities include the BPP and Doppler velocimetry, both of which are discussed in more detail later in this chapter. Sometimes, there may be identifiable and modifiable maternal conditions, such as acute hypovolemia or seizures that compromise of fetal oxygenation, and when these conditions are alleviated, fetal oxygenation may improve. In the presence of these conditions, attention is focused primarily on efforts to address the underlying cause of fetal compromise and not on additional testing. Similarly, the absence of accelerations coupled with the presence of prolonged, late, or repetitive variable FHR decelerations may indicate a fetus that is at increased risk for acute deterioration and warrants immediate evaluation for the need to expedite birth. This is particularly important if the decelerations are accompanied by a loss of variability.

In addition to its low predictive value for fetal hypoxia, another limitation of the NST is that it can take a significant amount of time to conduct. Loud external sounds and vibrations—referred to as acoustic or vibroacoustic stimulation (VAS)—have been used to elicit FHR accelerations. VAS is used to shorten the length of time needed for an NST or to stimulate accelerations in a fetus that has a nonreactive FHR monitoring strip in the initial 20–40 minutes of testing. This type of stimulation has been shown to significantly shorten the average time needed to achieve a reactive NST (Tan et al., 2013). Special caution is needed when interpreting the results of a NST in which accelerations are elicited via VAS, especially in the fetus with signs of possible compromised fetal oxygenation (e.g., decelerations or oligohydramnios). There is evidence that intense stimulation can provoke an acceleration in fetuses with scalp pH of <7.20; thus, it cannot be assumed that accelerations stimulated by the use of VAS are equivalent to spontaneous accelerations in predicting a well-oxygenated fetus (East et al., 2005). Maternal administration of glucose has also been used in an attempt to decrease both the amount of time needed to achieve a reactive NST and to decrease the rate of nonreactive NSTs in normal fetuses. However, research demonstrates that this practice does not achieve either of these goals (Esin et al., 2013).

Auscultated acceleration test (AAT): Accelerations of the FHR can be detected through auscultation (O'Leary et al., 1980). Fetal testing using manual plotting of auscultated accelerations has been proposed as an alternative to the NST (Paine, Johnson et al., 1986; Paine, Payton et al., 1986). During an AAT, the FHR is auscultated, and the number of beats in 5 seconds is counted and plotted in a grid that converts the beats in this 5-second period to beats per minute. This is done in alternating 5-second intervals for 3 minutes. If an acceleration of 2 bpm in a 5-second period associated with fetal movement is detected, the AAT is considered reactive. If no acceleration is detected in the first 3-minute period, an attempt is made to elicit fetal movement and the FHR is auscultated for another minute. If no acceleration with movement is detected in this additional minute, the process to elicit fetal movement is repeated and the FHR is auscultated for another 2 minutes. If no acceleration is detected in these additional 3 minutes of auscultation, then the AAT is

considered nonreactive. Nonrandomized studies have shown that the AAT produces comparable results to the NST (Daniels & Boehm, 1991) and may be a reasonable alternative to the NST, particularly in settings and/or situations where EFM is unavailable or impractical.

Key points on nonstress testing

- An FHR acceleration is an increase in the FHR of at least 15 bpm higher than baseline at its peak, and lasting 15 seconds or more from start to finish (10 bpm for 10 seconds or more if EGA is less than 32 weeks).
- Accelerations occur in association with fetal movement.
- The NST is based on the knowledge that FHR accelerations are a sign that the fetus is well oxygenated and neurologically intact.
- An NST is conducted by monitoring FHR for at least 20 minutes using a continuous EFM to look for FHR accelerations.
- After 20 minutes, the FHR monitoring strip is evaluated to look for accelerations and the test gets classified as reactive or nonreactive:
  - A reactive NST is one where there are two or more EGA-appropriate accelerations of the FHR in a 20-minute period.
    - A reactive NST correlates very highly with a fetus that is not acidotic (high **negative predictive value**).
  - A nonreactive NST is one in which either there is only one acceleration in a 20-minute period or there are no accelerations in a 20-minute period.
    - A nonreactive NST correlates poorly (poor positive predictive value) with a fetus who is acidotic.
- If an NST is nonreactive, additional testing is warranted before determining if intervention is warranted.
- The AAT is a reasonable alternative to the NST in settings or situations where EFM is not available or impractical.

Contraction Stress Test

A CST or oxytocin challenge test (OCT) is based on the premise that a fetus with compromised oxygenation will respond to the additional decrease in oxygenation resulting from contractions with compensatory mechanisms that result in a pattern of late FHR decelerations. A CST consists of provoking—three to five contractions in 10 minutes with oxytocin infusion or nipple stimulation and evaluating the FHR tracing for the presence of a pattern of late or repetitive variable decelerations. This test is undertaken in a location in which birth via cesarean section can be immediately conducted if necessary.

Results of a CST are interpreted as follows:

1. *Negative (normal)*—absence of late or significant (recurring and deep) variable FHR decelerations.
2. *Positive (abnormal)*—presence of recurrent (present in 50% or more of contractions) late decelerations or significant variable decelerations.
3. *Equivocal*—presence of intermittent late or variable decelerations, or recurrent FHR decelerations in the presence of uterine tachysystole.

Because CSTs are more invasive, require prolonged periods of time to conduct, and have the risk of creating complications such as preterm labor if conducted prior to term or tachysystole leading to fetal hypoxemia, the CST is not as commonly used as other tests of fetal oxygenation. This is especially true in settings that have other, more sensitive testing options such as Doppler velocimetry. There are, however, certain situations in which this test may be used to assess whether to proceed with an induction of labor or schedule a cesarean section in an individual at risk for fetal hypoxia.

Amniotic Fluid Volume Assessment

When a fetus is faced with prolonged periods of hypoxemia, one of its adaptive mechanisms is to redistribute cardiac output to selectively perfuse organs essential to survival—the placenta, heart, brain, and adrenal glands. This means that other organs, including the kidneys, have reduced circulation. Decreased renal perfusion results in decreased urine output. Fetal urine makes up most of the AFV during the end of second trimester and in the third trimester. Thus, a decrease in urine output leads to a decrease in AFV (oligohydramnios). This chain of events explains why the ultrasonographic measurement of AFV can be used to assess fetal oxygenation status. The assessment of AFV can also detect an excess of amniotic fluid (**polyhydramnios**), which can be due to decreased absorption or overproduction of amniotic fluid but can also be idiopathic. Decreased absorption usually results from inadequate fetal swallowing related to anatomic or neurogenic anomalies.

There are multiple methods that are used to quantify AFV. Table 14.3 describes these methods and their interpretation. Current evidence supports the use of a single maximum vertical pocket (MVP) of <2 cm as the threshold to diagnose oligohydramnios as this minimizes unnecessary intervention without adversely impacting perinatal outcomes (ACOG, 2021). See Chapter 34, *Amniotic Fluid and Fetal Growth Disorders*, for more detail on the diagnosis and management of disorders of amniotic fluid. Amniotic fluid volume is one of the components of both the BPP and the modified BPP that are further described in this chapter.

The Biophysical Profile and Modified BPP

The BPP uses sonography to look for multiple indicators of fetal well-being with the purpose of gaining a more accurate evaluation of fetal status than is possible with a single indicator such as FHR reactivity. The BPP is based on the knowledge that, in the absence of an anomaly, a fetus that is well oxygenated and neurologically intact will exhibit certain behavioral characteristics such as gross body movements and sufficient urine production to have an adequate amount of amniotic fluid. The indicators of well-being that are included in the BPP are (a) a reactive NST, (b) fetal breathing, (c) fetal movement, (d) fetal tone, and (e) AFV. Items a–d are considered acute measures of

Table 14.3 Ultrasound Methods to Estimate Amniotic Fluid Volume

Single deepest pocket
With the transducer at a right angle to the uterine contour, measure the vertical dimension of the largest pocket of amniotic fluid (without umbilical cord or fetal extremities/small parts). The horizontal dimension must be at least 1 cm.

Normal	Oligohydramnios	Polyhydramnios
Vertical depth: 2.1–8 cm	Vertical depth: 0–2 cm	Vertical depth: >8 cm

Two-diameter pocket technique
With the transducer at a right angle to the uterine contour, find the largest pocket of fluid (without umbilical cord or fetal extremities/small parts) and calculate the product of the vertical depth multiplied by the horizontal diameter.

Normal: 15.1–50 cm²	Oligohydramnios: 0–15 cm²	Polyhydramnios: >50 cm²

Amniotic fluid index (AFI)
Divide the uterus into four imaginary quadrants using the linea nigra for the right and left divisions and the umbilicus for the upper and lower quadrants. Calculate the AFI by measuring the maximum vertical amniotic fluid pocket diameter (without umbilical cord or fetal extremities/small parts) in each quadrant and adding the four measurements together.

Normal: 5–25 cm	Oligohydramnios: 0–5 cm	Polyhydramnios: >25 cm

The 2 × 1 cm pocket
The criterion for the biophysical profile (BPP) is to have at least one pocket of fluid with a measurement of 2 × 1 cm.

Source: Adapted from Chamberlain et al. (1984), Magann et al. (1992), Rutherford et al. (1987), and Manning et al. (1980).

fetal oxygenation because they are suppressed as an immediate response to fetal hypoxia, whereas decreased AFV is considered a chronic measure of fetal oxygenation because it takes a prolonged period of hypoxemia to produce **oligohydramnios**. The BPP, as initially described by Manning et al. (1980), is the most used BPP technique and is scored with each of the five components receiving a score of 2 if present and a score of 0 if absent. The maximum score for the BPP is 10/10. The scoring criteria for the Manning et al. method are described in Table 14.4.

A proposed modification to this scoring system gives a score of 1 when the fetus exhibits some activity in a component but does not meet the criteria to receive a score of 2, as originally described by Manning et al. (Vintzileos et al., 1983). This modified scoring system also includes placental grading as a sixth component of the BPP, which means that the maximum score for this version of the BPP is 12. The scoring for the Vintzileos et al. method is described in Table 14.5.

There are no large, randomized studies of the BPP. However, existing studies, including large observational studies, indicate that the BPP is effective at predicting the absence of fetal acidemia. The risk of fetal demise in the

Table 14.4   Biophysical Profile: Manning Method Scoring Criteria

Parameter	Scoring criteria
Movement	
Score 2	≥1 movement of limb from flexion to extension and back to flexion
Score 0	Limb extension with no return to flexion
Tone	
Score 2	≥3 gross body movements in 30 minutes
Score 0	<3 gross body movement in 30 minutes
Breathing	
Score 2	≥30 seconds of sustained fetal breathing movements in 30 minutes
Score 0	<30 seconds of sustained fetal breathing movements in 30 minutes
Amniotic fluid (AF)	
Score 2	≥1 AF pocket measuring ≥2 × 2 cm in two perpendicular planes
Score 0	No AF pockets measuring ≥2 × 2 cm in two perpendicular planes
Fetal heart rate (FHR)	
Score 2	≥2 FHR accelerations of >15 bpm lasting ≥15 seconds in a 40-minute period
Score 0	<2 FHR accelerations of >15 bpm lasting ≥15 seconds in a 40-minute period

Source: Adapted from Manning et al. (1980).

Table 14.5   Biophysical Profile: Vintzileos Method Scoring Criteria

Nonstress test (NST)

Score 2 (NST 2): five or more FHR accelerations of at least 15 bpm in amplitude and at least a 15-second duration associated with fetal movements (FMs) in a 20-minute period
Score 1 (NST 1): two to four accelerations of at least 15 bpm in amplitude and at least 15-second duration associated with FMs in a 20-minute period
Score 0 (NST 0): one or less acceleration in a 20-minute period

Fetal movements

Score 2 (FM 2): at least three gross (trunk and limbs) episodes of FMs within 30 minutes; simultaneous limb and trunk movements are counted as a single movement.
Score 1 (FM 1): one or two FMs within 30 minutes
Score 0 (FM 0): absence of FMs within 30 minutes
Fetal breathing movements (FBMs)
Score 2 (FBM 2): at least one episode of fetal breathing of at least 60-second duration within a 30-minute observation period
Score 1 (FBM 1): at least one episode of fetal breathing lasting 30–60 seconds within 30 within a 30-minute observation period
Score 0 (FBM 0): absence of fetal breathing of breathing lasting less than 30 seconds within a 30-minute observation period

Fetal tone

Score 2 (FT 2): at least one episode of extension of extremities with return to position of flexion and also one episode of extension of spine with return to position of flexion
Score 1 (FT 1): at least one episode of extension of extremities with return to position of flexion or one episode of extension of spine with return to flexion
Score 0 (FT 0): extremities in extension; FMs not followed by return to flexion; open hand

Amniotic fluid volume

Score 2 (AF 2): fluid evident throughout the uterine cavity; a pocket that measures greater than 2 cm in vertical diameter
Score 1 (AF 1): a pocket that measures less than 2 cm but more than vertical diameter
Score 0 (AF 0): crowding of fetal small parts; largest pocket less than 1 cm in vertical diameter

Placental grading

Score 2 (PL 2): placental grading 0, 1, or 2
Score 1 (PL 1): placenta posterior difficult to evaluate
Score 0 (PL 0): placental grading 3
Maximal score, 12; minimal score, 0

Source: Reproduced from Oyelese and Vintzileos (2011)/With permission from Elsevier.

week following a normal BPP is less than 1 in 1000 (Manning, 2002). Providers must keep in mind that the fetus at high risk for demise, such as a fetus with severe growth restriction, may have sudden and quick deterioration (Manning, 2009), limiting the ability to intervene in time to prevent a fetal death.

When making management decisions based on BPP results, the healthcare provider must take the full clinical picture into account. An acute change in maternal status, for example, could mean an acute change in fetal status that would require assessment or intervention regardless of the presence of a normal BPP within the past week. Additionally, when making decisions regarding the optimal timing for birth, maternal indicators for birth may supersede a reassuring BPP. A BPP score of 6, for example, may be managed quite differently in a fetus near term or early term when the risks of a slightly early birth may be outweighed by the risk of progressive fetal hypoxia, whereas a fetus far from term may face greater risks from a preterm birth.

The BPP is performed in a setting that has both EFM and ultrasound capabilities. In some settings or situations, the NST is conducted first, and the results of the NST are used to determine whether a full or modified BPP is performed (see textbox on BPP). In other settings or situations, the NST may be postponed until after the ultrasound portion of the BPP because, in the presence of all four ultrasound indicators of fetal well-being, the NST may not be necessary. The procedure for the NST is the same during a BPP as when it is done as an independent test. Ultrasound is used to look for the other four components of the BPP—movement, breathing, tone, and

Table 14.6 Interpretation and Management of Biophysical Score

Test result	Interpretation	Management
10/10 8/10 with normal fluid 8/8 without NST	The risk of fetal asphyxia is very low (1/1000 risk of perinatal death within 1 week if no intervention)	Manage based on clinical condition and factors
8/10 with abnormal fluid	Potential chronic fetal hypoxia	If membranes are intact and there is no known renal malfunction/abnormality, expedited birth is indicated if fetus is term. If <34-week gestation, increased surveillance may be preferred due to risks of prematurity
6/10 with normal fluid	Equivocal	Repeat test within 24 hours
6/10 with abnormal fluid	Possible fetal asphyxia	Deliver if fetus term. If <34-week gestation, consider clinical picture and whether increased fetal surveillance to prolong pregnancy is preferable to preterm birth
4/10	High likelihood of fetal asphyxia (91/1000 risk of perinatal death if no intervention within 1 week)	Deliver
2/10	Fetal asphyxia probable	Deliver
0/10	Fetal asphyxia nearly certain (600/1000 risk of perinatal death within 1 week if no intervention)	Deliver

Source: Adapted from Manning (1995).

amniotic fluid. As soon as a parameter is observed, it can be given a score of 2.

Continuous observation for 30 minutes is required before it can be determined that an indicator of well-being is absent and given a score of 0. This is to account for fetal sleep–wake cycles. At the end of the testing, the total score is calculated and interpreted, as shown in Table 14.6.

Research has demonstrated that the presence of normal AFV and a reactive NST is as accurate at ruling out fetal acidemia as is a score of 10 on a full BPP (Miller et al., 1996). To reduce the amount of time needed to conduct a BPP, therefore, it may be acceptable to conduct what is referred to as a "modified" BPP in which only the NST and AFV are obtained. If both assessments receive a score of 2, then fetal acidemia can be ruled out, but if one or both components receive a score of 0, then the full BPP is warranted (Figure 14.3).

It has also been demonstrated that if the four ultrasound parameters (AFV, movement, breathing, and tone) are present—that is, if the BPP score is 8/8—this is also as reliable at ruling out fetal acidemia as the full BPP or the modified BPP (Manning et al., 1987). If all ultrasound parameters receive a score of 2, the NST is not needed. If any parameter receives a 0, the NST is then performed. Similarly, achieving a score of 8/10 by any combination of parameters of the BPP is as effective at establishing fetal well-being as a score of 10/10 as long as the AFV is normal (Alfirevic & Neilson, 2000).

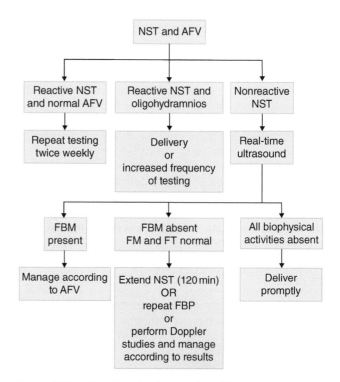

Figure 14.3 Algorithm for the use of modified BPP. AFV: amniotic fluid volume; FBM: fetal breathing movements; NST: nonstress test. Data from Hanley and Vintzileos (1988) and Vintzileos et al. (1991). Reproduced from Oyelese and Vintzileos (2011) /With permission from Elsevier.

> ### Key points on BPP
>
> - The BPP combines the NST and four ultrasound parameters (movement, tone, breathing movements, and AFV) to evaluate fetal oxygenation status.
> - Each of the five parameters receives a score of either 0 or 2 (present or not present).
> - A score of 10/10 indicates a fetus that is well oxygenated and has a low likelihood of dying in the seven days following testing.
> - There is no evidence to support the routine use of BPP in either low-risk or high-risk pregnancies.
> - The decision of whom to test and when to test must be made on a case-by-case basis determined by the clinical situation.
> - A modified BPP uses only the NST and the AFV, and a score of 4/4 on the modified BPP is as accurate as a score of 10/10 or 8/10 if AFV is normal on the full BPP in determining if a fetus is well oxygenated. If either the NST or the AFV are abnormal, the full BPP is indicated.
> - If the fetus is greater than 37 weeks of gestational age, and the score is anything less than 10/10 or 8/10 with normal AFV, then expedited birth may be indicated.
> - A patient at less than 37 weeks of gestation with a BPP of 8/10 with low fluid or with a BPP lower than 8/10 regardless of AFV should be transferred for medical management or managed in collaboration with a physician.

Doppler Ultrasonography

Doppler ultrasonography is the use of sound waves to examine the flow of blood in vessels. The flow through specific vessels of maternal and fetal circulation can be assessed for disruptions indicative of compromised placental circulation and/or deteriorating fetal status. Antenatal Doppler velocimetry allows the detection of placental resistance by measuring umbilical artery flow, the presence of "brain sparing" or preferential blood flow by measuring fetal middle cerebral artery flow, and fetal cardiac function by measuring the flow through the ductus venosus. Current evidence suggests that routine Doppler ultrasound examination in low-risk populations does not improve outcomes (Alfirevic et al., 2015), but that the use of Doppler ultrasound in the context of pregnancies at high risk for fetal demise can reduce the incidence of perinatal deaths and result in fewer obstetric interventions (Alfirevic et al., 2017; Berkley et al., 2012). Currently, therefore, this type of testing is most often used to optimize the timing of birth of fetuses in pregnant individuals who develop preeclampsia prior to 34 weeks of EGA or those who are preterm and have suspected or confirmed FGR and are at high risk for intrauterine demise.

While multivessel Doppler may be the most informative regarding overall fetal oxygenation, the assessment of individual vessels is also informative (Judd et al., 2020). The assessment of flow through the umbilical artery is probably the easiest and most widely used, and multiple studies have confirmed abnormal Doppler velocimetry of the umbilical artery as an accurate predictor of fetal hypoxia and acidemia.

There is an important role for antenatal testing, including Doppler ultrasound, in differentiating the fetus who is constitutionally small but achieving its growth potential, and thus not at increased risk for adverse outcomes, from the one that is truly growth restricted due to factors that increase the risk of intrauterine demise. Given that average fetal size at any given gestation may vary across populations, this differentiation is particularly important (Louis et al., 2015; Dubinsky & Sonneborn, 2020). Umbilical artery Doppler evaluation of the fetus with suspected FGR can help differentiate the hypoxic growth-restricted fetus that may benefit from intervention to expedite birth, from the constitutionally small fetus that is nonhypoxic and for whom intervention is not necessary. In the fetus who is growing normally, there is high-velocity diastolic flow in the umbilical artery, while in the growth-restricted fetus, umbilical arterial (UA) waveform shows decreased, absent, or even reversed end-diastolic flow. Fetuses with these Doppler abnormalities are at increased risk of demise (Alfirevic et al., 2013).

Doppler velocimetry of fetal vessels has also been used for the monitoring of fetal status in specific high-risk situations such as the evaluation of pregnancies with isoimmunization and fetal anemia. When an RhD-negative pregnant person is carrying an RhD-positive fetus and a critical titer of antibodies is reached or exceeded, the Doppler velocimetry of the middle cerebral artery peak systolic velocity (MCA-PSV) can be used to identify fetuses that may be severely anemic and minimize the number of fetal blood samples and the need for invasive procedures (Papantoniou et al., 2008).

The decisions of what test(s) to use in monitoring the fetus in a pregnancy at increased risk for poor outcome, when to initiate testing, and how often to repeat testing depends on the clinical picture. Other than in the context of postdate pregnancy, these decisions are often made in collaboration with an obstetrician or maternal–fetal medicine specialist. In general, testing is not begun when a fetus is at a gestational age that would preclude intervention—that is, if the fetus is so far from term that birth would not be an option. In pregnancies where there is an increased risk of stillbirth (Table 14.1), testing is usually initiated at approximately 32 weeks of gestation, except for testing for postdate pregnancy, which usually begins at 41 weeks of gestation. The testing modality and frequency may also be adapted based on gestational age or condition that puts the pregnancy at risk. Most clinical sites will conduct testing once or twice weekly; however, testing on a more frequent basis may be warranted in certain situations such as the preterm fetus with significant growth restriction who may have a rapid deterioration in status. The Doppler evaluation of the umbilical artery has been demonstrated to be a useful in reducing perinatal deaths in this context (ACOG, 2021).

In transient conditions, such as maternal respiratory distress due to an asthma exacerbation, testing may be repeated after the condition has been treated—particularly in the context of a preterm fetus. On the other hand, abnormal fetal testing in the context of a potentially quickly evolving situation, such as a pregnant patient with vaginal bleeding following a motor vehicle accident, may warrant immediate intervention. Additionally, the nature of the abnormal result (e.g., BPP of 0 versus 6 or reversed versus decreased end-diastolic flow) may also necessitate different responses in what may otherwise be similar clinical scenarios.

Providers and patients faced with abnormal fetal testing results may be confronted with difficult choices in which they will weigh the risks of intervention, such as the risks of premature birth or the need for cesarean birth, with those of nonintervention, such as the risk of preventable neurologic damage or fetal death. The optimal management of abnormal antenatal testing will depend on various factors including the clinical scenario, gestational age, and both the severity and likelihood of progression of the condition that is believed to be causing the abnormal results.

Most often, the antenatal surveillance of fetal well-being will provide reassurance that a fetus is well oxygenated and that, in the absence of other intervening factors, pregnancy can safely continue. However, when testing reveals compromised oxygenation, intervention to expedite birth may be indicated to optimize fetal outcomes. The decision on intervention is particularly difficult when there is abnormal testing in the setting of FGR in the fetus who is premature, particularly in cases of extreme prematurity. The decision to expedite birth in these situations puts the neonate at risk for known morbidity and mortality associated with prematurity, while failure to intervene can result in fetal demise in utero. The decision to expedite birth in a pregnancy with a near-term or term fetus may not pose the same medical risks but may be a difficult one, nonetheless, for the pregnant individual with a strong preference for physiologic labor and birth. In these situations, the healthcare provider will need to help the pregnant patient obtain as much information as they desire and is reasonably available and help them interpret this information in a way that promotes informed decision-making. Using decision support tools that provide statistics on outcomes in ways that consider varying degrees of health literacy can help this process. The "Extremely Preterm Birth Outcomes Tool" developed by the NICHD (https://www.nichd.nih.gov/research/supported/EPBO/use) is an example of such a tool. While it is often appropriate for providers to make recommendations for intervention, these recommendations should be made in the context of a shared decision-making process that recognizes that a pregnant individual who is a legally competent adult has the right to refuse intervention even when such refusal may endanger their life or the life of their fetus or neonate. Attempts to coerce or force intervention with measures such as appeals to conscience or use of court orders are considered unethical by the major professional organizations of prenatal care providers.

Education and Counseling

To optimize the effectiveness of any fetal surveillance plan, the pregnant patient must be considered as part of the team and counseled appropriately. Information on when and how to contact prenatal care providers including after hours and on weekends is provided. All pregnant persons are informed about normal fetal movement/behavior and counseled to be aware of fetal movement starting in the late second trimester and to immediately report a sudden decrease or cessation of fetal movement. The plan for antenatal testing and the patient education process is documented in the prenatal care record.

The following information is given to individuals undergoing fetal surveillance:

- indication for testing
- goals of testing
- testing method(s)
- testing frequency/schedule
- alternatives to testing
- potential outcomes of testing (including the possibility of emergent delivery)
- financial costs of testing

Pregnant persons and their families may develop unrealistic expectations of what antenatal fetal surveillance can achieve. This can lead to confusion and anger when there is a poor outcome despite reassuring testing or when emergent surgical birth is conducted, but there is no evidence of fetus compromise at birth. Thus, it is especially important that pregnant individuals be counseled on the limitations of antenatal fetal testing so that they know that many fetuses that have abnormal testing will have no evidence of compromise upon further testing or upon birth. Pregnant persons are made aware that fetal testing provides information on fetal status at the particular moment that the testing is conducted and reminded, therefore, that even if a test is reassuring, an acute event can lead to an acute change in fetal status. Individuals undergoing antenatal fetal surveillance for a severely growth-restricted fetus are at particular risk for sudden deterioration in fetal status and are to be counseled accordingly.

Cultural, Personal, and Family Considerations

Providers should be aware that in many families, the fetus is felt to be part of the family with whom parents, siblings, grandparents, and others will have bonded even before birth. The determination that a pregnancy is "high risk" and requires increased fetal surveillance is likely to be a source of anxiety and concern for these family members as well as the pregnant person.

There are some cultural, ethnic, and religious groups that may have restrictions on the use of technology either in general or on particular days of the week. For some of these individuals, the use of EFMs and ultrasound for fetal surveillance may be precluded. The initiation of fetal testing may be an issue that the pregnant individual will want to discuss with other family members and possibly with a religious leader before deciding on whether to consent to testing. Rather than making assumptions on what may or may not be acceptable for a particular person based on their religion or ethnic background, every person is asked if they have any concerns or limitations on the use of technology in pregnancy and use their response as a starting point for the conversation.

For those individuals who are uninsured, the need to undergo frequent fetal evaluation can mean a significant expense and one that they and their family may not be able to afford. Providers can help families find a testing site that provides free, reduced-cost, or sliding-scale fees. Local health departments may be able to help in identifying such services. It is important to refrain from making judgments about families that choose to forgo fetal testing for economic, religious, or other personal reasons. Once a person has received appropriate counseling on testing, it is their right to determine whether they will undergo the tests.

Health Disparities and Vulnerable Populations

The risk of poor perinatal outcomes is unevenly distributed among racial and ethnic groups in the United States. As discussed earlier, a Black pregnant person in the United States has more than twice the risk of experiencing a fetal death than a White pregnant person (MacDorman & Gregory, 2015; Pruitt et al., 2020). While many efforts to address these disparities are aimed at improving access to health services, the discrepancy in perinatal outcomes is due not only to inequalities in access but also to systemic inequities and discrimination that lead to differences in the prevalence of underlying risk factors including obesity, diabetes, and hypertensive disorders—all of which increase an individual's likelihood of experiencing poor pregnancy outcomes (Alhusen et al., 2016; Bryant et al., 2010; Willinger et al., 2009). While steps can be taken to ameliorate the effects of these risk factors on the fetus once a person is already pregnant, the biggest impact on these rates of complications will be achieved by improving the health of individuals prior to conception and addressing racism and inequality on a societal level.

Additionally, Black, Indigenous, and other People of Color (BIPOC) experience differential treatment within the healthcare system and are often impacted by discriminatory practices and biases (Blendon & Casey, 2019; Liu et al., 2018). Even when BIPOC patients have physical access to healthcare, their access to the full range of available services, including technologies to assess fetal well-being, within the system may not be equal. Providers can work to identify, acknowledge, and address such disparities. An example of an action is to eliminate the use of the term "noncompliant," which, in addition to presupposing that a successful healthcare exchange is defined as one in which the pregnant individual does as the provider recommends, also fails to take into account that an individual's ability to follow healthcare advice or to attend appointments may be impacted by barriers to care that are beyond their control and disproportionately distributed across races. A review of 40,113 history and physical notes from 18,459 patients for sentences containing a negative descriptor (e.g., resistant or noncompliant) of the patient or the patient's behavior found that compared with White patients, Black patients had 2.54 times the odds of having at least one negative descriptor in the history and physical notes (Sun et al., 2022). Evidence also suggests that protocols that define a standardized response to abnormal findings on fetal surveillance may help reduce bias in clinical decision-making (FitzGerald & Hurst, 2017; Narayan, 2019).

Legal and Liability Issues

The Doctors Company, the largest physician-owned medical malpractice insurer in the United States, conducted a review of 960 closed claims and 226 open claims reported between 2007 and 2015 which showed that the most common patient allegations in obstetrical claims is a delay in the treatment of fetal distress (17%), improper performance of vaginal delivery (16%), and improper management of pregnancy (12%). In the category of delays in the treatment of fetal distress and improper management of pregnancy are cases in which there was an alleged failure to test for fetal abnormalities, failure to recognize abnormal findings, and failure to address abnormal findings leading to adverse outcomes including fetal demise. An analysis of the cases related to management of pregnancy reveals several common contributors to claims including miscommunication among healthcare providers and lack of coordination of care.

These analyses of diagnosis-related claims are especially relevant when considering potential liability issues related to antenatal fetal surveillance. The most common issues identified in claims involving injury arising from the outpatient diagnostic process are:

- ordering of diagnostic/lab tests
- interpretation of tests
- history/physical and evaluation of symptoms
- management of referrals.

Follow-up and patient compliance with tests were also raised as recurring concerns in the outpatient diagnosis process.

The following are steps that may help reduce the medicolegal risks related to antenatal fetal surveillance:

1. Ensure that pregnant clients are offered screening for conditions that may warrant increased antenatal fetal surveillance.
2. Establish an appropriate fetal surveillance plan that is evidence-based and in line with current recommendations.
3. Ensure appropriate physician consultation, referral, and transfer of care for any of these conditions that are outside the scope of practice of the primary prenatal care provider.
4. Ensure that the fetal surveillance plan is documented in the chart.

5. Ensure adequate patient education and consent for tests and documentation of this process. It is especially important that pregnant persons and their families understand the limitations of the tests and any risks involved with testing or declining testing.
6. Put in place a clear and standardized process to ensure that there is timely review and follow-up of tests.

Summary

Despite the current widespread use of multiple tests of antenatal fetal well-being, there is still limited evidence to guide prenatal care providers on who to test, what tests to use, when to begin testing, or how often to test. There is observational evidence that the use of the tests described in this chapter coupled with immediate delivery when fetal acidemia is suspected can decrease the rates of stillbirth. There is also evidence to support the use of Doppler velocimetry to monitor the fetus with FGR. However, the impact of antenatal surveillance on neonatal mortality and significant morbidity such as cerebral palsy has not been conclusively established. Most guidelines are currently based on observational studies and consensus expert opinions. Given the risks associated with premature birth, the decision to deliver a fetus prior to term based on the results of antenatal testing is made with caution, especially considering the high rate of false positive results for many of the antenatal tests of fetal well-being. The decision to intervene for fetal indications at term is easier, but the risks to the pregnant individual associated with cesarean birth for both current and future pregnancies are taken into consideration.

In the absence of large, randomized trials to determine the optimal population, method, and timing for antenatal tests of fetal well-being, healthcare providers must create an individualized fetal surveillance plan considering maternal conditions, fetal conditions, obstetric history, and findings during routine prenatal assessments. Consultation, collaboration, or referral may be necessary in certain cases. In addition to providing pregnant clients with education and instructions on the why, how, when, and where of any recommended fetal testing, healthcare providers must also ensure that pregnant persons and their families understand both the benefits and the limitations of tests of fetal well-being. To reduce health disparities in fetal outcomes, providers must take purposeful steps to ensure equitable access to antenatal fetal surveillance and to eliminate the impact of harmful bias from decisions both to intervene and not intervene in response to the results of such surveillance.

Resources for Clients and Their Families

The AHRQ Question Builder website and app helps patients and caregivers prepare for medical appointments and maximize visit time: https://www.ahrq.gov/questions/question-builder/online.html

Resources for Healthcare Providers

National Institute of Child Health and Human Development Definitions and Classifications: Applications to Electronic Fetal Monitoring Interpretation https://www.nccwebsite.org/content/documents/cms/final_ncc_monograph_web-4-29-10.pdf

Perinatology.com. A website with access to clinical calculators and clinical decision-making support relevant to antenatal testing.

National Institute of Child Health and Human Development Extremely Premature Birth Outcomes Calculator: https://www.nichd.nih.gov/research/supported/EPBO/use

References

Alfirevic, Z., & Neilson, J. P. (2000). Biophysical profile for fetal assessment in high risk pregnancies. *Cochrane Database of Systematic Review, 2*, CD000038.

Alfirevic, Z., Stampalija, T., & Dowswell, T. (2017). Fetal and umbilical Doppler ultrasound in high-risk pregnancies. *Cochrane Database of Systematic Reviews, 6*, CD007529. https://doi.org/10.1002/14651858.CD007529.pub4

Alfirevic, Z., Stampalija, T., & Gyte, G. M. (2013). Fetal and umbilical Doppler ultrasound in high-risk pregnancies. *The Cochrane Library, 11*, CD007529. https://doi.org/10.1002/14651858.CD007529.pub3

Alfirevic, Z., Stampalija, T., & Medley, N. (2015). Fetal and umbilical Doppler ultrasound in normal pregnancy. *Cochrane Database of Systematic Reviews,* (4), CD001450. https://doi.org/10.1002/14651858.CD001450.pub4. PMID: 25874722; PMCID: PMC6464774

Alhusen, J. L., Bower, K. M., Epstein, E., & Sharps, P. (2016). Racial discrimination and adverse birth outcomes: An integrative review. *Journal of Midwifery & Women's Health, 61*(6), 707–720.

American College of Obstetricians and Gynecologists (ACOG). (2021). Antepartum fetal surveillance: ACOG practice bulletin, number 229. *Obstetrics and Gynecology, 137*(6), e116–e127.

Bailey, Z. D., Krieger, N., Agénor, M., Graves, J., Linos, N., & Bassett, M. T. (2017). Structural racism and health inequities in the USA: Evidence and interventions. *The Lancet, 389*(10077), 1453–1463.

Bellussi, F., Po,' G., Livi, A., Saccone, G., De Vivo, V., Oliver, E. A., & Berghella, V. (2020). Fetal movement counting and perinatal mortality: A systematic review and meta-analysis. *Obstetrics and Gynecology, 135*(2), 453–462. https://doi.org/10.1097/AOG.0000000000003645

Berkley, E., Chauhan, S. P., Abuhamad, A., & Society for Maternal-Fetal Medicine Publications Committee. (2012). Doppler assessment of the fetus with intrauterine growth restriction. *American Journal of Obstetrics and Gynecology, 206*(4), 300–308.

Blendon, R. J., & Casey, L. S. (2019). Discrimination in the United States: Perspectives for the future. *Health Services Research, 54*, 1467–1471.

Brown, R., Higgins, L. E., Johnstone, E. D., Wijekoon, J. H., & Heazell, A. E. (2016). Maternal perception of fetal movements in late pregnancy is affected by type and duration of fetal movement. *The Journal of Maternal-Fetal & Neonatal Medicine, 29*(13), 2145–2150.

Bryant, A. S., Worjoloh, A., Caughey, A. B., & Washington, A. E. (2010). Racial/ethnic disparities in obstetric outcomes and care: Prevalence and determinants. *American Journal of Obstetrics & Gynecology, 202*(4), 335–343.

Cetrulo, C. L., & Schifrin, B. S. (1976). Fetal heart rate patterns preceding death in utero. *Obstetrics & Gynecology, 48*(5), 521–527.

Chamberlain, P. F., Manning, F. A., Morrison, I., Harman, C. R., & Lange, I. R. (1984). Ultrasound evaluation of amniotic fluid volume. I. The relationship of marginal and decreased amniotic fluid volumes to perinatal outcome. *American Journal of Obstetrics & Gynecology, 150*(3), 245–249.

Coppens, M., Vindla, S., James, D. K., & Sahota, D. S. (2001). Computerized analysis of acute and chronic changes in fetal heart rate variation and fetal activity in association with maternal smoking. *American Journal of Obstetrics & Gynecology, 185*(2), 421–426.

Daniels, S. M., & Boehm, N. (1991). Auscultated fetal heart rate accelerations: An alternative to the nonstress test. *Journal of Nurse-Midwifery, 36*(2), 88–94.

Dubinsky, T. J., & Sonneborn, R. (2020). Trouble with the curve: Pearls and pitfalls in the evaluation of fetal growth. *Journal of Ultrasound in Medicine, 39*(9), 1839–1846.

East, C. E., Smyth, R., Leader, L. R., Henshall, N. E., Colditz, P. B., & Tan, K. H. (2005). Vibroacoustic stimulation for fetal assessment in labour in the presence of a nonreassuring fetal heart rate trace. *Cochrane Database of Systematic Reviews, 18*(2), CD004664.

Esin, S., Baser, E., Cakir, C., Ustun Tuncal, G. N., & Kucukozkan, T. (2013). Chocolate or orange juice for non-reactive non-stress test (NST) patterns: A randomized prospective controlled study. *The Journal of Maternal-Fetal & Neonatal Medicine, 26*(9), 915–919.

FitzGerald, C., & Hurst, S. (2017). Implicit bias in healthcare professionals: A systematic review. *BMC Medical Ethics, 18*(1), 1–18.

Flenady, V., Koopmans, L., Middleton, P., Frøen, J. F., Smith, G. C., Gibbons, K., Coory, M., Gordon, A., Ellwood, D., McIntyre, H. D., & Fretts, R. (2011). Major risk factors for stillbirth in high-income countries: A systematic review and meta-analysis. *Lancet, 377*(9774), 1331–1340.

Franks, Z., & Nightingale, R. (2014). Decreased fetal movements: A practical approach in a primary care setting. *Australian Family Physician, 43*(11), 782.

Gardosi, J., Kady, S. M., McGeown, P., Francis, A., & Tonks, A. (2005). Classification of stillbirth by relevant condition at death (ReCoDe): Population based cohort study. *BMJ, 331*(7525), 1113–1117.

Gardosi, J., Madurasinghe, V., Williams, M., Malik, A., & Francis, A. (2013). Maternal and fetal risk factors for stillbirth: Population based study. *BMJ, 346*, f108.

Grant, A., Valentin, L., Elbourne, D., & Alexander, S. (1989). Routine formal fetal movement counting and risk of antepartum late death in normally formed singletons. *Lancet, 334*(8659), 345–349.

Gregory, E. C., Valenzuela, C. P., & Hoyert, D. L. (2022). Fetal mortality: United States, 2020. *National Vital Statistics Reports: From the Centers for Disease Control and Prevention, National Center for Health Statistics, National Vital Statistics System, 71*(4), 1–20.

Grivell, R. M., Alfirevic, Z., Gyte, G. M. L., & Devane, D. (2010). Antenatal cardiotocography for fetal assessment. *Cochrane Database of Systematic Reviews, 1*, CD007863.

Hanley, M. L., & Vintzileos, A. M. (1988). *Antepartum and intrapartum fetal surveillance of fetal well being. Medicine of the fetus and mother* (2nd ed.). JB Lippincott.

Heazell, A. P., & Frøen, J. F. (2008). Methods of fetal movement counting and the detection of fetal compromise. *Journal of Obstetrics & Gynaecology, 28*(2), 147–154.

Hijazi, Z. R., & East, C. E. (2009). Factors affecting maternal perception of fetal movement. *Obstetrical & Gynecological Survey, 64*(7), 489–497.

Hutter, D., & Jaeggi, E. (2010). Causes and mechanisms of intrauterine hypoxia and its impact on the fetal cardiovascular system: A review. *International Journal Of Pediatrics, 2010*, 401323.

Judd, F. A., Haran, S. S., & Everett, T. R. (2020). Antenatal fetal wellbeing. *Obstetrics, Gynaecology & Reproductive Medicine, 30*(7), 197–204.

Khooshideh, M., Izadi, S., Shahriari, A., & Mirteymouri, M. (2009). The predictive value of ultrasound assessment of amniotic fluid index, biophysical profile score, nonstress test and foetal movement chart for meconium-stained amniotic fluid in prolonged pregnancies. *Journal of Pakistan Medical Association, 59*, 471–474.

Kingdom, J. C. P., & Kaufmann, P. (1997). Oxygen and placental villous development: Origins of fetal hypoxia. *Placenta, 18*(8), 613–621.

Kodama, Y., Sameshima, H., Ikeda, T., & Ikenou, T. (2009). Intrapartum fetal heart rate patterns in infants (≥34 weeks) with poor neurological outcome. *Early Human Development, 85*, 235–238.

Kontopoulos, E. V., & Vintzileos, A. M. (2004). Condition-specific antepartum fetal testing. *American Journal of Obstetrics & Gynecology, 191*(5), 1546–1551.

Liston, R., Sawchuck, D., Young, D., & Fetal Health Surveillance Consensus Committee. (2007). Fetal health surveillance: Antepartum and intrapartum consensus guideline. *Journal of Obstetrics & Gynaecology Canada, 29*(9), s1–s56.

Liston, R. M., Cohen, A. W., Mennuti, M. T., & Gabbe, S. G. (1982). Antepartum fetal evaluation by maternal perception of fetal movement. *Obstetrics & Gynecology, 60*(4), 424–426.

Liu, S. R., Kia-Keating, M., & Nylund-Gibson, K. (2018). Patterns of adversity and pathways to health among White, Black, and Latinx youth. *Child Abuse & Neglect, 86*, 89–99.

Louis, G. M. B., Grewal, J., Albert, P. S., Sciscione, A., Wing, D. A., Grobman, W. A., Newman, R. B., Wapner, R., D'Alton, M. E., Skupski, D., Nageotte, M. P., Ranzini, A. C., Owen, J., Chien, E. K., Craigo, S., Hediger, M. L., Kim, S., Zhang, C., & Grantz, K. L. (2015). Racial/ethnic standards for fetal growth: The NICHD Fetal Growth Studies. *American Journal of Obstetrics and Gynecology, 213*(4), 449.e1–449.e41.

Low, J. A., Pickersgill, H., Killen, H., & Derrick, E. J. (2001). The prediction and prevention of intrapartum fetal asphyxia in term pregnancies. *American Journal of Obstetrics & Gynecology, 184*, 724–730.

MacDorman, M. F., & Gregory, E. C. (2015). Fetal and perinatal mortality: United States, 2013. *National Vital Statistics Reports, 64*(8), 1–24.

Macones, G. A., Hankins, G. D., Spong, C. Y., Hauth, J., & Moore, T. (2008). The 2008 National Institute of Child Health and Human Development workshop report on electronic fetal monitoring: Update on definitions, interpretation, and research guidelines. *Journal of Obstetric, Gynecologic, & Neonatal Nursing, 37*(5), 510–515.

Magann, E. F., Nolan, T. E., Hess, L. W., Martin, R. W., Whitworth, N. S., & Morrison, J. C. (1992). Measurement of amniotic fluid volume: Accuracy of ultrasonography techniques. *American Journal of Obstetrics & Gynecology, 167*(6), 1533–1537.

Mangesi, L., Hofmeyr, G. J., Smith, V., & Smyth, R. (2015). Fetal movement counting for assessment of fetal wellbeing. *Cochrane Database of Systematic Reviews, (10)*, CD004909.

Manning, F. A. (1995). Dynamic ultrasound-based fetal assessment: The fetal biophysical profile score. *Clinical Obstetrics and Gynecology, 38*(1), 26–44.

Manning, F. A. (2002). Fetal biophysical profile: A critical appraisal. *Clinical Obstetrics and Gynecology, 45*(4), 975–985.

Manning, F. A. (2009). Antepartum fetal testing: A critical approach. *Current Opinion in Obstetrics and Gynecology, 21*, 348–352.

Manning, F. A., Morrison, I., Lange, I. R., Harman, C. R., & Chamberlain, P. F. (1987). Fetal biophysical profile scoring: Selective use of nonstress test. *American Journal of Obstetrics & Gynecology, 156*(3), 709–712.

Manning, F. A., Platt, L. D., & Sipos, L. (1980). Antepartum fetal evaluation: Development of a fetal biophysical profile. *American Journal of Obstetrics & Gynecology, 136*(6), 787–795.

Miller, D. A., Rabello, Y. A., & Paul, R. H. (1996). The modified biophysical profile: Antepartum testing in the 1990s. *American Journal of Obstetrics & Gynecology, 174*(3), 812–817.

Moore, T. R., & Piacquadio, K. (1989). A prospective evaluation of fetal movement screening to reduce the incidence of antepartum fetal death. *American Journal of Obstetrics and Gynecology, 160*(5 Pt. 1), 1075–1080.

Narayan, M. C. (2019). CE: Addressing implicit bias in nursing: A review. *AJN The American Journal of Nursing, 119*(7), 36–43.

Neldam, S. (1980). Fetal movements as an indicator of fetal wellbeing. *Lancet, 1*(8180), 1222–1224.

Norman, J. E., Heazell, A. E. P., Rodriguez, A., Weir, C. J., Stock, S. J. E., Calderwood, C. J., Burley, S. C., Frøen, J. F., Geary, M., Breathnach, F., Hunter, A., McAuliffe, F. M., Higgins, M. F., Murdoch, E., Ross-Davie, M., Scott, J., & Whyte, S., for the AFFIRM investigators(2018). Awareness of fetal movements and care package to reduce fetal mortality (AFFIRM): A stepped wedge, cluster-randomised trial. *The Lancet, 392*(10158), 1629–1638.

Ocak, V., Demirkiran, F., Sen, C., Colgar, U., Ocer, F., Kilavuz, O., & Uras, Y. (1992). The predictive value of fetal heart rate monitoring: A retrospective analysis of 2165 high-risk pregnancies. *European Journal of Obstetrics & Gynecology and Reproductive Biology, 44*, 53–58.

O'Leary, J., Mendenhall, H., & Andrinopoulos, G. (1980). Comparison of auditory versus electronic assessment and antenatal welfare. *Obstetrics & Gynecology, 56*(2), 244–246.

Olesen, A. G., & Svare, J. A. (2004). Decreased fetal movements: Background, assessment, and clinical management. *Acta Obstetricia et Gynecologica Scandinavica*, *83*(9), 818–826.

O'Neill, E., & Thorp, J. (2012). Antepartum evaluation of the fetus and fetal well-being. *Clinical Obstetrics and Gynecology*, *55*(3), 722–730.

O'Sullivan, O., Stephen, G., Martindale, E., & Heazell, A. E. P. (2009). Predicting poor perinatal outcome in women who present with decreased fetal movements. *Journal of Obstetrics & Gynaecology*, *29*(8), 705–710.

Oyelese, Y., & Vintzileos, A. M. (2011). The uses and limitations of the fetal biophysical profile. *Clinics in Perinatology*, *38*, 49.

Paine, L., Johnson, T. R. B., Turner, M. H., & Payton, R. G. (1986). Auscultated fetal heart rate accelerations part II. An alternative to the nonstress test. *Journal of Nurse-Midwifery*, *31*(2), 73–77.

Paine, L., Payton, R. G., & Johnson, T. R. B. (1986). Auscultated fetal heart rate accelerations part I. Accuracy and documentation. *Journal of Nurse-Midwifery*, *31*(2), 68–72.

Papantoniou, N., Daskalakis, G., Anastasakis, E., Marinopoulos, S., Mesogitis, S., & Antsaklis, A. (2008). Increasing the noninvasive management of rhesus isoimmunization. *International Journal of Gynecology & Obstetrics*, *101*(3), 281–284.

Pearson, J. F., & Weaver, J. B. (1976). Fetal activity and fetal wellbeing: An evaluation. *British Medical Journal*, *1*, 1305–1307.

Pillai, M., & James, D. (1990). The development of fetal heart rate patterns during normal pregnancy. *Obstetrics & Gynecology*, *76*(5 Pt. 1), 812–816.

Pruitt, S. M., Hoyert, D. L., Anderson, K. N., Martin, J., Waddell, L., Duke, C., Honein, M. A., & Reefhuis, J. (2020). Racial and ethnic disparities in fetal deaths—United States, 2015–2017. *Morbidity and Mortality Weekly Report*, *69*(37), 1277.

Rutherford, S. E., Phelan, J. P., Smith, C. V., & Jacobs, N. (1987). The four-quadrant assessment of amniotic fluid volume: An adjunct to antepartum fetal heart rate testing. *Obstetrics & Gynecology*, *70*(3 Pt. 1), 353–356.

Saastad, E., Winje, B. A., Israel, P., & Froen, J. F. (2012). Fetal movement counting—Maternal concern and experiences: A multicenter, randomized, controlled trial. *Birth*, *39*(1), 10–20.

Sadovsky, E., & Yaffe, H. (1973). Daily fetal movement recording and fetal prognosis. *Obstetrics & Gynecology*, *41*(6), 845–850.

Signore, C., Freeman, R. K., & Spong, C. Y. (2009). Antenatal testing—A reevaluation. *Obstetrics & Gynecology*, *113*(3), 687–701.

Sinha, D., Sharma, A., Nallaswarmy, V., Jayagopal, N., & Bhatti, N. (2007). Obstetric outcome in women complaining of reduced fetal movements. *Journal of Obstetrics & Gynaecology*, *27*(1), 41–43.

Sterpu, I., Pilo, C., Koistinen, I. S., Lindqvist, P. G., Gemzell-Danielsson, K., & Itzel, E. W. (2020). Risk factors for poor neonatal outcome in pregnancies with decreased fetal movements. *Acta Obstetricia et Gynecologica Scandinavica*, *99*(8), 1014–1021.

Sun, M., Oliwa, T., Peek, M. E., & Tung, E. L. (2022). Negative patient descriptors: Documenting racial bias in the electronic health record: Study examines racial bias in the patient descriptors used in the electronic health record. *Health Affairs*, *41*(2), 203–211.

Tan, K. H., Smyth, R. M., & Wei, X. (2013). Fetal vibroacoustic stimulation for facilitation of tests of fetal wellbeing. *Cochrane Database of Systematic Reviews*, (12), CD002963. https://doi.org/10.1002/14651858.CD002963.pub2

Tveit, J. V. H., Saastad, E., Stray-Pedersen, B., Bordahl, P. E., Flenady, V., Fretts, R., & Froen, J. F. (2009). Reduction of late stillbirth with the introduction of fetal movement information and guidelines—A clinical quality improvement. *BMC Pregnancy and Childbirth*, *9*(1), 32.

Velazquez, M. D., & Rayburn, W. F. (2002). Antenatal evaluation of the fetus using fetal movement monitoring. *Clinical Obstetrics and Gynecology*, *45*(4), 993–1004.

Vintzileos, A. M., Campbell, W. A., Igardia, C. J., & Nochimson, D. J. (1983). The fetal biophysical profile and its predictive value. *Obstetrics & Gynecology*, *62*(3), 271–278.

Vintzileos, A. M., Fleming, A. D., Scorza, W. E., Wolf, E. J., Balducci, J., Campbell, W. A., & Rodis, J. F. (1991). Relationship between fetal biophysical activities and umbilical cord blood gas values. *American Journal of Obstetrics & Gynecology*, *165*(3), 707–713.

Wang, E., Glazer, K. B., Howell, E. A., & Janevic, T. M. (2020). Social determinants of pregnancy-related mortality and morbidity in the United States: A systematic review. *Obstetrics & Gynecology*, *135*(4), 896.

Willinger, M., Ko, C. W., & Reddy, U. M. (2009). Racial disparities in stillbirth risk across gestation in the United States. *American Journal of Obstetrics & Gynecology*, *201*(5), 469.e1–469.e8.

15

Common Discomforts of Pregnancy

Robin G. Jordan and Anne Z. Cockerham

Relevant Terms

Anticipatory guidance—the preparation of a patient for an anticipated development and/or situation

Fibroadenomas—common, noncancerous breast lumps of fibrous and glandular tissue

Galactoceles—milk-filled cysts in the breast, common during lactation

Gastroesophageal reflux—a condition where stomach contents leak backward from the stomach to the esophagus

Hirsutism—excessive facial and body hair

Leukonychia—white spots on nail beds

Leukorrhea—excessive, often white vaginal discharge, nonirritating

Linea nigra—vertical line of skin on the abdomen that darkens during pregnancy

Lumbar lordosis—a condition in which the curve of the lumbar spine increases

Melasma—an increase in facial pigmentation generally over the cheeks and forehead

Melanonychia—brown or black spots on nail beds

Pelvic girdle—also called the bony pelvis, consists of the paired hipbones connected to the symphysis pubis anteriorly and the sacrum posteriorly, the ilium, ischium, and sacrum; forms the birth canal; transfers the weight of the upper body to the legs

Ptyalism—the excess secretion of saliva

Sleep hygiene—the term used to describe the set of behaviors used to control presleep and sleep environments

Striae gravidarum—atrophic linear scars specific to pregnancy, commonly known as stretch marks

Introduction

The common discomforts of pregnancy encompass a wide variety of physical and emotional signs and symptoms, occurring at various times throughout pregnancy. Almost all of them are due to the normal anatomical and physiological changes that occur during pregnancy, are self-limiting, and are benign to pregnancy outcome. Antepartum care providers must be well versed in the causes of, timing of, and relief measures for the common discomforts of pregnancy, as pregnant clients commonly report pregnancy symptoms that require further inquiry, knowledgeable discussion, and appropriate advice.

Some healthcare providers may refer to the common discomforts of pregnancy as temporary, minor, physical, or emotional changes; however, they are often not minor to the person who is experiencing them. While some physiologic changes may induce symptoms that are easily managed, other changes may cause symptoms that create profound discomfort and require alterations in lifestyle and, as a result, can be quite distressing. Individuals with numerous pregnancy-related physical symptoms can experience significant negative effects on life quality (Kazemi et al., 2017) and can develop depressive symptoms and low self-esteem (Kamysheva et al., 2009). Also, some physical symptoms can be a somatic manifestation of psychological or emotional concerns.

When a client reports a pregnancy-related symptom, it is important to ascertain that this symptom is indeed due to pregnancy and not pathology and is within the limits of normal for the symptom. While each symptom requires different questions, some symptoms share subjective data gathering components. Questions of onset, frequency and duration of the symptom, and anything that has made it worse or better are questions essential to almost all pregnancy discomforts that can quickly distinguish between normal and abnormal. The onset of a symptom can be an important diagnostic clue in determining whether the symptom falls into the category of a common discomfort or a pathology. Additionally, multiple symptoms can represent changes in a single body system or changes in more than one body system. The data obtained from a thorough symptom review guide which aspects of a physical examination are indicated.

Prenatal and Postnatal Care: A Person-Centered Approach, Third Edition. Edited by Karen Trister Grace, Cindy L. Farley, Noelene K. Jeffers, and Tanya Tringali.
© 2024 John Wiley & Sons Ltd. Published 2024 by John Wiley & Sons Ltd.
Companion website: www.wiley.com/go/grace/prenatal

> **Old Cart: A mnemonic for symptom review**
>
> **O**: onset
> **L**: location
> **D**: duration
> **C**: character
> **A**: aggravating/alleviating factors
> **R**: radiation
> **T**: timing

The manner in which these common pregnancy symptoms are viewed and presented is an important consideration when providing prenatal care. Most people report their symptoms to their healthcare provider and look for advice and information, but they also look for empathetic acknowledgment and active listening to their concerns. Traditional medical vernacular typically uses the title "Common Complaints of Pregnancy" and designates symptom reporting as "complaints." Rather than writing "complains of . . .," the more respectful phrase "reports symptoms of . . ." can be used when documenting. The word "complaining" implies whining, a negative behavior, and does not provide an accurate perspective on an individual's report of common changes experienced during pregnancy. Changing how these symptoms are viewed and communicated from common discomfort complaints to common discomfort symptoms can also allow individuals to feel more open to sharing their symptoms and seeking help from healthcare providers.

During prenatal care visits, it is essential to provide education about the normal changes occurring in the pregnant body. Pregnant people may perceive normal and benign symptoms as abnormal, promoting a reliance on medical care to interpret and resolve the discomfort. Prenatal **anticipatory guidance**, teaching, and reassurance of normalcy for pregnancy discomforts can normalize a person's perception of their body changes and promote self-knowledge of their body and pregnancy experience. All pregnant clients reporting common discomforts are informed of the physiological basis for their symptom(s), when they can expect relief, self-help measures to help ameliorate discomfort(s), and signs and symptoms to be alert for indicating a condition outside of the broad scope of normal when applicable.

Anticipatory guidance concerning common pregnancy discomforts and normal body changes requires a solid knowledge base of the normal maternal adaptations to pregnancy and recognition of the limits of normalcy. While most of the discomforts of pregnancy remain within the realm of normal, symptom characteristics that delineate normal from pathology should be considered.

This chapter is organized by topic alphabetically with sections on data gathering and relief measures included for each symptom. Many of the common discomforts of pregnancy can be alleviated with common-sense measures and "tincture of time"; others may require recommendations for treatment. A variety of relief measures, including more traditional or alternative remedies that have been used over time, are presented. For many pregnancy symptoms, reassurance of normal brings a measure of relief and ability to cope.

> **Health equity key points**
>
> - When suggesting relief and preventative measures for common discomforts, clinicians should be mindful and respectful concerning pregnant individuals' access to resources.
> - An empathetic, client-centered approach to evaluating and managing common discomforts provides an important opportunity to listen to pregnant individuals, particularly those from populations that have been marginalized. Clinicians who respond to individuals' concerns in a sensitive and caring way can build trust and reduce inequities in the care of all pregnant people. Conversely, clinicians contribute to barriers to optimal health by being dismissive and minimizing individuals' reports of common discomforts.
> - The presentation of many common prenatal skin changes differs among skin colors. Resources to aid in the identification of skin conditions manifesting on varying skin colors is essential for appropriate assessment and treatment.

Back Pain and Pelvic Girdle Pain

Back pain in pregnancy develops under the influence of progesterone and relaxin, which soften connective tissue including the ligaments and joints. Additionally, the shift in the individual's center of gravity as pregnancy progresses leads to postural changes that can contribute to back pain. Low back pain is common during pregnancy with 40% of pregnant individuals reporting pain in the first trimester and 44–70% in the third trimester (Backhausen et al., 2019). Lower backache is attributed to the **lumbar lordosis** required to counterbalance the weight of the growing uterus. Upper backache is caused by increasing weight of the breasts, postural factors, and employment requiring extended sitting.

Factors that increase the incidence of back pain are older age, higher parity, and occupations with heavy lifting or constant standing. Individuals who have experienced prior back pain while pregnant also have a higher incidence of back and **pelvic girdle** pain in subsequent pregnancies (Vermani et al., 2010). Back pain generally increases as pregnancy advances, and it can interfere with daily activities like carrying, cleaning, sitting, and walking. Back pain can become a barrier to work and sleep.

Sacroiliac joint pain is a type of pelvic girdle pain that may or may not be associated with lower back pain. It can be misdiagnosed as sciatica; however, only 1% of pregnant individuals actually have true sciatica (Richens et al., 2010). The etiology of pelvic girdle pain is thought to be the same as lower back pain; however, the presentation is different. The pain can radiate across the hip joints and the thigh bones, or close to the sacroiliac joints extending to the gluteal area. The pain can be described as shooting, pulsating, or burning. The pain often shoots into the symphysis pubis and is worse with movement, especially when walking or when bearing weight on one leg. A clicking, snapping sound, or grinding sensation within the symphysis pubis may accompany the pain. A waddling gait with short steps may develop to limit hip motion and avoid pain, and to provide more stability as weight is added to the anterior trunk (Ogamba et al., 2016).

The symphysis pubis of the anterior portion of the pelvis widens prenatally under hormonal influence in preparation for birth. The cartilage connecting the two halves of the pelvis at the symphysis pubis widens in all pregnant individuals, and in some, a separation of the bone from the cartilage occurs, creating a diastasis. Symphysis pubis diastasis is more common after birth; however, it can occur prenatally (Figure 15.1). Pain from symphysis separation can be significant and severely restrict capacity for sitting, standing, and walking.

Assessment

Subjective Data Gathering

The clinician should obtain the following information: the onset, location and description of symptoms, history of back problems before pregnancy or in prior pregnancies, associated activity, relief measures tried and effectiveness, presence of contractions, pelvic pressure, urinary tract infection (UTI) symptoms, and history of traumatic injury.

Objective Data Gathering

The goal of the physical examination is to rule out other causes of back pain and assess for disability. The clinician should observe posture, palpate the area for tenderness or signs of trauma, and perform additional assessments to rule out preterm labor or UTI as appropriate. The active straight leg test assesses for symphysis separation. The patient lies supine with straight legs and feet shoulder width apart. Ask the patient to raise one leg, then the other several feet off the table. Those with symptomatic separation feel pain upon this maneuver (Vleeming et al., 2008). The diagnosis of back and pelvic pain during pregnancy is often clinical, and imaging studies are typically not useful. Symphysis separation can be confirmed by ultrasound, though the degree of pain does not correlate with the degree of separation and does not change the management plan. Back pain that is consistent with expected, nonpathologic pregnancy discomforts should improve with rest. If the pain does not improve with rest or is severe and disabling, the clinician should consider more serious etiology, such as a herniated disc, additional evaluation, and possible referral.

Relief and Preventative Measures

Physical fitness prior to pregnancy reduces the incidence of back and pelvic pain during subsequent pregnancies (Vermani et al., 2010). Pelvic floor and pelvic tilt exercises help strengthen core body muscles and improve trunk stability, which can reduce back pain (Borg-Stein & Dugan, 2007), as these exercises involve the musculature that stabilizes the core and trunk (Table 15.1).

Swimming or aquatic therapy relieves joint and muscle pressure by providing a weightless environment and has been effective in relieving and reducing pregnancy-related back and pelvic girdle pain (van Benten et al., 2014). Some pregnant individuals report relief of low back pain from chiropractic manipulation (Conner et al., 2021). Practicing yoga for at least 1 hour per week has been shown to improve pelvic girdle and lower back pain (Martins & Pinto e Silva, 2014). Specific exercises under the guidance of a physical therapist can provide relief from back and pelvic girdle pain as well (Belogolovsky et al., 2015). Acupuncture is also useful for reducing low back pain and improving function during pregnancy (Bishop et al., 2019).

Symphysis Pubis Dysfunction

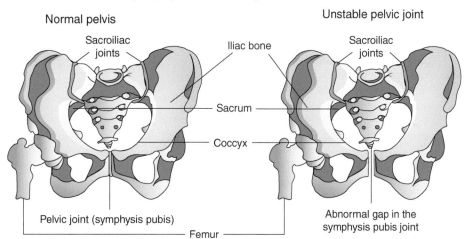

Figure 15.1 Symphysis separation.

Table 15.1 Instructions for Pelvic Floor and Pelvic Tilt Exercises

Pelvic floor exercises (Kegels)	Pelvic tilt exercises
• Squeeze and lift the muscles of the pelvic floor. If this is difficult, imagine you are trying to stop yourself from urinating or passing gas. • Hold these muscles in contraction for up to 10 seconds. • Relax the muscles slowly. Repeat. • Aim for 10 or more repetitions throughout the day.	• In the standing position: Lean against a wall with knees gently bent. Flatten the lower back against the wall as the abdominal muscles are contracted. • Repeat 5–10 times. • Aim for five or more repetitions throughout the day. • Continue to breathe during the movement. • In the hands/knees position: Keeping the head aligned with the body, straighten the back like a plank. Drop the lower back to a concave position. Return to the flat position.

Relief measures for pelvic girdle pain

Be aware of posture and stand straight with hips pulled forward.
Avoid standing for long periods of time.
Place one foot on a low stool if prolonged standing is unavoidable.
Use proper body mechanics when lifting.
Sleep on a mattress that offers support.
Sleep on the side with pillows propped under the uterus and between the knees.
Wear low-heeled shoes; avoid high heels as they strain the lower back muscles.
Pelvic tilt exercises help keep the back muscles stretched.
Acupuncture can be helpful.
Use supportive maternity belts, binders, or garments such as the BellyBra®.
Massage.
Warm pack to the affected area.
Sacroiliac belt that fits around the hips reduces symphysis pubis movement.
Short-term use of acetaminophen can be used in all trimesters of pregnancy. Typical doses are 325–650 mg po q4–6h prn up to a maximum of 3000 mg/day.

If pain is severe, pharmaceutical relief can be considered. It has been common practice to recommend acetaminophen for pain relief during pregnancy; however, new controversy over long-term effects has emerged. While not associated with teratogenicity, recent data suggest a modest but consistent association of acetaminophen use in pregnancy with possible neurodevelopmental problems in later childhood (Black et al., 2019). More research is needed to determine causation. Acetaminophen remains the analgesia of choice during pregnancy as needed, yet, as with all medications during pregnancy, should be used only when necessary and in the lowest effective dose.

Additional remedies can be advised and include relief for symphysis separation pain. A flexible pregnancy support belt provides the compression of the bony pelvis and lifts up the lower segment of the uterus, providing support and some pain relief and improvement in daily functioning (Morino et al., 2019). Kinesio taping, a noninvasive application of an elastic material to the patient's skin, is another modality that has shown promise in reducing low back pain (Xue et al., 2021). Individuals with severe back pain or possible separation of the symphysis pubis should undergo diagnostic imaging. Conservative treatment consists of pelvic binders, increased rest and limited or no physical work for the remainder of the pregnancy to achieve relief. Individuals with significant back or pelvic girdle pain unrelieved by common measures can benefit from physical therapy evaluation or referral to a physical medicine and rehabilitation physician (physiatrist).

Bleeding Gums

Estrogen increases blood flow to the mouth and gums and causes swelling of the gingival tissue. This is called gingivitis of pregnancy. The increase in small fragile blood vessels, hyperplasia, and edema can cause minor bleeding to occur while brushing or flossing teeth or when eating certain abrasive or rough foods. Approximately one-third of pregnant people will experience bleeding gums during pregnancy (Liu et al., 2016). During pregnancy, the increase in progesterone produces pH changes in the saliva that promote bacterial growth in the mouth (Nuriel-Ohayon et al., 2016). Additionally, there is a reduction of antimicrobial activity of peripheral neutrophils, essential components of periodontal tissues' immune defenses (Silva de Araujo Figueiredo et al., 2017). These pregnancy-related physiologic changes result in increased susceptibility to gingivitis. More rarely, pregnancy-related coagulopathies can also cause bleeding gums, such as gestational thrombocytopenia, idiopathic thrombocytopenic purpura, and HELLP syndrome.

Assessment

Subjective Data Gathering

The onset, nature and characteristics, predisposing or aggravating factors, oral hygiene practices, and prior history of dental disease are obtained.

Objective Data Gathering

Objective data gathering is an oral examination as indicated. See Chapter 16, *Oral Health*, for more detail on an oral health examination in pregnancy. If there is concern about low platelets as a potential etiology of bleeding gums, a CBC or platelet count will be important to review.

Relief and Preventative Measures

Clients experiencing bleeding gums should be reassured that this is a common and normal event in pregnancy because of estrogen effects and increased blood flow to the area. Periodic warm saltwater rinses can help ease irritation (one teaspoon salt to one cup of water). While dental hygiene activities can stimulate minor nonsignificant bleeding, regular flossing and brushing routines with a softer bristled brush and routine dental care should continue during pregnancy. Most common dental procedures can be done during pregnancy when needed. Preexisting gingivitis often worsens in pregnancy. If regular gingival bleeding occurs, oral examination for signs and symptoms of severe gingivitis and referral to a dentist is warranted. Periodontal disease can lead to systemic infection processes that are linked with an increase in preterm birth (PTB), preeclampsia, and low birth weight (Choi et al., 2021; Daalderop et al., 2018). However, there is insufficient evidence that the treatment of periodontal disease during pregnancy improves outcomes (Iheozor-Ejiofor et al., 2017).

Breast Tenderness

Breast tenderness is an almost universal symptom in pregnancy and can be one of its first physical signs. Initial acute breast tenderness typically begins four to six weeks after the last menstrual period (LMP). The body increases its levels of estrogen and progesterone, enabling the milk ducts and milk-producing cells to form in preparation for breastfeeding. Additional blood flow circulates in the breasts during this time, causing the swelling and tenderness typical of the first trimester. Layers of fat are deposited within the breasts, adding to the change in size and discomfort. Benign breast lumps, such as cysts, **galactoceles**, and **fibroadenomas**, normally enlarge in pregnancy under the influence of estrogen. Breast changes continue to occur throughout pregnancy; however, most individuals experience relief from acute tenderness by late first to mid-second trimester. Colostrum starts to form after 20 weeks of gestation and can produce nipple discharge in the latter half of pregnancy. Primigravidas are likely to experience more intense breast tenderness than multigravidas since the breast tissue is expanding in a new way.

Normal pregnancy breast symptoms

Increase in breast size by up to two cup sizes
Increase in areola size and darkening of the areola
Breast veins more prominent and visible
Highly sensitive nipples
Burning, tingling, or throbbing breast pain
Sensation of breast heaviness
Itchy breast skin and nipples
Throbbing or tingling breasts during sexual activity
Striae development on breasts
Leaking of colostrum in the latter half of pregnancy

Assessment

Subjective Data Gathering

The onset and characteristics of breast tenderness, prior history of breast problems, current lactation status, any nipple discharge, and its qualities should be obtained.

Objective Data Gathering

Inspection and palpation of the breast for infection, irritation, and masses are done as indicated. Color and odor of any discharge should be noted.

Relief and Preventative Measures

Reassurance that this is a normal and common pregnancy symptom and information regarding the physiology behind this symptom should be provided. Linking the changes to physiological preparation for lactation may help to cope with the discomfort (Johnson & Strube, 2011). Adequate support from clothing that limits breast movement is key to reducing the discomfort of breast tenderness. A diagnosis of breast cancer during pregnancy is very rare and found in approximately 1 in 3000 pregnant individuals (Rossi et al., 2019). Diagnosis can be challenging due to the normal pregnancy-related physiologic changes in the breast tissue.

Relief measures for pregnancy breast discomfort

Wear a well-fitting bra with adequate support and no underwire.
Choose cotton bras to help dissipate moisture.
Wear a sports bra that minimizes breast movement when exercising.
Apply a cool cloth to the breasts.
Avoid breast stimulation during sexual activity.
Pat breasts dry after bathing; no rubbing or stimulation.
Sleep in a bra if the breasts are tender at night.

Carpal Tunnel Syndrome

Carpal tunnel syndrome (CTS) is a frequently reported common discomfort of pregnancy in all trimesters, affecting an estimated 31–62% of pregnant individuals (Afshar & Tabrizi, 2021). CTS is caused by anything that compresses the median nerve, which runs from the forearm into the palm and the tendons in the carpal tunnel. The pathophysiology of CTS in pregnancy is primarily attributed to increased body fluid volume causing the compression of the median nerve. Median nerve compression occurs to some degree in all pregnant individuals; however, many remain asymptomatic. Common symptoms include numbness and/or tingling in the thumb, index finger, and middle fingers; wrist pain; and loss of grip strength and dexterity. It can occur in one or both hands, and impairment and discomfort can range from mild to severe. Symptoms are more pronounced after a period of rest or after a period of repetitive hand motions like typing. CTS symptoms are common during sleep when the wrist may be in a flexed position; this can contribute to disordered sleep and fatigue (Pflibsen et al., 2020).

CTS in pregnancy is most often a limited and benign discomfort. However, if left untreated, individuals experiencing severe symptoms may have permanent disability. Those who develop CTS during the first and second trimesters of pregnancy are more likely to have more severe symptoms and disability.

Diagnosis is made based on clinical symptom history and physical exam.

Assessment

Subjective Data Gathering

The onset, nature, characteristic and location of sensation, presence of pain, and degree of disability are obtained.

Objective Data Gathering

Carpal tunnel compression tests are specific and easy to perform in the office. A commonly used test consists of the examiner applying direct thumb pressure over the median nerve at the carpal tunnel and holding for 30 seconds. A positive test elicits paresthesias within this period. Another test consists of flexing the wrist downward while holding the elbow straight; the presence of paresthesias within 60 seconds of passive wrist flexion is positive for CTS. Diagnostic nerve conduction studies are often not necessary in pregnancy.

Relief and Preventative Measures

Treatment for most individuals during pregnancy is conservative as this condition may improve spontaneously within the first two weeks postpartum, when the body loses excessive pregnancy fluid.

Relief measures for CTS

Hand splint in neutral position worn at night and/or during the day as needed
Avoidance of extreme flexion or extension of the wrist
Decreased use of vibrating tools like lawn mowers
Decreased repetitive hand and wrist motions
Massage and gentle stretching of the fingers and wrist
Physical therapy or chiropractic manipulation

If CTS was present during pregnancy, a reassessment should be done at the six-week postpartum checkup. Although most symptoms resolve in the postpartum period, up to 49% of individuals report continuing symptoms and 11% continue to wear a splint at three years postpartum (Pflibsen et al., 2020). Individuals with severe pain due to CTS during pregnancy and those with persistent CTS symptoms several months after birth are referred to a hand specialist physician for possible corticosteroid injections.

Clinicians have advised pregnant patients for many years that acetaminophen (APAP, Tylenol) is safe in all the stages of pregnancy. However, a recent consensus statement urges caution as observational and animal studies have linked APAP with neurodevelopmental and other problems (Bauer et al., 2021). Other experts, including members of the Organization of Teratology Information Specialists (OTIS), contend that the studies included in the consensus statement do not provide clear evidence of causality and harm (Alwan et al., 2022). Additional research is needed. Until then, the American College of Obstetricians and Gynecologists (ACOG) and others advise that prudent, short-term use of APAP for relief of fever and acute pain is acceptable (ACOG, 2021).

Cervical Pain

Cervical lightning pain is a term informally coined by some pregnant people used to describe the sensation of sharp shooting pains felt within the vagina and cervix. The pain is typically very sudden and brief yet quite uncomfortable and typically occurs in the third trimester. Episodes may occur infrequently or several times a day. This transient pain is likely due to the increased pressure of the presenting part on the cervix, causing irritation of particular nerve endings. Because of the nature and location of the pain, some clients may be concerned that this pain could signal a problem. Reassurance can be provided that this episodic shooting pain is common during later gestation and likely due to fetal pressure on the cervix and is not known to be associated with any complications.

Constipation

Approximately 40% of pregnant individuals experience **constipation** during some point in pregnancy (Shin et al., 2015). Symptoms include difficult, painful defecation, hard stools, and feeling of incomplete evacuation. Pregnancy is a predisposing factor for constipation due to the rise in progesterone, delayed gastric motility, and mechanical changes with advancing pregnancy (Kuronen et al., 2021). Additional contributing factors may be diets low in fiber, decreased physical activity, prior history of constipation, and taking iron supplementation. Iron formulations high in elemental iron can produce significant constipation, and many will discontinue iron supplementation for this reason. Potential problems due to constipation are the development of hemorrhoids or anal fissures, both of which may cause pain and bleeding. Constipation can also induce abdominal pain, nausea, and poor appetite.

Assessment

Subjective Data Gathering

Areas to evaluate include the onset, usual bowel habits and current pattern, description of a typical stool, diet and fluid habits with particular attention to fiber intake, exercise patterns, medication history, self-help measures including over-the-counter (OTC) medication used to relieve constipation, and presence of abdominal pain or cramping. Ingestion of iron supplementation and the amount and type of iron in the prenatal vitamin is evaluated.

Objective Data Gathering

The clinician should palpate the abdomen for masses and bloating. A rectal exam may be appropriate in some situations. Stool can also be felt through the posterior vaginal wall during a pelvic exam.

Relief and Preventative Measures

In most situations, constipation is due to a combination of hormonal, dietary, and mechanical factors affecting normal gastrointestinal (GI) function. Generally, an explanation of the physiological basis, reassurance of normalcy, and self-treatment measures are all that is needed.

Information on high-fiber foods should be provided. If dietary and lifestyle changes do not produce relief from constipation, adding a bulking agent like two to four tablespoons of bran or psyllium may be all that is needed. It takes two to three days to feel the effects of bulk laxatives. Once desired results are achieved, the amount of supplementation is titrated to provide constipation prevention. Osmotic laxatives such as polyethylene glycol 8–25 mg/day and lactulose 15–30 mg/day are safe in pregnancy and are second-line measures if diet and bulk-forming laxatives are ineffective (Shin et al., 2015). They have the benefit of quicker relief; however, side effects such as diarrhea and abdominal discomfort may limit use (Rungsiprakarn et al., 2015). Self-administration of a Fleet type enema can also be offered as a safe and effective means of constipation relief (Table 15.2).

Dizziness/Syncope

It is estimated that approximately 28% of pregnant individuals experience dizziness, with almost 5% having an episode of syncope or loss of consciousness (Gibson et al., 2001). Syncope can occur during any trimester; however, it is more common in the late second and third trimesters. The normal physiologic changes promoting syncope include decreased systemic vascular resistance resulting in vasodilation and venous pooling in the legs. This leads to a drop in cardiac output and blood pressure, reducing cerebral blood flow, and causing the sensation of dizziness. Reports of dizziness or fainting while standing and waiting for periods of time during routine activities like waiting in the grocery checkout line or in the post office are common. Postural hypotension caused by a rapidly changing position from lying down to an upright position can also bring on dizziness. Hypoglycemic episodes in pregnancy can also lead to dizziness or syncope; a diet history can be done to determine if this is a factor. Lying supine, especially in the third trimester, causes the gravid uterus to put pressure on the inferior vena cava, causing decreased cardiac venous return, hypotension, and syncope.

Prevention and relief measures for constipation

Eat a high-fiber diet—25–30 g/day of dietary fiber is needed to prevent constipation. High-fiber foods include fruits, vegetables, breakfast cereals, whole grain breads, prunes, and bran.
Ensure adequate hydration—8–12 cups of water daily in combination with a high-fiber diet can provide enough bulk to promote regular bowel movement.
Exercise routinely—Daily walking, swimming, and other moderate exercise can help stimulate bowel activity.
Decrease, change, or eliminate iron supplements—Taking iron every third day can increase hematocrit and hemoglobin and reduce side effects. Changing iron supplement to a plant-based preparation like Floradix© can reduce constipation. Changing to a formula low in elemental iron can improve bowel function.
Defecate after meals—Bowel activity is increased at this time.
Avoid Valsalva straining during bowel movement—This is to prevent hemorrhoid formation.

Table 15.2 Remedies for Constipation

Laxative types and examples	Mechanism of action	Side effects
Bulk-forming laxatives Fiber supplements with psyllium, oat bran, or wheat fiber in pill, powder, liquid, or chewable form Citrucel, Metamucil, FiberCon, Benefiber	Increases stool transit time and frequency of bowel activity; must be taken with liquids to be effective	Bloating, cramping
Stool softeners/osmotic laxatives Miralax, Colace, Surfak, and pharmacy or store-branded products containing docusate	Prevents hardening of the feces by adding moisture	Bloating, cramping
Stimulant laxatives Oral stimulant (Senekot, senna) Rectal stimulant (bisacodyl) Castor oil should not be used to relieve constipation; gentler laxatives preferred	Causes intestinal contraction to expel stool	Abdominal pain, diarrhea, rectal irritation, electrolyte imbalance, colic; used with caution in pregnancy

Source: Adapted from Tharpe et al. (2022).

Assessment

Subjective Data Gathering

Assessment for possible injury and potential pathologic causes is key. This includes the onset, nature, and characteristics of symptoms, description of activity just prior to episode of dizziness or syncope, most recent food or fluid intake, environmental factors such as a heated or unventilated room, associated factors such as palpitations, headache or vomiting, and any significant medical history such as seizure disorder.

Objective Data Gathering

Observation for any signs of injury, blood pressure, and pulse measurements are obtained and heart auscultation performed as indicated. Gestational age is important as syncope in the early first trimester can be a sign of ectopic pregnancy.

Relief and Preventative Measures

Education on the physiology behind this symptom and the reassurance of normalcy are important elements of care. For dizziness due to postural hypotension, clients are advised to arise from bed slowly and to sit at the side of the bed for several moments.

Those who experience dizziness associated with chest pain or significant shortness of breath or loss of consciousness resulting in possible injury should be evaluated further. Cardiac disease complicates up to 4% of pregnancies and is the leading cause of death during pregnancy and the postpartum period, accounting for approximately 26% of maternal mortality (ACOG, 2019). Cardiac disease can be undiagnosed until pregnancy and is difficult to differentiate from common symptoms of pregnancy. An increase in adverse pregnancy outcomes and cardiac arrhythmias has been reported in pregnant individuals with syncope, especially if the episodes are in the first trimester (Chatur et al., 2019). For this reason, dizziness associated with chest pain or significant shortness of breath or loss of consciousness should be thoroughly explored and consultation or referral to a specialist care considered.

Prevention measures for pregnancy syncope

Arise from bed slowly.
Avoid extended periods of standing when possible.
Walk in place to promote venous return during those times when standing is unavoidable.
Eat small meals or snacks every few hours during the day.
Maintain adequate hydration.
Consider compression stockings when in an occupation requiring prolonged standing.
Avoid overheating.
Avoid closed-in areas with limited ventilation.
Avoid the supine position in the third trimester.

Edema

Total body fluids increase by 6–8 L in pregnancy, most of which is extracellular. Several liters of this fluid are found in the interstitial space, which is the space surrounding the body cells. When excessive fluid accumulates in the interstitial space, edema develops. This is a normal physiologic development in pregnancy. Dependent edema, the most common form of edema in pregnancy, affects most pregnant people to some degree. It is most noticeable in the legs in later pregnancy when the weight of the growing uterus interferes with venous return from the lower extremities. Edema of the hands is common in the morning and is likely postural. Edema can also be generalized over the entire body; this will present most notably as facial edema. Edema can produce symptoms of heaviness in the legs, discomfort, or pain and can limit mobility. It can also produce inconveniences such as tight or stuck rings and difficulty fitting into regular shoes. Severity of edema is assessed with a method such as the four-point scale (+1, slight, to +4, very marked); note any pitting quality, and note the height of the edema in the case of lower extremity edema.

Assessment

Subjective Data Gathering

Subjective data gathering consists of onset, location of edema, symptom description, and typical diet, noting water and salt intake. Potential symptoms of preeclampsia are especially noted, including headache and visual changes.

Objective Data Gathering

Objective data gathering consists of observation and inspection of edema, noting location, severity, presence of pitting, blood pressure, urine dip for protein, and weight gain pattern.

Relief and Preventative Measures

Water immersion provides a uniform compression and produces a natural pressure gradient and has been shown to effectively reduce peripheral edema in over 80% of cases (Smyth et al., 2015). Immersion should last at least 20 minutes and should be at least chest deep. Foot massage reduces edema and provides relief from discomfort (Van Kampen et al., 2015). Exercise involving the feet such as walking can reduce pedal edema (Mosti & Caggiati, 2021).

Relief measures for normal edema of pregnancy

Use water immersion for at least 20 minutes.
Exercise such as brisk walking or swimming improves venous return from the legs and reduces edema.
Apply compression stockings when first arising in the morning before dependent edema worsens.
Elevate the legs periodically throughout the day.
Drink plenty of fluids, especially water.
Perform a foot massage.
Avoid constrictive clothing such as knee-high socks.
Avoid heavily salted foods.

Rapid onset of edema or signs and symptoms, such as blurred vision, hypertension, and/or proteinuria, requires further evaluation for preeclampsia or deep vein thrombosis.

Emotional Changes

Pregnancy often brings a range of emotions throughout the prenatal course from joy and excitement to ambivalence, fear, and anxiety, sometimes all on the same day (see Chapter 23, *Psychosocial Adaptations in Pregnancy*). The physical changes and pregnancy discomforts and the tremendous hormonal influences play a role in a pregnant person's emotions. The very nature of creating a new life opens a person to loss and vulnerability in previously unknown ways and can manifest itself in anxieties about potential bodily harm to self and fetus. Reports of detailed and vivid dreams during pregnancy reflecting anxieties and concerns about pregnancy or parenting are common. These emotional changes are normal and universal across cultures during pregnancy. Most individuals cope well with their emotional changes and take them in stride. However, the clinician should remain alert for perinatal mood and anxiety disorders.

Assessment

Subjective Data Gathering

The onset, description of feelings and emotions, family member's reactions, sleep patterns, and usual diet are determined. Engage in dialogue with the individual; be curious about their daily life and feelings.

Objective Data Gathering

General affect and indicators of distress should be noted.

Relief and Preventative Measures

Active listening is the most helpful strategy a provider can implement in response to emotional issues. Reassurance that emotional changes are normal and expected can go a long way to help clients cope with this symptom. Encourage conversation with their partner and family members about their feelings to create an environment of support and safety. Ensuring adequate sleep and a nutritious diet can help maximize the ability to cope.

Normal emotional changes in pregnancy can sometimes mask the presence of depression, anxiety disorders, or chronic stress. Those who exhibit symptoms consistent with mood disorders, or those who are under severe and long-lasting stress, require additional screening and treatment options as indicated. See Chapter 47, *Mood and Anxiety Disorders,* for more detail.

Epistaxis

Approximately 20% of pregnant people will experience one or more episodes of nosebleed or epistaxis during pregnancy, more commonly in the third trimester (Singla et al., 2015). Individuals with a history of seasonal allergies and epistaxis before pregnancy have an increased risk of epistaxis during pregnancy (Dugan-Kim et al., 2009). A history of epistaxis increases the risk of postpartum hemorrhage, possibly due to factors related to clotting ability or abnormalities in vessel integrity that predispose to both conditions (Yousif & Anwer, 2021).

Assessment

Subjective Data Gathering

Often, bleeding occurs without warning; however, some symptoms that might precede an episode of epistaxis are itchy nose, dry nose, nasal congestion, sinus headache, or excessive sneezing or nose blowing. Inquire about typical nasal hygiene practices.

Relief and Preventative Measures

Reassurance that this is a common and typically harmless pregnancy symptom should be provided, along with instruction on the prevention of epistaxis and how to stop a nosebleed.

Measures to prevent pregnancy epistaxis

Use saline nasal spray, gel, or irrigation to lubricate nasal passages.
Drink plenty of fluids to hydrate nasal mucosa.
Increase room humidification, especially when sleeping.
Avoid vigorous nose blowing or nose picking.
Eat a nutritious diet to promote healthy tissue.

The vast majority of cases of epistaxis in pregnancy can be managed without medical intervention. Heavy and repeated epistaxis with significant blood loss is rare and can require nasal packing and/or surgical intervention. Nasal packing using petroleum laced gauze is effective in stopping blood loss (Abbas et al., 2020). Consultation for further evaluation is appropriate for those with frequent and prolonged episodes of epistaxis. Nasal granuloma gravidarum, an uncommon rapidly growing lesion, can cause torrential epistaxis and should be considered in individuals with recurrent or significant epistaxis (Ginat & Schatz, 2017). Pregnancy-related coagulopathies such as gestational thrombocytopenia, idiopathic thrombocytopenic purpura, and HELLP syndrome can cause epistaxis. If there is concern about low platelets as a potential etiology of epistaxis, a CBC or platelet count will be important to review. Clients should be advised to contact their healthcare provider if bleeding is significant, lasts more than 30 minutes, or they experience light headedness or difficulty breathing.

Measures to stop a nosebleed during pregnancy

Sit down and lean forward to stop the blood from running down the throat.
Pinch the nose firmly just under the bridge.
Maintain pressure for at least 10 minutes continuously.
Place an ice bag over the nose.
Avoid nose blowing for at least 12 hours to allow nasal mucosa healing.

Fatigue

Fatigue in the first trimester is one of the most common pregnancy symptoms and is due to the increase in progesterone. Although common, fatigue can have a negative impact on the pregnant individual's quality of life (Bai et al., 2016), and the clinician should use a caring approach to address the person's concerns without diminishing them. Differentiating normal pregnancy fatigue from fatigue due to pathology, such as anemia or depression, both of which are common in individuals of childbearing age, is essential. An efficient determination of normalcy of this symptom can be done with a few questions and a quick visual exam.

The most common symptom of anemia is fatigue and or weakness. Other signs and symptoms of anemia include shortness of breath, dizziness, headache, coldness in the hands and feet, and pale skin. Common signs and symptoms of depression are very similar to early pregnancy symptoms (see Chapter 47, *Mood and Anxiety Disorders*). These include a decrease of energy and/or motivation, insomnia, excessive sleeping, irritability, inability to concentrate or make decisions, and a feeling of sadness, heaviness, or apathy. While anemia and depression are fairly common in individuals of childbearing age, the most likely reason for fatigue in the first trimester is still the normal physiologic changes of pregnancy. Fatigue onset corresponding to five to seven weeks of gestation is the most significant clue as to the normal common discomfort of pregnancy or pathology. However, after ruling out the most common diagnoses, clinicians should broaden the differential diagnoses to consider other causes. Fatigue is a vague symptom associated with many conditions.

Assessment

Subjective Data Gathering

The onset and characteristics of fatigue, description of relief measures used, sleep habits, exercise habits, and prior history of anemia or depression are obtained.

Objective Data Gathering

The clinician should observe affect, and complete clinical assessments for anemia or depression as warranted.

Relief and Preventative Measures

The clinician should provide reassurance that fatigue is a normal and time-limited symptom, with most individuals experiencing relief around 12 weeks of gestation. It is especially important to encourage the pregnant individual to enlist help from their family and friends at this time, even writing a "prescription" for increased rest to show their family. Exercise during pregnancy can reduce fatigue and improve mood. Thirty minutes of walking or other aerobic exercise daily (Tella et al., 2011) and low to moderate muscle-strengthening exercises, such as biking, can help increase energy levels (Ward-Ritacco et al., 2016). Other strategies for dealing with early pregnancy fatigue are generally common-sense measures listed in the text box.

Relief measures for pregnancy fatigue

Take a daytime nap or rest if the schedule allows.
Get adequate night-time sleep.
Delegate household chores and modify a busy schedule.
Engage in 30 minutes of daily exercise.
Eat a diet adequate in protein and iron.
Eat every few hours to maintain blood glucose levels.

Flatulence

Flatulence is common in pregnancy and can occur during any trimester due to hormonal influence on the GI tract. The increase in progesterone and slowing of GI transit time allows for more gas formation in the gut. During the third trimester, the expanding uterus places increasing pressure on the intestines, slowing digestion further, and pressure on the rectum, decreasing muscle control and leading to increased flatulence. This may be an embarrassing pregnancy discomfort that clients are reluctant to discuss; therefore, it is prudent to ask about this discomfort so they can be informed about relief measures.

Assessment

Subjective Data Gathering

Information on the onset, amount, history of lactose intolerance or bowel disorders, usual diet habits, and level of distress over this symptom are obtained.

Objective Data Gathering

The abdomen is auscultated for bowel sounds and palpated for distention, although the enlarging uterus may make this exam difficult in late pregnancy.

Relief and Preventative Measures

Pregnancy-induced GI changes are explained. Emphasis is on prevention and relief measures.

Prevention and relief of flatulence

Eat six smaller meals per day to avoid digestive system overload.
Avoid gas-producing foods such as cabbage, beans, fried foods, and onions.
Avoid artificial sweeteners like sorbitol (common in diet soda) as they increase gas formation.
Avoid carbonated beverages.
Keep a food diary to identify patterns.
Eat slowly to reduce air swallowing.
Avoid using a straw or drinking from a bottle, which increases air swallowing.
Chew food thoroughly.
Lightly steaming vegetables can make them more easily digested than raw foods.
Take time to relax before eating, as tension can alter digestion.
Take a probiotic to balance bowel flora.

Increase dietary fiber to reduce gas formation.
Fresh ginger, carrot, celery, and apple juice may help calm the digestive tract.
Massage the abdomen in a clockwise rotation.
Side-lying position, knee-chest position, elevating hips above the head (hot air rises).
Yoga postures that promote intestinal circulation.
Brisk walking or exercise helps mobilize gas and provide relief.
Use OTC gas relief medication, such as Bean-o or Gas-X.

People who are especially distressed by this symptom may find relief with an OTC antiflatulence remedy. Those containing simethicone (e.g., Gas-X) are safe in pregnancy. Activated charcoal tablets should be avoided.

Headache

Most headaches during pregnancy are tension headaches, which usually respond to common relief measures. Abrupt elimination of caffeine is one benign and time-limited cause of headaches. Other benign causes of headache include sinus congestion, allergies, low blood sugar, or mild dehydration. Most individuals with a history of migraine headaches experience decreased frequency and severity of migraines during pregnancy (Ovadia, 2021). It is crucial to differentiate between benign headaches and those that herald pathologic conditions, particularly preeclampsia.

Assessment

Subjective Data Gathering

The onset, duration of headache, presence of aura, any associated symptoms, precipitating factors, location, bilateral or unilateral, occupational and activities of daily living (ADL) history, prior headache history, pattern of caffeine intake, diet and fluid intake, medication history, sleep adequacy, headache relief measures used, and their efficacy are assessed. Red flag symptoms include sudden onset, severe headache, pain lasting longer than 48 hours or taking much longer to resolve than normal, or headache associated with fever, seizures, or focal neurologic symptoms (Ovadia, 2021).

Objective Data Gathering

The clinician should assess the individual's general appearance, gestational age, blood pressure, weight, skin and mucosa for hydration, and presence of edema and proteinuria. Palpation of periorbital sinuses and funduscopic assessment are done as indicated.

Relief and Preventative Measures

If not associated with hypertension or other obvious medical issues, reassurance that most headaches in pregnancy are benign is appropriate. Keeping a headache diary with food consumed in the 24-hour period preceding the onset of a migraine can help determine food triggers. Exercise such as 30 minutes of brisk walking has been found effective in reducing headache (Bendtsen, 2015).

Individuals with sinus headache or additional symptoms of pharyngitis or fever will need further evaluation for appropriate pharmacological treatment. Specialty care should be sought for severe headache that does not respond to comfort measures and analgesia, new onset headache with neurological symptoms, headache with sudden onset that is severe (see Chapter 53, *Neurologic Disorders*), or if the headache is accompanied by an increase in blood pressure, proteinuria, or papilledema (see Chapter 36, *Hypertensive Disorders of Pregnancy*).

Relief and prevention measures for headache in pregnancy

Massage the head, neck, and back.
Get acupuncture therapy.
Use warm compress at the base of the head, neck, and forehead.
Relaxation exercises are helpful.
Increase rest.
Get regular exercise, such as walking.
Avoid environmental headache triggers (smoke, strong fragrances, skipping meals, stress, glaring lights, and excessive heat or cold).
Avoid food headache triggers (nitrates found in bacon, hot dogs, sulfites found in dried fruits and used as a preservative in packaged salads, artificial sweeteners, chocolate, and aged cheeses).

Heartburn

Heartburn, also called **gastroesophageal reflux** disease (GERD), is very common during pregnancy. Heartburn occurs when digested food from the stomach is pushed upward into the esophagus, causing a burning sensation that starts in the stomach and seems to rise into the lower throat. This feeling can range from mildly uncomfortable to extremely debilitating. Heartburn is estimated to occur in 30–50% of pregnancies and up to 80% occur during the third trimester (Thélin & Richter, 2020).

Two of the key factors most responsible for heartburn are pregnancy hormones and uterine growth. First, increased levels of estrogen and progesterone in pregnancy cause the lower esophageal sphincter (LES) to relax, which allows acid from the stomach to flow back up, causing burning and pain. In the second and third trimesters, LES pressure that keeps the esophagus closed gradually falls to approximately 30–50% of baseline values, reaching a nadir at 36 weeks of gestation (VanThiel et al., 1977). Second, as the uterus grows, it crowds the stomach and intestines, which causes the stomach and acid to back up into the esophagus. Contributors to heartburn are greasy or fatty foods, coffee and other drinks containing caffeine, onion, garlic or spicy foods, certain medications, overfilling the stomach, eating too quickly, and lying down after eating.

Individuals developing HELLP syndrome can report epigastric pain due to liver involvement that mimics heartburn. Common heartburn relief measures are not effective in these cases, which helps to differentiate.

Assessment

Subjective Data Gathering

The clinician should assess onset, description of symptoms, severity, frequency, associated symptoms, foods associated with heartburn, and relief measures used and their effectiveness.

Objective Data Gathering

Obtain blood pressure and palpate the abdomen as indicated by accompanying symptoms.

Relief and Preventative Measures

A stepwise approach should be followed, starting with the reassurance of normalcy in pregnancy. The clinician should then recommend lifestyle and dietary modifications to help alleviate heartburn during pregnancy (Quach et al., 2021).

Heartburn preventative measures

Encourage smaller meals. Eat five to six meals to facilitate digestion avoid overloading the stomach at one time.

Avoid drinking large amounts of fluids with meals; drink fluids between meals instead.

Avoid spicy, greasy, and fatty foods. Fats delay gastric emptying.

Choose low-fat or skim milk.

Avoid a large meal before bedtime.

Increase the length of time between the last meal of the day and bedtime.

Avoid caffeine.

Avoid lying down right after eating.

Gain appropriate pregnancy weight for body mass index (BMI). Excess weight exerts extra pressure on the abdomen, increasing potential for heartburn.

Wear nonrestrictive clothing around the abdomen.

Elevate the upper body on pillows when lying down.

For individuals who do not respond adequately to lifestyle modifications, the next step in the stepwise approach is generally antacids. Antacids containing magnesium hydroxide or magnesium trisilicate (Maalox, Mylanta) or sucralfate 1 g (a local cytoprotective agent) are commonly used in pregnancy to effectively treat heartburn. Antacids with sodium carbonate like Alka-Seltzer are avoided as they can cause maternal or fetal metabolic alkalosis. Antacids should not be taken with iron supplements or prenatal vitamins with iron because gastric acid facilitates iron absorption.

If symptoms persist, histamine 2-receptor antagonists comprise the next step. Medications in this category, including famotidine (Pepcid), are effective in treating heartburn and generally considered to be safe during pregnancy. As of 2021, one medication in this class, ranitidine (Zantac), is off the market due to Food and Drug Administration (FDA) concerns over impurities.

For pregnant individuals whose symptoms do not respond to other remedies, proton pump inhibitors (PPIs) comprise the next step in the stepwise approach. PPIs suppress the secretion of gastric acid and the class includes medications such as omeprazole (Prilosec) and esomeprazole (Nexium). Data concerning the safety of PPIs during pregnancy are limited, although there are some indications of an increased risk of congenital malformations associated with PPI use (Li et al., 2020).

Clinicians should advise clients to report the following:

- Heartburn that returns as soon as the medication wears off
- Heartburn that disrupts sleep
- Difficulty swallowing
- Weight loss
- Spitting up blood
- Black stools

Serious reflux complications are uncommon in pregnancy. Individuals who have evidence of GI bleeding or significant dysphagia require further evaluation for pharmacological or medical treatment.

Heart Palpitations

Pregnant individuals may report occasional heart palpitations. Heart palpitations can be perceived as a fluttering, a "flip-flop" feeling, an extra heartbeat, or a pause in the regular heartbeat, followed by rapid palpitations. Although this sensation can feel quite concerning to the pregnant individual, it is usually normal. Normal palpitations during pregnancy are related to the increase in blood volume and heart rate, which can stimulate ion channels in the cardiac walls (Wilson et al., 2018). Palpitations or ectopic beats are most commonly seen between 28 and 32 weeks of gestation, when the heart stroke volume peaks (Adamson & Nelson-Piercy, 2007). Sinus tachycardia is seen in the third trimester due to the physiologic increase in heart rate. Nonpathological ectopic beats or nonsustained arrhythmias are seen in the majority of pregnant individuals who undergo electrocardiogram for a report of palpitations (Adamson & Nelson-Piercy, 2007).

Assessment

Subjective Data Gathering

The onset, nature, and characteristics of symptom, precipitating events, associated symptoms, caffeine intake, medication history, and prior history of anxiety or depressive disorders and cardiac disease are assessed.

Objective Data Gathering

The clinician should note the individual's general affect, assess vital signs, and auscultate heart sounds.

Relief and Preventative Measures

Explanation of the physiologic basis and reassurance of normalcy is the most appropriate course of action. If the perception of palpitations is accompanied by dizziness, shortness of breath, or a history of cardiac problems, it is appropriate to facilitate an immediate evaluation by an obstetric or cardiac consultant.

Hemorrhoids

Hemorrhoids are swollen blood vessels in the lower rectum. They are clusters of vascular tissue and connective tissue beneath the normal epithelium of the anal canal that swell and often lead to itching, burning, and bleeding with the passage of stool. The incidence of hemorrhoids in pregnancy is not known; however, it is higher in pregnant individuals than in nonpregnant individuals and more commonly seen in the third trimester. Etiologies in pregnancy include decreased venous return, pressure of the enlarging uterus, increased progesterone causing decreased GI motility, and increased Valsalva pressure during defecation (Shirah et al., 2018). Symptoms include mild to severe pruritus, protrusion of vein through the anus, and rectal bleeding. Most hemorrhoids resolve spontaneously or with conservative medical therapy alone. However, complications can include thrombosis, secondary infection, ulceration, abscess, and fecal incontinence.

Assessment

Subjective Data Gathering

Evaluation consists of the quantity, color, amount, and timing of any rectal bleeding, usual diet, elimination habits, description of stool consistency, and prior history of constipation or inflammatory bowel disease.

Objective Data Gathering

A visual inspection of the rectum and a rectal digital exam are done if indicated.

Relief and Preventative Measures

First-line therapies are conservative measures to treat constipation and facilitate easier passage of stool with less strain. These include increased dietary fiber and the use of bulk and osmotic laxatives as needed (see the section, *Constipation*).

Relief measures for hemorrhoids in pregnancy

Increase dietary fiber.
Avoid prolonged toilet sitting.
Practice proper anal cleansing after bowel movement.
Use OTC pain relief preparations after bowel movement as directed (Preparation H or Anusol).
Use topical hydrocortisone cream or rectal suppositories as directed.
Do Kegel exercise to promote pelvic blood flow and muscle tone.
Use a warm-water Sitz bath.

If conservative measures provide no relief, further evaluation for possible hemorrhoid band ligation or injection sclerotherapy may be needed.

Increased Warmth and Perspiration

The increased blood flow through the skin during pregnancy makes most pregnant people feel warmer than usual. Blood volume starts to increase at about 6 weeks, and, by about 32 weeks, it can be as much as 50% more than what it would normally be. This increased blood flow combines with the relaxing effects of progesterone on cell walls to increase capillary vasodilatation. The basal metabolic rate during pregnancy increases by about 20%, contributing to higher body and skin temperature. Eccrine and sebaceous gland activity increases during pregnancy causing increased perspiration and other skin changes (Motosko et al., 2017). An explanation of the physiologic basis and simple measures can help individuals cope with this symptom.

Relief measures for increased warmth and perspiration

Wear light or layered clothing.
Ensure adequate hydration.
Lower the environmental temperature when possible.
Bathe or shower as often as needed for comfort.

Leukorrhea

Leukorrhea is the term used for the nonirritating vaginal discharge that starts in the first trimester of pregnancy. This is caused by the increase in pelvic blood flow. The secretions are clear to white in color, have a mild inoffensive odor, and can be thin and watery or more viscous. Estrogen causes the secretions to be more acidic in pregnancy, thereby providing some protection against infections.

Assessment

Subjective Data Gathering

The onset, nature, and characteristics of discharge, associated symptoms, sexual history, and condom use are evaluated.

Objective Data Gathering

If indicated by symptom presentation, a speculum exam and wet prep or point-of-care test for vaginitis may be done.

Relief and Preventative Measures

An explanation of the physiologic basis for the increase in vaginal discharge should be provided. Once the possibility of a sexually transmitted infection or vaginitis has been ruled out, clients can be advised that this is not a sign of infection, to avoid self-treatment with OTC medications, and to avoid douching. Other advice includes wearing absorbent cotton underwear, changing underwear several times daily, practicing daily perineal hygiene, and using unscented panty liners as desired. Vaginal discharge accompanied by itching, foul odor, or pain requires further evaluation for appropriate treatment.

Leg Cramps

Cramping of the calf and/or foot muscles is common in pregnancy. These cramps often occur at night after a period of inactivity and are more common during the second and third trimesters. The exact cause of leg cramps during pregnancy is unknown. One theory suggests a connection between leg cramps and the build-up of lactic and pyruvic acids (by-products of metabolizing dietary sugars and starches) that occurs as a result of impaired blood flow in the legs in pregnancy.

Assessment

Subjective Data Gathering

The onset, description of symptoms, occupational and ADL history, exercise patterns, relief measures used, and their efficacy are evaluated.

Objective Data Gathering

A visual inspection of the area is done along with palpation of lower extremities for edema, varicosities, and injury as indicated.

Relief and Preventative Measures

When a leg cramp strikes, standing up and stretching the affected leg and dorsiflexing the foot can ease the cramp (Figure 15.2). Reassurance should be provided that leg cramps are normal in pregnancy.

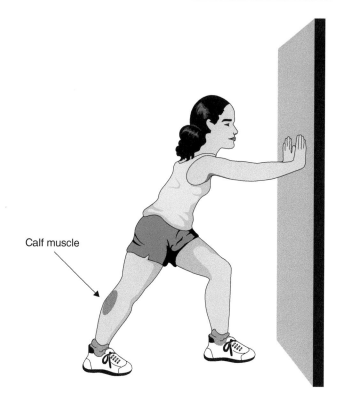

Figure 15.2   Stretching calf muscles to prevent leg cramps.

Methods to prevent pregnancy leg cramps

Exercise like walking promotes circulation of metabolic by-products that can cause cramping and keeps leg muscles stretched and pliant.
Drinking adequate fluids avoids dehydration.
Stretching the calf muscles before bed can help reduce legs cramps (Figure 15.2).
Avoid sitting or standing for prolonged periods of time.
Bathing in warm water before bed can relax leg muscles.

Theoretical physiologic explanations for prenatal leg cramps include low levels of vitamin B and disturbances in calcium–phosphorus–magnesium balance. Current research does not support the efficacy of magnesium supplements in reducing leg cramps (Araújo et al., 2020; Garrison et al., 2020).

Nasal Congestion

Pregnancy-induced or gestational rhinitis is clinically defined as nasal congestion in the last six weeks of pregnancy in the absence of allergy or infection that resolves within two weeks postpartum. Estrogen and placental growth hormone-induced nasal hyperemia are considered primary etiologies. The increased swelling and blood flow exert additional pressure on nasal mucosa, causing nasal congestion and predisposing the vessels to more easily erupt and bleed.

This pregnancy discomfort is experienced by approximately 20–30% of pregnant individuals and is higher in smokers and those exposed to secondhand smoke (Ridolo et al., 2016). Symptoms of pregnancy-induced rhinitis include persistent nasal congestion, possibly accompanied by clear nasal secretion, postnasal drip with no additional symptoms of a cold or seasonal allergy. Significant or prolonged nasal congestion can reduce sleep quality and increase snoring and the risk of sleep apnea (Kar, et al., 2021).

Pregnancy-induced rhinitis should be differentiated from allergic rhinitis, which manifests prior to pregnancy. Approximately one-third of clients with allergic rhinitis report an improvement in symptoms during pregnancy, with an equal number reporting either no change or worsening of symptoms (Carroll et al., 2019). Symptoms suggestive of allergic rhinitis or bacterial infection include cough, green nasal discharge, sinus headache, and pain and warrant additional evaluation and treatment. While pregnancy-induced rhinitis itself does not alter the course of pregnancy, it can cause snoring and mouth breathing, creating significant sleep disturbance with the associated potential for increased pregnancy complications.

Assessment

Subjective Data Gathering

The onset, nature, characteristics of symptom, signs and symptoms of upper respiratory infection, and the methods used for relief and efficacy are queried. History of smoking, allergies, and allergenic exposures is obtained.

Objective Data Gathering

Palpation of nasal sinuses and lymph nodes, inspection of nares as indicated, noting the presence of secretions, noting respirations, and auscultation and percussion of lung fields may be done.

Relief and Preventative Measures

An explanation of the physiologic basis for this symptom and the reassurance of its normalcy and transient nature should be provided. There is a lack of high-quality research on effective interventions for pregnancy-induced rhinitis (Lal et al., 2016).

Relief of nasal congestion of pregnancy

Increase room humidification.
Saline nasal drops, spray, gel, or irrigation can lubricate nasal passages.
Drinking hot beverages can liquefy secretions and provide temporary symptomatic relief.
Use temporary cotton nostril tamponade.
Use steam inhalation to liquefy secretions.
Sleep with head of the bed slightly elevated.
Avoid potential allergens and nasal irritants such as cigarette smoke.
Avoid medicated OTC nasal sprays.

While nasal spray decongestants can be immediately effective, pregnant clients should be advised to avoid the use of OTC nasal decongestant sprays or cold remedies as the rebound congestion that occurs once these are discontinued is often more severe than the original congestion. This often prompts an increase in dose in an effort to obtain relief, thereby entering a cycle of rebound congestion and higher dosing. For severe pregnancy-induced rhinitis, oral decongestants, such as chlorpheniramine, diphenhydramine, or pseudoephedrine, can be considered in normotensive individuals after the first trimester (Narayan, 2019). Corticosteroid nasal sprays have not been shown to be effective in pregnancy-induced rhinitis (Dubey, 2021). Symptoms suggestive of allergic rhinitis or bacterial infection such as cough, green nasal discharge, sinus headache, and pain warrant additional evaluation and treatment.

Nausea and Vomiting of Pregnancy

Nausea and vomiting of pregnancy (NVP) are common with a prevalence of 50–80% for nausea and 50% for vomiting (American College of Obstetricians and Gynecologists [ACOG] 2018). The etiology of NVP is attributed to endocrine factors such as human chorionic gonadotropin and estrogen. Increased levels of progesterone causing delayed gastric emptying also contribute to NVP. The presence of *Helicobacter pylori* has been implicated as an independent etiology of pregnancy vomiting (Grooten et al., 2017). Those with a personal history of nausea associated with motion, seasickness, migraine, contraceptives, and anesthesia, as well as those who have a family history of NVP, may be more susceptible (Laitinen et al., 2020). Symptoms vary widely from one individual to the next and from one pregnancy to the next. NVP

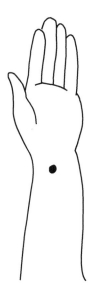

Figure 15.3 P6 acupressure point for relief of nausea. Located three fingerbreadths from the wrist.

typically starts around the sixth week of gestation, peaks at 9–11 weeks of gestation, and tends to subside by 12–14 weeks of gestation. It is resolved by 20 weeks of gestation for most individuals.

The term *morning sickness* can be misleading, as symptoms often occur throughout the day. Studies indicate that individuals who experience NVP suffer fewer miscarriages than those who do not have NVP (ACOG, 2018). Individuals with NVP also have lower rates of PTB and low birth weight, infants with congenital anomaly, and stillbirth (Koren et al., 2014). These positive outcomes can be reassuring and provide a positive perspective on this unpleasant symptom, although the reason for this association is unknown.

While nausea and vomiting are common early pregnancy symptoms, they may cause significant dehydration and contribute to poor nutrition. Additionally, even those who do not experience severe physiologic effects may have significant psychosocial consequences, including stress, anxiety, depression, fear that their symptoms might harm their baby, loss of time at work, and negative impact on relationships (Kramer et al., 2013). Important decision-making for the prenatal care provider includes when to escalate nonpharmacologic comfort measures to pharmacologic, and when to make the diagnosis of the pathologic hyperemesis gravidarum (see Chapter 40, *Hyperemesis Gravidarum*).

Assessment

Subjective Data Gathering

Evaluation begins with determining the onset, frequency, symptom characteristics, precipitating and aggravating factors, ability to carry out ADL and work activities, appetite, ability to keep food and liquids down, and relief measures tried and efficacy. Assessing the severity of NVP can be done by a relatively simple method known as the Pregnancy-Unique Quantification of Emesis (PUQE) scale (Table 15.3). This validated scale, in use since

Table 15.3   PUQE Scale

Pregnancy-Unique Quantification of Emesis and Nausea (PUQE) scoring system					
How many hours in the past 24 hours had you felt nauseated/sick to stomach?	Not at all (1)	1 hour or less (2)	2–3 hours (3)	4–6 hours (4)	more than 6 hours (5)
How many times in the past 24 hours did you vomit?	7 or more (5)	5–6 (4)	3–4 (3)	1–2 (2)	None (1)
How many times in the past 24 hours did you experience gagging, retching, or dry heaves?	None (1)	1–2 (2)	3–4 (3)	5–6 (4)	7 or more (5)

PUQE score: _____

How many hours have you slept out of 24 hours? Why? _____

On a scale of 0–10, how would you rate your well-being? 0 (worst possible) 10 (the best you felt before pregnancy) _____

Can you tell me what causes you to feel that way? _____

Source: From Ebrahimi et al. (2009)/With permission of Journal of Obstetrics and Gynaecology Canada.
The total score is the sum of points, noted in parentheses, awarded to each of the three questions. Nausea score: mild NVP = ≤6; moderate NVP = 7–12; severe NVP ≥ 13.

approximately 2002, allows prenatal care providers to efficiently evaluate NVP severity to aid in determining appropriate intervention (Koren & Cohen 2021).

While most reports of NVP are found to be within normal limits, it is appropriate to gather subjective information and to observe pertinent physical features, such as weight and skin turgor, to make sure that the clinical presentation has not crossed the line to pathology. Though this is an uncommon condition, 1–2% of pregnant individuals experience hyperemesis. Pertinent questions such as presence of **ptyalism**, frequency of vomiting, ability to function normally in daily routines as well as physical symptoms of dehydration, weight loss, and ketosis are important pieces of data gathering to initially decide if the individual is still within the realm of normal or not.

Objective Data Gathering

The clinician should obtain the individual's weight and note any change from baseline. Additionally, assess general appearance, skin turgor, mucosa, presence of ketonuria, presence of ptyalism, and signs of dehydration.

Relief and Preventative Measures

Prevention of NVP is the ideal goal. Several studies have found that those who are taking a prenatal vitamin at the time of conception experience less NVP, possibly due to adequate vitamin B stores (ACOG, 2018). For normal NVP that has minimal to moderate interference on ADL, relief measures should be instituted from least to most systemic. Clinicians should ensure that all individuals with NVP are aware of lifestyle and OTC measures so they can try various methods. What is effective varies from one person to the next and from one pregnancy to the next. Lifestyle and OTC measures are often enough to provide adequate relief. Table 15.4 describes NVP relief measures.

Although many of the dietary and lifestyle interventions have not been supported with clinical trials, they have significant anecdotal support and are unlikely to cause harm. OTC remedies are used for individuals who do not find relief with simple lifestyle and diet measures and for those presenting with moderate NVP. Ginger is effective in reducing nausea in some individuals but is less effective at reducing vomiting (ACOG, 2018). Ginger has not been associated with any adverse maternal or fetal outcomes (Ee et al., 2021). Typical dosage is 250 mg of ginger four times daily (ACOG, 2018). Acupressure at pressure point P6 (see Figure 15.3) has been shown to be successful in reducing NVP symptoms in some trials (National Institute for Health and Care Excellence [NICE] 2021; Solt Kirca & Kanza Gul, 2020).

Prescription pharmacologic measures are considered for individuals who report continuous, more severe, or disabling NVP. Doxylamine succinate/pyridoxine is commonly used as a first-line medication for NVP. Doxylamine is an H1 receptor agonist and is considered compatible with pregnancy, indicating that experience with human pregnancy has demonstrated very low or nonexistent embryo/fetal risk (Briggs et al., 2017). The initial starting dose is two tablets at bedtime and can be titrated up or down as needed. Because the primary potential side effects are somnolence and drowsiness, individuals should avoid activities such as driving until they know how they will react to the medication.

Clinicians should provide education about the physiology and the time-limited nature of NVP, and to eat whatever they can during the duration of this symptom. Instruction should be provided on reporting signs and symptoms of dehydration, unrelieved NVP, or inability to keep any food down for >24 hours. Medical consultation, intravenous (IV) fluid rehydration, and possible hospitalization are warranted in the case of severe and unrelenting NVP.

Ptyalism

Ptyalism is the excess secretion of saliva in the mouth. It is an unusual pregnancy discomfort and is more frequent in

Table 15.4 Relief Measures for Nausea and Vomiting of Pregnancy

Lifestyle measures	Rationale
Small frequent meals every 2–3 hours	Nausea may be worse with empty stomach
Increase periods of rest	NVP worse with fatigue
Sip clear carbonated or sour liquids	Reduces saliva, maintains hydration if taste of plain water is objectionable
Separate ingesting liquids from solid foods	Avoids expanding the stomach
Sip small amounts of fluids through the day	Avoids expanding the stomach, maintains hydration
Change prenatal vitamin to folic acid only until nausea resolves	Iron increases nausea
Suck on popsicles throughout the day	Cold food may be better tolerated, aids hydration
Decrease dietary fat	Fat is digested more slowly
Avoid strong-smelling foods and smoke	Can be a nausea trigger
Avoid highly spiced foods	Reduces gastric secretions
Increase intake of high-protein foods	Reduces gastric secretions
Increase intake of bland foods	Reduces gastric secretions
Eat something right before bed and upon rising	Nausea may be worse with empty stomach
Brush teeth between meals, not right after	Can be a nausea trigger, can induce gagging
Eat whatever seems appealing	A short-term nutrient imbalance is not harmful, keeping down some calories is the goal

Over-the-counter remedies	Administration	Comments
Acupressure at P6 of the Neiguan point	Seabands or self-administer	More effective for nausea See Figure 15.3—for P6 acupressure point
Ginger 1 g via capsule, tea, candy, soda	250 mg QID; ½ tsp grated rhizome in 1 cup tea X4; 1 × 1 in. pieces crystallized ginger × 2	Various forms to try; up to 1 g daily
Vitamin B_6 supplement	10–25 mg TID or QID; 50 mg BID	More effective for nausea
Vitamin B_6 plus doxylamine	10 mg vitamin B_6 and Unisom tablet (equals 12.5 mg doxylamine) 2 doses at bedtime and 1 dose morning and afternoon as needed **or** 20 mg vitamin B_6 and 1 Unisom tablet (equals 25 mg doxylamine) 1 dose at bedtime and 1 dose in the morning as needed	Significant nausea and vomiting relief. Safety is well established. No adverse fetal effects Initiate doxylamine at hs

Pharmacological measures	Administration	Comments
Initial pharmacologic options:		
• Doxylamine succinate and pyridoxine hydrochloride (Diclegis)	2 tablets at bedtime	Considered compatible with pregnancy; can cause drowsiness
If persistent symptoms, add one of the following:		
• Diphenhydramine (Benadryl)	25–50 mg po q4–6h	Considered compatible with pregnancy; can cause significant drowsiness
• Dimenhydrinate (Dramamine)	25–50 mg po q4–6h	Considered compatible with pregnancy
• Prochlorperazine (Compazine)	25 mg rectally q12h	Considered compatible with pregnancy; can cause significant drowsiness
• Promethazine (Phenergan)	12.5–25 mg po or per rectum q4–6	Considered compatible with pregnancy; can cause significant drowsiness
If symptoms persist after adding one of the above, consider the following:		
• Metoclopramide (Reglan)	5–10 mg q6–8h po or IM	Considered compatible with pregnancy
• Promethazine (Phenergan)	12.5–25 mg IM q4–6	Considered compatible with pregnancy; can cause significant drowsiness
• Ondansetron (Zofran)	4 mg po q8h	Briggs pregnancy recommendation: human data suggest risk; recent analyses are more reassuring that ondansetron is not associated with increased risks of malformations and embryonic/fetal loss

Source: Adapted from ACOG (2018), Briggs et al. (2017), Sakran et al. (2021), Dormuth et al. (2021), and Sun et al. (2021).

individuals with significant nausea with or without vomiting, particularly those diagnosed with hyperemesis of pregnancy. For individuals experiencing ptyalism associated with normal NVP, it tends to subside by 12–14 weeks of gestation. The etiology is unknown; however, it is theorized that it may be a combination of decreased swallowing in individuals with NVP, an increase in saliva production, and pregnancy hormonal influences.

Presenting symptoms may be a report of excessive saliva that is bitter tasting and/or extreme difficulty in swallowing the saliva. Patients may report that attempts to swallow their saliva prompt gagging and retching (Mchenga, 2021). The volume of saliva may be large, up to two liters per day (Bronshtein et al., 2018). Individuals with ptyalism will often carry tissues or a cup with them to spit into and report a decrease in appetite and food intake. Ptyalism can be a significant symptom as sleep is disturbed and work activities and social encounters are negatively affected.

Assessment

Subjective Data Gathering

This consists of the onset, description of the amount, and characteristics of saliva, and the presence of associated symptoms such as nausea.

Objective Data Gathering

An inspection of the oral cavity, observation of wiping the mouth frequently, and evaluation for signs and symptoms of dehydration may be done.

Relief and Preventative Measures

Relief measures for nausea and vomiting can also relieve ptyalism for some individuals, although relief measures for ptyalism are often unsuccessful (Suzuki et al., 2009). Ptyalism in pregnancy can cause psychological distress and interfere with normal daily activities. Unrelenting ptyalism may lead to dehydration and require further evaluation for care.

Comfort measures for ptyalism

Carry a spitting cup.
Place a towel under the face at night or while resting.
Lay in a side-lying position to facilitate flow of saliva.
Use soft flannel cloths to wipe the mouth to reduce skin chafing.
Rinse with mouthwash frequently to reduce the bitter taste.
Sour candies may improve the ability to swallow.

Restless Leg Syndrome

Restless leg syndrome (RLS) is a neurological and sensory motor disorder characterized by a strong urge to move the legs and typically occurs during the night during periods of inactivity. The prevalence of prenatal RLS is approximately two to three times higher than in the general population and thought to be related to hormonal changes and iron and folate status (Gupta et al., 2021; Srivanitchapoom et al., 2014). It is estimated that approximately one-third of pregnant people experience RLS, though it is widely considered to be underdiagnosed (Dunietz et al., 2017; Gupta et al., 2021). RLS is more common in the third trimester and is a major contributor to poor sleep quality and poor daytime functioning, which introduces risk for adverse perinatal outcome (see *Sleep Disturbances* section). Risk factors for RLS include a history of growing pains during childhood, a family history of RLS, multiparity, lack of exercise, and anemia in pregnancy (Dunietz et al., 2017; International Restless Leg Study Group, 2015). The majority of RLS diagnosed in pregnancy will be related to the pregnancy itself or to anemia. Depression is often a comorbid condition with RLS, and the administration of a depression inventory can be considered.

Assessment

Subjective Data Gathering

Diagnosis is made via four criteria experienced with RLS (Table 15.5). Clients will often use the words *creeping, itching, crawling, or gnawing* to refer to the sensation of RLS. Symptoms can range from mild to severe. Additional history includes onset, description of symptoms, symptoms prior to pregnancy, history of anemia, typical sleep patterns, history of insomnia, occupational and ADL history, and exercise patterns. Medication history

Table 15.5 RLS Diagnostic Criteria

Diagnostic criteria for RLS
These five features must be present for a diagnosis of restless legs syndrome:
1. There is an urge to move the legs, usually accompanied by or caused by uncomfortable and unpleasant sensations in the legs.
2. The urge to move the legs and any accompanying unpleasant sensations begin or worsen during periods of rest or inactivity such as lying or sitting.
3. The urge to move the legs and any accompanying unpleasant sensations are partially or totally relieved by movement, such as walking or stretching, at least as long as the activity continues.
4. The urge to move the legs and any accompanying or unpleasant sensations are worse in the evening or night than during the day or only occur in the evening or night.
5. The urge to move the legs and any accompanying unpleasant sensations are not solely accounted for by another condition, such as leg cramps, positional discomfort, leg swelling, or arthritis.

Source: Adapted from International Restless Leg Study Group. http://irlssg.org/diagnostic-criteria/

should be obtained. The General Sleep Disturbance Scale (GSDS) can be used to evaluate sleep quality and has been validated for use in pregnancy (Dunietz et al., 2017).

Objective Data Gathering

An inspection of the legs for lesions or varicosities is done, and a CBC with serum ferritin obtained as indicated.

Relief and Preventative Measures

Once RLS has been diagnosed, nonpharmaceutical measures should be tried first. For those with mild RLS, an explanation of the physiologic basis, sleep hygiene strategies, and reassurance may be adequate. One study noted improvement in RLS symptoms after using cold water immersion of the legs prior to sleep (Jafarimanesh et al., 2020). The treatment of anemia decreases the symptoms of RLS. Pregnant people diagnosed with RLS with serum ferritin levels <75 mcg/L are candidates for iron supplementation (Picchietti et al., 2015). Dopamine antagonists such as Benadryl, Reglan, and serotonergic antidepressants such as citalopram, escitalopram, and sertraline can make RLS worse and should be avoided. Avoiding RLS triggers, such as prolonged inactivity, caffeine, and alcohol, can reduce symptoms.

Relief measures for RLS in pregnancy

Treat underlying anemia.
Moderate intensity exercise such as aerobics.
Perform yoga positions that stretch the legs.
Massage legs if no varicosities are present.
Adequate sleep hygiene.
Discontinue strenuous activities after 4 p.m.
Eliminate caffeine-containing products.
Cold water immersion of the legs prior to bed.

There are no FDA-approved drugs to treat RLS during pregnancy. Gabapentin has been shown to be effective, although there is no consensus for use in pregnancy as the safety data is sparse. If gabapentin is used, folic acid supplementation must be given concurrently, as gabapentin depletes folate. Opioids such as oxycodone and tramadol are effective, currently have the best safety record for the treatment, and are reserved to limited use for individuals with severe, refractory RLS during pregnancy (Picchietti et al., 2015). If medication is prescribed, the lowest dose for the shortest duration should be used. Medical consultation for severe RLS requiring off-label use of these medications is appropriate.

Reassurance that there is often a marked decrease in RLS postpartum should be provided. Individuals who experience RLS during pregnancy have an increased risk of RLS in future pregnancies and for developing a form of RLS later in life (Prosperetti & Manconi, 2015).

Round Ligament Pain

This pregnancy symptom is commonly experienced in the late first trimester into the second trimester. The round ligaments suspend the uterus within the body. As the uterus expands in size and increases in weight, these ligaments are stretched like rubber bands. Nerve fibers that run next to the ligaments stretch along with them and can cause pain. This stretching can also produce a spasm of the round ligament that can result in sharp and sudden pain. Common symptoms are shooting pain after a sudden movement or sharp, knife-like pain in the lower abdomen or on one side, typically the right side, extending into the groin area. It can last a few seconds to a several minutes. Round ligament pain is often brought on by sudden movement, such as rising from a seated position or arising from bed first thing in the morning. Sometimes, turning over in bed can cause round ligament pain to awaken the individual during the night. Round ligament pain can be quite uncomfortable and worrisome, though it is benign (Figure 15.4).

Assessment

Subjective Data Gathering

The clinician should evaluate the onset, location of pain, presence of other associated symptoms, and relief measures used and effectiveness of each strategy.

Objective Data Gathering

The clinician should palpate the abdomen for tenderness, rebound tenderness, or masses, and should perform a pelvic examination to rule out ectopic pregnancy or preterm labor as indicated.

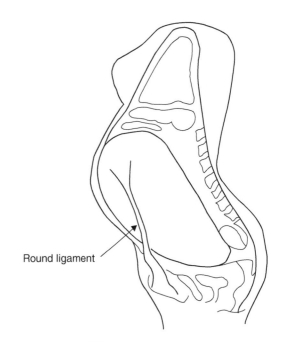

Figure 15.4   Round ligaments.

Relief and Preventative Measures

An explanation of the physiology of round ligament pain using a uterus model and reassurance of normalcy can facilitate understanding and coping with the pain. Clinicians should share methods to prevent and relieve round ligament pain.

Methods to prevent and relieve round ligament pain

Avoid sudden movement from sitting to standing.
Arise slowly from bed in the morning.
Support the uterus with a pillow under the abdomen and between the knees when side lying.
Wear an abdominal support garment or sling.
Apply a warm compress to the area.
During an episode of round ligament pain, sitting and flexing the knees to the abdomen shortens the ligaments and can provide relief, as can bending sideways toward the side that is painful.

Round ligament pain can mimic symptoms of ectopic pregnancy, preterm labor, threatened abortion, and appendicitis. Abdominal hernias and round ligament varicosities can occur in pregnancy. Careful history and additional exam will differentiate pathology from normal round ligament pain. Further evaluation should be done for those with increasing and unrelieved pain or additional symptoms indicative of possible pathology.

Shortness of Breath

Feeling short of breath is a common pregnancy discomfort of the first and third trimesters. The increase in progesterone starting in the first trimester causes an increase in respiratory capacity, tidal volume, and respiratory rate. This can result in feeling short of breath. In the late third trimester, the uterus compresses the diaphragm, mechanically decreasing capacity of the lungs to fully expand. This can increase shallow breathing, leading to a sensation of being short of breath. Once the fetus engages into the pelvis in late third trimester, the sensation of shortness of breath often decreases. Although lung function is more efficient during pregnancy, the sensation of feeling short of breath can escalate to a feeling of panic for some individuals.

Assessment

Subjective Data Gathering

The onset, nature and characteristics, predisposing or aggravating factors, and history of asthma or other respiratory illness are evaluated.

Objective Data Gathering

Observation of respirations at rest should be done, vital signs taken, and auscultation and percussion of the lung fields done as indicated by additional symptoms.

Relief and Preventative Measures

Reassurance that this is normal with explanation of physiologic basis goes a long way to coping with this sensation. Relief strategies include measures to expand lung capacity, such as good posture, lifting the arms over the head when shortness of breath occurs, and sleeping in a more upright position with pillow support.

Warning signs accompanying a feeling of shortness of breath include tachypnea, constant coughing, heart palpitations, chest pain, fever or chills, and faintness or dizziness. Pregnant people with obesity and those with asthma may experience heightened shortness of breath and need further assessment when presenting with this symptom.

Skin, Hair, and Nail Changes

Skin changes are nearly universal during pregnancy. Physiologic skin changes are numerous and include hypermelanosis or darkening of the skin, changes in the color of moles or nevi, development of spider angioma, and the appearance of striae. The increased production of estrogen, human placental growth factors, and melanin during pregnancy is primarily responsible for most changes. Many of the changes in the integumentary system start in the second trimester and progress in the third trimester. Skin changes in pregnancy that may indicate underlying pathology are covered in Chapter 54, *Dermatologic Disorders*.

Hyperpigmentation

Generalized hyperpigmentation can occur, but, more commonly, there is an accentuation of normally darker areas of skin. Increased pigmentation more significantly affects individuals with dark hair and skin due to a higher baseline level of melanin, compared with individuals with light hair and skin (Bieber et al., 2017). The anatomical areas most impacted include the areola, nipples, and genitalia. The axilla, inner thighs, and periumbilical areas also have a higher incidence of involvement. Freckles and scars may become darker. These pigmentation changes generally begin early in pregnancy and increase as the pregnancy advances. Even though hyperpigmentation tends to decrease after birth, the nipples, areola, and genital areas do not usually return to their prepregnant pigmentation (Nussbaum & Benedetto, 2006). Pregnant individuals with darker skin can have pigmentary demarcation lines on the outer, posterior portion of their legs and upper arms or darkening of vulvar skin (Tyler, 2015).

Melasma, also known as the mask of pregnancy or chloasma, is estimated to affect up to 70% of pregnant individuals to some degree, with individuals with darker skin experiencing higher rates (Motosko et al., 2017). A genetic component, along with rising levels of hormones, contributes to this condition. Melasma presents as uneven tan or brownish patches of darker skin on the forehead, temples, and cheeks. Melasma gradually fades and clears spontaneously over time after giving birth, though it is likely to recur in subsequent pregnancies.

Linea nigra begins to appear in the second trimester as a thin vertical line that extends from the umbilicus to the suprapubic area. The line gradually fades and disappears within a few months after giving birth.

Pigmented nevi or moles are growths on the skin that usually are flesh-colored, brown, or black. Nevi color changes are not common during pregnancy although some nevi can widen if they are on skin that stretches such as the abdomen or breasts (Motosko et al., 2017). Malignant melanoma has been reported to be the most common malignancy during pregnancy (Friedman et al. 2019); thus, changes in established mole size or color during pregnancy require evaluation by biopsy.

Breast skin changes are seen on the areola with the development of a line of pigmentation surrounding the areola. This is called the secondary areola and is less dark in color with its border merging with the surrounding skin. Small, oil-producing glands called Montgomery's tubercles become prominent around the edges of the areola. They make a protective secretion that keeps the nipple and areola supple and moist during breastfeeding.

Striae gravidarum develops on the abdomen, hips, thighs, and/or breasts in approximately 55–90% of pregnant individuals (Farahnik et al., 2017). Onset is usually in the mid to late second trimester and presents as pink and red lines with a shiny appearance (Figure 15.5). They may become raised, redder, and longer as pregnancy progresses.

The cause of striae gravidarum remains unknown, but a combination of genetics, the mechanical stretching of the skin, and hormonal factors are likely involved. Striae form due to structural connective tissue and collagen fiber changes. Lower levels of serum relaxin, which decreases the elasticity of connective tissues, are associated with a higher occurrence of striae gravidarum (Lurie

et al., 2011). Although striae gravidarum tends to occur in body areas experiencing extreme skin stretching, there is no correlation between degree of striae formation and extent of body enlargement in pregnancy, which supports hormonal involvement as an etiology. Individuals who develop stretch marks on their breasts are more likely to develop them elsewhere. The presence of striae has been associated with an increased risk of perineal tearing during birth, likely due to variations in elastic fiber component synthesis in the skin (Kapadia et al., 2016).

Molluscum fibrosum gravidarum are velvety flesh-colored skin tags that can develop or become exaggerated during pregnancy. These skin tags often develop near the neck, under the armpits, or under the breasts near the bra line, but can occur anywhere on the body. If developed during pregnancy, they commonly fall off within the first two months postpartum. Normal skin tags are differentiated from hyperpigmented, dark brown skin tags, called *acanthosis nigricans*. These occur more often in individuals with insulin resistance, metabolic syndrome, and diabetes and can be a marker for gestational diabetes in some individuals (Lauria & Saad, 2016).

Vascular Changes

Changing levels of estrogen and an increase in intravascular pressure account for vascular changes during pregnancy. These factors promote vasodilation and increase the development of spider angioma, palmar erythema, purpura and gingival edema, and hyperemia. Spider angiomas are tiny, dilated blood vessels that present as small bright red spots on the trunk, extremities, and occasionally on the face. There can be a central red dot with small radiating vessels on the periphery. Spider angiomas usually appear between 8 and 20 weeks of gestation. Spider angiomas fade or disappear after giving birth. Palmar erythema presents as either diffuse or mottling over the entire palm or mottling that is more concentrated over the thenar or hypothenar areas of the hand. Purpura appear as scattered petechia over the lower legs. Gingival edema and hyperemia are common findings in pregnancy; they appear initially in the first trimester and increase as the pregnancy progresses. Most vascular changes resolve without treatment following birth.

Hair and Nail Changes

Body hair changes during pregnancy as well. Because the estrogen-induced increase in the hair resting phase delays normal hair loss, many pregnant individuals notice an increase in hair thickness. Mild **hirsutism** is also commonly seen in pregnancy, especially on the face, including "peach fuzz" on the jawline and cheeks. This tends to be more pronounced in individuals with dark or abundant body hair (Motosko et al., 2017). Pregnant individuals may also notice fingernails and toenails growing faster than usual, and they may become brittle or soft. Other normal nail changes can include the development of transverse grooves, **leukonychia** or white spots on nail, **melanonychia** or brown or black pigmentation of nail, and thickening under the nail bed (Motosko et al., 2017).

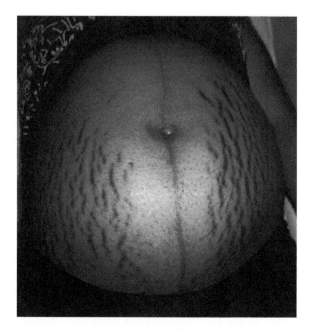

Figure 15.5   Striae gravidarum. Buchanan et al. (2010)/with permission from Elsevier.

Subjective Data Gathering

The onset, location of skin changes, characteristics of symptoms, presence of other associated symptoms such as pruritus or rash, spreading pattern, relief measures used and efficacy, sunscreen use habits, history of prior skin conditions, and presence of existing skin conditions are evaluated. If hair loss is reported, amount should be assessed.

Objective Data Gathering

A visual inspection of skin, nails, and hair patterns is done, and palpation or culture of skin lesions is performed as indicated. Changes in the size and shape of nevi or moles are noted and documented.

Relief and Preventative Measures

Although a benign condition, striae may become a cosmetic concern for some pregnant individuals. The cosmetic industry has sought to capitalize on this by marketing treatments claiming to prevent striae; however, their efficacy has not been demonstrated since the development of striae is not totally dependent on external skin stretching. Treatments such as olive oil, seaweed wraps, castor oil, glycolic acid, and zinc sulfate have been marketed, though there is no evidence to support these products for stretch mark prevention. Emollient creams are useful to decrease itching and dryness and can make the skin feel more pliable. Creams such as Trofolastin® that contain *Centella asiatica*, a medicinal herb thought to increase elastin and collagen fibers, have been successful in reducing stretch marks in some women (Farahnik et al., 2017). Striae do not completely disappear, though they fade into less noticeable smaller flesh-colored lines with time (Tyler, 2015).

Consistent use of sunscreen may prevent or reduce melasma of pregnancy. If melasma persists postpartum, creams containing a combination of tretinoin and glycolic acids and/or hydroquinone are often successful treatments. If nail brittleness or splitting occurs, nails should be kept short to reduce snagging.

Most skin, nail, and hair changes regress postpartum. Facial hair will gradually be lost, skin color will return to normal, and skin tags generally will fall off sometime postpartum. Moles that enlarge, darken, or change should have further evaluation. Increased hair loss postpartum is expected, as the stages of hair growth and loss return to their normal patterns. While there is no physical discomfort associated with most of these skin, nail, and hair conditions, pregnant individuals may regard them as conditions of concern. Understanding these normal skin changes provides the basis for education and reassurance.

Sleep Disturbances

Sleep disturbance is a common report during pregnancy regardless of parity and across all months of pregnancy and is characterized by periods of night-time waking, insomnia, daytime fatigue, restless legs, and difficulty maintaining a comfortable sleep (Mindell et al., 2015).

The optimal duration of sleep during pregnancy is unknown. Studies of sleep duration throughout pregnancy have found an increase in total sleep time and daytime sleepiness during the first trimester, which suggests that sleep needs may increase in early pregnancy. In contrast, the third trimester is characterized by a decrease in sleep time (Sedov et al., 2018).

There are two general indicators of sleep quality. Total sleep time is the actual time spent in sleep during the night, and wake after sleep onset (WASO) is the amount of time spent awake during the night after falling asleep. As pregnancy advances, WASO increases and becomes significant in the weeks prior to labor (Okun, 2019). This is especially pronounced in those who are overweight or obese prior to pregnancy and in those who gain excessive amounts of pregnancy weight (Gay et al., 2017). Sleep quality and time decreases from the first to the third trimester (Sedov et al., 2018).

Numerous factors contribute to poor sleep quality during pregnancy. Normal pregnancy physiologic changes, such as back pain, increased uterine size and physical discomforts, and increasing progesterone levels, contribute to poor sleep quality. Obesity is associated with disturbed sleep in both pregnant and nonpregnant women (Kalmbach et al., 2019). Snoring and restless legs increase in the third trimester and can interfere with sleep. Individuals with high levels of childbirth fear (tocophobia) can experience an increase in sleep deprivation and fatigue (Dencker et al. 2019). Individuals with prenatal depression can have less total sleep time and increased sleep disturbance, and disordered sleep can be a risk factor for depression (Field, 2017; Pauley et al., 2020).

Excessive fatigue from lack of sleep can affect ability to work and perform daily living activities. In addition, disordered sleep appears to play a role in adverse pregnancy outcomes. Chronic sleep loss can cause a hypothalamic–pituitary–adrenal mediated stress reaction in the pregnant person, which then activates proinflammatory pathways associated with adverse pregnancy outcomes (Chavan et al., 2015; Okun, 2019; Warland et al., 2018). Disordered sleep is associated with an increase in risk for PTB (Blair et al., 2015). The risk of PTB associated with poor sleep quality is higher in Black women, who exhibit a greater inflammatory response in pregnancy than White women due to higher levels of stress-induced inflammation related to systemic racism (Gillespie et al., 2017). Chronic prenatal sleep loss during pregnancy is also associated with gestational diabetes, increased pain perception in labor, prolonged labor, and cesarean section (Abd El-Razek et al., 2016; Okun, 2019; Li et al., 2017; Sedov et al., 2018). Sleep deprivation during pregnancy is a risk factor for developing postpartum depression (Okun, et al., 2018).

Women often hold multiple roles in today's society, with many employed fulltime while managing the majority of household and family responsibilities. Clients should be informed that sleep disturbances are more common in the last four weeks of pregnancy and strategies to obtain adequate sleep during this time should be discussed.

Assessment

Subjective Data Gathering

Screening for sleep quality is done for all clients at the first visit and at regular intervals throughout pregnancy. The onset, sleep patterns, **sleep hygiene** and routine, prior history of insomnia, presence of excessive anxiety or stress, and prior history of depression are evaluated. A formal tool such as the Pittsburgh Sleep Quality Index is commonly used to evaluate sleep quality, although it has not been validated for use during pregnancy. A depression inventory should be considered.

Objective Data Gathering

Observations are made for signs of sleep deprivation, such as lethargy and flat affect.

Relief and Preventative Measures

Education for pregnant individuals and their families about the importance of adequate rest during the prenatal period is essential to reduce poor outcomes associated with lack of sleep. Strategies to increase rest should be encouraged and supported by family members. Simple measures such as acupressure at pressure point H7 (heart 7 point), located on the inner side of the wrist crease in line with the little finger, have been reported to improve sleep quality in some pregnant women (Neri et al., 2016). Sleep hygiene measures and their rationale should be discussed with clients (Table 15.6). An at-home sleep-training program consisting of several weeks of audio relaxation exercises, readings, and daily sleep diaries is effective in improving sleep during pregnancy (Lee et al., 2016). Online delivery of cognitive behavioral therapy for insomnia has been shown to improve sleep quality and duration during pregnancy and postpartum (Kalmbach et al., 2020).

Relief measures for prenatal sleep disturbance

- Maintain a regular bedtime, use the bed only for resting and sleeping.
- Avoid any screen use for at least one hour prior to bedtime.
- Avoid cognitive or emotional arousal several hours prior to bedtime.
- Delegate chores and responsibilities.
- Modify diet prior to bedtime: avoid heavy meals (indigestion), spicy foods (heartburn), and drinking excessive liquids (nocturia).
- Use positioning aids to support the gravid uterus.
- Use relaxation aids such as relaxation exercises, visualization, music, aromatherapy, and warm bath.
- Prepare the sleep environment: darken the room and lower the room temperature by a few degrees.
- Use acupuncture.
- Use acupressure at H7 point.
- Consider cognitive therapy for insomnia.

Table 15.6 Evidence-based Sleep Hygiene Measures

Sleep hygiene recommendation	Summary of evidence
Avoid caffeine	• Caffeine intake close to bedtime disrupts sleep. • There is an inverse dose–response relationship with sleep. • Impact of morning and afternoon caffeine use is less clear. • Effects on sleep may be limited to caffeine-sensitive individuals. • Tolerance to effects on sleep develops within days.
Avoid nicotine	• Acute and chronic use disrupts sleep. • Night arousals increase temporarily during acute nicotine withdrawal.
Avoid alcohol	• Alcohol intake before bed decreases time getting to sleep but increases waking during second half of night. • There is an inverse dose–response relationship with sleep. • Tolerance to effects on sleep develops within days. • Sleep problems increase during acute withdrawal of dependent users.
Exercise regularly	• Regular or episodic exercise produces sleep improvements for those with and without sleep problems. • Current evidence does not support the claim that late-night exercise disrupts sleep.
Manage stress	• Psychosocial stress is associated with increased presleep arousal and impaired sleep. • Various stress management strategies have been shown to reduce presleep arousal and improve sleep. • Individual differences influence perception of stress and coping style.
Reduce bedtime noise	• Night-time noise increases arousals. • Tolerance to noise occurs, but EEG arousals persist. • Specific noise reduction strategies such as ear plugs and white noise can improve sleep.
Sleep timing regularity	• Regular sleep schedule can maximize synchrony among physiologic sleep drive, circadian rhythms, and sleep. • Irregular sleep schedules are associated with poor sleep.

Source: Adapted from Irish et al. (2015).

Sleep quality should be a routine assessment at various points in gestation. Lack of sleep can cause significant distress and a sympathetic listening ear is essential. It can be appropriate to initiate leave from work in the last one to two weeks of pregnancy to ensure that adequate rest is possible prior to labor, if this is economically feasible.

Supine Hypotension Syndrome

When a pregnant individual is in the supine position, the gravid uterus can compress the inferior vena cava; when the vena cava is compressed, the usual blood return to the heart from the lower half of the body is impeded. This compression decreases blood pressure, resulting in symptoms of intense dizziness, tachycardia, pallor, nausea, and sweating. Some individuals may lose consciousness. This is called vena cava syndrome or supine hypotension syndrome (SHS) and usually occurs in the second half of pregnancy as the uterus grows, and particularly in the third trimester when the uterus is at its largest. Changing position to the side quickly results in alleviation of symptoms.

Traditional advice during pregnancy has been not to exercise in the supine position after the first trimester; however, this advice has come under question. Since most pregnant individuals do not experience SHS, and the rhythmic movement of the legs during exercise increases blood flow to the heart, it is likely that most can safely exercise on their backs for short periods of time, at least until the beginning of the third trimester and perhaps longer. See Chapter 20, *Physical Activity and Exercise in the Perinatal Period,* for more detail. Pregnant individuals may have some misapprehension about inadvertently assuming the supine position during sleep; however, there is no evidence to indicate fetal or maternal harm. Importantly, individuals who become dizzy from SHS will naturally change position to alleviate symptoms.

Assessment

Subjective Data Gathering

The clinician should evaluate onset, frequency, description of symptoms, and associated symptoms.

Objective Data Gathering

Because this only occurs in the supine position, the observations are made during office visits or in labor if the individual assumes this position. Observe for signs of discomfort, anxiety, and restlessness.

Relief and Preventative Measures

Explanation and reassurance of normalcy are essential as this symptom can be frightening. SHS is immediately relieved by turning to the side-lying or sitting position. A flat supine position for should not be used for prenatal examinations. The head of the examination table should be elevated, and a lateral tilt can avoid compression of the vena cava, especially in the third trimester.

Urinary Frequency and Nocturia

During the first 12 weeks of pregnancy, the uterus is a pelvic organ. As the uterus grows, it may press on the bladder causing a sensation of bladder fullness and the urge to urinate. This often improves after 12 weeks of gestation as the uterus rises out of the pelvis and becomes an abdominal organ. In the later weeks of pregnancy when the fetal head descends into the pelvis, urinary frequency may occur again for the same reason. Resting in the lateral recumbent position facilitates venous return and increased urine output, resulting in nocturia, especially in the third trimester. It is important to differentiate physiologic urinary frequency from UTI.

Assessment

Subjective Data Gathering

This includes determining the onset, presence of dysuria, urgency, voiding small amounts, blood in urine, fluid intake habits, and prior history of UTIs.

Objective Data Gathering

Palpation of the suprapubic area for pain or tenderness, urine dip for nitrites, and/or urinalysis can be done. Culture and sensitivity tests are done, as indicated by other findings.

Relief and Preventative Measures

Liquids that are known bladder irritants, such as caffeine or carbonated beverages, can be eliminated to avoid exacerbating urinary frequency. An overfull bladder should be avoided. Suggestions include:

- Voiding soon after feeling the urge
- Voiding at scheduled intervals, every 2–3 hours
- Urinating before and after intercourse
- Reducing fluid intake in the later evening hours.

Clients should be informed of the physiologic basis for this symptom and that it tends to recur in the third trimester. Instructions on the warning signs of UTI are given. If frequency is accompanied by other signs of infection, further investigation is warranted (see Chapter 50, *Urinary Tract Disorders*).

Urinary Incontinence

The same hormonal and anatomical changes contributing to urinary frequency can lead to involuntary loss of urine, or urinary incontinence, during pregnancy. Increased pressure on the levator ani muscles from the gravid uterus and changes in the ureterovesical angles where the valve controlling urine flow from the bladder is located also contribute to involuntary loss of urine in pregnancy. Incontinence can range from the more common mild loss of several drops of urine while sneezing, laughing, or coughing to loss of copious amounts of urine requiring a change of clothing. It is estimated that approximately 40–75% of individuals experience some degree of urinary incontinence during pregnancy, typically a small amount of leakage occurring during the third trimester (Moossdorff-Steinhauser et al., 2021; Nigam et al., 2017). Urinary incontinence can sometimes be mistaken for rupture of membranes. Multigravida status, older age, and a prior history of incontinence in pregnancy, and those whose close family members experienced incontinence in pregnancy are more likely to experience this symptom; however, it should be noted that primiparous clients also experience urinary incontinence (Abdullah et al., 2016).

Assessment

Subjective Data Gathering

The onset of the symptom, frequency, predisposing events, characteristics of incontinence, description of the amount of urine lost, and effect on ADL and self-esteem are evaluated.

Objective Data Gathering

Visual inspection of a peripad for the amount of urine and evaluation for the odor of urine can be done if indicated.

Relief and Preventative Measures

Urinary incontinence can be a disturbing pregnancy sign. An explanation of the basis for this occurrence during pregnancy and reassurance that tone can be regained postpartum are essential. A program of regular pelvic floor exercises, also known as Kegel exercises, can reduce urinary incontinence during and after pregnancy (Torgbenu et al., 2021). A referral to a physical therapist knowledgeable in pelvic physiotherapy can be done during pregnancy or postpartum to provide instruction in strengthening pelvic floor musculature.

Relief measures for mild pregnancy urinary incontinence

- Empty the bladder frequently.
- Wear panty liners as needed.
- Do approximately 75–100/day Kegel exercises to increase muscle tone.

Small amounts of infrequent incontinence typically have minimal impact on the quality of life. While less common, significant prenatal urinary incontinence can cause distress and can negatively impact the quality of life. Incontinence lasting longer than six weeks postpartum should prompt a referral for further urogynecological evaluation.

Varicosities (Legs and Vulva)

Varicose veins, or varices, are abnormally enlarged superficial veins and are usually seen in the thigh, calf, and ankles. The veins in the legs are most commonly affected, as they are working against gravity. The relaxing effect of progesterone on vessel walls and valves makes them more pliable and is a major factor in the development of varicose veins during pregnancy. The increase in blood volume and compression of the gravid uterus on the iliac veins and pelvic vessels also leads to venous engorgement. Conditions that can predispose to varicosities and/or exacerbate existing varicosities are increased age, family history of varicose veins, obesity, prolonged standing, and existing leg trauma (Raetz et al., 2019). For those prone to varicosities of the leg or vulva, the varicosities will often worsen in size, shape, and symptoms with subsequent pregnancies.

Leg Varicosities

Common symptoms include pain, night cramps, numbness, or tingling in the area of the varicosities; the legs may feel heavy, achy, and may itch. As pregnancy progresses, the varicose veins are more engorged with blood and symptoms increase. Most individuals who develop varicosity of the leg veins will retain these varicosities after pregnancy, though they may decrease in size. During the third trimester and in the postpartum period, the varicose veins are at an increased risk of developing thrombophlebitis of superficial veins. Complications are not common, and most large superficial veins are solely a cosmetic nuisance. However, varicose veins in the legs can cause the following:

- Constant itching
- Pigmentation around the ankles
- Ulcers at the ankles
- Mild swelling of the feet
- Infection of the vein

Exercise may prevent varicose veins if started early in pregnancy. Instituting a program of regular walking before or at the onset of pregnancy and continuing throughout pregnancy can reduce the incidence of varicose veins (O'Flynn et al., 2014).

Subjective Data Gathering

History includes the onset, presence of symptoms, occupational and ADL history, exercise patterns, and relief measures used and efficacy, and history of varicosities and thrombophilias.

Objective Data Gathering

Physical assessment includes inspection of location, number and size of varicosities, redness, skin color, and palpation for areas of hardness, tenderness, and warmth.

Relief and Preventative Measures

While there is no cure for varicose veins, measures can reduce symptoms and possibly delay the worsening of existing varicose veins.

Elastic stockings can offer symptom relief and should have a gradient pressure, with the strongest pressure at the ankle and less pressure at more proximal points of the lower extremity. Compression hosiery is classified according to the pressure level applied at the ankle in three classes: class I = 20–30 mmHg; class II = 30–40 mmHg; and class III = 40–50 mmHg. There is no consensus on the class of compression needed for effective management of varicose veins. These garments should be put on upon first getting up in the morning before any swelling of the feet and legs occurs. They can be difficult to put on and may feel uncomfortably tight and hot. Periodic evaluation for continued use during pregnancy is recommended. Individuals with leg varicosities should be advised of signs and symptoms of venous thrombosis.

Relief measures for varicose veins in pregnancy

- Elevate the legs at any opportunity.
- Lie on the left side with the legs elevated on a pillow. This prevents the fetus from pressing on the vena cava, which is on the right side of the body, and decreases the chance of developing varicosities.
- Avoid standing for prolonged periods.
- Avoid crossing the legs when sitting down.
- Walk or exercise daily to stimulate muscles that promote venous return in the legs.
- Slightly raise the foot of the bed to elevate the legs at night.
- Avoid tight knee-high socks or stockings.
- Wear elastic compression stockings with pressure gradient.

Vulvar Varicosities

Pregnant individuals can develop varicosities in the vulva that may present as small, isolated protrusions, mainly in the labia majora, or as large masses, involving the vulvar area (Figure 15.6). Varicose veins in the vulvar and perivulvar area are estimated to occur in approximately 4% of pregnant individuals (Sueyoshi et al., 2018). Vulvar varicosities typically develop after 24 weeks of gestation and are more common in multigravidas. Vulvar varicosities are also associated with varicose veins down the inner or back part of the thigh. The risk of vulvar varicosities increases with the number of pregnancies.

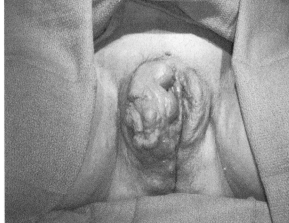

Figure 15.6   Vulvar varicosities. Used with permission from Elsevier.

The classical presentation of symptoms includes vulvovaginal swelling, a sensation of heaviness and pressure, and pain with prolonged standing (Gearhart et al., 2011). Pruritus, dyspareunia, and discomfort during walking may also be present. Some vulvar varicosities may be asymptomatic, though for some, the bulk, tension, and warmth of one or both labia majora can be extremely uncomfortable. Thrombosis and bleeding are rare but can occur. Vulvar varicosities typically do not interfere with normal vaginal birth. Unlike leg varicosities, vulvar varicosities disappear spontaneously by six weeks postpartum (Sueyoshi et al., 2018).

Subjective Data Gathering

The clinician should assess the onset, presence of symptoms, occupational and ADL history, exercise patterns, and relief measures used and effectiveness.

Objective Data Gathering

The clinician should perform a visual inspection of the perineal areas affected, including size, locations, and the approximate number of varicose veins. Ideally, the individual should be in the standing position to determine the extent of venous pooling; however, assessment can also be made while in a semirecumbent position.

Relief and Preventative Measures

The treatment of choice of vulvar varicosities during pregnancy is conservative and symptomatic. An explanation of the physiologic basis for these symptoms and reassurance that they will resolve postpartum can support coping with symptoms. While rare, vulvar varicosities presenting in the first trimester in a primigravida requires referral for further evaluation with Doppler studies to determine anatomical vein diameter and structure and any retrograde blood flow. Persistent vulvar varicosities after pregnancy also should prompt referral for evaluation and potential treatment with surgery or sclerotherapy.

Relief measures for vulvar varicosities

- Avoid prolonged periods of standing.
- Elevate the lower legs when sitting or lying down.
- Use a support device (such as V2® supporter) similar in appearance to an athletic scrotal supporter ("jock strap"). It is contoured to provide compressive support for the vulva, thus preventing the pooling of blood in the labial veins.
- Support garments such as bicycle shorts worn with peripads can put gentle counter pressure on vulvar varicosities.
- Support garments that lift the pregnant abdomen can reduce pressure on lower extremities.

Vision Changes

Due to some combination of hormonally mediated and fluid retention-related changes in the cornea, some pregnant individuals may perceive refractive changes

(Moshirfar et al., 2019; Wu et al., 2020). If present, these changes may prevent the usual degree of correction with glasses or contact lenses and contact lenses may become uncomfortable. Because these changes are temporary, it is wise to wait until several months postpartum before changing eye refraction prescriptions (Moshirfar et al., 2019).

Assessment

Subjective Data Gathering

The clinician should evaluate the onset, description of character of change in vision, history of diabetes, and associated symptoms.

Objective Data Gathering

This consists of obtaining blood pressure and performing an ophthalmoscopic eye exam as indicated. If needed, a visual assessment using a Snellen eye chart can be done.

Relief and Preventative Measures

The clinician should provide information about the physiologic basis and provide reassurance that this symptom is temporary. Individuals reporting blurry vision after approximately 20 weeks of gestation need immediate evaluation to rule out preeclampsia. Pregnant individuals with preexisting diabetes reporting eye changes should be referred for further evaluation, as diabetes-related retinopathy can progress during pregnancy.

Resources for Clients and Their Families

American College of Nurse-Midwives Share-with-Women—Back Pain during Pregnancy: https://onlinelibrary.wiley.com/doi/epdf/10.1111/jmwh.12597

American College of Nurse-Midwives Share-with-Women—Nausea & Vomiting during Pregnancy: https://onlinelibrary.wiley.com/doi/epdf/10.1111/jmwh.12451

American College of Obstetricians and Gynecologists—Frequently Asked Questions: Easing Back Pain during Pregnancy: http://www.acog.org/Patients/FAQs/Back-Pain-During-Pregnancy

American College of Obstetricians and Gynecologists—Frequently Asked Questions: Nausea and Vomiting: http://www.acog.org/Patients/FAQs/Morning-Sickness-Nausea-and-Vomiting-of-Pregnancy

American College of Obstetricians and Gynecologists—Frequently Asked Questions: Skin Conditions during Pregnancy: http://www.acog.org/Patients/FAQs/Skin-Conditions-During-Pregnancy

Resources for Healthcare Providers

- Childbirth Connections: Resources for Advocates and Professionals: http://www.childbirthconnection.org/resources/
- Common Dermatological Conditions in Skin of Color: https://pharmaceutical-journal.com/article/ld/common-dermatological-conditions-in-skin-of-colour

- StatPearls article: Stretch Marks (striae): https://www.ncbi.nlm.nih.gov/books/NBK436005/
- StatPearls article: Spider Angioma: https://www.ncbi.nlm.nih.gov/books/NBK507818/

References

Abbas, Y., Abdelkader, M., Adams, M., Addison, A., Advani, R., Ahmed, T., Alexander, V., Alli, B., Alvi, S., Amiraraghi, N., Ashman, A., Balakumar, R., Bewick, J., Bhasker, D., Bola, S., Bowles, P., Campbell, N., Can Guru Naidu, N., Caton, N., & Kwong, F. N. K. (2020). Nasal packs for epistaxis: Predictors of success. *Clinical Otolaryngology*, 45(5), 659–666. https://doi.org/10.1111/coa.13555

Abd El-Razek, A., Grobman, W. A., Reid, K. J., Parker, C. B., Hunter, S. M., & Silver, R. M. (2016). The relationship between sleep disturbance in late pregnancy and labor outcomes. *International Journal of Health*, 4, 12–16. https://doi.org/10.14419/ijh.v4i1.5559

Abdullah, B., Ayub, S. H., Zahid, A. M., Noorneza, A. R., Isa, M. R., & Ng, P. Y. (2016). Urinary incontinence in primigravida: The neglected pregnancy predicament. *European Journal of Obstetrics & Gynecology and Reproductive Biology*, 198, 110–115.

Adamson, D., & Nelson-Piercy, C. (2007). Managing palpitations and arrhythmias during pregnancy. *Heart (British Cardiac Society)*, 93, 1630–1036.

Afshar, A., & Tabrizi, A. (2021). Pregnancy-related hand and wrist problems. *The Archives of Bone and Joint Surgery*, 9(3), 345–349. https://doi.org/10.22038/abjs.2020.50995.2531

Alwan, S., Conover, E. A., Harris-Sagaribay, L., Lamm, S. H., Lavigne, S. V., Lusskin, S. I., Obican, S. G., Romeo, A. N., Scialli, A. R., & Wisner, K. L. (2022). Paracetamol use in pregnancy—Caution over causal inference from available data. *Nature Reviews. Endocrinology*, 18(3), 190. https://doi.org/10.1038/s41574-021-00606-x

American College of Obstetricians and Gynecologists. (2019). ACOG Practice Bulletin No. 212. Pregnancy and heart disease. *Obstetrics and Gynecology*, 133(5), e320–e356.

American College of Obstetricians and Gynecologists. (2021). *ACOG response to consensus statement on paracetamol use during pregnancy*. https://www.acog.org/news/news-articles/2021/09/response-to-consensus-statement-on-paracetamol-use-during-pregnancy

American College of Obstetricians and Gynecologists (ACOG). (2018). Practice Bulletin No. 189. Nausea and vomiting of pregnancy. *Obstetrics & Gynecology*, 131(1), e15–e30.

Araújo, C. A. L. D., Lorena, S. B. D., Cavalcanti, G. C. D. S., Leão, G. L. D. S., Tenório, G. P., & Alves, J. G. B. (2020). Oral magnesium supplementation for leg cramps in pregnancy—An observational controlled trial. *PLoS One*, 15(1), e0227497. https://doi.org/10.1371/journal.pone.0227497

Backhausen, M. G., Bendix, J. M., Damm, P., Tabor, A., & Hegaard, H. (2019). Low back pain intensity among childbearing women and associated predictors: A cohort study. *Women and Birth*, 32, e467–e476. https://doi.org/10.1016/j.wombi.2018.09.008

Bai, G., Korfage, I. J., Hafkamp-de Groen, E., Jaddoe, V. W., Mautner, E., & Raat, H. (2016). Associations between nausea, vomiting, fatigue and health-related quality of life of women in early pregnancy: The generation R study. *PLoS One*, 11(11), e0166133.

Bauer, A. Z., Swan, S. H., Kriebel, D., Liew, Z., Taylor, H. S., Bornehag, C.-G., Andrade, A. M., Olsen, J., Jensen, R. H., Mitchell, R. T., Skakkebaek, N. E., Jégou, B., & Kristensen, D. M. (2021). Paracetamol use during pregnancy—A call for precautionary action. *Nature Reviews. Endocrinology*, 17(12), 757–766. https://doi.org/10.1038/s41574-021-00553-7

Belogolovsky, I., Katzman, W., Christopherson, N., Rivera, M., & Allen, D. D. (2015). The effectiveness of exercise in treatment of pregnancy-related lumbar and pelvic girdle pain: A meta-analysis and evidence-based review. *Journal of Women's Health Physical Therapy*, 39(2), 53–64.

Bendtsen, L. (2015). Treatment guidelines: Implications for community-based headache treatment. *International Journal of Clinical Practice*, 69(S182), 13–16.

Bieber, A., Martires, K., Stein, J., Grant-Kels, J., Driscoll, M., & Pomeranz, M. (2017). Pigmentation and pregnancy: Knowing what is normal. *Obstetrics & Gynecology, 129*(1), 168–173. https://doi.org/10.1097/AOG.0000000000001806

Bishop, K. C., Ford, A. C., Kuller, J. A., & Dotters-Katz, S. (2019). Acupuncture in obstetrics and gynecology. *Obstetrical & Gynecological Survey, 74*(4), 241–251. https://doi.org/10.1097/OGX.0000000000000655

Black, E., Khor, K. E., Kennedy, D., Chutatape, A., Sharma, S., Vancaillie, T., & Demirkol, A. (2019). Medication use and pain management in pregnancy: A critical review. *Pain Practice: The Official Journal of World Institute of Pain, 19*(8), 875–899. https://doi.org/10.1111/papr.12814

Blair, L. M., Porter, K., Leblebicioglu, B., & Christian, L. M. (2015). Poor sleep quality and associated inflammation predict preterm birth: Heightened risk among African Americans. *Sleep, 38*(8), 1259.

Borg-Stein, J., & Dugan, S. A. (2007). Musculoskeletal disorders of pregnancy, delivery and postpartum. *Physical Medicine and Rehabilitation Clinics of North America, 18*(3), 459–476.

Briggs, G. G., Freeman, R. K., Towers, C. V., & Forinash, A. B. (2017). *Drugs in pregnancy and lactation: A reference guide to fetal and neonatal risk* (11th ed.). Wolters Kluwer.

Bronshtein, M., Gover, A., Beloosesky, R., Dabaja, H., Ginsberg, Y., Weiner, Z., & Khatib, N. (2018). Characteristics and outcomes of ptyalism gravidarum. *The Israel Medical Association Journal: IMAJ, 20*(9), 573–575.

Buchanan, K., Fletcher, H. M., & Reid, M. (2010). Prevention of striae gravidarum with cocoa butter cream. *International Journal of Gynecology & Obstetrics, 108*(1), 65–68. https://doi.org/10.1016/j.ijgo.2009.08.008

Carroll, M. P., Bulkhi, A. A., & Lockey, R. F. (2019). Rhinitis and sinusitis. In J. A. Namazy & M. Schwartz (Eds.), *Asthma, allergic and immunologic diseases during pregnancy* (pp. 61–86). Springer.

Chatur, S., Islam, S., Moore, L. E., Sandhu, R. K., Sheldon, R. S., & Kaul, P. (2019). Incidence of syncope during pregnancy: Temporal trends and outcomes. *Journal of the American Heart Association, 8*(10), e011608. https://doi.org/10.1161/JAHA.118.011608

Chavan, N., Ashford, K., Meints, L., McQuerry, K., McCubbin, A., Barnett, J., & O'Brien, J. (2015). 750: Changes in inflammatory cytokines with sleep disturbances in pregnancy. *American Journal of Obstetrics & Gynecology, 212*(1), S365.

Choi, S. E., Choudhary, A., Ahern, J. M., Palmer, N., & Barrow, J. R. (2021). Association between maternal periodontal disease and adverse pregnancy outcomes: An analysis of claims data. *Family Practice, 38*(6), 718–723. https://doi.org/10.1093/fampra/cmab037

Conner, S. N., Trudell, A. S., & Conner, C. A. (2021). Chiropractic care for the pregnant body. *Clinical Obstetrics and Gynecology, 64*(3), 602–610. https://doi.org/10.1097/GRF.0000000000000621

Daalderop, L. A., Wieland, B. V., Tomsin, K., Reyes, L., Kramer, B. W., Vanterpool, S. F., & Been, J. V. (2018). Periodontal disease and pregnancy outcomes: Overview of systematic reviews. *JDR Clinical & Translational Research, 3*(1), 10–27. https://doi.org/10.1177/2380084417731097

Dencker, A., Nilsson, C., Begley, C., Jangsten, E., Mollberg, M., Patel, H., Wigert, H., Hessman, E., Sjöblum, H., & Sparud-Lundin, C. (2019). Causes and outcomes in studies of fear of childbirth: A systematic review. *Women and Birth, 32*(2), 99–111. https://doi.org/10.1016/j.wombi.2018.07.004

Dormuth, C. R., Winquist, B., Fisher, A., Wu, F., Reynier, P., Suissa, S., Dahl, M., Ma, Z., Lu, X., Zhang, J., Raymond, C. B., Filion, K. B., Platt, R. W., Moriello, C., & Paterson, J. M. (2021). Comparison of pregnancy outcomes of patients treated with ondansetron vs alternative antiemetic medications in a multinational, population-based cohort. *JAMA Network Open, 4*(4), e215329. https://doi.org/10.1001/jamanetworkopen.2021.5329

Dubey, K. (2021). Pregnancy induced rhinitis: A systematic review. *European Journal of Biomedical and Pharmaceutical Sciences, 8*(1), 35–38.

Dugan-Kim, M., Connell, S., Stika, C., Wong, C. A., & Gossett, D. R. (2009). Epistaxis of pregnancy and association with postpartum hemorrhage. *Obstetrics & Gynecology, 114*(6), 1322–1325. https://doi.org/10.1097/AOG.0b013e3181bea830

Dunietz, G. L., Lisabeth, L. D., Shedden, K., Shamim-Uzzaman, Q. A., Bullough, A. S., Chames, M. C., Bowden, M. F., & O'Brien, L. M. (2017). Restless legs syndrome and sleep-wake disturbances in pregnancy. *Journal of Clinical Sleep Medicine, 13*(7), 863–870. https://doi.org/10.5664/jcsm.6654

Ebrahimi, N., Maltepe, C., Bournissen, F. G., & Koren, G. (2009). Nausea and vomiting of pregnancy: Using the 24-hour pregnancy-unique quantification of emesis (PUQE-24) scale. *Journal of Obstetrics and Gynaecology Canada, 31*(9), 803–807.

Ee, C., Levett, K., Smith, C., Armour, M., Dahlen, H. G., Chopra, P., Maroun, P., Rao, V. S., Avard, N., Grant, S., Keedle, H., Armour, S., Arentz, S., Cave, A. E., Sutcliffe, K., & Templeman, K. (2021). Complementary medicines and therapies in clinical guidelines on pregnancy care: A systematic review. *Women and Birth: Journal of the Australian College of Midwives, 35*(4), e303–e307. https://doi.org/10.1016/j.wombi.2021.08.003

Farahnik, B., Park, K., Kroumpouzos, G., & Murase, J. (2017). Striae gravidarum: Risk factors, prevention, and management. *International Journal of Women's Dermatology, 3*(2), 77–85.

Field, T. (2017). Prenatal depression risk factors, developmental effects and interventions: a review. *Journal of Pregnancy and Child Health, 4*(1), 301–307. https://doi.org/10.4172%2F2376-127X.1000301

Friedman, E. B., Scolyer, R. A., & Thompson, J. F. (2019). Management of pigmented skin lesions during pregnancy. *Australian Journal of General Practice, 48*(9), 621–624. https://doi.org/10.31128/AJGP-04-19-48952

Garrison, S. R., Korownyk, C. S., Kolber, M. R., Allan, G. M., Musini, V. M., Sekhon, R. K., & Dugré, N. (2020). Magnesium for skeletal muscle cramps. *Cochrane Database of Systematic Reviews*, (9). https://doi.org/10.1002/14651858.CD009402.pub3

Gay, C. L., Richoux, S. E., Beebe, K. R., & Lee, K. A. (2017). Sleep disruption and duration in late pregnancy is associated with excess gestational weight gain among overweight and obese women. *Birth, 00*, 1–8.

Gearhart, P., Levin, P., & Schimpf, M. (2011). Expanding on earlier findings: A vulvar varicosity grows larger with each pregnancy. *American Journal of Obstetrics & Gynecology, 204*(89), e1–e2.

Gibson, P. S., Powrie, R., & Peipert, J. (2001). Prevalence of syncope and recurrent presyncope during pregnancy. *Obstetrics & Gynecology, 97*(4), 1S–2S.

Gillespie, S. L., Neal, J. L., Christian, L. M., Szalacha, L. A., McCarthy, D. O., & Salsberry, P. J. (2017). Interleukin-1 receptor antagonist polymorphism and birth timing: Pathway analysis among African American women. *Nursing Research, 66*(2), 95–104.

Ginat, D. T., & Schatz, C. J. (2017). Nasal septum granuloma gravidarum. *Ear, Nose & Throat Journal, 96*(10–11), 412–414. https://doi.org/10.1177/0145561317096010-1118

Grooten, I., Den Hollander, W., Roseboom, T., Kuipers, E., Jaddoe, V., Gaillard, R., & Painter, R. (2017). Helicobacter pylori infection: A predictor of vomiting severity in pregnancy and adverse birth outcome. *American Journal of Obstetrics and Gynecology, 216*(5), 512–e1.

Gupta, R., Gupta, R., Kumar, N., Rawat, V. S., Ulfberg, J., & Allen, R. P. (2021). Restless legs syndrome among subjects having chronic liver disease: A systematic review and meta-analysis. *Sleep Medicine Reviews, 58*, 144–152. https://doi.org/10.1016/j.smrv.2021.101463

Iheozor-Ejiofor, Z., Middleton, P., Esposito, M., & Glenny, A. M. (2017). Treating periodontal disease for preventing adverse birth outcomes in pregnant women. *Cochrane Database of Systematic Reviews, 6*. https://doi.org/10.1002/14651858.CD005297

International Restless Leg Study Group. (2015). *Guidelines for first line treatment of RLS, prevention and treatment of augmentation.* http://irlssg.org/diagnostic-criteria/

Irish, L. A., Kline, C. E., Gunn, H. E., Buysse, D. J., & Hall, M. H. (2015). The role of sleep hygiene in promoting public health: A review of empirical evidence. *Sleep Medicine Reviews, 22*, 23–36.

Jafarimanesh, H., Vakilian, K., & Mobasseri, S. (2020). Effects of warm and cold footbath on sleep quality in pregnant women with restless legs syndrome. *The Iranian Journal of Obstetrics, Gynecology and Infertility, 23*(6), 51–60. https://doi.org/10.22038/ijogi.2020.16880

Johnson, T. S., & Strube, K. (2011). Breast care during pregnancy. *Journal of Obstetric, Gynecologic & Neonatal Nursing*, 40(2), 144–148. https://doi.org/10.1111/j.1552-6909.2011.01227.x

Kalmbach, D. A., Cheng, P., O'Brien, L. M., Swanson, L. M., Sangha, R., Sen, S., Guille, C., Cuamatzi-Castelan, A., Henry, A., Roth, T., & Drake, C. L. (2020). A randomized controlled trial of digital cognitive behavioral therapy for insomnia in pregnant women. *Sleep Medicine*, 72, 82–92. https://doi.org/10.1016/j.sleep.2020.03.016

Kalmbach, D. A., Cheng, P., Sangha, R., O'Brien, L. M., Swanson, L. M., Palagini, L., Brazen, L., Roth, T., & Drake, C. L. (2019). Insomnia, short sleep, and snoring in mid-to-late pregnancy: Disparities related to poverty, race, and obesity. *Nature and Science of Sleep*, 11, 301.

Kamysheva, E., Werthmeim, E., Skouteris, H., Paxton, S., & Milgrom, J. (2009). Frequency, severity, and effect on life of physical symptoms experienced during pregnancy. *Journal of Midwifery & Womens Health*, 54(1), 43–49.

Kapadia, S., Kapoor, S., Parmar, K., Patadia, K., & Vyas, M. (2016). Prediction of perineal tear during childbirth by assessment of striae gravidarum score. *International Journal of Reproduction, Contraception, Obstetrics and Gynecology*, 3(1), 208–212.

Kar, M., Bayar, M. N., & Negm, H. (2021). How should rhinitis be managed during pregnancy? In C. Cingi, N. Bayar Muluk, G. K. Scadding, & R. Mladina (Eds.), *Challenges in rhinology* (pp. 127–135). Springer. https://doi.org/10.1007/978-3-030-50899-9_15

Kazemi, F., Nahidi, F., & Kariman, N. (2017). Disorders affecting quality of life during pregnancy: A qualitative study. *Journal of Clinical and Diagnostic Research*, 11(4), QC06–QC10. https://doi.org/10.5664/jcsm.8248

Koren, G., & Cohen, R. (2021). Measuring the severity of nausea and vomiting of pregnancy; a 20-year perspective on the use of the pregnancy-unique quantification of emesis (PUQE). *Journal of Obstetrics and Gynaecology: The Journal of the Institute of Obstetrics and Gynaecology*, 41(3), 335–339. https://doi.org/10.1080/01443615.2020.1787968

Koren, G., Madjunkova, S., & Maltepe, C. (2014). The protective effects of nausea and vomiting of pregnancy against adverse fetal outcome—A systematic review. *Reproductive Toxicology*, 47, 77–80.

Kramer, J., Bowen, A., Stewart, N., & Muhajarine, N. (2013). Nausea and vomiting of pregnancy: Prevalence, severity and relation to psychosocial health. *MCN. The American Journal of Maternal Child Nursing*, 38(1), 21–27. https://doi.org/10.1097/NMC.0b013e3182748489

Kuronen, M., Hantunen, S., Alanne, L., Kokki, H., Saukko, C., Sjövall, S., Vesterinen, K., & Kokki, M. (2021). Pregnancy, puerperium and perinatal constipation—An observational hybrid survey on pregnant and postpartum women and their age-matched non-pregnant controls. *BJOG: An International Journal of Obstetrics and Gynaecology*, 128(6), 1057–1064. https://doi.org/10.1111/1471-0528.16559

Laitinen, L., Nurmi, M., Ellilä, P., Rautava, P., Koivisto, M., & Polo-Kantola, P. (2020). Nausea and vomiting of pregnancy: Associations with personal history of nausea and affected relatives. *Archives of Gynecology and Obstetrics*, 302(4), 947–955. https://doi.org/10.1007/s00404-020-05683-3

Lal, D., Jategaonkar, A. A., Borish, L., Chambliss, L. R., Gnagi, S. H., Hwang, P. H., Rank, M., Stankewitz, J., & Lund, V. J. (2016). Management of rhinosinusitis during pregnancy: Systematic review and expert panel recommendations. *Rhinology*, 54(2), 99. https://doi.org/10.4193/Rhino15.228

Lauria, M. W., & Saad, M. J. (2016). Acanthosis nigricans and insulin resistance. *New England Journal of Medicine*, 374(24), e31.

Lee, K. A., Gay, C. L., & Alsten, C. R. (2016). Sleep enhancement training for pregnant women. *Obstetrics & Gynecology*, 128(5), 964–971.

Li, C. M., Zhernakova, A., Engstrand, L., Wijmenga, C., & Brusselaers, N. (2020). Systematic review with meta-analysis: The risks of proton pump inhibitors during pregnancy. *Alimentary Pharmacology & Therapeutics*, 51(4), 410–420. https://doi.org/10.1111/apt.15610

Li, R., Zhang, J., Zhou, R., Liu, J., Dai, Z., Liu, D., Wang, Y., Zhang, H., Li, Y., & Zeng, G. (2017). Sleep disturbances during pregnancy are associated with cesarean delivery and preterm birth. *The Journal of Maternal-Fetal & Neonatal Medicine*, 30(6), 733–738.

Liu, P., Wen, W., Gao, X., Watt, R. M., & Wong, M. C. M. (2016). Oral health problems and oral health-related quality-of-life among pregnant women. *Journal of Dental Research*, 95(B).

Lurie, S., Matas, Z., Fux, A., Golan, A., & Sadan, O. (2011). Association of serum relaxin with striae gravidarum in pregnant women. *Archives of Gynecology and Obstetrics*, 283, 219–222.

Martins, R. F., & Pinto e Silva, J. L. (2014). Treatment of pregnancy-related lumbar and pelvic girdle pain by the yoga method: A randomized controlled study. *The Journal of Alternative and Complementary Medicine*, 20(1), 24–31.

Mchenga, N. L. (2021). My experience with ptyalism gravidarum during the COVID-19 pandemic. *Nursing for Women's Health*, 25(5), 400–402. https://doi.org/10.1016/j.nwh.2021.07.004

Mindell, J. A., Cook, R. A., & Nikolovski, J. (2015). Sleep patterns and sleep disturbances across pregnancy. *Sleep Medicine*, 16(4), 483–488.

Moossdorff-Steinhauser, H. F., Berghmans, B. C., Spaanderman, M. E., & Bols, E. M. (2021). Prevalence, incidence and bothersomeness of urinary incontinence in pregnancy: A systematic review and meta-analysis. *International Urogynecology Journal*, 1–20. https://doi.org/10.1007/s00192-020-04636-3

Morino, S., Ishihara, M., Umezaki, F., Hatanaka, H., Yamashita, M., Kawabe, R., & Aoyama, T. (2019). The effects of pelvic belt use on pelvic alignment during and after pregnancy: A prospective longitudinal cohort study. *BMC Pregnancy and Childbirth*, 19(1), 305. https://doi.org/10.1186/s12884-019-2457-6

Moshirfar, M., Rosen, D. B., Heiland, M. B., Ronquillo, Y. C., & Hoopes, P. C. (2019). Should I get LASIK if I'm breastfeeding? *Ophthalmology and therapy*, 8(3), 349–352. https://doi.org/10.1007/s40123-019-0195-5

Mosti, G., & Caggiati, A. (2021). The effects of water immersion and walking on leg volume, ankle circumference and epifascial thickness in healthy subjects with occupational edema. *Phlebology*, 36(6), 473–480.

Motosko, C. C., Bieber, A. K., Pomeranz, M. K., Stein, J. A., & Martires, K. J. (2017). Physiologic changes of pregnancy: A review of the literature. *International Journal of Women's Dermatology*, 3(4), 219–224. https://doi.org/10.1016/j.ijwd.2017.09.003

Narayan, K. V. (2019). Pregnancy and allergy. In J. Prasad, V. K. Jain, & N. Gupta (Eds.), *Clinical allergy* (pp. 355–362). Jaypee Brothers Clinical Publishers.

National Institute for Health and Care Excellence. (August 2021). *Antenatal care: Management of nausea and vomiting in pregnancy* [NICE Guideline NG201] https://www.nice.org.uk/guidance/ng201/evidence/r-management-of-nausea-and-vomiting-in-pregnancy-pdf-331305934365.

Neri, I., Bruno, R., Dante, G., & Facchinetti, F. (2016). Acupressure on self-reported sleep quality during pregnancy. *Journal of Acupuncture and Meridian Studies*, 9(1), 11–15.

Nigam, A., Ahmad, A., Gaur, D., Elahi, A. A., & Batra, S. (2017). Prevalence and risk factors for urinary incontinence in pregnant women during late third trimester. *International Journal of Reproduction, Contraception, Obstetrics and Gynecology*, 5(7), 2187–2191.

Nuriel-Ohayon, M., Neuman, H., & Koren, O. (2016). Microbial changes during pregnancy, birth, and infancy. *Frontiers in Microbiology*, 1031. https://doi.org/10.3389/fmicb.2016.01031

Nussbaum, R., & Benedetto, A. V. (2006). Cosmetic aspects of pregnancy. *Clinics in Dermatology*, 24(2), 133–141.

O'Flynn, N., Vaughan, M., & Kelley, K. (2014). Diagnosis and management of varicose veins in the legs: NICE guideline. *British Journal of General Practice*, 64(623), 314–315.

Ogamba, M. I., Loverro, K. L., Laudicina, N. M., Gill, S. V., & Lewis, C. L. (2016). Changes in gait with anteriorly added mass: A pregnancy simulation study. *Journal of Applied Biomechanics*, 32(4), 379–387.

Okun, M. L. (2019). Sleep disturbances and modulations in inflammation: Implications for pregnancy health. *Social and Personality Psychology Compass*, 13(5), e12451. https://doi.org/10.1111/spc3.12451

Okun, M. L., Mancuso, R. A., Hobel, C. J., Schetter, C. D., & Coussons-Read, M. (2018). Poor sleep quality increases symptoms of depression and anxiety in postpartum women. *Journal of Behavioral Medicine*, 41(5), 703–710. https://doi.org/10.1007/s10865-018-9950-7

Ovadia, C. (2021). Prescribing for pregnancy: Managing chronic headache and migraine. *Drug and Therapeutics Bulletin*, 59(10), 152–156. https://doi.org/10.1136/dtb.2021.000031

Pauley, A. M., Moore, G. A., Mama, S. K., Molenaar, P., & Symons Downs, D. (2020). Associations between prenatal sleep and psychological health: A systematic review. *Journal of Clinical Sleep Medicine*, 16(4), 619–630. https://doi.org/10.5664/jcsm.8248

Pflibsen, L. R., McCormick, B. A., Noland, S. S., & Kouloumberis, P. E. (2020). What came first-the chicken or the egg? Carpal tunnel syndrome and pregnancy. *Journal of Women's Health*, 29(7), 896–898. https://doi.org/10.1089/jwh.2020.8471

Picchietti, D. L., Hensley, J. G., Bainbridge, J. L., Lee, K. A., Manconi, M., McGregor, J. A., & International Restless Legs Syndrome Study Group. (2015). Consensus clinical practice guidelines for the diagnosis and treatment of restless legs syndrome/Willis-Ekbom disease during pregnancy and lactation. *Sleep Medicine Reviews*, 22, 64–77.

Prosperetti, C., & Manconi, M. (2015). Restless legs syndrome/Willis-Ekbom disease and pregnancy. *Sleep Medicine Clinics*, 10(3), 323–329. https://doi.org/10.1016/j.jsmc.2015.05.016

Quach, D. T., Le, Y.-L. T., Mai, L. H., Hoang, A. T., & Nguyen, T. T. (2021). Short meal-to-bed time is a predominant risk factor of gastroesophageal reflux disease in pregnancy. *Journal of Clinical Gastroenterology*, 55(4), 316–320. https://doi.org/10.1097/MCG.0000000000001399

Raetz, J., Wilson, M., & Collins, K. (2019). Varicose veins: Diagnosis and treatment. *American Family Physician*, 99(11), 682–688.

Richens, Y., Smith, K., & Leddington, S. (2010). Lower back pain during pregnancy: Advice and exercises for women. *British Journal of Midwifery*, 18(9), 562–566.

Ridolo, E., Caminati, M., Martignago, I., Melli, V., Salvottini, C., Rossi, O., Dama, A., Schiappoli, M., Bovo, C., Incorvaia, C., & Senna, G. (2016). Allergic rhinitis: Pharmacotherapy in pregnancy and old age. *Expert Review of Clinical Pharmacology*, 9(8), 1081–1089. https://doi.org/10.1080/17512433.2016.1189324

Rossi, L., Mazzara, C., & Pagani, O. (2019). Diagnosis and treatment of breast cancer in young women. *Current Treatment Options in Oncology*, 20, 86. https://doi.org/10.1007/s11864-019-0685-7

Rungsiprakarn, P., Laopaiboon, M., Sangkomkamhang, U. S., Lumbiganon, P., & Pratt, J. J. (2015). Interventions for treating constipation in pregnancy. *The Cochrane Database of Systematic Reviews*, 9, CD011448. https://doi.org/10.1002/14651858.CD011448.pub2

Sakran, R., Shechtman, S., Arnon, J., & Diav-Citrin, O. (2021). Pregnancy outcome following in-utero exposure to ondansetron: A prospective comparative observational study. *Reproductive Toxicology*, 99, 9–14. https://doi.org/10.1016/j.reprotox.2020.11.005

Sedov, I. D., Cameron, E. E., Madigan, S., & Tomfohr-Madsen, L. M. (2018). Sleep quality during pregnancy: A meta-analysis. *Sleep Medicine Reviews*, 38, 168–176. https://doi.org/10.1016/j.smrv.2017.06.005

Shin, G., Toto, E., & Schey, R. (2015). Pregnancy and postpartum bowel changes: Constipation and fecal incontinence. *The American Journal of Gastroenterology*, 110(4), 521–529.

Shirah, B. H., Shirah, H. A., Fallata, A. H., Alobidy, S. N., & Al Hawsawi, M. M. (2018). Hemorrhoids during pregnancy: Sitz bath vs. anorectal cream: A comparative prospective study of two conservative treatment protocols. *Women and Birth*, 31(4), e272–e277. https://doi.org/10.1016/j.wombi.2017.10.003

Silva de Araujo Figueiredo, C., Gonsalves Carvalho Rosalem, C., Costa Cantanhede, A. L., Abreu Fonseca Thomaz, E. B., da Cruz, F. N., & Carmen, M. (2017). Systemic alterations and their oral manifestations in pregnant women. *Journal of Obstetrics and Gynaecology Research*, 43(1), 16–22.

Singla, P., Gupta, M., Matreja, P. S., & Gill, R. (2015). Otorhinolaryngological complaints in pregnancy: A prospective study in a tertiary care centre. *International Journal of Otorhinolaryngology and Head Neck Surgery*, 1(2), 75–80.

Smyth, R., Aflaifel, N., & Bamigboye, A. (2015). Interventions for varicose veins and leg oedema in pregnancy. *Cochrane Database of Systematic Reviews*, 10, CD001066.

Solt Kirca, A., & Kanza Gul, D. (2020). Effects of acupressure applied to P6 point on nausea vomiting in pregnancy: A double-blind randomized controlled. *Alternative Therapies in Health and Medicine*, 26(6), 12–17.

Srivanitchapoom, P., Pandey, S., & Hallett, M. (2014). Restless legs syndrome and pregnancy: A review. *Parkinsonism & Related Disorders*, 20(7), 716–722. https://doi.org/10.3389/fnagi.2017.00171

Sueyoshi, M., Clevenger, S., & Hart, E. (2018). Large vaginal varicosities in the setting of pregnancy without known hepatic or vascular risks: A case report and review of the literature. *Case Reports in Obstetrics and Gynecology*, 2018, 2394695. https://doi.org/10.1155/2018/2394695

Sun, L., Xi, Y., Wen, X., & Zou, W. (2021). Use of metoclopramide in the first trimester and risk of major congenital malformations: A systematic review and meta-analysis. *PLoS One*, 16(9), e0257584. https://doi.org/10.1371/journal.pone.0257584

Suzuki, S., Igarashi, M., Yamashita, E., & Satomi, M. (2009). Ptyalism gravidarum. *North American Journal of Medical Sciences*, 1(6), 303–304.

Tella, B., Sokunbi, O., Akinlami, O., & Afolabi, B. (2011). Effects of aerobic exercise on the level of insomnia and fatigue in pregnant women. *International Journal of Gynecology & Obstetrics*, 15(1).

Tharpe, N. L., Farley, C. L., & Jordan, R. G. (2022). *Clinical practice guidelines for midwifery & women's health* (6th ed.). Jones & Bartlett Learning.

Thélin, C. S., & Richter, J. E. (2020). Review article: The management of heartburn during pregnancy and lactation. *Alimentary Pharmacology & Therapeutics*, 51(4), 421–434. https://doi.org/10.1111/apt.15611

Torgbenu, E. L., Aimakhu, C. O., & Morhe, E. K. (2021). Effect of Kegel exercises on pelvic floor muscle disorders in prenatal and postnatal women: A literature review. *Current Women's Health Reviews*, 17(3), 202–207. https://doi.org/10.2174/1573404816999200930161059

Tyler, K. H. (2015). Physiological skin changes during pregnancy. *Clinical Obstetrics and Gynecology*, 58(1), 119–124. https://doi.org/10.1097/GRF.0000000000000077

van Benten, E., Pool, J., Mens, J., & Pool-Goudzwaard, A. (2014). Recommendations for physical therapists on the treatment of lumbopelvic pain during pregnancy: A systematic review. *Journal of Orthopaedic & Sports Physical Therapy*, 44(7), 464–A15.

Van Kampen, M., Devoogdt, N., De Groef, A., Gielen, A., & Geraerts, I. (2015). The efficacy of physiotherapy for the prevention and treatment of prenatal symptoms: A systematic review. *International Urogynecology Journal*, 26(11), 1575–1586.

VanThiel, D. H., Gavaler, J. J., Joshi, S. N., Sara, R. K., & Stremple, J. (1977). Heartburn of pregnancy. *Gastroenterology*, 72, 668–678.

Vermani, E., Mittal, R., & Weeks, A. (2010). Pelvic girdle pain and low back pain in pregnancy: A review. *Pain Practice*, 10(1), 60–71.

Vleeming, A., Albert, H., Ostgaard, H., Sturesson, B., & Stuge, B. (2008). European guidelines on the diagnosis and treatment of pelvic girdle pain. *European Spine Journal*, 17(6), 794–819. https://doi.org/10.1007/s00586-008-0602-4

Ward-Ritacco, C., Poudevigne, M. S., & O'Connor, P. J. (2016). Muscle strengthening exercises during pregnancy are associated with increased energy and reduced fatigue. *Journal of Psychosomatic Obstetrics and Gynecology*, 37(2), 68–72.

Warland, J., Dorrian, J., Morrison, J. L., & O'Brien, L. M. (2018). Maternal sleep during pregnancy and poor fetal outcomes: A scoping review of the literature with meta-analysis. *Sleep Medicine Reviews*, 41, 197–219. https://doi.org/10.1016/j.smrv.2018.03.004

Wilson, J. L., Wilson, B. H., & Edwards, J. R. (2018). 13 weeks' gestation heart palpitations chest tightness Dx? *The Journal of Family Practice*, 67(8), E9–E11.

Wu, F., Schallhorn, J. M., & Lowry, E. A. (2020). Refractive status during pregnancy in the United States: Results from NHANES 2005–2008. *Graefe's Archive for Clinical and Experimental Ophthalmology*, 258(3), 663–667. https://doi.org/10.1007/s00417-019-04552-3

Xue, X., Chen, Y., Mao, X., Tu, H., Yang, X., Deng, Z., & Li, N. (2021). Effect of kinesio taping on low back pain during pregnancy: A systematic review and meta-analysis. *BMC Pregnancy and Childbirth*, 21(1), 712. https://doi.org/10.1186/s12884-021-04197-3

Yousif, T., & Anwer, R. N. A. D. (2021). Analysis of epistaxis of pregnancy and association with postpartum hemorrhage. *International Journal of Medicine and Pharmacy and Drug Research*, 5(3), 20–23. https://doi.org/10.22161/ijmpd.5.3.3

16

Oral Health

Julia Lange-Kessler

Relevant Terms

Caries—tooth decay, destruction of the hard outer layer or the enamel of teeth caused by the bacteria in plaque and the acids produced by plaque; can range in color from yellow to black

Early childhood caries—presence of one or more decayed, missing, or filled tooth surfaces due to tooth decay in any primary teeth between birth and 71 months of age

Enamel—the hard outer layer of the tooth that protects from chewing, biting, crunching, and grinding as well as potentially painful temperatures and chemicals

Enamel erosion—loss of tooth enamel over time due to the action of acid in the mouth, typically caused by bacteria, can also occur through frequent vomiting

Gingivitis—a mild form of gum disease that causes inflamed gums that may be red, tender, and sore

HEENOT—the abbreviation for examination of the head, eyes, ears, nose, oral cavity, and throat

Periodontitis—a severe form of gum disease that can affect both the hard and soft tissues surrounding the teeth and can contribute to tooth loss

Plaque—a sticky biofilm of bacteria that continually grows on tooth surfaces within the mouth, initially colorless but can develop pale yellow or brown hues

Pregnancy (pyogenic) granuloma—growth of small nodules in the oral cavity that develop from hormonal changes of pregnancy; these typically resolve spontaneously in the postpartum period

Introduction

Oral health is integral to systemic health and has profound effects during the childbearing year. Nonetheless, pregnancy and newborn complications from poor oral health have only recently been routinely recognized. Preventive dental hygiene, routine dental care, and education can help to ensure a healthy mouth, teeth, and gums. The postpartum time frame presents a critical opportunity for establishing positive mother/baby dyad oral health habits.

Up to 86% of women do not visit a dentist during pregnancy (Lange-Kessler, 2017). Two-thirds of Hispanic and non-Hispanic Black adults have an unmet need for dental treatment as do all people with lower incomes. The oral health status and barriers to dental care for transgender and gender nonbinary individuals remain understudied. A folklore adage claims that "for every baby, a tooth is lost," but this can be prevented with proper attention to the oral cavity and dentition by prenatal healthcare providers. This chapter will present information regarding the ease of performing an oral history and exam as well as the importance of recognition and management of systemic oral health before and during prenatal, postnatal, and newborn care.

Health equity key points

- Dental care is not accessible by many individuals; more people are unable to afford dental care than any other type of healthcare.
- Oral health assessment, education, and preventative services can be easily incorporated into routine prenatal care as one way to address inequities.
- Individuals in marginalized groups bear the greatest burden of oral disease.
- It is incumbent on prenatal healthcare providers to assess the oral health of their pregnant patients and to assist in securing dental services for those in need of dental care.

Prenatal and Postnatal Care: A Person-Centered Approach, Third Edition. Edited by Karen Trister Grace, Cindy L. Farley, Noelene K. Jeffers, and Tanya Tringali.
© 2024 John Wiley & Sons Ltd. Published 2024 by John Wiley & Sons Ltd.
Companion website: www.wiley.com/go/grace/prenatal

Anatomy of the Oral Cavity

The structures of the oral cavity are presented in Figure 16.1. There are eight different types of teeth in the 32 teeth of permanent dentition. Each tooth is anchored in the bony sockets of the mandible or maxilla, with the **enamel**-coated crown exposed. See Figure 16.2 for the internal anatomy of the tooth.

The roof of the oral cavity is formed by the hard and soft palates. The floor consists of soft tissues, which include the tongue. The lateral walls (cheeks) are muscular and merge anteriorly with the lips. The posterior oral cavity opens into the oral part of the pharynx.

Saliva balances the oral flora, helps in the maintenance of enamel, and prevents some oral infections with its antibacterial and antifungal properties. It is mainly produced

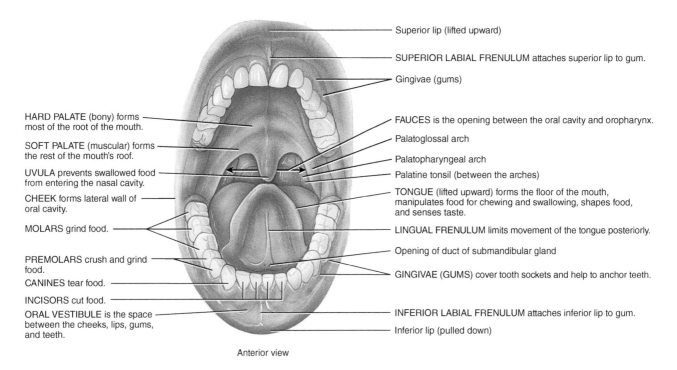

Anterior view

Figure 16.1 Structure of the mouth.

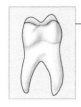
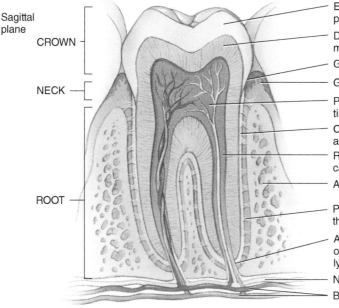

Sagittal section of a mandibular (lower) molar

Figure 16.2 A typical tooth and surrounding structures.

by three pairs of glands and contributes enzymes for the digestion of food.

Initial Assessment of the Oral Cavity

Oral Health History

Open-ended questions provide the most information regarding dental history and understanding of and attitudes toward oral health.

- How often do you brush your teeth?
- How often do you floss?
- Who is your dentist?
- Do you see the dentist for regular check-ups and cleanings?
- Have you seen a dentist or hygienist in the last six months?
- Are you in need of any dental treatment at this time?
- Have you ever had any disease or injury to the mouth or teeth?
- Do you have any dentures or partial plates?
- Do you have dental insurance?

Physical Exam

The first exam during pregnancy typically involves a head-to-toe exam. Many providers have changed the commonly used HEENT acronym (head, eyes, ears, nose, and throat) to **HEENOT** (head, eyes, ears, nose, oral cavity, and throat) so that the oral exam is not forgotten. An oral exam is easy and quick to perform and is conducted to determine the health status of the teeth and gums, and to note any precancerous or cancerous lesions.

Equipment needed for oral cavity examination

- Good light source
- Gloves
- Tongue blade
- Gauze (2 × 2) or (4 × 4)
- Mouth mirror (optional)

The face is examined for asymmetry or abnormal lesions. Lips must be thoroughly examined for evidence of herpes, impetigo, or angular cheilitis, which can also be caused by B_{12} deficiency, candidiasis, or poor-fitting dentures. Nonhealing lesions can indicate skin cancer and should be referred for further evaluation.

To inspect the mucosa and the gums, the insides of the lips are checked by folding the upper lip up and the lower lip down. A healthy mouth has smooth, pink, moist mucosa. Ulcerations or white to gray discolored patches are cause for concern. Gum inflammation and the presence of **plaque** or debris at the gum line or any gingival recession (gums shrinking away from teeth) are noted. This process is repeated for the inside of the cheeks, looking for the same evidence of smooth, pink, and moist mucosa and gums. Again, ulcerations are cause for

concern, particularly in someone who uses any type of tobacco (including smokeless and chewing). Education regarding regular dental visits as well as brushing/flossing is well suited to this part of the exam.

The anterior and posterior surfaces (if possible) of the teeth are examined, noting discoloration, **caries,** plaque, trauma, damaged, or missing teeth. If a mouth mirror is not available, the patient is instructed to tilt the head backward. With the head tilted back, the hard and soft palate are inspected, as these areas can be high-risk areas for oral cancers.

The tongue is an area that is common for the development of precancer or cancer and is often missed during an oral exam. The individual is asked to protrude the tongue in order to inspect the dorsum or anterior surface of the tongue. The tip of the tongue is grasped with the gauze and moved to one side while retracting the cheek with a tongue blade, finger, or mouth mirror in order to visualize posterior lateral margins of the tongue (a cancer-prone area) (NIH, 2021). As an alternative, the care provider can offer the gauze to the client and ask them to pull their tongue to each side so that the inspection can be performed. This process is repeated in the opposite direction for the opposite margin of the tongue.

The posterior pharynx is examined for the symmetry of size and the supporting structures are also examined. A tongue blade will help with holding down the tongue to assist with visualization. Any areas of erythema, exudate, or ulceration are noted. The person is asked to say "Ahhhh" to allow the observation of the movement of the uvula. The floor of the mouth is inspected and palpated by asking the person to lift their tongue to the roof of the mouth.

The observation of any white lesion in the mouth should be referred to a dentist or oral surgeon for further evaluation to rule out cancer. In 2020, oral cancer was ranked the 16th most common cancer globally according to the World Cancer Research Fund. In the United States, an estimated 54,000 cases are diagnosed each year (American Cancer Society, 2022; Oral Cancer Foundation, 2022). Finding oral cancers early allows for treatments that result in successful treatment. The large majority of oral cancers are advanced at the time of detection, leading to an estimated 11,230 deaths per year in the United States; however, it is rare in pregnancy and accounts for 2% of all cancers at this life stage (Sato et al., 2019). One person per hour will die from oral cancer every day (Brocklehurst et al., 2013; American Cancer Society, 2022; Oral Cancer Foundation, 2022). Early cancerous growth can be painless and unnoticed, thus increasing the risk of secondary primary tumors. Secondary primary tumor is the term used to indicate that a person has had a primary cancer in the past. The prognosis for a secondary cancer is poor (Lange-Kessler, 2017). Risk factors for oral and oropharyngeal cancer include the use of tobacco and alcohol as well as exposure to human papillomavirus type 16 (HPV-16). Oral squamous cell carcinoma (OSCC) is common in both the head and the neck. The five-year survival rate is only 50% making oral health a priority for all healthcare providers (Truong et al., 2018).

Dental Care during Pregnancy

All trimesters of pregnancy are safe for dental care (ADA, 2022; Merchant, 2015; CDC, 2022). If a client has not had a visit to the hygienist in the last six months, or if any unusual findings are noted during the oral exam, they should be referred for dental care. Dental X-rays and the use of local anesthetics and some medications are safe during pregnancy. If medications are prescribed, a consultation between the dentist and the prenatal care provider is common.

Influence of Oral Health on Pregnancy Outcomes

Associations have been established between oral health conditions and pregnancy disorders, including gestational diabetes, preeclampsia, preterm birth, and low birth weight (LBW) (Lange-Kessler, 2017). While the pathophysiology is not well understood, the fluctuating hormones of pregnancy are implicated in increased susceptibility to oral disease that in turn affects the pregnancy outcome (Wu et al., 2015).

Gingivitis

The early stage of periodontal disease is **gingivitis** (red and edematous gums). Swollen gums make oral hygiene more difficult. Pregnancy gingivitis is histologically the same as gingivitis in the nonpregnant adult. The inflammation of gums is exacerbated by the hormonal changes of pregnancy that support the development of plaque and is considered transient and resolves for most people in the postpartum period (Silk et al., 2018; Morelli et al., 2018). C-reactive proteins (CRPs) are inflammatory markers associated with chronic and acute infections. Higher levels of CRP have been found in women with gingivitis as well as women with both gingivitis and gestational diabetes together (Gogeneni et al., 2015). It has been suggested that maternal CRP levels in early pregnancy are associated with fetal growth restriction and increased risks of neonatal complications (Ernst et al., 2011; Vecchié et al., 2018; Zerbo et al., 2016). These findings have not been consistently demonstrated across studies (Ahmad et al., 2018). CRP levels are not part of routine prenatal lab tests; however, testing for CRP may be considered in selected cases.

Periodontitis

Left untreated, gingivitis develops into the worsening condition of **periodontitis**, which is a deep inflammation of the gums, ligaments, and bony structures. The gums pull away from the teeth, and supporting gum tissue is destroyed and can result in loose teeth that eventually fall out. Fifty percent of Americans aged 30 or older have some form of periodontitis (American Academy of Periodontology [AAP], 2022). Furthermore, the inflammation of the periodontal structures can provide an open pathway to the blood stream for the more than 150 bacteria that can reside in the mouth, including microbes that are sexually transmitted (see Chapter 56, *Sexually Transmitted Infections and Vaginitis*). Periodontitis is associated with systemic complications such as gestational diabetes mellitus (GDM) (Gogeneni et al., 2015) and preeclampsia (Silk et al., 2018). An association between periodontitis, LBW, and very low birth weight (VLBW) has also been demonstrated (Corbella et al., 2016).

Pregnancy (Pyogenic) Granuloma

Pregnancy (pyogenic) granuloma is a benign growth that is fairly common during pregnancy, affecting 1–5% of pregnant individuals (Kurien et al., 2013). It can develop during any trimester. Under hormonal influence, a highly vascular overgrowth of tissue usually located on the gums can range in size from a few millimeters to a couple of centimeters. It does not need to be treated unless it interferes with the intake of food. It typically resolves without treatment once the pregnancy has ended. While surgery can be performed, 72% of nodules will bleed extensively; this bleeding may be difficult to control when surgery is employed (Gondivkar et al., 2010).

Oral Health and Cultural Beliefs

Culturally influenced beliefs and behaviors affect oral hygiene practices and willingness to engage with dental health professionals. Lifestyle habits and dietary preferences also play a role in oral health and are often rooted in traditions handed down across generations. When caring for immigrants and refugees, it is important to note that many countries do not have dental healthcare systems and few, if any, dentists (World Cancer Research, 2022). For example, Haiti's population of 10 million has approximately 300 dentists, thus limiting dental care to a very few and to dental pain relief and emergency care, not preventative care (Adebayo, 2018).

Little is known about cultural beliefs surrounding oral health. Most information is extracted from epidemiology studies describing race and ethnic background related to incidence of oral disease. However, a literature review exploring oral health beliefs in selected African–American, Chinese, Hispanic, and Filipino groups in the Unites States found that commonalities including the fear of dentists, dental procedures without anesthesia, and previous negative experiences prevent individuals from seeking dental care for themselves and their children (Butani et al., 2008).

Pregnancy Conditions Affecting Oral Health

Certain pregnancy complications may necessitate delaying dental care until later in the pregnancy or until the postpartum period. For example, individuals who develop preeclampsia with severe features can be delayed in their normal dental care unless absolutely necessary for oral pain. People taking heparin for thrombophilia may be predisposed to excessive bleeding during dental procedures and are well advised to delay nonessential procedures until after birth. There is a relationship between glucose control and the health of the mouth. Periodontal changes are often an early clinical manifestation of diabetes. Pregnant people with prepregnancy diabetes and gestational diabetes will particularly benefit from routine and regular oral healthcare.

Prophylactic antibiotics during certain dental procedures that involve the manipulation of the gum tissues are recommended only for those individuals at high risk for developing infective endocarditis, such as those with cyanotic heart disease, a prosthetic heart valve, any prosthetic implant such as a knee replacement, or a prior history of infective endocarditis. During pregnancy, a benign functional heart murmur occurs in 90% of pregnant people and will resolve after pregnancy (see Chapter 5, *Physiologic Alterations during Pregnancy*). A functional heart murmur does not require antibiotics prior to dental treatment; current evidence suggests that antibiotics prior to a dental procedure are not beneficial to individuals with mild to moderate heart conditions and may be harmful (Nishimura et al., 2017). The maintenance of optimal oral health through daily oral hygiene is more important in reducing the risk of infective endocarditis than taking preventive antibiotics before a dental procedure.

Supine positions, such as in a reclining dental chair for a prolonged period of time, can cause a decrease in blood pressure and cardiac output and should be avoided in advanced pregnancy. The weight of the gravid uterus on the vena cava causes a decrease in cardiac output leading to hypotension, nausea, dizziness, and fainting. To prevent hypotensive syndrome, elevate the right hip 10–12 cm, or a 15% tilt can relieve pressure on the vena cava.

With hyperemesis gravidarum or frequent morning sickness, the stomach acids that reflux during vomiting can cause permanent damage to the enamel of the teeth. Rinsing with plain water or water mixed with baking soda (one teaspoon) will limit the damage to enamel.

As the hormone relaxin contributes to a loosening of the uterine ligaments, so too are the periodontal ligaments loosened, leading to possible periodontal disease in the mouth.

The use of tobacco, alcohol, and drugs during or outside of pregnancy can contribute to tooth discoloration, **enamel erosion**, dry mouth, and poor eating and dental hygiene habits, in addition to other serious behavioral and health consequences.

Dental concerns during pregnancy

- Dental care during pregnancy is safe during any trimester.
- Urgent procedures due to dental abscess, such as root canals and tooth extractions, should not be delayed.
- The use of lead aprons renders the risk of radiation exposure extremely low; dental X-rays can be done when indicated.
- Typical medications and anesthetics prescribed by dentists are not a risk to the fetus.
- Gums may bleed more easily during pregnancy, so a gentle approach to brushing and flossing is recommended.

Postpartum and Newborn Oral Health

The postpartum visit is an ideal time to discuss newborn oral health. In doing so, the provider help prevent future pain and suffering of the preventable infectious disease, **early childhood caries** (ECC) (Çolak et al., 2013). ECC is the most common and chronic childhood disease in the United States, affecting 40% of children from 2 to 11 years old (Meyer & Enax, 2018). Parents who are made aware of their influence on oral health for their children may be motivated to prioritize their children's oral health as well as their own. Oral hygiene, habits, and health can be perpetuated from one generation to the next (Shearer et al., 2011). Education and support from prenatal and postpartum care providers can help to promote optimal oral health.

Baby teeth are important for chewing, speaking, and smiling. They hold space in the jaw for permanent teeth. If they are lost too early, permanent teeth can drift, making it difficult for other teeth to find space or causing crooked or crowded teeth (ADA, 2023).

Teeth are susceptible to decay as soon as they erupt. Babies born by cesarean section are at higher risk for caries development. This is thought to be due to the lack of exposure to the maternal vaginal microbiome during the birth process (Smiles for Life, 2021). Evidence shows that parents transmit caries-causing bacteria to their newborns in the first two years of life (Smiles for Life, 2021). *Streptococcus mutans* and *Lactobacilli* species are the most common cariogenic bacteria.

Vertical transmission occurs through sharing food, spoons, or pacifiers. Unrestricted bottle-feeding and intake of fruit juices and sugary liquids can contribute to decay after the eruption of the first tooth. Unrestricted nocturnal breastfeeding can lead to an increased risk of caries (ADA, 2023). Children should be encouraged to drink from a cup by their first birthday to minimize retention of sugars in the oral cavity. Cleaning of the newborn mouth should start on day one of life. The aim is not only to keep the mouth clean but to establish a healthy routine.

How to perform newborn oral care

- Oral care is best done after breakfast and before bed.
- Wash hands thoroughly.
- Use a clean moist gauze or clean moist washcloth.
- Wrap the gauze or cloth around your finger.
- Gently put your finger inside baby's mouth wiping upper and lower gum pads once.
- Switch to a soft toothbrush at the eruption of the first teeth.

Inequities in Oral Health

The United States has a robust dental care system; however, it is not accessible by many individuals. More people are unable to afford dental care than any other type of healthcare (CDC, 2022). There is wide variability in dental coverage provided by private and public insurers, most affecting individuals of marginalized groups who bear the greatest burden of oral disease. Dental care is separated from primary healthcare services and yet oral health is integral to overall health. Oral health is one of the leading health indicators targeted by Healthy People 2030. Pregnant people often face a reluctance to be treated by dental professionals due to the fear of litigation. Oral health assessment, education, and preventative services can be easily incorporated into prenatal care as one way to address these inequities.

Summary

Awareness, treatment, appropriate referral, and education are the cornerstones to healthy parents and baby during the childbearing year, setting the stage for lifelong oral health habits. The provider has the opportunity to impact a positive oral health regimen and to empower current and future generations to achieve overall systemic health (NYU, 2003).

Resources for Pregnant People and Their Families

Pregnancy and teeth: https://www.mouthhealthy.org/life-stages/pregnancy

Babies' and kids' teeth: https://www.mouthhealthy.org/life-stages/babies-and-kids

American Academy of Pediatrics, *Protect Tiny Teeth Toolkit for Pregnant and New Moms.*

https://www.healthychildren.org/English/ages-stages/prenatal/Pages/Protect-Tiny-Teeth.aspx

Resources for Healthcare Providers

Oral Health and Primary Care Integration: https://bphc.hrsa.gov/technical-assistance/clinical-quality-improvement/oral-health-primary-care-integration

Oral Health Campaign Toolkit from the American Academy of Pediatrics: https://www.aap.org/en/newsroom/campaigns-and-toolkits/oral-health

References

Adebayo, Z. (2018) *Confronting oral health in Haiti*. The Borgen Project. https://borgenproject.org/oral-health-in-haiti

Ahmad, A., Nazar, Z., & Swaminathan, D. (2018). C-reactive protein levels and periodontal diseases during pregnancy in Malaysian women. *Oral Health and Preventive Dentistry, 16*(3), 281–289. https://pubmed.ncbi.nlm.nih.gov/30027167/

American Academy of Periodontology (AAP). (2022). *Gum disease risk factors*. https://www.perio.org/for-patients/gum-disease-information/gum-disease-risk-factors

American Cancer Society (ACS). (2022, January 12). *Key statistics for oral cavity and oropharyngeal cancers*. https://www.cancer.org/cancer/oral-cavity-and-oropharyngeal-cancer/about/key-statistics.html

American Dental Association (ADA). (2022). *Is it safe to go to the dentist during pregnancy?* Mouth Healthy. https://www.mouthhealthy.org/life-stages/pregnancy/pregnancy-dental-concerns.

American Dental Association (ADA). (2023). *Should I Worry about Cavities in Baby Teeth?* https://www.mouthhealthy.org/all-topics-a-z/baby-teeth

Brocklehurst, P., Kujan, O., O'Malley, L. A., Shepherd, S., & Glenny, A. M. (2013). Screening programs for the early detection and prevention of oral cancer. *Cochrane Database Systematic Reviews, 11*, CD004150. https://pubmed.ncbi.nlm.nih.gov/24254989

Butani, Y., Weintraub, J. A., & Barker, J. C. (2008). Oral health-related cultural beliefs for four racial/ethnic groups: Assessment of the literature. *BMC Oral Health, 8*(1), 1–13. https://doi.org/10.1186/1472-6831-8-26

Centers for Disease Control and Prevention [CDC]. (2022). *Disparities in oral health*. https://www.cdc.gov/oralhealth/oral_health_disparities/index.htm

Çolak, H., Dülgergil, Ç. T., Dalli, M., & Hamidi, M. M. (2013). Early childhood caries update: A review of causes, diagnoses, and treatments. *Journal of Natural Science, Biology, and Medicine, 4*(1), 29–38. https://www.ncbi.nlm.nih.gov/pmc/articles/PMC3633299

Corbella, S., Taschieri, S., Del Fabbro, M., Francetti, L., Weinstein, R., & Ferrazzi, E. (2016). Adverse pregnancy outcomes and periodontitis: A systematic review and meta-analysis exploring potential association. *Quintessence International Periodontology, 47*(3), 193–204. http://www.quintpub.com/userhome/qi/qi_47_3_corbella_p193.pdf

Ernst, G. D. S., de Jonge, L. L., Hofman, A., Lindemans, J., Russcher, H., Steegers, A., & Jaddoe, W. V. V. (2011). C-reactive protein levels in early pregnancy, fetal growth patterns, and the risk for neonatal complications: The generation R study. *American Journal of Obstetrics and Gynecology, 205*(2), 132.e1–132e12. https://doi.org/10.1016/j.ajog.2011.03.049

Gogeneni, H., Buduneli, N., Ceyhan-Ozturk, B., Gumus, P., Akcali, A., Zeller, I., Renaud, D., Scott, D. A., & Ozcaka, O. (2015). Increased infection with key periodontal pathogens during gestational diabetes mellitus. *Journal of Clinical Periodontology, 42*(6), 506–512. https://doi.org/10.1111/jcpe.12418

Gondivkar, S. M., Gadbail, A., & Chole, R. (2010). Oral pregnancy tumor. *Contemporary Clinical Dentistry, 1*(3), 190–192. https://doi.org/10.4103/0976-237X.72792

Kurien, S., Kattimani, V. S., Sriram, R. R., Sriram, S. K., Rao, V. K. P., Bhupathi, A., & Patil, N. (2013). Management of pregnant patient in dentistry. *Journal of International Oral Health: JIOH, 5*(1), 88–97. https://www.ncbi.nlm.nih.gov/pmc/articles/PMC3768073

Lange-Kessler, J. (2017). A literature review on women's oral health across the life span. *Nursing for Women's Health, 21*(2), 108–121. https://doi.org/10.1016/j.nwh.2017.02.010

Meyer, F., & Enax, J. (2018). Early childhood caries: Epidemiology, aetiology, and prevention. *International Journal of Dentistry, 2018*, 1415873, 7 pages. https://doi.org/10.1155/2018/1415873

Morelli, E. L., Broadbent, J. M., Leichter, J. W., & Thomson, W. M. (2018). Pregnancy, parity and periodontal disease. *Australian Dental Journal, 63*(3), 270–278. https://doi.org/10.1111/adj.12623

NIH National Cancer Institute. (2021). Lip and oral cavity cancer treatment (adult). https://www.cancer.gov/types/head-and-neck/patient/adult/lip-mouth-treatment-pdq

Nishimura, R. A., Otto, C. M., Bonow, R. O., Carabello, B. A., Erwin, J. P., Fleisher, L. A., Jneid, H., Mack, M. J., McLeod, C. J., O'Gara, P. T., Rigolin, V. H., Sundt, T. M., & Thompson, A. (2017). 2017 AHA/ACC focused update of the 2014 AHA/ACC guideline for the management of patients with valvular heart disease: A report of the American College of Cardiology/American Heart Association Task Force on Clinical Practice Guidelines. *Journal of the American College of Cardiology, 70*(2), 252–289. https://doi.org/10.1016/j.jacc.2017.03.011

NYU Dentistry. (2003). *The oral health system next door: A first-hand look at dental care in Cuba*. Global Health Nexus. https://dental.nyu.edu/aboutus/news/nexus/summer-2003/dental-care-in-cuba.html

Oral Cancer Foundation. (2022). *The oral cancer foundation*. http://oralcancerfoundation.org

Sato, K., Shimamoto, H., Mochizuki, Y., Hirai, H., Tomioka, H., Shimizu, R., Marukawa, E., Fukayama, H., Yoshimura, I., Ishida, H., & Harada, H. (2019). Treatment of oral cancers during pregnancy: A case-based discussion. *Journal of Otolaryngology-Head & Neck Surgery, 48*(1), 1–7. https://doi.org/10.1186/s40463-019-0331-1

Shearer, D. M., Thomson, W. M., Broadbent, J. M., & Poulton, R. (2011). Maternal oral health predicts their children's caries experience in adulthood. *Journal of Dental Research, 90*(5), 672–677. https://www.ncbi.nlm.nih.gov/pmc/articles/PMC3144114

Silk, H., Savageau, J. A., Sullivan, K., Sawosik, G., & Wang, M. (2018). An update of oral health curricula in US family medicine residency programs. *Family Medicine*, 50(6), 437–443. https://doi.org/10.22454/FamMed.2018.372427

Smiles for Life. (2021). *Caries risk transmission from mother to child.* https://www.smilesforlifeoralhealth.org/topic/caries-risk-transmission-from-mother-to-child/#:~:text=Mothers%20are%20the%20main%20source,tasting%20or%20pre%2Dchewing%20food.

Truong, M. T., Nadershah, M., Langmore, S. E., Kuno, H., Sakai, O., Salama, A., Arya, V., Jalisi, S., & Rubin, S. T. (2018). Advanced floor of mouth cancer. In R. B. Bell, R. P. Fernandes, & P. E. Andersen (Eds.), *Oral, head and neck oncology and reconstructive surgery* (pp. 428–457). Elsevier. https://doi.org/10.1016/B978-0-323-26568-3.00022-1

Vecchié, A., Bonaventura, A., Carbone, F., Maggi, D., Carloni, B., Andraghetti, G., Affinito Bonabello, L., Liberale, L., Dallegri, F.,

Montecucco, F., & Cordera, R. (2018). C-reactive protein levels at the midpregnancy can predict gestational complications. *BioMed Research International*, (2018). Article ID 1070151. https://www.hindawi.com/journals/bmri/2018/1070151/5

World Cancer Research. (2022). *Mouth and oral cancer statistics.* https://www.wcrf.org/cancer-trends/mouth-and-oral-cancer-statistics

Wu, M., Chen, S. W., & Jiang, S.-Y. (2015). *Relationship between gingival inflammation and pregnancy. Mediators of Inflammation*, 2015(623427), 1–11. https://doi.org/10.1155/2015/623427

Zerbo, O., Traglia, M., Yoshida, C., Heuer, L. S., Ashwood, P., Delorense, G. N., Hansen, R. L., Kharrazi, M., Van de Water, J., Yolken, R. H., Weiss, L. A., & Croen, L. A. (2016). Maternal mid-pregnancy C-reactive protein and risk of autism spectrum disorders: The early markers for autism study. *Translational Psychiatry*, 6, e783. https://doi.org/10.1038/tp.2016.46

17

Medication Use during Pregnancy

Katie McDevitt

The editors gratefully acknowledge Mary C. Brucker and Tekoa L. King, who were co-authors of the previous edition of this chapter.

Relevant Terms

Adverse drug effect—response to a drug that is noxious and unintended, and which occurs at doses normally used for prophylaxis, diagnosis, or therapy of disease or for the modification of physiological function

Background risk—risk that is unavoidable; in pregnancy, the background risk of a congenital anomaly is estimated at approximately 3–5%

Behind-the-counter drug—a subtype of over-the-counter drugs, behind-the-counter drugs are nonprescription but are not on open shelving due to potential for abuse after modification; the most common example is pseudoephedrine, which can be made into a type of amphetamine

Black box warning aka Boxed Warnings—a method that the US Food and Drug Administration uses to identify unusual harm associated with an agent; often, it is added to package inserts after postmarketing studies to identify unexpected risks

Botanicals—biologically based therapy using ingredients that are found in nature, including plants, herbs, food, and vitamins used for medicinal purposes

Brand name—a trademarked name assigned to a drug by the manufacturer

Clinical trials—any study that prospectively assigns human subjects to one or more interventions or drugs to ascertain effectiveness and safety

Controlled substance—pharmaceuticals listed in schedules found in Title 21 of the United States Code, section 802(32)(A); these agents include both opiates as well as nonopiates; focus is on agents that have a high risk of addiction, including those lacking valid medicinal use such as heroin and cocaine

Critical period—time in gestation that a particular organ or body part of the embryo or fetus is most susceptible to teratogenic damage

Cytochrome P450—a large family of enzymes involved with metabolism, especially of lipids, steroidal hormones, toxins, and various drugs; genetic variations within the subgroups of the family are often the etiology of drug–drug or drug–other agent interactions

Herbals—remedies that are derived from plants, sometimes considered a subset of botanicals and sometimes used interchangeably with the term botanicals

Nutritional/dietary supplements—food, vitamins, minerals, or herbs taken by mouth intended to restore nutrients to the body for health benefits

Off-label—the use of pharmaceutical drugs for an unapproved indication or in an unapproved age group, dosage, or route of administration

Over-the-counter drug—a drug available directly to consumers without a prescription

Pharmacogenetics—study of how specific variations in a gene can affect a person's response to a drug.

Pharmacogenomics—study of how all of a person's genes (genome) influence responses to drugs.

Pharmacodynamics—study of drug concentration and the recipient's response, including the drug's effects, duration, and magnitude of the physiologic response in relationship to the drug dose

Pharmacokinetics—process of drug absorption, distribution, metabolism, and elimination

Polypharmacy—the practice of treating individuals using multidrug regimens; generally accepted to mean administration of five or more drugs

Prescriptive authority—legal ability to prescribe drugs, medical devices, adjunct health/medical services, durable healthcare goods, and other equipment and supplies that are limited by state and federal law

Prescription drugs—agents that have been approved by the FDA in the United States, available by prescription only through a health professional with prescriptive authority

Teratogen—an agent (drug, virus, disease, or other) that causes a permanent congenital anomaly when taken during a critical period in embryonic or fetal development; from the Greek term for "monster"

Therapeutic window—plasma drug concentration in between the minimum effective concentration for obtaining the desired drug action and the mean toxic concentration

---

Prenatal and Postnatal Care: A Person-Centered Approach, Third Edition. Edited by Karen Trister Grace, Cindy L. Farley, Noelene K. Jeffers, and Tanya Tringali.
© 2024 John Wiley & Sons Ltd. Published 2024 by John Wiley & Sons Ltd.
Companion website: www.wiley.com/go/grace/prenatal

Introduction

Healthcare providers need solid diagnostic skills and a broad knowledge of effective therapeutic interventions, including nutrition, physical exercise, emotional support, and both pharmacologic and nonpharmacologic agents. Today, more than ever, healthcare providers must also be knowledgeable about the effects of medications. Office visits for healthcare result in the prescription of therapeutic drugs 68.7% of the time (Centers for Disease Control and Prevention [CDC], 2021a). The use of prescription medications during the first trimester has increased more than 60% over the last 30 years (CDC, 2020).

Clinically relevant pharmacologic information that is applicable to reproductive-aged people can be difficult to obtain because data about the pharmacologic effects of drugs on people who are pregnant or capable of becoming pregnant are limited. Drug trials often have a lower percentage of people who were assigned female sex at birth (AFAB) enrolled than people who were assigned male sex at birth (AMAB), and when AFAB people are included in drug trials, sex-specific analysis may not be conducted or published (Franconi et al., 2007). Sex differences in pharmacokinetics strongly predict sex-specific adverse drug reactions for AFAB people but not for AMAB participants (Zucker & Prendergast, 2020). The data are sparse with regard to pregnant and lactating people; however, it is well documented that there are physiologic changes between pregnant and nonpregnant people that impact drug efficacy (Patil et al., 2017; Scaffidi et al., 2016). Reasons for the lack of studies focusing on pregnant, postpartum, or lactating people include ethical dilemmas, potential fetal risks, or legal liability years after use. However, since approximately 4 million pregnant people give birth in the United States every year (Osterman et al., 2022), pharmacologic principles that apply to this population represent an essential body of knowledge for clinicians who care for pregnant and lactating people. In addition, structural racism affects many aspects of drug development, including which research gets funded, who receives a patent, and who is included in clinical trials. This is evident in the research and development of medications for patients, mostly White, who have cystic fibrosis versus the investment in research for sickle cell disease, in which most patients are Black (Krishtel, 2021). Medications may be indicated and should be used for the well-being of the patient and their offspring. This chapter reviews basic principles of prescribing and presents an overview of pregnancy-specific pharmacologic topics to assist providers when they engage in shared decision-making with pregnant patients.

Types of Pharmaceutical Agents

Pharmaceutical agents include all chemical substances used for the prevention, treatment, or cure of diseases. The majority of pharmaceutical agents are referred to as drugs or medications. Nonprescription agents include **over-the-counter (OTC) medicines**, **behind-the-counter (BTC) medicines**, and **herbals**, including **nutritional supplements**, **dietary supplements**, and **botanicals**. **Nonprescription agents** may be pharmacologically active and can be obtained directly without a prescription from a healthcare provider. **Prescription drugs** can only be dispensed if the medication is prescribed by a properly authorized clinician.

In addition to nonprescription and prescription drugs, individuals may be exposed to pharmaceuticals in other ways. For example, hormones and antimicrobials fed to animals enter the food chain. An analysis of water in the Great Lakes conducted in 2010 found that almost 35% of surface water contained traces of various pharmaceuticals (Klecka et al., 2010). Years ago, people were advised to discard out-of-date medications by flushing them down a toilet or washing them through the kitchen garbage disposal. These practices are no longer recommended due to concerns about environmental contamination. The current recommendation is to take unused medications to a local pharmacy or governmental agency that offers the disposal of pharmaceuticals (US FDA, 2020). Medications and their metabolites in the environment can have pharmacologic effects that result in endocrine disruptions, including abnormalities in menstrual cycles and neurodevelopmental disorders in children (Bennett et al., 2016).

Prescriptive Authority

Prescriptive authority is governed by state statute. Historically, physicians have had the broadest authority to prescribe drugs and medical devices; today, other healthcare providers also have various degrees of prescriptive authority, including dentists, midwives, nurse practitioners, podiatrists, psychologists, physician assistants, and veterinarians (Osborne, 2015; Plank, 2011). The type of prescriptive authority possessed by these clinicians varies by jurisdiction and may be limited by the discipline's professional scope of practice and evidence of successful completion of specific initial education and continuing education in pharmacology.

Governmental Oversight of Pharmaceutical Agents

Several different federal agencies regulate pharmaceutical agents. The US Food and Drug Administration (FDA) has authority to approve, monitor, and withdraw prescription and nonprescription agents, and monitor drug advertising.

Health equity key points

- Structural racism affects many aspects of drug development, including which research gets funded, who receives a patent, and who is included in clinical trials.
- Structural and institutional racism has decreased access to and affordability of medications for communities of color.
- Medications used to treat illnesses that disproportionately impact communities of color cost more, including medications for diabetes and some respiratory diseases.

An important exception concerns nutritional supplements and botanical agents. These products are not classified as drugs and are, therefore, not regulated by the FDA with regard to safety or efficacy. These agents can, however, have significant pharmacologic effects, including interactions with other prescribed drugs.

In addition to the FDA, other agencies that regulate pharmaceuticals include the Federal Trade Commission (FTC), which is authorized to monitor direct-to-consumer advertising of OTC medications. The Drug Enforcement Administration (DEA) regulates **controlled substance** drugs that have significant risks of addiction. These agents commonly are subdivided into five categories ranked from highest to lowest potential for addiction (Table 17.1). Agents in the first category (schedule I) include drugs rarely if ever prescribed for therapeutic reasons, such as heroin and cocaine. Agents in the last category (schedule V) may be indicated for therapeutic use and include cough suppressants that contain codeine in amounts no more than 200 mg of codeine per 100 mL or per 100 g (US Department of Justice and DEA, 2022). The DEA issues specific prescriber numbers to healthcare providers who are approved to write prescriptions for controlled substances. The agency monitors those prescriptions through DEA audits of provider records by Diversion Investigators. These audits may be complaint-driven or random to ensure compliance with laws and regulations governing the prescription of controlled substances. In some jurisdictions, the prescriptive authority of providers other than physicians may be limited based on controlled substance categories.

Of all the illicit or recreational drugs in popular use, marijuana is the most common. An increasing number of states are legalizing this drug for medicinal or recreational use. As this book goes to press, 18 states and the District of Columbia (DC) have legalized marijuana for recreational use and 38 states and DC for medical use. Concerns have been raised regarding the safety of marijuana use during pregnancy and lactation (Berke et al., 2022; Volkow et al., 2017). There is a misconception that if marijuana is legal, it must be safe; increasing use in pregnancy has been noted with the legalization of marijuana. See Chapter 18, *Substance Use during Pregnancy,* for detailed information on marijuana and other substances in pregnancy and lactation.

Premarketing Drug Testing

When a pharmaceutical company seeks FDA approval to market a drug for the treatment of a specific condition, they conduct preapproval studies that are designed to demonstrate the drug's efficacy and safety. In the past

Table 17.1 Schedules for Controlled Substances

Schedule	Definition/examples
I	Substances in this schedule have a high potential for abuse, have no currently accepted medical use for treatment in the United States, and there is a lack accepted safety for use of the drug or other substance under medical supervision. Some examples of substances listed in schedule I are heroin, lysergic acid diethylamide (LSD), marijuana (cannabis)[a], peyote, methaqualone, and 3,4-methylenedioxymethamphetamine ("Ecstasy").
II/IIN	Substances in this schedule have a high potential for abuse, which may lead to severe psychological or physical dependence. Schedule II narcotic substances include combination products containing less than 15 mg of hydrocodone per dosage unit (Vicodin®), hydromorphone (Dilaudid®), methadone (Dolophine®), meperidine (Demerol®), oxycodone (OxyContin®), and fentanyl (Sublimaze® or Duragesic®). Examples of schedule IIN stimulants include amphetamines (Dexedrine®, Adderall®), methamphetamine (Desoxyn®), and methylphenidate (Ritalin®). Other schedule II substances include cocaine, amobarbital, glutethimide, and pentobarbital.
III	Substances in this schedule have less potential for abuse than substances in schedules I or II, and abuse may lead to moderate or low physical dependence or high psychological dependence. Examples of schedule III narcotics include products containing not more than 90 mg of codeine per dosage unit (Tylenol with Codeine®). Also included are buprenorphine products (Suboxone® and Subutex®) used to treat opioid addiction. Examples of schedule III nonnarcotics include benzphetamine (Didrex®), phendimetrazine, ketamine, and anabolic steroids such as Depo® (Testoterone).
IV	Substances in this schedule have a low potential for abuse relative to substances in schedule III. Examples of schedule IV narcotics are alprazolam (Xanax®), carisoprodol (Soma®), clonazepam (Klonopin®), clorazepate (Tranxene®), diazepam (Valium®), lorazepam (Ativan®), midazolam (Versed®), temazepam (Restoril®), and triazolam (Halcion®).
V	Substances in this schedule have a low potential for abuse relative to substances listed in schedule IV and consist primarily of preparations containing limited quantities of certain narcotics. These are generally used for antitussive, antidiarrheal, and analgesic purposes. Examples include cough preparations containing not more than 200 mg of codeine per 100 mL or per 100 g (Robitussin AC® and Phenergan with Codeine), and ezogabine.

Source: Adapted from: US Department of Justice and Department of Drug Enforcement Administration (2022).
[a] Since the establishment of the Controlled Substances Act (CSA) in 1970, marijuana has been listed as a schedule I controlled substance. The inclusion of marijuana as a schedule I controlled substance has implications for research, legal consequences, and business funding. In 2016, the DEA and the FDA rejected two petitions to move marijuana to a less-restrictive schedule under the CSA (Sacco, 2022).

few years, there have been concerns that drug manufacturers might selectively report only **clinical trials** that were favorable to their products. Today, all clinical trials are required to be registered with the FDA (US National Institutes of Health [NIH], 2022). Clinical trials with human subjects occur in three phases. Phase I trials study healthy individuals to determine the **pharmacokinetics** and **pharmacodynamics** of an agent. Phase II trials enroll small numbers of persons with the disorder of interest to determine the initial efficacy of a medication. Phase III trials enroll larger numbers of individuals to see if the initial efficacy is statistically and clinically significant. The FDA's Center for Drug Evaluation and Research (CDER) evaluates the results of these clinical trials and recommends or denies approval of the medication. Despite this three-tiered system, some adverse effects of medications are not discovered until large groups of individuals use it for a length of time after it has been approved.

It is important to note that a drug can be prescribed to treat a disorder that the drug is not specifically approved to treat. **Off-label** prescriptions are legal and common; it is estimated that one in five prescriptions written today are for off-label uses. An example of off-label prescribing is the use of misoprostol (Cytotec®), a drug that has the FDA approval for the indication of treating an individual with ulcers but is used off-label for cervical ripening prior to induction of labor and as part of regimens for medication abortion.

The Prescription: Essential Components

Historically, prescriptions have been written on a paper pad of preprinted blanks and given to a consumer who took the paper to a pharmacy where the medication was dispensed. These prescription pads had important components essential for security and prevention of fraud such as anticopy watermarks, ink that turns a copy black upon photocopying, colored backgrounds to prevent erasures, unique batch numbers, and even UV fibers similar to US currency embedded in the paper on which the prescription is written. Today, electronic methods of prescribing (e-prescribing) provide technological protections from fraud and have the additional advantage of minimizing medical errors from illegible handwriting. Drop-down menus of standard drug dosages help to eliminate erroneous prescriptions. e-prescribing is promoted as a component of electronic health records through federal campaigns including Medicare. In 2020, 84% of all prescriptions were sent electronically. 89% of noncontrolled substances were electronically prescribed and 58% of controlled substances. The COVID-19 pandemic increased the rate of electronic prescribing due to the increase in telehealth (Surescripts, LLC., 2021). Effective in 2013, Center for Medicaid and Medicare Services (CMS) established its e-prescribing rule, which is a part of their "meaningful use" incentive program to encourage more efficient and higher quality healthcare systems.

In 2022, CMS released the Fee Schedule Rule that implements phase 2 of Section 2003 of the SUPPORT Act. The Rule requires electronic prescriptions for schedule II, III, IV, and V controlled substances under Medicare Part D (CMS, 2021a). With the implementation of such legislation and the increased accuracy with e-prescribing, the number of prescriptions sent electronically will continue to increase.

Regardless of whether the prescription is handwritten or electronic, several essential components are required. These include the name, address, and phone number of the provider. If a provider is in a group practice, a listing of all members may be included, but the individual prescriber should be indicated. Prescriptions also include the consumer's name, age, address, and current date; generic or brand name of medication; dose; amount to be dispensed; and number of times the medication can be refilled. The letters "RX" or "R" are included to signify the "recipe" and to verify that this is a drug prescription; the provider's signature or e-signature, license number, and National Provider Identifier (NPI) or DEA number are included. The CMS issues the NPI, which is a unique identifier for healthcare providers that does not disclose any information about the provider (CMS, 2021b). The DEA number is a unique number created using a standardized coding method that identifies the type of provider through a letter prefix. The DEA is charged with monitoring the prescription of controlled substances only. Since May 2013, the NPI number is required on all prescriptions for controlled and noncontrolled substances (CMS, n.d.).

The use of the generic name for a particular medication on the prescription allows the pharmacist to dispense a less expensive formulation if one is available. Some prescribers will choose to request a particular **brand name** and indicate in writing that no substitution should be given. Some medications have variable biologic effects in different formulations. When this is the case, a specific brand name may be necessary to ensure a consistent effect. In those unusual situations, a note clarifying why the brand is medically indicated should be placed in the health record. Access to affordable generic and, when indicated, brand name medications is essential for all patients; however, structural and institutional racism has decreased access to and affordability of medications for communities of color. In addition, many medications used to treat illnesses that disproportionately impact communities of color cost more, including medications for diabetes and some respiratory diseases (Kogut, 2020).

Unintended distortion in writing a prescription can have severe consequences. With the vast array of pharmaceutical agents available, many with similar sounding or looking names, attention should be devoted to error prevention at each instance of prescribing. Because many distortions arise from misunderstood translations of symbols or abbreviations, they are also some of the most remediable sources of medical errors. Components of safe prescription writing are listed in the text box.

Safe prescription writing

Specify drug name. Be sure to spell correctly.

Specify exact dose to be taken.

Specify exact quantities to be dispensed. For example, 30 tablets.

Specify the therapeutic duration.

Specify route of administration. For example, by mouth.

Specify how many doses are taken at one time. For example, 2 tablets.

Specify the number of times per day or hour intervals. For example, every eight hours.

Specify how drug should be taken. For example, with food.

Use a zero before the decimal point if dosage is < one unit. For example, 0.25 mcg.

Avoid trailing zeros. For example, 250 mg, **not** 250.0 mg.

Avoid abbreviations. For example, spell out units instead of abbreviating.

Specify the number of refills.

Include the date and signature by a legal prescriber.

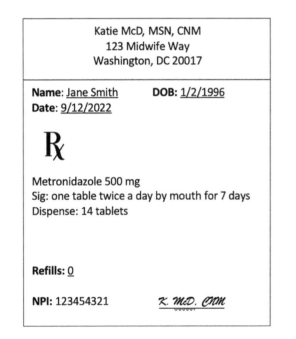

FDA Categories for Drugs in Pregnancy

In 1979, the FDA published a pregnancy-specific categorization of drugs in an attempt to facilitate the recognition of teratogenic drugs, so the agents could be avoided or at least used judiciously (US FDA, 1979). The five categories (A, B, C, D, and X) were replaced in 2015 with a newer and more extensive narrative system. Although a new law required that the old categories be removed from drug labels by 2018, they remain in use today.

The older letter categories were not well defined and not useful for clinical practice. For example, few drugs were able to meet the rigor required to be a category A drug, meaning that adequate research has demonstrated no risk to the fetus in the first trimester or later trimesters. Therefore, a large number of agents such as vitamins,

anti-infectives, and pharmaceuticals used to treat common conditions such as headache were listed in category B, even though most clinicians and researchers described them as safe. Drugs assigned to categories D and X are known **teratogens**, but the two categories are divided on the basis of whether or not the clinical indication for the drug outweighs the risk of using it, requiring clinical acumen of the provider. For example, some commonly used anticonvulsants were classified as category D because the risk of teratogenicity was not absolute, and the pregnant person's need for the drug could be significant. In contrast, isotretinoin (Accutane) was a category X agent because there are no known situations in which the treatment of acne outweighs the potential teratogenic risk. FDA category C contained the most complex array of medications and because of this, it is the most confusing. Category C drugs included drugs that cause teratogenic effects in animals but have no apparent untoward effects in humans. The prototypical drug for this class is a corticosteroid that is linked to birth defects in rabbits but has not been linked to abnormalities in humans. Additionally, drugs for which no data on safety during pregnancy exist are assigned to category C. Most pharmaceutical agents fall into this subcategory of the larger category C. Therefore, the fewest number of drugs were found in categories A and X, yet those categories had definitions that are the most useful for clinical decision-making. Drugs from any category can also carry a [black] boxed warning, which alerts health care providers and consumers to the increased risk of serious adverse reactions associated with the use of the drug or restrictions to the use of the drug (Clinical info HIV.gov, n.d.).

Adding to confusion with the letter system, the FDA developed and published the categorization method, but drug manufacturers were responsible for assigning a drug to a specific category. Since there are few well-controlled studies on therapeutic drugs in pregnant people, most information about drug safety during pregnancy is derived from animal studies, uncontrolled studies, and postmarketing surveillance.

In large part because of controversies about the overly simplistic system, risks of inaccurate interpretation, and emerging data provided by new research, the FDA approved a new labeling system in 2015, termed the FDA Pregnancy/Lactation Labeling Rule (PLLR). This system focuses on the reproductive safety of drugs for individuals in one of three categories: (a) people who are pregnant; (b) people who are lactating; and (c) people who are of reproductive age (US FDA, 2021). The labeling rule is found within the section of the law pertaining to drug labeling in general, and specifically under the section titled *Special Populations*.

Although the newer system is more comprehensive, it does not answer all the problems a clinician faces when assessing the effectiveness and safety of a particular drug. The narrative approach means clinicians are responsible to carefully read the narrative information, consider the research, and share the data with a person considering use of the drug. The PLLR promotes pregnancy drug registries that providers must be aware of and use when appropriate. The new PLLR labeling is being introduced gradually. All drugs that have been approved since 2001 (brand and generics) must have the new system in place. Drugs approved before June 2001 do not need to immediately implement the rule, although as of 2018, these older drugs can no longer use the older ABCDX categories in their labeling. In addition, this rule does not apply to OTC drugs, BTC drugs, botanicals, herbals, or nutritional supplements. A 2020 review found that while many new therapeutics complied with the PLLR regulation, more than a one-third of labels remain out of compliance, and less than 20% of new product labeling contained human data on pregnancy and lactation (Bryne et al., 2020).

Medication Use during Pregnancy

The use of medications during pregnancy has increased over the past three to four decades, including use during the first trimester. According to the CDC, about 90% of pregnant people take at least one drug, 70% take at least one prescription medication, and a growing number of pregnant people take four or more drugs (CDC, 2020). The most commonly used medications by pregnant people include acetaminophen (19.9%), antiemetics or gastrointestinal agents (34.3%), and antibiotics (25.5%) by pregnant people (Haas et al., 2018).

In addition to prescription-only and OTC drugs, the estimate for pregnant people using herbal medications, such as *Echinacea purpurea,* ginger, cranberry, or raspberry leaves, to treat a common discomfort of pregnancy ranges from 10% to 73% in the United States (Sarecka-Hujar & Szulc-Musioł, 2022).

Teratology

A major concern about the use of medications during pregnancy is the risk of harm to the fetus, which in many cases is unknown. For the pregnant person and their healthcare provider, this can be a complex challenge as they weigh the risks versus benefits of pharmacologic treatment. For example, a pregnant person with a seizure disorder may be at risk of experiencing status epilepticus with significant oxygen deprivation for themselves and their fetus, or, if treated with an anticonvulsant, they may have an increased risk of a specific birth defect for the fetus. The likelihood of adverse events if a disorder is untreated should be weighed against the likelihood of adverse effects of the drug for the pregnant person and/or fetus. The identification of the fetal risk associated with individual drugs is difficult because few clinical trials have included pregnant participants. In addition, the identification of fetal harm may take several years to become apparent.

Drugs used by a pregnant person can cause direct harm to the fetus in two ways: teratogenesis and/or fetotoxicity. Teratogens cause permanent change in structure, function, or growth. Most of the well-known teratogenic drugs interfere with organogenesis during the embryonic period, which results in birth defects such as a cleft palate, cardiac anomaly, facial abnormality, or other dysmorphic effects. Fetotoxic agents, like tetracycline, exert effects on growth or fetal development in the second and third trimesters such as fetal growth restriction (FGR). Fetotoxic agents can also be teratogens.

The first teratogen discovered was not of pharmaceutical origin but was viral—rubella. Congenital rubella syndrome was identified in the early 1940s by Norman Gregg, an Australian ophthalmologist, who noticed that there was an increase in neonatal cataracts after an outbreak of rubella some months before (Dunn, 2007). Gregg's discovery was counter to the then prevailing theory that the placenta provided an impenetrable barrier that protected the fetus, and therefore, any birth defect must be solely inheritable. This observation changed the understanding about the risk to the fetus from environmental exposures. More recently, the Zika RNA virus has been identified as a viral teratogen, associated with birth defects that include microcephaly, neurodevelopmental abnormalities, brain anomalies, eye anomalies, and hearing loss (Benavides-Lara et al., 2021). The COVID-19 virus has not been associated with birth defects; however, cohort studies are underway to see if there are developmental effects.

In the United States, the public became aware of the risk of drugs in pregnancy when mass media widely publicized the dangers of thalidomide. In the late 1950s, thalidomide, produced in Germany, was prescribed as a sedative and antiemetic and marketed primarily as a treatment for people with nausea and vomiting of pregnancy. Data regarding teratogenic effects emerged in Europe, while the FDA was scrutinizing the agent for approval in the United States. The data revealed that thalidomide interrupts limb formation such that exposed embryos are born with various limb deformities. Although the drug was never FDA approved for use in pregnancy, it was estimated that several thousand pregnant people residing in the United States took thalidomide via the samples provided to physicians in anticipation of FDA approval. After the thalidomide tragedy was recognized, the FDA imposed stricter regulations for the approval of new drugs. A result of the thalidomide tragedy was a general shift to the public belief that all drugs are potential teratogens until disproven, and the misconception that drugs are the most common etiology for birth effects.

Etiology of Congenital Anomalies

The **background risk** of congenital anomalies secondary to unknown causes is approximately 3–5% of all births (MotherToBaby, 2021). An estimated 65–70% of anomalies are idiopathic with no known etiology (Jacobs et al., 1974; Koren, 2011). Additionally, about 25% of anomalies are identified as having a genetic cause. As illustrated in Figure 17.1, drugs and chemicals account for about 1% of all identified anomalies. The other causes of congenital anomalies include perinatal diseases, bacterial and viral infections, radiation, chemicals, and various environmental insults.

Although the number of medications prescribed during pregnancy has increased during recent years, the

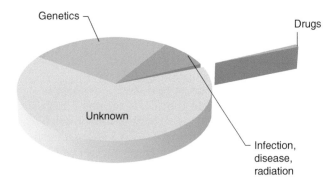

Figure 17.1 Causes of congenital anomalies. Adapted from: Jacobs et al. (1974) and Koren (2011).

number of known teratogenic drugs has remained remarkably small with only a few new discoveries in recent decades. In addition, even though the number of congenital anomalies due to pharmaceutical agents also is limited, the emphasis on teratogenic drugs remains important because any drug-associated birth defect can potentially be avoided entirely if the drug is not taken during pregnancy.

Mechanisms of Teratogenic Drugs

Contemporary to the thalidomide event, embryologist Wilson identified six principles of teratology that continue to be relevant today (Friedman, 2010; Wilson, 1959, 1977; Table 17.2). In the first principle, Wilson noted the importance of host susceptibility, which explains why not all fetuses have the same reaction to a specific teratogen.

The second principle provides credence to the concept of the **critical period**. When critical periods are discussed, publications often report the stage of pregnancy in weeks after fertilization as opposed to gestational weeks, which are calculated from the date of the last normal menses. Embryologists describe gestational age using the date of conception as the starting point for calculating the age of the conceptus (postconception dating). In contrast, healthcare providers usually calculate the number of gestational weeks from the first day of the last menstrual period (menstrual age or gestational age). Thus, in the area of teratology, it is important to know which type of dating is in use in order to identify critical periods.

With regard to the risk of damage from exposure to a teratogenic agent, pregnancy is subdivided into three time periods: pre-embryonic (between fertilization and implantation), embryonic (between implantation and nine postconception weeks), and the fetal period (after nine postconception weeks). Exposure to a teratogen during the pre-embryonic period usually results in an "all or none" effect. Since the tissue is undifferentiated, either the pregnancy is lost or there is no teratogenic effect at all. The lack of differentiation at this stage is also illustrated with the technique of preimplantation genetic diagnosis. This type of early embryo assessment used with *in vitro* fertilization consists of removing a few cells with the knowledge that the remaining cells will compensate without evidence of harm.

The embryonic period is the period of greatest concern for exposure to pharmaceuticals. The fetal period is the time when the fetus is most susceptible to FGR and developmental or behavioral abnormalities. Figure 17.2 is a classic illustration of the critical periods in human development from the viewpoint of an embryologist using postconceptional dating. Some organ systems are susceptible for a few days, whereas the central nervous system develops over a period of months and therefore has a longer period of vulnerability.

Wilson's third principle addresses the mechanisms of teratology. A review of drugs in pregnancy identified the mechanisms of most teratogens to be one of folate antagonism, neural crest cell disruption, endocrine disruption of sex hormones, oxidative stress, vascular disruption, or specific receptor- or enzyme-mediated reactions (van Gelder et al., 2010). Genetic predisposition may also play a role in some drug-related teratogenic effects (Cassina et al., 2017). Newer research regarding mechanisms eventually may result in some changes in the design of drugs to prevent teratogenic effects or possibly create antidotes.

The last two principles proposed by Wilson reflect the potency and type of teratogen. High doses of a potent teratogen logically would have the potential for causing a more severe effect than lower doses of a less potent drug.

Identification of a Teratogen

Unlike a laboratory diagnosis of a condition like diabetes mellitus or a bacterial infection, the identification of a

Table 17.2 Wilson's Six Principles of Teratology

Principle 1	Susceptibility to teratogenesis depends on the genotype of the conceptus and the manner in which this interacts with environmental factors.
Principle 2	Susceptibility to teratogenic agents varies with the developmental stage at the time of exposure.
Principle 3	Teratogenic agents act in specific ways (mechanisms) on developing cells and tissues to initiate abnormal embryogenesis (pathogenesis).
Principle 4	The final manifestations of abnormal development are death, malformation, FGR, and functional disorder.
Principle 5	The access of adverse environmental influences to developing tissues depends on the nature of the influences (agent).
Principle 6	Manifestations of deviant development increase in degree as dosage increases from no-effect to a totally lethal level.

Source: Adapted from: Wilson (1977).

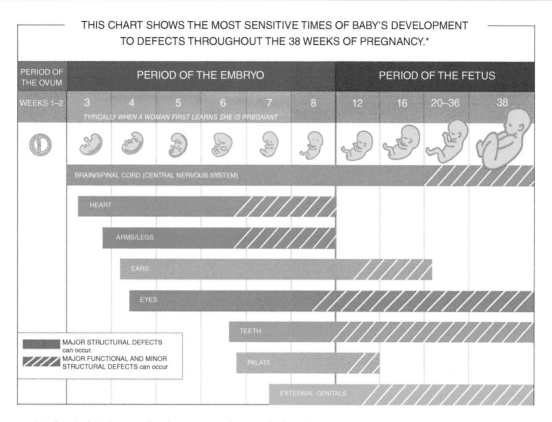

Figure 17.2   Critical periods in human development. MotherToBaby (2021), https://mothertobaby.org/factsheets/critical-periods-development/pdf/

teratogen is quite difficult. Most teratogenic drugs are not identified as such before being approved by the FDA. The initial animal studies done in preapproval testing may not demonstrate any teratogenic effects. Although potentially helpful, information from animal studies is not definitive as the effect of a drug on an animal is not always the same as the effect on humans.

The randomized clinical trials (RCTs) conducted with human participants to test safety and efficacy prior to FDA approval for marketing are not able to identify rare harms for three reasons. First, these trials typically do not have enough participants to detect conditions that only occur once in several thousand births. Second, these trials usually exclude people capable of pregnancy, people who take other medications, and people who have comorbid conditions that might interfere with the drug's effects. Thus, the safety and efficacy data obtained under controlled research conditions are not necessarily generalizable to a larger population. Third, RCTs only document immediate effects, as they generally do not follow participants for long periods after the exposure. Preapproval drug RCTs are helpful to determine immediate drug benefits, side effects, and adverse effects but are poor at detecting long-term harms (Vandenbroucke & Psaty, 2008).

Unfortunately, teratogenicity, like other rare **adverse drug effects**, is a post hoc phenomenon and is revealed only after children are affected. Among the factors for consideration when a drug is being evaluated as a teratogen includes an exploration of an increase in the frequency of the congenital anomaly in the exposed group of pregnant people compared to general population. The likelihood of teratogenicity is strengthened if the congenital anomaly is rare and if a similar finding is apparent in animal models. The presence of two specific effects, namely, dose response and threshold, also serve to validate the probability of a teratogen (Friedman & Polifka, 1994).

Although teratogens are occasionally first identified as such after years of use in the general marketplace, an agent may also be mislabeled as a teratogen by the public without scientific foundation. The ease with which information is placed on the Internet and shared on social media sites can cause unfounded opinions to become accepted as fact. Some historically marginalized groups may have lower health literacy and less access to options that include shared decision-making due to inequitable distribution of resources, structural racism and discrimination (National Academies of Sciences, Engineering, and Medicine, 2020). People may reasonably question agents that have little or no scientific data about teratogenicity. During the COVID-19 pandemic, misinformation regarding vaccine efficacy and safety has been shared on social media sites or inappropriately translated and shared via applications such as WhatsApp (Blisten, 2021; Vijaykumar et al., 2021).

More recently, pregnancy registries have been developed to help identify fetotoxic and teratogenic effects of drugs (Sinclair et al., 2016). These registries are prospective observational studies that collect postmarketing information about drug exposure and pregnancy outcomes. Information is collected longitudinally through childhood, based on data provided by healthcare providers and exposed individuals. A drug manufacturer may develop a pregnancy registry itself or a registry may be required by a regulating agency. The FDA maintains a website that lists the current pregnancy registries, and it is recommended that all perinatal care providers be aware of these registries and participate in data collection.

Selected Teratogens

A major difficulty with determining harm from drugs used during pregnancy is the difficulty in differentiating the cause of a congenital anomaly between the general background risk and risk related to the use of a specific drug. Older drug studies, in particular, were contaminated by problems such as **polypharmacy** used by the pregnant person, not recognizing adverse fetal effects of an untreated disorder, and use of observational research methodologies. Table 17.3 contains a list of selected teratogens or common agents proposed to have teratogenic effects. The majority of teratogens have been known for decades. The most recent additions to the list are some of the newer antidepressants, although it seems likely they are weak teratogens and require more study.

Conversely, lack of evidence of teratology does not indicate that an agent is safe. For example, the daughters of people who were prescribed diethylstilbesterol (DES) during pregnancy (prescribed between 1940 and 1971 to prevent

Table 17.3 Selected Known and Possible Teratogens

Teratogen	Time of exposure	Possible effects
Angiotensin converting enzyme inhibitors (ACEI) and angiotensin II antagonists	Questionable adverse effect in first trimester, most apparent in late pregnancy due to hemodynamic effects	Possible cardiovascular, central nervous system (CNS) defects, intrauterine renal insufficiency, oligohydramnios with complications (e.g., limb contractures, lung hypoplasia), prematurity, fetal death, neonatal hypotension
Antidepressants (e.g., fluoxetine, sertraline, paroxetine) Note: If severe depression is untreated, it may result in low birth weight, malnutrition, and other poor outcomes	First trimester (although several studies are contradictory in findings)	If teratogenic, considered low potency; however, several studies have associated use of paroxetine with cardiac defects
Antineoplastic agents	First-trimester exposure	Significant increase in congenital anomalies in general and spontaneous pregnancy loss
Antithyroid drugs (propylthiouracil [PTU], methimazole); if untreated, increased risk of congenital anomalies, preterm birth, and FGR may result	Less risk with PTU in first trimester, but higher risk of liver disease Methimazole is recommended after the first trimester due to prevent liver damage	PTU is associated with fetal hypothyroidism and, rarely, aplasia cutis Methimazole associated with fetal hypothyroidism in a dose-dependent fashion and is commonly associated with fetal anomalies such as aplasia cutis, esophageal atresia, and choanal atresia
Benzodiazepines (e.g., diazepam [Valium])	First-trimester exposure	No link with significant teratogenic effects; conflicting findings about link to cleft palate; some studies report an increased chance for preterm delivery, low birth weight, and/or smaller head circumference; neonates may exhibit withdrawal symptoms after birth, including breathing problems, jitteriness, excessive crying, and trouble maintaining body temperature. Some newborns may experience lax muscle tone at birth
Carbamazepine (anticonvulsant/mood stabilizer)	First-trimester exposure	1% risk for open neural tube defect (10X baseline), increased risk of cardiovascular defects, syndrome similar to that with hydantoins reported
Corticosteroids	*Possibly* first trimester	Cleft lip or palate in older studies
Coumadin /Warfarin	First trimester (4–7 postconceptional weeks) Some defects are found in half of pregnancies when coumadin derivative is given during any trimester	Fetal warfarin syndrome (nasal hypoplasia and epiphyseal defects); also associated with FGR, CNS delays, ophthalmic issues and hearing loss, pregnancy loss Risk of CNS damage due to hemorrhage after the first trimester

Table 17.3 (*Continued*)

Teratogen	Time of exposure	Possible effects
Diethylstilbestrol (DES; synthetic nonsteroidal estrogen); *No longer marketed in United States*	Exposure prior to 16 postconceptional weeks	Increased risk of pregnancy loss and preterm birth (ironically the indication for which it was initially administered); first discovered as a teratogen when "DES daughters" were found to have a high rate of vaginal clear cell carcinoma. There is questionable influence on children of the DES daughters also. DES often used as example of an agent in use for decades before teratogenicity was discovered
Ethanol/alcohol	Throughout pregnancy; some indication of dose relationship although threshold and critical periods remain unclear	Fetal alcohol spectrum disorders (FASD) that include FGR, facial changes, cleft palate, cardiac defects, and developmental delays
Folic acid antagonists (e.g., aminopterin and methotrexate—both chemotherapeutics)	First trimester (most likely 6–8 postconceptional weeks)	Fetal aminopterin-methotrexate syndrome: FGR, CNS defects, cranial/facial defects, cardiovascular abnormalities, developmental delay, intellectual disability
Hormones (especially sex hormones such as estrogen, progesterone, androgens)	First-trimester *potential*	No strong evidence of teratogenic effects; *possible* association between progesterone and male virilization of female genitalia; *possible* association of hypospadias and pseudohermaphrodism with androgens; association, although not strong, between combined oral contraceptives and vertebral, anal, cardiac, tracheoesophageal, renal, and limb defects
Hydantoins (phenytoin [Dilantin]—anticonvulsant and antiarrhythmic)	First trimester	Fetal hydantoin syndrome that includes craniofacial abnormalities, hypoplasia of distal phalanges and nails, FGR, mental deficiency, and cardiac defects
Lithium (mood stabilizer)	First trimester	Cardiac defects, especially Ebstein anomaly, although absolute numbers are small
Methimazole (Tapazole)	First trimester	Dysmorphia, choanal atresia, urinary system abnormalities
Misoprostol (prostaglandin)	First trimester	Mobius syndrome (facial paralysis) and limb defects; may have pregnancy loss with large doses
Retinoids (e.g., isotretinoin [Accutane], megadoses of vitamin A)	Appears to be primarily first trimester; consumer education mandates two forms of contraception for at least one month prior to starting method and two months after discontinuing; also instructs patient not to donate blood while on drug	Potent teratogen with structural and behavioral risks; retinoic acid embryopathy that includes craniofacial dysmorphology, cardiac defects, abnormalities of thymus, and alterations in CNS development; estimated 40% risk of pregnancy loss
Tetracyclines (anti-infective)	After 17 weeks postconception. Late third trimester	Discoloration of teeth. Risk of staining of permanent teeth
Thalidomide (primarily listed as sedative, limited availability in the United States)	34–50 days after LMP	Predilection for mesodermal tissue, resulting in limb reduction, and defects of gut, ears, and cardiovascular systems; drugs. There is also a chance of other problems such as missing or small eyes, paralysis of the face, and defects in the heart, kidney, genitals (sex organs), and gastrointestinal tract (stomach and intestines)
Valproic acid (mood stabilizer and anticonvulsant [Depakene])	First trimester, between the 17th and 30th day after fertilization	Neural tube defects (including meningomyelocele), lumbar disorders, cardiovascular malformations, and hypospadias; some studies indicate possible fetal valproate syndrome: craniofacial defects, cardiovascular defects, long digits, abnormal fingernails and cleft lip; neurobehavioral changes

Source: Adapted from: Briggs et al. (2022), Koren (2011), Feldcamp et al. (2015), CDC (2022), and MotherToBaby (2020, 2021).

miscarriage, preterm labor, and related complications of pregnancy) did not demonstrate reproductive system cancers until they were postpubescent (National Cancer Institute, 2021; Troisi et al., 2016). However, many drugs have been used extensively in a wide array of populations for decades, and there is no compelling reason to prohibit their use, assuming that a need for the medication exists.

Boxed Warnings

The FDA **boxed warnings**, formerly known as **black boxed warnings**, highlights for prescribers the following situations. These warnings are surrounded by a box that contains the word "WARNING" followed by information on the safety risk (Cheng et al., 2010).

1. These warnings indicate that an adverse reaction so serious in proportion to the potential benefit from the drug that it is essential that it be considered in assessing the risks and benefits of using the drug.
2. There is a serious adverse reaction that can be prevented or reduced in frequency or severity by appropriate use of the drug.
3. FDA approved the drug with restrictions to ensure safe use because FDA concluded that drug can be safely used only if distribution or use is restricted (US FDA, 2011).

Boxed warnings are generally based on observed serious adverse reactions, but may be placed when there is anticipated harm, such as drugs that pose a serious risk of developmental toxicity during pregnancy (US FDA, 2011).

Isotretinoin (Accutane®) contains the following boxed warning, "causes birth defects, do not get pregnant." There is an extremely high risk that severe birth defects will result if pregnancy occurs (Roche, 2008). Metoclopramide (Reglan®)'s boxed warning advises that treatment can cause tardive dyskinesia, which increases with duration of treatment and total cumulative dose (ANI Pharmaceuticals, Inc., 2011).

Boxed warnings are an important tool for providers and patients. While the FDA's Med-Watch maintains notifications for boxed warnings released from 1996 to present, there is no official list of drugs with FDA boxed warnings (Cheng et al., 2010).

Pharmacokinetics in Pregnancy

Pharmacokinetics refers to how the body acts on drugs and includes absorption, distribution, metabolism, and elimination. The normal physiologic changes of pregnancy directly influence pharmacokinetics. For example, because plasma volume expands approximately 50% during pregnancy, higher doses of antibiotics are necessary to achieve the optimal plasma levels needed to obtain a therapeutic effect. Thus, higher doses of antibiotics are needed for pregnant people. Table 17.4 provides an overview of the most common pharmacokinetic changes that occur during pregnancy.

Pharmacogenetics

Pharmacogenetics refers to the differences in drug responses among groups of unrelated individuals and the relationship to specific genes or genomic loci based on population-based studies. The efficacy of drugs in pregnancy may be impacted by genetic factors in addition to pharmacokinetic changes. Pharmacogenetics influences the variability in drug response, both in therapeutic and adverse effects, including drug classes that are commonly prescribed in pregnancy (Betcher & George, 2020). For example, the CYP2D6, a liver enzyme important in drug metabolism, is induced throughout the course of pregnancy. Pregnant patients who have certain SNPs in CYP2D6 are poor metabolizers and therefore, may not receive adequate pain relief from codeine as it is not converted to the active metabolite (Haas, 2014).

Common Medications Used during Pregnancy

Fortunately, most commonly used drugs in pregnancy have wide **therapeutic windows,** and little customization in route, dosing, or administration is needed. For some medications, adjustments in dose can be needed to account for the changes in pharmacokinetics during pregnancy. This information can be found in the PLLR labeling system described earlier. Table 17.5 displays selected medications used during pregnancy with

Table 17.4   Physiologic Changes in Pregnancy and Pharmacokinetics

Pharmacokinetics and pregnancy	Clinical implications
Changes in absorption	
Intestinal motility increases	Delayed or absent drug response/changes in absorption
Gestational nausea and vomiting are possible	Drug absorption is delayed due to decreased time in GI system
Gastric pH increased/decreased gastric acidity (by second trimester)	Changes in stomach absorption of oral drugs and increased ionization of weak acids
Slower gastric emptying	Delayed peak concentration of drugs that are absorbed in the intestine
Respiratory minute volume increases approximately 50%	Absorption of inhaled drugs increases through lungs, resulting in potential therapeutic effects at lower dosage
Skin perfusion, skin hydration, and perfusion to muscles increase	Intramuscular absorption of drugs increased; transcutaneous absorption of lipophilic and hydrophilic drugs increase
Routine simultaneous use of certain oral agents	Inactivation of absorption (e.g., calcium and iron in some prenatal combination multivitamins and minerals)

Table 17.4 (*Continued*)

Pharmacokinetics and pregnancy	Clinical implications
Changes in distribution	
Plasma volume increases by approximately 50%	Potential need to increase dosage of hydrophilic drugs because of decreased concentration in plasma (dilutional effect) Increased volume of distribution that may include fetal compartment
Hypoalbuminemia	Hypoalbuminemia may result in higher levels of free drug that can reach receptor for drugs that are normally highly protein bound
Hepatic blood flow increases	Higher hepatic blood flow will result in increased first-pass effect
Changes to regional blood flow	Decreased concentration of drug at the receptor site
Body fat stores increase by 3–4 kg	Long-term use of lipophilic drugs increases accumulation in body fat
Plasma albumin concentrations decrease (dilutional effect with increased plasma volume), resulting in less protein bound drugs	Increased incidence of free drugs if agents are highly protein bound. Drugs that are highly protein bound will have more pharmacologic activity in a pregnant person
Changes in metabolism	
Cytochrome P450 enzyme activity changes due to increased estrogen and progesterone levels (e.g., decreased CYP1A2; increased CYP 3A4 and CYP2C9)	Some drugs are more rapidly metabolized, and others will be metabolized at a slower rate relative to nonpregnant patients Profound changes in metabolism of some drugs, including tripling of half-life of caffeine and increased half-life of other agents such as sertraline (Zoloft®)
Changes in elimination	
Cardiac output increases 30–50%; Increase in stroke volume and heart rate; Changes to regional blood flow; Increased respiration rate; Decreased functional reserve capacity	More rapid clearance of drugs
Glomerular filtration rate increases throughout pregnancy by 50% at term	Decreased effect of renal drugs because of rapid clearance of such agents
Addition of fetal compartment	
Unique addition of fetal compartment influences pharmacokinetics, especially in area of distribution	Drugs that are highly lipophilic; low molecular weight and low protein binding can accumulate in fetal compartment. Majority of drugs in the fetal compartment are approximately 50–100% maternal concentration
Fetal circulation is more acidic than maternal circulation	Drugs that are of basic pH can concentrate in fetal compartment because of ion trapping
Fetal albumin plasma concentration increases throughout pregnancy until at term approximately 20% higher than maternal concentrations	Drugs highly bound to albumin accumulate in the term fetus; drugs can promote displacement or lack of binding of bilirubin, resulting in neonatal jaundice/kernicterus

Source: Adapted from: Lassiter & Manns-James (2017) and Patil et al. (2017).

Table 17.5 Selected Drugs Commonly Used during Pregnancy[a]

Medication class	Select summary comments (See Each Drug FDA Information Sheet for Full Summary)
Pain relievers	
Acetaminophen (Tylenol®)	An ingredient in many cold, flu, and allergy medicines. Recent studies link prenatal use of acetaminophen with an increased risk of neurodevelopmental, reproductive and urogenital disorders. Methodologies prevent reliable conclusions, recommendations unchanged. Use only when necessary in lowest dose for shortest time (Andrade, 2016; Bauer et al., 2021; Food and Drug Administration (FDA), 2016).
NSAIDS *Examples*: Naproxen sodium (Aleve®) Ibuprofen (Motrin®), Diclofenac (Voltaren), Celecoxib (Celebrex®)	Avoid NSAID use during third trimester, as it may cause premature closure of the ductus arteriosus. Not recommended in people capable of pregnancy who are attempting to conceive as may impair fertility. *Ibuprofen*: extremely low levels in human milk, short half-life and safe use in infants in doses much higher than those excreted in human milk, is a preferred choice as an analgesic or anti-inflammatory agent in lactating parents. *Naproxen*: Low levels in human milk, has a long half-life and reported serious adverse reaction in a neonate fed with human milk, other agents may be preferred while nursing a newborn or preterm infant. *Diclofenac*, drug has a short half-life, considered acceptable during lactation. *Celecoxib*: Low levels in human milk, considered acceptable for lactation.

(*Continued*)

Table 17.5 (*Continued*)

Medication class	Select summary comments (See Each Drug FDA Information Sheet for Full Summary)
Aspirin, acetylsalicylic acid ASA	No formal assignment, though it was considered category D by the FDA if full dose is taken in the third trimester. ASA is associated with increased maternal and fetal bleeding risk. High-dose aspirin (2 g/day) is associated with adverse perinatal outcomes. Low dose (81 mg/day) is recommended for pregnant patients with risk factors for pre-eclampsia. It should be initiated between 12 and 28 weeks, ideally at 16 weeks, and continued until delivery (US Preventive Task Force, 2021).
Opioids	
Buprenorphine (Subutex)	Buprenorphine is a potent narcotic agonist and antagonist that has been used during human pregnancy for analgesia and for the maintenance treatment of opioid dependence. It is about 33 times more potent than morphine (0.3-mg buprenorphine is equivalent to 10-mg morphine in analgesic and respiratory depressant effects). Neonatal withdrawal has occurred, but the symptoms are usually less than that expected with methadone. Animal studies have demonstrated dose-related embryo-fetal developmental toxicity. The American College of Obstetricians and Gynecologists recommends that both methadone and buprenorphine should be considered as options for opioid treatment. Buprenorphine is excreted into human milk but is poorly absorbed orally. Breast/chest feeding an infant with Neonatal Opioid Withdrawal Syndrome (NOWS) may decrease the severity of NOWS, shorten the neonatal intensive care unit stay, and decrease the pharmacotherapy required for the infant.
Methadone	The reported use in pregnancy of methadone is almost exclusively related to the treatment of heroin addiction, but the drug also is used in patients addicted to other opioid agonists. The National Birth Defects Prevention Study found evidence that opioid use during organogenesis is associated with a low absolute risk of congenital birth defects. A second study also found a similar association. Because patients taking methadone usually consume a wide variety of drugs, it is not always possible to separate completely the effects of methadone from the effects of other agents. Neonatal narcotic withdrawal and low birth weight appear to be major problems. Methadone is excreted into breast milk and claims have been made that it could prevent withdrawal in addicted infants. It is important to assess for use of other drugs when encouraging lactation for a patient prescribed methadone. Breast/chest feeding an infant with Neonatal Opioid Withdrawal Syndrome (NOWS) may decrease the severity of NOWS, shorten the neonatal intensive care unit stay, and decrease the pharmacotherapy required for the infant.
Oxycodone	The National Birth Defects Prevention Study found evidence that opioid use during organogenesis is associated with a low absolute risk of congenital birth defects. Use for prolonged periods or in high doses at term has the potential to cause neonatal abstinence syndrome or respiratory depression in the newborn. If a lactating patient is receiving oxycodone, the nursing infant should be monitored for sedation and other adverse effects, such as gastrointestinal effects and changes in feeding patterns. Prolonged use increases the risk of adverse side effects, including increased sleepiness, difficulty breastfeeding, breathing difficulties, or limpness.
Antacids	
Calcium Carbonate (Tums®)	Considered safe during pregnancy and lactation.
Cimetidine (Tagamet HB®)	There are no controlled data in human pregnancy. Cimetidine has been used safely during pregnancy. Considered compatible with lactation by the American Academy of Pediatrics.
Famotidine (Pepcid®)	Considered safe during pregnancy and lactation.
Antifungals	
Clotrimazole (Gyne-Lotrimin®) topical	Systemic absorption is minimal following topical or vaginal administration. There are no data on the excretion into human milk, use considered acceptable.
Miconazole (Monistat®) topical	Considered safe in pregnancy by the FDA.
Fluconazole (Diflucan®) oral	A single 150 mg tablet dose for vaginal candidiasis is considered low risk of teratogenicity. Should not be prescribed at higher doses or for longer term use. Considered safe with lactation.

Table 17.5 (*Continued*)

Medication class	Select summary comments (See Each Drug FDA Information Sheet for Full Summary)
Antivirals	
Acyclovir (Zovirax®) Valacyclovir (Valtrex®) oral	There are no controlled data in human pregnancy. There is no evidence of an association between first trimester use of these agents and major groups of malformations.
Antibiotics	
Amoxicillin (Amoxil®)	Animal studies have failed to reveal evidence of teratogenicity, impaired fertility, or fetal harm. There are no controlled data in human pregnancy. Penicillin is considered low risk at any stage of pregnancy. However, one large study found that exposure to amoxicillin during organogenesis was associated with a small risk of oral clefts.
Amoxicillin Clavulanate (Augmentin®)	Small risk for cleft lip and palate in the first trimester. Small risk for necrotizing enterocolitis (NEC) in the third trimester.
Azithromycin (Zithromax®)	Animal models have failed to reveal evidence of teratogenicity. There are no controlled data in human pregnancy.
Cefazolin (Ancef®, Kefzol®)	Animal studies have failed to reveal evidence of fetal harm or impaired fertility. This drug crosses the placental barrier into cord blood and amniotic fluid. There are no controlled data in human pregnancy. No adverse fetal effects have been reported. A positive direct and indirect antiglobulin (Coombs) test may occur in neonates of mothers who received cephalosporins before delivery.
Cephalexin (Keflex)	Animal models have failed to reveal evidence of impaired fertility and fetal harm. There are no controlled data in human pregnancy.
Ciprofloxacin (Cipro®)	There are no controlled data in human pregnancy. Substantial teratogenic risk is unlikely using therapeutic doses; data insufficient to state that there is no risk. Use is acceptable in lactating patients with monitoring of the infant for possible effects on the gastrointestinal flora, such as diarrhea or candidiasis.
Clindamycin (Cleocin®)	There are no controlled data in human pregnancy. Can alter breastfed infant's gastrointestinal flora.
Erythromycin (E-Mycin) ®	There are no controlled data in human pregnancy. Considered compatible with lactation by the American Academy of Pediatrics.
Metronidazole (Flagyl®)	There are no controlled data in human pregnancy. Opinions vary among experts on long-term metronidazole use while lactating. Oral metronidazole is excreted in large amounts in human milk; however, the dose is lower than the dose given to treat young infants.
Nitrofurantoin (Macrodantin®)	Contraindicated at term (38–42 weeks of gestation) due to possible fetal hemolytic anemia. Low levels in human milk, can be used while breastfeeding older infants, alternate drugs are preferred in lactating parents of infants under 8 days of age, or infants with G-6-PD deficiency of any age.
Penicillin G (Procaine®)	There are no controlled data in human pregnancy. There is no evidence of an association between first trimester use of these agents and major groups of malformations. Acceptable use during lactation.
Antihypertensives	
Hydralazine (Apresoline®)	Should be avoided during the first two trimesters of pregnancy.
Labetalol (Trandate®)	Low levels in human milk, unlikely to have any adverse effects in full-term infants. Risk of neonatal beta-blockade symptoms if used by pregnant person in late third trimester, which generally pass by three days of age.
Nifedipine (Procardia®)	Large, retrospective study did not find association between the use of nifedipine and congenital anomalies. Risks unknown. There are low levels in human milk, unlikely to have any adverse effects in infants.
Methyldopa (Aldomet®; oral)	Animal studies have failed to reveal evidence of teratogenicity or fetotoxicity. There are low levels in human milk, unlikely to have any adverse effects in infants.
Medications for insomnia and nausea	
Diphenhydramine (Benadryl®)	Animal studies have failed to reveal teratogenicity, no associated teratogenicity in large retrospective study; is excreted into human milk, can inhibit lactation. Manufacturer recommends that due to the potential for serious adverse reactions in infants, a decision should be made to discontinue lactation or discontinue the drug.
Doxylamine (Unisom®)	No formal assignment, though, is considered safe in pregnancy by the FDA.
Doxylamine/Pyridoxine (Diclegis®)	The single most studied pharmacologic agent for use in pregnancy. Studies with hundreds of thousands of exposed pregnant people have not found that use during pregnancy increases the chances of birth defects. It is considered the first line treatment for nausea and vomiting of pregnancy.

(*Continued*)

Table 17.5 (Continued)

Medication class	Select summary comments (See Each Drug FDA Information Sheet for Full Summary)
Zolpidem (Ambien)	There are no controlled data in human pregnancy. Chronic use of hypnotics during late pregnancy may be associated with neonatal withdrawal symptoms. Use only when necessary. Low levels in human milk; considered compatible with lactation.
Antiemetics	
Metoclopramide (Reglan®)	Risk of tardive dyskinesia. Should be avoided in pregnant people with a history of major depression.
Ondansetron (Zofran®)	In the first trimester, small increase (1%) in cleft palate and cardiac defects. Person taking the medication may develop heart rhythm problem, QT interval prolongation, and in severe cases develop Torsades de Pointes.
Prochlorperazine (Compazine®)	There is inadequate evidence of the safety in human pregnancy. There is evidence of harmful effects in animals. Extrapyramidal and withdrawal symptoms such as agitation, abnormally increased or decreased muscle tone, tremor, sleepiness, severe difficulty breathing, and difficulty in feeding have been reported in exposed neonates.
Promethazine (Phenergan®)	There are no controlled data in human pregnancy. There is no evidence of increased risk of congenital malformations in humans.
Steroids	
Betamethasone	There are no controlled studies in human pregnancy. Recommended for use during pregnancy when there are no alternatives and benefit outweighs risk. Use 3–9 days prior to preterm birth might decrease postpartum milk production in some people. Local injections would not be expected to cause adverse effects in infants fed with human milk.
Prednisone	There are no controlled data in human pregnancy. Avoid in first trimester due to possible increased risk of cleft palate.
Antihistamines	
Cetirizine (Zyrtec®)	Considered safe in pregnancy and lactation.
Fexofenadine (Allegra®)	Considered safe in pregnancy and lactation.
Loratadine (Claritin®)	One study showed that first-trimester use demonstrated a small increase in risk for hypospadias.
Constipation management	
Docusate sodium (Colace®)	Considered safe in pregnancy and lactation when the recommended amount is taken. One study noted decreased magnesium levels in a neonate when taking higher than the recommended amount.
Osmotic laxatives, including magnesium hydroxide (Milk of Magnesia®) and sodium bisphosphate (OsmoPrep®), and sugars, such as lactulose and polyethylene glycol (Miralax®)	Considered safe in pregnancy and lactation when using the lowest effective dose for the shortest period of time. Not well absorbed by the intestine, so little gets in the bloodstream.
Fiber or bulk laxatives include psyllium (Metamucil®) and methylcellulose (Citrucel®).	Considered safe in pregnancy and lactation when using the lowest effective dose for the shortest period of time. Generally do not pass through the bloodstream.

Source: Andrade (2016), Avella-Garcia et al. (2016), Briggs et al. (2022), http://Drugs.com (2022), Kinnunen (2019), MotherToBaby (2021), and Rizk (2019).

[a]This list is not comprehensive and is only provided to give the reader a general overview of some medications most often used by pregnant people.

components of the PLLR safety narrative and safety data from other sources.

Vaccines during Pregnancy

Three vaccines—the COVID-19 vaccines, inactivated influenza, and the combination vaccine that includes tetanus toxoid, reduced diphtheria toxoid, and acellular pertussis (Tdap)—are recommended for use by all pregnant people by the National Center for Immunization and Respiratory Diseases (CDC, 2021b). All people who are or will be pregnant during flu season should receive the influenza vaccination. Pregnant people are more likely to become severely ill with COVID-19; therefore, the COVID-19 vaccines, including the booster, are recommended in pregnancy if not previously received. Other vaccines such as cholera, rabies, hepatitis A, and hepatitis B may be given during pregnancy if the risk of infection is substantial. Live-attenuated vaccines should be avoided by people who are or may become pregnant, due to a theoretical risk that a live-attenuated vaccine may cause subclinical placental and neonatal infection. For example, rubella vaccine is a live-attenuated vaccine and not recommended for use during pregnancy. However, occasionally, this vaccine is inadvertently administered to a person prior to pregnancy being recognized. No neonatal defects have been attributed to in-utero exposure to rubella vaccine, and people who were vaccinated during early pregnancy are not advised to terminate pregnancy based solely on this theoretical risk. Table 17.6 lists specific information about vaccines during the childbearing year.

Rational Use of Drugs in Pregnancy

No specific guidelines exist to aid clinicians when choosing a medication for a pregnant person in order to avoid fetal risk. However, there are some general strategies that can be used, including choosing drugs listed in Table 17.5 when possible. Additionally, a medication that is older and well known should be used rather than one that is newly approved. When considering dosing, the initial choice should be a dose in the lowest therapeutic range, taking into account the altered pharmacokinetics during pregnancy. Higher doses may be necessary for some drugs to achieve a therapeutic effect. Drugs that have not been proven to be safe for use during organogenesis should be avoided during the first trimester when possible. The use of a single agent is preferred over a combination of drugs to avoid polypharmacy and potential drug interactions. Lastly, pregnant people should be counseled that OTC, herbs, nutritional supplements, and botanicals should be regarded as drugs and discussed with a healthcare professional before self-administration.

The one exception to the recommendation of a single agent concerns prenatal vitamins, which have a combination of vitamins in one pill. In low- to middle-income countries, a daily multiple micronutrient agent is found to have positive influence on pregnancy outcomes (Haider & Bhutta, 2015), but no similar findings have been reported for the United States. Folic acid is associated with a lower risk for neural tube defects and is well established as a therapeutic agent, especially when taken during the first trimester. Thus, people who are planning a pregnancy should take it daily as soon as they start trying to conceive. There is less indication for folic acid later in pregnancy. Vitamin D supplementation is associated with a decrease in pre-eclampsia, gestational diabetes, and severe postpartum hemorrhage and probably reduces the risk of a baby with low birth weight. Vitamin D supplementation alone may make little or no difference in the risk of having preterm birth. Administration with calcium likely reduces the risk of pre-eclampsia but may increase the risk of

Table 17.6   Vaccines during Pregnancy and Postpartum

Vaccine	During pregnancy	After pregnancy	Type of vaccine
Influenza	Yes, during flu season	Yes	Inactivated
Tdap	Yes, in each pregnancy	Yes	Toxoid/inactivated
COVID-19	Yes	Yes	mRNA, inactivated
Td	May be recommended, Tdap preferred	May be recommended, Tdap preferred	
Hepatitis A	May be recommended	May be recommended	Inactivated
Hepatitis B	May be recommended	May be recommended	Inactivated
Meningococcal	Inadequate data to recommend	May be recommended	Inactivated
Pneumococcal	Inadequate data to recommend	May be recommended	Inactivated
Human papillomavirus	No	May be recommended through age 45	Inactivated
Measles Mumps Rubella	No	May be recommended	Live
Varicella	No	May be recommended	Live

Source: Adapted from: CDC (2020) and Rasmussen et al. (2014).

Table 17.7   Common Ingredients in Prenatal Vitamin/Mineral Supplements

Calcium	200–300 mg
Folate (folic acid or B$_9$)	0.4 mg (400 mcg)
Iron	30 mg
Niacin B$_3$	20 mg
Riboflavin B$_2$	2 mg
Thiamine	3 mg
Vitamin A	2000 IU
Vitamin B$_{12}$	6 mcg
Vitamin B$_6$	2 mg
Vitamin C	50–70 mg
Vitamin D	400 IU
Vitamin E	10 mg
Zinc	15 mg
Omega-3 fatty acids (DHA)	200–300 mg

Source: Adapted from Duerbeck et al. (2014).

preterm birth, while the effect on gestational diabetes and low birth weight is uncertain (De-Regil et al., 2016; Palacios et al., 2019). Docosahexaenoic acid (DHA), an omega-3 fatty acid, is suggested as a supplement in prenatal vitamins during the pregnancy and lactation as it is a critical building block of the brain and retina in the fetus and neonate (Gázquez & Larqué, 2021). Some combinations such as calcium or iron can cause drug–drug interactions. Therefore, the optimal composition of a prenatal multivitamin/mineral remains elusive. The common ingredients in prenatal vitamins are listed in Table 17.7.

Summary

Healthcare providers are challenged to stay current with advances in pharmacology, especially when caring for pregnant people and their offspring. Pharmaceutical agents should be recommended or prescribed when they are needed with knowledge about pharmacokinetic changes in pregnancy and how an individual medication works. Drugs used in pregnancy must be scrutinized as to effects (including therapeutic, side, and adverse) as well as embryonic and fetal risks. Issues such as cost, accessibility, and **pharmacogenomics** are also important considerations. Perhaps most importantly, new information about existing drugs and new medications is rapidly emerging, emphasizing the importance of being current in practice.

Resources for Clients and Their Families

Connecting world-renowned experts in the field of birth defects research to the general public: https://mothertobaby.org/

Most recent drug labeling information submitted to the FDA and currently in use: https://dailymed.nlm.nih.gov/dailymed

FDA drug safety information for consumers and healthcare providers: https://www.fda.gov/Drugs/DrugSafety/PostmarketDrugSafetyInformationforPatientsandProviders/default.htm

Resources for Healthcare Providers

A brief overview of the PLLR: https://www.fda.gov/drugs/labeling-information-drug-products/pregnancy-and-lactation-labeling-drugs-final-rule

Drugs and Lactation Database (LactMed), a free online database with information on drugs and lactation: https://www.ncbi.nlm.nih.gov/books/NBK501922

FDA: List of pregnancy exposure registries: https://www.fda.gov/science-research/womens-health-research/list-pregnancy-exposure-registries

MedWatch: The FDA Safety Information and Adverse Event Reporting Program: https://www.fda.gov/safety/medwatch-fda-safety-information-and-adverse-event-reporting-program

MotherToBaby provides information for patients and healthcare providers on the risks and safety of medications during pregnancy and lactation: http://www.mothertobaby.org

The National Library of Medicine (NLM) has integrated the Toxnet information into other NLM products and services. Access specific information from the free online databases on toxicology chemical, pharmaceuticals, environmental health, and toxic releases: https://www.nlm.nih.gov/toxnet/index.html

References

Andrade, C. (2016). Use of acetaminophen (paracetamol) during pregnancy and the risk of autism spectrum disorder in the offspring. *The Journal of Clinical Psychiatry, 77*(2), e152–e154.

ANI Pharmaceuticals, Inc. (2011). *Reglan* [medication guide]. https://www.accessdata.fda.gov/drugsatfda_docs/label/2011/017854s058lbl.pdf

Avella-Garcia, C. B., Julvez, J., Fortuny, J., Rebordosa, C., García-Esteban, R., Galán, I. R., Tardón, A., Rodríguez-Bernal, C. L., Iñiguez, C., Andiarena, A., Santa-Marina, L., & Sunyer, J. (2016). Acetaminophen use in pregnancy and neurodevelopment: Attention function and autism spectrum symptoms. *International Journal of Epidemiology, 45*(6), 1987–1996. https://doi.org/10.1093/ije/dyw115

Bauer, A. Z., Swan, S. H., Kriebel, D., Liew, Z., Taylor, H. S., Bornehag, C. G., Andrade, A. M., Olsen, J., Jensen, R. H., Mitchell, R. T., Skakkebaek, N. E., Jégou, B., & Kristensen, D. M. (2021). Paracetamol use during pregnancy—A call for precautionary action. *Nature Reviews. Endocrinology, 17*(12), 757–766. https://doi.org/10.1038/s41574-021-00553-7

Benavides-Lara, A., la Paz Barboza-Arguello, M., González-Elizondo, M., Hernández-deMezerville, M., Brenes-Chacón, H., Ramírez-Rojas, M., Ramírez-Hernández, C., Arjona-Ortegón, N., Godfred-Cato, S., Valencia, D., Moore, C. A., & Soriano-Fallas, A. (2021). Zika virus-associated birth defects, Costa Rica, 2016–2018. *Emerging Infectious Diseases, 27*(2), 360–371. https://doi.org/10.3201/eid2702.202047

Bennett, D., Bellinger, D. C., Birnbaum, L. S., Bradman, A., Chen, A., Cory-Slechta, D. A., Engel, S. M., Fallin, M. D., Halladay, A., Hauser, R., Hertz-Picciotto, I., Kwiatkowski, C. F., Lanphear, B. P., Marquez, E., Marty, M., McPartland, J., Newschaffer, C. J., Payne-Sturges, D., Patisaul, H. B., . . . National Medical Association. (2016). Project TENDR: Targeting environmental neuro-developmental risks the

TENDR consensus statement. *Environmental Health Perspectives*, *124*(7), A118–A122. https://doi.org/10.1289/EHP358

Berke, J., Gal, S, & Lee, Y.J. (2022, May 27). *Marijuana legalization is sweeping the US. See every state where cannabis is legal*. Insider. https://www.businessinsider.com/legal-marijuana-states-2018-1

Betcher, H. K., & George, A. L., Jr. (2020). Pharmacogenomics in pregnancy. *Seminars in Perinatology*, *44*(3), 151222. https://doi.org/10.1016/j.semperi.2020.151222

Blisten, J. (2021, May 3). *John Oliver debunks Covid-19 vaccine skepticism on 'Last Week Tonight'*. Rolling Stone. https://www.rollingstone.com/tv/tv-news/john-oliver-covid-19-vaccine-skeptics-joe-rogan-1164129

Briggs, G. G., Towers, C. V., & Forinash, A. B. (2022). *Briggs drugs in pregnancy and lactation: A reference guide to fetal and neonatal risk* (12th ed.). Lippincott Williams & Wilkins.

Byrne, J. J., Saucedo, A. M., & Spong, C. Y. (2020). Evaluation of drug labels following the 2015 pregnancy and lactation labeling rule. *JAMA Network Open*, *3*(8), e2015094. https://doi.org/10.1001/jamanetworkopen.2020.15094

Cassina, M., Cagnoli, G. A., Zuccarello, D., Di Gianatonio, E., & Clementi, M. (2017). Human teratogens and genetic phenocopies. Understanding pathogenesis through human genes mutation. *European Journal of Medical Genetics*, *60*(1), 22–31.

Centers for Disease Control and Prevention (CDC). (2020). *Pregnant or thinking of getting pregnant?* https://www.cdc.gov/pregnancy/meds/treatingfortwo/facts.html

Centers for Disease Control and Prevention (CDC). (2021a). *Therapeutic drug use*. https://www.cdc.gov/nchs/fastats/drug-use-therapeutic.htm

Centers for Disease Control and Prevention (CDC). (2021b). *Vaccines during and after pregnancy*. https://www.cdc.gov/vaccines/pregnancy/vacc-during-after.html

Centers for Disease Control and Prevention (CDC). (2022). *Fetal alcohol spectrum disorders (FASD)*. https://www.cdc.gov/ncbddd/fasd/index.html

Centers for Medicare & Medicaid Services (CMS). (2021a). *E-Prescribing*. https://www.cms.gov/Medicare/E-Health/Eprescribing

Centers for Medicare & Medicaid Services (CMS). (2021b). *National provider identifier standard*. https://www.cms.gov/Regulations-and-Guidance/Administrative-Simplification/NationalProvIdentStand

Centers for Medicare & Medicaid Services (CMS). (n.d.). *Prescribers be aware: The NPI is here. The NPI is now. Do you have one? Are you using it?* https://www.cms.gov/Regulations-and-Guidance/Administrative-Simplification/NationalProvIdentStand/Downloads/NPI-Requirements-for-Prescribers.pdf

Cheng, C. M., Guglielmo, B. J., Maselli, J., & Auerbach, A. D. (2010). Coverage of FDA medication boxed warnings in commonly used drug information resources. *Archives of Internal Medicine*, *170*(9), 831–833. https://doi.org/10.1001/archinternmed.2010.91

Clinical Info HIV.gov. (n.d.). *HIV/AIDS Glossary*. https://clinicalinfo.hiv.gov/en/glossary/boxed-warning#:~:text=The%20strongest%20form%20of%20warning,on%20use%20of%20a%20drug.

De-Regil, L. M., Palacios, C., Lombardo, L. K., & Peña-Rosas, J. P. (2016). Vitamin D supplementation for women during pregnancy. *Cochrane Database of Systematic Reviews*, *1*, CD008873.

Drugs.com. (2022). *Find drugs and conditions*. Retrieved September 3, 2022 from https://www.drugs.com

Duerbeck, N. B., Dowling, D. D., & Duerbeck, J. M. (2014). Prenatal vitamins: What is in the bottle? *Obstetrical and Gynecological Survey*, *69*(12), 777–788.

Dunn, P. M. (2007). Perinatal lessons from the past: Sir Norman Gregg, ChM, MC, of Sydney (1892–1966) and rubella embryopathy. *Archives of Disease in Childhood. Fetal and Neonatal Edition*, *92*(6), F513–F514.

Feldcamp, M. L., Botto, L. D., & Carey, J. C. (2015). Reflections on the etiology of structural birth defects: Established teratogens and risk factors. *Birth Defects Research*, *103*(8), 652–655.

Franconi, F., Brunelleschi, S., Steardo, L., & Cuomo, V. (2007). Gender differences in drug responses. *Pharmacological Research*, *55*(2), 81–95.

Friedman, J., & Polifka, J. (1994). *Teratogenic effects of drugs, a resource for health care providers (TERIS)*. Johns Hopkins University Press.

Friedman, J. M. (2010). The principles of teratology: Are they still true? *Birth Defects Research Part A, Clinical and Molecular Teratology*, *88*(10), 766–768.

Gázquez, A., & Larqué, E. (2021). Towards an optimized fetal DHA accretion: Differences on maternal DHA supplementation using phospholipids vs. triglycerides during pregnancy in different models. *Nutrients*, *13*(2), 511. https://doi.org/10.3390/nu13020511

Haas, D. M. (2014). Pharmacogenetics and individualizing drug treatment during pregnancy. *Pharmacogenomics*, *15*(1), 69–78. https://doi.org/10.2217/pgs.13.228

Haas, D. M., Marsh, D. J., Dang, D. T., Parker, C. B., Wing, D. A., Simhan, H. N., Grobman, W. A., Mercer, B. M., Silver, R. M., Hoffman, M. K., Parry, S., Iams, J. D., Caritis, S. N., Wapner, R. J., Esplin, M. S., Elovitz, M. A., Peaceman, A. M., Chung, J., Saade, G. R., & Reddy, U. M. (2018). Prescription and other medication use in pregnancy. *Obstetrics & Gynecology*, *131*(5), 789–798. https://doi.org/10.1097/AOG.0000000000002579

Haider, B. A., & Bhutta, Z. A. (2015). Multiple-micronutrient supplementation for women during pregnancy. *Cochrane Database of Systematic Reviews.*, *11*, CD004905.

Jacobs, P. A., Melville, M., Ratcliffe, S., Keay, A. J., & Syme, J. (1974). A cytogenetic survey of 11,680 newborn infants. *Annals of Human Genetics*, *37*(4), 359.

Kinnunen, M., Piirainen, P., Kokki, H., Lammi, P., & Kokki, M. (2019). Updated clinical pharmacokinetics and pharmacodynamics of oxycodone. *Clinical Pharmacokinetics*, *58*(6), 705–725. https://doi.org/10.1007/s40262-018-00731-3

Klecka, G., Persoon, C., & Currie, R. (2010). Chemicals of emerging concern in the Great Lakes Basin, an analysis of environmental exposures. *Reviews of Environmental Contamination and Toxicology*, *207*, 1–93.

Kogut, S. J. (2020). Racial disparities in medication use: Imperatives for managed care pharmacy. *Journal of Managed Care & Specialty Pharmacy*, *26*(11), 1468–1474. https://doi.org/10.18553/jmcp.2020.26.11.1468

Koren, G. (2011). Fetal risks of maternal pharmacotherapy, identifying signals. *Handbook of Experimental Pharmacology*, *205*, 285–294.

Krishtel, P. (2021, February 22). *Building a bigger table for a more equitable drug development system*. Kaiser Permanente: Institute for Health Policy. https://www.kpihp.org/blog/building-a-bigger-table-for-a-more-equitable-drug-development-system

Lassiter, N. T., & Manns-James, L. (2017). Pregnancy. In T. L. King & M. C. Brucker (Eds.), *Pharmacology for women's health* (2nd ed., pp. 1025–1065). Jones and Bartlett Learning.

MotherToBaby. (2020, April 1). *Metronidazole*. https://mothertobaby.org/fact-sheets/metronidazole-flagyl-pregnancy/pdf

MotherToBaby. (2021, March 1). *Critical periods of development*. https://mothertobaby.org/fact-sheets/critical-periods-development/pdf

National Academies of Sciences, Engineering, and Medicine. (2020). *Birth settings in America: Outcomes, quality, access, and choice*. National Academies Press. https://doi.org/10.17226/25636

National Cancer Institute. (2021). *Diethylstilbestrol (DES) exposure and cancer*. https://www.cancer.gov/about-cancer/causes-prevention/risk/hormones/des-fact-sheet

Osborne, K. (2015). Regulation of prescriptive authority for certified nurse-midwives and certified midwives, 2015 national overview. *Journal of Midwifery and Women's Health*, *60*(5), 519–533.

Osterman, M. J., Hamilton, B. E., Martin, J. A., & Valenzuela, C. P. (2022). Births: Final data for 2020. *National Vital Statistics Reports*, *70*(17), 1–15. https://www.cdc.gov/nchs/data/nvsr/nvsr70/nvsr70-17.pdf

Palacios, C., Kostiuk, L. K., & Peña-Rosas, J. P. (2019). Vitamin D supplementation for women during pregnancy. *The Cochrane Database of Systematic Reviews*, *7*(7), CD008873. https://doi.org/10.1002/14651858.CD008873.pub4

Patil, A. S., Sheng, J., Dotters-Katz, S. K., Schmoll, M. S., Onslow, M., & Pierson, R. C. (2017). Fundamentals of clinical pharmacology with application for pregnant women. *Journal of Midwifery & Women's Health*, *62*(3), 298–307. https://doi.org/10.1111/jmwh.12621

Plank, L. S. (2011). Governmental oversight of prescribing medications, history of the US food and drug administration and prescriptive authority. *Journal of Midwifery & Women's Health*, *56*(3), 198–204.

Rasmussen, S. A., Watson, A. K., Kennedy, E. D., Broder, K. R., & Jamieson, D. J. (2014). Vaccines and pregnancy: Past, present, and future. *Seminars in Fetal and Neonatal Medicine, 19*(3), 161–169.

Rizk, A. H., Simonsen, S. E., Roberts, L., Taylor-Swanson, L., Lemoine, J. B., & Smid, M. (2019). Maternity care for pregnant women with opioid use disorder: A review. *Journal of Midwifery & Women's Health, 64*(5), 532–544. https://doi.org/10.1111/jmwh.13019

Roche. (2008). *Accutane* [medication guide]. https://www.accessdata.fda.gov/drugsatfda_docs/label/2008/018662s059lbl.pdf

Sacco, L. (2022). *The schedule I status of marijuana*. Congressional Research Service. https://crsreports.congress.gov/product/pdf/IN/IN11204

Sarecka-Hujar, B., & Szulc-Musioł, B. (2022). Herbal medicines-are they effective and safe during pregnancy? *Pharmaceutics, 14*(1), 171. https://doi.org/10.3390/pharmaceutics14010171

Scaffidi, J., Mol, B. W., & Keelan, J. A. (2016). The pregnant woman as a drug orphan: A global survey of registered clinical trials of pharmacological interventions in pregnancy. *BJOG, 124*(1), 132–140. https://doi.org/10.1111/1471-0528.14151

Sinclair, S. M., Miller, R. K., Chambers, C., & Cooper, E. M. (2016). Medication safety during pregnancy: Improving evidence-based practice. *Journal of Midwifery & Women's Health, 61*(1), 52–67.

Surescripts, LLC. (2021). *2020 national progress report*. https://surescripts.com/docs/default-source/national-progress-reports/2020-national-progress-report.pdf?sfvrsn=8f9171ca_6

Troisi, R., Hatch, E. E., Palmer, J. R., Titus, L., Robboy, S. J., Strohsnitter, W. C., Herbst, A. L., Adam, E., Hyer, M., & Hoover, R. N. (2016). Prenatal diethylstilbestrol exposure and high-grade squamous cell neoplasia of the lower genital tract. *American Journal of Obstetrics and Gynecology, 215*(3), 322.e1–322.e8.

US Department of Justice & Drug Enforcement Administration. (2022). *Controlled substance schedules*. Retrieved on September 4, 2022 from https://www.deadiversion.usdoj.gov/schedules

US Food and Drug Administration (FDA). (1979). Specific requirements on content and format of labeling for human prescription drugs. *Federal Register, 44*, 37434–37467.

US Food and Drug Administration (FDA). (2016). *FDA drug safety communication: FDA has reviewed possible risks of pain medication during pregnancy*. https://www.fda.gov/Drugs/DrugSafety/ucm429117.htm

US Food and Drug Administration (FDA). (2020). *Disposal of unused medications: What you should know*. https://www.fda.gov/drugs/safe-disposal-medicines/disposal-unused-medicines-what-you-should-know

US Food and Drug Administration (FDA). (2021). *Pregnancy and lactation labeling (drugs): Final rule*. http://www.fda.gov/Drugs/DevelopmentApprovalProcess/DevelopmentResources/Labeling/ucm093307.htm

US Food and Drug Adminstration (FDA). (2011). Guidance for industry. *Warnings and precautions, contraindications, and boxed warning sections of labeling for human prescription drug and biological products – content and format*. https://www.fda.gov/files/drugs/published/Warnings-and-Precautions--Contraindications--and-Boxed-Warning-Sections-of-Labeling-for-Human-Prescription-Drug-and-Biological-Products--—-Content-and-Format.pdf

US National Institutes of Health (NIH). (2022). *FDAAA 801 and the final rule*. https://clinicaltrials.gov/ct2/manage-recs/fdaaa

US Preventive Services Task Force. (2021). Aspirin use to prevent preeclampsia and related morbidity and mortality: US preventive services task force recommendation statement. *JAMA, 326*(12), 1186–1191. https://doi.org/10.1001/jama.2021.14781

van Gelder, M. M. H. J., van Rooij, I. A. L. M., Miller, R., Zielhuis, G. A., de Jong-van den Berg, L. T. W., & Roeleveld, N. (2010). Teratogenic mechanisms of medical drugs. *Human Reproduction Update, 16*(4), 378–394.

Vandenbroucke, J. P., & Psaty, B. M. (2008). Benefits and risks of drug treatments, how to combine the best evidence on benefits with the best data about adverse effects. *JAMA: The Journal of the American Medical Association, 300*, 2417–2418.

Vijaykumar, S., Rogerson, D. T., Jin, Y., & de Oliveira Costa, M. S. (2021). Dynamics of social corrections to peers sharing COVID-19 misinformation on WhatsApp in Brazil. *Journal of the American Medical Informatics Association: JAMIA, 29*(1), 33–42. https://doi.org/10.1093/jamia/ocab219

Volkow, N. D., Han, B., Compton, W. M., & Blanco, C. (2017). Marijuana use during stages of pregnancy in the United States. *Annals of Internal Medicine, 166*(10), 763–764. https://doi.org/10.7326/L17-0067

Wilson, J. (1959). Experimental studies on congenital malformations. *Journal of Chronic Diseases, 10*(2), 111–130.

Wilson, J. (1977). Current status of teratology, general principles and mechanisms derived from animal studies. In J. Wilson & F. Fraser (Eds.), *Handbook of teratology* (pp. 47–74). Springer.

Zucker, I., & Prendergast, B. J. (2020). Sex differences in pharmacokinetics predict adverse drug reactions in women. *Biology of Sex Differences, 11*(1), 32. https://doi.org/10.1186/s13293-020-00308-5

18

Substance Use during Pregnancy

Signy Toquinto

The editors gratefully acknowledge Daisy J. Goodman and Kelley A. Bowden who co-authored the previous edition of this chapter.

Relevant Terms

Binge drinking—consumption of alcohol that brings blood alcohol concentration to about 0.08% or above, typically four or more alcohol servings on a single occasion, for people assigned female at birth

Detoxification—medically supervised withdrawal from physiologic dependence on a substance

Harm reduction approach—a philosophy, set of clinical practices, or policies aimed at reducing negative consequences associated with substance use

Illicit or illegal substance use—use of cannabis (in some states), cocaine, methamphetamine, heroin, illegally acquired prescription drugs (fentanyl, opioids, benzodiazepines, and amphetamines), hallucinogens (psilocybin, LSD)

Licit or legal substance use—use of alcohol, tobacco, cannabis (in some states), prescription opioids, prescription amphetamines, prescription benzodiazepines

Medication for opioid use disorder or medication-assisted treatment or opioid replacement therapy—treatment of opioid use disorder with a longer acting opioid agonist medication, typically methadone or buprenorphine

Motivational interviewing—nonjudgmental, neutral approach to promote dialogue and enhance motivation to change behavior

Neonatal opioid withdrawal syndrome or neonatal abstinence syndrome—the constellation of signs and symptoms displayed by a neonate with chronic prenatal opioid exposure

Physiologic dependence—physiologic increase in tolerance of the effects of a substance and presence of withdrawal symptoms upon abrupt cessation

Primary mental health disorders—a mental health condition that is not secondary to a general medical illness or side effect from medication.

Substance use disorder—recurrent use of a substance causing clinically significant impairment, including health problems, disability, and failure to meet major responsibilities at work, school, or home. May or may not include physiologic dependence and withdrawal

Substance use—the use of any substance (e.g., alcohol, tobacco, and cocaine) by any mode of administration (e.g., drinking, smoking, and injection drug use)

Abbreviations

AA	Alcoholics Anonymous	FGR	fetal growth restriction
ATOD	alcohol, tobacco, and other drugs	IDU	injection drug use
AUD	alcohol use disorder	IOPs	intensive outpatient programs
CBT	cognitive-behavioral therapy	IUFD	intrauterine fetal demise
CDC	Centers for Disease Control and Prevention	IUGR	intrauterine growth restriction
CPS	Child Protection Services	LBW	low birth weight
CUD	cannabis use disorder	MAT	medication-assisted treatment
FAS	Fetal Alcohol Syndrome	MI	motivation interviewing
FASD	Fetal Alcohol Spectrum Disorder	MOUD	medications for opioid use disorder

---

Prenatal and Postnatal Care: A Person-Centered Approach, Third Edition. Edited by Karen Trister Grace, Cindy L. Farley, Noelene K. Jeffers, and Tanya Tringali.

NAS	neonatal abstinence syndrome	SAMHSA	Substance Abuse and Mental Health Services Administration
NOWS	neonatal opioid withdrawal syndrome	SBIRT	screening, brief intervention, referral to treatment
NRT	nicotine-replacement therapy		
PDMP	prescription drug monitoring programs		
PrEP	pre-exposure prophylaxis	SSRIs	selective serotonin reuptake inhibitors
PPROM	preterm prelabor rupture of membranes	STI	sexually transmitted infections
PTB	preterm birth	SUD	substance use disorder
PTSD	post-traumatic stress disorder	SUID	sudden unexpected infant death

Introduction

Substance use during pregnancy is an ongoing social phenomenon that fosters controversy around healthcare management and treatment, legal and public health policy, criminalization and punishment, and parental rights. While concern regarding substance use and pregnancy is not new, it has recently increased as a result of the opioid epidemic's impact on pregnant people and their infants, as well as the general population (Patrick & Schiff, 2017). This chapter focuses on historical and contemporary substance use policies and trends in the United States, but many aspects of this content are applicable to global settings.

Substance use disorders (SUDs) are increasing among pregnant and birthing people and, when untreated, increase perinatal morbidity and mortality, pose risks to fetal and neonatal health, and increase healthcare costs. Additionally, bias, judgment, and scrutiny for substance use during pregnancy, especially from healthcare workers, reduce the willingness and ability of many people to seek healthcare and support. Roughly one in five maternal deaths are a result of opioid overdose in the United States (Metz et al., 2016; Schiff et al., 2018), exceeding deaths from hemorrhage, emboli, preeclampsia, and sepsis (Centers for Disease Control and Prevention [CDC], 2016). With the introduction of synthetic opioids like fentanyl to the nationwide drug supply, overdose increased 16% from 2018 to 2019 (CDC, 2021b). Pharmacotherapy for opioid use disorder (OUD) is a proven and successful safety and prevention strategy, but to be successful, pregnant and birthing people must have access to these therapeutics. Black, Indigenous, and people of color have greater risk of life-threatening health issues compared to White people when their pregnancies are complicated by SUD (Admon & Winkelman, 2019), which can likely be attributed to systemic and structural racism (Powell, 2008), thus highlighting a need for explicitly antiracist perinatal health practices that include screening and assessment for substance use and SUD as well as treatment.

There are many barriers to safe, effective, and patient- and family-centered care to pregnant and parenting people who use substances or have SUDs, including knowledge gaps among inpatient and outpatient obstetric and pediatric providers and staff, gaps in care coordination and communication, stigma and prejudice toward pregnant and parenting people, and inadequate capacity to meet the treatment and recovery needs of pregnant and parenting people who use substances (California Maternal Quality Care Collaborative [CMQCC], 2021). To avoid perpetuating harmful biases and stigma related to substance use and pregnancy, this chapter will first discuss both harm reduction and reproductive justice frameworks. These frameworks will be continuously referenced throughout the chapter as critical approaches to the topic, management, and treatment of substance use in pregnancy.

Health equity key points

- Increase the number of healthcare providers of color who provide perinatal substance use treatment to provide racially and linguistically concordant care to communities of color.
- Incorporate explicitly antiracist harm reduction clinical protocols and practices for the management of substance use and SUD in pregnancy.
- Increase accessibility of naloxone, safer drug use supplies, and harm reduction programs within communities of color that specifically target and support pregnant and parenting people.
- Increase programs that support the pregnant parent and infant dyad, that aim to keep families together despite substance use or SUD, and to eliminate racially discriminant CPS removal of infants and children of color.

Harm Reduction Approach to Perinatal Substance Use

The most promising approach to respond to substance use is harm reduction (Lie et al., 2022). The harm reduction philosophy is a 50-year-old movement for social justice that understands substance use as a complex, multifaceted phenomenon and prioritizes quality of life and well-being, honors and accepts personal agency and choice, and aims to minimize the harmful effects associated with substance use rather than promote abstinence (Harm Reduction Coalition, 2016). Examples of pragmatic harm reduction programs include syringe exchange, peer-to-peer outreach, controlled drinking programs, **medications for opioid use disorder (MOUD)** or **medication-assisted treatment (MAT)**, and safe consumption sites (Boyd et al., 2017; Wright et al., 2012).

Practically speaking, policies that discourage pregnant people from seeking prenatal care or treatment for substance use increase the risk of overdose, injury, sexually transmitted infection (STI) transmission, and other devastating outcomes that could be mitigated by supportive care. In contrast to approaches based on a perceived antagonism between a substance-using pregnant person's actions and the safety and well-being of their fetus, sometimes referred to as a "maternal-fetal conflict" (Fasouliotis & Schenker, 2000), harm reduction approaches strive to support the birthing parent *and* child as a unit and not two opposing entities with separate interests. While complete abstinence from substance use during pregnancy is a goal that may or may not be attainable, every action that reduces risk is recognized as a positive for the dyad. A **harm reduction approach** encourages pregnant people to engage with healthcare and supports collaboration between a pregnant person and their prenatal care provider toward a mutual goal of healthy pregnancy. While the harm reduction approach is criticized as legitimizing or supporting illegal activity, it is a proven strategy with documented positive outcomes (Wright et al., 2012). And while total abstinence may be the safest strategy during pregnancy and breastfeeding, harm reduction understands that some people have trouble achieving abstinence or are simply not ready. A harm reduction approach recognizes that SUDs are often relapsing and remitting conditions that are impacted by racism, poverty, stigma, discrimination, trauma, and social injustice.

Reproductive Justice Approach to Perinatal Substance Use

Reproductive justice is an intersectional framework that situates reproductive health and rights within human rights and social justice frameworks (Ross, 2006; Ross & Solinger, 2017). It is an interdisciplinary theory that requires the consideration of "nonbiological issues"—such as immigration, gentrification, and incarceration—and externally imposed policies and practices that directly impact pregnancy and parenting (Ross & Solinger, 2017). Reproductive justice places attention on aspects of privilege and oppression in healthcare systems (Eagen-Torkko, 2015), and recognizes the criminalization of pregnancy and pathologization of "risky" or "harmful" behaviors—such as substance use—as reproductive oppression aimed at subjugating the reproductive lives of people of color and people experiencing poverty (National Women's Law Center, 2013).

Reproductive justice is based on three interconnected tenets: "(a) the right to have a child under the conditions of one's choosing; (b) the right not to have a child using birth control, abortion, or abstinence; and (c) the right to parent children in safe and healthy environments free from violence by individuals or the state" (Ross, 2017, p. 290).

Reproductive injustice is evident in the pregnancy, birthing, and parenting experiences of people of color who use substances or have SUDs. While White people use drugs at higher rates than people of color (Ritchie, 2017) and White and Black people use alcohol at similar rates (Chasnoff et al., 1990), Black pregnant people are more likely to be screened or tested for substance use in pregnancy (Harp & Buntig, 2020) and 10 times more likely to be reported to child welfare authorities for substance use during pregnancy (Roberts & Nuru-Jeter, 2012; Roberts & Sangoi, 2018). Black families are also more likely to be reported to the child abuse hotline and investigated for child abuse and neglect, more likely to have their children removed from their care, and less likely to regain custody of their children (Roberts & Nuru-Jeter, 2010; Roberts & Sangoi, 2018).

It is critical that perinatal healthcare incorporate a reproductive justice approach to caring for pregnant and birthing people who use substances or have SUDs and their infants, to reduce harm, provide equitable and just care, and to eliminate the current practice of criminalizing and pathologizing people of color and their pregnancies. The approach to care should employ collaboration and transparency with and accountability to people and communities of color who use substances or have SUDs.

Prevalence of Prenatal Substance Use

Alcohol use during pregnancy is relatively common—21% report any alcohol use, 13.5% report current use, and 5.2% report **binge drinking** (Godsin et al., 2022; Lange et al., 2017). In 2019, CDC researchers found that about one in nine pregnant people reported drinking alcohol in the past 30 days, and about one-third of those who consumed alcohol reported binge drinking (Denny et al., 2019). According to data from the 2016 National Vital Statistics System, approximately 7.2% of women reported smoking cigarettes during pregnancy (Drake et al., 2018), and among women who quit during pregnancy, 31% started smoking again within six months after delivery (Sohrab & Seyed, 2021). On the 2018 National Survey on Drug Use and Health, cannabis was the most widely used substance during pregnancy in the United States, after tobacco and alcohol; 5.4% of pregnant people reported past month use, while less than 1% reported past month use of opioids and less than 0.5% reported past month use of cocaine (Substance Abuse and Mental Health Services Administration [SAMHSA], 2019). Daily or almost daily cannabis use was reported by 1.7% of pregnant people. An increase in prenatal cannabis use has been associated with the COVID-19 pandemic (Young-Wolff et al., 2021). Concurrent use of cannabis and other substances is common. Alcohol, tobacco, and other drug use was less common in the second and third trimester compared to the first trimester (SAMHSA, 2014). The National Institute on Drug Abuse (NIDA) estimates that the rate of **illicit drug use** and recreational use of prescription drugs among pregnant people is 5.4% overall, ranging from 14.6% for ages 15–17 to 3.2% for ages 26–44

(Forray, 2016). The number of opioid-related diagnoses, including OUD, at the time of birth increased 131% from 2010 to 2017 (Hiari et al., 2021). According to self-reported data from 2019, 7% of pregnant people reported any use of prescription opioids during pregnancy, and of those, 20% report recreational use of prescription opioids (CDC, 2021c; Ko et al., 2020b).

Between 2010 and 2019, 11.4% of perinatal deaths were drug-related and the overall maternal mortality ratios from drug use increased from 2.7 to 7.8 per 100,000 live births, a 190% relative increase (Margerison et al., 2022). Overdose deaths from prescription analgesics increased more than 400% among women between 1999 and 2010 (US Office on Women's Health [USOWH], 2017), and heroin use among women increased by 100% between 2002 and 2013 (US Substance Abuse and Mental Health Services Administration (SAMHSA), Center for Behavioral Health Statistics and Quality, 2011). The highest risk of morbidity and mortality related to relapse and overdose is during the postpartum period, with the highest overdose rate 7–12 months after delivery (Schiff et al., 2018).

Terminology

The American Psychiatric Association (APA)'s Diagnostic and Statistical Manual of Mental Disorders (DSM) is regarded as the defining standard for mental health diagnoses, including SUD. Terminology and diagnostic criteria for SUDs were revised in 2013 with the release of the fifth edition of the DSM (DSM-5) to better reflect current scientific knowledge. Whereas SUDs were previously described as manifestations of underlying primary psychopathology, they are now identified as **primary mental health disorders.** This change reflects a socially responsible and more medically accurate paradigm shift in the medical, moral, and legal conceptualizations of substance use (Robinson & Adinoff, 2016).

The term **addiction** is commonly used by the general public to describe SUDs and often confused with **physiologic dependence**. Historically, the term became enmeshed with moral judgment and intentionally inextricably linked with non-White communities, immigrants, impoverished workers, and criminal behavior (Robinson & Adinoff, 2016). In 1952, the DSM-I first conceptualized SUDs as personality disorders that had sociopathic aspects (Robinson & Adinoff, 2016). In 1980, the DSM-III acknowledged, for the first time, the cultural acceptability of substance use, moving away from pathology and realigning with a more medical approach with the inclusion of diagnostic criteria of SUD, distinguishing between use and physiologic dependence, and separately diagnosing SUD from other mental health conditions (Robinson & Adinoff, 2016). The term addiction does not even appear in the DSM-5 because of stigmatizing and negative connotations (APA, 2013); however, it is still commonly used in healthcare today. The American Society for Addiction Medicine (ASAM) offers the following definition of the term *addiction*:

> ### ASAM definition of addiction
>
> "Addiction is a treatable, chronic medical disease involving complex interactions among brain circuits, genetics, the environment, and an individual's life experiences. People with addiction use substances or engage in behaviors that become compulsive and often continue despite the consequences. Prevention efforts and treatment approaches for addiction are generally as successful as those for other chronic diseases."
>
> Source: ASAM (2019)/American Society of Addiction Medicine, Inc.

The distinction between substance use, physiologic dependence, and SUDs of any severity is a critical one for perinatal healthcare providers to understand. A basic knowledge of diagnostic criteria is important in assessing and assisting pregnant people to access an appropriate level of care. The DSM-5 removed the abuse-dependence paradigm in its revision and instead categorizes SUD by severity, using mild (two to three symptoms endorsed), moderate (four to five symptoms endorsed), and severe (six or more symptoms endorsed). Additionally, the DSM-5 further categorizes SUD into a number of more specific singular disorders (e.g., alcohol use disorder [AUD]). Table 18.1 depicts the APA's diagnostic criteria for SUDs.

SUDs should be distinguished from physiologic dependence, defined as the increased tolerance of its effects as well as the presence of withdrawal symptoms upon abrupt cessation. Although tolerance and withdrawal may be present as symptoms and are listed under pharmacologic criteria for SUDs, they are not diagnostic and may be associated with any chronic use of a substance causing physiologic dependence, such as the treatment of pain (APA, 2013). For example, an individual prescribed opioids for cancer pain would likely be physically dependent but would only receive a diagnosis of SUD if other diagnostic criteria were met.

Given the stigma surrounding substance use, especially substance use in pregnancy, healthcare providers should consistently utilize harm reduction language. Use "person-first" or humanizing language when describing or discussing people who use substances. An example of this is: "people who use cannabis" as opposed to "cannabis users." Avoid using stigmatizing and judgment-laden language, such as referring to something or someone as "clean" or "dirty" (often used when referring to the result of urine toxicology testing). Instead, the results of urine toxicology testing should be described with the clinically appropriate terms "negative" or "positive." Avoid referring to someone or their actions as substance abuser/abuse or misuser/misuse. In the past, the term "substance misuse" was used to refer to the use of substances in a harmful and/or dangerous manner, however, this did not equate with meeting diagnostic criteria for a SUD. However, there is no clinical consensus around what constitutes harmful use; thus, this term has been subjectively applied by the person using it. Instead, refer to a person's substance use as simply "use," and if they do not

Table 18.1   Criteria to Diagnose SUDs[a]

DSM-V diagnostic criteria
1. Opioids are often taken in larger amounts or over a longer period than was intended.
2. There is a persistent desire or unsuccessful efforts to cut down or control opioid use.
3. A great deal of time is spent in activities necessary to obtain the opioid, use the opioid, or recover from its effects.
4. There is craving, or a strong desire or urge to use opioids.
5. Recurrent opioid use results in a failure to fulfill major role obligations at work, school, or home.
6. Opioid use continues despite having persistent or recurrent social or interpersonal problems caused or exacerbated by the effects of opioids.
7. Important social, occupational, or recreational activities are given up or reduced because of opioid use.
8. Opioid use recurs in situations in which it is physically hazardous.
9. Opioid use continues despite knowledge of having a persistent or recurrent physical or psychological problem that is likely to have been caused or exacerbated by the substance.
10. Tolerance is manifested, as defined by either of the following[b]:   1. A need for markedly increased amounts of opioids to achieve intoxication or desired effect.   2. A markedly diminished effect with continued use of the same amount.
11. Withdrawal is manifested by either of the following: 1. The characteristic opioid withdrawal syndrome.   2. Opioids (or a closely related substance) are taken to relieve or avoid withdrawal symptoms.

Source: Adapted from APA (2013).
[a] Opioids are specified here, but the criteria are appropriate to diagnose other SUDs.
[b] This may also be true for those taking prescribed opioids for a medical indication, in which case this should not be considered diagnostic of OUD.

meet diagnostic criteria for a SUD, describe the frequency, amount of use, or how the use impacts daily activities. Evidence indicates that harmful language increases stigma related to substance use and reduces the quality of care patients receive and decreases public support for evidence-based strategies which reduce substance-related harm (Ashford et al., 2019; McGinty & Barry, 2020; NIDA, 2022).

Historical Approaches to Prenatal Substance Use

Pregnant people who use substances or have SUDs have been victims of significant stigma and punitive actions by both healthcare providers and the criminal justice system; this approach continues to be evident today. This history is often well understood by Black and Indigenous and increasingly Latine communities, whose pregnancies have disproportionately been subjugated and criminalized. Healthcare providers must be informed of this history and accountable for how inequitable injustices continue to operate today.

From the 1870s to the early 1900s, the first antidrug laws were passed in the United States specifically targeting communities of color and immigrant communities (Drug Policy Alliance, 2022). In 1971, US President Richard Nixon declared a "war on drugs" generating repressive drug laws and draconian sentencing policies (such as mandatory minimum sentencing), which were unequally enforced on communities and people of color (Drug Policy Alliance, 2022). An example includes the "100:1

rule," referring to a 1980s Act of Congress that disproportionately criminalizes crack cocaine compared to powder cocaine; the 100:1 ratio references the amount of powder cocaine versus crack cocaine needed to trigger mandatory prison sentences, which specifically criminalized and punished cocaine use specifically among Black and low-income communities (Vagins & McCurdy, 2006). This was not ameliorated until 2010 with the passage of the Fair Sentencing Act (ACLU, 2012). Additionally, the drug war's scripted racist archetypal propaganda portrayed people who use drugs, especially Black, Indigenous, and other communities of color and people experiencing poverty, as uncontrollable, self-destructive, lacking individual agency, and criminals in need of punishment (Walker, 2017). The moral panic around crack cocaine in the 1980s produced the image of the "monstrous crack-smoking mother" and fostered in many Americans a sense that deviant unruly women—the majority poor and Black (Roberts, 1997)—are responsible for generations living "at-risk" (Murphy & Rosenbaum, 1999; Roberts, 1997).

During the 1980s, concerns about a perceived epidemic of fetal exposure to crack cocaine (and the derogatory term *crack babies*) led to nonconsensual drug testing and the illegal release of confidential patient information to law enforcement (Wolff, 2011), a practice that the US Supreme Court eventually identified as a constitutional violation in 2001 (Metzl & Roberts, 2014). Between 1980 and 2000, over 200 women in 30 states were arrested and charged for alleged drug use and related actions during pregnancy (Metzl & Roberts, 2014). Some cases were successfully argued in favor of the defendants as violations of the Fourteenth Amendment guarantee of freedom from unreasonable search, but in others, women served long sentences and lost custody of their children (Lewis, 2016). The prosecution for substance use in pregnancy has disproportionately targeted Black, Indigenous, and increasingly Latine and other communities of color and low-income pregnant and parenting people (Guttmacher Institute, 2022; Paltrow & Flavin, 2013).

The legal landscape in the United States varies by state. Currently, 24 states and the District of Columbia consider substance use during pregnancy to be child abuse and three states consider it to be grounds for civil commitment, where a person may be forced into inpatient treatment programs (Guttmacher Institute, 2022). In 2014, Tennessee became the first state to pass a law criminalizing drug use during pregnancy, effectively permitting the incarceration of pregnant people and parents for their drug use (Angelotta & Appelbaum, 2017). However, it was determined that the law deterred pregnant people from seeking prenatal care and impeded access to medical treatment, and the law has not been in effect since 2016 (ACLU, 2016). Additionally, at least 13 states have passed legislation requiring some form of drug testing or screening for applicants or recipients of public assistance, and many other states have proposed legislation (Center for Law and Social Policy, 2019). Selective drug testing of any defined population (including pregnant people) is considered by health and substance use experts to be discriminatory and unethical.

Punitive drug-testing policies result in pregnant people reporting fear of incarceration, forced abortion, loss of healthcare services, and loss of custody of their children, which cause pregnant people to avoid prenatal care, attempt to stop using drugs before attending, or to delay or forgo prenatal care entirely (Roberts & Nuru-Jeter, 2010; Roberts & Pies, 2011; Stone, 2015). These adverse consequences disproportionately affect communities of color and people experiencing poverty. Extensive literature documents the disproportionate burden, structural violence, and racism that Black, Indigenous, and other communities of color have experienced related to drug policy, criminalization, and pathologization of substance use (Drug Policy Alliance, 2016; Netherland & Hansen, 2016; Ritchie, 2017; Roberts, 1997). The American Academy of Pediatrics (AAP) makes the strong statement that "punitive measures taken toward pregnant people, such as criminal prosecution and incarceration, have no proven benefits for infant health policy" (Patrick & Schiff, 2017), and nonpunitive approaches are specifically endorsed by the American College of Obstetricians and Gynecologists (ACOG, 2015), the American College of Nurse-Midwives (ACNM, 2013), and the American Society of Addiction Medicine (ASAM, 2020a, 2020b).

Criminalization of Substance Use in Pregnancy and Impact on Child Welfare

Of the serious legal and social consequences of biological toxicology testing from the expansion of state surveillance of substance use in pregnancy, the identification of substance use leading to child removal by child protective services (CPS) has become the most common reason for child removal from their family in the United States (SAMHSA, 2016).

Around the same time as the war on drugs was escalating, the Child Abuse Prevention and Treatment Act (CAPTA) (initially passed by Congress in 1974), encouraged states to enact mandatory reporting laws requiring certain professionals to report child abuse. With the criminalization and pathologization of substance use, mandated reporters began making reports to child welfare about parental substance use. During the era of increased crack cocaine use, the number of children taken from their parents and placed in foster care increased over 100% (Movement for Family Power, 2020). The increase in child removal related to substance use evolved from the exaggerated perception of harm from substance exposure in utero, much of this originating from medical, social, and scientific propaganda of the effects of substance use on pregnancy and parenting and the stigmatization and criminalization in general. Substance use became viewed as the antithesis of proper parenting (Murphy & Rosenbaum, 1999) and "quantifiable markers of poor mothering" (Knight, 2015, pp. 88–89). Conflicting research has challenged some of these assumptions; while there are immediate risks associated with the use of cocaine in pregnancy (low birth weight [LBW] and preterm labor), recent systemic reviews and meta-analyses show that specific long-term effects of cocaine exposure have not been established (Betancourt et al., 2011; Cestonaro et al., 2022) and instead suggest that socioeconomic and environmental factors contribute to neurodevelopmental outcomes equally or greater than cocaine (Cressman et al., 2014). While substance use during pregnancy has documented risks to both the pregnant person and the fetus—much like other known chronic health conditions, such as diabetes or high blood pressure—research continues to document the further harm caused by stigmatizing and criminalizing use in pregnancy.

Substance use screening and reporting and involvement of child welfare disproportionately impacts Black, Indigenous, and other people of color, as a result of structural and systemic racism. This has ongoing community impacts including increased use of substances among parents affected, housing instability, mental distress, and trauma and related sequelae (Kenny et al., 2015; Kenny et al., 2021). In order to address the devastating harms originating from biases and structural racism, perinatal healthcare providers need re-education, re-evaluation of policies and practices, and to create systems of care that compassionately support pregnant people using substances while keeping families intact to prevent further trauma.

Prenatal Screening

Substance use screening can provide pregnant people with meaningful interventions including possibilities for prevention, early diagnosis and intervention, counseling, and treatment in people of reproductive age.

Universal verbal substance use screening in perinatal care lessens the stigma associated with use and provides opportunity for health education/counseling, **motivational interviewing** (MI), and early intervention as needed. Reducing substance use can benefit pregnancy outcomes, an individual's long-term health, and the health of their infants. Screening and early identification of use may also reduce immediate and long-term economic costs to society (Berger, 2002). Pregnancy is socially and medically viewed as a window of opportunity, or "teachable moment," where pregnant people may be highly motivated to make changes that support improving their health and the health of their fetus (Arabin & Baschat, 2017; Bloch & Parascandola, 2014; Forray, 2016).

Universal substance use screening in pregnancy (verbal screening for alcohol, tobacco, cannabis, and other drug use) is recommended by the ACNM, the ACOG, AAP, and the United States Preventive Services Task Force (USPSTF) (ACNM, 2017, 2018; ACOG, 2011a; ACOG, 2017a, reaffirmed 2021; ACOG, 2020; Patrick & Schiff, 2017; USPSTF, 2018; USPSTF, 2021). Barriers to screening during prenatal care include being overwhelmed by the amount of screening, feeling inadequately trained for handling a positive screen, doubt about the benefits of screening, and the belief that one's patients do not use substances (Wright et al., 2016). When patients do not disclose their use, this should be considered a missed opportunity on behalf of the clinic or provider, not the patient's attempt to deceive the provider. It is the responsibility of the healthcare provider to create a safe environment for disclosure. Many people who use substances in pregnancy report willingness to disclose and high acceptability for the verbal screening (Toquinto et al., 2020).

Before screening, providers should carefully consider if they are prepared to adequately support the pregnant person in their recovery or treatment; if not, screening may only serve the purpose of reporting and child welfare involvement, which can be detrimental to the health and well-being of the pregnant person and infant. Research documents that healthcare providers are biased in drug use screening/testing and disproportionately screen, test, and make reports to CPS when the pregnant person is a person of color or living in poverty (Roberts & Nuru-Jeter, 2010). Mandatory universal or standardized substance use screening and testing protocols in perinatal care aim to reduce racial biases in provider screening, but fail to address CPS reporting disparities, reflecting provider bias and systemic racism (Roberts & Nuru-Jeter, 2010; Roberts et al., 2015; Wright et al., 2016).

Universal verbal screening for substance use allows the healthcare provider to discuss the risks of substance use with *every* pregnant person. Early screening at the first prenatal visit enables timely intervention and referral to treatment for pregnant people with a SUD and maximizes efforts at harm reduction. Screening should be done with a nonjudgmental and respectful approach using a validated screening instrument (see *Resources for Healthcare Providers*). The use of a structured approach increases the number of pregnant people who receive

treatment (Chang et al., 2011; Stockton-Joreteg & Griffin, 2020). Integrating substance use screening and intervention into routine prenatal care is effective and is associated with decreases in preterm birth (PTB), placental abruption, and intrauterine fetal demise (Goler et al., 2008; Wright et al., 2016).

Harm reduction approach to universal verbal screening

Normalize the conversation:
"This is something I ask everyone/all patients. . ."

State WHY you are asking:
"I would like to ask you about past and current substance use. I am asking because many people use alcohol, tobacco, cannabis, and other drugs before and during pregnancy. Substance use can affect your health and maybe you have questions about it."

Transparency! Discuss what happens if they disclose:
"I want you to know if you choose to disclose any substance use to me today, my goal would be to talk about: your use, how it impacts you, and your goals around your use during pregnancy"
"I will not have any judgment of you and this will in no way impact the quality of care you receive."
"My goal is to listen to you and your needs. To discuss how substance use can impact pregnancy. And to work with you to reduce any harms associated with substance use."
"If you disclose substance use today, this does NOT mean that I will ask to test your urine for drugs or substances."

Acknowledging the harms of the system:
"I want to acknowledge that there is a long history of the healthcare system punishing pregnant people for their substance use. I want to name this and recognize the harm caused. My goal is to reduce the harms of the healthcare system. To be an advocate for you. To help you navigate this system in the least harmful way."

Standardized Verbal Screening Tools

Several interview-based and self-administered screening instruments have been developed and tested for use with pregnant people. These include the T-ACE, TWEAK, and AUDIT-C, which screen for alcohol use, and the 5Ps Plus, NIDA Quick Screen-ASSIST and CRAFFT, which screen more generally for substance use. The T-ACE tool identifies lower levels of alcohol consumption than the TWEAK tool and is the preferred tool for use in pregnancy (ACOG, 2011a, reaffirmed 2021). However, the AUDIT-C is more precise in determining alcohol use quantity and patterns (Dawson et al., 2005) and can also be scored based on preconceptional use, to identify individuals who may return to higher use patterns postpartum, even if they are able to stop during pregnancy. (See *Resources for Healthcare Providers* for the AUDIT-C scoring algorithm). The 5Ps Plus consists of seven questions (related to parents, peers, partners, past use, use during pregnancy) and is considered positive if there was an affirmative response, the NIDA Quick Screen-ASSIST is a two part screening tool that classifies use by risk level and assesses use of specific substances, and the CRAFT is a validated screening tool for adolescents aged 12–21 (Coleman-Cowger et al., 2019; Ondersma et al., 2019).

Biological Toxicology Testing

Biological toxicology testing includes the testing of biological sampling (maternal: urine, blood, or hair; or neonatal: urine, meconium, or umbilical cord sampling) for the purposes of identifying alcohol or other drug use. Universal prenatal urine toxicology testing is routinely performed in many prenatal practices and has been promoted as an approach to reducing racial and economic biases. Because of ongoing prejudice in reporting of positive tests of pregnant and parenting people who are Black, Indigenous, and people of color, despite universal testing, this practice should be scrutinized and avoided. Urine toxicology testing should never replace verbal screening for alcohol, tobacco, cannabis, and other drugs. Currently, no professional organizations recommend universal urine toxicology testing.

There are many limitations and drawbacks to using urine toxicology testing as a screening tool. Standard urine toxicology tests have limited ability to detect intermittent use, may not reflect the types of drugs prevalent in a particular community, and do not routinely include testing for the metabolites of alcohol. Institutions and providers should be aware of specificity and sensitivity of the modalities they are using (CMQCC, 2021). Most urine toxicology tests are only able to detect recent use, generally one to five days for most substances or in the cases of daily cannabis use up to 30 days. In addition, high false positive rates of rapid urine tests require that a more expensive confirmatory test (gas chromatography–mass spectrometry or liquid chromatography–mass spectrometry) be performed for accuracy (Heit, 2016). Commonly used medications such as diphenhydramine, metformin, promethazine, sertraline, bupropion, and other antidepressants can produce false positives for amphetamines and benzodiazepines in rapid immunoassay tests. Additionally, care should be taken when collecting urine samples during a hospital admission to thoroughly document what medications have been given to the patient, especially opioid analgesics, prior to the sample collection. Recent research has also shown that the use of fentanyl in a labor epidural can impact both maternal and neonatal toxicology tests, thus, it should be considered as a possible etiology of a positive test (Siegel et al., 2022). A positive urine toxicology test does not provide information on the nature or extent of drug use and a negative test does not rule out drug use (Wright et al., 2016). A positive test is not a tool for assessing or diagnosing the severity or frequency of use or if the person has a SUD. A negative test does not rule out substance use or SUD—it does not capture 100% of all substance use. A positive test does not indicate a person's capacity to parent and should not be utilized to make this determination.

Perinatal urine toxicology testing can identify newborns exposed to both **licit** and **illicit** substances and should be utilized if the results of the test will change the management and care of the newborn. However, the reliance on and the routine use of urine toxicology testing have the potential to do significant harm and disrupt the therapeutic relationship between the patient and the provider. The utilization of urine toxicology testing communicates to patients that healthcare providers do not trust their honest disclosure of substance use. Additionally, copious research indicates that a proportion of pregnant people report that universal toxicology testing would discourage them from attending prenatal care, indicating that universal drug screening policies can have negative effects on maternal–child health (Tucker Edmonds et al., 2017).

Due to high cost, limited sensitivity and specificity, and ethical issues involved, urine toxicology is not recommended as a screening method for substance use by pregnant people. When urine toxicology testing is performed, it is essential to provide explicit informed consent (written consent should be considered when possible). It is the responsibility of the healthcare provider to provide a clear explanation of why testing is being recommended, the benefits and risks of testing, including the potential legal, criminal, and child welfare considerations. Every patient has the right to withhold consent or decline testing without assumptions of use and repercussions and without use of coercive language (CMQCC, 2021). It is also the responsibility of the healthcare provider to provide anticipatory guidance about the possibility, potential, or likelihood of neonatal biological testing postpartum and if any potential risks exist as a result of declining testing.

Brief Intervention

Screening, brief intervention, and referral to treatment (SBIRT) was originally developed as a public health model designed for the universal screening for alcohol, tobacco, cannabis, or other drug use (ATOD) in primary care settings (SAMHSA, 2022). There is substantial evidence of its effectiveness in reducing alcohol consumption in the general population (SAMHSA, 2011), but limited evidence about its use in pregnancy. Although substance use screening can identify a person *at risk* for perinatal effects of ATOD, it does not diagnose a SUD. Further subjective data gathering is essential following a positive screen to explore the extent and type of a person's substance use, for example, by utilizing the NIDA assessment tool or ASSIST, to determine whether criteria for a SUD are met (Table 18.1). Exploring a person's readiness to address this issue and goals for their use, pregnancy, and parenting will also guide care and referrals. Perinatal outcomes are improved for substance-affected pregnancies when substance use screening and treatment are integrated with prenatal care (Goler et al., 2008, 2012). Figure 18.1 illustrates the level of care decisions based on the person's substance use and care preferences.

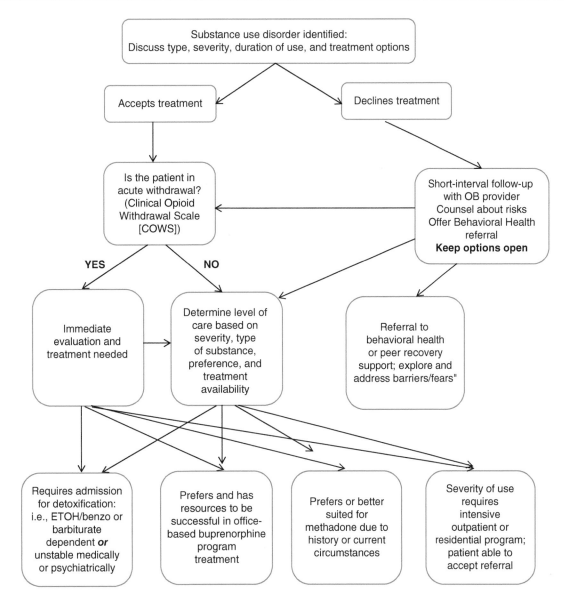

Figure 18.1   Algorithm for discussing levels of care for SUD. Daisy Goodman CNM WHNP-BC, used with permission.

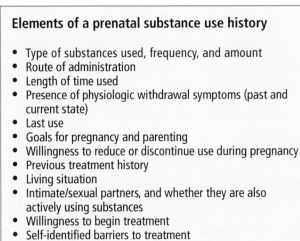

Elements of a prenatal substance use history

- Type of substances used, frequency, and amount
- Route of administration
- Length of time used
- Presence of physiologic withdrawal symptoms (past and current state)
- Last use
- Goals for pregnancy and parenting
- Willingness to reduce or discontinue use during pregnancy
- Previous treatment history
- Living situation
- Intimate/sexual partners, and whether they are also actively using substances
- Willingness to begin treatment
- Self-identified barriers to treatment
- Self-identified supports to the success of their recovery

MI techniques can facilitate conversation and information gathering about substance use in pregnancy. Facility with MI requires training and practice and is strongly recommended for all healthcare professionals; see the *Resources for Healthcare Providers* section. However, there are some elements of the approach that can be incorporated into brief interventions even without formal training (Table 18.2), including asking permission, assessing existing knowledge/providing information, evoking readiness for change, and building partnership.

Instead of giving directions or making accusations, the brief intervention should identify what patient goals for pregnancy, parenting, and their substance use are and should include accurate information about maternal and fetal risks specifically associated with the substance use. A harm reduction approach is essential for any meaningful conversation that supports a pregnant person's ability to

Table 18.2   Brief Substance Use Intervention Steps

Intervention step	Rationale	Example
Asking permission	Promotes engagement and trust	"Thank you for sharing that with me. Can I ask you how you are thinking or feeling in regards to your [substance] use now that you are pregnant?" "What are your hopes or goals for this pregnancy regarding your [substance] use?"
Assessing existing knowledge/ providing information	Respects that both clinician and patient have expertise	"What do you know or have heard about [substance] use and its effects during pregnancy? May I give you some information about what we know about the effects of using [substance] during pregnancy?" (Share information without conveying judgment. If there is insufficient evidence available, state this, and also that this does not mean that the substance is safe to use.)
Evoking readiness for change	Reflecting/summarizing patient's thoughts and eliciting patient's motivations	"I hear you say that you are concerned about how the use of [substance] has impacted or will impact your pregnancy. It sounds like you've identified some motivations to make some changes in your use of [substance] or how you use [substance]."
Building partnership	Provides tangible care and support	"Thank you for being willing to talk about this, and your openness to the information I gave you. What can I do for you today? What can we do to help you have the pregnancy experience you desire? What can we do to help support your goals for parenting?" If they indicated a desire for assistance: ". . . I have referred many of my patients who use [substance] for counseling [or other treatment]. Is this something you might be interested in? Would you be willing to try this?"

make changes. Appropriate options for treatment based on the type of substance(s) used are provided at this time. Ambivalence on the part of the pregnant person is normal, and it is most important to leave the conversation open so that it can be revisited at a later encounter. Always maintain nonjudgmental care regardless of where the pregnant person is in their recovery and regularly affirm the mutual goal of a healthy pregnancy and ensuring safety for the pregnant person, fetus, and newborn. A supportive, pragmatic approach is central to exploring options in partnership. Providers should understand that a pregnant person may either seek to minimize their use, based on fear of stigma, embarrassment, and self-blame, or, conversely, be forthcoming and relieved that help is available. It is the provider's responsibility to create an environment where the pregnant person feels safe to disclose substance use and details regarding use. In turn, the provider has an ethical obligation to be knowledgeable and transparent about current evidence regarding risks, and about institutional policy and state law regarding prenatal substance use, including the states' or counties' laws and customary practice of reporting to child welfare services.

If a pregnant person is not ready or unable to seek treatment, it is critical that they feel safe and comfortable returning to prenatal care. Perinatal care providers should maintain a readily accessible and up-to-date list of treatment resources. Warm hand offs with treatment providers or supportive resources should be provided when possible.

Treatment Types

For pregnant people with identified SUDs meeting DSM-5 criteria, referral to treatment is recommended. Treatment for OUDs is designed at different levels of intensity and duration, as indicated by the severity of the use disorder (Figure 18.1). Access to person-centered treatment that accepts Medicaid is often limited and varies widely by region. Some programs do not accept pregnant people or allow children to accompany their parents to treatment, creating inequitable barriers for pregnant and parenting people.

ASAM has developed a classification system for substance use treatment options which fall into four general categories:

1. **Office-based treatment** includes behavioral treatment for substance use with or without medication. For OUD, medication may consist of buprenorphine/naloxone, buprenorphine monotherapy, or naltrexone.
2. **Methadone maintenance programs** combine behavioral treatment with daily observed treatment with methadone.
3. **Intensive outpatient programs (IOPs)** offer substance use treatment several days of the week for a standard number of hours on an outpatient basis.
4. **Residential treatment programs** offer daily, intensive substance use treatment in a residential setting. Some residential programs are gender specific. A few residential programs are also equipped to accommodate children whose parents are seeking treatment.

Identifying the appropriate level of treatment is a shared decision-making process, which requires a frank discussion about barriers and facilitators for treatment retention, prior history of treatment success or failure, social/environmental risks such as partners who are actively using, safe storage of medications (if applicable), and other risks or threats to recovery. The choice about appropriate treatment is especially complex for parenting people, who will often choose a lower level of care than would be most helpful to them, in order to remain with their children. Utilizing a harm reduction approach is critical to meeting the person where they are at, in terms of their readiness, their goals, and what type of treatment works in their life. The shared goal is to help facilitate the engagement in ongoing treatment and prenatal care.

Pregnant people using substances frequently disclose guilt about being unable to discontinue and require significant reassurance regarding the progress of their pregnancies (Jessup & Brindis, 2005). Regular participation in substance use counseling is an important component of treatment for SUD but should never be a requirement of treatment, as some people may be successful in their recovery with only the use of MOUD. Ideally, pregnant people with complex SUDs have access to integrated treatment programs capable of delivering co-located psychiatric, substance use, and prenatal care. However, such programs are relatively rare in most regions of the United States. Thus, prenatal healthcare providers are often in the position of coordinating services.

Common Factors Affecting People Who Use Substances

Mental Health

Pregnant people with SUDs have a high prevalence of concurrent mental health conditions. Rates of mood and anxiety disorders have been found to increase during pregnancy in pregnant people with OUD (Carter & Kostaras, 2005) and SUD, and rates of prenatal and postpartum depression are increased (Arnaudo et al., 2017; Forray, 2016). In one study, high scores on a depression scale correlated with double the rate of alcohol use during pregnancy (Harrison & Sidebottom, 2009). Post-traumatic stress disorder (PTSD) is a common comorbidity for pregnant, substance-using people, which impacts both engagement in prenatal care and treatment success (Bell & Seng, 2013). The majority of opioid-dependent pregnant people report PTSD symptoms rooted in histories of sexual and physical abuse as children and adults (Andrews et al., 2011; Arnaudo et al., 2017; Helmbrecht & Thiagarajah, 2008; Jessup & Brindis, 2005; Velez et al., 2006). Untreated depression is particularly associated with dependence on opioids, with a prevalence rate over 50% in some studies (Carrà et al., 2019; Moylan et al., 2001; Eggleston et al., 2009). Depression screening for people reporting substance use is essential, and for people who screen positive, treatment through either primary care or mental health services should be facilitated.

Social/Structural Determinants of Health

Physical, sexual, and emotional trauma, including adverse childhood experiences (ACEs), are associated with increased risk of SUD, and this risk is further increased when it intersects with bias and discrimination (Hansen et al., 2022).

Intimate partner violence (IPV) among people with SUDs is highly prevalent (Dillon et al., 2013; Engstrom et al., 2012; Schneider et al., 2009). Additionally, IPV is associated with increased risk of subsequent substance use and SUDs (Ogden et al., 2022). There is a strong correlation between substance use in people with current or past physical and sexual trauma, and other significant ACEs (Horrigan et al., 2000; Leza et al., 2021). A trauma-informed approach to screening and discussing IPV and substance use during pregnancy is critical. Providers should provide education around healthy relationships and discuss available supportive resources related to IPV without requiring a pregnant person to disclose their trauma to avoid retraumatization. Substance use may be a coping mechanism for current or past trauma (Asberg & Renk, 2012). The prevalence of IPV among people with SUDs may complicate a person's ability to seek and continue treatment, especially when the partner is also substance using (Velez et al., 2006; Terplan et al., 2015).

People who are using substances may experience homelessness, unstable housing, poverty, and food insecurity (Davis et al., 2019; Schmitz et al., 2016). People experiencing the effects of poverty should be offered social work, case management, and other supportive resources for housing, food, and Women, Infants, and Children (WIC) benefits.

The criminalization of **illicit substances** increases the risks that pregnant people who use drugs may be court involved (may have a history of or current incarceration). The racist war on drugs has caused the disproportionate policing, punishment, incarceration, and hypercriminalization of communities of color. The inequitable and unjust punishment of people of color who use drugs leads people to fear service engagement and is a barrier for people seeking treatment and supportive services. Additionally, immigrant people who use drugs may be hesitant to engage in treatment services for the very realistic fear of detention and deportation (Lopez et al., 2022).

Other Medical Conditions

Perinatal substance use is associated with potential significant medical risks, which are related to type of substance used, mode of administration, and potential harmful behaviors while a person is under the influence. Chief among these is the risk for infectious disease transmission and overdose. Hepatitis C, which is associated with drug use, is the most common blood-borne illness in the United States and is associated with high mortality when untreated (CDC, 2016; Denniston et al., 2014; Ly et al., 2020). Condomless sex, sex with multiple partners, and the prevalence of transactional sex or sex work among people with SUDs increases the risk of STIs, HIV, and hepatitis B and C. Providers should utilize a harm reduction approach when discussing safe sex education and offer safe sex supplies, like condoms and pre-exposure prophylaxis (PrEP).

Syringe sharing and recurrent use of used syringes increases the transmission risk of hepatitis B and C and HIV, cellulitis, needle-site abscess, tissue loss and necrosis, and increasing rates of fungal and bacterial endocarditis. Risk for colonization with multidrug-resistant organisms such as methicillin-resistant *Staphylococcus aureus* (MRSA) is increased. Thrombophlebitis, deep vein thrombosis, and resulting emboli are frequent sequelae of injection drug use. Rh isoimmunization even in nulligravid persons is a pregnancy-specific risk of sharing needles with consequences. People who inject drugs should be referred to syringe exchange sites and local harm reduction programs.

Smoking or inhaling substances have risks specific to the method of use. Sharing pipes or mouthpieces for the consumption of drugs can increase risks for infections transmitted through sores or burns, such as HIV, hepatitis C, tuberculosis, and herpes zoster. Healthcare providers should refer a person to harm reduction sites to obtain pipe or rubber stem covers to reduce infectious disease transmission. Inhaling or snorting substances can cause bleeding from the inside of the nose; thus, people should use their own straws or inhalation devices and not share to reduce the transmission of hepatitis C (Fernandez et al., 2016).

Polysubstance use, high doses of opioids, co-occurring mental health conditions, and adulterated fentanyl increases a person's risk for overdose. All pregnant people who report any opioid use should be routinely prescribed naloxone for overdose prevention. Given increasing rates of fentanyl in other recreational drugs, such as cocaine and methamphetamine, pregnant people who believe they are using nonopioid drugs should also be recommended and prescribed naloxone; they should also be referred to syringe exchange sites where they can obtain fentanyl test strips to check their supply. People should be encouraged to avoid using drugs alone, as this increases a person's risk for fatal overdose.

Undernutrition is prevalent among people with SUDs and may cause osteopenia, osteoporosis, anxiety, and depression (Jeynes & Leigh-Gibson, 2017). Poor nutritional status can impair placental development, including reduction in placental size and blood flow and can impair the delivery of nutrients to the fetus which can increase risks for PTB, LBW, and fetal growth restriction (FGR) (Hendrixson et al., 2021). Prenatal vitamins should be encouraged for people with SUDs and nutritional counseling and food pantry programs should be offered.

Commonly Used Substances, Pregnancy Implications, and Recommended Treatment

Alcohol

Alcohol use during pregnancy is the leading preventable cause of developmental disabilities and birth defects in the United States (National Institute on Alcohol Abuse and Alcoholism, 2021). There is no known safe level of prenatal alcohol exposure; therefore, it is recommended for pregnant people to abstain (Bandoli et al., 2019; CDC, 2021a). The severity of alcohol's effects on a fetus primarily depends on the amount of alcohol consumed, the frequency of use, and the timing of use (National Institute on Alcohol Abuse and Alcoholism, 2021). Significant alcohol exposure in the first trimester is associated with facial and major structural anomalies (Feldman

Table 18.3 Fetal Alcohol Spectrum Disorder Diagnoses

Diagnosis	Characteristics
Fetal alcohol syndrome (FAS)	Growth deficiency, CNS problems with developmental disability or brain damage, and characteristic facial dimorphisms of short philtrum, thin upper lip, and short distance between the inner and outer eye canthus
Alcohol-related neurodevelopmental disorders (ARND)	Intellectual, behavioral, and learning disabilities and problems with behavior and learning, characterized by academic difficulties with math, memory, attention, judgment, and poor impulse control
Alcohol-related birth defects (ARDB)	Cardiovascular, renal, and/or skeletal abnormalities
Neurobehavioral disorder associated with prenatal alcohol exposure (ND-PAE)	Problems with thinking and memory, behavior, and activities of daily living

Source: Adapted from CDC (2022).

et al., 2012), whereas exposure in the second trimester is associated with spontaneous abortion; exposure in the third trimester predominantly affects fetal weight and brain growth and is associated with increased risk for FGR, PTB, and stillbirth (Bailey & Sokol, 2011; Senturias et al., 2019).

Alcohol exposure during pregnancy is widely recognized as teratogenic and associated with a range of specific conditions with mild to severe phenotypes grouped together as fetal alcohol spectrum disorders (FASDs) (though not every pregnant person with alcohol exposure will have an affected fetus). Irreversible central nervous system (CNS) effects are the primary feature of FASD (Riley et al., 2011). There are four identifiable diagnoses associated with prenatal alcohol exposure under the FASD umbrella, described in Table 18.3. Fetal alcohol syndrome (FAS) is the most severe of the conditions, affecting multiple structures in the brain and other organs. The duration of alcohol exposure, especially into the third trimester, is associated with cognitive-behavioral problems in childhood (ACOG, 2011a, reaffirmed 2021). Cessation of alcohol use at any point in pregnancy is beneficial, as children born to parents who stop drinking even late in pregnancy have better outcomes than those born to parents who drink throughout pregnancy (ACOG, 2011a, reaffirmed 2021).

Treatment of Alcohol Use and AUD in Pregnancy

There are many approaches to treatment for people who are ready to change their drinking or abstain from alcohol use entirely. The quantity and quality of alcohol a person uses should be carefully assessed, and providers should work closely with pregnant people who continue to use alcohol to determine the level of support needed to help them stop. Healthcare providers should offer and refer pregnant people to individual counseling and/or group therapy; some patients may benefit from 12 Step meetings such as Alcoholics Anonymous (AA) or other community meetings; however, given that alcohol use during pregnancy is highly stigmatized, a group setting with other nonpregnant people may not feel supportive to all patients.

Standard medications for the treatment of alcohol dependence include naltrexone tablets or injections, acamprosate, disulfiram, and gabapentin; however, there is not good evidence on the safety of these medications during pregnancy. If abstinence is not achieved without the use of medications, the risks of continued drinking likely outweigh the possible adverse effects of medication (DeVido et al., 2015). One small study suggested no clear association between acamprosate and poor maternal or fetal outcomes (Kelty et al., 2019). Naltrexone is likely safe as it has been used more widely for the treatment of SUD in pregnancy (Kelty et al., 2021). Disulfiram, when used in the first trimester, has been associated with increased risk for fetal malformations; however, the continued use of alcohol and its risks and pregnancy should be weighed against the risks of medication (DeVido et al., 2015). Pregnant people who are physiologically dependent on alcohol require medically supervised withdrawal described as **detoxification**, which frequently must be managed in the inpatient setting.

Tobacco and Nicotine

The use of tobacco products is one of the most modifiable causes of adverse maternal, fetal, and neonatal outcomes in the United States (ACOG, 2020). Cigarettes are the most commonly used tobacco product during pregnancy, but e-cigarettes/vaporizers, cigars, and hookahs are becoming increasingly common. Nicotine is a potent adrenergic stimulant that increases the release of dopamine and is also a toxin that is easily absorbed and transfers readily to the brain, crosses the placenta to the fetus, and is found in fetal blood, amniotic fluid, and breastmilk. Tobacco exposure is associated with increased risk of intrauterine growth restriction (IUGR), preterm premature rupture of membranes (PPROM), placental abruption, LBW, stillbirth, and perinatal mortality in a dose-dependent relationship (ACOG, 2020; Bailey et al., 2012; CDC, 2020; Varner et al., 2014). Nicotine is also a known risk factor for cervical dysplasia and cervical cancer. Cigarette use in people of childbearing age is associated with reduced fertility and an increased risk of ectopic pregnancy (ACOG, 2020; Xuan et al., 2016). Harm from smoking in pregnancy results from effects on fetal oxygenation, development, and toxin exposure (Rodriguez, 2022a). The neurotoxic effects of nicotine and of carbon monoxide in smoke, as well as vasoconstriction, compromise placental function (McDonnell & Regan, 2019). Carbon monoxide is transferred through the placenta to the fetus and reduces fetal oxygenation (Rodriguez, 2022a), resulting in numerous fetal, neonatal, and childhood sequelae.

Chronic in utero exposure to nicotine also leads to neonatal withdrawal, intensifying symptoms associated with **Neonatal Opioid Withdrawal Syndrome** (NOWS) (Choo et al., 2004). Nicotine has a direct inhibitory effect on lung tissue maturation and reduces the infant's ability to respond during episodes of hypoxia, contributing to the higher incidence of sudden unexpected infant death (SUID) among nicotine-exposed infants (Zhang & Wang, 2013). Nicotine use is associated with physiologic dependence and commonly co-occurs with other SUDs.

Complications related to nicotine exposure

Neonatal/childhood complications associated with nicotine exposure	Perinatal complications associated with nicotine exposure
Cleft lip and palate	Spontaneous abortion
Musculoskeletal defects (clubfoot, craniosynostosis)	Ectopic pregnancy
Gastrointestinal defects (gastroschisis, hernia)	Placental abruption
Asthma and other atopic diseases	Preterm premature rupture of membranes
Type 2 diabetes	Placenta previa
Otitis media	Preterm birth
Neurological development deficits	Fetal growth restriction
Sudden unexpected infant death	Low birth weight
Reduced head circumference	Stillbirth
Altered brainstem development	
Cognitive, emotional, and behavioral problems	
Altered lung structure	
Cerebral palsy	
Tourette Syndrome	

Source: ACOG (2020), Anderka et al. (2010); Hackshaw et al. (2011), Rodriguez (2022a), and Wehby et al. (2011).

Treatment of Tobacco Use Disorder during Pregnancy

Optimally, tobacco cessation should occur prior to conception; however, many people are still actively smoking when they become pregnant. Tobacco cessation, reduction of use, avoidance of second-hand smoke, and prevention of relapse should be part of perinatal counseling. Individual psychosocial interventions—MI or cognitive-behavioral therapy (CBT)—have shown positive effects on reducing tobacco use in pregnancy (Chamberlain et al., 2017; Patnode et al., 2015). Provider advice to quit, accompanied by self-help materials, has been shown to increase abstinence from tobacco almost twofold (AHRQ, 2020). Counseling approaches to decrease cigarette smoking reduce the risks of SUID (Anderson et al., 2019). The "5 As" approach may be used to address smoking during pregnancy and is simple to remember (AHRQ, 2020) (see *Resources for Healthcare Providers* for this and other resources). Referral to smoking cessation programs within the patient's community is important. There is insufficient evidence on the effectiveness of mindfulness, hypnosis, or acupuncture on smoking cessation (Barnes et al., 2019; Maglione et al., 2017; White et al., 2014), but emerging research (not with pregnant people) on the use of psilocybin-facilitated smoking cessation is associated with long-term abstinence (Johnson et al., 2017; Martinez, 2021). Providers should always individualize care plans with patients and offer psychological, behavioral, and/or pharmacologic interventions.

For pregnant people who report heavy nicotine use or have difficulty reducing or ceasing use, pharmacotherapy, such as bupropion or nicotine-replacement therapy (NRT), is recommended (ACOG, 2020).

Nicotine-Replacement Therapy

NRT is a reasonable option for pregnant people either in conjunction with cessation counseling or on its own. NRT is a harm reduction method, and while it contains nicotine, the risks from exposure to pure nicotine is smaller than exposure to nicotine with other cigarette toxins, such as carbon monoxide and ammonia. The benefits of using nicotine replacement likely outweigh the risks of continuing cigarette smoking (Apelberg et al., 2010). There are some data that NRT may be associated with lower rates of PTB and LBW (Taylor et al., 2021). In a 2020 meta-analysis, among smokers, NRT was not associated with higher rates of miscarriage, stillbirth, PTB, LBW, congenital abnormalities, neonatal intensive care unit (NICU) admissions, or neonatal death compared to placebo (Claire et al., 2020). NRT used in adjunct with behavioral therapy also increases the likelihood of smoking cessation later in pregnancy (Claire et al., 2020).

The goal of NRT is to provide a level of nicotine just above that associated with withdrawal symptoms and to deliver nicotine at a constant rate, thereby reducing craving. It is essential that the dose administered is sufficient to be successful. The transdermal patch is the more commonly prescribed NRT in pregnancy as it provides low, long-lasting, steady concentrations of nicotine (Clark & Nakad, 2011). The transdermal patches come in 21-mg and 14-mg formulations with the higher doses used for individuals smoking more than 24 cigarettes daily. It is recommended that the lowest effective dose of the NRT transdermal patch be prescribed in pregnancy (Rodriguez, 2022b). In the case of very heavy tobacco use, both daily patches and "as needed" use of 2-mg gum or lozenges may be required initially. If NRT is not effective, it should be discontinued. NRT should be used during any hospitalizations, including labor; this is an important harm reduction tool that may assist a person in receiving care when they are not permitted to smoke during a hospitalization.

Some pregnant people may attempt to reduce their cigarette smoking by utilizing electronic nicotine delivery systems (ENDS), such as e-cigarettes or vaporizers ("vaping"). In a survey of pregnant people who use ENDS, 75% perceived these products to be safer than cigarettes (Mark et al., 2015). It is important to assess what a person is vaping; some products contain very high concentrations of nicotine, while others do not contain any. There are insufficient data on the safety and use of ENDS as a harm reduction strategy or nicotine-replacement strategy in pregnant people, however, in a recent randomized control trial there were improved rates of smoking cessation in pregnant people using ENDS compared to traditional NRT (Hajek et al., 2022).

Bupropion (Zyban®, Wellbutrin®)

An antidepressant that increases release and decreases reuptake of dopamine and norepinephrine and targets nicotinic receptors has been shown to be effective in decreasing smoking and is an approved for the promotion of smoking cessation in nonpregnant adults (Kranzler et al., 2021). Bupropion crosses the placenta and metabolites are found in umbilical cord and amniotic fluid (Fokina et al., 2016). There is limited evidence on its use in pregnancy; however, most suggests that it has low risk (ACOG, 2020; Kranzler et al., 2021). There are no known risks of fetal anomalies or adverse pregnancy outcomes (Louik et al., 2014; Turner et al., 2019). A recent retrospective study using birth cohort data from Quebec found an association between the use of bupropion and increased smoking cessation and reduced rate of PTB (Berard et al., 2016). Bupropion is a first-line agent typically used in individuals who have been unable to quit with cessation counseling alone or in addition to NRT, or for people with contraindications or who decline NRT (Rodriguez, 2022b). It is recommended to wait until after the first trimester as there are conflicting data on the risks of congenital malformations, yet evidence suggests that the bupropion does not increase overall risk (Turner et al., 2019). A pregnant person may initiate 150 mg once daily for three days and then increase to 150 mg twice daily (Rodriguez, 2022b). At this dose, low levels have been detected in breastmilk but have not been shown to cause adverse effects in infants (LactMed, 2022b).

Varenicline (Chantix®)

Varenicline is a partial agonist for nicotine receptors in the brain (ACOG, 2020). There is insufficient information on the safety of varenicline use in pregnancy, but several small studies have not demonstrated teratogenicity (Richardson et al., 2017). A 2019 systematic review of varenicline use in pregnancy found no increased risk of congenital anomalies, PTB, or LBW (Turner et al., 2019). Given the lack of evidence on safety of varenicline in pregnancy, it is not frequently utilized for pregnant or lactating people and alternative therapies are preferred (ACOG, 2020).

Nicotine-replacement therapy

Delivery	Strength	Dosing
Nicotine patch	14 mg patch (≤10 cigarettes/day) 21 mg patch (>10 cigarettes/day)	Apply one new patch daily Rotate application site Tapering dose not required
Nicotine gum	4 mg 2 mg	1 piece q 1–2 hours Maximum dose 24 pieces/day
Nicotine lozenges	4 mg 2 mg	1 lozenge q 1–2 hours Maximum dose 20 lozenges/day or 5 lozenges/6 hours

Source: Rigotti (2021), Rodriguez (2022).

General principles of prescribing medications during pregnancy should be followed when using pharmaceutical agents for smoking cessation. These include using the lowest dose necessary to achieve success to minimize fetal exposure and delaying therapy until the second trimester to avoid the period of embryogenesis.

Cocaine

Cocaine is a stimulant that can be used either in the form of powder or rock, which is often referred to as "crack cocaine." Cocaine blocks dopamine transporters in the brain and crosses the placenta causing vasoconstriction (Plessinger & Woods, 1993) and can also be found in meconium (D'Avila and Limberger, 2016).

The risks of cocaine use in pregnancy are not well studied, and many of the existing studies have methodological shortcomings that include not controlling for the impacts of socioeconomic factors, other ATOD use, and maternal age (Chang, 2022). In the few adequately controlled reports, the impact of cocaine is related to the dose and stage of pregnancy (Chang, 2022). In a 2011 meta-analysis, the use of cocaine during pregnancy was associated with PTB, LBW, and small for gestational age (SGA) (Gouin et al., 2011); another study found increased risk of spontaneous abortion, placental abruption, FGR, and fetal demise (Cain et al., 2013). Cocaine does not act independently as a structural teratogen (Cressman et al., 2014). The use of cocaine can cause stress on the heart and circulatory system, which can cause hypertension and mimic preeclampsia (Chang, 2022). Hydralazine was previously the preferred hypertension treatment for pregnant people who use cocaine (Kuczkwoski, 2007); however, there are emerging arguments that beta blockers should be offered as part of the standard care to pregnant people using stimulants (Wilson et al., 2022). There is no evidence of teratogenicity despite previous case reports of cardiac and genitourinary abnormalities (Battin et al., 1995; Behnke

et al., 2001; Briggs et al., 2017). There is no evidence of neonatal withdrawal, although some infants may exhibit temporary neurobehavioral abnormalities in the first 48–72 hours of life, including tremors, irritability, high pitched cry, excess suck, hyper alertness, and apnea or tachypnea (Bauer et al., 2005; Eyler et al., 2001; Hudak & Tan, 2012). There are no differences in long-term outcomes of children exposed to cocaine in utero compared to children who were not exposed (Betancourt et al., 2011; Cressman et al., 2014); another study found that there may be language delays in adolescents with cocaine exposure in utero (Landi et al., 2017).

Treatment of Cocaine Use Disorder in Pregnancy

CBT is currently the only evidence-based treatment for cocaine or stimulant use disorders, although research to identify pharmacological agents that can reduce cravings is ongoing. Clonidine, topiramate, and baclofen have been used off-label with some success in small studies, but further research is needed (Jobes et al., 2011). Pregnant people with moderate to severe cocaine use disorder may be offered residential treatment; shared decision-making should be utilized. A national study that did not include pregnant people found that providing monetary incentives to people using either cocaine or methamphetamine successfully increased abstinence (Petry et al., 2005). Referring people using cocaine to harm reduction community programs is also beneficial for accessing pipes, pipe covers, and other supplies that can reduce the harms of using cocaine.

Benzodiazepines

Benzodiazepines (diazepam, alprazolam, lorazepam, and clonazepam) are among the most used recreational prescription drugs. Prescribed for the management of anxiety, sleep, and seizures, this class of CNS depressants can produce high tolerance and physical dependence. Abrupt discontinuation after chronic use causes severe anxiety and may precipitate seizure activity similar to withdrawal from alcohol. When used concurrently with opioids or alcohol, which is common (Votaw et al., 2019), benzodiazepines enhance respiratory depression and can lead to fatal overdose.

Benzodiazepines cross the placenta and can impact the fetus, although specific data about the implications of benzodiazepine use during pregnancy are variable. Some studies have found an increased risk of cleft lip or palate (Zwink & Ekkehart, 2018); however, a systematic review found no increased risk of congenital malformations (Grigoriadis et al., 2019). Benzodiazepines are associated with increased risk for PTB and LBW (Shyken et al., 2019). Regular use during pregnancy has been associated with withdrawal in infants (ACOG, 2008; Wikner et al., 2007). There are conflicting data on the impact on infant neurobehavioral outcomes (ACOG, 2008; Gentile, 2010); a recent meta-analysis concluded that it is not currently possible to determine the effect of benzodiazepines on neurodevelopmental outcomes in children exposed in utero given confounding variables, variability in timing of exposure and duration, and unreliability of studies where neurodevelopment was assessed by a nonclinical assessor (Wang et al., 2022).

Pregnant people who are using recreational benzodiazepines may be self-treating anxiety and should be referred to mental health specialists for assessment. The management of benzodiazepine dependence includes either medically assisted taper or maintenance treatment (Brett & Murnion, 2015).

Cannabis

Cannabis is the most used drug among pregnant people (SAMHSA, 2019). Reported prevalence rates of cannabis use during pregnancy vary from a low of 5.4% (SAMHSA, 2019) to a high of 29.3% (Mark et al., 2016); however, daily use is much less common during pregnancy (1.7%; SAMHSA, 2019). Cannabis is still considered a Schedule 1 substance by the federal government (Food and Drugs, 2011); however, 21 states and the District of Columbia have legalized recreational use and 38 states have legalized medical use as of April 2023 (National Conference of State Legislatures, 2023). The most common reasons cited for use during pregnancy are to relieve nausea/vomiting, anxiety, pain, insomnia, or cope with stress or trauma (Ko et al., 2020a; Woodruff et al., 2021; Young-Wolff et al., 2019). The principal active component of cannabis is tetrahydrocannabinol (THC), which is highly lipophilic and readily crosses the placenta. It is likely that the route of consumption (smoking versus ingested), frequency of use, and amount used results in different exposures for the fetus (Grant et al., 2018).

Data about the potential effects of cannabis use during pregnancy are variable in quality as well as interpretation—many of the studies inadequately controlled for poverty, polysubstance use, and tobacco smoking (Woodruff et al., 2021). A recent study showed correlation between cannabis use and PTB; however, this study was unable to control for participants who were also smoking tobacco/nicotine (Corsi et al., 2019); most reports do not correlate cannabis and PTB (ACOG, 2017b; Conner et al., 2016; Warshak et al., 2015). In a 2016 meta-analysis, using cannabis in pregnancy less than weekly did not impact rates of LBW, though using weekly or more had higher rates (Conner et al., 2016). Some studies have found associations with THC exposure and neurocognitive outcomes (Sharapova et al., 2018), including deficits in attention span (Astley & Little, 1990; Volkow et al., 2017). Again, these data should be cautiously interpreted given the potential confounding impact of environmental factors including maternal nutrition, poverty, and other substance exposure (Mark et al., 2016). A more recent systematic review of prenatal cannabis exposure found that children who were exposed had normal cognitive functioning refuting prior research claims (Torres et al., 2020).

Healthcare providers should discuss cannabis use with pregnant people to assess their reasons for use. If a person is using cannabis to self-treat pregnancy symptoms such as nausea or insomnia, offer alternative antiemetics or sleep aids. One study noted that most pregnant people stopped cannabis use during pregnancy with prenatal counseling on the potential perinatal effects (Mark et al., 2016). Additionally, some pregnant people use cannabis as a harm reduction tool to abstain or decrease use of other drugs.

Amphetamines/Methamphetamines

Amphetamines, such as dextroamphetamine, are commonly prescribed for the treatment of attention deficit/hyperactivity disorder, whereas methamphetamine is an illicit manufactured substance. Both are stimulants that can lead to stimulant or amphetamine use disorder. Synthetic cathinones, or "bath salts," are beta-ketone amphetamine analogs, which have a similar mechanism of action to methamphetamine (Kampman, 2021). The effects of bath salts on pregnancy are unknown, but pregnant people should be discouraged from using them. Potential health complications include arrythmias, hypertension, aortic dissection, and stroke (Schürer et al., 2017).

Amphetamines are known to cross the placenta (Jones et al., 2009); however, no fetal anomalies are associated with prenatal amphetamine exposure (ACOG 2011a, 2011b, reaffirmed 2021; Andrade, 2018; Huybrechts et al., 2018; Oei et al., 2021). Perinatal adverse outcomes include higher risks of FGR (Nguyen et al., 2010), gestational hypertension, PTB (Wright et al., 2015), preeclampsia, placental abruption, fetal demise, and neonatal and infant death (Gorman et al., 2014). In a recent meta-analysis, prenatal methamphetamine exposure led to LBW, shorter body length, and smaller head circumference (Harst et al., 2021). There is conflicting evidence and very limited data about whether infants experience withdrawal after amphetamine exposure, as occurs in adults. The evidence on neurodevelopmental outcome for children exposed to amphetamines in utero may be confounded by other factors including poverty and polysubstance use (Chu et al., 2020; Eze et al., 2016; Jansson, 2021a). In a study with 45 participants, children with prenatal methamphetamine exposure exhibited learning and memory difficulties (Kwiatkowski et al., 2018). In a longitudinal study of children who were exposed to prenatal methamphetamine exposure, no behavioral problems at ages 3, 5, and 7.5 were noted (Chu et al., 2020).

All pregnant people using amphetamines/methamphetamines during pregnancy should be counseled and offered supportive resources to reduce to discontinue their use (ACOG, 2011b, reaffirmed 2021). Cessation of use during pregnancy reduced the risk of LBW and PTB and improved birth outcomes (Wright et al., 2015). Currently, there are no FDA-approved medications for stimulant (or methamphetamine) use disorder. There are some studies on off-label medication and prescription amphetamine use for nonpregnant people with methamphetamine use disorders, and in some cases, these treatments were found to be helpful (National Harm Reduction Coalition, 2020). CBT should be offered; some people also find 12-step or mutual support programs helpful.

Some people benefit from intense treatment in a residential treatment setting. There is evidence that contingency management interventions or providing incentives in exchange for engaging in treatment/care or maintain abstinence has been effective (Roll et al., 2006).

Opioids

OUD has become a major public health issue in the United States, and rates have significantly increased among pregnant people in the last decade (Ecker et al., 2019). The estimated number of maternal OUD diagnoses increased from 3.5 per 1000 delivery hospitalizations in 2010 to 8.2 in 2017 (a 131% increase; Hiari et al., 2021). It is predicted that 1 in 300 opioid-naïve people who have cesarean deliveries will become persistent users of opioids (after being prescribed opioids for pain management; Bateman et al., 2016). Additionally, an epidemic of overdose deaths related to fentanyl and synthetic opioids has become a major public health concern (Boyd et al., 2022). Multiple states have identified opioid-related deaths as a major contributor to pregnancy-associated deaths (accounting for as much as 11–20%; Schiff et al., 2018). From 2015 to 2017, synthetic opioid fatalities increased by 361% for Black adults and 350% for Latine adults compared to 192% increase for White adults (El-Bassel et al., 2021; CDC, 2019; Lopez et al., 2022), reflecting a lack of resources devoted to marginalized communities (Lie et al., 2022).

There are four general sources of opioid dependence that have variable pregnancy outcomes: untreated OUD, chronic pain management, recreational use of fentanyl or synthetic opioids, and MOUD. Untreated chronic use of recreational opioids is associated with lack of prenatal care, IUGR, placental abruption, and PTB (ACOG, 2017a). In a recent large cohort study, the risk of PTB was 14.0% compared to 6.0% in nonopioid users (Corsi et al., 2019). Untreated OUDs are strongly associated with concurrent polysubstance use and tobacco exposure, making it difficult to determine the impact of opioid exposure alone. As with the consumption of any substance, the method of use (IDU, inhaling, or smoking) has associated risks.

There is limited evidence on the risks of opioid use for the treatment of chronic pain during pregnancy—however, prescription opioids for the treatment of acute or chronic pain appear to be relatively safe and have not been linked to fetal malformations (Babb et al., 2010). In a recent meta-analysis, there was some association with prenatal opioid exposure and oral clefts, club foot, and atrial septal defects; however, the authors note substantial concerns about the quality of included studies (Lind et al., 2017). The long-term outcomes in children exposed to opioids (including illicit opioids) appear similar to children who are not exposed (Academy of Perinatal Harm Reduction, 2022; Behnke et al., 2013). In studies, oxycodone use was associated with PTB (Kelly et al., 2011) and hydrocodone was associated with SGA (Smith et al., 2015). Chronic prescription opioid use during pregnancy is associated with NOWS. Some pregnant people may consider a slow titration to a lower dosage over the course of

pregnancy; however, this should be managed by or with a pain specialist (Ecker et al., 2019).

The intentional and unintentional use of illicit fentanyl poses unique risks for pregnant and parenting people. In recent years, fentanyl and other synthetic analogs have been added as adulterants to heroin, cocaine, methamphetamine, and counterfeit pills, causing high rates of drug-related overdose deaths (Han et al., 2019). Many people are unaware of their fentanyl use and may not report it (Daniulaityte et al., 2019); however, the introduction of illicitly made fentanyl has slowly replaced heroin (Kral et al., 2021), and in some cases, there is an increasing preference for fentanyl (Ickowicz et al., 2022; Morales et al., 2019). There are very limited data on the use of recreational fentanyl during pregnancy.

Pain management, including during labor and postpartum, for pregnant people who are taking opioids for chronic pain or who have OUD requires a multidisciplinary approach, and it is highly recommended to refer the person for an anesthesia consultation prior to birth (Ecker et al., 2019). People with prolonged use of opioids have a high tolerance for opioids and many experience opioid-induced hyperalgesia (Tompkins & Campbell, 2011). For these reasons, epidural or combined spinal–epidural may be recommended during labor. Nalbuphine and butorphanol are contraindicated during childbirth because they can precipitate acute opioid withdrawal due to their antagonist effects. Mu-agonist opioid analgesics can be safely used (e.g., fentanyl during labor; oxycodone and hydromorphone postoperatively).

Medication for Opioid Use Disorders in Pregnancy

MOUD (also referred to as MAT) is the standard of care treatment for pregnant people with OUD (ASAM, 2020a, 2020b; Ecker et al., 2019). Shared decision-making should be utilized when electing the type of treatment for OUD. MOUD is frequently used for moderate to severe OUD or when a person has physical dependence. Pregnant people with OUD should also be offered referral to behavioral health for CBT or psychotherapy; additionally, some people benefit from contingency management or 12 step programs like Narcotics Anonymous. However, MOUD can be successful without these other interventions. Some treatment programs that also provide housing and case management have demonstrated success (Hansen et al., 2022), and Indigenous communities in Canadian First Nations have integrated buprenorphine treatment with organized healing sessions, fishing, hunting, and community gardening which have high rates of treatment retention (Mamakwa et al., 2017). All pregnant persons with OUD should be counseled on overdose risks and given naloxone. Referral to harm reduction programs and syringe access sites should be highly considered.

The goal of MOUD is to provide entry to recovery, and to reduce or abstain from use of recreational opioids, facilitate prenatal care, reduce risk of overdose, and prevent pregnancy and neonatal complications. MOUDs are life-saving medications that decrease overdose deaths by 70% (Klaman et al., 2017). They have also been found to increase retention in prenatal care and recovery treatment, decrease the risk of HIV and hepatitis B and C, and decrease fetal demise, IUGR, and PTB (Klaman et al., 2017). A recent retrospective cohort study found that for each additional week a pregnant person used MOUD overdose decreased by 2%, PTB decreased by 1%, and postpartum MOUD continuation increased by 95% (Krans et al., 2021).

Medically supervised opioid withdrawal is also an alternative for pregnant people, but it is not recommended given evidence of low completion rates, high rates of relapse (59% to 90%; Saia et al., 2016), and limited data regarding the effect of **detoxification** on maternal and neonatal outcomes beyond delivery (Jones et al., 2010; Terplan et al., 2018). Initial studies from the 1970s demonstrated fetal distress with withdrawal (Zuspan et al., 1975); however, more recent data show that withdrawal management can be safe for the fetus (Bell et al., 2016).

There are three types of MOUD used in pregnancy: methadone, buprenorphine, and buprenorphine-naloxone.

Methadone

Methadone is a highly effective, evidence-based treatment for OUD. It is a full agonist for the mu-opioid receptor, which must be administered by a federally accredited opioid treatment program and is generally dosed once daily under direct observation (Ecker et al., 2019). Methadone has been the standard of care for the treatment of OUDs during pregnancy since the 1970s, and the federal law requires that pregnant people receive priority admission to methadone treatment centers. Typical starting dose is 20–30 mg, and because pregnant people metabolize methadone more quickly, they generally require higher daily doses (80–120 mg or more). It is likely that this dose may need to be split for twice-daily or more dosing, particularly later in pregnancy (Meyer et al., 2015).

Buprenorphine and Buprenorphine-Naloxone

Buprenorphine is a partial agonist for the mu-opioid receptor and is becoming increasingly used for the treatment of OUD in pregnancy because of its safety, efficacy, and ability to be prescribed by primary care and perinatal providers, thereby reducing some of the barriers to treatment associated with methadone, particularly the daily dosing schedule. Data indicate that buprenorphine to treat OUD during pregnancy has comparable or better outcomes compared with methadone treatment (Meyer et al., 2015; Zedler et al., 2016).

In 2016, the passage of the Comprehensive Addiction Recovery Act allowed nurse practitioners and physicians' assistants to obtain Drug Enforcement Administration (DEA) waivers to prescribe buprenorphine. In 2018, the ability was expanded to include certified nurse-midwives, clinical nurse specialists, and certified registered nurse anesthetists. On January 12, 2023, SAMSHA and the DEA announced the elimination of the x-waiver; granting any clinician with a current DEA registration that includes Schedule III authority ability to prescribe buprenorphine for OUD.

Buprenorphine is available as a monoproduct or in combination with naloxone. There is increasing evidence that buprenorphine-naloxone is safe in pregnancy (Lund et al., 2013). The goal is to reach a dose that is high enough to block cravings. People need to be in mild to moderate withdrawal when initiating buprenorphine to avoid experiencing precipitated withdrawal, a common reason for discontinuing treatment. If a person is not in withdrawal, consider prescribing to allow the person to self start at home once in mild-moderate withdrawal. Starting dose is 8–16 mg, which can be titrated upon initiation to achieve a therapeutic level. Dosage often needs to be increased particularly in the second and third trimesters due to normal physiologic changes during pregnancy (Ecker et al., 2019). Typically dosing in pregnancy is 16–24 mg or more, and split dosing is often used due to the accelerated metabolic clearance of pregnancy (Ecker et al., 2019).

Treatment with Methadone versus Buprenorphine

The decision between methadone and buprenorphine requires careful consideration and should be individualized for each pregnant person. Available options, patient preference, patient's prior experiences, severity of OUD, social supports, and intensity of treatment needed should be considered. If the pregnant person has been stabilized on either medication prior to pregnancy, it is reasonable to continue with the same medication. Other practical considerations such as access, transportation, employment, and childcare may guide treatment decisions. Recent studies suggest buprenorphine is associated with less PTB, higher birth weight (Suarez et al., 2022), and larger head circumference (Zedler et al., 2016); it is also associated with lower rates of NOWS compared to methadone (Noormohammadi et al., 2016; Suarez et al., 2022). An infant with NOWS after buprenorphine exposure in utero typically has shorter NICU hospitalizations (10 days compared to 17.5 for methadone) and requires less morphine supplementation for the treatment of NOWs (1.1 mg compared to 10.4 mg for methadone) (Jones et al., 2010). Racial disparities impact the treatment of OUD, Latine pregnant people are typically diagnosed with OUD 37 days later than their white counterparts, Black and Latine pregnant people are less like to receive, continue, and report consistent use of MOUD and are typically treated with lower doses of methadone compared to white pregnant women (Gao et al., 2022). Historically, buprenorphine was only covered by private insurance and was disproportionately marketed to White communities, whereas methadone became more associated with communities of color (Hansen et al., 2013; Hatcher et al., 2018; Netherland & Hansen, 2017); buprenorphine is now more widely available and covered by public insurance; however, it is still more often prescribed for patients who are White (Lie et al., 2022).

While a MOUD provider will likely be managing most aspects of treatment, the prenatal care provider (if different from MOUD provider) should be aware of the importance of evaluating a pregnant person in recovery, including assessing for opioid craving and/or potential opioid withdrawal symptoms.

Whether the pregnant person is using methadone or buprenorphine, factors associated with prenatal care are largely similar. Ideally, a pregnant person should be referred for consultation with a pediatric provider who will monitor and care for the infant with NOWS, to give anticipatory guidance about NICU assessments, care, length of stay, etc. Patients should also be given counseling and anticipatory guidance on the recommendation to continue MOUD at least one year postpartum to prevent risk of relapse and overdose deaths (Ecker et al., 2019; Schiff et al., 2018).

See "Resources for Healthcare Providers" for more information on MOUD management.

Perinatal Care of Pregnant and Birthing People with SUDs

Perinatal care for pregnant and birthing people who use substances or have SUDs should be a routine component of care provided by midwives, nurse practitioners, and physicians who care for people with other chronic conditions. Because midwives and advanced practice nurses are trained to provide care for pregnant and birthing people in the context of family and community, they are well prepared to coordinate a multidisciplinary treatment approach that addresses pregnancy, medical, psychiatric, and social needs. Prenatal care should be delivered in collaboration with a consulting obstetrician or maternal-fetal medicine (MFM) specialist, as well as an addiction medicine specialist, a licensed substance use counselor, and, ideally, a mental health provider. Social services and public health nursing services are involved whenever possible.

The overall goal of treatment is to improve outcomes for both the pregnant/birthing person and baby by minimizing perinatal risk, increasing participation in perinatal care, and assisting the pregnant person to access the services needed to ensure a safe and stable environment for the dyad. Harm reduction should be a guiding principle for the perinatal care of pregnant and birthing people with SUDs.

Pregnancy Dating

Accurate pregnancy dating is an important component of managing substance-exposed pregnancies for a variety of reasons. Some people who use substances may experience amenorrhea or oligomenorrhea, which might contribute to both late entry to care and uncertainty about timing of conception. As much pregnancy dating precision as possible is important given the risk of PTB and possible need for labor induction in cases of IUGR or other complications. Pregnancy dating ultrasound should be offered upon entry to care.

Pregnancy Options Counseling

All pregnant people, including those with SUDs, should be offered options counseling with the confirmation of pregnancy. The healthcare provider should assess if the pregnant person desires to continue the pregnancy or to end the pregnancy; they should also assess if the pregnant person desires to parent or not to parent. Decisions regarding pregnancy and parenting should never be assumed by the healthcare provider.

Prenatal Laboratory Testing

In addition to routine prenatal labs and HIV testing, pregnant people with SUDs should be screened for hepatic function, and tuberculosis. HIV, hepatitis B and C viruses, and gonorrhea and chlamydia testing should be repeated in the third trimester as indicated (Gopman, 2014). Urine toxicology testing should only be performed with the explicit written consent of the pregnant person. Informed consent includes a clear explanation of why testing is being recommended, the benefits and risks of testing, including the potential legal, criminal, and child welfare considerations (CMQCC, 2021).

Psychosocial Assessment

As discussed, pregnant people who use substances or have SUDs have high rates of anxiety, depression, and trauma. Assessment and treatment for depression and anxiety should be routine, as well as IPV screening and discussion of healthy relationships. Screening for physical, sexual, and emotional trauma, PTSD, and ACEs should also be completed. Consider referral to case management, social work, and behavioral health as needed.

Screening for Social-Structural Determinants

Pregnant people who use substances or have SUDs may be impacted by a range of social-structural determinants. Discrimination based on race, ethnicity, LGBTQ status, and gender increase risk of SUD (Hansen et al., 2022). Homelessness and unstable housing may cause challenges to retention in care and treatment. Pregnant people should be asked about additional barriers to care, including lack of transportation, childcare, and access to essential resources such as food and shelter. Validated screening tools for social determinants are available (National Association of Community Health Centers, 2016). Healthcare providers should screen for and discuss protective and supportive factors, such as peer and community support and faith-based organizations and offer nutritional resources, including registered dietician, WIC benefits, and food pantry programs. Clinicians should consider the flexibility of their schedule to accommodate lateness and offer drop-in and telehealth appointments.

Concurrent Medications

Drug interactions are important to consider for people on MOUD who are also receiving psychiatric medications. Metabolism of buprenorphine and methadone may be altered by selective serotonin reuptake inhibitors (SSRIs). Concurrent treatment with fluoxetine and fluvoxamine has been found to increase serum concentrations of methadone due to the inhibition of opioid metabolism, although this has not been demonstrated to date with buprenorphine (Jones et al., 2010; Maremmoni et al., 2019). When possible, avoid ondansetron among people using methadone as it causes QTc interval prolongation and ventricular arrythmias. Potentially lethal interactions exist between MOUDs, benzodiazepines and alcohol. Prescription drug monitoring programs (PDMPs) should be monitored periodically during pregnancy to verify prescribed medications and inform clinical practice as needed. Finally, naloxone prescription and education on overdose and naloxone rescue should be discussed with all pregnant patients who are using substances.

Fetal Assessment

Little data are available on which to base protocols for fetal assessment for substance-exposed pregnancies. A level II anatomy scan between 18 and 20 weeks is recommended when polysubstance use or use of substances with known teratogenic effects is suspected. Fetal surveillance during the second half of pregnancy should be individualized, and serial growth ultrasounds may be recommended. Antenatal testing (NST and amniotic fluid assessment) may be recommended starting at 32–36 weeks. When fetal testing is performed, it is important to recognize that peak methadone levels occurring in the first few hours after dosing alters fetal heart rate variability and can also reduce fetal breathing motion on biophysical profile (Jansson et al., 2005).

Anticipatory Guidance

Pregnant people with SUDs often experience significant guilt and anxiety regarding impending hospitalization, labor, and birth. Anticipatory guidance in the antepartum period is essential, and providers have the ethical responsibility to discuss hospital substance use policies honestly and transparently. Education includes options for management of labor pain, hospital policies about parental and neonatal urine toxicology testing or other biological testing, continuation of MOUD, breastfeeding, protection of patient confidentiality, and smoking. When antenatal substance use carries risk for NOWS, patients and their families should be provided with accurate information about observation periods, diagnosis, and treatment of NOWS prior to admission, so expectations are accurate. Perinatal providers should consider patient consults with the pediatric team to assist with anticipatory guidance. Written institutional policies regarding breastfeeding for people with substance use should be discussed. Perinatal providers have an ethical obligation to be familiar with relevant state and federal rules regarding mandated reporting to CPS, and these should be openly discussed.

Communication and Coordination of Care

Integrated care models provide both maternity care and substance use treatment in the same location or in close coordination. Pregnant people enrolled in programs integrating maternity care and substance use treatment attend more prenatal visits and are less likely to use illicit drugs at the time of birth than those who are untreated (Sweeney et al., 2000). Additional benefits include increased prenatal care attendance, increased length of gestation, decreased length of hospitalization for infants, increased access to family planning services, and decreased costs to the healthcare system. Participants in integrated programs express increased satisfaction with care, and appreciation for consistent, supportive relationships with caregivers (Goler et al., 2012; Lefebvre et al., 2010; Haug et al., 2014).

Neonatal Opioid Withdrawal Syndrome and Neonatal Abstinence Syndrome

NOWS and Neonatal Abstinence Syndrome (NAS) are complex constellations of signs and symptoms that occur after chronic exposure to substances in utero (Jansson, 2021b). Whereas NOWS is specific to opioid exposure, NAS refers to the withdrawal of other substances including nicotine, benzodiazepines, SSRIs, or polysubstance use. The incidence of NAS has increased from 4.0 per 1000 birth hospitalizations in 2010 to 7.3 per 1000 birth hospitalizations in 2017 (Hirai et al., 2021). The rate varies by state, for example, West Virginia has the highest rate of NOWS at 49.6 per 1000 hospital births, compared to Hawaii at 1.3 per 1000 hospital births (Healthcare Cost and Utilization Project, 2022). NOWS is a complex disorder that primarily involves the central and autonomic nervous systems, and the gastrointestinal system. If NOWS occurs, symptoms typically present 24–72 hours after birth, although they can be delayed until five to seven days of age (Patrick et al., 2020). Signs and symptoms include sleep–wake cycle disturbance, alterations in tone (tremors, jitteriness, and hypertonicity), autonomic dysfunction (sweating, sneezing, fever, nasal stuffiness, and frequent yawning), and easy overstimulation, sensitivity, and hyperarousal (irritability, crying) (Jansson, 2021b; Ko et al., 2017). Some infants may have difficulties feeding leading to poor weight gain, and some have gastrointestinal symptoms (gassiness, vomiting, and loose stools) (Jansson, 2021b).

NOWS occurs in approximately 40–60% of neonates who were exposed to MOUD during pregnancy (Ecker et al., 2019; Jones et al., 2010). There is no correlation between NOWS and dosage of MOUD (Ecker et al., 2019; Patrick et al., 2020) or maternal opioid dose (O'Connor et al., 2016). Co-occurrent use of other substances, such as cigarettes, benzodiazepines, and gabapentin, may influence severity and onset of NOWS (Patrick et al., 2020). Birthing parents should be counseled to reduce or eliminate cigarette smoking to reduce the severity of NOWS. Breastfeeding is encouraged for infants exposed prenatally to opioids and may reduce the severity of NOWS; it also decreases the length of NICU admissions (Ecker et al., 2019).

Toxicology testing, including urine, meconium, or umbilical cord, should only be done if it will inform clinical management of NOWS/NAS. Several scoring tools exist to assess an infant's symptoms of NOWS/NAS (the most widely used being the Finnegan scale) and the progression or alleviation of those symptoms. Typically, the use of the Finnegan scale results in close monitoring in the NICU and pharmacologic treatment with a drug from the same class as that causing withdrawal—morphine and methadone are commonly used.

More recently, a new tool has emerged, called Eat, Sleep, Console (ESC), which measures the infant's ability to eat ≥1 oz, sleep ≥1 hour, and be consoled/soothed (Patrick et al., 2020). Nonpharmacological interventions are also utilized, such as keeping infants in a quiet and dimly lit room, swaddling, holding/rocking, skin-to-skin care, limiting visitors, clustering care, rooming in with the postpartum parent, and breastfeeding. ESC has been found to decrease the need for pharmacological intervention, the length of hospitalization, and the overall cost (Grisham et al., 2019).

The length of stay for infants with NOWS will vary by prenatal exposures and need for pharmacological treatment. The length of stay for infants not requiring pharmacological treatment may be as short as four days, while those requiring treatment may anticipate a stay of 12–23 days.

Postpartum Care

Close postpartum follow-up is recommended for people with SUDs. There are significant stressors during the postpartum period; additionally, people with SUDS may experience difficulties accessing to care, potential child welfare involvement, and potential infant hospitalization for NOWS (Ecker et al., 2019). Resumption of substance use is possible, and postpartum parents are at exceptionally high rates of overdose in the first 12 months following birth (Ecker et al., 2019; Schiff et al., 2018); thus, postpartum parents with OUD should be encouraged to continue MOUD for at least 12 months after birth. People with SUDs are at increased risk for postpartum depression and should be followed closely, treated appropriately, and/or referred to behavioral health or specialists in the treatment of co-occurring psychiatric disorders. When antidepressant therapy is indicated, potential drug interactions should be considered.

All postpartum parents should be offered and counseled on contraceptive options. The use of contraceptives should be guided by patients' preference and their goals for interpregnancy spacing and family size. While long-acting reversible contraception (LARC) should be offered, people should never be coerced. Contraceptive counseling should be about meeting the patient where they are by utilizing reflective listening and shared decision-making.

Transition to a primary care provider is important in continuing progress toward the person's goals for their health, their SUD management, and the management of any other chronic health conditions.

Breastfeeding[1] and Substance Use

Human milk and breastfeeding have numerous benefits both for the birthing parent and infant. Birthing people who use substances or have SUDs should be given evidence-based information about potential benefits and risks of breastfeeding to make informed decisions together with the perinatal healthcare provider, lactation consultant(s), and infant provider(s).

Breastfeeding can be a protective factor for infants born to birthing parents with SUDs, who may be at risk for health and developmental difficulties (Reece-Stremtan & Marinelli, 2015) since breastfeeding decreases the incidence of child abuse and neglect (Strathearn et al., 2009), increases bonding and attachment, reduces experiences with physical and emotional stress, and increases cognitive ability in children (Krol & Grossmann, 2018). Birthing parents who are receiving MOUD should be encouraged to breastfeed.

Historically, pregnant people with SUDs exhibit low rates of breastfeeding. It is difficult to determine to what extent this is related to individual choice or clinician recommendation. There is limited evidence on the risks of exposure to illicit substances in human milk, but significant misinformation that lacks scientific support is common. Table 18.4 summarizes evidence regarding specific substances and breastfeeding. Transfer of medications and/or illicit substances from serum into human milk depends on a variety of factors, including lipid solubility, molecular weight, and half-life. Healthcare providers should also consider the potential risks of discouraging breastfeeding, including that early interruption may prevent the possibility of breastfeeding in the future (Thompson, 2019).

Although substance use carries potential risk to the infant, it is not necessarily a contraindication to breastfeeding (WHO, 2014); each person should be evaluated for type of substance used, amount of time since last use, and frequency of use (Rad et al., 2020). In response to the limited guidance available about breastfeeding and substance use, the Academy of Breastfeeding Medicine (ABM) developed guidelines for breastfeeding in substance-using birthing people (ABM, 2015). Unless other contraindications exist, birthing people engaged in substance use treatment, who have received consistent prenatal care, and have abstained from **illicit substance use** in the 90 days prior to birth, should be encouraged to breastfeed (ABM, 2015). According to ABM, pregnant and birthing people who are not currently or not planning to engage in substance use treatment as well as those who have used substances in the 30 days prior to birth should be discouraged from breastfeeding. Additionally, if the pregnant or birthing person desires to breastfeed, the ABM recommends forming a prenatal care plan that includes preparation for breastfeeding, SUD treatment, instruction if relapse occurs during lactation regarding potential for donor milk and formula preparation, and should breastfeeding become contraindicated (ABM, 2015). (See *Resources for Healthcare Providers*.)

---

[1] The author recognizes that not all lactating persons identify as having breasts or breastfeeding; some may refer to this as chestfeeding or body feeding.

Table 18.4 Specific Substances and Breastfeeding

Substance	Comments
Alcohol	• The use of minimal amounts of alcohol, such as one glass of wine or beer, is not likely to cause problems for the breastfeeding infant (D'apolito, 2013; Haastrup et al., 2014; LactMed, 2022a). • The amount of alcohol in human milk is 5–6% of the weight-adjusted parental dose and is similar to maternal blood levels (Mennella & Beauchamp, 1991). • Parents should be advised to wait at least 2–4 hours per drink to breastfeed as peak alcohol levels in breastmilk occur shortly after ingestion. • Daily use of larger amounts of alcohol can decrease milk production; however, the long-term effects of daily alcohol on infants are unclear (LactMed, 2022a). Some evidence indicates it may be associated with impaired infant growth and motor function and may interfere with parenting skills (LactMed, 2022a). • Alcohol test strips are available in most drugstores that can be used to test human milk prior to providing milk to the baby.
Amphetamines	• In regularly prescribed doses, breastfeeding does not appear to be contraindicated. Breastfeeding is discouraged when the parent is actively using methamphetamines (ACOG, 2011b, reaffirmed 2021). • Methamphetamine is excreted in human milk at concentrations 2.88 to 7.5 times higher than maternal plasma (ACOG 2011b; Bartu et al., 2009) • Stimulants can decrease milk supply (Bartu et al., 2009).
Benzodiazepines	• Breastfeeding is not explicitly contraindicated if the medications are taken as prescribed (Hale, 2010). • Take as low a dose of benzodiazepines as possible to achieve a therapeutic dose. • Not all benzodiazepines are the same regarding safety with lactation, for example, lorazepam is safer than diazepam (LactMed, 2021b; LactMed, 2021c). • These medications and their metabolites pass freely into breastmilk and cause sedation, breastfeeding difficulty, and poor weight gain (LactMed, 2021c).
Cannabis	• Current data is insufficient to evaluate long-term effects of cannabis use on infants. Many professional groups either urge caution or discourage cannabis use while breastfeeding (CMQCC, 2021). • THC is excreted into human milk in small quantities, estimates suggest the infant receive 0.8% of maternal weight-adjusted dose (LactMed, 2021a), dosage peaking at 1 hour after smoking and decreased within 4 hours (Baker et al., 2018) and may be present in higher concentrations than in maternal serum due to its high lipophilicity (Hale, 2010).
Cocaine	• ABM suggests that pregnant people who use cocaine should generally not breastfeed, unless they have negative urine toxicology at time of birth, have been abstinent for 90 days, and are in a treatment program with plans to continue postpartum (Reece-Stremtan & Marinelli, 2015). • A breastfeeding abstinence period for 24 hours may be considered for parents who occasionally use cocaine to allow for elimination (Cressman et al., 2012; LactMed, 2020). • Cocaine is excreted in human milk (LactMed, 2020). • Stimulants can decrease milk supply (Bartu et al., 2009). • Infants may be exposed to significant amounts of cocaine through breastmilk (Winecker et al., 2001). • Serious adverse reactions include vomiting, diarrhea, and seizures (Chasnoff et al., 1987).
Illicit opioids	• When used in excess, infants can experience lethargy and breathing difficulties. • Breastfeeding is generally discouraged in people using nonprescribed opioids.
MOUD	• People who received methadone, buprenorphine, or buprenorphine-naloxone maintenance during pregnancy and are stable in treatment should be encouraged to breastfeed regardless of what dose is being taken (Sachs et al., 2013). • NOWS is an expected outcome. Eat, sleep, console/soothe is an evidence-based approach for reducing symptoms of NOWS that includes promoting breastfeeding (Patrick et al., 2020). • About 2% of total methadone dose has been found in human milk (Montgomery et al., 2012). There are negligible amounts of buprenorphine in human milk and infants absorb even less because buprenorphine is not well absorbed in the stomach (Ilett et al., 2012; Lindemalm, 2009).
Nicotine/tobacco	• Breastfeeding is not contraindicated. • Cigarette smoking reduces milk supply, lowers milk fat concentration, and may cause milk to dry up earlier (Letsen et al., 2002). • Nicotine and other cigarette chemicals can pass into human milk (Primo et al., 2013). • Parents smoking cigarettes should be encouraged to: (a) smoke away from the baby, preferably outdoors, (b) smoke right after nursing sessions, (c) smoke as few cigarettes as possible; infant risks such as respiratory allergy and SUID increase with smoking more than 20 cigarettes a day, (d) NRT may be helpful, and (e) be aware that reduction in milk supply, inhibition of the let-down reflex, and physical symptoms in the baby, such as nausea, abdominal cramps, vomiting, and diarrhea, may occur (Reece-Stremtan & Marinelli, 2015).

Summary

Substance use during pregnancy continues to be a perinatal health concern as the use of prescription drugs, opioids, and cannabis continues to rise among pregnant people. All forms of prenatal substance use carry maternal and fetal risk. Universal verbal screening for substance use with validated verbal screening tools, followed by brief intervention and referral to treatment (SBIRT), is an emerging standard of care and provides a framework for a population-based approach. Outcomes are improved with early identification of substance use, referral, and, when indicated, MAT.

Harm reduction approaches to perinatal care for pregnant people who use substances or have SUDs should be consistently utilized as they reduce risks associated with substance use, increase retention in care, facilitate successful treatment, and improve patient care experiences. The disproportionate criminalization and pathologization of people of color who use substances or have SUDs and their pregnancies—reflections of structural and systemic racism—highlight the need for explicitly antiracist perinatal care protocols and practices to strive for equity and justice.

Perinatal clinicians are ideally positioned to care for pregnant people with SUDs due to the high motivation for self-care experienced by many people during pregnancy, and the longitudinal relationship developed with perinatal care providers. Perinatal care providers have a unique opportunity and an ethical responsibility to provide evidence-based, supportive, and nonjudgmental care to this highly vulnerable patient population. Substance use care is ideally continued through the postpartum year to reduce relapse rates, prevent overdose, and improve sexual and reproductive health. Pregnant and birthing people who use substances are equally deserving of patient- and family-centered care that honors their autonomy, promotes partnership, and supports them in attaining authentic and healthy lives.

Resources for Clients and Families

CA BRIDGE: Eat, Sleep, Soothe: https://obgyn.ucsf.edu/sites/obgyn.ucsf.edu/files/CA%20BRIDGE%20-%20PATIENT%20MATERIALS%20-%20Prevent%20%20treat%20opioid%20withdrawal%20in%20your%20baby%20-%20September%202020.pdf

National Advocates for Pregnant Women Birth Rights: https://www.nationaladvocatesforpregnantwomen.org/birth-rights-a-resource-for-everyday-people-to-defend-human-rights-during-labor-and-birth-2

National Advocates for Pregnant Women: https://www.nationaladvocatesforpregnantwomen.org/issues/pregnancy-and-drug-and-alcohol-use

National Harm Reduction Coalition Pregnancy and Substance Use: A Harm Reduction Approach: https://www.perinatalharmreduction.org/toolkit-pregnancy-substance-use

SAMHSA: Buprenorphine Practitioner Locator: https://www.samhsa.gov/medication-assisted-treatment/find-treatment/treatment-practitioner-locator

SAMHSA: Methadone Treatment Locator: https://dpt2.samhsa.gov/treatment/directory.aspx

SAMHSA: Treating Babies Who Were Exposed to Opioids Before Birth: https://store.samhsa.gov/sites/default/files/d7/priv/sma18-5071fs3.pdf

Resources for Healthcare Providers

ABM Clinical Protocol #21: Guidelines for Breastfeeding and Substance Use and Substance Use Disorder, Revised 2015: https://www.ncbi.nlm.nih.gov/pmc/articles/PMC4378642

ACEs Aware: Do No Harm: Building Trust and Keeping Families Together: https://www.acesaware.org/wp-content/uploads/2021/12/DoNoHarmFinal.pdf

ACOG Substance Use Disorders in Pregnancy: Clinical, Ethical, and Research Imperatives of the Opioid Epidemic: https://www.ajog.org/article/S0002-9378(19)30500-9/fulltext

Alliance for Innovation for Maternal Health Obstetric Care for Women with OUD: https://saferbirth.org/psbs/care-for-pregnant-and-postpartum-people-with-substance-use-disorder

ASAM: Substance Use and Substance Use Disorder Among Pregnant and Postpartum People: https://www.asam.org/advocacy/public-policy-statements/details/public-policy-statements/2022/10/12/substance-use-and-substance-use-disorder-among-pregnant-and-postpartum-people

ASAM: Appropriate Use of Drug Testing in Clinical Addiction Medicine: https://www.asam.org/quality-care/clinical-guidelines/drug-testing

ASAM Buprenorphine X-waiver Course: https://elearning.asam.org/buprenorphine-waiver-course

AUDIT-C screening tool scoring system: http://www.integration.samhsa.gov/images/res/tool_auditc.pdf

California BRIDGE: Buprenorphine Quick Start in Pregnancy: https://cabridge.org/resource/buprenorphine-quick-start-in-pregnancy

CMQCC: The Mother & Baby Substance Exposure Toolkit: https://www.cmqcc.org/resources-toolkits/toolkits/mother-baby-substance-exposure-initiative-toolkit

MGH: Microdosing and Extended Release Buprenorphine: https://mghcme.org/app/uploads/2021/02/DeWeese_Mico-PTT-1.pdf

National Advocates for Pregnant Women Confronting Pregnancy Criminalization: https://www.nationaladvocatesforpregnantwomen.org/wp-content/uploads/2022/06/1.Confronting-Pregnancy-Criminalization_6.22.23-1.pdf

National Harm Reduction Coalition Pregnancy and Substance Use: A Harm Reduction Approach: https://harmreduction.org/wp-content/uploads/2020/10/09.17.20_Pregnancy-and-Substance-Use-2.pdf

NIDA Quick Screen-ASSIST: https://nida.nih.gov/nidamed-medical-health-professionals/screening-tools-resources/chart-screening-tools

SAMSHA: Clinical Guidelines for Treating Pregnant and Parenting Women with OUD and their Infants: https://store.samhsa.gov/sites/default/files/d7/priv/sma18-5054.pdf

SAMSHA: Approach to the Treatment of Pregnant Women with OUD: https://ncsacw.samhsa.gov/files/Collaborative_Approach_508.pdf

Smoke Free Tools and Tips: https://smokefree.gov/

The Council on Patient Safety in Women's Healthcare: Patient Safety Bundle: Obstetric Care for Women with Opioid Use Disorder: https://safehealthcareforeverywoman.org/wp-content/uploads/Obstetric-Care-for-OUD-Bundle.pdf

WHO: Substance use and Substance Use Disorders in Pregnancy: http://apps.who.int/iris/bitstream/handle/10665/107130/9789241548731_eng.pdf?sequence=1

WHO: Toolkit for Delivering the 5As Brief Tobacco Interventions: https://apps.who.int/iris/bitstream/handle/10665/112835/9789241506953_eng.pdf

Equity

Amnesty International: Criminalizing Pregnancy: Policing Pregnant Women Who Use Drugs in the USA: https://www.amnesty.org/en/documents/amr51/6203/2017/en

APHA: Racism: The Ultimate Underlying Condition: https://www.apha.org/events-and-meetings/webinars/racial-equity/webinar-1-recording

APHA: A Path to Reproductive Justice: Research, Practice, and Policies: https://www.apha.org/events-and-meetings/webinars/racial-equity/webinar-2-recording

Bixby Center for Global Reproductive Health: Advancing Equity and Justice in SRH: https://www.innovating-education.org/course/structures-self-advancing-equity-and-justice-in-sexual-and-reproductive-healthcare

Black Families Matter: How the Child Welfare System Punishes Poor Families of Color: https://theappeal.org/black-families-matter-how-the-child-welfare-system-punishes-poor-families-of-color-33ad20e2882e

Movement for Family Power: How the Foster System Has Become Ground Zero for the U.S. War on Drugs: https://static1.squarespace.com/static/5be5ed0fd274cb7c8a5d0cba/t/5eead939ca509d4e36a89277/1592449422870/MFP+Drug+War+Foster+System+Report.pdf

Substance Use, Pregnancy, and Lactation

ABM Clinical Protocol #21: Guidelines for Breastfeeding and Substance Use and Substance Use Disorder, Revised 2015: https://www.ncbi.nlm.nih.gov/pmc/articles/PMC4378642

ACOG: Marijuana Use During Pregnancy and Lactation: https://www.acog.org/clinical/clinical-guidance/committee-opinion/articles/2017/10/marijuana-use-during-pregnancy-and-lactation

ACOG: Methamphetamine Abuse in Women of Reproductive Age: https://www.acog.org/clinical/clinical-guidance/committee-opinion/articles/2011/03/methamphetamine-abuse-in-women-of-reproductive-age

ACOG: Opioid Use Disorder in Pregnancy: https://www.acog.org/clinical/clinical-guidance/committee-opinion/articles/2017/08/opioid-use-and-opioid-use-disorder-in-pregnancy

ASAM: Compassionate Care for Neonatal Abstinence Syndrome: https://50f378edf9ff4c9f6f9f-30f035c9227b07afda0d0be1818388ef.ssl.cf1.rackcdn.com//1201075-95062-001.pdf

California BRIDGE: Eat, Sleep, Soothe: https://obgyn.ucsf.edu/sites/obgyn.ucsf.edu/files/CA%20BRIDGE%20-%20PATIENT%20MATERIALS%20-%20Prevent%20%20treat%20opioid%20withdrawal%20in%20your%20baby%20-%20September%202020.pdf

CDC: Substance Use During Pregnancy: https://www.cdc.gov/reproductivehealth/maternalinfanthealth/substance-abuse/substance-abuse-during-pregnancy.htm

Elephant Circle: Fetal Exposure to Cannabis: https://static1.squarespace.com/static/57126eff60b5e92c3a226a53/t/5af4d0fe575d1fcc6ea0ac60/1525993733216/Cannabis+in+Pregnancy+-+a+summary+of+the+scientific+literature.pdf

References

Academy of Breastfeeding Medicine (ABM). (2015). ABM clinical protocol #21: Guidelines for breastfeeding and substance use or substance use disorder. *Breastfeeding Medicine*, 10(3), 135–141.

Academy of Perinatal Harm Reduction. (2022). *Pregnancy and substance use: A harm reduction toolkit*. https://www.perinatalharmreduction.org/toolkit-pregnancy-substance-use

Admon, L., & Winkelman, T. (2019). *IHPI brief: Substance use and pregnancy: What we know and what we can do*. Institute for Healthcare Policy & Innovation University of Michigan. https://ihpi.umich.edu/sites/default/files/2019-04/0124_Substance-Use-Pregnancy_BoE_FINAL-042419.pdf

Agency for Healthcare Research and Quality. (2020). *Treating tobacco use and dependence: 2008 update*. https://www.ahrq.gov/prevention/guidelines/tobacco/index.html

American Civil Liberties Union (ACLU). (2012). *Fair sentencing act*. https://www.aclu.org/issues/criminal-law-reform/drug-law-reform/fair-sentencing-act

American Civil Liberties Union (ACLU). (2016). *Drug use and pregnancy in Tennessee*. https://www.aclu-tn.org/wp-content/uploads/2016/09/Fetal-Assault-Direct-Impact.pdf

American College of Nurse-Midwives. (2017). *Position statement: Screening and brief intervention to prevent alcohol-exposed pregnancy*. American College of Nurse-Midwives. http://www.midwife.org/acnm/files/ACNMLibraryData/UPLOADFILENAME/000000000309/ScreeningBriefInterventionPreventAlcoholExposedPregnancyMay2017.pdf

American College of Nurse-Midwives. (2018). *Position statement: Substance use disorders in pregnancy*. American College of Nurse-Midwives. http://www.midwife.org/acnm/files/acnmlibrarydata/uploadfilename/000000000052/PS-Substance-Use-Disorders-in-Pregnancy-FINAL-20-Nov-18.pdf

American College of Nurse-Midwives (ACNM). (2013). *Position statement: Addiction in pregnancy*. American College of Nurse-Midwives. http://www.midwife.org/ACNM/files/ACNMLibraryData/UPLOADFILENAME/000000000052/Addiction%20in%20Pregnancy%20May%202013.pdf

American College of Obstetricians and Gynecologists (ACOG). (2008). Practice bulletin: Clinical management guidelines for obstetrician-gynecologists number 92. Use of psychiatric medications during pregnancy and lactation. *Obstetrics & Gynecology, 111*(4), 1001–1020.

American College of Obstetricians and Gynecologists (ACOG). (2011a, reaffirmed 2021). At-risk drinking and alcohol dependence: Obstetric and gynecologic implications. Committee opinion no. 496. *Obstetrics & Gynecology, 18*, 383–388.

American College of Obstetricians and Gynecologists (ACOG). (2011b, reaffirmed 2021). Methamphetamine abuse in women of reproductive age. Committee opinion no. 479. *Obstetrics & Gynecology, 117*(3), 751–755.

American College of Obstetricians and Gynecologists (ACOG). (2015, reaffirmed 2021). Alcohol abuse and other substance use disorders: Ethical issues in obstetric and gynecologic practice. ACOG Committee opinion no. 633. *Obstetrics & Gynecology, 125*, 1529–1537.

American College of Obstetricians and Gynecologists (ACOG). (2017a, reaffirmed 2021). Opioid use and opioid use disorder in pregnancy. Committee opinion no. 711. *Obstetrics & Gynecology, 130*, 81–94.

American College of Obstetricians and Gynecologists (ACOG). (2017b, reaffirmed 2021). Marijuana use during pregnancy and lactation. Committee opinion no. 722. *Obstetrics & Gynecology, 130*, 205–209.

American College of Obstetricians and Gynecologists (ACOG). (2020). Tobacco and nicotine cessation during pregnancy. ACOG Committee opinion no. 807. *Obstetrics & Gynecology, 135*(5), 221–229.

American Psychiatric Association (APA). (2013). *Diagnostic and statistical manual of mental disorders (DSM-5)* (5th ed.). American Psychiatric Publishing.

American Society of Addiction Medicine. (2020a). National practice guideline for the treatment of opioid use disorder. Focused update. *Journal of Addiction Medicine: March/April 2020, 14*(2S), 1–91.

American Society of Addiction Medicine (ASAM). (2019). *Definition of addiction.* https://www.asam.org/Quality-Science/definition-of-addiction

American Society of Addiction Medicine (ASAM). (2020b). Substance use and substance use disorder among pregnant and postpartum people. https://www.asam.org/advocacy/public-policy-statements/details/public-policy-statements/2022/10/12/substance-use-and-substance-use-disorder-among-pregnant-and-postpartum-people

Anderka, M., Romitti, P. A., Sun, L., Druschel, C., Carmichael, S., & Shaw, G. (2010). Patterns of tobacco exposure before and during pregnancy. *Acta Obstetricia et Gynecologica Scandinavica, 89*(4), 505–514.

Anderson, T., Lavista Ferres, J., You Ren, S., Moon, R., Goldstein, R., Ramirez, J., & Mitchell, E. (2019). Maternal smoking before and during pregnancy and the risk of sudden unexpected infant death. *Pediatrics, 143*(4), 1–8.

Andrade, C. (2018). Risk of major congenital malformations associated with the use of methylphenidate or amphetamines in pregnancy. *Journal of Clinical Psychiatry, 79*(1). https://pubmed.ncbi.nlm.nih.gov/29370484

Andrews, C., Cao, D., Marsh, J. C., & Shin, H. C. (2011). The impact of comprehensive services in substance abuse treatment for women with a history of intimate partner violence. *Violence Against Women, 17*(5), 550–567.

Angelotta, C., & Appelbaum, P. S. (2017). Criminal charges for child harm from substance use in pregnancy. *The Journal of the American Academy of Psychiatry and the Law, 45*(2), 193–203.

Apelberg, B. J., Onicescu, G., Avila-Tang, E., & Samet, J. M. (2010). Estimating the risks and benefits of nicotine replacement therapy for smoking cessation in the United States. *American Journal of Public Health, 100*(2), 341–348.

Arabin, B., & Baschat, A. A. (2017). Pregnancy: An underutilized window of opportunity to improve long-term maternal and infant health-An appeal for continuous family care and interdisciplinary communication. *Frontiers in Pediatrics, 5*, 69.

Arnaudo, C. L., Andraka-Christou, B., & Allgood, K. (2017). Psychiatric co-morbidities in pregnant women with opioid use disorders: Prevalence, impact, and implications for treatment. *Current Addiction Reports, 4*(1), 1–13.

Asberg, K., & Renk, K. (2012). Substance use coping as a mediator of the relationship between trauma symptoms and substance use consequences among incarcerated females with childhood sexual abuse histories. *Substance Use & Misuse, 47*(7), 799–808.

Ashford, R. D., Brown, A. M., & Curtis, B. (2019). "Abusing addiction": Our language still isn't good enough. *Alcoholism Treatment Quarterly, 37*(2), 257–272.

Astley, S. J., & Little, R. E. (1990). Maternal marijuana use during lactation and infant development at one year. *Neurotoxicology and Teratology, 12*, 161–168.

Babb, M., Koren, G., & Einarson, A. (2010). Treating pain during pregnancy. *Canadian Family Physician Medecin de Famille Canadien, 56*(1), 25–27.

Bailey, B. A., McCook, J. G., Hodge, A., & McGrady, L. (2012). Infant birth outcomes among substance using women: Why quitting smoking during pregnancy is just as important as quitting illicit drug use. *Maternal and Child Health Journal, 16*(2), 414–422.

Bailey, B. A., & Sokol, R. J. (2011). Prenatal alcohol exposure and miscarriage, stillbirth, preterm delivery, and sudden infant death syndrome. *Alcohol Research & Health: The Journal of the National Institute on Alcohol Abuse and Alcoholism, 34*(1), 86–91.

Baker, T., Datta, P., Rewers-Felkins, K., Thompson, H., Kallem, R. R., & Hale, T. W. (2018). Transfer of inhaled cannabis into human breast milk. *Obstetrics & Gynecology, 131*(5), 783–788.

Bandoli, G., Coles, C. D., Kable, J. A., Wertelecki, W., Yevtushok, L., Zymak-Zakutnya, N., Wells, A., Granovska, I. V., Pashtepa, A. O., Chambers, C. D., & CIFASD. (2019). Patterns of prenatal alcohol use that predict infant growth and development. *Pediatrics, 143*(2), 1–10.

Barnes, J., McRobbie, H., Dong, C. Y., Walker, N., & Hartman-Boyce, J. (2019). Hypnotherapy for smoking cessation. *The Cochrane Database of Systematic Reviews, 2019*(6), CD001008.

Bartu, A., Dusci, L. J., & Ilett, K. F. (2009). Transfer of methylamphetamine and amphetamine into breast milk following recreational use of methylamphetamine. *British Journal of Clinical Pharmacology, 67*(4), 455–459. https://doi.org/10.1111/j.1365-2125.2009.03366.x

Bateman, B. T., Franklin, J. M., Bykov, K., Avorn, J., Shrank, W. H., Brennan, T. A., Landon, J. E., Rathmell, J. P., Huybrechts, K. F., Fischer, M. A., & Choudhry, N. K. (2016). Persistent opioid use following cesarean delivery: Patterns and predictors among opioid-naïve women. *American Journal of Obstetrics and Gynecology, 215*(3), 353.e1–353.e18. https://doi.org/10.1016/j.ajog.2016.03.016

Battin, M., Albersheim, S., & Newman, D. (1995). Congenital genitourinary tract abnormalities following cocaine exposure in utero. *American Journal of Perinatology, 12*(6), 425.

Bauer, C. R., Langer, J. C., Shankaran, S., Bada, H. S., Lester, B., Wright, L. L., Krause-Steinrauf, H., Smeriglio, V. L., Finnegan, L. P., Maza, P. L., & Verter, J. (2005). Acute neonatal effects of cocaine exposure during pregnancy. *Archives of Pediatric & Adolescent Medicine, 159*(9), 824.

Behnke, M., Eyler, F. D., Garvan, C. W., & Wobie, K. (2001). The search for congenital malformations in newborns with fetal cocaine exposure. *Pediatrics, 107*(5), E74.

Behnke, M., & Smith, V. C., Committee on Substance Abuse, & Committee on Fetus and Newborn(2013). Prenatal substance abuse: Short- and long-term effects on the exposed fetus. *Pediatrics, 131*(3), e1009–e1024. https://doi.org/10.1542/peds.2012-3931

Bell, J., Towers, C. V., Hennessy, M. D., Heitzman, C., Smith, B., & Chattin, K. (2016). Detoxification from opiate drugs during pregnancy. *American Journal of Obstetrics and Gynecology, 215*(3), 374.e1–374.e3746. https://doi.org/10.1016/j.ajog.2016.03.015

Bell, S. A., & Seng, J. (2013). Childhood maltreatment history, posttraumatic relational sequelae, and prenatal care utilization. *Journal of Obstetric, Gynecologic, & Neonatal Nursing, 42*(4), 404–415.

Berard, A., Zhao, J., & Sheehy, O. (2016). Success of smoking cessation interventions during pregnancy. *American Journal of Obstetrics and Gynecology, 633*, e1–e8.

Berger, L. M. (2002). Estimating the benefits and costs of a universal screening and treatment referral policy for pregnant women. *Journal of Social Service Research*, 29(1), 57–84.

Betancourt, L. M., Yang, W., Brodsky, N. L., Gallagher, P. R., Malmud, E. K., Giannetta, J. M., Farah, M. J., & Hurt, H. (2011). Adolescents with and without gestational cocaine exposure: Longitudinal analysis of inhibitory control, memory, and receptive language. *Neurotoxicology and Teratology*, 33(1), 36–46.

Bloch, M., & Parascandola, M. (2014). Tobacco use in pregnancy: A window of opportunity for prevention. *The Lancet. Global Health*, 2(9), e489–e490.

Boyd, J., Maher, L., Austin, T., Lavalley, J., Kerr, T., & McNeil, R. (2022). Mothers who use drugs: Closing the gaps in harm reduction response amidst the dual epidemics of overdose and violence in a Canadian urban setting. *American Journal of Public Health*, 112(S2), S191–S198.

Boyd, S., Murray, D., & MacPherson, D. (2017). Telling our stories: Heroin-assisted treatment and SNAP activism in the Downtown Eastside of Vancouver. *Harm Reduction Journal*, 14(27), 1–14.

Brett, J., & Murnion, B. (2015). Management of benzodiazepine misuse and dependence. *Australian Prescriber*, 38(5), 152–155.

Briggs, G. G., Freeman, R. K., Yaffe, S. J., Tower, C. V., & Forinash, A. B. (2017). *Drugs in pregnancy and lactation* (11th ed.). Lippincott, Williams & Wilkins.

Cain, M. A., Bornick, P., & Whiteman, V. (2013). The maternal, fetal, and neonatal effects of cocaine exposure in pregnancy. *Clinical Obstetrics and Gynecology*, 56(1), 124–132.

California Maternal Quality Care Collaborative (CMQCC). (2021). *Mother and baby substance exposure toolkit*. https://nas-toolkit-prod.s3.amazonaws.com/pdfs/mbsei_toolkit_2021-02-17.pdf

Carrà, G., Bartoli, F., Galanter, M., & Crocamo, C. (2019). Untreated depression and non-medical use of prescription pain relievers: Findings from the National Survey on drug use and health 2008–2014. *Postgraduate Medicine*, 131(1), 52–59.

Carter, D., & Kostaras, X. (2005). Psychiatric disorders in pregnancy. *BCMJ*, 47(2), 96–99.

Center for Law and Social Policy. (2019). *Drug testing and public assistance. Report/Brief*. Washington, D.C. https://www.clasp.org/wp-content/uploads/2022/01/2019_drug-testing-and-public-_0.pdf

Centers for Disease Control and Prevention. (2016). Increased hepatitis C virus (HCV) detection in women of childbearing age and potential risk for vertical transmission—United States and Kentucky, 2011–2014. *MMWR Morbidity and Mortality Weekly Report*, 65(28). https://www.cdc.gov/mmwr/volumes/65/wr/pdfs/mm6528a2.pdf

Centers for Disease Control and Prevention. (2019). Racial/ethnic and age group differences in opioid and synthetic opioid-involved overdose deaths among adults aged ≥18 years in metropolitan areas—United States, 2015–2017. *MMWR Morbidity and Mortality Weekly Report*, 68(43), 967–973.

Centers for Disease Control and Prevention. (2020). *Smoking during pregnancy*. https://www.cdc.gov/tobacco/basic_information/health_effects/pregnancy/index.htm

Centers for Disease Control and Prevention. (2021a). *Fetal alcohol spectrum disorders: Alcohol use during pregnancy*. https://www.cdc.gov/ncbddd/fasd/alcohol-use.html

Centers for Disease Control and Prevention. (2021b). *Opioids: Fentanyl*. https://www.cdc.gov/opioids/basics/fentanyl.html

Centers for Disease Control and Prevention. (2021c). *About opioid use during pregnancy*. https://www.cdc.gov/pregnancy/opioids/basics.html

Centers for Disease Control and Prevention. (2022). *Basics About FASDs*. https://www.cdc.gov/ncbddd/fasd/facts.html#:~:text=Fetal%20alcohol%20spectrum%20disorders%20(FASDs)%20are%20a%20group%20of%20conditions,problems%20with%20behavior%20and%20learning

Cestonaro, C., Menozzi, L., & Terranova, C. (2022). Infants of mothers with cocaine use: Review of clinical and medico-legal aspects. *Children*, 9(67), 1–17.

Chamberlain, C., O'Mara-Eves, A., Porter, J., Coleman, T., Perlen, S. M., Thomas, J., & McKenzie, J. E. (2017). Psychosocial interventions for supporting women to stop smoking in pregnancy. *Cochrane Database of Systemic Reviews 2017*, (2). Art. No.: CD001055

Chang, C. (2022). Substance use in pregnancy: An overview of selected drugs. In C. J. Lockwood, A. J. Saxon, & K. Eckler (Eds.), *UpToDate*. Available from https://www.uptodate.com/contents/substance-use-during-pregnancy-overview-of-selected-drugs#H1735652429

Chang, G., Orav, E. J., Jones, J. A., Buynitsky, T., Gonzalez, S., & Wilkins-Haug, L. (2011). Self-reported alcohol and drug use in pregnant young women: A pilot study of associated factors and identification. *Journal of Addiction Medicine*, 5(3), 221–226.

Chasnoff, I. J., Landress, H. J., & Barrett, M. E. (1990). The prevalence of illicit-drug or alcohol use during pregnancy and discrepancies in mandatory reporting in Pinellas County, Florida. *The New England Journal of Medicine*, 322(17), 1202–1206.

Chasnoff, I. J., Lewis, D. E., & Squires, L. (1987). Cocaine intoxication in a breast-fed infant. *Pediatrics*, 80(6), 836–838.

Choo, R. E., Huestis, M. A., Schroeder, J. R., Shin, A. S., & Jones, H. E. (2004). Neonatal abstinence syndrome in methadone-exposed infants is altered by level of prenatal tobacco exposure. *Drug and Alcohol Dependence*, 75, 253–260.

Chu, E. K., Smith, L. M., Derauf, C., Newman, E., Neal, C. R., Arria, A. M., Huestis, M. A., DellaGrotta, S. A., Roberts, M. B., Dansereau, L. M., & Lester, B. M. (2020). Behavior problems during early childhood in children with prenatal methamphetamine exposure. *Pediatrics*, 146(6), 1–8.

Claire, R., Chamberlain, C., Davey, M. A., Cooper, S. E., Berlin, I., Leonardi-Bee, J., & Coleman, T. (2020). Pharmacological interventions for promoting smoking cessation during pregnancy. *Cochrane Database Systemic Review 2020*, 3. CD010078

Clark, S. M., & Nakad, R. (2011). Pharmacotherapeutic management of nicotine dependence in pregnancy. *Obstetrics & Gynecology Clinics of North America*, 38(2), 297–311.

Coleman-Cowger, V. H., Oga, E. A., Peters, E. N., Trocin, K. E., Koszowski, B., & Mark, K. (2019). Accuracy of three screening tools for prenatal substance use. *Obstetrics & Gynecology*, 133(5), 952–961.

Conner, S. N., Bedell, V., Lipsey, K., Macones, G. A., Cahill, A. G., & Tuuli, M. G. (2016). Maternal marijuana use and adverse neonatal outcomes: A systematic review and meta-analysis. *Obstetrics & Gynecology*, 128(4), 713–723.

Corsi, D. J., Walsh, L., Weiss, D., Hsu, H., El-Chaar, D., Hawken, S., Fell, D. B., & Walker, M. (2019). Association between self-reported prenatal cannabis use and maternal, perinatal, and neonatal outcomes. *JAMA*, 322(2), 145–152. https://doi.org/10.1001/jama.2019.8734

Cressman, A. M., Koren, G., Pupco, A., Kim, E., Ito, S., & Bozzo, P. (2012). Maternal cocaine use during breastfeeding. *Canadian family physician Medecin de famille canadien*, 58(11), 1218–1219.

Cressman, A. M., Natekar, A., Kim, E., Koren, G., & Bozzo, P. (2014). Cocaine abuse during pregnancy. *Obstetrics and Gynaecology Canada*, 36(7), P628–P631.

Daniulaityte, R., Carlson, R. R., Juhascik, M. P., Strayer, K. E., & Sizemore, I. E. (2019). Street fentanyl use: Experiences, preferences, and concordance between self-reports and urine toxicology. *International Journal of Drug Policy*, 71, 3–9.

D'apolito, K. (2013). Breastfeeding and substance abuse. *Clinical Obstetrics and Gynecology*, 56(1), 202–211.

D'Avila, F. B., & Limberger, R. P. & Fröehlich, P. E. (2016). Cocaine and crack cocaine abuse by pregnant or lactating mothers and analysis of its biomarkers in meconium and breast milk by LC-MS-A review. *Clinical Biochemistry*, 49(13–14), 1096.

Davis, J. P., Diguiseppi, G., De Leon, J., Prindle, J., Sedano, A., Rivera, D., Henwood, B., & Rice, E. (2019). Understanding pathways between PTSD, homelessness, and substance use among adolescents. *Psychology of Addictive Behaviors*, 33(5), 467–476.

Dawson, D., Grant, B., Stinson, F., & Zhou, Y. (2005). Effectiveness of the derived alcohol use disorder identification test (AUDIT-C) in screening for alcohol use disorders and risky drinking the US general population. *Alcohol Clinical and Experimental Research*, 29(5), 844–854.

Denniston, M. M., Jiles, R. B., Drobeniuc, J., Klevens, R. M., Ward, J. W., McQuillan, G. M., & Holmberg, S. D. (2014). Chronic hepatitis C virus infection in the United States, national health and nutrition examination survey 2003 to 2010. *Annals of Internal Medicine*, *160*(5), 293–300.

Denny, C. H., Acero, C. S., Naimi, T. S., & Kim, S. Y. (2019). Consumption of alcohol beverages and binge drinking among pregnant women aged 18–44 years—United States, 2015–2017. *MMWR Morbidity and Mortality Weekly Report, 68*, 365–368.

DeVido, J., Bogunovic, O., & Weiss, R. D. (2015). Alcohol use disorders in pregnancy. *Harvard Review of Psychiatry, 23*(2), 112–121.

Dillon, G., Hussain, R., Loxton, D., & Rahman, S. (2013). Mental and physical health and intimate partner violence against women: A review of the literature. *International Journal of Family Medicine, 2013*, 313909.

Drake, P., Driscoll, A.K., & Mathews, T.J. (2018). *Cigarette smoking during pregnancy: United States, 2016. NCHS Data Brief, no 305*. National Center for Health Statistics.

Drug Policy Alliance. (2016). *The drug war and mass deportation*. https://drugpolicy.org/sites/default/files/DPA%20Fact%20Sheet_The%20Drug%20War%20and%20Mass%20Deportation_%28Feb.%202016%29.pdf

Drug Policy Alliance. (2022). *A history of the drug war*. https://drugpolicy.org/issues/brief-history-drug-war

Drugs and Lactation Database (LactMed). (2022a). *Alcohol*. National Library of Medicine. https://www.ncbi.nlm.nih.gov/books/NBK501469

Drugs and Lactation Database (LactMed). (2022b). *Bupropion*. National Library of Medicine. https://www.ncbi.nlm.nih.gov/books/NBK501184

Drugs and Lactation Database (LactMed). (2021a). *Cannabis*. National Library of Medicine. https://www.ncbi.nlm.nih.gov/books/NBK501587

Drugs and Lactation Database (LactMed). (2021b). *Clonazepam*. National Library of Medicine. https://www.ncbi.nlm.nih.gov/books/NBK501209

Drugs and Lactation Database (LactMed). (2021c). *Diazepam*. National Library of Medicine. https://www.ncbi.nlm.nih.gov/books/NBK501214

Drugs and Lactation Database (LactMed). (2020). *Cocaine*. National Library of Medicine. https://www.ncbi.nlm.nih.gov/books/NBK501588

Eagen-Torkko, M. (2015). *Compliance and concordance: Prevalence and predictors of breastfeeding in survivors of childhood abuse*. [Doctoral dissertation, University of Washington Bothell].

Ecker, J., Abuhamad, A., Hill, W., Bailit, J., Bateman, B. T., Berghella, V., Blake-Lamb, T., Guille, C., Landau, R., Minkoff, H., Prabhu, M., Rosenthal, E., Terplan, M., Wright, T., & Yonkers, K. A. (2019). Substance use disorders in pregnancy: Clinical, ethical, and research imperatives of the opioid epidemic: A report of a joint workshop of the Society for Maternal-Fetal Medicine, American College of Obstetricians and Gynecologists, and American Society of Addiction Medicine. *SMFM Special Reports, 221*(1), PB5-B28.

Eggleston, A. M., Calhoun, P. S., Svikis, D. S., Tuten, M., Chisolm, M. S., & Jones, H. E. (2009). Suicidality, aggression, and other treatment considerations among pregnant substance-dependent women with posttraumatic stress disorder. *Comprehensive Psychiatry, 50*, 415–423.

El-Bassel, N., Shoptaw, S., Goodman-Meza, D., & Ono, H. (2021). Addressing long overdue social and structural determinants of the opioid epidemic. *Drug & Alcohol Dependence, 222*, 108679.

Engstrom, M., El-Bassel, N., & Gilbert, L. (2012). Childhood sexual abuse characteristics, intimate partner violence exposure, and psychological distress among women in methadone treatment. *Journal of Substance Abuse Treatment, 43*(3), 366–376.

Eyler, F. D., Behnke, M., Garvan, C. W., Woods, N. S., Wobie, K., & Conlon, M. (2001). Newborn evaluations of toxicity and withdrawal related to prenatal cocaine exposure. *Neurotoxicology & Teratology, 23*(5), 399.

Eze, N., Smith, L. M., LaGasse, L. L., Derauf, C., Newman, E., Arria, A., Huestis, M. A., Della Grotta, S. A., Dansereau, L. M., Neal, C., & Lester, B. M. (2016). School-aged outcomes following prenatal methamphetamine exposure: 7.5-year follow up from the infant development, environment, and lifestyle study. *Journal of Pediatrics, 170*, 34.

Fasouliotis, S. J., & Schenker, J. G. (2000). Maternal-fetal conflict. *European Journal of Obstetrics & Gynecology and Reproductive Biology, 89*(1), 101–107.

Feldman, H. S., Jones, K. L., Lindsay, S., Slymen, D., Klonoff-Cohen, H., Kao, K., Rao, S., & Chambers, C. (2012). Prenatal alcohol exposure patterns and alcohol-related birth defects and growth deficiencies: A prospective study. *Alcoholism: Clinical & Experimental Research, 36*(4), 670.

Fernandez, N., Towers, C. V., Wolfe, L., Hennessy, M. D., Weitz, B., & Porter, S. (2016). Sharing of snorting straws and hepatitis C virus infection in pregnant women. *Obstetrics & Gynecology, 128*(2), 234–237.

Fokina, V. M., West, H., Oncken, C., Clark, S. M., Ahmed, M. S., Hankins, G. D., & Nanovskaya, T. N. (2016). Bupropion therapy during pregnancy: The drug and its major metabolites in umbilical cord plasma and amniotic fluid. *American Journal of Obstetrics & Gynecology, 497*, e1–e7.

Food and Drugs, 21 U.S.C. §811. (2011). https://www.govinfo.gov/content/pkg/USCODE-2011-title21/html/USCODE-2011-title21-chap13-subchapI-partB.htm

Forray, A. (2016). Substance use during pregnancy. *F1000 Research, 5*, 1–9.

Gao, Y. A., Drake, C., Krans, E. E., Chen, Q., & Jarlenski, M. P. (2022). Explaining racial-ethnic disparities in the receipt of medication for opioid use disorder during pregnancy. *Journal of Addiction Medicine, 16*(6), e356–e365.

Gentile, S. (2010). Neurodevelopmental effects of prenatal exposure to psychotropic medications. *Depression and Anxiety, 27*(7), 675.

Godsin, L. K., Deputy, N. P., Kim, S. Y., Dang, E. P., & Denny, C. H. (2022). Alcohol consumption and binge drinking during pregnancy among adults aged 18–49 years—United States, 2018–2020. *MMWR Morbidity and Mortality Weekly Report, 71*, 10–13.

Goler, N., Armstrong, M., Caughey, A., Haimowits, M., Hung, Y., & Osejo, V. (2012). Early start, a cost-beneficial perinatal substance abuse program. *Obstetrics & Gynecology, 19*(1), 102–110.

Goler, N., Armstrong, M., Taillac, C., & Osejo, V. (2008). Substance abuse treatment linked with prenatal visits improves perinatal outcomes: A new standard. *Journal of Perinatology, 28*, 597–603.

Gopman, S. (2014). Prenatal and postpartum care of women with substance use disorders. *Obstetrics & Gynecology Clinics, 41*(2), 213–228.

Gorman, M. C., Orme, K. S., Nguyen, N. T., Kent, E. J., & Caughey, A. B. (2014). Outcomes in pregnancies complicated by methamphetamine use. *American Journal of Obstetrics & Gynecology, 211*(4), 429–e1.

Gouin, K., Murphy, K., & Shah, P. S. (2011). Effects of cocaine use during pregnancy on low birthweight and preterm birth: Systematic review and meta-analyses. *American Journal of Obstetrics & Gynecology, 204*(4), 340–e1.

Grant, K. S., Petroff, R., Isoherranen, N., Stella, N., & Burbacher, T. M. (2018). Cannabis use during pregnancy: Pharmacokinetics and effects on child development. *Pharmacology & Therapeutics, 182*, 133–151.

Grigoriadis, S., Graves, L., Peer, M., Mamisashvili, L., Dennis, C., Vigod, S. N., Steiner, M., Brown, C., Cheung, A., Dawson, H., Rector, N., Guenette, M., & Ritcher, M. (2019). Benzodiazepine use during pregnancy alone or in combination with an antidepressant and congenital malformations: Systematic review and meta-analysis. *Journal of Clinical Psychiatry, 80*(4), e1–e12.

Grisham, L. M., Stephen, M. M., Coykendall, M. R., Kane, M. F., Maurer, J. A., & Bader, M. Y. (2019). Eat, sleep, console approach: A family-centered model for the treatment of neonatal abstinence syndrome. *Advances in Neonatal Care, 19*(2), 138–144.

Guttmacher Institute, (2022). *Substance use during pregnancy*. https://www.guttmacher.org/state-policy/explore/substance-use-during-pregnancy

Haastrup, M. B., Pottegård, A., & Damkier, P. (2014). Alcohol and breastfeeding. *Basic & Clinical Pharmacology & Toxicology, 114*(2), 168–173.

Hackshaw, A., Rodeck, C., & Boniface, S. (2011). Maternal smoking in pregnancy and birth defects: A systematic review based on 173,687 malformed cases and 11.7 million controls. *Human Reproduction Update, 17*(5), 589.

Hajek, P., Phillips-Waller, A., Przulji, D., Pesola, F., Myers Smith, K., Bisal, N., Li, J., Parrott, S., Sasieni, P., Dawkins, L., Ross, L., Goniewicz, M., Wu, Q., & McRobbie, H. J. (2019). A randomized trial of e-cigarettes versus nicotine-replacement therapy. *New England Journal of Medicine*, 380(7), 629.

Hajek, P. Przulj, D., Pesola, F., Griffiths, C., Walton, R., McRobbie, H., Coleman, T., Lewis, S., Whitemore, R., Clark, M., Ussher, M., Sinclair, L., Seager, E., Cooper, S., Bauld, L., Naughton, F., Sasieni, P., Manyonda, I., & Myers Smith, K. (2022). Electronic cigarettes versus nicotine patches for smoking cessation in pregnancy: a randomized controlled trial. *Nature Medicine*, 28, 958–964.

Hale, T. (2010). *Medications and mothers' milk*. Hale Publishing.

Han, Y., Yan, W., Zheng, Y., Khan, M. Z., Yuan, K., & Lu, L. (2019). The rising crisis of illicit fentanyl use, overdose, and potential therapeutic strategies. *Translational Psychiatry*, 9, 282.

Hansen, H., Jordan, A., Plough, A., Alegria, M., Cunningham, C., & Ostrovsky, A. (2022). Lessons for the opioid crisis integrating social determinants of health into clinical care. *American Journal of Public Health*, 112(S2), S109–S111.

Hansen, H. B., Siegel, C. E., Case, B. G., Bertollo, D. N., DiRocco, D., & Galanter, M. (2013). Variation in use of buprenorphine and methadone treatment by racial, ethnic, and income characteristics of residential social areas in New York City. *Journal of Behavioral Health Services & Research*, 40(3), 367–377.

Harm Reduction Coalition. (2016). *Principles of Harm Reduction*. Oakland, CA. http://harmreduction.org/about-us/principles-of-harm-reduction/

Harp, K. L., & Buntig, A. M. (2020). The racialized nature of child welfare policies and the social control of black bodies. *Social Politics*, 27(2), 258–281.

Harrison, P., & Sidebottom, A. (2009). Alcohol and drug use before and during pregnancy: An examination of use patterns and predictors of cessation. *Maternal and Child Health Journal*, 13, 386–394.

Harst, L., Deckert, S., Haarig, F., Reichert, J., Dinger, J., Hellmund, P., Schmitt, J., & Rudiger, M. (2021). Prenatal methamphetamine exposure: Effects on child development–a systematic review. *Deutsches Ärzteblatt International*, 118(18), 313.

Hatcher, A. E., Mendoza, S., & Hansen, H. (2018). At the expense of a life: Race, class, and the meaning of buprenorphine in pharmaceuticalized "care". *Substance Use & Misuse*, 53(2), 301–310.

Haug, N. A., Duffy, M., & McCaul, M. E. (2014). Substance abuse treatment services for pregnant women: Psychosocial and behavioral approaches. *Obstetrics and Gynecology Clinics of North America*, 41(2), 267–296.

Healthcare Cost and Utilization Project (HCUP). (2022). *HCUP fast stats – Map of neonatal abstinence syndrome (NAS) among newborn hospitalizations*. Agency for Healthcare Research and Quality. https://www.hcup-us.ahrq.gov/faststats/NASMap

Heit, H. (2016). *Urine drug testing: Facts you should know!* [Powerpoint slides]. Providers' Clinical Support System for Medication Assisted Treatment. http://pcssmat.org/wp-content/uploads/2014/06/Heit-ASAM-PCSS-MAT-Online-Module-2.pdf

Helmbrecht, G. D., & Thiagarajah, S. (2008). Management of addiction disorders in pregnancy. *Journal of Addiction Medicine*, 2(1), 1–16.

Hendrixson, D. T., Manary, M. J., Trehan, I., & Lewis, W. (2021). Undernutrition in pregnancy: Evaluation, management, and outcome in resource limited areas. *UpToDate*. https://www.uptodate.com/contents/undernutrition-in-pregnancy-evaluation-management-and-outcome-in-resource-limited-areas?search=nutrition%20pregnancy&topicRef=453&source=see_link

Hiari, A. H., Ko, J. Y., Owens, P. L., Stocks, C., & Patrick, S. W. (2021). Neonatal abstinence syndrome and maternal opioid-related diagnoses in the US, 2010–2017. *JAMA*, 325(2), 146.

Horrigan, T., Schroeder, A., & Schaffer, R. (2000). The triad of substance abuse, violence and depression are interrelated in pregnancy. *Journal of Substance Abuse Treatment*, 18, 55–58.

Hudak, M., & Tan, R. (2012). Neonatal drug withdrawal. *Pediatrics*, 129(2).

Huybrechts, K. F., Bröms, G., Christensen, L. B., Einarsdóttir, K., Engeland, A., Furu, K., Gissler, M., Hernandez-Diaz, S., Karlsson, P., Karlstad, Ø., Kieler, H., Lahesmaa-Korpinen, A. M., Mogun, H., Nørgaard, M., Reutfors, J., Sørensen, H. T., Zoega, H., & Bateman, B. T. (2018). Association between methylphenidate and amphetamine use in pregnancy and risk of congenital malformations:

A cohort study from the international pregnancy safety study consortium. *JAMA Psychiatry*, 75(2), 167–175.

Ickowicz, S., Kerr, T., Grant, C., Milloy, M. J., Wood, E., & Hayashi, K. (2022). Increasing preference for fentanyl among a cohort of people who use opioids in Vancouver, Canada, 2017–2018. *Substance Abuse*, 43(1), 458–464.

Ilett, K. F., Hackett, L. P., Gower, S., Doherty, D. A., Hamilton, D., & Bartu, A. E. (2012). Estimated dose exposure of the neonate to buprenorphine and its metabolite norbuprenorphine via breastmilk during maternal buprenorphine substitution treatment. *Breastfeeding Medicine: The Official Journal of the Academy of Breastfeeding Medicine*, 7, 269–274.

Jansson, L., DiPietro, J., & Elko, A. (2005). Fetal response to maternal methadone administration. *American Journal of Obstetrics & Gynecology*, 193, 611–617.

Jansson, L. M. (2021a). Infants with prenatal substance exposure. *UpToDate*. https://www.uptodate.com/contents/infants-with-prenatal-substance-use-exposure?sectionName=Cocaine&search=cocaine%20pregnancy&topicRef=128152&anchor=H16&source=see_link#H20

Jansson, L. M. (2021b). Neonatal abstinence syndrome. *UpToDate*. https://www.uptodate.com/contents/neonatal-abstinence-syndrome?search=neonatal%20opioid%20withdrawal&source=search_result&selectedTitle=1~25&usage_type=default&display_rank=1#H3

Jessup, M., & Brindis, C. (2005). Issues in reproductive health and empowerment in perinatal women with substance use disorders. *Journal of Addictions Nursing*, 16, 97–105.

Jeynes, K. D., & Leigh-Gibson, E. (2017). The importance of nutrition in aiding recovery from substance use disorders: A review. *Drug and Alcohol Dependence*, 179, 229–239.

Jobes, M., Ghitza, U., Epstein, D., Phillips, K., Heishman, S., & Preston, K. (2011). Clonidine blocks stress-induced craving in cocaine users. *Psychopharmacology*, 218(1), 83–88.

Johnson, M. W., Garcia-Romeu, A., & Griffiths, R. R. (2017). Long-term follow-up of psilocybin-facilitated smoking cessation. *American Journal of Drug & Alcohol Abuse*, 43(1), 55–60.

Jones, H. E., Kaltenbach, K., Heil, S. H., Stine, S. M., Coyle, M. G., Arria, A. M., & Fischer, G. (2010). Neonatal abstinence syndrome after methadone or buprenorphine exposure. *The New England Journal of Medicine*, 363, 2320–2331.

Jones, J., Rios, R., Jones, M., Lewis, D., & Plate, C. (2009). Determination of amphetamine and methamphetamine in umbilical cord using liquid chromatography-tandem mass spectrometry. *Journal of Chromatography B: Analytical Technologies in the Biomedical and Life Sciences*, 877(29), 3701.

Kampman, K. (2021). Approach to treatment of stimulant use disorder in adults. *UpToDate*. https://www.uptodate.com/contents/approach-to-treatment-of-stimulant-use-disorder-in-adults?search=bath%20salts&source=search_result&selectedTitle=2~23&usage_type=default&display_rank=2#H4138207814

Kelly, L., Dooley, J., Cromarty, H., Minty, B., Morgan, A., Madden, S., & Hopman, W. (2011). Narcotic-exposed neonates in a first nations population in northwestern Ontario: Incidence and implications. *Canadian Family Physician*, 57(11), e441–e447.

Kelty, E., Terplan, M., Greenland, M., & Preen, D. (2021). Pharmacotherapies for the treatment of alcohol use disorders during pregnancy: Time to reconsider? *Drugs*, 81(7), 739–748.

Kelty, E., Tran, D., Lavin, T., Preen, D. B., Hulse, G., & Harvard, A. (2019). Prevalence and safety of acamprosate use in pregnant alcohol-dependent women in New South Wales, Australia. *Addiction*, 114(2), 206.

Kenny, K. S., Barrington, C., & Green, S. L. (2015). "I felt for a long time like everything beautiful in me had been taken out": Women's suffering, remembering, and survival following the loss of child custody. *International Journal of Drug Policy*, 26(11), 1158–1166.

Kenny, K. S., Krüsi, A., Barrington, C., Ranville, F., Green, S. L., Bingham, B., Abrahams, R., & Shannon, K. (2021). Health consequences of child removal among indigenous and non-indigenous sex workers: Examining trajectories, mechanisms and resiliencies. *Sociology of Health & Illness*, 43(8), 1903–1920.

Klaman, S. L., Isaacs, K., Leopold, A., Perpich, J., Hayashi, S., Vender, J., Campopiano, M., & Jones, H. E. (2017). Treating women who are pregnant and parenting for opioid use disorder and the concurrent care of their infants and children: Literature review to support national guidance. *Journal of Addiction Medicine, 11*(3), 178–190.

Knight, K. (2015). *addicted.pregnant.poor.* Duke University Press.

Ko, J. Y., Coy, K. C., & Haight, S. C. (2020a). Characteristics of marijuana use during pregnancy—Eight states, pregnancy risk assessment monitoring system. *MMWR Morbidity and Mortality Weekly Report, 69*, 1058–1063.

Ko, J. Y., D'Angelo, D. V., Haight, S. C., et al. (2020b). *Vital signs:* Prescription opioid pain reliever use during pregnancy—34 U.S. jurisdictions. *MMWR Morbidity and Mortality Weekly Report, 69*(28), 897–903.

Ko, J. Y., Wolicki, S., Barfield, W. D., Patrick, S. W., Broussard, C. S., Yonkers, K. A., Naimon, R., & Iskander, J. (2017). CDC grand rounds: Public health strategies to prevent neonatal abstinence syndrome. *MMWR Morbidity and Mortality Weekly Report, 66*(9), 242–245.

Kral, A. H., Lambdin, B. H., Browne, E. N., Wenger, L. D., Bluthenthal, R. N., & Davidson, P. J. (2021). Transition from injecting opioids to smoking fentanyl in San Francisco, California. *Drug and Alcohol Dependence, 227*, 109003.

Krans, E. E., Kim, J. Y., Chen, Q., Rothenberger, S. D., James Ill, A. E., Kelley, D., & Jarlenski, M. P. (2021). Outcomes associated with the use of medications for opioid use disorder during pregnancy. *Addiction, 6*(12), 3504–3514.

Kranzler, H., Washio, Y., Zindel, L., Wileyto, E., Srinivas, S., . . . Schnoll, R. (2021). Placebo-controlled trial of bupropion for smoking cessation in pregnant women. *American Jounral of Obstetrics & Gynecology Maternal Fetal Medicine, 3*(6), 100315.

Krol, K. M., & Grossmann, T. (2018). Psychological effects of breastfeeding on children and mothers. *Bundesgesundheitsblatt, Gesundheitsforschung, Gesundheitsschutz, 61*(8), 977–985.

Kuczkwoski, K. M. (2007). The effects of drug abuse on pregnancy. *Current Opinion in Obstetrics & Gynecology, 19*(6), 578.

Kwiatkowski, M. A., Donald, K. A., Stein, D. J., Ipser, J., Thomas, K. G. F., & Roos, A. (2018). Cognitive outcomes in prenatal methamphetamine exposed children aged six to seven years. *Comprehensive Psychiatry, 80*, 24.

Landi, N., Avery, T., Crowley, M. J., Wu, J., & Mayes, L. (2017). Prenatal cocaine exposure impacts language and reading into late adolescence: Behavioral and ERP evidence. *Developmental Neuropsychology, 42*(6), 369.

Lange, S., Probst, C., Gmel, G., Rehm, J., Burd, L., & Popova, S. (2017). Global prevalence of fetal alcohol spectrum disorder among children and youth: A systematic review and meta-analysis. *JAMA Pediatrics, 171*, 948–956.

Lefebvre, L., Midmer, D., Boyd, J. A., Ordean, A., Graves, L., Kahan, M., & Pantea, L. (2010). Participant perception of an integrated program for substance abuse in pregnancy. *Journal of Obstetric, Gynecologic & Neonatal Nursing, 39*, 46–52.

Letsen, G. W., Rosenberg, K. D., & Wu, L. (2002). Association between smoking during pregnancy and breastfeeding at about 2 weeks of age. *Journal of Human Lactation, 18*(4), 368.

Lewis, M. S. (2016). Criminalizing substance abuse and undermining *roe v. Wade:* The tension between abortion doctrine and the criminalization of prenatal substance abuse. *William & Mary Journal of Women & Law, 23*, 185.

Leza, L., Siria, S., López-Goñi, J. J., & Fernández-Montalvo, J. (2021). Adverse childhood experiences (ACEs) and substance use disorder (SUD): A scoping review. *Drug and Alcohol Dependence, 221*, 108563.

Lie, A. K., Hansen, H., Herzberg, D., Mold, A., Jauffret-Roustide, M., Dussauge, I., Greene, J., & Campbell, N. (2022). The harms of constructing addiction as a chronic, relapsing brain disease. *American Journal of Public Health, 112*(S2), S104–S108.

Lind, J. N., Interrante, J. D., Ailes, E. C., Gilboa, S. M., Khan, S., Frey, M. T., Dawson, A. L., Honein, M. A., Dowling, N. F., Razzaghi, H., Creanga, A. A., & Broussard, C. S. (2017). Maternal use of opioids during pregnancy and congenital malformations: A systematic review. *Pediatrics, 139*(6), e20164131.

Lindemalm, S. (2009). Transfer of buprenorphine into breast milk and calculation of infant drug dose. *Journal of Human Lactation, 25*(2), 199–205.

Lopez, A. M., Thomann, M., Dhatt, Z., Dhatt, Z., Ferrera, J., Al-Nassir, M., Ambrose, M., & Sullivan, S. (2022). Understanding racial inequities in the implementation of harm reduction initiatives. *American Journal of Public Health, 112*(S2), S173–S181.

Louik, C., Kerr, S., & Mitchell, A. A. (2014). First-trimester exposure to bupropion and risk of cardiac malformations. *Pharmacoepidemiology Drug Safety, 23*, 1066–1075.

Lund, I. O., Fischer, G., Welle-Strand, G. K., O'Grady, K. E., Debelak, K., Morrone, W. R., & Jones, H. E. (2013). A comparison of buprenorphine + naloxone to buprenorphine and methadone in the treatment of opioid dependence during pregnancy: Maternal and neonatal outcomes. *Substance Abuse: Research and Treatment, 7*, 61–74.

Ly, K., Miniño, A., Liu, S., Roberts, H., Hughes, E., Ward, J., & Jiles, R. (2020). Deaths associated with hepatitis C virus infection among residents in 50 states and the district of Colombia, 2016–2017. *Clinical Infectious Disease, 71*(5), 1149–1160.

Maglione, M. A., Maher, A. R., Ewing, B., Colaiaco, B., Newberry, S., Kandrack, R., Shanman, R. M., Sorbero, M. E., & Hempel, S. (2017). Efficacy of mindfulness meditation for smoking cessation: A systematic review and meta-analysis. *Addictive Behaviors, 69*, 27–34.

Mamakwa, S., Kahan, M., Kanate, D., Kirlew, M., Folk, D., Cirone, S., Rea, S., Parsons, P., Edwards, C., Gordon, J., Main, F., & Kelly, L. (2017). Evaluation of 6 remote first nations community-based buprenorphine programs in northwestern Ontario: Retrospective study. *Canadian Family Physician, 63*(2), 137–145.

Maremmoni, A., Pacini, M., & Maremmoni, I. (2019). What we have learned from methadone maintenance treatment of dual disorder heroin use disorder patients. *International Journal of Environmental Research and Public Health, 16*(3), 447.

Margerison, C. E., Roberts, M. H., Gemmill, A., & Goldman-Mellor, S. (2022). Pregnancy-associated deaths due to drugs, suicide, and homicide in the United States, 2010-2019. *Obstetrics and gynecology, 139*(2), 172–180.

Mark, K., Desai, A., & Terplan, M. (2016). Marijuana use and pregnancy: Prevalence, associated characteristics, and birth outcomes. *Archives of Women's Mental Health, 19*(1), 105–111

Mark, K. S., Farquhar, B., Chisolm, M. S., Coleman-Cowger, V. H., & Terplan, M. (2015). Knowledge, attitudes, and practice of electronic cigarette use among pregnant women. *Journal of Addiction Medicine, 9*(4), 266.

Martinez, M. (2021). *John's Hopkins receives first federal grant for psychedelic treatment research in 50 years.* Hub. https://hub.jhu.edu/2021/10/20/first-nih-grant-for-psychedelics-in-50-years

McDonnell, B. P., & Regan, C. (2019). Smoking in pregnancy: Pathophysiology of harm and current evidence for monitoring and cessation. *The Obstetrician & Gynecologist, 21*, 169–175.

McGinty, E. E., & Barry, C. L. (2020). Stigma reduction to combat addiction crisis—Developing an evidence base. *New England Journal of Medicine, 382*, 1291–1292.

Mennella, J. A., & Beauchamp, G. K. (1991). The transfer of alcohol to human milk. Effects on flavor and the infant's behavior. *New England Journal of Medicine, 325*(14), 981.

Metz, T. D., Rovner, P., Hoffman, M. C., Allshouse, A. A., Beckwith, K. M., & Binswanger, I. A. (2016). Maternal deaths from suicide and overdose in Colorado, 2004–2012. *Obstetrics & Gynecology, 128*(6), 1233–1240.

Metzl, J. M., & Roberts, D. E. (2014). Structural competency meets structural racism: Race, politics, and the structure of medical knowledge. *American Medical Association Journal of Ethics, 16*(9), 674–690.

Meyer, M. C., Johnston, A. M., Crocker, A. M., & Heil, S. H. (2015). Methadone and buprenorphine for opioid dependence during pregnancy: A retrospective cohort study. *Journal of Addiction Medicine, 9*(2), 81.

Mitra, A., Brandt, J., Rossen, T., Ananth, C., & Schuster, M. (2020). Opioid use disorder: A poorly understood cause of maternal mortality in the United States. *Obstetrics & Gynecology, 135*, 56S.

Montgomery, A., Hale, T. W., & Academy of Breastfeeding Medicine. (2012). ABM clinical protocol #15: Analgesia and anesthesia for the breastfeeding mother, revised 2012. *Breastfeeding Medicine: The Official Journal of the Academy of Breastfeeding Medicine, 7*(6), 547–553.

Morales, K. B., Nyeong Park, J., Glick, J. L., Rouhani, S., Green, T. C., & Shernman, S. G. (2019). Preference for drugs containing fentanyl from a cross-sectional survey of people who use illicit opioids in three United States cities. *Drug and Alcohol Dependence, 204*, 107547.

Movement for Family Power. (2020). *"Whatever they do, I'm her comfort, I'm her protector." How the foster system has become ground zero for the U.S. drug war.* https://static1.squarespace.com/static/5be5ed0fd274cb7c8a5d0cba/t/5eead939ca509d4e36a89277/1592449422870/MFP+Drug+War+Foster+System+Report.pdf

Moylan, P. L., Jones, H. E., Haug, N. A., Kissim, W. B., & Svikis, D. S. (2001). Clinical and psychosocial characteristics of substance-dependent pregnant women with and without PTSD. *Addictive Behaviors, 26*(3), 469–474.

Murphy, S., & Rosenbaum, M. (1999). *Pregnant women on drugs: Combating stereotypes and stigma.* Rutgers University Press.

National Association of Community Health Centers. (2016). *Protocol for responding to and assessing patients' assets, risks and experience (PRAPARE).* https://prapare.org/wp-content/uploads/2023/01/PRAPARE-English.pdf

National Conference of State Legislatures. (2023). *State medical cannabis laws.* https://www.ncsl.org/health/state-medical-cannabis-laws

National Harm Reduction Coalition. (2020). *Pregnancy and substance use: A harm reduction toolkit.* https://harmreduction.org/wp-content/uploads/2020/10/09.17.20_Pregnancy-and-Substance-Use-2.pdf

National Institute for Drug Abuse (NIDA). (2022). *Your words matter – Language showing compassion and care for women, infants, families, and communities impacted by substance use disorder.* https://nida.nih.gov/nidamed-medical-health-professionals/health-professions-education/words-matter-language-showing-compassion-care-women-infants-families-communities-impacted-substance-use-disorder

National Institute on Alcohol and Alcoholism. (2021). *Fetal alcohol exposure.* https://www.niaaa.nih.gov/publications/brochures-and-fact-sheets/fetal-alcohol-exposure

National Women's Law Center. (2013). *If you really care about criminal justice, you should care about reproductive justice!* https://nwlc.org/wp-content/uploads/2015/08/yp_criminal_justice_reproductive_justice_factsheet_09-18-13.pdf

Netherland, J., & Hansen, H. (2017). White opioids: Pharmaceutical race and the war on drugs that wasn't. *BioSocieties, 12*(2), 217–238.

Netherland, J., & Hansen, H. B. (2016). The war on drugs that wasn't: Wasted whiteness, 'dirty doctors,' and race in media coverage of prescription opioid misuse. *Culture, Medicine, and Psychiatry, 40*(4), 664–686.

Nguyen, D., Smith, L. M., Lagasse, L. L., Derauf, C., Grant, P., Shah, R., Arria, A., Huestis, M. A., Haning, W., Strauss, A., Della Grotta, S., Liu, J., & Lester, B. M. (2010). Intrauterine growth of infants exposed to prenatal methamphetamine: Results from the infant development, environment, and lifestyle study. *Journal of Pediatrics, 157*(2), 337.

Noormohammadi, A., Forinash, A., Yancey, A., Crannage, E., Campbell, K., & Shyken, J. (2016). Buprenorphine versus methadone for opioid dependence in pregnancy. *The Annals of Pharmacotherapy, 50*(8), 666–672.

O'Connor, A., O'Brien, L., Alto, W., & Wong, J. (2016). Does concurrent in utero exposure to buprenorphine and antidepressant medications influence the course of neonatal abstinence syndrome? *Journal of Maternal Fetal Neonatal Medicine, 29*(1), 112–114.

Oei, J. L., Kingsbury, A., Dhawan, A., Burns, L., Feller, J. M., Clews, S., Falconer, J., & Abdel-Latif, M. E. (2021). Amphetamines, the pregnant woman and her children: A review. *Journal of Perinatology, 32*(10), 737.

Ogden, S. N., Dichter, M. E., & Bazzi, A. R. (2022). Intimate partner violence as a predictor of substance use outcomes among women: A systematic review. *Addictive Behaviors, 127*, 107214.

Ondersma, S. J., Chang, G., Blake-Lamb, T., Gilstad-Hayden, K., Orav, J., Beatty, J. R., Goyert, G. L., & Yonkers, K. A. (2019). Accuracy of five self-report screening instruments for substance use in pregnancy. *Addiction, 114*(9), 1683–1693.

Paltrow, L. M., & Flavin, J. (2013). Arrests of and forced interventions on pregnant women in the United States, 1973–2005: Implications for women's legal status and public health. *Journal of Health Politics, Policy and Law, 38*(2), 299–343.

Patnode, C.D., Henderson, J.T., Thompson, J.H., Senger, C.A., Fortmann, S.P., Whitlovk, E.P. (2015). *Behavioral counseling and pharmacotherapy interventions for tobacco cessation in adults, including pregnant women: A review of reviews for the U.S. Preventive Services Task Force* [Internet]. Agency for Healthcare Research and Quality (Evidence Syntheses, No. 134) https://www.ncbi.nlm.nih.gov/books/NBK321744

Patrick, S., & Schiff, S. (2017). A public health response to opioid use in pregnancy. Policy statement of the American Academy of Pediatrics. *Pediatrics, 139*(3), 1–7.

Patrick, S. W., Barfield, W. D., & Poindexter, B. B. AAP committee on fetus and newborn, committee on substance use and prevention(2020). Neonatal opioid withdrawal syndrome. *Pediatrics, 146*(5), e2020029074.

Petry, N. M., Peirce, J. M., Stitzer, M. L., Blaine, J., Roll, J. M., Cohen, A., Obert, J., Killeen, T., Saladin, M. E., Cowell, M., Kirby, K. C., Sterling, R., Royer-Malvestuto, C., Hamilton, J., Booth, R. E., Marilyn, M., Liebert, M., Rader, L., Burns, R., . . . Li, R. (2005). Effect of prize-based incentives on outcomes in stimulant abusers in outpatient psychosocial treatment programs: A National Drug Abuse Treatment Clinical Trials Network study. *Archives of General Psychiatry, 62*(10), 1148–1156.

Plessinger, M. A., & Woods, J. R. (1993). Maternal, placental, and fetal pathophysiology of cocaine exposure during pregnancy. *Clinical Obstetrics and Gynecology, 36*(2), 267.

Powell, J. A. (2008). Structural racism: Building upon the insights of John Calmore. *North Carolina Law Review, 86*, 791–816.

Primo, C. C., Ruela, P. B., Brotto, L. D., Garcia, T. R., & Lima, E. (2013). Effects of maternal nicotine on breastfeeding infants. *Revista Paulista de Pediatria: Orgao Oficial da Sociedade de Pediatria de Sao Paulo, 31*(3), 392–397.

Rad, J., Tesfalul, M., Leza, M., & Flood, P. (2020). *Encourage breastfeeding for women with opioid use disorder.* CMQCC mother and baby substance use exposure toolkit. https://nastoolkit.org/explore-the-toolkit/best-practice/9#authors

Reece-Stremtan, S., & Marinelli, K. A. (2015). AMB clinical protocol #21: Guidelines for breastfeeding and substance use or substance use disorder, revised 2015. *Breastfeeding Medicine, 10*(3), 135–141.

Richardson, J. L., Stephens, S., Yates, L. M., Diav-Citrin, O., Arnon, J., Beghin, D., Kayser, A., Kennedy, D., Cupitt, D., Te Winkel, B., Peltonen, M., Kaplan, Y. C., & Thomas, S. H. (2017). Pregnancy outcomes after maternal varenicline use; analysis of surveillance data collected by the European network of teratology information services. *Reproductive Toxicology, 67*, 26–34.

Rigotti, N. A. (2021). Pharmacotherapy for smoking cessation in adults. *UpToDate.* https://www.uptodate.com/contents/pharmacotherapy-for-smoking-cessation-in-adults?search=nicotine%20replacement%20therapy&source=search_result&selectedTitle=2~149&usage_type=default&display_rank=1#H13311131

Riley, E. P., Infante, M. A., & Warren, K. R. (2011). Fetal alcohol spectrum disorders: An overview. *Neuropsychology Review, 21*(2), 73–80.

Ritchie, A. (2017). Policing paradigms and criminalizing webs. In *Invisible No More: Police Violence against Black Women and Women of Color* (pp. 61–87). Beacon Press.

Roberts, D. (1997). *Killing the black body: Race, reproduction, and the meaning of liberty.* Vintage Books.

Roberts, D. & Sangoi, L. (2018). *Black families matter: How the child welfare system punishes poor families of color.* The appeal. https://theappeal.org/black-families-matter-how-the-child-welfare-system-punishes-poor-families-of-color-33ad20e2882e

Roberts, S. C., & Nuru-Jeter, A. (2010). Universal alcohol/drug screening in prenatal care: A strategy for reducing racial disparities? Questioning the assumptions. *Maternal Child Health Journal, 15*, 1127–1134.

Roberts, S. C., & Nuru-Jeter, A. (2012). Universal screening for alcohol and drug use and racial disparities in child protective services reporting. *Journal of Behavioral Health Services Research, 39*(1), 1199–1216.

Roberts, S. C. M., & Pies, C. (2011). Complex calculations: How drug use during pregnancy becomes a barrier to prenatal care. *Journal of Maternal Child Health, 15*, 333–341.

Roberts, S. C. M., Zahnd, E., Sufrin, C., & Armstrong, M. A. (2015). Does adopting a prenatal substance use protocol reduce racial disparities in CPS reporting related to maternal drug use? A California case study. *Journal of Perinatology, 35*, 146–150.

Robinson, S. M., & Adinoff, B. (2016). The classification of substance use disorders: Historical, contextual, and conceptual considerations. *Behavioral Sciences, 6*(3), 18.

Rodriguez, D. (2022a). Cigarette and tobacco products in pregnancy: Impact on pregnancy in the neonate. *UpToDate.* https://www.upto date.com/contents/cigarette-and-tobacco-products-in-pregnancy-impact-on-pregnancy-and-the-neonate

Rodriguez, D. (2022b). Tobacco and nicotine use in pregnancy: Cessation strategies and treatment options. *UpToDate.* https://www.uptodate.com/contents/tobacco-and-nicotine-use-in-pregnancy-cessation-strategies-and-treatment-options?search=treatment%20for%20tobacco%20use&topicRef=16634&source=see_link#H3292840660

Roll, J. M., Petry, N. M., Stitzer, M. L., Brecht, M. L., Peirce, J. M., McCann, M. J., Blaine, J., MacDonald, M., DiMaria, J., Lucero, L., & Kellogg, S. (2006). Contingency management for the treatment of methamphetamine use disorders. *The American Journal of Psychiatry, 163*(11), 1993–1999.

Ross, L. (2006). *Understanding reproductive justice.* SisterSong Women of Color Reproductive Justice Collective. https://d3n8a8pro7vhmx.cloudfront.net/rrfp/pages/33/attachments/original/1456425809/Understanding_RJ_Sistersong.pdf?1456425809

Ross, L. (2017). Reproductive justice as intersectional feminist activism. *Souls, 19*(3), 286–314.

Ross, L., & Solinger, R. (2017). *Reproductive justice: An introduction.* University of California Press.

Sachs, H. C., Committee on Drugs, Frattarelli, D. A. C., Galinkin, J. L., Green, T. P., Johnson, T., Neville, K., Paul, I. M., & Van den Anker, J. (2013). The transfer of drugs and therapeutics into human breast milk: An update on selected topics. *Pediatrics, 132*(3), e796–e809.

Saia, K. A., et al. (2016). Caring for pregnant women with opioid use disorder in the USA: Expanding and improving treatment. *Current Obstetrics and Gynecology Reports, 5*(3), 257–263.

Schiff, D. M., Nielsen, T., Terplan, M., Hood, M., Bernson, D., Diop, H., Bharel, M., Wilens, T. E., LaRochelle, M., Walley, A. Y., & Land, T. (2018). Fatal and nonfatal overdose among pregnant and postpartum women in Massachusetts. *Obstetrics and Gynecology, 132*(2), 466–474.

Schmitz, J., Kral, A., Chu, D., Wenger, L., & Bluthenthal, R. (2016). Food insecurity among people who inject drugs in Los Angeles and San Francisco. *Public Health Nutrition, 19*(12), 2204–2212.

Schneider, R., Burnette, M. L., Ilgen, M. A., & Timko, C. (2009). Prevalence and correlates of intimate partner violence victimization among men and women entering substance use disorder treatment. *Violence and Victims, 24*(6), 744–756.

Schürer, S., Klingel, K., Sandri, M., Majunke, N., Besler, C., Kandolf, R., Lurz, P., Luck, M., Hertel, P., Schuler, G., Linke, A., & Mangner, N. (2017). Clinical characteristics, histopathological features, and clinical outcome of methamphetamine-associated cardiomyopathy. *JACC Heart Failure, 5*(6), 435.

Senturias, Y. S., Weitzman, C. C., & Amgott, R. (2019). Fetal alcohol spectrum disorders. In M. Augustyn & B. Zuckerman (Eds.), *Zuckerman Parker handbook of developmental and behavioral pediatrics for primary care* (4th ed., pp. 539–553). Wolters Kluwer.

Sharapova, S. R., Phillips, E., Sirocco, K., Kaminski, J. W., Leeb, R. T., & Rolle, I. (2018). Effects of prenatal marijuana exposure on neuropsychological outcomes in children aged 1–11 years: A systematic review. *Paediatric & Perinatal Epidemiology., 32*(6), 512–532.

Shyken, J., Babbar, S., Babbar, S., & Forinash, A. (2019). Benzodiazepines in pregnancy. *Clinical Obstetrics and Gynecology, 62*(1), 156–167.

Siegel, M., Mahowald, G., Uljon, S., James, K., Leffert, L., Sullivan, M., Hernandez, S., Gray, J., Schiff, D., & Bernstein, S. (2022). Fentanyl in the labor epidural impacts the results of intrapartum and postpartum maternal and neonatal toxicology tests. *American Journal of Obstetrics and Gynecology, S0002-9378*(22), 02185–02188.

Smith, M. V., Costello, D., & Yonkers, K. A. (2015). Clinical correlates of prescription opioid analgesic use in pregnancy. *Maternal Child Health Journal, 19*(3), 548–556.

Sohrab, A., & Seyed, S. (2021). Smoking and smoking relapse in postpartum: A systematic review and meta-analysis. *Addictive Disorders and Their Treatment, 20*(4), 486–499.

Stockton-Joreteg, C. & Griffin, C. (2020). *Use validated verbal screening and assessment tools to evaluate all pregnant women for substance use disorders* CMQCC Mother & Baby Substance Exposure Toolkit Best Practice No. 1. https://nas-toolkit-prod.s3.amazonaws.com/pdfs/best_practice_1_2020-09-04.pdf

Stone, A. M. (2015). Pregnant women and substance use: Fear, stigma, and barriers to care. *Health and Justice, 3*(2), 1–15.

Strathearn, L., Mamun, A. A., Najman, J. M., & O'Callaghan, M. J. (2009). Does breastfeeding protect against substantiated child abuse and neglect? A 15-year cohort study. *Pediatrics, 123*(2), 483–493.

Suarez, E. A., Huybrechts, K. F., Straub, L., Hernández-Díaz, S., Jones, H. E., Connery, H. S., Davis, J. M., Gray, K. J., Lester, B., Terplan, M., Mogun, H., & Bateman, B. T. (2022). Buprenorphine versus methadone for opioid use disorder in pregnancy. *The New England Journal of Medicine, 387*(22), 2033–2044.

Substance Abuse and Mental Health Services Administration (SAMHSA). (2011). *Screening brief intervention and referral to treatment (SBIRT) in behavioral care.* https://www.samhsa.gov/sites/default/files/sbirtwhitepaper_0.pdf

Substance Abuse and Mental Health Services Administration (SAMHSA). (2014). *Results from the 2013 National Survey on Drug Use and Health: Summary of national findings, NSDUH Series H-48, HHS Publication No. (SMA) 14-4863.* https://www.samhsa.gov/data/sites/default/files/NSDUHresultsPDFWHTML2013/Web/NSDUHresults2013.pdf

Substance Abuse and Mental Health Services Administration (SAMHSA). (2016). *Results from the 2015 National Survey on Drug Use and Health: Detailed tables.* https://www.samhsa.gov/data/sites/default/files/NSDUH-DetTabs-2015/NSDUH-DetTabs-2015/NSDUH-DetTabs-2015.pdf

Substance Abuse and Mental Health Services Administration (SAMHSA). (2019). *Key substance use and mental health indicators in the United States: Results from the 2018 National Survey on Drug Use and Health (NSDUH) (HHS Publication No. PEP19-5068, NSDUH Series H-54).* Center for Behavioral Health Statistics and Quality, Substance Abuse and Mental Health Services Administration. https://www.samhsa.gov/data/sites/default/files/cbhsq-reports/NSDUHNationalFindingsReport2018/NSDUHNationalFindingsReport2018.pdf

Substance Abuse and Mental Health Services Administration (SAMHSA). (2022). *Screening brief intervention and referral to treatment (SBIRT).* https://www.samhsa.gov/sbirt

Substance Abuse and Mental Health Services Administration (SAMHSA), Center for Behavioral Health Statistics and Quality. (May 12, 2011). *Trends in emergency department visits for drug-related suicide attempts among females: 2005 and 2009.* Rockville, MD.

Sweeney, P. J., Schwartz, R. M., Mattis, N. G., & Vohr, B. (2000). The effect of integrating substance abuse treatment with prenatal care on birth outcome. *Journal of Perinatology, 20*(4), 219.

Taylor, L., Claire, R., Campbell, K., Coleman-Haynes, T., Leonardi-Bee, J., Chamberlain, C., Berlin, I., Davey, M. A., Cooper, S., & Coleman, T. (2021). Fetal safety of nicotine replacement therapy in pregnancy: Systematic review and meta-analysis. *Addiction, 116*(2), 239.

Terplan, M., Laird, H. J., Hand, D. J., Wright, T. E., Premkumar, A., Martin, C. E., Meyer, M. C., Jones, H. E., & Krans, E. E. (2018). Opioid detoxification during pregnancy: A systematic review. *Obstetrics and Gynecology, 131*(5), 803–814.

Terplan, M., Longinaker, N., & Appel, L. (2015). Women-centered drug treatment services and need in the United States, 2002–2009. *American Journal of Public Health, 105*, e50–e54.

Thompson, H. (2019). *Drug use and human milk: Child welfare considerations.* The elephant circle. https://static1.squarespace.com/static/57126eff60b5e92c3a226a53/t/5cd9e8819140b7ba382598a4/1557784705180/Substances+and+Lactation+fact+sheet.pdf

Tompkins, D. A., & Campbell, C. M. (2011). Opioid-induced hyper-algesia: Cinically relevant or extraneous research phenomenon? *Current Pain and Headache Reports, 15*(2), 129–136.

Toquinto, S. M., Berglas, N. F., McLemore, M. R., Delgado, A., & Roberts, S. C. M. (2020). Pregnant women's acceptability of alcohol, tobacco, and drug use screening and willingness to disclose use in prenatal care. *Women's Health Issues, 30*(5), 345–352. https://doi.org/10.1016/j.whi.2020.05.004

Torres, C., Medina-Kirchner, C., O'Malley, K. Y., & Hart, C. L. (2020). Totality of the evidence suggests prenatal cannabis exposure does not lead to cognitive impairments: A systematic and critical review. *Frontiers in Psychology, 11*(816), 1–28. https://www.frontiersin.org/articles/10.3389/fpsyg.2020.00816/full#:~:text=Conclusions%3A%20The%20current%20evidence%20does,clinically%20significant%20cognitive%20functioning%20impairments

Tucker Edmonds, B., Mckenzie, F., Austgen, M. B., Carroll, A. E., & Meslin, E. M. (2017). Women's opinions of legal requirements for drug testing in prenatal care. *The Journal of Maternal-Fetal & Neonatal Medicine, 30*(14), 1693–1698.

Turner, E., Jones, M., Vaz, L. R., & Coleman, T. (2019). Systematic review and meta-analysis to assess the safety of bupropion and varenicline in pregnancy. *Nicotine & Tobacco Research, 21*(8), 1001.

United States Office on Women's Health. (2017). *Final report: Opioid use, misuse, and overdose among women.* US Department of Health and Human Services. https://owh-wh-d9-dev.s3.amazonaws.com/s3fs-public/documents/final-report-opioid-508.pdf

United States Preventative Services Task Force (USPSTF). (2018). *Unhealthy alcohol use in adolescents and adults: Screening and behavioral counseling interventions.* https://www.uspreventiveservicestaskforce.org/uspstf/recommendation/unhealthy-alcohol-use-in-adolescents-and-adults-screening-and-behavioral-counseling-interventions

United States Preventative Services Task Force (USPSTF). (2021). *Tobacco smoking cessation in adults, including pregnant women: Behavioral and pharmacotherapy interventions.* https://www.uspreventiveservicestaskforce.org/uspstf/recommendation/tobacco-use-in-adults-and-pregnant-women-counseling-and-interventions

Vagins, D., & McCurdy, J. (2006). *Cracks in the system: Twenty years of unjust federal crack cocaine law.* American Civil Liberties Union (ACLU). https://www.aclu.org/other/cracks-system-twenty-years-unjust-federal-crack-cocaine-law?redirect=criminal-law-reform/cracks-system-twenty-years-unjust-federal-crack-cocaine-law

Varner, M. W., Silver, R. M., Hogue, C. J. R., Willinger, M., Parker, C. B., Thorsten, V. R., Goldenberg, R. L., Saade, G. R., Dudley, D. J., Coustan, D., Stroll, B., Bukowski, R., Koch, M. A., Conway, D., Pinar, H., Reddy, U. M., & Kennedy Shriver, U. (2014). Association between stillbirth and illicit drug use and smoking during pregnancy. *Obstetrics & Gynecology, 123*(1), 113.

Velez, M. L., Montoya, I. D., Jansson, L. M., Walters, V., Svikis, D., Jones, H. E., & Campbell, J. (2006). Exposure to violence among substance-dependent pregnant women and their children. *Journal of Substance Abuse Treatment, 30*, 31–38.

Volkow, N. D., Compton, W. M., & Wargo, E. M. (2017). The risks of marijuana use during pregnancy. *JAMA, 317*(2), 129–130.

Votaw, V. R., Geyer, R., Rieselbach, M. M., & McHaugh, R. K. (2019). The epidemiology of benzodiazepine misuse: A systematic review. *Drug and Alcohol Dependence, 200*, 95–114.

Walker, I. (2017). *High: Drugs, desires, and a nation of users.* University of Washington Press.

Wang, X., Zhang, T., Ekheden, I., Chang, Z., Hellner, C., Hasselström, J., Jayaram-Lindström, N., D'Onofrio, B., Larsson, H., Mataix-Cols, D., & Sidorchuk, A. (2022). Prenatal exposure to benzodiazepines and Z-drugs in humans and risk of adverse neurodevelopmental outcomes in offspring: A systemic review. *Neuroscience & Biobehavioral Reviews, 137*, 1–16.

Warshak, C. R., Regan, J., Moore, B., Magner, K., Kritzer, S., & Van Hook, J. (2015). Association between marijuana use and adverse obstetrical and neonatal outcomes. *Journal of Perinatology, 35*(12), 991–995.

Wehby, G. L., Prater, K., McCarthy, A. M., Castilla, E. E., & Murray, J. C. (2011). The impact of maternal smoking during pregnancy on early child neurodevelopment. *Journal of Human Capital, 5*(2), 207–254.

White, A. R., Rampes, H., Liu, J. P., Stead, L. F., & Campbell, J. (2014). Acupuncture and related interventions for smoking cessation. *The Cochrane Database of Systematic Reviews, 1*, CD000009.

Wikner, B. N., Stiller, C. O., Bergman, U., Asker, C., & Källén, B. (2007). Use of benzodiazepines and benzodiazepine receptor agonists during pregnancy: Neonatal outcome and congenital malformations. *Pharmacoepidemiology and Drug Safety, 16*(11), 1203.

Wilson, T., Pitcher, I., & Bach, P. (2022). Avoidance of beta-blockers in patients who use stimulants is not supported by good evidence. *CMAJ. Canadian Medical Association Journal, 194*(4), E127–E128.

Winecker, R. E., Goldberger, B. A., Tebbett, I. R., Behnke, M., Eyler, F. D., Karlix, J. L., Wobie, K., Conlon, M., Phillips, D., & Bertholf, R. L. (2001). Detection of cocaine and its metabolites in breast milk. *Journal of Forensic Sciences, 46*(5), 1221–1223.

Wolff, K. (2011). Panic in the ER: Maternal drug use, the right to bodily integrity, privacy, and informed consent. *Politics and Policy, 39*(5), 679–714.

Woodruff, K., Scott, K., & Roberts, S. C. M. (2021). Pregnant people's experiences discussing cannabis use with prenatal care providers in a state with legalized cannabis. *Drug and Alcohol Dependence, 227*, 108998.

World Health Organization [WHO]. (2014). *Guidelines for the identification and management of substance use and substance use disorders in pregnancy.* World Health Organization. https://apps.who.int/iris/bitstream/handle/10665/107130/9789241548731_eng.pdf

Wright, T., Terplan, M., Ondersma, S., Boyce, C., Yonkers, K., Chang, M. D. G., & Creanga, A. (2016). The role of screening, brief intervention, and referral to treatment in the perinatal period. *American Journal of Obstetrics & Gynecology, 215*(5), 539–547.

Wright, T. E., Schuetter, R., Fombonne, E., Stephenson, J., & Haning, W. F. (2012). Implementation and evaluation of a harm-reduction model for clinical care of substance using pregnant women. *Harm Reduction Journal, 9*, 5.

Wright, T. E., Schuetter, R., Tellei, J., & Sauvage, L. (2015). Methamphetamines and pregnancy outcomes. *Journal of Addiction Medicine, 9*(2), 111–117.

Xuan, Z., Zhongpeng, Y., Yanjun, G., Jiaqi, D., Yuchi, Z., Bing, S., & Chenghao, L. (2016). Maternal active smoking and risk of oral clefts: A meta-analysis. *Oral Surgery, Oral Medicine, Oral Pathology and Oral Radiology, 122*(6), 680–690.

Young-Wolff, K. C., Ray, G. T., Alexeeff, S. E., Adams, S. R., Does, M. B., Ansley, D., & Avalos, L. A. (2021). Rates of prenatal cannabis use among pregnant women before and during the COVID-19 pandemic. *JAMA, 326*(17), 1745–1747.

Young-Wolff, K. C., Sarovar, V., Tucker, L. Y., Avalos, L. A., Alexeeff, S., Conway, A., et al. (2019). Trends in marijuana use among pregnant women with and without nausea and vomiting in pregnancy, 2009–2016. *Drug & Alcohol Dependence., 196*, 66–70.

Zedler, B. K., Mann, A. L., Kim, M. M., Amick, H. R., Joyce, A. R., Murrelle, E. L., & Jones, H. E. (2016). Buprenorphine compared with methadone to treat pregnant women with opioid use disorder: A systematic review and meta-analysis of safety in the mother, fetus and child. *Addiction, 111*(12), 2115–2128.

Zhang, K., & Wang, X. (2013). Maternal smoking and increased risk of sudden infant death syndrome: A meta-analysis. *Legal Medicine, 15*(3), 115–121.

Zuspan, F. P., Gumpel, J. A., Mejia-Zelaya, A., Madden, J., & Davis, R. (1975). Fetal stress from methadone withdrawal. *American Journal of Obstetrics and Gynecology, 122*(1), 43–46.

Zwink, N., & Ekkehart, J. (2018). Maternal drug use and the risk of anorectal malformations: Systematic review and meta-analysis. *Orphanet Journal of Rare Diseases, 13*(75), 1–23.

19

Culture and Community

Cindy L. Farley and Raven Fulton

The editors gratefully acknowledge Cindy L. Farley and Michal Wright, who were co-authors of the previous version of this chapter called Diversity and Inclusion.

Relevant Terms

Community—a social group whose members share a common government, geographic location, culture, heritage, or interest

Culture—the learned and shared knowledge that specific groups use to generate their behavior and interpret their experience of the world

Cultural appreciation—the earnest seeking of knowledge about a cultural group to explore and honor their beliefs and practices

Cultural appropriation—the inappropriate or unacknowledged adoption of cultural customs and practice by those outside that cultural group; typically done by majority groups in a disrespectful or exploitative manner

Cultural competence—a set of congruent behaviors, attitudes, and policies that come together in a system, agency, or among professionals and enable that system, agency, or those professionals to work effectively in cross-cultural situations

Cultural humility—openness to what others have determined is their personal expression of their heritage and culture, laying aside one's own ethnocentric beliefs

Cultural sensitivity—awareness that cultural differences and similarities between people exist without assigning them a value—positive or negative, better or worse, right or wrong

Emic—viewpoint of a member of a social group on that group

Etic—viewpoint of someone outside a social group on that group

Ethnicity—a population group whose members identify with each other on the basis of common nationality or shared cultural traditions

Ethnocentrism—the belief that one's own group or culture is better or more important than others

Generalization—reasoning from detailed facts to general principles for broad groups of people or things; must keep in mind that all members of a group may not adhere to the generalization made

Prelacteal feeds—food other than breast milk provided to the newborn prior to initiation of breastfeeding

Stereotype—oversimplified attitudes people hold toward those outside one's own experience who are different, typically a result of incomplete or distorted information accepted as fact without question

---

Introduction

"The greatness of a community is most accurately measured by the compassionate actions of its members."
—Coretta Scott King

The **culture** in which we are born and raised provides the lens through which we first learn to interpret the world. We are shaped by genetics and biology and by relationships and experiences. The nature versus nurture debate regarding the importance of each to human development is an enduring discussion. This chapter considers culture and community and their influence on how childbirth is viewed and what behaviors are enacted by pregnant individuals and their families. Healthcare as a culture is discussed and you are asked to reflect on your role within this culture and how that shapes the childbirth experience of the people you serve.

It is vital to remember that individuals have personal, social, and cultural identities. Personal and social identities evolve over time. These identities are an outgrowth of the questions "Who am I?" and "How do others see me?" Cultural identities tend to be more enduring, although culture is not static. A person may belong to a primary cultural group, but also belong to various subcultures with values and behaviors that may not be congruent (Scheepers & Ellemers, 2019). For example, an individual employed in

Prenatal and Postnatal Care: A Person-Centered Approach, Third Edition. Edited by Karen Trister Grace, Cindy L. Farley, Noelene K. Jeffers, and Tanya Tringali.
© 2024 John Wiley & Sons Ltd. Published 2024 by John Wiley & Sons Ltd.
Companion website: www.wiley.com/go/grace/prenatal

the technology sector may desire a technology-free birth experience. A person's childbirth preferences and behaviors cannot be assumed from their sociocultural circumstances. Luckily, there is an easy solution—simply ask. Ask in a straightforward and accepting manner.

Childbirth is an important event in an individual's life, but it is also important to a **community**. For a community to enrich the lives of its members, there needs to be a shared sense of trust, connection, and caring for one another. A sense of community connection was challenged in the lockdowns initiated during the early days of the global COVID-19 pandemic. For example, loneliness was identified as an influence on people's health during this time (McQuaid et al., 2021). The risk of loneliness rises during transitional periods in life, such as in pregnancy and parenthood. This perceived lack of a social community is implicated in many negative health outcomes, such as higher levels of stress and inflammation and an increase in mental health disorders and chronic diseases. It is critical to connect parents and newborns to their community in order to optimize perinatal health.

Rituals are a way of providing social acknowledgment of important life events and fostering a connection to the community. Ceremonies and traditions to recognize the pregnancy and honor the birth are done to welcome the newborn and support the growing family (Cheyney & Davis-Floyd, 2021). Such traditions give the new family a sense of belonging and offer both tangible and emotional assistance during this time of adjustment. Knowledge of cultural practices is handed down through generations and strengthens communities.

Health equity key points

- The structural roots of the current system of care for childbearing people are heavily influenced by White, patriarchal, and medical cultures and offer little room to incorporate culturally valued traditions into pregnancy and birth experience.
- Building a diverse perinatal workforce will help provide culturally concordant care, particularly important in the development of trust for individuals from marginalized groups.

A grassroots revival of traditional birth work is taking place as the recognition of ancestral healing and caring methods grows (Farrell, 2022). For example, Canada's evacuation policy of moving geographically remote Indigenous childbearing people to cities for hospital birth in their last month of pregnancy has been deemed harmful and exposes individuals to bias, racism, and trauma (National Council of Aboriginal Midwives [NACM], 2019). It places people in situations where they lack resources and skills to navigate day-to-day living at a very vulnerable time with no support from their community of origin. This policy is being challenged and changed by Indigenous and professional organizations in Canada.

Culture and community are becoming recognized at a systems level as being essential to human flourishing and optimal health.

Healthcare System Culture

The healthcare system itself is a culture constructed from beliefs about the nature of disease and the human body. Cultural issues are central to the structure and delivery of health services, treatment, and preventive interventions. The ways in which people experience pregnancy and birth have been substantively changed by the biomedical model applied to childbirth. This was enabled by the movement of birth from the home into the hospital, when, in the early twentieth century, birth practices came under the control of White male physicians. The social model of childbirth that was practiced through a gathering of women who were considered healers and midwives in the culture was denigrated. As science advanced, these healers and midwives were excluded from new knowledge and practices, and attempts were made to eradicate midwives or control their practice through restrictive legislation and regulation (Dawley, 2000).

The dominant biomedical culture of healthcare faces a paradox of trying to technologically control pregnancy and birth, which are fundamentally physiologic processes that are resistant to such control (Liese et al., 2021). In order to justify this control, the label of "high risk" is applied to many prenatal conditions and internalized by pregnant and birthing people to conceptualize the pregnant body as defective and in need of tests and medical procedures to assure a safe outcome. Legal and financial incentives contribute to providers' needs to orchestrate the pregnancy and birth processes to minimize litigation risk and maximize economic return. Thus, this culture becomes self-reinforcing and blind to its own shortcomings, leading to **ethnocentrism**.

However, there are those birthing people and providers who see birth through a different cultural lens (Cheyney & Davis-Floyd, 2021; Davis-Floyd, 1990). They view the pregnant body as uniquely powerful and healthy in its own right and the birth process as a physiologic function of this power. The care required is that of support rather than control. Procedures to control this process are seen as dehumanizing, disempowering, and inherently risky. These dichotomous cultural views of childbearing promote different care strategies.

Prenatal healthcare providers need to examine their own background and biases to appreciate and support the many cultures that the people they serve bring to care encounters. Providers have a role to play in the equitable provision of services. At a systems level, barriers to culturally appropriate care can be identified and action plans created to rectify noted disparities for childbearing persons and their families. At the individual level, respectful education and options are given according to stated needs and preferences, making space for cultural rituals and traditions as desired. Additionally, healthcare providers can share their enthusiasm for the care of childbearing families and recruit people from marginalized communities to consider entering the health professions as a career path. Clinicians can invite individuals from underrepresented groups to shadow for a day as the authentic experience of observing care providers interact with clients may encourage a career path in perinatal healthcare. Support for organizations that create pathways to health professional education for people from marginalized communities is also essential (see *Resources for Healthcare Providers*). Building a diverse workforce will provide greater access to culturally concordant care, particularly important in the development of trust for individuals from marginalized groups. Keeping current with the latest theories, research, and best practices to reduce health disparities is essential for all healthcare providers.

The dominant culture in the United States is a White, Eurocentric, patriarchal system; this is reflected in the healthcare culture (Liese et al., 2021). This dominant culture is blind to its own inequities, believing its practices are best. Indeed, many White people do not consider White as a culture (DeLibertis, 2015; Drew & Reis, 2020). However, some normative features of White culture correspond to the medical model of care prevalent in the care of childbearing people, such as paternalism, and time as a commodity (Jones & Okun, 2000). The majority of healthcare providers in prenatal and birth care are White (American College of Nurse-Midwives [ACNM], 2019; López et al., 2021), conferring privileges of the dominant group that are invisible and, therefore, unexamined (McIntosh, 1989).

A consequence of the dominant healthcare system is the perpetuation of inequities in health outcomes. This can happen through explicit and implicit **bias** and ethnocentrism. For example, as pregnancy and birth care has become increasingly medicalized, there is homogenization of care practices with little to no room for incorporation of meaningful traditions that help childbearing people connect to their own cultural community. When faced with truths about racial inequities perpetuated by systems perceived as normative, some White people will become defensive and engage in denial, rationalization, and anger, known as White fragility (Okun, 2013). Dismantling the legacy of systemic and institutional racism takes individual and collective work; it is not easy, and it will take ongoing effort.

Generalizations versus Stereotyping

No two people experience or express their culture in the same way. It is vital to remember that while the concept of culture refers to specific groups about which broad **generalizations** can be made, healthcare is provided to individuals who may not ascribe to all the beliefs and behaviors of their cultural reference group. It is vitally important not to **stereotype** an individual based on assumptions about their age, gender, sexuality, religion, race, **ethnicity**, geographic origin, or other categorization. Individuals are part of multiple and intersecting sociocultural groups; some of these groups can support opposing beliefs. Healthcare decisions by the individual can vary from the

norms of an affiliation group. A key ingredient in **cultural competence** is meaningful dialogue with the person presenting for care—respectful questioning and active listening with **cultural sensitivity** and **cultural humility**. One way to ask about this would be, "Are there any traditions important to you to include in your care or at your birth?" The understanding generated through this discussion is then translated into a culturally inclusive plan of care. *Ask and listen* are simple tenets to apply in the care of people from any culture.

4C Questions to elicit cultural beliefs

- What do you **C**all your condition?
- What do you think **C**aused your problem?
- How do you **C**ope with your condition?
- What **C**oncerns do you have regarding your condition?

Source: Galanti (2015) / University of Pennsylvania Press.

Developing Cultural Competence, Sensitivity, and Humility

Values, attitudes, and beliefs are rooted in the culture of the society and the subgroups to which individuals belong. Culture comprises beliefs about reality, how people should interact with each other, what they know about the world, and how they should respond to the social and material environments in which they find themselves. It is reflected in their religions, morals, customs, technologies, and survival strategies. It affects how they work, parent, love, marry, and understand health, mental health, wellness, illness, disability, and death (Table 19.1). Childbearing

Table 19.1   Selected Health Belief Models

Magico-religious	These beliefs arise from conditions that appear unpredictable and uncontrollable as people try to manage fear and make sense of these conditions by ascribing causality to supernatural forces or the action of God. Illness is viewed as a punishment for transgression. Human action may or may not return an individual to a healthy state. Healing is aimed at acceptance of God's will or through supplication of supernatural forces.
Holistic	Health is viewed as a positive state of well-being attained by harmony of physical and metaphysical elements within the individual. Illness is viewed as a state of imbalance in natural forces. Healing is aimed at restoring balance.
Biomedical	The body is a machine controlled by anatomic and biochemical processes. Health is reflected in the proper functioning of these elements, while illness is a state of malfunction of these structures and processes. Healing is aimed at restoring function of the body through surgery or medication.

Source: Galanti (2015)/University of Pennsylvania Press.

Table 19.2 Key Attributes of Cultural Humility

Openness	Receptive to engaging in cross-cultural interactions, and to new ideas
Self-awareness	Mindful of one's own strengths, challenges, values, beliefs, and behavior
Egoless	Displays humbleness and modesty and believes that all people are equal
Supportive interaction	Engages in social relations with others that result in positive dialogues
Self-reflection and critique	Considers aspects of self through ongoing deep introspection

Source: Foronda et al. (2016)/With permission of SAGE Publication.

individuals bring values and attitudes about healthcare, pregnancy, birth, and infant care that come from different traditions and life experiences.

Healthcare providers bring their own unique backgrounds to care encounters. Their values and beliefs about health are shaped by their education and socialization into their profession and are affected by the cultures of mainstream and alternative healthcare groups. Developing **cultural competence** is a professional responsibility that requires engagement in cultural knowledge and experience, as well as self-assessment of one's own biases. However, the term cultural competence implies an end point of cultural knowledge and skills, which is not possible to achieve. This has led to the term cultural humility being favored. Cultural humility implies an attitude of openness and lifelong learning with the intent to rectify the power imbalances in the patient-provider relationship (Foronda et al., 2016). See Table 19.2 and selected self-assessment tools designed to assist in reflecting on one's own cultural journey in the *Resources for Healthcare Providers* at the end of this chapter.

Communication

According to the US Census Bureau (2015), there are at least 350 languages spoken in homes in the United States. Encountering cultural differences and language barriers does not require travel to a different country; it happens in local practices serving diverse populations. Millions of US citizens are bilingual. It is projected that the United States will become the country with the largest Spanish speaking population in the world within the next few years (Anderson, 2022). Misunderstandings can arise due to different meanings ascribed to same word spellings. Consider what the common written prescription advice "Take once daily" might mean to an individual who speaks Spanish (once = 11 times) compared to English (once = 1 time) and the potential for harm if not clearly understood. Individuals from some cultures may not be comfortable or familiar with anatomic language often used by clinicians and may use different words to describe their physical concerns.

Voice recognition and translator apps are inexpensive, portable, and very useful in many situations. Over 70 language translation apps are currently available for use with smartphones. Other tools include phone-in translation services and person-to-person interpreter services. Some healthcare providers learn a second language to better serve selected populations under their care. Looking at the person rather than the translator when conversing via an intermediary will help to engage that person directly in the conversation. Use of relatives as interpreters and clinic staff who are not certified medical interpreters is discouraged. The method of communication with patients with limited English should be documented in the medical record (e.g., "interviewed in Spanish" or "used German translator #1234").

Nonverbal behavior is culturally influenced and can be misinterpreted by those outside the culture. Healthcare providers should have an awareness of cultural differences in communication patterns. For example, people from some cultures are less verbally expressive and will not question healthcare providers. And because no questions are raised, the healthcare provider may assume that the message was received correctly. Asking the individual to explain or rephrase the message back to the provider is one way to evaluate comprehension.

Cultural Appreciation versus Appropriation

Cultural appreciation is needed by healthcare providers in order to make space for personally meaningful traditions in the care of childbearing individuals. Learning about other cultures to broaden one's perspective and learn how to interact respectfully is the mark of a positive global citizen. However, the use of one culture's symbols, artifacts, rituals, or tools by another culture is considered **cultural appropriation.** It often occurs without permission, acknowledgment, or payment, especially when the person using the cultural practice is in a higher position of power and privilege. Culture is not stagnant; it changes over time and as cultural groups intermingle. There can be debate about whether an adopted practice from another culture is appreciation or appropriation from both an **emic** and an **etic perspective**.

The Dine/Navajo Blessingway is an example of a tradition that has been adopted and altered in modern societies by those outside the Dine/Navajo culture (Burns, 2015). Individuals attempting to reject the commercialism of baby showers and "gender reveal" parties and interested in honoring the spiritual nature of childbirth are hosting ceremonies and calling them Blessingways. Rather than gifts and games, this ritual "blesses the way" for the pregnant individual and spiritually celebrates the impending birth and changes in the family. Is this appreciation or appropriation? Modern versions actually bear little resemblance to traditional Dine/Navajo ceremony which incorporates chants, songs and sand paintings and can continue over several days. The Navajo use the Blessingway in a number of different ceremonies to seek harmonious balance between the individual and the natural world (Burns, 2015). Out of respect for the historical significance and the sacred nature of the Blessingway to Dine/Navajo people, other terms, such as "Birth Blessing," can be used (Figure 19.1).

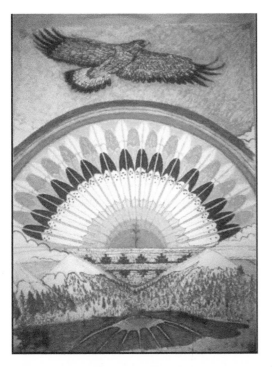

Figure 19.1 An image by Dine/Navajo Wayne representing the cosmic universe in the Dine/Navajo tradition used at some Dine/Navajo Blessingway ceremonies. Dine′ Navajo Wayne/Wikimedia Commons/CC BY-SA 4.0.

Food and Culture in Childbearing

Food is an important aspect of culture, as unique to a culture as its language. Traditional foods and cultural rituals at meals confer a sense of identity and belonging (Farley & Jacobwitz, 2019). Certain foods have been incorporated into cuisines over time and have become associated with an area or a cultural group. Specific foods have special meaning and are used to signify celebrations, transitional life events, and communal experiences. Family celebrations to welcome the newborn and support the childbearing person are common in many cultures. For example, in the Netherlands, a traditional food served announcing the sex or status of the newborn is called "biscuits with mice". It consists of rusks covered with candy-coated anise seeds (Atlas Obscura, 2022). Pink seeds are used to indicate female sex, blue seeds indicate male sex, and orange seeds indicate royalty.

Nutrition is an important area of discussion throughout pregnancy, postpartum, and lactation. Food provides the building blocks for nourishing the pregnant person and their fetus, supporting breastfeeding success, and optimizing newborn health. There are many cultural prescriptions and prohibitions regarding what foods people may or may not eat before, during, and after pregnancy. In some cultures, pregnancy is considered a "hot" state, and foods are prescribed to provide balance. "Hot" and "cold" classifications of food are based on intrinsic and functional qualities, may have no relationship to actual temperatures or spice levels, and vary among cultural groups. For example, vegetables, fruits, and foods high in water content are often considered cold. In contrast to the hot state of pregnancy, postpartum is seen as a cold state by many groups, and foods considered warm or hot are encouraged to correct imbalances. For example, in some communities in India, morning sickness is believed to be related to an excess of body heat from the pregnancy; "cold" foods, such as yogurt and most fruits and vegetables, may be recommended (Iradukunda, 2020). A hearty Colombian stew called Sancocho may be served during the cuarentena, a 40-day postpartum period where rest and warm, comforting foods promote healing and bonding (Waugh, 2011). Assessment and counseling around food choices may be more effective when taking into account individual preferences and cultural values.

Cultural Traditions in the Childbearing Year

A number of childbirth traditions are anchored in the history of the culture and may not be practiced today. However, some people may incorporate these traditions without informing the provider, out of fear of judgment, embarrassment, or a perceived lack of interest by the healthcare provider. Cultural practices should be welcomed into the plan of care to the extent that the person desires.

Pregnancy

The Western structure of contemporary prenatal care is widely adopted throughout the United States and is generally regarded as essential to positive outcomes. However, prenatal care has primarily evolved into a series of biomedical checkpoints through tests and information sharing, with little time left for the dialogue and relationship building valued by the individual and necessary for healthcare providers to understand and respond to their needs. According to a review of experiences with prenatal care, women of color had a number of suggestions for improving the current system of prenatal care to better respond to their needs (Altman et al., 2020; Shepherd et al., 2018). These suggestions include relationship-based continuity of care and racial concordance with healthcare staff (Kathawa et al., 2022). Other models of care are needed to better respond to cultural differences.

Pregnancy and birth are processes that were historically mysterious and poorly understood, leading to a number of protective practices based in magico-religious belief systems. The evil eye or other symbols of danger are appeased through avoidance behaviors, such as limited or no preparation for the baby and no compliments about the pregnancy or the baby. Positive protection is assured through prayer, wearing of amulets, and rituals designed to invoke spiritual guardians.

Pregnancy is deemed a state of health, as it often is, and medical care is not needed, according to some cultures. For example, people of the Amish culture typically have large families, and particularly after the first pregnancy, may not attend prenatal visits according to Western prenatal care schedules (Anderson & Potts, 2020). Many Amish prefer midwives, professionally or traditionally educated, for prenatal and birth care and often choose low intervention style births in the hospital setting or choose home or birth center settings.

Labor and Birth Care

Childbirth pain is a phenomenon toward which much thought and anticipation are invested on the part of the pregnant person and their care providers. Pain in other circumstances usually signals that something is going wrong, but in labor, pain is often a sign of progress. Pain in labor also has an end point—the much-anticipated arrival of the baby. Because pain is a physiologically mediated sensation that is interpreted cognitively, culture and individual characteristics play a role in how pain is perceived and what behaviors are expressed (Cheyney & Davis-Floyd, 2021). Studies have shown that fear of childbirth and perception of childbirth pain varies across cultures (Whitburn et al., 2019). The fear–tension–pain cycle is mediated by sociocultural expectations. Culture and individual characteristics also play a role in what measures are considered appropriate to use in childbirth, who should be at the birth, and which providers are sought (Cheyney & Davis-Floyd, 2021). Prenatal care providers need to work with those professionals and other attendants who will be present at birth to develop care plans that include and support cultural traditions.

Some rituals are enacted at or shortly after birth. For example, some Muslim families incorporate the Adhan prayer into their birth. This brief prayer is usually whispered by the father or a respected member of the local community into the newborn's ear and is intended to be the first sound the newborn hears (Gatrad & Sheikh, 2001). The individuals must be present at the birth to conduct this ceremony. Birth care providers can provide care quietly to respect this ritual; some individuals will prefer a few minutes of privacy to conduct this ceremony. It is a declaration of faith, an initiation into Islam, and an important ritual to many Muslim families.

Postpartum

Postpartum is viewed as a time of rest and recuperation by most cultures and generally extends for several weeks to months. Interestingly, the typical American 6-week postpartum visit is at 42 days, following a similar time frame of many postpartum cultural prescriptions and proscriptions, restrictions, and community aids to the new family. However, the US healthcare system is lacking in supportive services for postpartum individuals, making community support very important in the successful transition of the family. Additionally, the pressures of modern society can create difficulties in stepping away from jobs or typical responsibilities in the postpartum period. Rest can be limited and undervalued as postpartum people seek to return to preexisting routines. Postpartum care is largely neglected, underfinanced, and underused across many cultures and in both high- and low-income countries (Finlayson et al., 2020). Barriers to postpartum care are

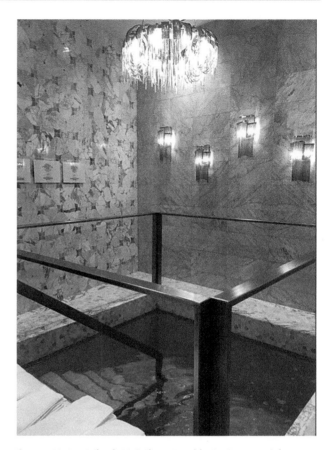

Figure 19.2 Mikvah Mei Chaya Mushka in Crown Heights, Brooklyn, USA. Mk17b / Wikimedia Commons / CC BY-SA 4.0.

linked to sociocultural and economic factors. Postpartum care needs to include the consideration of the adaptations the childbearing families make within the context of their own culture as they adapt their identities and relationships to their new circumstances.

In contrast to the *hot* state of pregnancy, postpartum is seen as a *cold* state by many groups, particularly in some Asian and Hispanic cultures (Wilson, 2012). In an illustrative example, a common practice in hospitals is to have a pitcher of ice water on the bedside table to encourage hydration. This goes against the belief of restoring balance to maintain health in the postpartum period. Understanding this can lead to simple solutions, such as offering tepid drinking water for those who hold to this tradition.

Postpartum people are deemed *unclean* in some cultures, often reflecting the timing of lochial flow. Cleansing rituals are believed to restore a state of purity and readiness to rejoin the community or resume sexual relations. For example, the practice in Orthodox Judaism called mikvah, a ritual bath with a source of naturally collected water, such as a river, stream, or lake water, after which contact with spouses can resume (Semenic et al., 2004; Figure 19.2). Contemporary postpartum education often includes advice regarding resumption of sexual intercourse and birth control measures. Cultural beliefs are influential in these practices and should be considered during these discussions.

Infant Care

Newborns are welcomed into their families and communities with a variety of celebrations and rituals at different time points, some occurring in the first minutes after birth and others occurring days, weeks, or months later. Some practices are thought to have a basis in historical conditions that led to high rates of infant death. For example, delayed naming traditions or prohibition of complimenting the child are thought to protect from evil spirits that would take the baby away. Under conditions of high infant mortality, these traditions can have a protective psychological distancing effect.

A number of traditions related to newborn care continue in some cultures that are either unsafe or of questionable health value. People from geographically disparate areas hold the belief that colostrum is weak or harmful to the neonate. Customs of avoiding colostrum are associated with higher rates of infant diarrheal diseases, a significant contributor to infant morbidity and mortality worldwide (Mose et al., 2021). **Prelacteal feeds** of various substances, such as date purée or honey-infused water, may be practiced. Honey is not recommended for infants under 12 months of age due to a rare but serious risk of botulism from spores that may be in the honey (Centers for Disease Control and Prevention [CDC], 2022). It should be noted that delay of breastfeeding in such cultures does not preclude a high degree of breastfeeding success once the transition to mature milk begins.

Some traditional methods of cord care can be harmful and include application of ash, breastmilk, ghee, cow dung, and saliva (Karumbi et al., 2013). A change in contemporary healthcare practice regarding cord management is delayed cord clamping. In the extreme, lotus birth is nonseverance of the umbilical cord. This choice is made by parents who believe this is a natural and nonviolent approach to cord care (Hayes, 2019). Typically, the placenta in lotus birth is dried and treated with salts and herbs and wrapped in plastic or a diaper. The cord is allowed to dry and separate naturally; this usually takes about a week. While there is a body of scientific evidence supporting the benefits of delayed cord clamping, there is limited evidence on the safety of lotus birth. Concerns are raised regarding the possibility of infection, though case reports document the lack of harm for infants (Hayes, 2019).

Female genital cutting (FGC) is the culturally perpetuated practice of cutting off parts of the clitoris and/or labia, narrowing the vaginal opening, or surgical alteration to external genitalia for the purpose of controlling sexuality, enhancing marriageability, and increasing partners' sexual pleasure (US Department of Health and Human Services, Office on Women's Health [HHS-OWH], 2021). It is typically done to infants in the first two weeks after birth, although it can be done later. It is not condoned by any religion, although it is associated with northern and sub-Saharan African areas with large Muslim populations. FGC is illegal in the United States and many parts of the world. FGC may have consequences for labor and birth, depending on the degree of cutting and vaginal obstruction. Prenatal care providers should be aware of the cultural context of this practice (American College of Nurse-Midwives [ACNM], 2022).

Summary

There are 195 countries across the globe, hundreds of ethnic and Indigenous groups, 11 major religions, many smaller religious sects, and multiple birthing subcultures that make up the patchwork quilt of beliefs, rituals, and traditions surrounding childbearing. There are themes regarding pregnancy and birth that recur across time, across borders, and across cultures. There are both unique and universal qualities and experiences to pregnancy and birth that create bonds among those who have children and those who care for them. To honor this bond, healthcare providers are called to give care that is individualized and respectful of all cultures and must commit to ongoing learning and self-reflection that includes cultural sensitivity and humility training.

> For all our differences and disagreements, we can live in a world of peace. In opposing every attempt to create a rigid uniformity, we can and must build unity on the basis of our diversity of languages, cultures and religions, and lift our voices against everything which would stand in the way of such unity.
>
> —Pope Francis, 9/11 Memorial, September 25, 2015

Resources for Clients and Their Families

Office of Minority Health. https://www.minorityhealth.hhs.gov

Resources for Healthcare Providers

Midwifery in Color provides mentorship and support for student and new graduate midwives of color: https://www.midwiferyincolor.org

National Black Midwives Alliance provides funding and mentorship for Black student midwives: https://blackmidwivesalliance.org

Cultural and Linguistic Competence Health Practitioner Assessment (CLCHPA): http://www.clchpa.org

Office of Minority Health: https://www.minorityhealth.hhs.gov/omh/browse.aspx?lvl=1&lvlid=6

National Standards for Culturally and Linguistically Appropriate Services in Health and Healthcare: https://thinkculturalhealth.hhs.gov/clas/standards

World Health Organization Care of Girls & Women Living with Female Genital Mutilation: A Clinical Handbook: https://apps.who.int/iris/bitstream/handle/10665/272429/9789241513913-eng.pdf?sequence=1&isAllowed=y

References

Altman, M. R., McLemore, M. R., Oseguera, T., Lyndon, A., & Franck, L. S. (2020). Listening to women: Recommendations from women of color to improve experiences in pregnancy and birth care. *Journal of Midwifery & Women's Health*, 65(4), 466–473. https://doi.org/10.1111/jmwh.13102

American College of Nurse-Midwives (ACNM). (2019). *Midwifery educational trends report* 2019. https://www.midwife.org/acnm/files/acnmlibrarydata/uploadfilename/000000000321/Midwifery_Education_Trends_Report_2019_Final.pdf

American College of Nurse-Midwives (ACNM). (2022). *Female genital cutting.* https://www.midwife.org/acnm/files/acnmlibrarydata/uploadfilename/000000000068/2022_ps_female-genital-cutting.pdf?mc_cid=a7c37480c1&mc_eid=f604fe943f

Anderson, C., & Potts, L. (2020). The Amish health culture and culturally sensitive health services: An exhaustive narrative review. *Social Science & Medicine, 265*, 113466. https://www.ncbi.nlm.nih.gov/pmc/articles/PMC8431948

Anderson, R. (2022). From "foreign languages" to "world languages" within US institutions: Abandoning misleading terminologies. *Critical Internationalization Studies Review, 1*(1), 3–5. https://doi.org/10.32674/cisr.v1i1.4869

Atlas Obscura. (2022). *Biscuits with mice.* https://www.atlasobscura.com/foods/beschuit-met-muisjes

Burns, E. (2015). The blessingway ceremony: Ritual, nostalgic imagination and feminist spirituality. *Journal of Religion and Health, 54*(2), 783–797. https://doi.org/10.1007/s10943-014-9991-3

Centers for Disease Control and Prevention (CDC). (2022). *Botulism.* https://www.poison.org/articles/dont-feed-honey-to-infants

Cheyney, M., & Davis-Floyd, R. (2021). Rituals and rites of childbirth across cultures. In S. Han & C. Tomori (Eds.), *The Routledge handbook of anthropology and reproduction* (pp. 480–493). Routledge. ISBN10 - 1138612871

Davis-Floyd, R. E. (1990). The role of obstetrical rituals in the resolution of cultural anomaly. *Social Science & Medicine, 31*(2), 175–189. https://doi.org/10.1016/0277-9536(90)90060-6

Dawley, K. (2000). The campaign to eliminate the midwife. *AJN The American Journal of Nursing, 100*(10), 50–56.

DeLibertis, J. (2015). *Shifting the frame: A report on diversity and inclusion in the American College of Nurse-Midwives.* American College of Nurse-Midwives. http://www.midwife.org/acnm/files/ccLibraryFiles/Filename/000000005329/Shifting-the-Frame-June-2015.pdf

Drew, M. L., & Reis, P. (2020). Black lives matter: A message and resources for midwives. *Journal of Midwifery & Women's Health, 65*(4), 451–458. https://doi.org/10.1111/jmwh.13155

Farley, C. L., & Jacobwitz, J. (2019). Cooking up a delicious experiential learning activity. *Nurse Education Today, 77*, 24–26. https://doi.org/10.1016/j.nedt.2019.03.003

Farrell, M. V. (2022). Why restoring birth as ceremony can promote health equity. *AMA Journal of Ethics, 24*(4), 326–332. https://journalofethics.ama-assn.org/article/why-restoring-birth-ceremony-can-promote-health-equity/2022-04

Finlayson, K., Crossland, N., Bonet, M., & Downe, S. (2020). What matters to women in the postnatal period: A meta-synthesis of qualitative studies. *PLoS One, 15*(4), e0231415. https://doi.org/10.1371/journal.pone.0231415

Foronda, C., Baptiste, D. L., Reinholdt, M. M., & Ousman, K. (2016). Cultural humility: A concept analysis. *Journal of Transcultural Nursing, 27*(3), 210–217. https://doi.org/10.1177/1043659615592677

Galanti, G. A. (2015). *Caring for patients from different cultures* (5th ed.). University of Pennsylvania Press.

Gatrad, A. R., & Sheikh, A. (2001). Muslim birth customs. *BMJ: Archives of Disease in Childhood—Fetal and Neonatal Edition, 84*(1). https://fn.bmj.com/content/fetalneonatal/84/1/F6.full.pdf

Hayes, E. H. (2019). Placentophagy, lotus birth, and other placenta practices: What does the evidence tell us? *The Journal of Perinatal & Neonatal Nursing, 33*(2), 99–102. https://doi.org/10.1097/JPN.0000000000000402

Iradukunda, F. (2020). Food taboos during pregnancy. *Health Care for Women International, 41*(2), 159–168. https://doi.org/10.1080/07399332.2019.1574799

Jones, K., & Okun, T. (2000). *Dismantling racism: A workbook for social change groups.* dRworks.

Karumbi, J., Mulaku, M., Aluvaala, J., English, M., & Opiyo, N. (2013). Topical umbilical cord care for prevention of infection and neonatal mortality. *The Pediatric Infectious Disease Journal, 32*(1), 78.

Kathawa, C. A., Arora, K. S., Zielinski, R., & Low, L. K. (2022). Perspectives of doulas of color on their role in alleviating racial disparities in birth outcomes: A qualitative study. *Journal of Midwifery & Women's Health, 67*(1), 31–38. https://doi.org/10.1111/jmwh.13305

Liese, K. L., Davis-Floyd, R., Stewart, K., & Cheyney, M. (2021). Obstetric iatrogenesis in the United States: The spectrum of unintentional harm, disrespect, violence, and abuse. *Anthropology & Medicine, 28*(2), 188–204. https://doi.org/10.1080/13648470.2021.1938510

López, C. L., Wilson, M. D., Hou, M. Y., & Chen, M. J. (2021). Racial and ethnic diversity among obstetrics and gynecology, surgical, and nonsurgical residents in the US from 2014 to 2019. *JAMA Network Open, 4*(5), e219219–e219219. https://doi.org/10.1001/jamanetworkopen.2021.9219

McIntosh, P. (1989). *White privilege: Unpacking the invisible knapsack.* https://psychology.umbc.edu/files/2016/10/White-Privilege_McIntosh-1989.pdf

McQuaid, R. J., Cox, S. M., Ogunlana, A., & Jaworska, N. (2021). The burden of loneliness: Implications of the social determinants of health during COVID-19. *Psychiatry Research, 296*, 113648. https://doi.org/10.1016/j.psychres.2020.113648

Mose, A., Dheresa, M., Mengistie, B., Wassihun, B., & Abebe, H. (2021). Colostrum avoidance practice and associated factors among mothers of children aged less than six months in Bure District, Amhara region, north west, Ethiopia: A community-based cross-sectional study. *PLoS One, 16*(1), e0245233. https://doi.org/10.1371/journal.pone.0245233

National Council of Aboriginal Midwives (NACM.). (2019). *Position statement on evacuation for birth.* https://indigenousmidwifery.ca/wp-content/uploads/2019/05/PS_BirthEvac.pdf

Okun, T. (2013). *White supremacy culture.* https://collectiveliberation.org/wp-content/uploads/2013/01/White_Supremacy_Culture_Okun.pdf

Scheepers, D., & Ellemers, N. (2019). Social identity theory. In K. Sassenberg & M. L. W. Vliek (Eds.), *Social psychology in action* (pp. 129–143). Springer. https://doi.org/10.1007/978-3-030-13788-5_9

Semenic, S. E., Callister, L. C., & Feldman, P. (2004). Giving birth: The voices of Orthodox Jewish women living in Canada. *Journal of Obstetrics Gynecology & Neonatal Nursing, 33*(1), 80–87. https://doi.org/10.1177/0884217503258352

Shepherd, S. M., Willis-Esqueda, C., Paradies, Y., Sivasubramaniam, D., Sherwood, J., & Brockie, T. (2018). Racial and cultural minority experiences and perceptions of health care provision in a mid-western region. *International Journal for Equity in Health, 17*(33). https://doi.org/10.1186/s12939-018-0744-x

US Census Bureau. (2015, November 3). *Census bureau reports at least 350 languages Spoken in U.S. Homes.* https://content.govdelivery.com/accounts/USCENSUS/bulletins/122dd88

US Department of Health and Human Services, Office on Women's Health (HHS-OWH). (2021). *Female genital cutting fact sheet.* https://www.womenshealth.gov/a-z-topics/female-genital-cutting

Waugh, L. J. (2011). Beliefs associated with Mexican immigrant families' practice of la cuarentena during postpartum recovery. *Journal of Obstetric, Gynecologic & Neonatal Nursing, 40*(6), 732–741. https://doi.org/10.1111/j.1552-6909.2011.01298.x

Whitburn, L. Y., Jones, L. E., Davey, M. A., & McDonald, S. (2019). The nature of labour pain: An updated review of the literature. *Women and Birth, 32*(1), 28–38. https://doi.org/10.1016/j.wombi.2018.03.004

Wilson, L. (2012). Cultural competence: Implications for childbearing practices. *International Journal of Childbirth Education, 27*(1), 10–17. https://www.thefreelibrary.com/Culturalcompetence:implicationsforchildbearingpractices.-a0302298434

20

Physical Activity and Exercise in the Perinatal Period

Meghan Garland and Tanya Tringali

Relevant Terms

Counting talk test (CTT)—maximum number of integers counted in a single breath while at rest. 33–50% of CTT is considered moderate intensity

Exercise—energy expenditure resulting from planned recreation

Functional fitness—an exercise modality that emphasizes movements patterns that mimic movement used in activities of daily living

High-intensity interval training (HIIT)—brief, intermittent bursts of vigorous activity at near maximal levels, interspersed by periods of rest or low-intensity exercise

Intensity—(moderate to vigorous) activity that increases respiration and heart rate above baseline (e.g. brisk walking [>2.5 mph], jogging, dancing, gardening, or yard work)

Mobility—ability of a joint to move through its range of motion. It requires a combination of flexibility (i.e., the ability for a muscle to lengthen) and strength

Physical activity (PA)—energy expenditure resulting from activities of daily living including leisure, transportation, household, and occupational activities

Progressive overload—the gradual increase of the variables used in fitness training (i.e., repetitions, sets, weight/load, speed, distance, and training frequency)

Repetition—each individual exercise movement (i.e., one squat or bicep curl)

Resistance training—a type of exercise in which the person aims to build muscle using their own body weight, bands, free weights, or machines

Sedentary behavior—activities done while sitting or lying down

Set—consecutive repetitions (i.e., 10 squats or bicep curls)

Talk test—a measure of moderate exercise intensity (i.e., the person can talk but not sing during exercise)

Introduction

Prenatal exercise is one of the most effective interventions to improve pregnancy health and reduce complications of pregnancy and birth (Berghella & Saccone, 2017). The benefits of regular exercise during pregnancy for pregnancy health and throughout the life course for both parent and fetus outweigh the minimal risks of strains or sprains for almost all pregnant people. Only the small fraction of pregnant people with hemodynamically unstable or restrictive cardiovascular disease (CVD) may need to modify **physical activity** (PA) during pregnancy, but this caution is based on consensus opinion, not evidence (Berghella & Saccone, 2017). Despite clear benefits of regular exercise and significant risks to **sedentary behavior**, only about 15% of pregnant people report achieving the recommended levels of 150 minutes weekly of moderate-intensity exercise throughout pregnancy and 60% of pregnant women report no leisure time PA (Hesketh & Evenson, 2016). The 2018 Physical Activity Guidelines for Americans and the American College of Obstetrician Gynecologists (ACOG) recommend that pregnant women engage in both aerobic and strength training throughout pregnancy (Piercy et al., 2018; ACOG, 2020). Ongoing assessment of PA and sedentary behavior during pregnancy with the goal of assisting pregnant people to maintain or increase activity and reduce sedentary behavior is a cost-effective intervention to improve pregnancy outcomes. Body mass index (BMI) cannot be used to gauge PA participation or sedentary behavior. Many factors contribute to low rates of PA. Pregnant people report numerous exercise barriers including pregnancy-related symptoms and limitations, limited time, perceptions of already being active, lack of motivation, safety concerns for self and fetus, lack of advice and information, lack of social support, adverse weather, and lack of resources (Coll et al., 2017). These estimates of moderate-intensity **exercise** (planned recreation) do not include all forms of PA (physical energy expenditure in leisure, transportation, household, and occupational activities) or light-intensity activity that make significant contributions to overall energy expenditure. Clinicians can assist pregnant people to identify barriers and support self-confidence to overcome barriers to pregnancy PA. Very little research has examined PA participation and determinants of PA behavior among pregnant people of color (Garland et al., 2019). It is unknown how experiences of discrimination affect pregnancy PA.

Estimates suggest that pregnant people spend more than 50% of their time in sedentary behaviors (activities done while sitting or lying down; Fazzi et al., 2017). Time spent in sedentary behavior is associated with CVD and type 2 diabetes, and the link between behavior and impaired glucose tolerance is stronger for people assigned female at birth than for people assigned male (Dunstan et al., 2010; Hu et al., 2003; Katzmarzyk et al., 2009). The link between sedentary behavior and gestational diabetes mellitus (GDM) and hypertensive disorders of pregnancy is less clear, but reducing sedentary time has benefits beyond pregnancy (Fazzi et al., 2017; Lin et al., 2021). Increased time in sitting behaviors is associated with increased age-adjusted mortality across all BMI categories (Katzmarzyk et al., 2009). Studies of people with restricted activity, such as bedrest, experience adverse changes in cardiac output and stroke volume, glucose tolerance, and triglyceride clearance. Adults who spend 50% or more of their waking hours in sitting behaviors have an increased risk of mortality.

Health equity key points

- It is unknown how experiences of discrimination affect pregnancy PA. Research is needed.
- PA participation should be evaluated and encouraged in all people throughout pregnancy.
- Social determinants of health affect PA engagement. Appropriate referrals to community resources may facilitate increased pregnancy PA.
- Structured fitness training and classes may be cost prohibitive or not located within communities of color and rural communities.
- Ineffective counseling and support are sources of health inequity. Successful pregnancy PA counseling is tailored to the individual, incorporates an exercise prescription, is delivered face-to-face, and incorporates behavioral components such as goal setting and self-monitoring.

Physiologic Changes during Pregnancy and Physical Activity

Pregnancy has effects on body systems that are directly affected during PA including cardiovascular, metabolic, respiratory, musculoskeletal, and thermoregulatory systems. Physiologic responses to PA during pregnancy include increased cardiac workload, increased oxygen consumption, and redistribution of blood flow away from the viscera and myometrium into the skin and skeletal muscle. Several compensatory mechanisms preserve fetal oxygen availability during PA. The decrease in blood flow to the placenta is much lower than the decrease to the myometrium due to selective distribution mechanisms. Additionally, sustained PA during pregnancy is associated with increased placental villous size and volume. Biophysical profile and umbilical artery blood flow before and after 30 minutes of strenuous PA demonstrates that PA is well tolerated in the fetuses of active and inactive people (American College of Obstetricians and Gynecologists [ACOG], 2020). Maternal hematocrit rises during PA, thus increasing oxygen carrying capacity. Uterine oxygen uptake also increases during PA. The normal changes in respiratory function in pregnancy are the same as those during mild to moderate PA in the nonpregnant state. Respiratory rate during light PA is greater than that of nonpregnant people, but this difference ceases during moderate PA. Gas exchange is not altered by pregnancy, and PA-induced acid–base balance is similar to nonpregnant people.

PA significantly increases muscle glucose uptake that extends 2–3 hours into the postexercise period. Enhanced insulin sensitivity can last up to 48 hours after PA. The physiologic mechanisms responsible for increased insulin sensitivity are not solely dependent on insulin-dependent metabolic pathways affected by GDM and type 2 diabetes. PA is an alternate pathway to increase glucose uptake and decrease hyperglycemia in insulin-resistant individuals (Dipla et al., 2021). Strength training increases muscle mass and stimulates glucose uptake. Alone or combined with aerobic PA, strength training is associated with significant reductions in insulin needed to treat GDM (Dipla et al., 2021). Aerobic and strength training are associated with reduced incidence of GDM, improved glucose control in the presence of GDM and reduced incidence of CVD, type 2 diabetes, and elevated BMI later in life for both parent and child (Doi et al., 2020; Nagpal & Mottola, 2020)

PA is associated with increased heat production and body temperature and may alter fetal heat dissipation. However, most people tolerate moderate PA with no change in core body temperature. The ability of pregnant people to dissipate heat generated during PA increases as pregnancy progresses.

Physiologic changes during exercise in pregnancy

Increased:
- Cardiac workload
- Oxygen consumption
- Oxygen carrying capacity
- Uterine oxygen uptake
- Skeletal muscle glucose uptake
- Heat production and body temperature
- Ability to dissipate heat

Redistribution of blood flow away from viscera and myometrium to skin and skeletal muscle

Preferential distribution of blood to placenta

Benefits of Physical Activity and Exercise in Pregnancy

Healthy pregnant people as well as those with risk factors such as BMI ≥ 30, history of type 1 and type 2 diabetes, chronic hypertension, and a history of preterm birth benefit from pregnancy PA (ACOG, 2020). A habit of engaging in regular PA and exercise during pregnancy may be one of the most effective ways to ameliorate a wide range of pregnancy discomforts, reduce risk for complications, and improve lifelong cardiovascular and metabolic health. Pregnant people who achieve higher levels of PA have better self-rated health, fewer symptoms of depression, lower rates of excessive gestational weight gain, and fewer unplanned cesarean births (DiPietro et al., 2019; Meander et al., 2021). Pregnancy PA does not contribute to preterm birth and may lead to shorter labors and more vaginal births (Bauer et al., 2020; Haakstad & Bø, 2020; Table 20.1). Aerobic exercise and strengthening back and abdominal muscles during exercise decreases back and pelvic discomforts and reduces the risk of falls due to pregnancy-associated anatomical changes (Hrvatin & Rugelj, 2021; Marín-Jimenez et al., 2019).

Regular moderate to vigorous PA leads to a dramatic reduction in rates of GDM and preeclampsia that substantially increase the lifetime risk of type 2 diabetes and CVD (Kris-Etherton et al., 2021). Pregnant people who engage in at least 150 minutes weekly of moderate-intensity exercise throughout pregnancy reduce their risk of GDM by 25% and preeclampsia by 38% (Davenport, Ruchat, et al., 2018). PA promotes changes in blood vessels and muscle cells that affect the utilization of blood glucose leading to better fasting and postprandial blood glucose levels thus delaying or preventing the need for insulin therapy (Dipla et al., 2021; Nagpal & Mottola, 2020).

There are substantial fetal and neonatal benefits of PA during pregnancy that also affect adult health. Both small for gestational age (SGA) and large for gestational age (LGA) infants are at higher risk of adult obesity, type 2 diabetes, and CVD related to the intrauterine environment (hyperglycemia, inflammation, altered vascularization, and epigenetic changes) (Nagpal & Mottola, 2020; Rasmussen & Jamieson, 2020). Prenatal PA reduces the risk of LGA infants by 39% and does not increase the risk of infants born SGA (Davenport, Meah, et al., 2018). Institutional racism is associated with adverse pregnancy outcomes by reinforcing White/Black disparities in income, employment status, education, and access to healthcare (Loggins Clay et al., 2018). Chronic stress from race-based discriminatory experiences and institutionalized racism has been associated with Black pregnant people experiencing disproportionately more preterm and SGA infants compared to White pregnant people (Giurgescu et al., 2011). The effects of pregnancy PA on pregnancy-related morbidity disproportionately

Table 20.1 Myths about Physical Activity in Pregnancy Versus Evidence

Myth	Evidence
There is no high-quality evidence supporting the safety of pregnancy PA.	Level-1 evidence from over 50 RCTs demonstrates the safety of pregnancy PA.
Pregnant people should moderate the intensity of pregnancy PA or not exercise more than prepregnancy.	Moderate-intensity PA is recommended for all healthy adults regardless of pregnancy status or PA habits prepregnancy.
Strenuous exercise is harmful.	There is no evidence of harm in those who continue strenuous exercise.
Pregnant people with a history of preterm birth (PTB) or a short cervix in the current pregnancy should moderate activity.	Pregnancy PA decreases the risk of PTB. There is no increased risk of PTB in the presence of short cervix or cerclage. Sedentary behavior is associated with increased risk of PTB.
Pregnant people with multifetal pregnancies should moderate activity.	No evidence of harm from pregnancy PA in multifetal pregnancies. There is harm from sedentary behavior (bedrest).
Pregnant people experiencing vaginal bleeding or placenta previa should moderate activity.	No high-quality evidence of harm from pregnancy PA with vaginal bleeding or placenta previa. There is evidence of harm from sedentary behavior (bedrest).
Pregnant people diagnosed with chronic hypertension (CHTN), preeclampsia, and gestational hypertension should moderate activity.	Pregnancy PA reduces the incidence of pregnancy hypertensive disorders in people with and without diagnosed CHTN. Limited evidence does not demonstrate harm from moderate-intensity activity in the presence of gestational hypertension and preeclampsia. There is evidence of harm from sedentary behavior for prevention and treatment of hypertensive disorders.
Pregnant people should walk, swim, or do yoga for recreation during pregnancy.	Pregnant people can participate in all types of recreation including high-impact activities such as running. However, scuba diving, contact sports and sports with a high risk of falling (boxing/sky diving) may lead to injury.

Source: Berghella and Saccone (2017) and ACOG (2020).

experienced by Black pregnant people have not been well studied (Raper et al., 2021). Neonates in a small study of 30 non-Hispanic Black people in a structured prenatal exercise program weighed, on average, 40 g more than nonexercise controls representing 20% of the average 200 g weight disparity between Black and White neonates (Raper et al., 2021).

Assessing Sources of Energy Expenditure and PA Intensity

Estimating sources of PA. Energy is expended from many sources, not only planned leisure exercise. Most pregnant people engage in significant amounts of light- to moderate-intensity PA that should not be overlooked as contributors to overall energy expenditure and may have associated health benefits. Walking for transportation, occupation, or leisure is the most commonly reported PA during pregnancy (Connolly et al., 2019). Other significant contributors to moderate energy expenditure reported by pregnant people are childcare and household activities (Yeo & Logan, 2014). Several studies have noted significant health benefits from yoga and stretching including lower rates of preterm birth, and an inverse association with GDM and preeclampsia (Pais et al., 2021; Yeo et al., 2008; Yeo & Kang, 2021). All activity, regardless of **intensity**, is associated with health benefits. Clinicians should encourage PA and low-intensity exercise that may be more desirable or attainable for some people (Yeo & Kang, 2021). The lowest threshold for benefit for pregnancy PA is not known. Pregnant people should be encouraged to increase activity by any amount of time or intensity and reduce sedentary time by any amount that can be achieved and sustained.

Estimating moderate to vigorous PA intensity. Moderate to vigorous activity intensity is sufficient to increase respiration and heart rate above baseline. Examples of moderate to vigorous physical activities include brisk walking (>2.5 mph), jogging, dancing, gardening, or yard work. The **"talk test"** (the ability to converse during exercise) can be used to approximate the ventilatory threshold (the inflection point when ventilation rapidly increases during exercise; Reed & Pipe, 2016). Pregnant people can learn to estimate PA intensity using the **counting talk test** (CTT). While at rest, the person counts integers until they need to take a second breath. During moderate to vigorous exercise, pregnant people should be able to count 33–50% of their resting CTT. For example, if a person were able to count to 10 with a single breath while at rest, they have achieved moderate intensity when they are able to say 5 integers in a single breath and vigorous activity when only able to say 3 words.

Estimating sedentary behavior. Sedentary behavior is an independent risk factor for metabolic and CVD regardless of other PA behaviors (Katzmarzyk et al., 2009). Examples of sedentary behavior include activities done while sitting including working at a desk, riding in a car, or playing video games. Clinicians should assess sedentary time independently of PA. Although the harm of bedrest is well-known, the threshold for adverse pregnancy outcomes from sedentary behavior is unknown. In studies of nonpregnant adults, people who spend more than 50% of their time in sedentary behavior are at increased risk of death from all causes and CVD (Katzmarzyk et al., 2009). Pregnant people should be encouraged to limit their time spent sitting throughout the day.

Benefits of PA during pregnancy

Pregnancy PA decreases:

- Hypertensive disorders of pregnancy
- GDM
- Preterm birth
- Total weight gain
- Length of labor
- Pregnancy discomforts
- Symptoms of depression
- LGA and SGA infants
- Cesarean births
- Metabolic and cardiovascular disorders across the lifespan for both birthing people and their offspring

Source: ACOG (2020), DiPietro et al. (2019), Haastad and Bø (2020), and Kris-Etherton et al. (2021).

Motivation for Physical Activity

Pregnancy is a time of profound change and may provide incentive for people to engage in healthier behaviors, including PA. However, evidence suggests that the adoption of new behaviors during pregnancy is not easy. Social determinants of health contribute to health inequities and poor outcomes. Social, economic, environmental, and interpersonal forces all affect behaviors like PA that contribute to pregnancy health and downstream risk of CVD (Kris-Etherton et al., 2021). Numerous interventions have attempted to improve pregnancy PA; those that incorporate theory-based behavior change techniques are more likely to be effective (Currie et al., 2013). Health promotion and behavior change are complex topics. A recent review of interventions to increase pregnancy PA found that increased confidence to overcome PA barriers and encouragement to be active were associated with increased PA (Chan et al., 2019). Education about the benefits and suggested target activity levels were also effective intervention components (Chan et al., 2019). Successful interventions incorporate a structured exercise component such as a class, though attending exercise classes may be less feasible for people who have barriers related to families, work, transportation, or cost. A meta-analysis of interventions to increase PA in healthy adults found that successful interventions were tailored to the individual, incorporate an exercise prescription or goal, are delivered face-to-face, and incorporate behavioral components such as goal setting and self-monitoring (Conn et al., 2011).

Both the ACOG and the American Heart Association recommend using the motivational counseling tool for lifestyle-related behavior change counseling, the Five As (assess, advise, agree, assist, arrange; Table 20.2; ACOG, 2020; Kris-Etherton et al., 2021). **Assess** involves screening for nonmedical, health-related social needs and social determinants of health (housing instability, food insecurity, transportation needs, utility needs, interpersonal safety), psychosocial stressors and social factors including beliefs and motivation for behavior change. **Advise** and **Agree** applies principles of shared decision-making to develop a lifestyle activity goal that is achievable in the pregnant person's current circumstances. **Assist** applies principles of motivational interviewing by encouraging patients to identify their own barriers using non-judgemental and empathetic language. The clinician uses open-ended questions to assist the pregnant person to identify strategies to overcome barriers that will work for them rather than the clinician offering solutions. **Arrange** involves the clinician making appropriate referrals to social workers or community services to address unmet needs. There is clear guidance for healthcare providers and pregnant people about target levels of PA, how to engage in PA safely, and strategies to achieve a threshold of PA consistent with recommendations. PA behavior should be assessed on a regular basis, similar to asking about the presence of fetal movement or adequacy of diet.

Table 20.2   The Five As for Lifestyle-related Behavior Change Counseling

Assess	Screen for nonmedical, health-related social needs and social determinants of health including: Housing instability Food insecurity Transportation and utility needs Interpersonal safety Psychosocial stressors and social factors including: Beliefs Motivation for behavior change Communication strategies: Nonjudgmental and open-ended questions Reflective language Summarizing statements
Advise and agree	Apply principles of shared decision-making to develop a lifestyle activity goal that is achievable in the pregnant person's current circumstances
Assist	Encouraging patients to identify their own barriers Assist the pregnant person to identify barriers to PA and realistic strategies to overcome barriers Avoid offering solutions OR ask permission before offering solutions
Arrange	Make appropriate referrals to social workers or community services and resources to address unmet needs

Assisting Pregnant People to Meet Their PA Goals

Like all health behaviors, the goals of the pregnant person should be centered in the care plan. Patient communication frameworks such as motivational interviewing may be employed to assist the patient in problem-solving. The clinician should avoid lecturing about the benefits of PA and instead tailor information to what is needed or desired for goal setting. Assessing health goals for the person and their fetus may help the clinician to align those goals with increasing PA or reducing sedentary behavior. Some motivations may be more clearly linked to PA, such as a desire to continue existing PA habits, and others may seem more tangential. For example, a person who identifies wanting to protect their fetus from harm may be motivated to increase PA if they are aware of the decreased risk of preterm birth associated with meeting PA guidelines. In addition to short-term pregnancy-related goals, assessing long-term health goals may also assist pregnant people to align values with behavior. Pregnant people who identify avoiding type 2 diabetes and CVD as long-term health goals may be motivated to decrease sedentary time if they are aware that spending less than half their time sitting during daily activities is associated with a reduced risk of these diseases.

Assessing barriers to maintaining or increasing PA and reducing sedentary behavior is essential. Once healthcare goals have been established and information about pregnancy PA tailored to those goals is provided, clinicians should assess barriers. Open-ended questions that encourage patients to identify their unique barriers help keep the patient at the center of the conversation. Using reflective language and summarizing statements assures the person you are listening and prevents misunderstanding. For example, the clinician may say "Getting more exercise would help you meet your goal of preventing type 2 diabetes. What happens during your week that keeps you from being more physically active?" Asking patients about past PA behavior may be helpful. If a person was physically active in the past but their activity has decreased, exploring the reasons why may identify current barriers. For people without a history of PA, inquiring about any barriers that dampened motivation may highlight current barriers. Inquiring about what the pregnant person enjoyed about their past PA behavior may elucidate additional benefits not directly related to pregnancy health such as social aspects of PA. For many clinicians, it is tempting to offer solutions to pregnancy PA barriers, but this practice should be avoided because it removes the patient from the center of care. The use of open-ended questions such as "What do you think would be helpful?" or "What do you think you could do?" keeps the patient at the center of the conversation and encourages problem-solving. If the person is unable to identify any way to overcome a barrier to PA, the clinician should ask permission before offering any solutions.

Once current PA and sedentary behavior levels have been assessed, healthcare goals and pregnancy PA benefits have been aligned, barriers have been identified, and the pregnant person has identified potential ways to overcome these barriers, the patient should set a realistic goal. Unrealistic outcome expectations may lead to disappointment and inhibit PA over time (Garland et al., 2021). PA goals should be short-term, attainable, and should be assessed at the next prenatal visit. Goals may be to increase the time spent engaged in PA at any intensity, decreasing by any amount the time spent in sedentary behavior, increasing the frequency of PA, or increasing the activity intensity using the CTT. Once a plan has been developed, the clinician should verbalize the plan to assure mutual agreement. Finally, providing encouragement to the pregnant person, acknowledging their ability to overcome barriers and to meet their PA goals may help foster patient confidence.

General advice for exercising in pregnancy

- People who do not regularly engage in exercise prior to pregnancy should begin
- People can anticipate feeling slightly short of breath during exercise related to normal respiratory changes during pregnancy
- People who wish to engage in safe moderate to vigorous PA should not be discouraged
- Avoid exercising in the fasting state and in very hot and humid conditions
- Ensure adequate hydration during exercise
- Exercise in comfortable clothing that allows heat dissipation and evaporation of sweat
- Strength/resistance training should be incorporated into all phases of pregnancy and throughout the lifespan
- Stationary exercise in the supine or standing positions for long periods (yoga, for example) may cause hypotension
- Avoid exercise that carries a high risk of falls or abdominal trauma

---

Exercise Prescription for Gestational Diabetes

Types of activities that have demonstrated efficacy to improve glycemic control for GDM are large muscle aerobic activities performed at moderate to vigorous intensity (fast walking, cycling, and water aerobics at 33–50% of CTT) as well as resistance training using weights and resistance bands (Dipla et al., 2021). Exercise should be performed at moderate to vigorous intensity. For treating GDM, large muscle aerobic and strength training bouts should take place five times weekly, lasting 40–60 minutes (Dipla et al., 2021). This is roughly double the number of weekly minutes recommended for nonpregnant adults.

Exercise helps to normalize blood glucose levels in all people and all life stages. Given the increased lifetime risk for developing type 2 diabetes, it is important that people with GDM return to PA in the postpartum period, a process for which will be discussed later in this chapter.

Common Conditions that Impact Adherence to Exercise

Only 50% of pregnant people receive guidance on exercise during pregnancy from their healthcare providers and approximately 15% are told to stop exercising (Rudin et al., 2021); additionally, many clinicians (32%) report not feeling comfortable providing exercise guidance due to a lack of knowledge and safety concerns (McGee et al., 2018). Many active pregnant people will experience one or more common complaints of pregnancy that can impact their desire or ability to engage in PA. They may also experience musculoskeletal changes that can lead to pain, discomfort, and ultimately questions directed to their healthcare team about how best to proceed. Except in the case of medical contraindications, which are uncommon, clients need reassurance, guidance, and support. Remaining active, with modifications to exercise volume, load, and intensity, is generally all that is needed to promote continued PA during pregnancy. Understanding the various strategies and modifications that can be used in the perinatal period for conditions that commonly occur may provide clinicians with new language and tools and ultimately greater confidence in helping clients meet their fitness goals during the perinatal period.

Additionally, there are increasing numbers of high-performing athletes in their childbearing years including elite athletes (i.e., collegiate, regional, and national athletes and Olympians). During postpartum recovery, high-performing athletes may derive parts of their identity from their fitness endeavors. Increased frequency and intensity of exercise can lead to challenges that differ from people who engage in exercise more recreationally. They may have a real or perceived sense of urgency to return to a prior level of ability, athleticism, or body composition. These may be felt by any postpartum person; however, in the context of athleticism in the perinatal period, we are referring to the athletes' desire to push themselves harder than may be appropriate for a given stage of recovery. Pushing too hard, too soon, can increase one's risk for injury or impact other aspects of the postpartum experience and new parenthood (i.e., increased vaginal bleeding, delayed wound healing, less time spent resting/sleeping, etc.).

Fatigue

Fatigue is a common complaint in the first trimester of pregnancy and largely related to hormonal and anatomical changes as well as increased metabolic demands of pregnancy (*see Chapters 5 and 6 to review Physiologic Alterations during Pregnancy and the Postnatal Period*). Many pregnant people report feeling more fatigue during exercise than before pregnancy and may be surprised or even frightened by this. Reminding clients that fatigue is common and expected may give them permission to self-modify, while others may need reassurance that it is safe to continue. Clinicians can provide anticipatory guidance by explaining that it is also common and expected for one's exercise routine to evolve throughout pregnancy. It may also change significantly from day to day based on how they are feeling. They can choose to modify any or all exercise variables including frequency, duration, intensity, volume, and load as needed. Finally, they may need to be reminded that fatigue is temporary and that they will have more energy again soon. It is recommended to exercise in a thermoneutral environment and avoid prolonged exposure to heat (ACOG, 2020).

Nausea and Vomiting of Pregnancy

Nausea will cause most people to reduce their level of activity. People experiencing this need the standard education and management (see Chapter 15, *Common Discomforts of Pregnancy*), and a close assessment of their daily caloric intake and hydration status may be needed to assure adequacy as people engaging in regular exercise may need to make additional adjustments. A light snack shortly before and after exercise may help to minimize or prevent nausea from occurring during a workout.

Musculoskeletal Changes

Symptoms associated with joint laxity include an anterior pelvic tilt, lordosis, changes in center of gravity affecting balance, and widening and flattening of the feet (Bø et al., 2016). Although not yet well understood, joint laxity seems to explain why some people assigned female at birth experience a higher incidence of knee osteoarthritis and other orthopedic complaints more frequently than people assigned male at birth and parous people more than nulliparous people (Chu et al., 2019). These complaints linger well beyond six weeks postpartum (Chu et al., 2019) and for some, up to three months after weaning (Goom et al., 2019).

Pregnant people are two to three times more likely to fall and be injured than the general population (Bø et al., 2016), and people who are sedentary during pregnancy fall more often than people who engage in exercise (Cakmak et al., 2016). Therefore, it is thought that exercise may help to mitigate this. Clients experiencing symptoms can continue strength training while emphasizing stability and balance in their workouts. Encouraging them to shorten their range of motion may provide a greater sense of control, reduce fear, and prevent pain. Certain movements such as single-leg exercises can be modified by holding onto a stable object such as a dowel, chair, or wall. If the client is concerned about the risk of falls, movements such as running and jumping can be replaced with other more stable options, such as walking, step-ups, or the use of equipment such as an elliptical machine.

Research has shown that those who engage in regular PA report less back pain during pregnancy (Clinton et al., 2017). Exploring different postures, shortening the length of time spent sitting, modifying movements that cause pain, or, in some cases, avoiding them altogether,

while continuing to strengthen the core in the seated, kneeling, or upright positions may help pregnant people remain active during pregnancy.

Pelvic girdle pain (PGP), including symphysis pubis dysfunction (SPD), affects approximately 50% of pregnant people (Varley & Hunter, 2019). PGP can present as mild to severe and may be exacerbated by certain activities of daily living (ADLs) and exercises. SPD is less common but described as more debilitating by many who have experienced it. It can be exacerbated by the most common and necessary ADLs such as walking or getting in and out of a car. Additionally, movements that involve hip abduction, a split leg stance, or single-leg movements should be modified or discontinued in those reporting PGP (Walters et al., 2018). Common examples of these movements include Cossack squats, lunges, clamshells, and single-leg deadlifts (Figure 20.1). Likewise, exercises that focus on strengthening the gluteus and hip adductors may help to improve symptoms in some pregnant and postpartum individuals. The use of a pelvic support belt while walking or during exercise can also provide relief and help some to stay active (Walters et al., 2018).

Intra-abdominal pressure (IAP) is the pressure contained within the abdominal cavity. Pressure changes with phase of breathing (i.e., inhalation versus exhalation), position, bodily functions such as coughing, sneezing, urination, and defecation as well as with all forms of PA. One's ability to manage their IAP is thought to be a factor in pelvic floor disorders such as stress urinary incontinence (SUI), pelvic organ prolapse (POP), and diastasis recti (DR). Strenuous strength training and impact activities such as running and jumping are thought to have the greatest effect on increases in IAP possibly affecting the integrity of the pelvic floor musculature (Bø & Nygaard, 2020). This has led many to believe that there are "safe" and "unsafe" exercises for pregnant and postpartum people. However, research has not consistently shown this to be true. Current methods for measuring IAP have limitations that affect accuracy of results, variability between study participants is high, and some exercises associated with higher IAP have been found to produce lower pressures than certain ADLs in the research setting (Bø & Nygaard, 2020; Tian et al., 2017).

Providing anticipatory guidance early in pregnancy can prepare people for these changes and encourage them to modify movements as opposed to stopping exercise altogether.

Returning to Physical Activity and Exercise in the Postpartum Period

People engage in PA in the early postpartum period for a variety of reasons including childcare, household chores, lifestyle activities, employment as well as resuming health and leisure-related PA. Some people engage in moderate to vigorous PA in the early postpartum period; however, this tends to occur in short durations, as little as 5–10 minutes at a time with walking and toning exercises being among the most popular (Wolpern et al., 2021). However,

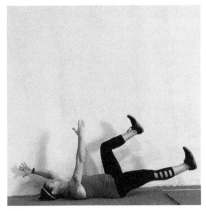
(A)

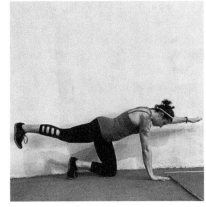
(B)

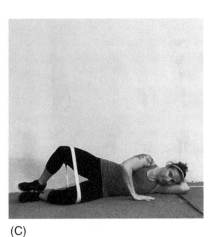
(C)

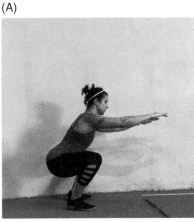
(D)

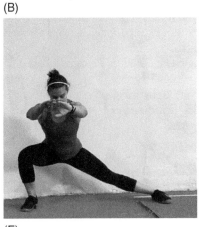
(E)

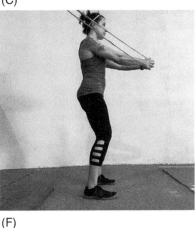
(F)

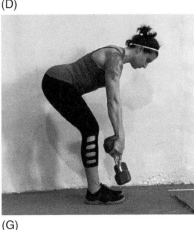
(G)

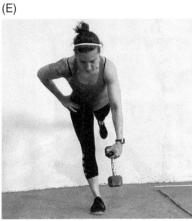
(H)

A. Dead bugs
B. Bird dog
C. Clam shells
D. Squat
E. Cossack squat
F. Paloff press
G. Deadlift
H. Single-leg deadlift

Figure 20.1 Examples of pregnancy and postpartum exercises to improve strength and balance.

returning to PA is challenging for many postpartum people. According to one systematic review, the most common barriers to PA in the postpartum period include lack of sleep, unpredictable routines and schedules, domestic responsibilities, lack of support, weather, and breastfeeding (Edie et al., 2021). Other reasons reported include a lack of motivation, low energy, appearance, employment, and finances.

As little as 15–30 days of not exercising contributes to significant muscle atrophy (Bø et al., 2017). While there are very little data about how the pelvic floor is affected by returning to vigorous exercise in the early postpartum

period, there is also no evidence of harm (Bø et al., 2017). Muscles, nerves, and connective tissue are actively healing during this time; therefore, current expert opinion suggests that one's return to fitness be gradual. This may begin as early as one to two weeks postpartum with breathing exercises and an emphasis on **mobility**, i.e., the movement of a joint, ideally through its full range of motion. This requires a balance of strength and flexibility, which is the ability for a muscle to lengthen. People in the early postpartum period often complain that their shoulders, neck, thoracic spine, and hip flexors feel tight. This is likely related to long periods of time spent sitting, resting, and feeding their infants. The posture of new parents is commonly head forward, shoulders rounded, anterior pelvic tilt, lumbar lordosis, with tight hamstrings, hip flexors and weak abdominals, back extensors, and gluteus muscles (Gaikwad & Shinde, 2019).

Many postpartum people anxiously await their six-week postpartum visit as they are eager to return to their prepregnant levels of PA. Whether stated explicitly or implicitly, many clients who have been "cleared" at their six-week visit believe that they should be able to easily return to their prepregnancy PA levels immediately. Clinicians should provide clear guidance and reasonable expectations about the typical return to exercise including acceptable forms of PA in the first six weeks, information on the range of normal, and when and how to seek additional support. Ideally, this support begins during pregnancy and continues through the fourth trimester. However, as many as 40% of people do not attend their six-week postpartum visit (ACOG et al., 2018); therefore, healthcare providers should not rely on this visit as the only opportunity to discuss PA. Likewise, people who exercise in the perinatal period may have difficulty determining the most appropriate modifications for themselves. On the one hand, this can lead to longer periods of physical inactivity, while on the other, it can lead to doing too much too quickly. In the early months of one's postpartum return to exercise, remaining symptom-free during PA should be paramount. Professional support may help people learn how to modify movements while maintaining the intended stimulus. A lack of information, advice, and encouragement is a barrier to successfully starting or returning to exercise postpartum (Edie et al., 2021). Expert guidance from physical therapists (PTs) and specialized fitness trainers and coaches who have additional training and expertise in exercise throughout the perinatal period can be helpful (see *The Multidisciplinary Team* below and *Resources for Healthcare Providers and Clients*).

High-performing and elite athletes may choose to resume PA as early as the first week postpartum. They should be supported by their healthcare providers while also working closely with a multidisciplinary team including a pelvic floor physical therapist (PFPT) and their coach (Jackson et al., 2021).

0–2 Weeks Postpartum

Encourage clients to focus on sleep and their physical recovery, regardless of the mode of birth. Some who are highly motivated to return to previous fitness levels will begin reconnecting their breath to their core and pelvic floor during this time. The goal is to find and engage the transverse abdominis (TA) while gently lifting the pelvic floor (Kegel). These muscles contract slightly during exhalation and relax again upon inhalation (Emerich Gordon & Reed, 2020). This can be practiced in supine, prone, sitting, and hands and knees positions and provides an opportunity to incorporate mobility exercises. These sessions can be brief, lasting as little at

5–10 minutes. One strategy is to exhale slowly and completely while placing fingertips on the TA just above the pubic symphysis. They will feel it firm up under the fingertips similarly to the way healthcare providers assess the strength of a contraction at the uterine fundus.

2–4 Weeks Postpartum

The core is comprised of muscles on all sides of the body. It is shaped like a canister and is surrounded by the TA and rectus abdominis anteriorly, the internal and external obliques laterally, the erector spinae posteriorly with the diaphragm at the top, and the pelvic floor at the bottom (Figure 20.2). With a more holistic view of the core, it becomes easier to see how the movement of the limbs originates from and depends upon a strong, stable yet flexible core. For example, the hip flexors originate at various points within the pelvis and the latissimus dorsi originates along the thoracic spine and inserts into the humerus. This makes low demand yet multijoint movements an accessible starting place for the early postpartum period. Common examples include bird dog and dead bugs (Figure 20.1).

Adequate sleep should remain a top priority in this phase, but for clients who are eager to return to exercise, they can gently increase demand on the trunk stabilizers while recognizing that strength and coordination depend in part upon the shortening of the abdominal muscles that were lengthened during pregnancy. These muscles do not return to their prepregnancy length immediately postpartum, and research has shown that this can take up to four months (Fukano et al., 2021). They may also choose to add additional exercises in the form of common ADLs such as squats to the height of a chair or the deadlift, a hip hinging movement that along with the squat is a common functional movement for ADLs such as picking

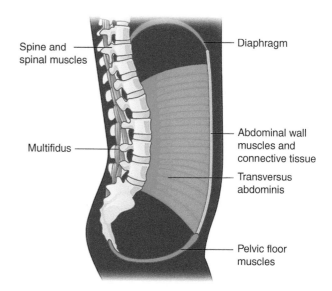

Figure 20.2 Transverse abdominis, diaphragm, and pelvic floor (sagittal view). Image used with permission from Pelvic Guru®, LLC as a member of the Global Pelvic Health Alliance. www.pelvicglobal.com.

things up from the floor (i.e., grocery bags or babies). Other exercises, such as glute bridges, can be helpful as the posterior chain, or the backside of the body is often weakened during pregnancy and postpartum due to an anterior pelvic tilt. People who have had a cesarean birth should avoid excessive stretching on the incision and can lift light objects while engaging their TA muscles. Those healing from a perineal tear or episiotomy should avoid excessive hip abduction until they are well healed.

4–6 Weeks Postpartum

For those who are progressing well and remaining symptom-free (i.e., no vaginal pressure, pelvic/low back pain, or leaking), some will feel ready to gradually begin returning to aerobic activities, commonly in the form of longer walks. People who maintained a higher level of intensity throughout pregnancy may feel ready to add inclines such as stairs or hills, circuits of various body weight movements such as lunges and squats, as well as the use of resistance bands and light weights. The use of weight is highly dependent upon what the person was accustomed to before and during pregnancy. Initially, all people should reduce weight used while focusing on rehabilitation of the core and pelvic floor. This is a good time to focus on proper technique. People can increase their training volume (i.e., weights, sets, reps, speed, etc.) according to their previous experience and capacity.

6–12 Weeks Postpartum

Those who have been steadily increasing volume are likely feeling ready to begin increasing intensity, speed, and/or weight with the goal of improving both strength and/or aerobic capacity. They should continue their focus on technique while remaining patient with themselves as abdominal muscles can take six months to one year to return to prepregnancy strength (Deering et al., 2018). Individualization is key to progress at this stage and is highly dependent upon the sport being trained, the level of fitness previously achieved, as well as the unique circumstances of one's pregnancy, birth, and postpartum recovery including both physical and mental health.

Lactation and Exercise

Moderate- to high-intensity exercise during lactation does not affect the overall quantity or composition of human milk or impact infant growth (Be'er et al., 2020). Moderate- or high-intensity exercise during lactation does not impede infant acceptance of human milk consumed postexercise (Wright et al., 2002). While vigorous exercise does not affect supply or composition, the monitoring of hydration status is important for lactating people (ACOG, 2020).

Although not yet well understood, some people experience joint laxity for up to three months after they have stopped lactating. Joint laxity can increase the risk for injury and pelvic floor dysfunction (Goom et al., 2019). While some people will feel completely recovered at six weeks postpartum, others may not feel recovered until after they have stopped lactating. Consider a referral to physical therapy for clients with persistent or worsening symptoms of PGP and continue to provide education and reassurance, as discussed in *Musculoskeletal Changes* above.

Common Postpartum Conditions that Complicate Physical Activity

Some people who experience SUI will avoid PA altogether (Al-Shaikh et al., 2018). Others will choose to wear dark clothing, absorbent pads, or underwear and continue PA despite SUI. Those experiencing SUI may feel reluctant to speak with healthcare providers or their coaches and trainers, as some do not see this as problematic but rather as inevitable. Clinicians should screen for and offer treatment options and referrals for SUI and POP.

SUI can present with or without POP. Weight loss, smoking cessation, constipation management, and pelvic floor exercises are considered first-line conservative management; however, pessaries are increasingly being used to treat POP and SUI and are an excellent option for people who experience these conditions with vigorous exercise (Al-Shaikh et al., 2018).

DR, a midline separation of the rectus abdominis muscles at the linea alba, the fibrous connective tissue formed at the midline junction of the right and left rectus abdominis muscles, is another common condition that can complicate one's postpartum return to exercise. DR can extend from the xiphoid process to the pubic symphysis or occur in only one part of the abdomen (Figure 20.3). Historically, only the inter-rectus diameter has been measured clinically; however, the use of ultrasound in current research has led to an increased interest in understanding other characteristics of DR such as the depth of diastasis, the degree of tissue stiffness, elasticity, and muscle thickness (He et al., 2021). The role of DR in low back pain, lumbopelvic pain, SUI, POP, and abdominal strength is still unclear (Benjamin et al., 2019). There is currently no consensus on the most appropriate abdominal exercises to prevent or treat DR (Bø et al., 2017). Even the "drawing in" exercise commonly used to activate the TA has been shown to widen rather than narrow the gap when assessed by ultrasound (Benjamin et al., 2019). As previously described, current guidance suggests that postpartum people progress slowly, allowing time for the muscles to shorten while exploring breath and movement strategies that may require individualization and the expertise of a PFPT or coach with specialized training. Over time, they will become more able to increase demand by moving from the supine and prone positions to sitting, standing, and ultimately increasing load and range of motion.

Excessive breast motion during exercise can be uncomfortable and even painful. Exercise may be more comfortable if breasts are not overly full and when wearing a supportive bra. Compression bras flatten the breasts and distribute the mass evenly across the chest. They may

Variations of Diastasis Recti

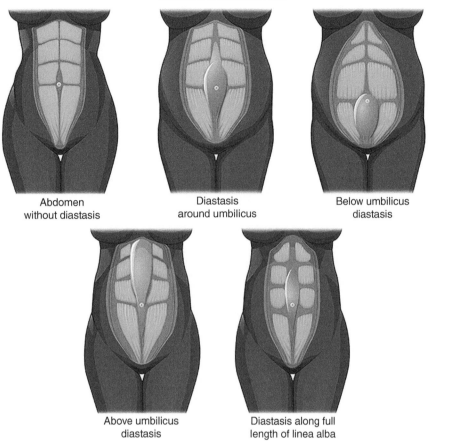

| Abdomen without diastasis | Diastasis around umbilicus | Below umbilicus diastasis |

Above umbilicus diastasis

Diastasis along full length of linea alba

Figure 20.3   Diastasis recti variations. Image used with permission from Pelvic Guru, LLC as a member of the Global Pelvic Health Alliance. www.pelvicglobal.com.

be more comfortable for people with smaller breasts. Encapsulation bras support the breasts individually and may be more helpful in reducing vertical movement of the breasts. These are preferred by people with larger breasts and with increasing age (Brown et al., 2014).

Healthcare providers should be prepared to address the full range of barriers and discomforts with their clients, acknowledging the challenges of returning to PA and exercise postpartum, helping problem solve, and referring clients to a broad interdisciplinary team, and additional support services can go a long way toward supporting clients' goals.

Common Questions and Concerns for Selected Activities

Running/Jogging

During pregnancy, most runners, both competitive and recreational, voluntarily and without professional advice choose to reduce their training volume during pregnancy, especially in the third trimester (Bø et al., 2016). Given this decline, the focus for most will be on how and when to return to running in the postpartum period.

There are currently no guidelines for returning to running postpartum; however, based on the best available

evidence, an expert panel concluded that the most appropriate time to return to high-impact activities such as running is between three to six months postpartum (Goom et al., 2019). This allows time for pelvic floor rehabilitation, shortening of the levator ani, connective tissues, nerves, and tissue remodeling. Strength training is encouraged in the earlier postpartum months (Goom et al., 2019). Reminding clients to use the "three Ps" (pain, pressure, and peeing) as a guide to what is appropriate for them is one easy way to expand upon the age-old, yet vague wisdom of, "Listen to your body."

Approximately 35% of people report pain when they return to running postpartum, predominantly in the low back, pelvis, and hips (Christopher et al., 2020). According to an expert panel of PTs, weakness of the abdominal muscles, hips, and pelvic floor may contribute to pain as can tight hip flexors, which are common in both runners and postpartum people (Christopher et al., 2020). Muscular imbalances, or asymmetries, are a risk factor for pain in postpartum runners; thus, runners may benefit from a thorough assessment by a PT and a retraining regimen that focuses on muscular strength and stability.

Fatigue is a known risk factor for injury among runners, and lack of sleep is common among new parents. Therefore, providers should discuss the importance of sleep with clients who want to return to running. If a new parent is getting too few hours of sleep, suggesting a lower intensity activity or a rest day may be helpful.

Some postpartum people will take up running for the first time in the postpartum period. Novice runners are more likely to become injured than seasoned runners; however, runners who use a structured program such as the "Couch to 5K" (see *Resources for Clients*) have lower injury rates (Christopher et al., 2020). Runners should consider three variables: frequency, duration, and intensity in their programming as they practice the mechanics of running. A history of previous injury is a risk factor for reinjury. A common strategy used to help postpartum people return to running involves short intervals of running followed by longer periods of walking and/or other body weight movements. Over time and to tolerance, they can slowly increase the duration of each run interval and shorten the duration of each walk/strength interval. Walking uphill or on an incline is another common strategy.

High-Intensity Interval Training

High-intensity interval training (HIIT) is a popular fitness option, defined as brief, intermittent bursts of vigorous activity at near maximal levels, interspersed by periods of rest or low-intensity exercise (MacInnis & Gibala, 2017). A meta-analysis of sedentary women showed that sessions lasting 18–30 minutes three times per week over a four-week period improved aerobic capacity and cardiovascular fitness (Syamsudin et al., 2021). Other studies have shown similar benefits with as little as 12-minute sessions (Nayor et al., 2020). Despite numerous studies showing a positive effect on cardiovascular health, weight management, and metabolic profiles, certain movements commonly seen in HIIT workouts can trigger pelvic floor symptoms among the general population of pregnant and postpartum people (i.e., the three Ps mentioned above). Running, jumping, and weightlifting are common examples of triggering activities seen in HIIT workouts (Poli de Araújo et al., 2020). Pregnant people will often slow their movements, effectively reducing intensity, and should be supported in their desire to stay active by encouraging modifications. For example, a standard push-up can be done on a raised surface such as a bench, box, or at the wall. Postpartum people can attempt shorter bursts of intensity, attempting to stay below their symptom threshold as they slowly rebuild their capacity. Over time, they will likely notice that they are able to sustain longer periods of intensity without triggering symptoms.

Strength Training

Strength training (i.e., resistance training, weightlifting, powerlifting, and Olympic lifting) is the third most common form of exercise that pregnant people engage in (Prewitt-White et al., 2018). During pregnancy, many fitness professional and PTs recommend reducing load as pregnancy progresses, and certain lifts may be eliminated for a variety of reasons such as avoiding changes to one's technique, preventing unnecessary strain on the linea alba, or irritation to the pubic symphysis or sacroiliac joints. While individualization is key, current wisdom is that pregnancy is not the ideal time to attempt maximal lifts. As the fetus grows, it becomes more common to favor the use of dumbbells and kettlebells over the barbell to avoid contact with the abdomen. Given the time spent working with lighter loads and time away from lifting in the early weeks of one's postpartum recovery, athletes returning to lifting should be encouraged to focus on technique while exploring breath patterns and learning to manage IAP. This can be frustrating to athletes for whom these strategies were once intuitive.

Functional Fitness

Functional fitness is a mixed modality that incorporates HIIT, bodyweight training, weightlifting, and, in some cases, gymnastics movements. At the root of functional fitness is a desire for the workouts to improve the quality of life and ability to remain completely independent in ADLs (i.e., squatting and deadlifting mimic movements used to pick up objects or children from the floor, overhead pressing movements mimic those used to put an item on a high shelf, etc.). CrossFit® (CF) is a company that popularized this style of fitness. It has been closely scrutinized by both the fitness and medical industries as it was once considered less safe than other forms of exercise, a claim that resulted in litigation ultimately supporting the safety of CF (CrossFit, 2019).

The use of vigorous exercise that involves strength training has not been adequately studied in a pregnant population. However, a study of 22 pregnant people who participated in CF for at least six months during their pregnancies found benefits related to community support, confidence, and perceptions of easier pregnancies, more energy, less fatigue and better mood, appropriate weight gain and loss, and improved physical functioning postpartum (Prewitt-White et al., 2018).

There are additional considerations for gymnastics movements. One common example of this is the pull-up. Much like overhead pressing movements, this puts significant tension on the linea alba and challenges the athlete to manage IAP, which becomes increasingly difficult as pregnancy progresses. This continues into the postpartum period when the muscles of the abdominal wall are still lengthened. Coaches and clients may watch for bulging, often called coning or doming, at the midline of the abdomen. This may indicate excess IAP that the person is still learning to manage and can provide helpful information to people as they make decisions about when to begin modifying movements in pregnancy and reintroducing higher demand movements in the postpartum period. Athletes can always substitute lower demand movements for the more common higher demand movements such as an inverted row or ring rows in place of pull ups (Christensen, 2017).

The Multidisciplinary Team

Most healthcare providers are aware of the benefits of exercise during pregnancy. However, clinicians have reported a lack of time, knowledge, and training as barriers to the promotion of PA (Wattanapisit et al., 2018). In a study of physicians' counseling practices, the majority correctly counseled clients on aerobic exercise in the first trimester, incorrectly counseled clients on strength training and maximum heart rate in the third trimester, and also failed to counsel their sedentary clients on exercise (McGee et al., 2018). Despite overwhelming evidence in support of exercise throughout the perinatal period, clinicians remain concerned about the potential for injury, and some believe that it can be harmful to the pregnant person and developing fetus (Rudin et al., 2021).

Clinicians must become competent and confident in their ability to provide support and guidance in helping people meet their personal health goals. Minimally, they should be able to provide evidence-based information, motivational counseling, and anticipatory guidance throughout the lifespan but particularly in the perinatal period where fear and myths are more common. This task need not fall entirely upon those providing perinatal care as they should utilize a broader interprofessional referral team that may include fitness professionals such as coaches and trainers, especially those with perinatal expertise, as well as PTs, particularly those with pelvic floor health expertise.

Pelvic Floor Physical Therapists

PFPTs are licensed physical therapy professionals who chose to continue their education via focused continuing education courses and additional certifications that include the treatment of specific obstetrical, gynecological, and musculoskeletal conditions that commonly present with and contribute to pelvic pain (i.e., endometriosis and vulvodynia). They are skilled at treating pelvic floor conditions that are associated with pregnancy and the postpartum period including low back pain, sciatica, urinary and fecal incontinence, POP, and DR. These conditions are commonly seen and diagnosed by perinatal healthcare providers, but their treatment requires collaboration and referral as most are not trained in the various manual therapies and treatments or the individualized rehabilitative exercises. Physical therapy with a pelvic floor specialist should be offered to clients with any of these conditions including pelvic floor and other musculoskeletal complaints.

Perinatal clinicians are encouraged to form relationships with PFPTs in their communities whenever possible for consultation, collaboration, and referral. Studies show that manual therapy is a safe, relatively noninvasive strategy that reduces symptoms and avoids medication and surgery for an array of pelvic floor concerns including urinary frequency and urgency for which PFPTs are sometimes overlooked (Adams et al., 2015). While there

Table 20.3 Example of Progressive Overload

Increasing weight	Increasing repetitions
Week 1 : 3 sets of 10 reps body weight only squats Week 2 : 3 sets of 8 reps goblet squats with 10-pound dumbbell Week 3 : 3 sets of 6 reps goblet squats with 15-pound dumbbell	Goblet Squats Week 1 : 3 sets of 8 reps 10-pound dumbbell Week 2 : 3 sets of 12 reps 10-pound dumbbell Week 3 : 3 sets of 16 reps 10-pound dumbbell

are still large parts of the country without access to this specialty, the profession is growing and can be provided through telehealth (Da Mata et al., 2021).

Fitness Professionals Specializing in the Perinatal Period

There are currently no national or state licensing requirements for fitness professionals in the United States. However, numerous organizations now certify personal trainers in this area of specialization throughout the United States, Canada, and Europe. Some fitness professionals use a brief screening tool that helps clients self-identify the need for additional screening, clearance, and guidance. One of the skills learned during basic personal trainer certification is called **progressive overload**, the gradual increase of the variables used in fitness training (i.e., **repetitions**, sets, weight/load, speed, distance, and training frequency). Having a general understanding of progressive overload, its function and how it is implemented, can be helpful when discussing fitness strategies with clients, especially in their return to exercise in the postnatal period (Table 20.3). Organizations that offer programs for pregnant and postpartum people as well as additional training for both health and fitness professionals are listed in the resources section of this chapter.

Additional Tools for Healthcare Providers

Online Resources

Mobile applications or "apps" have become ubiquitous in our daily lives and are increasingly being used by pregnant people to improve their nutrition and increase PA (Sandborg et al., 2021). A recent review of apps intended to improve pregnancy and/or postpartum PA available in the United States concluded that none of those currently available are likely to enable pregnant people to achieve recommended levels of PA due to low-quality, low-perceived impact, lack of evidence-based information in accordance with guidelines, and/or high price-point (Tinius, Polston, et al., 2021). Despite these limitations, apps may be helpful in assisting women who cite barriers to becoming physically active including rural location, childcare needs, or safety concerns (Tinius, Duchette, et al., 2021). A 2019 review of PA apps in nonpregnant adults found that those with web-based social support from other users were associated with improved PA and app engagement compared to apps without a web-based support component (Petersen et al., 2019). In one Australian study of 410 pregnant people, 75% used two to four pregnancy-related apps during their pregnancies (Lupton & Pedersen, 2016). Social media and apps have become an important source of information for pregnant people. Unfortunately, misinformation is common and only 35% of participants rated the apps they were using as trustworthy (Tinius, Polston, et al., 2021). Pregnant people are inundated with contradictory images and messages about how to stay "fit" during pregnancy and how to "get your body back" after the birth of a baby. To the extent possible, clinicians should be cognizant of this when clients present with questions or concerns and help them to identify evidence-based and body-positive resources. An open line of communication among the interprofessional team can facilitate this process and streamline the messaging received by shared clients.

The Internet is a great source of free content for clients who want or need to exercise at home. Clients can explore an array of time domains, styles, and modalities including yoga and Pilates-based workouts, aerobic, HIIT, body weight, and other forms of strength training for those who own and have a comfort level with equipment such as dumbbells, kettlebells, and barbells. Advise clients that they can skip any movement that causes discomfort or that they do not feel confident or safe completing and that they can and should rest anytime. They should not feel pressured to keep up with the instructor. As they gain more experience with a particular style or instructor, they will increase their strength and stamina.

There are also many affordable flat-rate programs available on the market, several of which have been designed by PFPTs and trainers that specialize in the perinatal period (see *Resources for Clients*). Clients can be advised to look for programs that offer several modifications for each movement, which serves as evidence that the program has been designed to accommodate the changing body and various levels of ability and athleticism.

Summary

Pregnant and postpartum people benefit from confidence to overcome PA barriers and support from family, friends, and the healthcare team to reach their PA goals. Pregnant people who experience pain, pressure, or urine leakage should be offered referral to a knowledgeable coach and/or PT. Open communication among interdisciplinary team members facilitates safe pregnancy PA that is medically appropriate, tailored to the client's medical and obstetrical history and each team member's scope of practice. Healthcare providers do not need a high level of fitness knowledge to provide evidence-based support. Resources, a deeper understanding of the roles and functions of other team members, and an expanded view on collaboration are all that is needed to better support clients and build a toolkit that will grow with time and exposure. The clinician should focus on applying the Five

As aligning the patient's values and healthcare goals with increased pregnancy PA and decreased sedentary behavior, using therapeutic communication techniques such as motivational interviewing to assist clients to identify and overcome barriers and develop confidence to increase pregnancy PA.

Resources for Healthcare Providers

Exercise is Medicine—includes provider's action guide and patient handouts (not specific to perinatal period) https://www.exerciseismedicine.org/eim-in-action/health-care/health-care-providers

Julie Wiebe Free course for healthcare providers https://courses.juliewiebept.com/p/physicians-midwives-nurse-practitioners-resource-tool-kit

Park Rx America https://parkrxamerica.org/providers

Pelvic Guru: A worldwide network of health and fitness professionals, tools and resources https://pelvicguru.com

POP UP: An uplifting resource—for people with pelvic organ prolapse https://www.popuplifting.com

Motivational Interviewing Network of Trainers—a resource for those seeking information on motivational interviewing https://motivationalinterviewing.org

Resources for Clients

Expecting and Empowered: Exercise Programs and app: https://www.expectingandempowered.com/

Pregnancy and Postpartum Athleticism, Brianna Battles (See fitness programs) https://www.briannabattles.com

Julie Wiebe https://www.juliewiebept.com/products/online-courses

Munira Hudani: For people with DR https://www.munirahudanipt.com/online-progams

Pelvic Guru (Worldwide directory of pelvic health professionals) https://pelvicguru.com/directory

POP UP: An uplifting resource—For healthcare professionals https://www.popuplifting.com

Move your way: Community Resources https://health.gov/our-work/nutrition-physical-activity/move-your-way-community-resources

Couch to 5K: https://www.nhs.uk/live-well/exercise/running-and-aerobic-exercises/get-running-with-couch-to-5k/#:~:text=What%20is%20Couch%20to%205K,each%20of%20the%209%20weeks

Pregnancy: A practical guide for scaling (Downloadable PDF from the CrossFit Journal, Christensen, 2017) https://journal.crossfit.com/article/cfj-pregnancy-a-practical-guide-for-scaling

Fitness Programs for Clients and Additional Training for Healthcare Providers

BirthFit https://birthfit.com

Girls Gone Strong (Molly Galbraith): https://www.girlsgonestrong.com

Pregnancy and Postpartum Athleticism, Brianna Battles (See coaching certifications, resources, or find a coach) https://www.briannabattles.com

References

Adams, S., Dessie, S., Dodge, L., Mckinney, J., Hacker, M., & Elkadry, E. (2015). Pelvic floor physical therapy as primary treatment of pelvic floor disorders with urinary urgency and frequency-predominant symptoms. *Female Pelvic Medicine & Reconstructive Surgery*, 21(5), 252–256. https://doi.org/10.1097/SPV.0000000000000195

Al-Shaikh, G., Syed, S., Osman, S., Bogis, A., & Al-Badr, A. (2018). Pessary use in stress urinary incontinence: A review of advantages, complications, patient satisfaction, and quality of life. *International Journal of Women's Health*, 10, 195–201. https://doi.org/10.2147/IJWH.S152616

American College of Obstetricians & Gynecologists (ACOG). (2020). Physical activity and exercise during pregnancy and the postpartum period. Committee opinion no. 804. *Obstetrics & Gynecology*, 137(2), e135–e142.

American College of Obstetricians and Gynecologists, Stube, A., Auguste, T., & Gulati, M. (2018). Optimizing postpartum care. *Obstetrics & Gynecology*, 131(5), e140–e150.

Bauer, I., Hartkopf, J., Kullmann, S., Schleger, F., Hallschmid, M., Pauluschke-Fröhlich, J., Fritsche, A., & Preissl, H. (2020). Spotlight on the fetus: How physical activity during pregnancy influences fetal health: A narrative review. *BMJ Open Sport & Exercise Medicine*, 6(1). https://doi.org/10.1136/bmjsem-2019-000658

Be'er, M., Mandel, D., Yelak, A., Gal, D. L., Mangel, L., & Lubetzky, R. (2020). The effect of physical activity on human milk macronutrient content and its volume. *Breastfeeding Medicine*, 15(6), 357–361. https://doi.org/10.1089/bfm.2019.0292

Benjamin, D. R., Frawley, H. C., Shields, N., van de Water, A. T. M., & Taylor, N. F. (2019). Relationship between diastasis of the rectus abdominis muscle (DRAM) and musculoskeletal dysfunctions, pain and quality of life: A systematic review. *Physiotherapy*, 105(1), 24–34. https://doi.org/10.1016/j.physio.2018.07.002

Berghella, V., & Saccone, G. (2017). Exercise in pregnancy! *American Journal of Obstetrics & Gynecology*, 216(4), 335–337. https://doi.org/10.1016/j.ajog.2017.01.023

Bø, K., Artal, R., Barakat, R., Brown, W., Davies, G. A. L., Dooley, M., Evenson, K. R., Haakstad, L. A. H., Henriksson-Larsen, K., Kayser, B., Kinnunen, T. I., Mottola, M. F., Nygaard, I., Van Poppel, M., Stuge, B., & Khan, K. M. (2016). Exercise and pregnancy in recreational and elite athletes: 2016 evidence summary from the IOC expert group meeting, Lausanne. Part 1—Exercise in women planning pregnancy and those who are pregnant. *British Journal of Sports Medicine*, 50(10), 571–589. https://doi.org/10.1136/bjsports-2016-096218

Bø, K., Artal, R., Barakat, R., Brown, W. J., Davies, G. A. L., Dooley, M., Evenson, K. R., Haakstad, L. A. H., Kayser, B., Kinnunen, T. I., Larsén, K., Mottola, M. F., Nygaard, I., Van Poppel, M., Stuge, B., & Khan, K. M. (2017). Exercise and pregnancy in recreational and elite athletes: 2016/17 evidence summary from the IOC expert group meeting, Lausanne. Part 3—Exercise in the postpartum period. *British Journal of Sports Medicine*, 51(21), 1516–1525. https://doi.org/10.1136/bjsports-2017-097964

Bø, K., & Nygaard, I. E. (2020). Is physical activity good or bad for the female pelvic floor? A narrative review. *Sports Medicine*, 50(3), 471–484. https://doi.org/10.1007/s40279-019-01243-1

Brown, N., White, J., Brasher, A., & Scurr, J. (2014). An investigation into breast support and sports bra use in female runners of the 2012 London Marathon. *Journal of Sports Sciences*, 32(9), 801–809. https://doi.org/10.1080/02640414.2013.844348

Cakmak, B., Ribeiro, A. P., & Inanir, A. (2016). Postural balance and the risk of falling during pregnancy. *The Journal of Maternal-Fetal & Neonatal Medicine*, 29(10), 1623–1625. https://doi.org/10.3109/14767058.2015.1057490

Chan, C. W., Au Yeung, E., & Law, B. M. (2019). Effectiveness of physical activity interventions on pregnancy-related outcomes among pregnant women: A systematic review. *International Journal of Environmental Research and Public Health*, 16(10), 1840. https://doi.org/10.3390/ijerph16101840

Christensen, N. (2017). *Pregnancy: A practical guide to scaling*. CrossFit Journal. https://journal.crossfit.com/article/cfj-pregnancy-a-practical-guide-for-scaling

Christopher, S. M., Garcia, A. N., Snodgrass, S. J., & Cook, C. (2020). Common musculoskeletal impairments in postpartum runners: An international Delphi study. *Archives of Physiotherapy*, 10(1), 1–19. https://doi.org/10.1186/s40945-020-00090-y

Chu, S. R., Boyer, E. H., Beynnon, B., & Segal, N. A. (2019). Pregnancy results in lasting changes in knee joint laxity. *PM&R*, 11(2), 117–124. https://doi.org/10.1016/j.pmrj.2018.06.012

Clinton, S. C., Newell, A., Downey, P. A., & Ferreira, K. (2017). Pelvic girdle pain in the antepartum population: Physical therapy clinical practice guidelines linked to the international classification of functioning, disability, and health from the section on women's health and the orthopaedic section of the American Physical Therapy Association. *Journal of Women's Health Physical Therapy*, 41(2), 102–125. https://doi.org/10.1097/JWH.0000000000000081

Coll, C. V., Domingues, M. R., Gonçalves, H., & Bertoldi, A. D. (2017). Perceived barriers to leisure-time physical activity during pregnancy: A literature review of quantitative and qualitative evidence. *Journal of Science and Medicine in Sport*, 20(1), 17–25. https://doi.org/10.1016/j.jsams.2016.06.007

Conn, V. S., Hafdahl, A. R., & Mehr, D. R. (2011). Interventions to increase physical activity among healthy adults: Meta-analysis of outcomes. *American Journal of Public Health*, 101(4), 751–758. https://doi.org/10.2105/AJPH.2010.194381

Connolly, C. P., Conger, S. A., Montoye, A. H., Marshall, M. R., Schlaff, R. A., Badon, S. E., & Pivarnik, J. M. (2019). Walking for health during pregnancy: A literature review and considerations for future research. *Journal of Sport and Health Science*, 8(5), 401–411. https://doi.org/10.1016/j.jshs.2018.11.004

CrossFit. (2019). Major victory for CrossFit: Judge orders terminating and massive monetary sanctions against the NSCA. CrossFit. (2019, December 5). https://www.crossfit.com/battles/major-victory-for-crossfit-judge-orders-terminating-and-massive-monetary-sanctions-against-the-nsca

Currie, S., Sinclair, M., Murphy, M., Madden, E., Dunwoody, L., & Liddle, D. (2013). Reducing the decline in physical activity during pregnancy: A systematic review of behavior change interventions. *PLoS One*, 8(6), e66385. https://doi.org/10.1371/journal.pone.0066385

da Ueda, Mata, K. R., Costa, R. C. M., Carbone, E. D. S. M., Maria Gimenez, M., Augusta, M., Bortolini, T., Castro, R. A., & Faní Fitz, F. (2021). Telehealth in the rehabilitation of female pelvic floor dysfunction: A systematic literature review. *The International Urogynecological Association*, 32, 249–259. https://doi.org/10.1007/s00192-020-04588-8

Davenport, M. H., Meah, V. L., Ruchat, S. M., Davies, G. A., Skow, R. J., Barrowman, N., Adamo, K. B., Poitras, V. J., Gray, C. E., Jaramillo Garcia, A., Sobierajski, F., Riske, L., James, M., Kathol, A. J., Nuspl, M., Marchand, A. A., Nagpal, T. S., Slater, L. G., Weeks, A., . . . Mottola, M. F. (2018). Impact of prenatal exercise on neonatal and childhood outcomes: A systematic review and meta-analysis. *British Journal of Sports Medicine*, 52(21), 1386–1396. https://doi.org/10.1136/bjsports-2018-099836

Davenport, M. H., Ruchat, S. M., Poitras, V. J., Garcia, A. J., Gray, C. E., Barrowman, N., Skow, R. J., Meah, V. L., Riske, L., Sobierajski, F., James, M., Kathol, A. J., Nuspl, M., Marchand, A. A., Nagpal, T. S., Slater, L. G., Weeks, A., Adamo, K. B., Davies, G. A., . . . Mottola, M. F. (2018). Prenatal exercise for the prevention of gestational diabetes mellitus and hypertensive disorders of pregnancy: A systematic review and meta-analysis. *British Journal of Sports Medicine*, 52(21), 1367–1375. https://doi.org/10.1136/bjsports-2018-099355

Deering, R., Cruz, M., Senefeld, J., Pashibin, T., Eickmeyer, S., & Hunter, S. (2018). Impaired trunk flexor strength, fatigability, and steadiness in postpartum women. *Medicine and Science in Sports and Exercise*, 50(8), 1558–1569. https://doi.org/10.1249/MSS.0000000000001609

DiPietro, L., Evenson, K. R., Bloodgood, B., Sprow, K., Troiano, R. P., Piercy, K. L., Vaux-Bjerke, A., & Powell, K. E. (2019). Benefits of physical activity during pregnancy and postpartum: An umbrella review. *Medicine & Science in Sports & Exercise*, 51(6), 1292–1302. https://doi.org/10.1249/mss.0000000000001941

Dipla, K., Zafeiridis, A., Mintziori, G., Boutou, A. K., Goulis, D. G., & Hackney, A. C. (2021). Exercise as a therapeutic intervention in gestational diabetes mellitus. *Endocrine, 2*(2), 65–78. https://doi.org/10.3390/endocrines2020007

Doi, S. A., Furuya-Kanamori, L., Toft, E., Musa, O. A., Mohamed, A. M., Clark, J., & Thalib, L. (2020). Physical activity in pregnancy prevents gestational diabetes: A meta-analysis. *Diabetes Research and Clinical Practice, 168*, 108371. https://doi.org/10.1016/j.diabres.2020.108371

Dunstan, D. W., Barr, E. L., Healy, G. N., Salmon, J., Shaw, J. E., Balkau, B., Magliano, D. J., Cameron, A. J., Zimmet, P. Z., & Owen, N. (2010). Television viewing time and mortality: The Australian diabetes, obesity and lifestyle study (AusDiab). *Circulation, 121*(3), 384–391. https://doi.org/10.1161/CIRCULATIONAHA.109.894824

Edie, R., Lacewell, A., Streisel, C., Wheeler, L., George, E., Wrigley, J., Pietrosimone, L., & Figuers, C. (2021). Barriers to exercise in postpartum women: A mixed-methods systematic review. *Journal of Women's Health Physical Therapy, 45*(2), 83–92. https://doi.org/10.1097/JWH.0000000000000201

Fazzi, C., Saunders, D. H., Linton, K., Norman, J. E., & Reynolds, R. M. (2017). Sedentary behaviours during pregnancy: A systematic review. *International Journal of Behavioral Nutrition and Physical Activity, 14*(1), 1–13. https://doi.org/10.1186/s12966-017-0485-z

Fukano, M., Tsukahara, Y., Takei, S., Nose-Ogura, S., Fujii, T., & Torii, S. (2021). Recovery of abdominal muscle thickness and contractile function in women after childbirth. *International Journal of Environmental Research and Public Health, 18*, 2130. https://doi.org/10.3390/ijerph18042130

Gaikwad, A., & Shinde, S. (2019). Postural impairments in primi-para women after one year of delivery. *International Journal of Innovative Knowledge Concepts, 7*(2), 1–7.

Garland, M., Wilbur, J., Fogg, L., Halloway, S., Braun, L., & Miller, A. (2021). Self-efficacy, outcome expectations, group social support, and adherence to physical activity in African American women. *Nursing Research, 70*(4), 239–247. https://doi.org/10.1097/NNR.0000000000000516

Garland, M., Wilbur, J., Semanik, P., & Fogg, L. (2019). Correlates of physical activity during pregnancy: A systematic review with implications for evidence-based practice. *Worldviews on Evidence-Based Nursing, 16*(4), 310–318. https://doi.org/10.1111/wvn.12391

Giurgescu, C., McFarlin, B. L., Lomax, J., Craddock, C., & Albrecht, A. (2011). Racial discrimination and the black-white gap in adverse birth outcomes: A review. *Journal of Midwifery & Women's Health, 56*(4), 362–370. https://doi.org/10.1111/j.1542-2011.2011.00034.x

Goom, T., Donnelly, G., & Brockwell, E. (2019). *Returning to running postnatal -guidelines for medical, health and fitness professionals managing this population*. https://doi.org/10.13140/RG.2.2.35256.90880/2 https://www.researchgate.net/publication/335928424_Returning_to_running_postnatal_-_guidelines_for_medical_health_and_fitness_professionals_managing_this_population/link/5de13bca4585159aa453d963/download

Gordon, K., & Reed, O. (2020). The role of the pelvic floor in respiration. *Journal of Voice, 34*(2), 243–249. https://doi.org/10.1016/j.jvoice.2018.09.024

Haakstad, L. A. H., & Bø, K. (2020). The marathon of labour—Does regular exercise training influence course of labour and mode of delivery? *European Journal of Obstetrics & Gynecology and Reproductive Biology, 251*, 8–13. https://doi.org/10.1016/j.ejogrb.2020.05.014

He, K., Zhou, X., Zhu, Y., Wang, B., Fu, X., Yao, Q., Chen, H., & Wang, X. (2021). Muscle elasticity is different in individuals with diastasis rectus abdominis than healthy volunteers. *Insights into Imaging, 12*(87). https://doi.org/10.1186/s13244-021-01021-6

Hesketh, K. R., & Evenson, K. R. (2016). Prevalence of US pregnant women meeting 2015 ACOG physical activity guidelines. *American Journal of Preventive Medicine, 51*(3), e87–e89. https://doi.org/10.1016/j.amepre.2016.05.023

Hrvatin, I., & Rugelj, D. (2021). Risk factors for accidental falls during pregnancy—A systematic literature review. *The Journal of Maternal-Fetal & Neonatal Medicine*, 1–10. https://doi.org/10.1080/14767058.2021.1935849

Hu, F. B., Li, T. Y., Colditz, G. A., Willett, W. C., & Manson, J. E. (2003). Television watching and other sedentary behaviors in relation to risk of obesity and type 2 diabetes mellitus in women. *JAMA, 289*(14), 1785–1791. https://doi.org/10.1001/jama.289.14.1785

Jackson, T., Bostock, E. L., Hassan, A., Greeves, J. P., Sale, C., & Elliott-Sale, K. J. (2021). *The legacy of pregnancy*. Ovid Technologies (Wolters Kluwer Health). https://doi.org/10.1249/jes.0000000000000274

Katzmarzyk, P. T., Church, T. S., Craig, C. L., & Bouchard, C. (2009). Sitting time and mortality from all causes, cardiovascular disease, and cancer. *Medicine & Science in Sports & Exercise, 41*(5), 998–1005.

Kris-Etherton, P. M., Petersen, K. S., Després, J.-P., Braun, L., de Ferranti, S. D., Furie, K. L., Lear, S. A., Lobelo, F., Morris, P. B., & Sacks, F. M. (2021). Special considerations for healthy lifestyle promotion across the life span in clinical settings: A science advisory from the American Heart Association. *Circulation, 144*(24). https://doi.org/10.1161/cir.0000000000001014

Lin, Y., Liu, Q., Liu, F., Huang, K., Li, J., Yang, X., Wang, X., Chen, J., Liu, X., Cao, J., Shen, C., Yu, L., Lu, F., Wu, X., Zhao, L., Li, Y., Hu, D., Lu, X., Huang, J., & Gu, D. (2021). Adverse associations of sedentary behavior with cancer incidence and all-cause mortality: A prospective cohort study. *Journal of Sport and Health Science, 10*(5), 560–569. https://doi.org/10.1016/j.jshs.2021.04.002

Loggins Clay, S., Griffin, M., & Averhart, W. (2018). Black/white disparities in pregnant women in the United States: An examination of risk factors associated with black/white racial identity. *Health & Social Care in the Community, 26*(5), 654–663. https://doi.org/10.1111/hsc.12565

Lupton, D., & Pedersen, S. (2016). An Australian survey of women's use of pregnancy and parenting apps. *Women and Birth: Journal of the Australian College of Midwives, 29*(4), 368–375. https://doi.org/10.1016/j.wombi.2016.01.008

MacInnis, M. J., & Gibala, M. J. (2017). Physiological adaptations to interval training and the role of exercise intensity. *The Journal of Physiology, 595*(9), 2915–2930. https://doi.org/10.1113/JP273196

Marín-Jiménez, N., Acosta-Manzano, P., Borges-Cosic, M., Baena-García, L., Coll-Risco, I., Romero-Gallardo, L., & Aparicio, V. A. (2019). Association of self-reported physical fitness with pain during pregnancy: The GESTAFIT project. *Scandinavian Journal of Medicine & Science in Sports, 29*(7), 1022–1030. https://doi.org/10.1111/sms.13426

McGee, L. D., Cignetti, C. A., Sutton, A., Harper, L., Dubose, C., & Gould, S. (2018). Exercise during pregnancy: Obstetricians' beliefs and recommendations compared to American Congress of Obstetricians and Gynecologists' 2015 guidelines. *Curēus, 10*(8), Article e3204. https://doi.org/10.7759/cureus.3204

Meander, L., Lindqvist, M., Mogren, I., Sandlund, J., West, C. E., & Domellöf, M. (2021). Physical activity and sedentary time during pregnancy and associations with maternal and fetal health outcomes: An epidemiological study. *BMC Pregnancy and Childbirth, 21*(1), 1–11. https://doi.org/10.1186/s12884-021-03627-6

Nagpal, T. S., & Mottola, M. F. (2020). Physical activity throughout pregnancy is key to preventing chronic disease. *Reproduction, 160*(5), R111–R118. https://doi.org/10.1530/REP-20-0337

Nayor, M., Shah, R. V., Miller, P. E., Blodgett, J. B., Tanguay, M., Pico, A. R., Murthy, V. L., Malhotra, R., Houstis, N. E., Deik, A., Pierce, K. A., Bullock, K., Dailey, L., Velagaleti, R. S., Moore, S. A., Ho, J. E., Baggish, A. L., Clish, C. B., Larson, M. G., . . . Lewis, G. D. (2020). Metabolic architecture of acute exercise response in middle-aged adults in the community. *Circulation, 142*(20), 1905–1924. https://doi.org/10.1161/CIRCULATIONAHA.120.050281

Pais, M., Pai, M. V., Kamath, A., Bhat, R., Bhat, P., & Joisa, G. H. (2021). A randomized controlled trial on the efficacy of integrated yoga on pregnancy outcome. *Holistic Nursing Practice, 35*(5), 273–280. https://doi.org/10.1097/HNP.0000000000000472

Petersen, J. M., Prichard, I., & Kemps, E. (2019). A comparison of physical activity mobile apps with and without existing web-based social networking platforms: Systematic review. *Journal of Medical Internet Research, 21*(8), e12687. https://doi.org/10.2196/12687

Piercy, K. L., Troiano, R. P., Ballard, R. M., Carlson, S. A., Fulton, J. E., Galuska, D. A., George, S. M. & Olson, R. D. (2018). The physical activity guidelines for Americans. *Jama, 320*(19), 2020–2028.

Poli de Araújo, M., Brito, L. G., Rossi, F., Garbiere, M., Vilela, M., & Bittencourt, V. (2020). Prevalence of female urinary incontinence in Crossfit practitioners and associated factors: An internet population-based survey. *Female Pelvic Medicine & Reconstructive Surgery, 26*(2), 97–100. https://doi.org/10.1097/SPV.0000000000000823

Prewitt-White, T., Connolly, C. P., Feito, Y., Bladek, A., Forsythe, S., Hamel, L., & McChesney, M. R. (2018). Breaking barriers: Women's experiences of CrossFit training during pregnancy. *Women in Sport & Physical Activity Journal*, 26(1), 33–42. https://doi.org/10.1123/wspaj.2017-0024

Raper, M. J., McDonald, S., Johnston, C., Isler, C., Newton, E., Kuehn, D., Collier, D., Broskey, N. T., Muldrow, A., & May, L. E. (2021). The influence of exercise during pregnancy on racial/ethnic health disparities and birth outcomes. *BMC Pregnancy and Childbirth*, 21(1). https://doi.org/10.1186/s12884-021-03717-5

Rasmussen, S. A., & Jamieson, D. J. (2020). Caring for women who are planning a pregnancy, pregnant, or postpartum during the COVID-19 pandemic. *JAMA*, 324(2), 190–191. https://doi.org/10.1001/jama.2020.8883

Reed, J. L., & Pipe, A. L. (2016). Practical approaches to prescribing physical activity and monitoring exercise intensity. *Canadian Journal of Cardiology*, 32(4), 514–522.

Rudin, L. R., Dunn, L., Lyons, K., Livingston, J., Waring, M. E., & Pescatello, L. S. (2021). Professional exercise recommendations for healthy women who are pregnant: A systematic review. *Women's Health Reports*, 2(1), 4–412. http://online.liebertpub.com/doi/10.1089/whr.2021.0077

Sandborg, J., Söderström, E., Henriksson, P., Bendtsen, M., Henström, M., Leppänen, M. H., Maddison, R., Migueles, J. H., Blomberg, M., & Löf, M. (2021). Effectiveness of a smartphone app to promote healthy weight gain, diet, and physical activity during pregnancy (HealthyMoms): Randomized controlled trial. *JMIR mHealth & uHealth*, 9(3), e26091. https://doi.org/10.2196/26091

Syamsudin, F., Wungu, C. D. K., Qurnianingsih, E., & Herawati, L. (2021). High-intensity interval training for improving maximum aerobic capacity in women with sedentary lifestyle: A systematic review and meta-analysis. *Journal of Physical Education and Sport*, 21(4), 1788–1797. https://doi.org/10.7752/jpes.2021.04226

Tian, T., Budgett, S., Smalldridge, J., Hayward, L., Stinear, J., & Kruger, J. (2017). Assessing exercises recommended for women at risk of pelvic floor disorders using multivariate statistical techniques. *International Urogynecology Journal*, 29(10), 1447–1454. https://doi.org/10.1007/s00192-017-3473-6

Tinius, R., Duchette, C., Beasley, S., Blankenship, M., & Schoenberg, N. (2021). Obstetric patients and healthcare providers' perspectives to inform mobile app design for physical activity and weight control during pregnancy and postpartum in a rural setting. *International Journal of Women's Health*, 13, 405. https://doi.org/10.2147/IJWH.S296310

Tinius, R. A., Polston, M., Bradshaw, H., Ashley, P., Greene, A., & Parker, A. N. (2021). An assessment of mobile applications designed to address physical activity during pregnancy and postpartum. *International Journal of Exercise Science*, 14(7), 382. https://doi.org/10.2147/IJWH.S296310

Varley, M., & Hunter, L. (2019). How does pelvic girdle pain impact on a woman's experience of her pregnancy and the puerperium? *Evidence Based Midwifery*, 17(2), 60–70.

Walters, C., West, S., & Nippita, T. (2018). Pelvic girdle pain in pregnancy. *The Royal Australian College of General Practitioners*, 47(7), 439–444. https://doi.org/10.31128/AJGP-01-18-4467

Wattanapisit, A., Tuangratananon, T., & Thanamee, S. (2018). Physical activity counseling in primary care and family medicine residency training: A systematic review. *BMC Medical Education*, 18(1), 159. https://doi.org/10.1186/s12909-018-1268-1

Wolpern, A. E., Bardsley, T. R., Brusseau, T. A., Byun, W., Egger, M. J., Nygaard, I. E., Wu, J., & Shaw, J. M. (2021). Physical activity in the early postpartum period in primiparous women. *Journal of Science and Medicine in Sport*, 24(11), 1149–1154. https://doi.org/10.1016/j.jsams.2021.06.009

Wright, K. S., Quinn, T. J., & Carey, G. B. (2002). Infant acceptance of breast milk after maternal exercise. *Pediatrics*, 109, 585–589. https://doi.org/10.1542/peds.109.4.585

Yeo, S., Davidge, S., Ronis, D. L., Antonakos, C. L., Hayashi, R., & O'Leary, S. (2008). A comparison of walking versus stretching exercises to reduce the incidence of preeclampsia: A randomized clinical trial. *Hypertension in Pregnancy*, 27(2), 113–130. https://doi.org/10.1080/10641950701826778

Yeo, S., & Kang, J. H. (2021). Low-intensity exercise and pregnancy outcomes: An examination in the Nurses' health study II. *Women's Health Reports*, 2(1), 389–395. https://doi.org/10.1089/whr.2021.0011

Yeo, S. A., & Logan, J. G. (2014). Preventing obesity. *Journal of Perinatal & Neonatal Nursing*, 28(1), 17–25. https://doi.org/10.1097/jpn.0000000000000000

21

Sexuality

Jenna Benyounes and Tanya Tringali

Relevant Terms

Asexual—a persistent lack of sexual attraction to others. People who identify as asexual experience romantic attraction and may engage in sexual activities

Consensual nonmonogamy—the practice of engaging in multiple concurrent sexual, intimate, and/or romantic relationships with agreement among all partners

Cognitive distraction—more commonly known as "spectatoring"; the observing and monitoring of one's behavior during sex which may distract from sexual sensations and cues

Gender identity—a person's individual experience of gender which may not be in alignment with their sex assigned at birth

PLISSIT model—Permission, Limited Information, Specific Suggestions, Intensive Therapy. A framework to aid clinicians in introducing and creating a safe space for discussion, narrowing the client's concern, and offering counseling or treatment

Polyamory—desiring or engaging in more than one romantic relationship

Sexual orientation—emotional, romantic, and/or sexual attraction to other people

Spontaneous desire—desire that is present without being provoked

Responsive desire—there is a cue or cues that lead to an increase in desires. It is influenced by context, society, and culture

Biopsychosocial approach—approach to care that considers the biological, psychological, and social factors that influence clients

---

Introduction

Sexual health is sometimes referred to as another vital sign as it may provide insight into one's overall health status (Kingsberg et al., 2019). Unfortunately, clinicians and clients often avoid addressing sexual health issues due to social taboos, stigma, shame, embarrassment, and misconceptions associated with sex (Table 21.1). Avoiding these conversations perpetuates the myth that concerns, such as a lack of interest in sex or painful penetration, are not modifiable. Likewise, when a client has a negative experience discussing sexual health with a healthcare provider, it can contribute to a perception that the provider believes sexuality is unimportant or that they do not value their client's experiences (Kingsberg et al., 2019). When surveyed, two-thirds of healthcare providers stated that they routinely ask about sexual activity but only 40% ask about concerns and 29% about satisfaction (Sobecki et al., 2012).

Current studies indicate that approximately half of all women suffer from sexual dysfunction at some point in their lives (Yeniel & Petri, 2014). The frequency among pregnant women in the United States ranges from 31% to 58% (Vannier & Rosen, 2017). An improved understanding of sexuality through the lifespan, comfort with the topic, communication skills, and knowledge regarding treatment options is needed to better serve clients. This chapter provides an overview of human sexuality, as the field of study has evolved over the past century, and defines the various types of sexual dysfunctions. The primary focus is on sexuality in the perinatal period with the goal of providing clinicians with insights into common questions, concerns, and experiences of pregnant and postpartum people. The goal of this chapter is to assist clinicians in supporting clients who are experiencing the unique physical and psychological issues that commonly contribute to or exacerbate sexual dysfunctions during this life stage.

Finally, it is important to note that commonly used diagnoses in sexual health include the designation "female" and "male." However, these diagnoses can be used for all people and should be used to describe a person's current anatomy rather than that assigned at birth (APA, 2022).

Prenatal and Postnatal Care: A Person-Centered Approach, Third Edition. Edited by Karen Trister Grace, Cindy L. Farley, Noelene K. Jeffers, and Tanya Tringali.
© 2024 John Wiley & Sons Ltd. Published 2024 by John Wiley & Sons Ltd.
Companion website: www.wiley.com/go/grace/prenatal

Table 21.1 Barriers to Effective Sexual Healthcare

Patient	Provider
Social stigma	Time constraints
Fear of broaching the subject	Lack of training about
Low awareness of conditions and/or available treatments	diagnostic tools and treatment options
Misperceptions about treatments	Costs, coverage, and regulatory issues

Source: Adapted from Kingsberg et al. (2019).

Health equity key points

- Black, brown, and LGBTQI+ people are underrepresented in sexuality and sexual dysfunction literature.
- A lack of knowledge and personal biases affect the frequency and ways in which clinicians engage in discussions of sexual health with their clients.
- Treatment for sexual health problems can be cost prohibitive for many clients.

Historical Context

The early twentieth century ushered in a new era of groundbreaking research and interest in the field of sexology. In the 1920s, Katherine Davis (1929) published research on "normal" female sexuality. She surveyed both married and unmarried women and explored sexual practices and experiences previously not discussed in the literature. Maslow's (1943) hierarchy of needs, a motivational theory (Figure 21.1), mentions sex twice: first, in the physiological needs tier for procreation and again in the love/belonging tier as sexual intimacy. Alfred Kinsey founded the Institute for Sex Research in 1947 and wrote the best sellers, *Sexual Behavior in the Human Male* and *Sexual Behavior in the Human Female* (Indiana University, 2020a). These researchers paved the way for Masters and Johnson's work in the 1960–1970s on human four-stage model of sexual response (excitement, plateau, orgasm, and resolution) with the addition of desire as the first stage in the linear model in 1977.

While the study of human sexuality has led to greater bodily autonomy, access to contraception, and the decriminalization of the same sex relationships, it is not without its shameful contributions to racist injustice, including the promotion of eugenicist ideas and forced sterilizations (Cullen & Gotell, 2002). Like much of the research of these earlier years, the knowledge gained was based on the lived experiences of White, middle-class Americans while systematically excluding Black and poor or working-class people (Cullen & Gotell, 2002).

Human Sexuality

Sexuality exists along a spectrum, including **gender identity** and **sexual orientation**, and is commonly referred to as being **fluid**, or having the potential to change over time. This term describes both expression and identity and acknowledges that sexuality is not a choice, a static state, or binary.

Romantic attraction and relationship styles also exist along a continuum. A person who identifies as **asexual** may experience romantic attraction to one or both sexes and may or may not remain celibate (Herbitter et al., 2021). On the other end of the spectrum, one in five people reports ever having practiced some form of **consensual nonmonogamy** and may identify as polyamorous or report being in an open relationship (Herbitter et al., 2021).

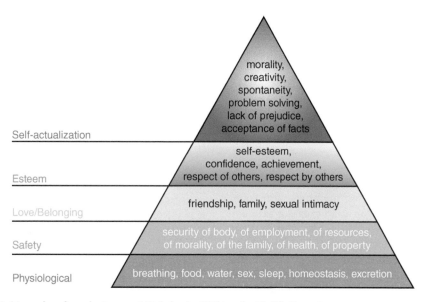

Figure 21.1 Maslow's hierarchy of needs. Source: J. Finkelstein / Wikipedia / Public Domain.

Taking a Sexual History in the Perinatal Period

The perinatal period presents unique challenges and opportunities for clients and their partners. It is a time of frequent healthcare visits and an optimal time to discuss sexual health concerns. Screening for sexual health concerns should occur at routine visits to identify issues while also destigmatizing the discussion of sexual health (Kingsburg et al., 2019). Taking a sexual history allows providers an opportunity to assess their client's comfortability with the topic and provides insights into how they experience their own sexuality. While not all clients will feel comfortable discussing this the first time they are asked, being thorough and revisiting this topic periodically sets the stage for open and honest conversations as pregnancy progresses and into the postpartum period.

A thorough sexual history should be included at the initial prenatal visit or upon transfer of care. For existing clients, the initial prenatal visit is a time to review their sexual history in the same manner that it should be reviewed at each annual exam. It is important to avoid assumptions about gender, sexual orientation, or relationship style and to give clients the opportunity to discuss any changes in sexual function that may have occurred since their previous visit. The elements of a sexual history remain the same regardless of pregnancy. To learn more about taking a sexual history, see *Resources for Healthcare Providers*.

Elements of a sexual history

CDC's 5 Ps + 3

5 Ps
Partners
Practices
Pregnancy intention
Protection from STIs
Past STIs

Plus 3
Pain
Pleasure
Past or present trauma

Source: Adapted from CDC (2022).

Trauma-informed sexual healthcare begins before the client enters the exam room. All the interactions with staff can impact one's experience and openness. This begins with knowing how the clients would like to be addressed and their pronouns. Providing staff members with training in trauma-informed care can help create a safe and comfortable environment. To begin the conversation about sexual health, introduce the topic, explain why the questions are important, and obtain consent to continue discussing sexual health. Typically, more personal questions are completed later in the visit after a rapport has been established.

Examples of how to start the conversation

If it is ok with you, I am going to ask you some questions about your sexual health and sexual practices. I ask these questions of all my patients because these questions are as important as the questions about other areas of your physical and mental health.

I am going to ask you some questions about your sexual health that I ask all my patients. I understand that these questions are personal but they are important for your overall health which is why I ask. Like the rest of our visits, this information is kept in strict confidence unless you or someone else is being hurt or is in danger.

Source: Adapted from CDC (2022).

Even when they do not have overt sexual disorders, clients commonly have questions and concerns, particularly in the perinatal period. However, owing to a lack of time, education, and training, clinicians may not always know how to start the conversation or how best to respond to questions. This is not a reason to skip these questions as many clients express that they want clinicians to initiate the conversation. In some instances, clinicians have the knowledge but need more time with clients, while in others, their knowledge or skillset is not robust. The International Society for the Study of Women's Sexual Health (ISSWSH) created a four-step model for addressing sexual health concerns to aid clinicians who are not sexual health experts meet the expectation that universal screening for sexual concerns be incorporated into routine care and to help guide further assessment and treatment (Parish et al., 2019).

ISSWSH four-step model for addressing sexual health concerns

Step 1: Elicit the story
Create space and time for the clients to tell their story and to explain how the concern is impacting them. This allows the clinician to ask questions, preferably open-ended ones, clarify concepts with the client, and assess the magnitude of distress.

Step 2: Name and reframe
Validate the importance of their sexual concern rather than simply offer a diagnosis. Clinicians should be aware that sometimes, the concern initially shared with staff at the time of scheduling is not the actual concern. When this occurs, the clinician can say "it seems to me that in addition to your <initial complaint>, what you've told me about your <sexual concern> is just as painful, important, and worthy of attention." For the client, this demonstrates to them that the clinician sees the concern and the importance of it, thus creating a therapeutic space.

Step 3: Empathetic witnessing
While it may seem small, this is the first step in treatment for clients. Empathetic witnessing is hearing what the client has

experienced and commending them for what they have done to address their concern.

Step 4: Referral for assessment and treatment

This final step offers two possible pathways based upon on the clinician's ability to evaluate and treat. When the clinician does not have the training or knowledge to thoroughly address the clients' concern, the recommendation is to refer them to a sexual health specialist (Parish et al., 2019). Clients with sexual health concerns commonly see multiple clinicians without obtaining proper treatment or a resolution to their problem. To prevent the client from feeling hopeless when referring a client to another, more knowledgeable provider, language is important. A formula that can be utilized is to first acknowledge the importance of the concern and then inform the client that their concern would be better addressed by a specialist. Example: "*The painful penetration you are experiencing is real and not in your head. This is impacting your life in big ways so a clinician who specializes and knows how to treat this is what you deserve. I want you to get the best care so I'd like to refer you to Sally who has treated many of my patients with similar concerns.*"

***In other instances, clinicians have the knowledge to evaluate and treat the client but may not have time that day. Start by acknowledging the importance of the concern. Let the client know that it deserves more time and how they should follow up. Example: "*I'm so glad you told me about the pain you are experiencing. This discussion deserves more time than we have today, so I'd like you to come back Friday for a longer appointment, so we have plenty of time to address your concern.*"

Source: Adapted from Parish et al. (2019).

The **Permission, Limited Information, Specific Suggestions, Intensive Therapy (PLISSIT) model** (Table 21.2) is another framework that aids clinicians in discussing sexual health concerns, creating a safe space, narrowing the client's concern, and offering counseling or treatment. The goal is not necessarily to develop a diagnosis and treatment plan but to be able to listen carefully and provide the support they need and refer out when indicated (Annon, 1976).

Table 21.2   PLISSIT Model

PLISSIT model	Examples
P: Permission	"Many clients I see have concerns about sexual health, do you have any concerns or questions that you would like to discuss?"
LI: Limited information	"Using a lubricant with sex can make it more comfortable."
SS: Specific suggestions	"I would recommend a water-based lubricant since that will be safe with the dilator kit you are using."
IT: Intensive Therapy	That is, referral to a specialist (sex therapist, pelvic floor physical therapist, sexual health practitioner, etc.)

Source: Adapted from Annon (1976).

Sexual Response

Clinicians and clients alike should understand the sexual response cycle as this knowledge can prove extremely helpful for couples as they navigate common challenges that arise in the perinatal period. While these models are not intended to explain the nuances of pregnancy or the postpartum period, understanding the range of normal human sexuality is key and may help couples better understand the changes that are occurring.

Linear Sexual Response Models

The four-stage model of human sexual response was developed by Masters and Johnson in 1966. In their research, they noted four distinct phases that occurred in order and are, thus, described as "linear." These phases were identified by recording the physiologic responses of 10,000 participants (Rowland & Gutierrez, 2017). They include excitement, plateau, orgasm, and resolution, occurring one after the other, thus, "linear." In 1979, Helen Singer Kaplan added "desire" as the starting point of her linear model (Rowland & Gutierrez, 2017).

Linear models, while novel in their time, imply that sexual response is spontaneous, do not account for the often more complex patterns that describe female sexual response, and do not acknowledge psychology, relational, and other contexts (Rowland & Gutierrez, 2017) that can alter sexual responses in individuals.

Basson Model

The Basson Model was created in 2005 to address the fact that linear models do not always apply to female sexuality. It was also one of the first models to not focus on orgasm as an outcome and incorporated emotional satisfaction that can be an outcome and motivator for intimacy or sex (Basson et al., 2001). This model highlights two ways people can experience desire: **spontaneous** and **responsive**.

Dual Control Model

The dual control model posits that there are physiologic and psychological factors that either inhibit or excite sexual response (Indiana University, 2020b). The imbalance between the two is what creates the motivation or inhibition of sex. When inhibitions are higher than excitement, hypoactive sexual desire may occur. The dual control model is a clinically helpful framework that utilizes a **biopsychosocial approach** in the assessment and treatment of clients with sexual dysfunction(s). Nagoski (2021) explains the dual control model using the analogy of the gas (excitatory) and brake (inhibitory) pedals of a car. Clinicians and clients can use it to determine if they need less inhibition, more excitement or both.

Clinicians have a responsibility to assess, diagnose, and treat gynecological conditions that may be contributing to pain but must also be willing to inquire about the impact that decreased sexual functioning may have on their client's relationships and quality of life and how fear and anxiety may impact sexual functioning, and to provide simple advice (i.e., use of lubricants and position changes).

Sexual Dysfunctions

The Diagnostic and Statistical Manual of Mental Health Disorders, 5th edition text revision, offers four possible diagnoses for female sexual dysfunction, including sexual interest arousal disorder, orgasmic disorder, genitopelvic pain/penetration disorder, and substance/medication-induced sexual dysfunction (APA, 2022). More research is needed to better understand sexual dysfunction in gender fluid and trans people (APA, 2022). Except for substance/medication-induced disorder, symptoms need to be present for six months or more and lead to personal distress in order to diagnose dysfunction. Other causes, such as nonsexual mental health disorder (a medical condition), severe relationship distress, and other significant life stressors, need to be ruled out. Multiple diagnoses of sexual dysfunction can be present simultaneously.

Genitopelvic pain/penetration disorder also includes vulvodynia, dyspareunia, and vaginismus, three distinct diagnoses that usually have a physiologic origin that can be treated if the underlying pathology is identified. Many clients with genitopelvic pain/penetration disorder develop anxiety secondary to the pain that they are experiencing. If clinicians are unable to find the underlying cause(s), they should refer to specialists that can be identified through the ISSWSH, the International Pelvic Pain Society, and the National Vulvodynia Association. A comprehensive team includes the client, a clinician (nurse practitioner, midwife, physician or physician's assistant), a pelvic floor physical therapist (PFPT), and a counselor/therapist (Dias-Amaral & Marques-Pinto, 2018; Parish et al., 2019). Clinicians can also choose to obtain additional training and learn to evaluate and treat these conditions themselves.

Diagnoses associated with painful sex

Vulvodynia—umbrella term for pain of the vulva; this diagnosis requires a detailed evaluation to determine the underlying cause of the pain

Dyspareunia—painful penetration

Vaginismus—involuntary guarding, contracting, or clenching of the pelvic floor, especially with attempts at penetration

---

Sexuality during Pregnancy

Pregnancy is a season in life full of change, physically, hormonally, psychologically, and socially, all of which can alter how people feel about themselves as sexual beings. Some studies have shown pregnancy to be associated with more negative body image, while others have shown it to be protective, a time where people embrace their changing bodies and selves (Pascoal et al., 2019). For many, sexual frequency decreases as gestation increases. One study, including 237 women (54% White and 46% Black), showed an 18% decrease per week from conception to 11 weeks of gestation followed by a 3% increase each week

---

Diagnostic criteria for sexual dysfunction

Sexual interest arousal disorder

Lack of, or significantly reduced, sexual interest/arousal, as manifested by at least three of the following:

- Absent/reduced interest in sexual activity
- Absent/reduced sexual/erotic thoughts or fantasies
- No/reduced initiation of sexual activity and typically unreceptive to a partner's attempts to initiate
- Absent/reduced sexual excitement/pleasure during sexual activity in almost all or all (approximately 75–100%) sexual encounters
- Absent/reduced sexual interest/arousal in response to any internal or external sexual/erotic cues (e.g., written, verbal, and visual)
- Absent/reduced genital or nongenital sensations during sexual activity in almost all or all (approximately 75–100%) sexual encounters

Orgasmic disorder

- Delayed, infrequent, or absent orgasm or markedly decreased intensity of orgasm after a normal sexual arousal phase on all or almost all occasions of sexual activity

Genitopelvic pain/penetration disorder

- Persistent or recurrent difficulties with one or more of the following:
  - Vaginal penetration during intercourse
  - Vulvovaginal or pelvic pain during vaginal intercourse or attempts at penetration
  - Fear or anxiety about vulvovaginal or pelvic pain in anticipation of, during, or as a result of vaginal penetration
  - Tightening or tensing of the pelvic floor muscles during attempted vaginal penetration

Substance/medication-induced sexual dysfunction

- Occurs secondary to the use of substances or medications.

Source: APA (2022) and Rothblum et al. (2020).

until 21 weeks and finally a 6% decrease per week that continued until the birth (Blumenstock & Barber, 2022).

A recent prospective longitudinal study, one of the first of its kind, showed that sexual problems (i.e., interest, arousal, orgasm, lubrication, and dissatisfaction) increase during pregnancy and remain elevated for the first few months postpartum before declining again and may be more common in people experiencing comorbid anxiety and depressive symptoms (Asselmann et al., 2016). The frequency of sexual problems also increased between study points, which occurred at 22–24 weeks of gestation until 4 months postpartum and then decreased again between 4 and 16 months postpartum.

Research has shown that as many as one in five women experiences pain with vaginal intercourse, and the majority do not seek treatment (Rossi et al., 2019); specifically, only 29–46% of pregnant women have discussed sexual activity with their healthcare providers (Rossi et al., 2019). Genitopelvic pain can begin before pregnancy and can be related to a preexisting physical pathology. It can also present for the first time during pregnancy as a result of edema, varicosities, or muscular and connective tissue changes. Pain is complex and can be caused by neurological (i.e., previous physical injuries and unknown causes) and psychological conditions, such as depression or fear of harming the pregnancy. In some cases, pain that begins during pregnancy will resolve on its own without intervention, but for others, pain can persist well into the postpartum period (Rossi et al., 2019). Some may avoid sex all together as a means of avoiding the potential for experiencing pain.

Unlike a reduced desire to engage in sexual activity as gestation advances, pain with sexual activity should not be considered normal. Clinicians should consider the possible reasons for genitopelvic pain and should be prepared to discuss them with clients. This includes the effects on sexual function related to perinatal mood and anxiety disorders, relationship issues, body dissatisfaction, and **cognitive distraction** (Pascoal et al., 2019). Genitopelvic pain during pregnancy is a risk factor for postpartum genitopelvic pain and depression (Rossi et al., 2019). One of the most common concerns people have about birth is regarding potential effects on sexual function. Some people express desire for planned cesarean births in an effort to preserve sexual function, though there is a lack of evidence and conflicting results in this area (Spiach et al., 2020). A study of 522 women showed that sexual function declined significantly at three and six months postpartum but recovered close to prepregnancy levels for all the participants regardless of the mode of delivery (Spaich et al., 2020). This study also found that breastfeeding can have a negative effect on sexual function, and participants who anticipated negative effects were more likely to experience them.

Genitopelvic pain can be a significant source of distress. Clinicians should be aware that some people will become pregnant without engaging in penetrative intercourse via ejaculate deposited on the vulva or may request intrauterine insemination due to genitopelvic pain. Likewise, some people with this symptom will benefit from an epidural during labor and birth to help them avoid dissociation and be present for the birth of their baby.

With the pregnant person's explicit permission, partners should be included in discussions about sexuality in pregnancy because they may also have sexual concerns. For example, they may fear harming the fetus by engaging in penetrative sex during pregnancy. Reviewing anatomy can be reassuring. Providing advice on sexual positions that may be more comfortable for the pregnant person should be offered as well as suggestions such as the importance of viewing what is considered sex more broadly, i.e., alternatives to penetrative sex. People who have experienced vaginal bleeding following intercourse during pregnancy, or who fear causing vaginal bleeding or other symptoms, may also avoid sex. In the first trimester alone, as many as 25% of people experience vaginal bleeding, though the connection between early pregnancy bleeding and miscarriage is not established (Hasan et al., 2010). Clinicians should review physiologic changes of pregnancy that contribute to bleeding, evaluate clients promptly when bleeding occurs, and provide reassurance when appropriate.

Wondering if one's feelings and experiences are normal is a common concern. It is the responsibility of healthcare providers to engage clients in discussions that normalize common experiences for pregnant people and their partners. This can play a crucial role in their understanding of human sexuality during this transformative time. Anticipatory guidance regarding pregnancy-related discomforts during sex and information regarding effective treatments may help clients feel comfortable bringing concerns to their providers' attention.

Sexuality in the Postpartum Period

Postpartum people and their partners frequently are concerned about how to safely resume sexual activity, how to avoid pregnancy, changes in body image, and sexual desire. Sexual concerns and decreased intimacy contribute to a decline in relationship satisfaction. Both are common in the postpartum period, further highlighting the importance of early intervention, a more active role, and proactive approaches to sexual healthcare in the perinatal period (Schlagintweit et al., 2016).

Most common postpartum sexual concerns of new parents

- Frequency of sexual intercourse
- When to resume sexual intercourse (safely and comfortably)
- Impact of changes to birthing parent's body image
- Impact of sleep deprivation and breastfeeding on sexual desire
- Physical recovery from childbirth

Source: Adapted from Schlagintweit et al. (2016).

Table 21.3 Strategies for Reestablishing Intimacy in Romantic Relationships in the Postpartum Period

- Open and honest communication about fears and barriers *ex: fear of pain or exhaustion*
- Discuss taking certain sexual acts "off the table" *ex: No touching of breasts or no vaginal penetration*
- Nonsexual touch *ex: Holding hands, hugging, slow dancing*
- Be patient with yourself/your partner. *ex: Waiting for desire, arousal and explicit permission to take the next step*
- Discuss mutual physical, emotional, and relational needs *ex: Feeling seen, appreciated, attractive, helping with household responsibilities*

Clients may be apprehensive about having intercourse for the first time after the birth of a baby, regardless of when they choose to resume sexual activity. It may be helpful to offer strategies to reengage in intimacy without feeling pressured to have intercourse (Table 21.3). Common causes of pain and discomfort in the postpartum period include postpartum atrophic vaginitis and vaginal dryness caused by low estrogen levels in breastfeeding people, scar tissue from lacerations and episiotomies, pelvic organ prolapse, and various other pelvic floor dysfunctions. These conditions can be effectively treated. Anticipatory guidance should be provided on what to expect when resuming sexual activity and instructions to call the provider if pain or discomfort persists after the first few attempts at resuming sexual activity or with experience of severe pain at any point.

Screening Tools

Written questionnaires can be used clinically to screen clients for sexual concerns or dysfunction as well as evaluate the effects of treatment. While verbal follow-up discussion is encouraged, questionnaires can be used for preappointment screening or as adjunct to clinical conversations.

Female Sexual Function Index

The Female Sexual Function Index (FSFI) is a 19-question questionnaire to evaluate six different components of female sexual dysfunction, including desire, arousal, lubrication, orgasm, satisfaction, and pain (Rosen et al., 2000). The FSFI has been cross validated for use in multiple languages, in adolescence through menopause, and during pregnancy, in those with more than one sexual dysfunction diagnosis, and chronic medical issues (Rehman et al., 2015).

Female Sexual Distress Scale-Revised

The Female Sexual Distress Scale-Revised (FSDS-R) is used to help providers determine if a client meets criteria according to the DSM V for sexual dysfunction. The FSDS measures distress experienced as a result of sexual dysfunction (DeRogatis et al., 2008).

Brief Sexual Symptom Checklist for Women

While not a validated tool, the Brief Sexual Symptom Checklist for Women (BSSC-W) is a quick and easy screening tool that was created by the International Consultation in Sexual Medicine. It starts with the initial question, "Are you satisfied with your sexual function?" If the client answers yes, screening is completed. If they answer no, there are 11 more questions about what is dissatisfying, how bothersome the symptoms are, and if the patients are interested in discussing it with their provider (Dawson et al., 2017).

Evaluation and Treatment

A thorough evaluation starts with a physical examination to identify underlying causes (Table 21.4). While all sexual and reproductive health providers can diagnose and treat these conditions, PFPTs are trained to treat the physical manifestations, including pain or lack of sensation. People suffering from sexual dysfunction can have underlying mental health conditions or may have experienced abuse or trauma. Cognitive behavioral therapists and sex therapists are an equally important part of the team, each playing a unique role in helping people achieve higher levels of sexual functioning and satisfaction. Referral to these specialists is an important component of prenatal and postnatal care.

Laboratory testing, microscopy, and imaging can be useful in the diagnosis of underlying gynecological etiology, but once that is ruled out, such testing is rarely needed. There are some medications available to treat low libido and even genitopelvic pain, but most are contraindicated in pregnancy and breastfeeding.

Availability and receipt of sexual health education varies greatly by race, gender identity, and sexual orientation. In a qualitative study of Black women's concerns with sexual and reproductive health services by Thompson et al. (2022), many participants felt that they did not receive sexual health information that was relevant to their lives, fewer resources were offered, and more of their care was provided by trainees. People of color are underrepresented in sexual health research, although organizations and researchers have begun addressing this. LGBTQI+ people experience heightened risk of sexual violence and yet experience more barriers to healthcare. Clinicians must identify and address their own biases and avoid assumptions about their clients' gender, sexuality, relationship status, and style and consider literacy and numeracy in every interaction.

Table 21.4 Underlying Gynecological Causes of Sexual Dysfunction

- Sexually Transmitted Infections
- Recurrent vaginitis (yeast and bacterial vaginosis)
- Scar tissue (perineal lacerations, episiotomies, and cesarean sections)
- Pelvic organ prolapse
- Atrophic vaginitis (related to low estrogen levels in breastfeeding people)
- Medications
- Vaginismus
- Endometriosis
- Ovarian cysts
- Uterine fibroids

Finally, access to care and to insurance coverage can present barriers to sexual healthcare. Billing codes are not always applicable for sexual health problems, which can impact third-party reimbursement. Because sexual health is multifactorial, longer and more frequent visits are often needed, but not always reimbursed. Specialists in sexual health may be out of network or may have long waitlists (Mettenbrink et al., 2015).

Summary

Primary care clinicians, including nurse practitioners and midwives, who engage in long-term relationships with their clients should use standardized sexual health screening tools and discussion techniques, such as the PLISSIT model, which can help clinicians start the conversation. However, some clinicians will benefit from engaging in continuing education to improve comfort with and knowledge about sexual health. The use of communication skills and strategies, including shared decision-making, open-ended questions, greeting clients while they are still fully dressed, sitting at eye level with clients, expressing empathy, and being nonjudgmental, is essential to legitimizing the client's experience and building trust.

Resources for Clients

Books

Casperson, K. J. (2022). *You are not broken: Stop "shoulding" all over your sex life*. YANB Media.

Foley, S., Kope, S. A., & Sugrue, D. P. (2012). *Sex matters for women: A complete guide to taking care of your sexual self*, 2nd ed. Guilford Press.

Goldstein, A., Pukall, C. F., & Goldstein, I. (2011). *When sex hurts: A woman's guide to banishing sexual pain*. Da Capo Press.

Mintz, L. B. (2018). *Becoming cliterate: Why orgasm equality matters–and how to get it*. HarperOne, an imprint of HarperCollins Publishers.

Nagoski, E. (2021). *Come as you are: The surprising new science that will transform your sex life*. Simon and Schuster Paperbacks.

Websites

International Society for the Study of Women's Sexual Health https://www.isswsh.org

National Vulvodynia Association https://www.nva.org

Resources for Clinicians

American Association of Sexuality Educators, Counselors and Therapists (ASSECT) https://www.aasect.org

International Society for the Study of Women's Sexual Health (ISSWSH) https://www.isswsh.org

International Society of Sexual Medicine (ISSM) https://www.issm.info

International Pelvic Pain Society (IPPS) https://www.pelvicpain.org

International Society for the Study of Vulvovaginal Disease (ISSVD) https://www.issvd.org

Klein Sexual Orientation Grid (online tool) https://bi.org/en/klein-grid

Moscrop A. (2012). Can sex during pregnancy cause a miscarriage? A concise history of not knowing. *The British journal of general practice: the journal of the Royal College of General Practitioners, 62*(597), e308–e310. https://doi.org/10.3399/bjgp12X636164

Sexuality Training Institute – offers training in which clinicians are encouraged to challenge their own assumptions, beliefs, and feelings about human sexuality through exposure to group discussions and media images https://www.sexualitytraininginstitute.org/live-sexual-attitude-reassessment

The Guttmacher Institute https://www.guttmacher.org

References

American Psychiatric Association (APA). (2022). *Diagnostic and statistical manual of mental disorders* (5th ed., text revision). American Psychiatric Association Publishing. https://doi.org/10.1176/appi.books.9780890425787

Annon, J. S. (1976). The PLISSIT model: A proposed conceptual scheme for the behavioral treatment of sexual problems. *Journal of Sex Education and Therapy, 2*(1), 1–15.

Asselmann, E., Hoyer, J., Wittchen, H., & Martini, J. (2016). Sexual problems during pregnancy and after delivery among women with and without anxiety and depressive disorders prior to pregnancy: A prospective longitudinal study. *The Journal of Sexual Medicine, 13*, 95–104. https://doi.org/10.1016/j.jsxm.2015.12.005

Basson, R., Berman, J., Burnett, A., Derogatis, L., Ferguson, D., Fourcroy, J., et al. (2001). Report of the international consensus development conference on female sexual dysfunction: Definitions and classifications. *Journal of Sex and Marital Therapy, 27*(2), 83–94. https://doi.org/10.5603/GP.2020.0062

Blumenstock, S., & Barber, J. (2022). Sexual intercourse frequency during pregnancy: Weekly surveys among 237 women from a random population-based sample. *The Journal of Sexual Medicine, 19*(10), 1–12. https://doi.org/10.1016/j.jsxm.2022.07.006

Centers for Disease Control and Prevention. (2022). *A guide to taking a sexual history*. https://www.cdc.gov/std/treatment/SexualHistory.htm

Cullen, D., & Gotell, L. (2002). From orgasms to organizations: Maslow, women's sexuality, and the gendered foundations of the needs hierarchy. *Gender, Work and Organization, 9*(5), 537–555. https://doi.org/10.1111/1468-0432.00174

Davis, K. B. (1929). *Factors in the sex life of twenty-two hundred women*. Harper & Brothers. https://wellcomecollection.org/works/ym92nz52/items?canvas=9

Dawson, M. L., Shah, N. M., Rinko, R. C., Veselis, C., & Whitmore, K. E. (2017). The evaluation and management of female sexual dysfunction: Patients often fail to bring it up, and physicians may be reluctant to discuss it, but ignoring sexual dysfunction can disrupt a woman's most intimate relationships. *Journal of Family Practice, 66*(12), 722–729.

DeRogatis, L., Clayton, A., Lewis-D'Agostino, D., Wunderlich, G., & Fu, Y. (2008). Validation of the female sexual distress scale-revised for assessing distress in women with hypoactive sexual desire disorder. *The Journal of Sexual Medicine, 5*(2), 357–364.

Dias-Amaral, A., & Marques-Pinto, A. (2018). Female genito-pelvic pain/penetration disorder: Review of the related factors and overall approach. *Revista Brasileira de Ginecologia e Obstetrícia, 40*, 787–793.

Hasan, R., Baird, D. D., Herring, A. H., Olshan, A. F., Jonsson Funk, M. L., & Hartmann, K. E. (2010). Patterns and predictors of vaginal bleeding in the first trimester of pregnancy. *Annals of Epidemiology, 20*(7), 524–531. https://doi.org/10.1016/j.annepidem.2010.02.006

Herbitter, C., Vaughan, M., & Pantalone, D. (2021). Mental health provider bias and clinical competence in addressing asexuality, consensual non-monogamy, and BDSM: A narrative review. *Sexual and Relationship Therapy*, 1-24. https://doi.org/10.1080/14681994.2021.1969547

Indiana University. (2020a). *Learn our history*. Kinsey Institute. https://kinseyinstitute.org/about/history/index.php

Indiana University. (2020b). *The dual control model of sexual response*. Kinsey Institute. https://kinseyinstitute.org/research/dual-control-model.php

Kingsberg, S. A., Schaffir, J., Faught, B. M., Pinkerton, J. V., Parish, S. J., Iglesia, C. B., Gudeman, J., Krop, J., & Simon, J. A. (2019). Female sexual health: Barriers to optimal outcomes and a roadmap for improved patient-clinician communications. *Journal of Women's Health*, 28(4), 432–443. https://doi.org/10.1089/jwh.2018.7352

Maslow, A. H. (1943). A theory of human motivation. *Psychological Review*, 50(4), 430–437.

Mettenbrink, C., Al-Tayyib, A., Eggert, J., & Thrun, M. (2015). Assessing the changing landscape of sexual health clinical service after the implementation of the Affordable Care Act. *Sexually Transmitted Diseases*, 42(12), 725–730.

Nagoski, E. (2021). *Come As You Are: The Surprising New Science that Will Transform Your Sex Life*. Simon and Schuster Paperbacks.

Parish, S. J., Hahn, S. R., Goldstein, S. W., Giraldi, A., Kingsberg, S. A., Larkin, L., Minkin, M. J., Brown, V., Christien, K., Hartzell-Cushanick, R., Kelly-Jones, A., Rullo, J., Sadovsky, R., & Faubion, S. S. (2019). The International Society for the Study of Women's sexual health process of care for the identification of sexual concerns and problems in women. *Mayo Clinic Proceedings*, 94(5), 842–856. Elsevier. https://doi.org/10.1016/j.mayocp.2019.01.009

Pascoal, P., Rosa, P., & Coelho, S. (2019). Does pregnancy play a role? Association of body dissatisfaction, body appearance, cognitive distraction, and sexual distress. *The Journal of Sexual Medicine*, 16, 551–558. https://doi.org/10.1016/j.jsxm.2019.01.317

Rehman, K. U., Asif Mahmood, M., Sheikh, S. S., Sultan, T., & Khan, M. A. (2015). The female sexual function index (FSFI): Translation, validation, and cross-cultural adaptation of an Urdu version "FSFI-U". *Sexual Medicine*, 3(4), 244–250. https://doi.org/10.1002/sm2.77

Rosen, R., Brown, C., Heiman, J., Leiblum, S., Meston, C., Shabsigh, R., Ferguson, D., & D'Agostino, R., Jr. (2000). The female sexual function index (FSFI): A multidimensional self-report instrument for the assessment of female sexual function. *Journal of Sex & Marital Therapy*, 26(2), 191–208. https://doi.org/10.1080/009262300278597

Rossi, M., Mooney, K., Binik, Y., & Rosen, N. (2019). A descriptive and longitudinal analysis of pain during intercourse in pregnancy. *The Journal of Sexual Medicine*, 16, 1996–1977. https://doi.org/10.1016/j.jsxm.2019.09.011

Rothblum, E. D., Krueger, E. A., Kittle, K. R., & Meyer, I. H. (2020). Asexual and non-asexual respondents from a US population-based study of sexual minorities. *Archives of Sexual Behavior*, 49(2), 757–767.

Rowland, D., & Gutierrez, B. R. (2017). Phases of sexual response cycle. *Psychology Faculty Publications*, 62. https://scholar.valpo.edu/psych_fac_pub/62

Schlagintweit, H., Bailey, K., & Rosen, N. (2016). A new baby in the bedroom: Frequency and severity of sexual concerns and their associations with relationship satisfaction in new parent couples. *The Journal of Sexual Medicine*, 13, 1455–1465. https://doi.org/10.1016/j.jsxm.2016.08.006

Sobecki, J. N., Curlin, F. A., Rasinski, K. A., & Lindau, S. T. (2012). What we don't talk about when we don't talk about sex: Results of a national survey of U.S. obstetricians/gynecologists. *The Journal of Sexual Medicine*, 9, 1285–1294. https://doi.org/10.1111/j.1743-6109.2012.02702.x

Spiach, S., Link, G., Ortiz Alvarez, S., Weiss, C., Sutterlin, M., Tuschy, B., & Berlit, S. (2020). Influence of peripartum expectations, mode of delivery, and perineal injury on women's postpartum sexuality. *The Journal of Sexual Medicine*, 17, 1312–1325. https://doi.org/10.1016/j.jsxm.2020.04.383

Thompson, T. M., Young, Y., Bass, T. M., Baker, M. S., Njoku, O., Norwood, J., & Simpson, M. (2022). Racism runs through it: Examining the sexual and reproductive health experience of black women in the south. *Health Affairs*, 41(2), 195–202. https://doi.org/10.1377/hlthaff.2021.01422

Vannier, S. A., & Rosen, N. O. (2017). Sexual distress and sexual problems during pregnancy: Associations with sexual and relationship satisfaction. *The Journal of Sexual Medicine*, 14(3), 387–395. https://doi.org/10.1016/j.jsxm.2016.12.239

Yeniel, A. O., & Petri, E. (2014). Pregnancy, childbirth, and sexual function: Perceptions and facts. *International Urogynecology Journal*, 25(1), 5–14. https://doi.org/10.1007/s00192-013-2118-7

22

Occupational and Environmental Health in Pregnancy

Katie Huffling

The editors gratefully acknowledge Meghan Garland, who authored portions of the previous edition of this chapter.

Relevant Terms

Body burden—the amount of a toxic of a substance present in the human body and is influenced by the rate of absorption and excretion

Critical window of vulnerability—a limited and often unknown time period when exposure to environmental contaminants can disrupt or interfere with the normal physiology of a cell, tissue, or organ

Cumulative impacts—the total burden of stressors, both chemical and nonchemical, that can impact health and quality of life outcomes

Endocrine disruptors—chemicals that either mimic or antagonize the effects of endogenous hormones in the endocrine system

Environmental justice—a movement addressing: (a) the historical exclusion of people of color and other marginalized groups from decision-making around policies, projects, and regulations that impact the environmental health of their communities; and (b) environmental racism that disproportionately exposes Black, Indigenous, and other people of color to environmental hazards or diminished environmental quality

Environmental justice communities of concern—a neighborhood or community, composed predominantly of persons of color or a substantial proportion of persons with low income that have been historically excluded from decision-making around policies, projects, and regulations that impact the environmental health of their communities; these communities have experienced environmental racism that disproportionately exposes them to environmental hazards or diminished environmental quality

Fenceline communities—neighborhoods located next to polluting industries

Reference dose—an amount determined to be safe based on available toxicity information; used to provide a basis for establishing safety standards and guidelines

Shift work—an employment practice of providing service over a 24-hour period, requiring workers to cover various segments of time of work; the term includes both regular night shifts and work schedules in which employees change or rotate shifts

---

Introduction

The purpose of this chapter is to introduce environmental and occupational health into the clinician's consciousness and offer a guide to appropriate resources to improve care. The environment plays a crucial role in the complex process of disease formation. The incidence of acute and chronic health conditions, such as asthma, obesity, infertility, developmental disorders, and certain types of cancers, has increased significantly since the 1970s. Working pregnant people can face issues that have the potential to impact their physical and mental health such as inadequate rest, toxic workplace exposures, occupational tasks that become difficult with the physiologic changes of pregnancy, and workplace discrimination. Listening to clients about concerns that affect their daily lives at home and in the workplace and then assisting them to navigate through issues to promote pregnancy health are essential components of comprehensive prenatal care.

Prenatal and Postnatal Care: A Person-Centered Approach, Third Edition. Edited by Karen Trister Grace, Cindy L. Farley, Noelene K. Jeffers, and Tanya Tringali.
© 2024 John Wiley & Sons Ltd. Published 2024 by John Wiley & Sons Ltd.
Companion website: www.wiley.com/go/grace/prenatal

Environmental Exposures

All persons are exposed to a variety of chemical exposures on a daily basis in the home, workplace, and neighborhood, and these exposures are often influenced by social, economic, and cultural factors (e.g., income, housing, and food sources and preparation). The ubiquitous and growing nature of these exposures is highlighted in an analysis of data from the Environmental influences on Child Health Outcomes (ECHO) program that tested for 89 analytes (79 individual chemicals and 10 composites) in pregnant people and found that 36 analytes were present in over half of the population studied and 19 analytes were found in ≥90% of the population (Buckley et al., 2022). The researchers also found demographic differences in concentrations of analytes showing higher exposures in people of color, indicating that they bear a disproportionate burden of toxic chemical exposure.

Pregnancy is an especially vulnerable time with regard to toxic exposure. The first trimester is a sensitive period for the developing embryo or fetus; exposure to drugs and chemicals during this time can range from no effect to lethal anomalies. Heavy metals such as lead and mercury, organic solvents, pesticides, air pollution, secondhand smoke, water contaminants (nitrates, arsenic, and industrial byproducts), persistent organic pollutants (POP), bisphenols, phthalates, perflourinated compounds (PFOS and PFOA), alcohol, and ionizing radiation are confirmed environmental teratogens; exposures can contribute to pregnancy loss, stillbirth, fetal growth restriction (FGR), preterm birth (PTB), and congenital anomalies (Nieuwenhuijsen et al., 2013). All of these substances are readily found in contemporary environments—homes, food sources, and workplaces.

All employees face some workplace risks to their health. Very few chemicals used in the workplace are adequately tested for safety during pregnancy. There is limited or no toxicological information for the majority of chemicals used in industry and in household cleaners. Certain occupations and exposures are linked to specific adverse pregnancy outcomes. Efforts should be made to identify, eliminate, or reduce the risks associated with each pregnant employee's duties. The changing nature of employment has caused new workplace hazards for people of reproductive age. However, care should be taken not to raise undue fear or worry about the risks associated with work. Several clinical factors need to be considered before tentative conclusions can be drawn regarding the teratogenicity of environmental exposures. These include gestational age at the time of exposure, the amount of toxin reaching the developing embryo/fetus, the duration of exposure, the impact of other factors or substances to which the pregnant person or fetus is simultaneously exposed, and the overall health of the pregnant person and fetus.

While the threshold for harm is often unknown, even small amounts of substance exposures during a **critical window of vulnerability** can lead to adverse birth outcomes and higher risk for disease and disability across the lifespan. Environmental contaminants harmful to reproductive health disproportionately affect low-income and underserved communities, making people from these communities more vulnerable to adverse reproductive outcomes (American College of Obstetricians and Gynecologists [ACOG], 2021).

There is growing recognition of the unequal burden of environmental contamination experienced by many communities of color and people with lower incomes. These may include **fenceline communities**, neighborhoods located next to polluting industries. Many of the residents within these communities face added burdens of lack of jobs, poor schools and decreased access to education, unsafe neighborhoods, and other social determinants of health (Prochaska et al., 2014). **Environmental justice communities of concern** are communities that have historically had unequal access to decision-making around policies, projects, and regulations that impact the environmental health of their communities and that experience environmental racism, which is "the institutional rules, regulations, policies or government and/or corporate decisions that deliberately target certain communities for locally undesirable land uses and lax enforcement of zoning and environmental laws, resulting in communities being disproportionately exposed to toxic and hazardous waste based upon race" (Green Action, n.d.). This results in communities that have been disadvantaged now facing disproportionate burdens of exposure from resource extraction (i.e., fossil fuel industries) and land use (i.e., landfills and other heavily polluting industries). For many communities, environmental racism began with segregation and redlining (discriminatory practices in real estate and mortgage lending) in the early twentieth century and continues today in communities such as Flint, MI, where a predominantly Black, low-income population was exposed to lead in drinking water and Mossville, LA, a community founded by free Blacks in the 1700s, where more than a dozen chemical plants have been built (Clarke, 2016; Reiss, 2021). The residents of Mossville were ultimately forced to accept buyouts for their homes to escape the toxic pollution, ending this vibrant 300-year-old community. The recognition of environmental injustice is now leading to a movement to address **cumulative impacts**, from both chemical and nonchemical sources, in order to holistically address the environmental and social burdens facing these communities.

Inclusion into Practice

Historically, pregnant people have been assessed for environmental exposures during the first prenatal visit, when questions about substance and tobacco use, occupation, and medication usage are asked. However, assessing for exposures only after a person is pregnant misses an opportunity to prevent exposures that may occur during periods of vulnerability in early pregnancy. By assessing for environmental exposures during preconception and periodically across the lifespan, healthcare providers can have a significant impact on reducing exposures and negative health impacts.

Healthcare providers are responsible for understanding environmental health and how to use this knowledge in practice. As healthcare providers generally have strong credibility with the public, they have both the opportunity and the responsibility to aid in the prevention of problems related to exposure to environmental toxins. Additionally, as healthcare providers have multiple visits with clients during pregnancy and provide continuity of care before, between, and after pregnancies, they are in a prime position to have a positive effect on the health of childbearing people and children. Careful history taking and physical evaluation, laboratory screening, and anticipatory guidance are all tools to identify and treat problems.

In 2021, the American College of Obstetricians and Gynecologists updated their 2013 Committee Opinion recognizing reduction of environmental exposures as a "critical area of intervention" for reproductive healthcare professionals and emphasizing the positive role they can play in reducing exposures and improving the health of their clients. The American College of Nurse-Midwives (2015) has also affirmed that midwives and reproductive healthcare professionals have an ethical and professional responsibility to address environmental exposures in their clients due to the increasing evidence of health impacts from these exposures.

Healthcare providers implement environmental health practice in the clinical setting through anticipatory guidance, counseling, and referral. The majority of clinical practices utilize electronic health records (EHRs); thus, an opportunity exists to streamline the assessment of environmental exposures and provide anticipatory guidance. For example, EHR systems can facilitate medical history taking and a decision tree can be created to direct the provider to ask follow-up questions if an exposure is identified, provide referrals, and automatically print out teaching sheets for the client. The use of this technology can help increase provider confidence and encourage the incorporation of environmental health into standard practice.

Environmental Exposures

Making an Environmental Exposure Assessment

There are numerous challenges in assessing exposures in pregnant people, including the availability and sensitivity of laboratory analyses, the pharmacokinetics of individual chemicals (such as short half-life or fat solubility), the altered pharmacokinetics during pregnancy, and the cost of chemical analyses. Healthcare providers should also be familiar with toxic environmental contaminants specific to their geographic area.

The assessment of risk, which includes a health history, should be made at initial healthcare visits and updated at subsequent visits as indicated (see Table 22.1). Questions about the client's environment are basic to their health history. This is particularly true for people who might become pregnant or who have unexplained symptoms. Preconception visits should always include environmental screening, because the effects of exposure to environmental toxins vary depending on the developmental stage of the fetus.

Environmental exposures can trigger illnesses or cause exacerbations of underlying medical conditions. For example, in respiratory illnesses such as asthma and other airway diseases, environmental tobacco smoke (ETS) is the most commonly associated environmental toxin. Most often, because symptoms may not immediately suggest an environmental cause, it is important to actively consider the environment when presented with a case that has atypical symptoms or that is unresponsive to treatment.

Suggested questions to evaluate symptoms related to environmental exposures are similar to those used to evaluate other symptoms. See box below.

Evaluation for environmental exposure

Are the symptoms present or worse in certain locations (e.g., the workplace)?

What is the timing of the symptoms (e.g., every day, only during the week, and only on weekends)?

When did the symptoms begin?

Is there something else associated with the symptoms (e.g., a particular activity)?

Does anyone else that you know have the same symptom(s)?

If yes, who are they or how are they associated with you?

Table 22.1   Contents of Healthcare Visits Relative to Environmental Health

	Environmental history	Focused environmental history	Anticipatory guidance	Focused physical exam[a]	Laboratory/ procedures	Consultation or referral
Visit type						
Preconception	X		X	X	X	X
Initial prenatal	X		X	X	X	X
Prenatal		X	X	X	X	X
Interconceptional	X		X	X	X	X
Post-childbearing	X		X	X	X	X
Illness	X		X	X	X	X

An "X" indicates that these visits should include the particular action.
[a] Includes appropriate screenings for cancer depending on age, history, family history, and other factors, such as breast examination and mammogram.

Specific information about employment including tasks performed, chemicals in the environment including metals and solvents, as well as other potential exposures should be obtained at the preconception visit or first prenatal visit. The Agency for Toxic Substances and Disease Registry (ATSDR) suggests the mnemonic, I PREPARE, to guide evaluation of and response to environmental exposures (Paranzino et al., 2005). This tool is especially useful in eliciting information about possible workplace exposures.

I PREPARE

I—Investigate potential exposures
P—Present work

- Are you exposed to solvents, dust, fumes, radiation, loud noise, pesticides, or other chemicals?
- Are work clothes worn at home?
- Do you wear personal protective gear?
- Do your coworkers have similar health problems?

R—Residence
E—Environmental concerns
P—Past work

- What are your past work experiences?
- Have you ever been in the military, worked on a farm, or done seasonal work?

A—Activities
R—Referrals and resources
E—Educate

Source: Paranzino et al. (2005)/SAGE Publications.

If exposure is identified, the healthcare provider should gather further detailed history on route, timing, and duration of exposure. The use of protective equipment, such as gloves or masks, should be noted. Clients may not know the names of chemicals used in their workplace. The Occupational Health and Safety Administration (OSHA) mandates that the names and health effects of all chemicals be available to workers on site via the material safety data sheet (MSDS). Clients should be informed of their right to access MSDSs for any potential workplace toxicants and to access their employer's occupational health nurse to discuss personal protective equipment and other environmental exposure mitigants (OSHA, 2019). However, it should be noted that MSDSs do not have to include exempt ingredients, such as fragrance mixtures or ingredients below a certain percentage within the product, so they may not provide a complete picture of potential exposures.

Laboratory

Laboratory testing is of limited value in environmental health, particularly in the primary healthcare setting. Specific laboratory tests that identify exposures are not available for many suspected toxins, nor would they be useful in guiding practice. Many of these tests are extremely expensive and are unlikely to be covered by insurance. Exceptions include tests for lead and mercury levels and per- and polyfluorinated alkyl substances, although normal blood levels do not exclude mercury poisoning. Even if such tests were readily available, few, if any, treatments exist that can effectively eliminate toxins from the body or mitigate their short- or long-term effects.

Diagnosis, Treatment, and Referral

Depending on the type of exposure, the Pediatric Environmental Health Specialty Units (PEHSUs) are an excellent resource on the health impacts, diagnosis, and management of exposures (see *Resources for Health Providers*). There are PEHSUs located throughout the United States and provide guidance, education, and referrals for environmental health issues from preconception, pregnancy, postnatally (including breastfeeding related issues), and throughout childhood. The local or state health department is another resource for information on particular environmental hazards and individual exposures (thus aiding in diagnosis). Health department staff can also assist with locating appropriate consultants. As with any diagnosis when environmental risks are present, a plan should be developed that includes further testing, consultation, referral, and other interventions, as appropriate.

Anticipatory Guidance

Many of the toxins to which people of reproductive age are exposed have no treatment other than the prevention of further exposure. Therefore, anticipatory guidance is the key intervention in clinical practice. Guidance depends on the reason for the healthcare visit and individual characteristics such as childbearing status. For example, a preconception visit would focus on past and present environmental risks such as chemical exposures and ways to avoid exposures at home and the workplace. The client could be counseled on risks to the fetus associated with chemical exposures and given tools and resources to decrease these exposures. Sensitivity to the emotional issues raised in the inadvertent or unintentional exposure to potentially fetotoxic substances is essential. Keep in mind that much of the time, a known exposure may be brief, and often, reassurance is an appropriate part of the plan of care, but this should be tempered with prognostic uncertainties.

To address the realities of a busy practice as well as the enormity of discussion or intervention for possible environmental exposures, practices may develop a packet of information about environmental exposures. There are many scientifically accurate resources already developed that could be added to such a packet and Web resources such as those provided at the end of the chapter.

Common environmental exposures are noted in Table 22.2, and several selected contaminants are discussed in more detail below.

Table 22.2   Substances, Sources, and Adverse Health Effects

Chemical/substance	Source	Health effects
Lead	Occupations with battery manufacturing and recycling, water from lead pipes, gun cleaning and shooting, soldering, imported ceramics and cosmetics, lead paint, and contaminated soil	Neurodevelopmental delays Behavioral issues and attention deficits Increased allergies Alterations in **DNA methylation**
Mercury	Seafood consumption	Decreased cognitive function Impaired neurodevelopment Neural tube and craniofacial defects
Pesticides	Farms, communities, and homes	Decreased cognitive function Impaired neurodevelopment Fetal growth restriction Childhood cancer
Arsenic	Is a carcinogen, toxicant and **endocrine disruptor**; found in groundwater, arsenic treated lumber in landfills, arsenic-based pesticide runoff, released by coal-fired power plants	Pregnancy hypertension Spontaneous abortion Stillbirth Neonatal mortality Alterations in DNA methylation
Bisphenols (A, F, S)	Food and product packages	Neurodevelopmental disorders Reproductive disorders Obesity Diabetes
Organic solvents	The largest category of chemical production in the United States; used in plastics, resins, nylon, synthetic fibers, rubber, lubricants, detergents, carpet pesticides, glues, and many other applications	Spontaneous abortion Fetal loss
Phthalates	Found in many products such as building materials, cleaning products, cosmetics, personal care products, food wrapping, and toys	Preterm birth Higher oxidative stress markers Penis/testicle congenital anomalies Decreased head circumference
Per- and Poly- fluorinated alkyl substances (PFAS)	Water contamination, firefighting foam, nonstick cookware, stain and water-resistant fabrics, some food packaging	Low birth weight Gestational hypertension Decreased immune response to vaccines
Formaldehyde	Wood adhesives, building materials, household pesticides, fungicides, personal care products	Spontaneous abortion Low birth weight
Air pollution	Nitrogen dioxide, carbon dioxide and benzene are primary air pollutants found in urban areas, dry cleaners, industrial areas	Preterm birth Reduced birth weight Stillbirth Birth defects
Halogenated flame retardants	Flame-retardant materials, furniture, carpeting, plastics, electronics	Neurodevelopment disorders Preterm birth Reduced birth weight
Anesthetic gases	Inhaled in healthcare and veterinary settings	Congenital anomalies Spontaneous abortion
Ethylene oxide	Inhaled in healthcare settings where instruments are sterilized	Spontaneous abortion Preterm and postterm birth

Source: Bornehag et al. (2015), Kim et al. (2020), La-Llave-León et al. (2016), Polanska et al. (2016), Quansah et al. (2015), ACOG (2021), and Bekkar et al. (2020).

Mercury

Sources of Exposure

Mercury is a neurotoxic heavy metal. It occurs in three forms: the metallic element, inorganic salts, and organic compounds, of which the most dangerous is methylmercury. In the metallic form, mercury has industrial uses that include thermometers, batteries, and fluorescent lighting. Exposure to elemental mercury is primarily by fume inhalation after an accidental spill. Inorganic mercury salts are found in some over-the-counter drugs and herbal remedies.

The primary source of environmental mercury in the United States is combustion of coal for energy production. Steel production and waste incinerators also contribute (US Environmental Protection Agency [EPA], 2022b). Mercury is released into the air and then deposited onto land and water surfaces, where it remains indefinitely. Methylmercury, the most toxic organic form, is produced by environmental interaction with carbon; the most common exposure of humans to methylmercury is from eating contaminated fish (EPA, 2022b).

A **reference dose** (RfD) is an amount determined to be safe based on available toxicity information and used to provide a basis for establishing safety standards and guidelines. The mercury RfD is based on mercury levels in the cord blood of children in the Faroe Islands (the population of these islands has a relatively high level of fish consumption); levels at or below this RfD are recommended to prevent neurodevelopmental effects from fetal and childhood exposures. The current RfD for mercury is 0.1 μg/kg per day (Rice, et al., 2003).

Diagnosis

Diagnosis of mercury poisoning is made by history and physical examination. Some signs and symptoms are tremors, impaired vision and hearing, paralysis, insomnia, emotional instability, developmental deficits during fetal development, and attention deficit and developmental delays during childhood. Laboratory testing may demonstrate elevated blood mercury, although normal blood levels do not exclude mercury poisoning (American Academy of Pediatrics Council on Environmental Health, 2019). Pregnant people with elevated mercury levels may not exhibit any symptoms, and in these people, it is only through a diet or environmental health history that exposures will be discovered.

Treatment

The treatment for exposure to mercury is to eliminate the source. Although chelating agents have been used for the treatment of elemental and inorganic mercury poisoning, it is not clear whether this treatment helps. There is no chelating agent approved by the US Food and Drug Administration (FDA) that is effective for organic (methylmercury) poisoning (Risher & Amler, 2005).

Preventing mercury intake is the only way to prevent its effects. As there are potential neurotoxic risks to the fetus and child, fish consumption advisories for pregnant people, for people with capacity for pregnancy, and for children are in place in the United States. Fish intake during pregnancy is encouraged, due to the positive impacts of omega-3 fatty acids on fetal neurodevelopment, but pregnant people should be advised to choose seafood sources lower in mercury. The FDA and the EPA advise women of childbearing age, pregnant and nursing women, and young children to avoid some types of fish and shellfish (see *Resources for Clients and Families*).

Impact on Health, Including Pregnancy, Lactation, and the Fetus

Mercury attacks the central nervous system, kidneys, and lungs. Ingested methylmercury (via fish consumption) crosses the placenta easily, causing decreased IQ levels and adverse neurobehavioral effects (American Academy of Pediatrics Council on Environmental Health, 2019). Organic mercury, a powerful teratogen, causes the disruption of the normal patterns of neuronal migration and nerve cell histology in the developing brain. Among the gradually developing symptoms are psychomotor retardation, blindness, deafness, and seizures. In 2013, the EPA estimated that 1.4 million people who could become pregnant had blood mercury concentrations high enough to place their future children at risk of learning disabilities (EPA, 2022b).

Lead

Lead is a naturally occurring element. Blood levels are low in the absence of industrial activities or other environmental sources.

Sources of Exposure

Lead is a neurotoxic agent that is ubiquitous in the environment. Lead exposure occurs commonly in work environments that involve lead smelting, soldering, mining, welding, brass foundries, stained glass manufacture, construction and demolition, battery storage, printing, painting, shipping, and automobile manufacture (La-Llave-León et al., 2016; Sathyanarayana et al., 2012). Hobbies such as stained glass and ceramics may involve lead. The most common route of workplace exposure is through the inhalation of lead dust from these activities. Environmental exposure can also occur through the ingestion of contaminated foods or water. Lead poisoning is less common since leaded gasoline was banned in 1996. Lead paint remains a possible exposure source, as does water supplied through lead pipes in older homes (La-Llave-León et al., 2016). Subpopulations such as people who work in battery factories, people who ingest certain nonfood substances (pica), and recent immigrants who use traditional folk remedies or emigrated from countries with inadequate regulation of lead pollution may benefit from lead screening (Sathyanarayana et al., 2012).

Levels of Exposure for Concern

In 2010, the Centers for Disease Control and Prevention (CDC) issued "Guidelines for the Identification and Management of Lead Exposure in Pregnant and Lactating Women." While there has been a significant decrease in US blood lead levels, 1% of pregnant people still have blood lead levels (BLL) 5 mcg/dL or more. All pregnant people should be screened for exposures, and blood lead levels should be checked if a risk is identified. The CDC guidelines provide several examples of screening tools created by health departments that can be modified based on a practice's client population. Routine testing for most populations is not recommended.

Key recommendations for healthcare providers for the management of pregnant and lactating people with blood lead levels ≥5 µg/dL

For pregnant people with prenatal blood lead levels ≥5 µg/dL,

- Attempt to determine source(s) of lead exposure and counsel clients on avoiding further exposure, including the identification and assessment of pica behavior.
- Assess nutritional adequacy and counsel on eating a balanced diet with at least the recommended daily intake of iron and calcium.
- Perform confirmatory and follow-up blood lead testing according to the recommended schedules.
- For occupationally exposed people, review the proper use of personal protective equipment and consider contacting the employer to encourage reducing exposure.
- Encourage breastfeeding consistent with CDC recommendations.

For pregnant people with prenatal blood lead levels of 10–14 µg/dL, ALL OF THE ABOVE, PLUS:

- Notify Lead Poisoning Prevention Program of local health department if BLLs ≥10 µg/dL are not reported by laboratory.
- Refer occupationally exposed people to occupational medicine specialists and remove from workplace lead exposure.

For pregnant people with prenatal blood lead levels of 15–44 µg/dL, ALL OF THE ABOVE, PLUS:

- Support environmental risk assessment by the corresponding local or state health department with subsequent source reduction and case management.

For pregnant people with prenatal blood lead levels ≥45 µg/dL, ALL OF THE ABOVE, PLUS:

- Treat as high-risk pregnancy and consult with an expert in lead poisoning on chelation and other treatment decisions.

Source: CDC (2010)/US Department of Health and Human Services/Public Domain.

Ways to Minimize Exposure

The public should know the lead level in local tap water sources. If lead pipes are present, water filters that address lead should be used for water for drinking and cooking. This is especially important for infants who are being fed formula reconstituted with tap water. Additionally, the prevention of ingestion or inhalation of lead-based paint chips and fuels is important. People with capacity for pregnancy can be encouraged to consume adequate amounts of calcium, iron, and zinc and vitamins C, D, and E in order to minimize lead absorption from the environment and release of lead from bony body stores (American College of Obstetricians and Gynecologists [ACOG], 2012). Pregnant people should also be screened for pica behavior, because cases of lead poisoning have been reported in women consuming lead-contaminated pottery and soil (CDC, 2010). Ensuring adequate intake of vitamin C, iron, and calcium may be of even greater importance in these people, because it may minimize further lead exposure from endogenous and exogenous sources.

Impact on Pregnancy, Lactation, the Fetus, and Children

In high enough doses, exposure to lead is toxic to every organ system. Prenatal exposure can cause delayed development, reduced intelligence, and behavioral problems in offspring. Lead is stored in teeth and bones. It is theorized that the mobilization of maternal calcium stores during pregnancy may increase lead levels in the blood. Low blood lead concentrations (between 5 and 10 µg/dL) in pregnant people have been associated with spontaneous abortion, gestational hypertension, or preeclampsia, PTB, premature rupture of the membranes, and low birth weight (LBW; La-Llave-León et al., 2016).

Lead levels in human milk are low. Laws enacted in the 1970s that banned lead in gasoline and paint have led to substantial decreases in blood lead levels. Fatal lead encephalopathy has virtually disappeared. However, while lead poisoning is less common, it still occurs, particularly in infants and children living in older and substandard housing, in those who emigrated from parts of the world where lead exposures are high, and in pregnant people who engage in pica behavior.

Pesticides

The US industrialized food system is largely dependent on the application of pesticides and fertilizers. Pesticide use has grown considerably since the 1940s, with approximately 0.2 million tons used globally per year in the 1950s to more than 5 million tons being used annually by 2000 (Tudi et al., 2021). Pesticide is a broad term that includes insecticides, fungicides, herbicides, rodenticides, and fumigants. Many classes of compounds are used as pesticides. Some compounds rapidly degrade in the environment after a few hours, and others linger in the environment for years (Sathyanarayana et al., 2012).

Sources of Exposure

Exposure can occur through three routes: inhalation, ingestion, and dermal. Agricultural workers and pesticide applicators need to be especially careful when using pesticides and wear appropriate protective equipment. By law, an MSDS, which provides information on proper handling, use, and protective equipment needed, must be available for employees for each chemical being used. Pesticides can spread beyond crops into the wider environment where they contaminate the air, water, and soil. Exposure can also come from home or commercial pesticide use, professional lawn services, use on pets, and from residues on home or commercially grown produce.

Impact on Pregnancy, Lactation, the Fetus, and Children

Studies suggest an increased risk of fetal harm associated with pesticides in general and with maternal employment in agricultural industries. Exposure to pesticides in pregnancy has been shown to increase the risk of poor prenatal growth, birth defects, leukemia, and impaired neurodevelopment. Pesticides act on the central nervous system and could affect a developing fetus. Forty percent of US children have enough cumulative exposure to pesticides to potentially impact their brains and nervous systems (Sutton et al., 2011). Prenatal exposure to organophosphates may affect neurodevelopment, behavior, cognitive, and motor function (González-Alzaga et al., 2014). Exposure to pesticides and insecticides before and during pregnancy increases the risk of FGR, congenital anomalies, childhood lymphoma and leukemia, and poor performance on neurodevelopmental testing (Omidakhsh et al., 2017; Sathyanarayana et al., 2012). In one study, women who were exposed to pesticides during pregnancy were 1.7 times more likely to experience PTB than women who were not exposed to pesticides during pregnancy (Anand et al., 2019). Pesticide exposures have also been linked to breast cancer, lymphoma, decreased sperm counts, endocrine disruption, and difficulty conceiving (Woodruff et al., 2008).

Ways to Minimize Exposure

Providers should recommend the following to minimize exposure to pesticides:

- Household members who work with or around pesticides should be instructed not to wear their work shoes into the home, and their clothes should be washed and stored separately from others' in the household. The Migrant Clinicians Network has a number of resources for clinicians, including assessment and management tools for acute pesticide exposures and education materials especially geared toward agricultural workers and their families (see *Resources for Clients and Families*).
- Encourage use of integrated pest management (IPM) in the home and workplace. IPM can even be used in the healthcare setting. It is a common-sense approach that focuses on keeping food and water away from pests, keeping pests out, and using the least toxic pesticides if needed. For non- and low-toxic pest management techniques, see Beyond Pesticides in *Resources for Clients and Families*.
- If the client has to use pesticides in the home (i.e., individuals living in apartment buildings that spray periodically), they should make sure that all food, food-preparation items, and toys are stored (not on counters). Especially during pregnancy, they should try to stay out of the home for at least 24 hours. They should wash all the counters when they return.
- Some fruits and vegetables contain higher levels or greater numbers of pesticides than others. Washing

fruits and vegetables is usually not enough to remove the pesticides. If possible, clients should be encouraged to buy organic varieties of fruits and vegetables that have the highest levels of pesticides, while buying conventionally grown varieties of produce that have the lowest pesticide levels. The Environmental Work Group has created guidance to help with these decisions (see *Resources for Clients and Families*).

Per- and Polyfluoroalkyl Substances

Per- and polyfluoroalkyl substances (PFAS) are a group of over 12,000 synthetic chemicals that are found in thousands of products including firefighting foam, nonstick cookware, food packaging, water and soil resistant fabrics, and many industrial products. The properties that make them so useful in products, such as oil and water repellency and friction reduction, make them difficult to break down in the environment, giving them the moniker "forever chemicals."

Sources of Exposure

Due to the widespread use and broad environmental contamination from this class of chemicals, virtually all Americans are now shown to have been exposed to PFAS (CDC, 2018). Exposure to PFAS chemicals predominantly occurs through contaminated drinking water, eating fish caught from contaminated water, eating food packaged with PFAS chemicals, or using consumer products containing PFAS (Agency for Toxic Substances and Disease Registry [ATSDR], 2022). Water contamination in the United States is pervasive, with over 2800 sites contaminated (EWG, 2022). It is estimated that the drinking water supplies of over 100 million people are contaminated with PFAS (EWG, 2018).

Levels of Concern

In 2016, the EPA set nonenforceable health advisory limits for PFAS in drinking water of 70 parts per trillion (ppt). In October 2021, the EPA announced a Strategic Roadmap, in which they committed to establishing enforceable drinking water standards by 2023 (EPA, 2022a). In June 2022, the EPA set new limits for two types of PFAS—PFOS 0.02 ppt and for PFOA 0.004 ppt (EPA, 2022c). This is in recognition of the significant health and environmental risks posed by these chemicals. However, there is concern that, for many water systems, the technology is not available to be able to reduce PFAS levels that low.

Impact on Pregnancy, Lactation, the Fetus and Children

In 2022, the National Academies of Science, Engineering, and Medicine (NASEM) produced the first report to date providing a robust analysis of health effects from PFAS exposure and clinical guidance. Their analysis found strong evidence of decreased antibody response to vaccines, dyslipidemia, decreased growth in infants and children, and increased risk of kidney cancer. They also found moderate levels of association with the risk of breast cancer, liver enzyme changes, increased risk of gestational hypertension and preeclampsia, risk of testicular cancer, thyroid disease, and risk of ulcerative colitis.

Clinical Management

The NASEM report (2022) recommends all clients suspected of PFAS exposure be offered PFAS blood testing. They provide recommendations on tests to be ordered and clinical guidance for management if PFAS is found. For pregnant clients, this includes screening for hypertensive disorders of pregnancy at all prenatal visits if PFAS blood serum levels are greater than 2. PFAS has been found in breastmilk. Current clinical guidance does not recommend testing breastmilk for PFAS and for most breastfeeding people to continue breastfeeding even if PFAS exposure is found due to the health benefits of breastfeeding (ATSDR, 2021).

Anticipatory Guidance

- Avoid nonstick cookware. Use cast iron instead.
- Avoid microwave popcorn.
- Avoid stain resistant coatings on fabric and carpets.
- Be aware of water advisories in the community. If there is PFAS contamination, use water filters rated for PFAS for drinking and cooking.
- Be aware of fish advisories and do not eat fish from PFAS contaminated waterways.
- Use PFAS-free dental floss.

Polyvinyl Chloride Plastic, Phthalates

Polyvinyl chloride (PVC) is a chlorinated plastic. The use of PVC plastic leads to environmental contamination by dioxin and di-2-ethylhexyl phthalate (DEHP), each of which has different toxic effects. Phthalates are antiandrogenic endocrine-disrupting chemicals (EDCs). They can impact hormone levels, lower the age of puberty in people assigned female at birth, and increase the risk of pregnancy loss (Wang & Qian, 2021). Male infants exposed to phthalates in utero appear to be especially sensitive to the endocrine-disrupting effects with an increased risk of decreased ano-genital distance and cryptorchidism.

Sources of Exposure for Dioxin and DEHP (Phthalates)

Dioxin is created when PVC is manufactured and when materials that contain chlorine are burned. Long-term exposure to dioxin is linked to impaired immune functioning, endocrine disruption, reproductive effects, and neurologic impacts (World Health Organization [WHO], 2016). The WHO International Agency for Research on Cancer (IARC) has classified dioxin as a known human carcinogen.

PVC plastic is made soft and flexible for most applications by the addition of DEHP. It is widely used by the food and construction industries, as well as in healthcare. Some common sources of dioxin and/or DEHP are:

- Building products (wall and floor coverings, carpet backing, piping, and vinyl shower curtains)

- Personal care products—phthalates are added as a fragrance stabilizer (lotions, cosmetics, hair products, nail polish, and perfume)
- Children's toys (teething rings and children's meal toy products)
- Food preparation and packaging (plastic wraps, plastic containers, and vinyl gloves for food workers)
- Medical products such as intravenous bags and tubing, and other tubing used in dialysis, cardiopulmonary bypass, and enteral and total parenteral nutrition (TPN; the packaging for the product should state if the product contains DEHP.)

Routes of Contamination

Humans ingest dioxin in food after particles are released via incineration into the atmosphere and distributed by wind and rain. These particles become lodged in soil, lakes, and rivers and settle on plants. When humans consume contaminated fish, meat, and dairy products, the bioaccumulative dioxin dose that an animal incurred over its lifespan and stored in its fatty tissue is also ingested. Additionally, the fats in human milk can store dioxin. Inhalation of airborne dioxin particles can also lead to exposure.

DEHP plasticizer is not chemically bound to PVC. During medical procedures with DEHP-containing products, the chemical can be absorbed into the human body when in contact with fluids such as blood, plasma, and drug solutions, or it can be released and migrate when the device is heated. The rate of migration depends on the storage conditions (temperature of the fluid contacting the device, the amount of fluid, the contact time, the extent of shaking, or flow rate of the fluid) and the lipophilicity of the fluid (Koopman-Esseboom et al., 1996).

Levels of Exposure for Concern

Dioxin is a potent carcinogen at very low levels of exposure, and even daily exposures of dioxin measured in picograms or nanograms can cause toxic effects, including endocrine disruption. In 2012, the EPA released an RfD of dioxin of 0.7 pg/kg/day (EPA, 2012). Dioxin levels are falling due to regulatory improvements; however, they still are not at safe levels (Vogt et al., 2012).

Daily human exposure to DEHP in the United States is significant, with biomonitoring indicating widespread exposure. They have also found people of color, especially non-Hispanic Black people, have the highest levels of DEHP and other phthalates (CDC, 2021). This disparity is thought to be caused in part by higher levels of these chemicals in personal care products marketed to Black women (Zota & Shamasunder, 2017).

Impact on Pregnancy, Lactation, the Fetus and Children

There is no known way to lower **body burdens** of toxins generated by PVCs other than to avoid exposure. Thus far, the infant morbidity attributable to exposure to these compounds is believed to come from prenatal exposure to maternal body burden rather than from exposure through breast milk. Some nursing infants may be exposed to dioxin levels at high concentrations. However, the long-term impact of exposure to dioxin from breast milk seems to be minimal. While shorter-term studies have shown an association between breast milk intake and adverse cognitive function from dioxin exposure, longer-term studies have not. Long-term studies following breast-fed and formula-fed infants have found an association between pregnancy maternal body burden and poorer cognitive function, but no association between type of feeding and dioxin-related damage (Mead, 2008; WHO, 2016). Therefore, there is no recommendation to avoid breast-feeding infants due to dioxin exposure in the breastfeeding person. Rather, the emphasis should be on reducing the body burden by minimizing exposure to these chemicals.

Ways to Minimize Exposure to Dioxin and DEHP

The 2008 Consumer Product Safety Improvement Act prohibited the use of DEHP and certain other phthalates in children's toys and products. To avoid exposure to PVC, dioxin, and phthalates, recommendations include:

- Choose products not made with vinyl for children's toys, food containers, car seats, crib bumpers, wallpaper, wall coverings, and flooring. If a vinyl product must be used, choose one that is phthalate free.
- Avoid burning PVC (#3) plastic.
- Avoid cooking/microwaving food in plastic containers or with plastic cling wrap.
- Avoid putting plastic in the dishwasher.
- Eat fewer fatty foods (e.g., cheese, red meats, and whole milk).
- Avoid personal care products made with phthalates. Avoid all personal care products with "fragrance" on the ingredient list as these fragrance blends often contain phthalates. And limit the total number of products used.

Flame Retardants

Halogenated flame retardants (HFRs) are a group of chemicals added to products to make them more resistant to heat and flames, such as polybrominated diphenyl ethers (PBDEs), chlorinated tris, hexabromocyclododecane (HBCD), and tetrabromobisphenol A (TBBPA). HFRs are added to a wide range of products, including electronics, furniture, appliances, building materials, and childcare products. The levels of HFRs in the US population are up to 20 times higher than in other countries, and biomonitoring studies have found flame retardants in almost all of the US population (Shaw, 2010). Besides the toxicity inherent in these chemicals, they also produce dioxins and furans across their entire lifecycle. Both are toxic chemicals that build up in the environment and have been linked to chloracne, hyperlipidemia, cancer, and reproductive effects (CDC, 2017).

HFRs tend to be lipophilic and bioaccumulative, building up in the body over time. HFRs have been shown to have a number of harmful human health effects. These include (Shaw, 2010):

- Neurodevelopmental effects: Children exposed in utero are at increased risk for autism, attention deficit hyperactivity disorder (ADHD), decreased IQ, and poor motor development.
- Endocrine-disrupting effects: People in homes with higher HFR levels were found to have lower thyroid hormone levels and lower prolactin levels. People assigned male at birth may have lower testosterone levels and children whose mothers have high PBDE levels during pregnancy had lower thyroid hormone levels. There is also an increased risk of diabetes and obesity.
- Reproductive issues: HFRs may decrease sperm counts, increase time to conception, and increase risk of cryptorchidism. There is also an increased risk of poor pregnancy outcomes including LBW, preterm delivery, and stillbirth.
- Cancer.

Sources of Exposure

Due to the widespread use of HFRs, they are ubiquitous in the environment and are found in air, dust, soil, and food. House dust and food are significant sources of exposure. When HFRs are burned, such as in a house fire, they produce dioxins. The elevated cancer rates among firefighters are thought to be related to dioxin exposure (Shaw, 2010).

Routes of Contamination

The most common route of ingestion is through food and accidental ingestion of house dust. Exposure through house dust is of particular concern for children who are more likely to be crawling and playing on the floor and because of their hand-to-mouth activities. Many of the HFRs are lipophilic and are excreted during breastfeeding. A 2005 study found US human milk PBDE levels to be 35–500 times higher than in other countries (Kotz et al., 2005). The two main types of PBDEs were removed from the market in 2005 due to health concerns, and if the experiences of other countries that removed PBDE from use are an indication, breast milk levels will decline significantly over time. HFR exposure is also an **environmental justice** issue. HFRs are found in higher levels in low-income and Hispanic and Black populations. This is exemplified by a study of women in California that found low-income and African American and Latina women had the highest levels of HFRs worldwide (Zota et al., 2011). This may be due to disproportionate exposure through the workplace and at home, including having older furniture that have higher levels of HFRs (Orta et al., 2020).

Levels of Exposure for Concern

US residents are exposed to significant amounts of HFRs every day. While there are ways to minimize these exposures, regulatory action must be taken that does not require the use of toxic chemicals in order to pass flammability standards. Public engagement is also needed to pressure manufacturers to discontinue the use of these toxic chemicals.

Ways to Minimize Exposure

There are a number of ways to reduce exposures:

- Vacuum frequently and use a high-efficiency particulate-arresting (HEPA) filter.
- Wet mop floors and damp dust furniture regularly.
- Wash hands frequently and always before eating.
- Look for the TB 117-2013 label on polyurethane foam products and buy those marked "contains no added flame-retardant chemicals." If the label is not marked, contact the manufacturer and inquire. Do not buy products with flame retardants added to the foam. This is especially true for infant and child products, such as nursing pillows, changing pads, and strollers.
- Replace furniture with crumbling foam cushions and make sure foam is covered by fabric.

Climate Change

Climate change is one of the greatest global public health threats we currently face. Climate change is the result of global warming caused by an excess of greenhouse gas emissions, predominantly due to the burning of fossil fuels for energy production and transportation. Other important sources of greenhouse gas emissions include large-scale animal production, chlorofluorocarbons that are used as refrigerants, and waste anesthetic gases.

Due to the changing climate, the planet now experiences more frequent extreme weather events such as flooding and drought, heat waves, more intense hurricanes and storms, and wildfires. The ranges of vector-borne diseases are expanding, and in many areas, air quality is falling. Extreme heat and air pollution are impacting cardiovascular and respiratory health (see Figure 22.1). Childbearing persons, children, the elderly, and lower income populations are groups that are disproportionately affected by the health impacts of climate change (US Global Research Change Program [USGRCP], 2016).

Just as seen with other structural inequities faced by communities of color, a 2021 report by the US Environmental Protection Agency found that American Indian and Alaska Natives, Black, Hispanic and Latino, and Asian individuals are most likely to live in areas that are experiencing the greatest impacts from climate change. They may also have the least number of resources to be resilient in the face of the changing climate such as lack of access to air conditioning, funds to evacuate during extreme weather events, and resources to rebuild after events. Many segregated Black and immigrant neighborhoods in cities, created through redlining, are located in

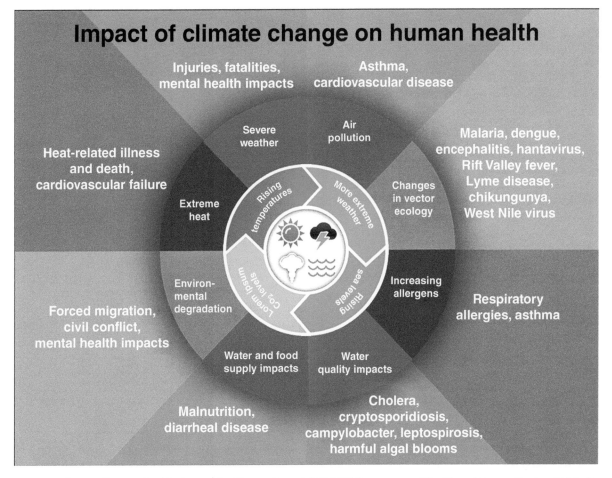

Figure 22.1 Climate effects on health. Centers for Disease Control (2022)/US Department of Health and Human Services/Public Domain.

areas that are prone to the flooding that will be increasing as the climate changes (Capps & Cannon, 2021).

Air Pollution

Climate change and air pollution go hand in hand. Besides producing greenhouse gases such as carbon dioxide and nitrous oxide, burning of fossil fuels also produces ground-level ozone and other air pollutants like sulfur dioxide and particulate matter. There is a strong link between poor pregnancy outcomes and exposure to air pollution. Air pollutants can cross the placenta and impair fetal growth. Negative respiratory and cardiac impacts from air pollutants can also impact placental function, leading to compromised fetal development (Sorensen et al., 2018). Pregnant persons exposed to air pollution are at increased risk of PTB, LBW, and stillbirth (Bekkar et al., 2020). Prepregnancy exposure to air pollution is also associated with infertility (Guidice et al., 2021). Particulate matter exposure is also an increased concern in areas now experiencing more frequent and severe wildfires.

Heat

As the climate changes, more areas of the United States will experience extreme heat days. Physiologic changes make pregnant persons less efficient at cooling and more likely to experience negative impacts from extreme heat events. Higher temperatures are associated with increases in PTB, LBW, and stillbirth (Bekkar et al., 2020). Fetal impacts include heart defects and cataracts, and prenatal exposures have been associated with decreased cognitive abilities (Guidice et al., 2021).

For pregnant people who work outside, such as farm-workers and construction workers, high heat days can pose a pregnancy risk. Due to physiologic changes during pregnancy, pregnant people can have a harder time staying cool, resulting in increased risk of heat exhaustion or stroke. It can also be challenging for pregnant people to stay hydrated during extreme heat events, leading to dehydration and increased risk of preterm labor (PTL). Counseling clients on the importance of breaks and hydration is key. Avenues for workplace accommodations should also be explored. However, for jobs like farm work, that pay by the amount picked, it can be challenging for pregnant persons to take adequate breaks needed to reduce negative pregnancy outcomes.

Vector-Borne Diseases

As the temperature increases, many vectors, such as disease-carrying mosquitoes and ticks, are finding expanded geographic homes. Due to the physiologic changes of pregnancy, including increased carbon dioxide production and increased peripheral blood flow, pregnant people are more susceptible to mosquito-transmitted diseases such as malaria, zika, and dengue fever (see Chapter 55, *Infectious Diseases*). During pregnancy, there can be a decreased immune response to infections, leading to more severe disease. For example, pregnant people

are at three times greater risk of having severe malaria than nonpregnant persons (Sorensen et al., 2018).

Extreme Weather Events

These events may include hurricanes and cyclones, localized heavy rains that produce flooding, drought, and wildfire. These events can cause short- and long- term displacement of communities, lack of access to food and water, lack of access to healthcare, and increased stress (USGRCP, 2016). People who give birth during these events have increased risk of preeclampsia and LBW (Sorensen et al., 2018). Extreme weather events can also be a time of greater risk for intimate partner violence and child abuse. Pregnant people are also at higher risk for depression during these events.

Anticipatory guidance includes:

- Ways to reduce exposure to air pollution such as monitoring outdoor conditions through http://Airnow.gov and adjusting activities accordingly
- Utilizing cooling stations. If they are not available go to library, mall, or other air-conditioned facilities
- Hydration during extreme heat events
- Connect with services for reduced/no cost air conditioning and assistance for electric bills
- Provide copy of prenatal records if an extreme weather event is forecasted
- Assess for intimate partner violence and potential for child abuse
- Primary prevention for mosquito and tick-borne illnesses: long pants and shirts, DEET or lemon/eucalyptus repellants, tick checks, avoid outdoor activities at times mosquitoes active
- Assess for depression and provide support, referrals, and pharmacological support as needed

The Workplace and Pregnancy

More than three-quarters of pregnant people in the United States will continue to work outside the home, and 80% of them will work until the last month of pregnancy (Gao & Livingston, 2015). The effect of specific work tasks on pregnancy outcomes is a difficult phenomenon to study. People who work may be healthier than those who cannot, making working people less likely to experience adverse pregnancy outcomes. Conversely, people from low-income communities may have to work during pregnancy and may be more likely to experience adverse pregnancy outcomes unrelated to work (van Beukering et al., 2014). Many occupational activities involve multidimensional mental and physical tasks rather than an isolated metric such as only standing or only lifting.

Shift Work

There may be a statistical association between adverse pregnancy outcomes, rotating shifts, and working the night shift, but the evidence is inconsistent and not conclusive (Chau et al., 2014). In a systematic review by Cai et al. (2019), the authors found long shifts, over 40 hours per week, were associated with PTB and small for gestational age. They also found that pregnant people who worked rotating shifts had an increased risk of PTB and preeclampsia when compared to those who worked set shifts. The mechanisms that may contribute to poor pregnancy outcomes related to **shift work** are not completely understood, though the disruption of the circadian rhythm, psychosocial stress, and disturbed sleep have been proposed (Lin et al., 2011). Shift work has a negative effect on several physiologic pathways, including neuroendocrine (disruptions in melatonin production), behavioral (stress response), immune, and vascular mechanisms (Bonzini et al., 2011). There may be additional differences between nulliparous and multiparous pregnant people. There is limited evidence suggesting that stress related to higher work and life burden can affect pregnancy outcomes for people working night shift who must care for children during the day (Chau et al., 2014).

A small increase in the risk of preterm labor due to shift work alone exists, but when combined with other environmental risks, the effects are compounded (Bonzini et al., 2011). The risk appears to be more pronounced for pregnant persons' work schedules that do not change over the course of pregnancy. There may be an association between spontaneous abortion and working night shift, but results should be drawn with caution due to methodological flaws and conceptual inconsistencies (Chau et al., 2014). It is prudent for employers to make reasonable workplace accommodations for pregnant persons regarding workloads, opportunities to rest when fatigued, and reduced exposure to shift and night work. These accommodations can be encouraged or prescribed by the healthcare provider as needed. Providers can also encourage their clients to exercise, maintain a healthy diet, and ensure adequate sleep, to improve prenatal health.

Heavy Lifting and Long Work Hours

As an isolated risk factor, heavy lifting (defined as heavy or repetitive load carrying, lifting, manual labor, or significant exertion) is not a risk factor for FGR or PTB. However, pregnant people who combine two or more physically demanding tasks at work may be at greater risk of PTB (van Beukering et al., 2014). Standing, bending, lifting, and working long hours is not associated with poor pregnancy outcomes in the majority of studies, but the evidence is inconsistent (Salihu et al., 2012). Mandatory occupational restrictions in pregnancy are not supported by current evidence. Falls related to slippery floors, hurried pace, or carrying objects are the most common type of work-related injury. Pregnancy can contribute to falls through changes in gait and center of gravity, which, combined with physically demanding work, could lead to injury, although the outcomes of work-related falls in pregnancy have not been studied (Salihu et al., 2012). It is prudent to advise pregnant people to limit engagement in such activities, especially in late pregnancy when fatigue is increased, and joint laxity is more pronounced.

Fatigue associated with work outside the home as a potential cause of adverse perinatal outcome has also been examined. Fatigue is linked to adverse health outcomes such as cardiovascular disease, metabolic syndrome, and depression in other populations (Okun et al., 2012). Poor sleep quality is common across all months of pregnancy, characterized by periods of nighttime waking, insomnia, daytime fatigue, restless legs, and difficulty maintaining a comfortable sleep position (Mindell et al., 2015). Chronic sleep loss can cause a hypothalamic–pituitary–adrenal mediated stress reaction in the pregnant person, which, in turn, activates inflammatory pathways (Palagini et al., 2014). These physiologic events can influence pregnancy outcomes. Chronic lack of sleep is associated with an increase in risk for gestational diabetes (Alghamdi et al., 2016), PTB, prolonged labor, and cesarean birth (Li et al., 2017; Okun et al., 2012).

Noise Exposure

Sound is transmitted from the air over the abdominal wall and the uterus to the fetus during pregnancy. Fetal hearing begins to develop around 16 weeks of gestation, and after that time, noise stimulates the fetal inner ear through a soft tissue conduction route. Excessive noise can potentially affect the hearing of the fetus by damaging inner and outer hair cells within the cochlea, especially since the maturing cochlea is more sensitive to disruption than those of adults (Chordekar et al., 2012). Both animal and human experimental studies show that the attenuation of noise through the passage of the abdominal wall and the uterus is strongly dependent on the frequency of the noise. The fetus is well protected against high-frequency noise; however, low-frequency sounds can be amplified as the sound moves through the amniotic fluid (Chordekar et al., 2012). A prospective population-based study in Sweden with over 1 million participants found that offspring of women who work in environments where they are exposed to >85 dB (equivalent to a household blender) are at increased risk for hearing loss (Selander et al., 2016). This suggests that pregnant persons should not be exposed to high levels of noise at work. The work environment assessment should include gathering information about noise in the workplace and working with clients to reduce high-decibel noise exposure during pregnancy.

Psychosocial Stress and Employment

The potential impact of workplace stress on pregnancy outcomes is an important concern. Conflicting role obligations, inadequate time for rest, financial issues, workplace discrimination, and physiologic body habitus changes affecting work performance are some of the concerns that can increase stress in the workplace. Stress and emotional symptoms such as anxiety are associated with a shorter length of gestation, PTB, and LBW (Littleton et al., 2010; Loomans et al., 2013). Elevated cortisol levels appear to be linked to poor pregnancy outcomes. Stress during pregnancy is associated with significantly elevated cortisol levels, which, in turn, can trigger PTB

(Kane et al., 2014). Maternal cortisol also acts directly on the fetus and its developing nervous system and is linked to behavioral and physiological disorders in infants and children (Davis et al., 2011).

Several associated factors seem to compound workplace stress and to increase the risk of poor pregnancy outcomes. Problems encountered in the workplace that cause maternal stress, such as harassment, discrimination, bullying, or bad job fit, and working more than 40 hours per week, have been linked with adverse perinatal outcomes (Naik et al., 2017). Poor social support and a perception of little control in the work environment are both associated with PTB and LBW (Loomans et al., 2013).

The ability to modify work responsibilities and increase flexibility in the workplace during pregnancy may change the degree to which work-related stress influences pregnancy outcomes. These issues should be discussed with each working pregnant person and avenues for modification explored.

Pregnancy Discrimination in the Workplace

The Pregnancy Discrimination Act (PDA), enacted in 1978, mandates that employers treat pregnant employees the same as all other employees. People cannot legally be fired, demoted, or penalized in the workplace for being pregnant or while they are on maternity leave. The PDA was the first federal law to explicitly protect pregnant workers. Despite the clarity of the mandate, pregnancy discrimination in the workplace continues to be a problem in the United States, across all industries, ethnicities, and states (Equal Employment Opportunity Commission [EEOC], n.d.). Being fired while pregnant is the most common reason pregnancy discrimination cases are filed. This is followed by discriminatory workplace situations such as being denied accommodations like more frequent bathroom breaks or being allowed to carry a water bottle, and by being denied time off (National Partnership for Women and Families, 2022). The most economically vulnerable people are disproportionally affected by workplace pregnancy discrimination (Brake & Grossman, 2013). Cultural and gender bias underpinnings in organizational environments promote the perception of a pregnant person as far from meeting the ideal (stereotypical male) worker norm of being flexible and singularly committed to the job (Byron & Roscigno, 2014).

Generally, pregnant persons are not limited in their personal lives or work activities due to pregnancy. There are times, however, when some workplace accommodations are needed. Pregnancy raises difficult questions regarding the interaction of policies regarding sex discrimination in the workplace and policies regarding disabilities. Healthcare providers can help pregnant persons become aware of their rights.

Workplace Exposures

Below are a couple of examples of workplace exposures that were not described in the previous general exposure section.

Organic Solvents

Organic solvents, such as benzene, toluene, hydrogen sulfide, carbon tetrachloride, aliphatic hydrocarbons, phenols, and phthalates, are carbon-containing liquids that can dissolve or disperse other substances. Organic solvents are found in some paints, varnishes, glues, and cleaning/degreasing agents, and in the production of dyes, printer inks, plastics, textiles, and agricultural products. Occupational exposures are an important source of exposure. Pregnant persons may be more susceptible to inhalation of organic solvents due to increased respiratory rate and oxygen consumption. Organic solvent exposure in the first two weeks after conception is linked to an increased risk of spontaneous abortion (Red et al., 2011). Toluene is an organic solvent of special concern because of its potential to be used recreationally (Red et al., 2011). People who recreationally use toluene-containing products such as paints, varnishes, lacquers, glues, and enamels during pregnancy have increased risks of PTB, perinatal death, and FGR (Red et al., 2011). In a study assessing for occupational and hobby exposures during pregnancy, two-thirds of participants reported being regularly exposed to organic solvents (Zachek et al., 2019). Clients should be counseled on the use of proper personal protective equipment for the chemicals they are using in the workplace and how to report unsafe workplace practices.

Assessing Occupational Conditions

During the health history and physical at the first prenatal visit, the types of occupational activities performed and the number of hours worked should be determined. In certain occupations, it may be appropriate to evaluate the level of noise exposure. The person's feelings about their work should be assessed. Do they have adequate social support, transportation, or childcare to engage in work outside the home? Do they see themselves as a valued and autonomous employee? Do they have control over their work environment? Their plan for continued employment during and after pregnancy and plans for time off with their newborn should be evaluated. This can provide an opportunity to facilitate information about rights regarding pregnancy and the workplace and disability and maternity leave.

Supporting Pregnancy Health in the Workplace

Clients with low social support can be directed to community services to help with transportation and childcare. Some employers have employee stress reduction and assistance programs. Using validated antenatal depression tools in clients with low levels of control in their work environments or who present with psychosomatic reports such as disturbed sleep may also be useful to identify those at risk for poor perinatal outcomes. Some clients can modify their work schedule or take personal days to catch up on rest, especially in the first and third trimesters. Discuss ways to obtain periods of rest during the workday. Encourage sleep for a minimum of seven or eight hours nightly. By optimizing sleep hygiene, utilizing cognitive behavioral therapy, and employing measures to reduce pregnancy-related discomfort, heartburn, and nocturia, clinicians can help clients improve their sleep (see Chapter 15, *Common Discomforts of Pregnancy*).

Clients in physically demanding jobs can be encouraged to modify their work as pregnancy progresses. In some cases, providing a pregnancy accommodation letter for clients who perform certain tasks or to modify working hours is necessary. Examples of modification include restricting the work week to 40 hours or less and shift duration to 8 hours, increasing frequency of work breaks, limiting pounds lifted, and avoiding repetitive motions if musculoskeletal overuse injury is a concern. Healthcare providers should be cognizant of legal rights and unique issues pregnant people face in the workplace and facilitate appropriate work accommodations as needed.

Resources for Clients and Families

Beyond Pesticides. Low and nontoxic pesticide resources. www.beyondpesticides.org

Environmental Work Group (EWG). Advocacy organization that produces excellent resources for consumers and has a number of tools to help consumers choose safe products. www.ewg.org

Getting Ready for Baby. —Safe baby products guide. www.gettingready4baby.org

Food and Drug Administration (FDA). Provides information on medications, food safety, breast pumps, and more. https://www.fda.gov/consumers/women/womens-health-topics

March of Dimes Birth Defects Foundation provides fact sheets, brochures, and an exposure screening checklist. http://www.marchofdimes.org/pregnancy/is-it-safe.aspx

National Institute of Occupational Safety and Health (NIOSH) conducts research and makes recommendations on preventing work-related injury and illness. Specific information about reproductive health and work for pregnant people is available. http://www.cdc.gov/niosh

National Institutes of Health (NIH) provides a Consumer Product Information Database. https://www.whatsinproducts.com/

The US Equal Employment Opportunity Commission (EEOC) provides information to pregnant persons and employers on nondiscrimination during pregnancy. http://www.eeoc.gov/laws/types/pregnancy.cfm

US Environmental Protection Agency and Food and Drug Administration Fish Consumption Guidelines. https://www.fda.gov/media/102331/download

Women's Voices for the Earth is a grassroots environmental health and justice organization. Reports and fact sheets with specific information on risks of household products and exposures are available. http://www.womensvoices.org

Resources for Healthcare Providers

Agency for Toxic Substances and Disease Registry (ATSDR). Resources for healthcare providers. These include case studies that are self-instructional continuing education primers and excellent information on the toxicity of specific chemicals. http://www.atsdr.cdc.gov

Alliance of Nurses for Healthy Environments. Nursing organization focusing on environmental health. Website resources include: assessment tools, eTextbook, information on environmental contaminants and health impacts, and can be used to connect with other nurses interested in environmental health. www.envirn.org

Association of Occupational and Environmental Clinics. The website links to resources about environment and occupational medicine and a directory of environmental medicine clinics in the United States. http://www.aoec.org/about.htm

Breast Cancer Prevention Partners. Dedicated to preventing breast cancer by exposing and eliminating environmental causes of breast cancer. https://www.bcpp.org

Collaborative on Health and the Environment. International collaborative whose mission is to maintain a dialogue and foster collaboration on environmental factors affecting human health. www.healthandenvironment.org

Healthcare Without Harm (HCWH). Has a wide array of publications, information, and programs on many of the health hazards encountered in healthcare. www.noharm.org

Migrant Clinicians Network. Tools for assessment and management of acute pesticide exposure, client materials. www.migrantclinician.org

Mother to Baby. Website that is a service of the Organization of Teratology Information Specialists (OTIS), a nonprofit organization of physicians, genetics counselors, and others dedicated to dissemination of information about environmental risks during pregnancy. http://mothertobaby.org

National Institute of Environmental Health Sciences (NIEHS). Funds research on environmental health and provides resources for scientists, healthcare providers, and the public. Informational materials for children and adults are also provided http://www.niehs.nih.gov

National Library of Medicine (NLM) LactMed database has extensive information on drugs and chemicals and their impacts on breastfeeding. https://www.ncbi.nlm.nih.gov/books/NBK501922/?report=classic

NLM PubChem. Large chemical database that includes toxicology information. https://pubchem.ncbi.nlm.nih.gov

Pediatric Environmental Health, 4th Edition. Policy manual geared toward the pediatrician, although also very relevant to sexual and reproductive healthcare providers. Provides lists of toxins and discussion of communication of risk to clients as well as how to advocate for environmental policy. https://shop.aap.org/pediatric-environmental-health-4th-edition-paperback

Pediatric Environmental Health Specialty Units (PEHSU). A national network of experts in the prevention, diagnosis, management, and treatment of health issues that arise from environmental exposures from preconception through adolescence. https://www.pehsu.net

Case Studies in Environmental Medicine. http://www.atsdr.cdc.gov/csem/csem.html

Program on Reproductive Health and the Environment. Website links to sample environmental exposure questionnaires for use in pregnancy and numerous resources about environmental and workplace toxicants. https://prhe.ucsf.edu

US Environmental Protection Agency. Excellent website and publications relevant to almost all aspects discussed in this chapter, including environmental justice, pregnancy and children's health, reproductive health, and endocrine disruptor screening program. http://www.epa.gov

Environmental Justice. http://www.epa.gov/environmentaljustice

Endocrine Disruptor Screening Program. https://www.epa.gov/endocrine-disruption

Office of Children's Health Protection. http://www.epa.gov/children

References

Agency for Toxic Substances and Disease Registry. (2021). *PFAS and breastfeeding*. https://www.atsdr.cdc.gov/pfas/health-effects/pfas-breastfeeding.html

Agency for Toxic Substances and Disease Registry. (2022). *Per- and polyfluoroalkyl substances (PFAS) and your health*. https://www.atsdr.cdc.gov/pfas/health-effects/overview.html

Alghamdi, A. A., Al Afif, N. A., Law, G. R., Scottand, E. M., & Ellison, G. T. (2016). Short sleep duration is associated with an increased risk of gestational diabetes: Systematic review and meta-analysis. *The Proceedings of the Nutrition Society, 75*(OCE1), 1. https://doi.org/10.1017/S0029665115004383

American Academy of Pediatrics Council on Environmental Health. (2019). Mercury. In R. A. Etzel (Ed.), *Pediatric environmental health* (4th ed., pp. 585–600). American Academy of Pediatrics.

American College of Nurse-Midwives. (2015). *The effect of environmental toxins on reproductive and developmental health*. https://www.midwife.org/acnm/files/ACNMLibraryData/UPLOADFILENAME/000000000292/Environmental-Toxins-June-2015.pdf

American College of Obstetricians and Gynecologists, & Committee on Obstetric Practice. (2012). Lead screening during pregnancy and lactation: ACOG Committee Opinion, Number 533. *Obstetrics and Gynecology, 120*, 416–420.

American College of Obstetricians and Gynecologists, & Committee on Obstetric Practice. (2021). Reducing prenatal exposure to toxic environmental agents: ACOG Committee opinion, number 832. *Obstetrics and Gynecology, 138*(1), e40–e54.

Anand, M., Singh, L., Agarwal, P., Saroj, R., & Taneja, A. (2019). Pesticides exposure through environment and risk of pre-term birth: A study from Agra city. *Drug and Chemical Toxicology, 42*(5), 471–477.

Bekkar, B., Pacheco, S., Basu, R., & DeNicola, N. (2020). Association of air pollution and heat exposure with preterm birth, low birth weight, and stillbirth in the US: A systematic review. *JAMA Network Open, 3*(6), e208243. https://doi.org/10.1001/jamanetworkopen.2020.8243

Bonzini, M., Palmer, K., Coogan, D., Carungo, M., Cromi, A., & Ferrario, M. (2011). Shift work and pregnancy outcomes: A systematic review and meta-analysis of currently available epidemiological studies. *BJOG: An International Journal of Obstetrics & Gynecology, 118*(12), 1429–1437.

Bornehag, C. G., Carlstedt, E., Jönsson, B. A., Lindh, C. H., Jensen, T. K., Bodin, A., Jonsson, C., Janson, S., & Swan, S. H. (2015). Prenatal phthalate exposures and anogenital distance in Swedish boys. *Environmental Health Perspectives, 123*(1), 101. https://doi.org/10.1289/ehp.1408163

Brake, D. L., & Grossman, J. L. (2013). Unprotected sex: The pregnancy discrimination act at 35. *Duke Journal of Gender Law and Policy, 12*, 67–123.

Buckley, J. P., Kuiper, J. R., Bennett, D. H., Barrett, E. S., Bastain, T., Breton, C. V., Chinthakindi, S., Dunlop, A. L., Farzan, S. F., Herbstman, J. B., Karagas, M. R., & Woodruff, T. J. (2022). Exposure to contemporary and emerging chemicals in commerce among pregnant women in the United States: The Environmental influences on Child Health Outcome (ECHO) program. *Environmental Science & Technology, 56*(10), 6560–6573. https://doi.org/10.1021/acs.est.1c08942

Byron, R. A., & Roscigno, V. J. (2014). Relational power, legitimation, and pregnancy discrimination. *Gender & Society, 28*(3), 435–462.

Cai, C., Vandermeer, B., Khurana, R., Nerenberg, K., Featherstone, R., Sebastianski, M., & Davenport, M. H. (2019). The impact of occupational shift work and working hours during pregnancy on health outcomes: A systematic review and meta-analysis. *American Journal of Obstetrics and Gynecology, 221*(6), 563–576.

Capps, K., & Cannon, C. (2021, March 15). *Redlined, now flooding*. Bloomberg. https://www.bloomberg.com/graphics/2021-flood-risk-redlining

Centers for Disease Control and Prevention. (2010). *Guidelines for the identification and management of lead exposure in pregnant and lactating women*. http://www.cdc.gov/nceh/lead/publications/leadandpregnancy2010.pdf

Centers for Disease Control and Prevention. (2017). *Dioxins, furans and dioxin-like polychlorinated biphenyls factsheet*. https://www.cdc.gov/biomonitoring/DioxinLikeChemicals_FactSheet.html

Centers for Disease Control and Prevention. (2018). *Fourth national report on human exposure to environmental chemicals, updated tables, March 2018*. https://www.cdc.gov/exposurereport/pdf/archives/WhatsNewArchive_March2018-508.pdf

Centers for Disease Control and Prevention. (2021). *Phthalates factsheet*. https://www.cdc.gov/biomonitoring/Phthalates_FactSheet.html

Chau, Y., West, S., & Mapedzahama, V. (2014). Night work and the reproductive health of women: An integrated literature review. *Journal of Midwifery & Women's Health, 59*(2), 113–126.

Chordekar, S., Kriksunov, L., Kishon-Rabin, L., Adelman, C., & Sohmer, H. (2012). Mutual cancellation between tones presented by air conduction, by bone conduction and by non-osseous (soft tissue) bone conduction. *Hearing Research, 283*(1), 180–184.

Clarke, K. (2016). *The environmental racism flowing in Flint*. Open Society Foundations. https://www.opensocietyfoundations.org/voices/environmental-racism-flowing-flint

Consumer Product Safety Improvement Act of. 2008. PUBLIC LAW 110–314. https://www.govinfo.gov/app/details/PLAW-110publ314

Davis E., Glynn L., Waffarn E, & Sandman C., (2011). Prenatal maternal stress programs infant stress regulation. *Journal of Child Psychology and Psychiatry, 52*, 119–129.

Environmental Working Group. (2018). *Report: Up to 110 million Americans could have PFAS-contaminated drinking water*. https://www.ewg.org/research/report-110-million-americans-could-have-pfas-contaminated-drinking-water

Environmental Working Group. (2022). *Mapping the PFAS contamination crisis: New data show 2,858 sites in 50 states and two territories*. https://www.ewg.org/interactive-maps/pfas_contamination

Equal Employment Opportunity Commission (EEOC). (n.d.). *Pregnancy discrimination charges FY 2010 - FY 2021*. https://www.eeoc.gov/data/pregnancy-discrimination-charges-fy-2010-fy-2021

Gao, G. & Livingston, G. (2015). *Working while pregnant is much more common than it used to be*. Pew Research Center. http://www.pewresearch.org/fact-tank/2015/03/31/working-while-pregnant-is-much-more-common-than-it-used-to-be

Giudice, L. C., Llamas-Clark, E. F., DeNicola, N., Pandipati, S., Zlatnik, M. G., Decena, D. C. D., Woodruff, T. J., Conry, J. A., & FIGO Committee on Climate Change and Toxic Environmental Exposures. (2021). Climate change, women's health, and the role of obstetricians and gynecologists in leadership. *International Journal of Gynecology & Obstetrics, 155*(3), 345–356. https://doi.org/10.1002/ijgo.13958

González-Alzaga, B., Lacasaña, M., Aguilar-Garduño, C., Rodríguez-Barranco, M., Ballester, F., Rebagliato, M., & Hernández, A. (2014).

A systematic review of neurodevelopmental effects of prenatal and postnatal organophosphate pesticide exposure. *Toxicology Letters*, *230*(2), 104–121.

Green Action. (n.d.). *Environmental justice & environmental racism*. https://greenaction.org/what-is-environmental-justice

Kane, H. S., Schetter, C. D., Glynn, L. M., Hobel, C. J., & Sandman, C. A. (2014). Pregnancy anxiety and prenatal cortisol trajectories. *Biological Psychology*, *100*, 13–19.

Kim, J. J., Kumar, S., Kumar, V., Lee, Y. M., Kim, Y. S., & Kumar, V. (2020). Bisphenols as a legacy pollutant, and their effects on organ vulnerability. *International Journal of Environmental Research and Public Health*, *17*(1), 112. https://doi.org/10.3390/ijerph17010112

Koopman-Esseboom, C., Weisglas-Kuperus, N., de Ridder, M. A., Van der Paauw, C. G., Tuinstra, L. G., & Sauer, P. J. (1996). Effects of poly-chlorinated biphenyl/dioxin exposure and feeding type on infants' mental and psychomotor development. *Pediatrics*, *97*(5), 700–706.

Kotz, A., Malisch, R., Kypke, K., & Oehme, M. (2005). PBDE, PBDD/F and mixed chlorinated-brominated PXDD/F in pooled human milk samples from different countries. *Organohalogen Compounds*, *67*, 1540–1544.

La-Llave-León, O., Salas Pacheco, J., Estrada Martínez, S., Esquivel Rodríguez, E., Castellanos Juárez, F., Sandoval Carrillo, A., Lechuga Quiñones, A., Vázquez Alanís, F., García Vargas, G., Méndez Hernández, E., & Duarte Sustaita, J. (2016). The relationship between blood lead levels and occupational exposure in a pregnant population. *BMC Public Health*, *16*(1), 1–9.

Li, R., Zhang, J., Zhou, R., Liu, J., Dai, Z., Liu, D., Wang, Y., Zhang, H., Li, Y., & Zeng, G. (2017). Sleep disturbances during pregnancy are associated with cesarean delivery and preterm birth. *The Journal of Maternal-Fetal & Neonatal Medicine*, *30*(6), 733–738.

Lin, Y. C., Chen, M. H., Hsieh, C. J., & Chen, P. C. (2011). Effect of rotating shift work on childbearing and birth weight: A study of women working in a semiconductor manufacturing factory. *World Journal of Pediatrics*, *7*(2), 129–135.

Littleton, H., Bye, K., Buck, K., & Amacker, A. (2010). Psychosocial stress during pregnancy and perinatal outcomes: A meta-analytic review. *Journal of Psychosomatic Obstetrics and Gynecology*, *31*(4), 219–228.

Loomans, E. M., Van Dijk, A. E., Vrijkotte, T. G., Van Eijsden, M., Stronks, K., Gemke, R. J., & Van den Bergh, B. R. (2013). Psychosocial stress during pregnancy is related to adverse birth outcomes: Results from a large multi-ethnic community-based birth cohort. *The European Journal of Public Health*, *23*(3), 485–491.

Mead, M. N. (2008). Contaminants in human milk: Weighing the risks against the benefits of breastfeeding. *Environmental Health Perspectives*, *116*(10), A427–A434.

Mindell, J. A., Cook, R. A., & Nikolovski, J. (2015). Sleep patterns and sleep disturbances across pregnancy. *Sleep Medicine*, *16*(4), 483–488.

Naik, K., Nayak, V., & Ramaiah, R. (2017). Pregnancy outcome in working women with work place stress. *International Journal of Reproduction, Contraception, Obstetrics and Gynecology*, *6*(7), 2891–2896.

National Academies of Sciences, Engineering, and Medicine (NASEM). (2022). *Guidance on PFAS exposure, testing, and clinical follow-up*. The National Academies Press. https://doi.org/10.17226/26156

National Partnership for Women and Families. (2022). *Pregnancy discrimination*. http://www.nationalpartnership.org/issues/fairness/pregnancy-discrimination.html

Nieuwenhuijsen, M., Dadvand, P., Grellier, J., Martinez, D., & Vri-jheid, M. (2013). Environmental risk factors of pregnancy outcomes: A summary of recent meta-analyses of epidemiological studies. *Environmental Health*, *12*(1). https://doi.org/10.1186/1476-069X-12-6

Occupational Safety and Health Administration (OSHA). (2019). *Workers' rights- OSHA 3021-12R 2019*. https://www.osha.gov/Publications/osha3021.pdf

Okun, M., Luther, J., Wisniewski, S., Sit, D., Prairie, B., & Wisner, K. (2012). Disturbed sleep, a novel risk factor for preterm birth? *Journal of Women's Health*, *21*(1), 54–60.

Omidakhsh, N., Ganguly, A., Bunin, G. R., von Ehrenstein, O. S., Ritz, B., & Heck, J. E. (2017). Residential pesticide exposures in pregnancy and the risk of sporadic retinoblastoma: A report from the Children's Oncology Group. *American Journal of Ophthalmology*, *176*, 166–173.

Orta, O. R., Wesselink, A. K., Bethea, T. N., Henn, B. C., McClean, M. D., Sjödin, A., Baird, D. D., & Wise, L. A. (2020). Correlates of plasma concentrations of brominated flame retardants in a cohort of US Black women residing in the Detroit, Michigan metropolitan area. *Science of the Total Environment*, *714*, 136777.

Palagini, L., Gemignani, A., Banti, S., Manconi, M., Mauri, M., & Riemann, D. (2014). Chronic sleep loss during pregnancy as a determinant of stress: Impact on pregnancy outcome. *Sleep Medicine*, *15*(8), 853–859.

Paranzino, G. K., Butterfield, P., Nastoff, T., & Ranger, C. (2005). I PREPARE: Development and clinical utility of an environmental exposure history mnemonic. *AAOHN Journal*, *53*(1), 37–42.

Polanska, K., Ligocka, D., Sobala, W., & Hanke, W. (2016). Effect of environmental phthalate exposure on pregnancy duration and birth outcomes. *International Journal of Occupational Medicine and Environmental Health*, *29*(4), 683–697. https://doi.org/10.13075/ijomeh.1896.00691

Prochaska, J. D., Nolen, A. B., Kelley, H., Sexton, K., Linder, S. H., & Sullivan, J. (2014). Social determinants of health in environmental justice communities: Examining cumulative risk in terms of environmental exposures and social determinants of health. *Human and Ecological Risk Assessment: An International Journal*, *20*(4), 980–994. https://doi.org/10.1080/10807039.2013.805957

Quansah, R., Armah, F., Essumang, D., Luginaah, I., Clarke, E., Marfo, K., Cobbina, S., Nketiah-Amponsah, E., Namujju, P., Obiri, S., & Dzodzomenyo, M. (2015). Association of arsenic with adverse pregnancy outcomes-infant mortality: A systematic review and meta-analysis. *Environmental Health Perspectives*, *123*(5), 412. https://doi.org/10.1289/ehp.1307894

Red, R., Richards, S., Torres, C., & Adair, C. (2011). Environmental toxicant exposure during pregnancy. *Obstetrical & Gynecological Survey*, *66*(3), 159–169.

Reiss, J. (2021, December 20). Touring Louisiana's chemical ghost town. *The New Yorker*. https://www.newyorker.com/magazine/2021/12/20/touring-louisianas-chemical-ghost-town

Rice, D. C., Schoeny, R., & Mahaffey, K. (2003). Methods and rationale for derivation of a reference dose for methylmercury by the US EPA. *Risk Analysis: An International Journal*, *23*(1), 107–115.

Risher, J. F., & Amler, S. N. (2005). Mercury exposure: Evaluation and intervention the inappropriate use of chelating agents in the diagnosis and treatment of putative mercury poisoning. *Neurotoxicology*, *26*(4), 691–699.

Salihu, H., Myers, J., & August, E. (2012). Pregnancy in the workplace. *Occupational Medicine*, *62*(2), 88–97.

Sathyanarayana, S., Focareta, J., Dailey, T., & Buchanan, S. (2012). Environmental exposures: How to counsel preconception and prenatal patients in the clinical setting. *American Journal of Obstetrics & Gynecology*, *207*(6), 463–470.

Selander, J., Albin, M., Rosenhall, U., Rylander, L., Lewne, M., & Gustavsson, P. (2016). Maternal occupational exposure to noise during pregnancy and hearing dysfunction in children: A nationwide prospective cohort study in Sweden. *Environmental Health Perspectives*, *124*(6).

Shaw, S. (2010). Halogenated flame retardants: Do the fire safety benefits justify the risks? *Reviews on Environmental Health*, *25*(4), 261–306.

Sorensen, C., Murray, V., Lemery, J., & Balbus, J. (2018). Climate change and women's health: Impacts and policy directions. *PLoS Medicine*, *15*(7), e1002603. https://doi.org/10.1371/journal.pmed.1002603

Sutton, P., Wallinga, D., Perron, J., Gottlieb, M., Sayre, L., & Woodruff, T. (2011). Reproductive health and the industrialized food system: A point of intervention for health policy. *Health Affairs*, *30*(5), 888–897.

Tudi, M., Daniel Ruan, H., Wang, L., Lyu, J., Sadler, R., Connell, D., Chu, C., & Phung, D. T. (2021). Agriculture development, pesticide application and its impact on the environment. *International Journal of Environmental Research and Public Health*, *18*(3), 1112.

US Environmental Protection Agency. (2012). *2,3,7,8-Tetrachlorodibenzo-p-dioxin*. IRIS. https://cfpub.epa.gov/ncea/iris2/chemicalLanding.cfm?substance_nmbr=1024

US Environmental Protection Agency. (2021). *Climate change and social vulnerability in the United States. A focus on six impacts*. https://www.epa.

gov/system/files/documents/2021-09/climate-vulnerability_september-2021_508.pdf

US Environmental Protection Agency. (2022a). *PFAS Strategic Roadmap: EPA's commitments to action 2021-2024.* https://www.epa.gov/pfas/pfas-strategic-roadmap-epas-commitments-action-2021-2024

US Environmental Protection Agency. (2022b). *How people are exposed to mercury.* http://www.epa.gov/mercury/how-people-are-exposed-mercury

US Environmental Protection Agency. (2022c). *2022 interim updated PFOA and PFOS health advisories.* https://www.epa.gov/sdwa/drinking-water-health-advisories-pfoa-and-pfos

US Global Change Research Program. (2016). *The impacts of climate change on human health in the United States: A scientific assessment.* https://doi.org/10.7930/J0R49NQX

van Beukering, M., van Melick, M., Mol, B., Frings-Dresen, M., & Hulshof, C. (2014). Physically demanding work and preterm delivery: A systematic review and meta-analysis. *International Archives of Occupational and Environmental Health, 87*(8), 809–834.

Vogt, R., Bennett, D., Cassady, D., Frost, J., Ritz, B., & Hertz-Picciotto, I. (2012). Cancer and non-cancer health effects from food contaminant exposures for children and adults in California: A risk assessment. *Environmental Health, 11*(1), 1–14.

Wang, Y., & Qian, H. (2021). Phthalates and their impacts on human health. *Healthcare, 9*(5), 603. https://doi.org/10.3390/healthcare9050603

Woodruff, T. J., Carlson, A., Schwartz, J. M., & Giudice, L. C. (2008). Proceedings of the summit on environmental challenges to reproductive health and fertility: Executive summary. *Fertility and Sterility, 89*(2), 281–300.

World Health Organization. (2016). *Dioxins and their effects on human health.* https://www.who.int/news-room/fact-sheets/detail/dioxins-and-their-effects-on-human-health

Zachek, C. M., Schwartz, J. M., Glasser, M., DeMicco, E., & Woodruff, T. J. (2019). A screening questionnaire for occupational and hobby exposures during pregnancy. *Occupational Medicine, 69*(6), 428–435.

Zota, A. R., Park, J. S., Wang, Y., Petreas, M., Zoeller, R. T., & Woodruff, T. J. (2011). Polybrominated diphenyl ethers, hydroxylated polybrominated diphenyl ethers, and measures of thyroid function in second trimester pregnant women in California. *Environmental Science & Technology, 45*(18), 7896–7905.

Zota, A. R., & Shamasunder, B. (2017). The environmental injustice of beauty: Framing chemical exposures from beauty products as a health disparities concern. *American Journal of Obstetrics and Gynecology, 217*(4), 418–e1.

23

Psychosocial Adaptations in Pregnancy

Cindy L. Farley

The editors gratefully acknowledge Cindy L. Farley, Eva M. Fried, and Amy R. Chavez, who were coauthors of the previous edition of this chapter.

Relevant Terms

Active listening—communication process whereby the listener fully concentrates without distraction, withholds judgment, seeks to understand, and responds reflectively used to build rapport, understanding, and trust in relationships

Adaptation—the process of making necessary accommodations to changing circumstances while maintaining a coherent identity

Anxiety—a state of uneasiness and apprehension about a real or imagined threat

Attachment—a lasting psychological connectedness between human beings

Attitude—a relatively enduring organization of beliefs, feelings, and behavioral tendencies toward socially significant objects, groups, events, or symbols

Body image—a subjective awareness and attitude toward one's body and its parts that may or may not correspond to objective measures

Coping—the process of dealing with internal or external demands that are perceived to be threatening or overwhelming

Culture—the sum total of ideas, beliefs, values, material goods and tools, and nonmaterial aspects that individuals make as members of a society

Disorganized attachment—a relationship that emerges when parental response to infant distress is disrupted, mismatched, or abusive, creating and not soothing infant fears, resulting in an approach/avoidance paradox with long-lasting effects

Expectation—a strong belief that something will happen or be the case in the future

Family—a group of people related by blood, legal document, or choice, traditionally with the primary function of raising children to the age of maturity; variations in family structure and composition exist

Fear—a psychophysiologic response to a perceived threat that is consciously recognized as danger

Gender—the socially constructed aspects of a person's biological sex or personal identity; may not correspond with their sex assigned at birth.

Maternal identity—an internalized view of one's self as mother

Pain—a complex and subjective interaction of multiple physiologic and psychologic factors on an individual's interpretation of noxious stimuli

Paternal identity—an internalized view of one's self as father

Perception—cognitive processes that organize sensory information and interpret its meaning

Psychophysiologic—pertaining to cognitive, emotional, and behavioral phenomenon as related to and revealed through physiologic processes and events

Role—a pattern of expected behaviors associated with a particular position or status in a social system

Self-esteem—a person's overall self-evaluation or appraisal of self-worth

Sex—biologic classification as female, male, or intersex based on chromosomes, genitalia, and reproductive organs

Sexuality—how people experience and express themselves as sexual beings

Stress—a psychophysiologic response to perceived pressure, demands, challenging tasks, adverse events, or negative experiences

Tokophobia—extreme fear of childbirth, classified as a Specific Phobia within the category of anxiety disorders

---

Introduction

Pregnancy, labor, and birth are **psychophysiologic** processes embedded in a sociocultural context. Many profound changes occur within the pregnant individual and within their **family** structure during the childbearing year. These changes call for an approach to care that is concerned with more than just screening for pathology. These changes call for an approach to care that is based on

Prenatal and Postnatal Care: A Person-Centered Approach, Third Edition. Edited by Karen Trister Grace, Cindy L. Farley, Noelene K. Jeffers, and Tanya Tringali.
© 2024 John Wiley & Sons Ltd. Published 2024 by John Wiley & Sons Ltd.
Companion website: www.wiley.com/go/grace/prenatal

a relationship of trust and mutual respect between care providers and the people they serve, and a provision of services that address psychologic, social, and spiritual needs in addition to biological needs.

Prenatal care offers a unique opportunity to get to know a person and their family over time. Beyond meeting the individual's healthcare needs, the provider works in the context of a developing relationship to support the achievement of optimal health and honor the pregnant person's preferences, and facilitate the safe conduct of labor and birth. In addition to assessing the physiologic course of pregnancy at each visit, the assessment of the changes and development in psychosocial **attachment** and **adaptation** processes must occur as well. Providers of prenatal care seek not only safe passage through pregnancy, labor, and birth for the birthing person and their baby but also the promotion of psychological health and resiliency that will assist in facing the challenges of the long process of raising their newborn child to maturity.

Time spent in dialogue is an essential element in the development of a relationship. While rapport (an affinity or sympathetic understanding) with an individual can be developed in the early minutes of a first meeting, developing a therapeutic relationship of mutuality and trust takes time–time to listen to and honor their life stories, time to respond with support and acceptance, and time to reconvene, reconnect, and follow-up on previous conversations.

In order to actualize relationship-based care, it is important to deliberately structure generous amounts of time for initial and return prenatal visits and to provide continuity of care with the same clinician or set of clinicians to foster the development of a therapeutic relationship. It is an ongoing struggle to allow for unhurried client encounters in an era of productivity measures applied to healthcare. Productivity tends to be defined as seeing a certain number of clients in a truncated amount of time. Effective, high-quality, humanistic prenatal care requires focus and engagement in the moment with the person who is in front of you now.

The psychological mechanisms, theories, and care practices presented in this chapter give the prenatal care provider a structure for exploring a variety of psychosocial issues important to healthy adaptation, attachment, and **maternal, paternal, or parental role development** in the pregnant person. These issues are best explored over several visits and in the context of a developing relationship of mutual dialogue and trust. The prenatal visit offers opportunity for casual but concentrated conversation in which to hear the pregnant individual's stories while examining the pregnant abdomen. The prenatal care provider can encourage sharing of important information through **active listening**, liberal use of affirmations and probes, and a warm, caring, and nonjudgmental attitude. While prenatal care providers are not psychological therapists per se, much of the information, counseling, and support provided during prenatal care will prove reassuring and therapeutic to the pregnant person.

Because much of the research and theories discussed in this chapter are derived from studying gender-specific roles, gendered language will be used more frequently in this chapter than in other areas of the book. Additionally, it is important to note that bisexual, queer, trans, and **gender**-diverse parent families remain understudied family types, especially in terms of attachment and adaptations in the childbearing year. However, what contemporary research has clearly demonstrated is that although the family structure does not affect the development of children with sexual and/or gender minority parents, discrimination and stigmatization against their family do. For more details on the preconception, pregnancy, and postpartum care of LGTBQ+ individuals, see Chapter 25, *Preconception, Pregnancy, and Postpartum Care of LGBTQ+ Individuals.*

Health equity keys points

- Black motherhood exists at the intersection of race and gender; prenatal psychosocial adaptations can be complicated by racist assumptions and discriminatory treatment.
- Attachment of the newborn to their primary caretaker is universal, but culturally dependent, shaped by culturally specific forms of adaptation and development.
- Weight stigma around weight gain and loss in the childbearing year is prevalent and can contribute to negative outcomes for pregnant and postpartum individuals.

Attachment and Adaptation

The attachments individuals form with a small circle of family and friends can give meaning and direction to their lives. Joys, sorrows, triumphs, and challenges are shared; information and tangible aids are given and received through these important social relationships. Mental and physical health processes and outcomes are mediated by psychosocial connections (Eick et al., 2018). Perhaps no single relationship in life is as important as that between a primary caregiver and child in setting the stage for later life. Parental-infant bonding has its roots in early life experiences and circumstances surrounding the current pregnancy. Attachment to the fetus and adaptation of the pregnant person and their family during pregnancy are processes that can be evaluated by the prenatal care provider. Interventions, education, support, and referrals can be made to ameliorate problems and to promote psychosocial health.

There are many interesting questions raised regarding basic processes underlying the origins and transmission of gender-role attitudes and structures, many of which begin in the prenatal period (Zosuls et al., 2011). For example, how does choosing to know the **sex** of the fetus by ultrasound or genetic tests early in pregnancy shape parental behavior and **expectations** and ultimately the socialization of the child? Our understanding of issues related to the role of gender in shaping individuals, relationships, and social institutions is evolving.

Adaptation to the pregnancy and attachment to the fetus are critical to the survival of the newly born baby and to the ongoing health of the mother or birth parent (Robakis et al., 2016). Prenatal attachment to the fetus is associated with positive postnatal bonding and decreased maternal anxiety and depression in the postpartum period (Dubber et al., 2015, Pisoni et al., 2014). Healthy adaptation and attachment are evidenced by the mother or birth parent's physical caretaking and emotional attentiveness to their baby's needs; this is enacted during pregnancy as self-care measures, such as avoiding alcohol and teratogens. Emotional attentiveness may manifest in other behaviors, such as giving the fetus a nickname, talking to the fetus, and playing music for the fetus. Failure to adapt and attach can lead to a variety of disorders after birth; for the mother or birth parent, these can include postpartum depression, detached parenting, abusive parenting, social isolation, and deterioration of self-care practices; for the baby, these can include failure to thrive without organic cause, risk of abuse, and inability to form social bonds with others (Hornor, 2019).

Pregnancy as a transitional event in the life of an individual and their family has been conceptualized from two overarching psychosocial perspectives: (a) pregnancy as a crisis; and (b) pregnancy as a developmental life phase. Each perspective informs theoretical relationships and care strategies. Paradoxically, both perspectives may operate jointly or alternately in the individual's experience of pregnancy. For the prenatal care provider, conceptual frameworks, philosophical tenets, and approaches to care logically follow from each perspective. Therefore, each perspective will be considered here.

The word *crisis* derives from Greek and literally translates "to decide." While the word typically is used to express more negative connotations of disaster or the likelihood of a poor outcome, it has also been interpreted as a turning point or opportunity. A crisis is said to occur whenever an event or circumstance disrupts normal functioning or perspectives. The individual enters a state of disequilibrium and must find new methods of problem-solving in order to reach an altered yet effective state of functioning. Pregnancy necessitates physical and psychosocial adjustments in functioning and perspectives by the pregnant individual and their family, meeting the definition of crisis. Whether this crisis is resolved in a positive or negative manner depends on such factors as the meaning of the pregnancy to the person, the support and resources available to deal with the pregnancy, and the resiliency and emotional management systems that the individual can access (Sahin, 2022).

Pregnancy has also been conceptualized as a developmental phase or challenge from a life course perspective. In this worldview, pregnancy is seen as a maturational stage that most people able to become pregnant in the United States will experience in their lives. However, population trends show that adults voluntarily choosing not to have children are rising; these individuals and couples are called child-free to distinguish them from those who are childless and struggling with infertility (Neal & Neal, 2022). The changes inherent in the developmental phase of pregnancy are tasks that must be mastered in order to move to a new level of functioning. A developmental phase can lead to growth or decline in individual or family functioning. Importantly, in either paradigm of pregnancy, the pregnant individual and their family are open to the services and ministrations of a professional to assist them in this process of transition and change.

Attachment Theory

A number of theoreticians have contributed to modern understandings of attachment and adaptation in the childbearing year (Bowlby, 1978; Brazelton, 1973; Kennell & Klaus, 1976). John Bowlby, a British psychoanalyst, described attachment theory from his observations working with maladapted adolescents (Bowlby, 1978). He noted that the presence of the mother or a primary caretaker was a key variable in healthy personality development for an individual. His premise is that the mother and the infant are biologically preprogrammed to form a strong attachment relationship, but their roles are different. The baby's role is to lead the relationship through behavioral cues, and the mother's role is to respond to these cues in a timely and sensitive manner. Infant behavior, such as cooing and crying, is designed to attain and maintain proximity to the mother. Evidence supports Bowlby's contention that early child–caregiver attachment influences the individual's ability to form and maintain close relationships throughout life (Liu, 2019; Pallini et al., 2014).

Mary Ainsworth was a protégé and colleague of John Bowlby. She theorized that maternal sensitivity to her infant gave the child a secure base from which to explore the environment (Van Rosmalen et al., 2016). She created a psychological tool to explore security and attachment in children called "the strange situation." A mother and her infant were brought into a room with a stranger. After several minutes, the mother unobtrusively exited the room. The infant's behavior upon recognition of the absence of the mother was observed and was considered a reflection of the degree of attachment. This test is still used in research in the area of attachment psychology. Bowlby and his associates focused more on delineating infant behaviors; their work served as a foundation for Kennell and Klaus in their development of a theory of maternal–infant bonding that revolutionized thinking about prenatal and birth practices in America in the 1970s and beyond (Kennell & Klaus, 1976; Klaus et al., 1995).

Marshall Kennell and John Klaus, physicians in neonatal intensive care units (NICUs), noted that premature babies who spent extended periods of separation from their mothers after birth would graduate from the nursery to the home environment once they were considered healthy and growing. However, a disproportionate number of these children would return to the emergency department, victims of abuse, or nonorganic failure to thrive (Klaus & Klaus, 1976; Klaus et al., 1995). Mothers became emotionally detached from these fragile infants due to limited to no contact with their infants, as was the custom in NICUs at the time. These mothers harbored feelings of **fear** that their babies did not belong to them and would not live long. The mothers also had few authentic skills in handling or providing care for their babies and, therefore, had little confidence that they could nurture their babies. Their lack of mothering skills and emotional stamina during this transition led to conditions under which their infants did not grow and develop properly.

Kennell and Klaus (1976) began to examine neonatal intensive care practices that exacerbated this emotional disconnect for mothers, which led to the investigation of birth practices for both preterm and term infants. Kennell and Klaus observed births in Guatemala in environments where the laboring woman was continuously attended by a female support person and where the baby was never separated from its mother. They found that both the mother and the baby are in a special sensitive period immediately postbirth, in which postpartum physiology and prolonged physical contact lead to profound connections between the mother and the neonate. The affective quality of maternal behaviors toward the newborn was gentler and more responsive in women who had the opportunity for skin-to-skin and prolonged contact. This sensitive period has been called the Golden Hour, referring to the hour immediately following birth. The Golden Hour is being recognized as many hospitals are altering their routine practices to include uninterrupted skin-to-skin contact and postpartum rooming-in in order to facilitate maternal–infant bonding.

Mothers follow a specific and universal pattern of behavior in becoming acquainted with their newborn (Kennell & Klaus, 1976). The tendency is to touch with fingertips first starting at the face, followed by gentle rubbing motion using the palms. They will align their face with their baby's face in the *en face* position to establish eye contact and for full visual exploration of their newborn. A high-pitched voice is used as they softly speak to their newborn. Maternal behavior such as this tends to elicit satisfying responses from the baby, which, in turn, stimulates the release of oxytocin and prolactin in the mother and affirms her mothering skills, leading to beneficial health effects for postpartum recovery. Postbirth bonding processes are important to review in the prenatal period with the pregnant person as some birth routines persist that do not honor the reciprocal interaction of the birth parent and the baby (Bergman & Bergman, 2013).

Prenatal preparation for postbirth bonding

1. Obtain the services of providers whose labor and birth practices are person-centered and baby friendly.
2. Attend childbirth education classes.
3. Articulate preferences for the conduct of labor, birth, and immediate postpartum in a written birth plan.
4. Arrange for continuous labor support with sensitive family, friends, a doula, or a midwife.
5. Have baby placed skin to skin immediately postbirth and leave undisturbed for a prolonged period of time.
6. Delay nonurgent procedures, such as cord clamping, injections, weighing, bathing, and eye prophylaxis.
7. Allow generous amounts of time for the baby to breastfeed and interact with the family.

Infant Contributions to Attachment

The contribution of newborn behavior to the establishment of the early mother–infant bond was not acknowledged until the past few decades (Brazelton, 1973). T. Berry Brazelton was a pediatrician who led this body of work by calling attention to the remarkable behaviors and resiliency of the newborn. Prior to this, the neonate was considered a "*tabla rasa,*" a blank slate that was primarily a product of the environment and, therefore, did not evolve a personality until after birth. However, it has become apparent that temperament and capabilities are inborn and evolve. Individual differences in fetal reactivity and regulation can be identified in the in-utero period and have been associated with infant temperament (Pingeton et al., 2021). Neonatal behaviors, such as crying, rooting, and gazing, call forth maternal responses, such as singing, nursing, and comforting.

A critical concept for prenatal care practice is that as fetal sensorimotor capabilities develop, the fetus is acting, reacting, and learning in the intrauterine environment. Sharing the developing wonder of what the fetus is capable of and experiencing at various gestational weeks are important teaching points during prenatal care and can support the development of maternal and parental fetal attachment. Inviting the pregnant person to feel what the clinician is palpating during Leopold maneuvers is a powerful and interactive teaching moment (Nishikawa & Sakakibara, 2013). Additionally, preparing the family for the range of normal early newborn activities, including the various newborn states, such as sleep, drowsiness, quiet alert, activeness, excitability, and crying, will give them tools for interpreting and interacting with their newborn's behavior.

Prenatal teaching regarding fetal growth and development

1. Share the average weight and length of the fetus for gestational age at each visit, easily available on gestational wheels or prenatal apps.
2. Motor capabilities develop in the late embryonic phase at seven to eight weeks of gestation and change in quality and pattern as nerves and muscles mature.
3. Fetal reactivity to touch and pressure begins early, at 10–12 weeks of estimated gestational age.
4. Fetal hearing develops at 23–24 weeks; the fetus will respond to sound.
5. Fetal vision is the last sense to develop; eyes unfuse at 24–26 weeks and sight matures over time.

Source: Blackburn (2018)/Elsevier.

Neurobiology of Attachment

Early activation of maternal behavior and infant response is influenced not only by social expectations and behavioral norms, but also by hormones, such as oxytocin and prolactin, and by brain circuitry, such as the hypothalamic–midbrain–limbic–paralimbic–cortical circuits of the brain (Bjelica et al., 2018). Inborn neural pathways are shaped by early experiences and set by repetitive patterns that lead to various types of attachments and emotional regulation. While the neural networks of the brain exhibit plasticity (i.e., the ability to change and adapt), it is important to support the foundational formative experiences that set the stage for developing and maintaining positive relationships over a lifetime.

The reciprocal physiologic interaction of maternal–infant attachment is most striking in the early hours after birth. Processes are interrelated, coordinated, and mutually regulated between mother and baby to optimize outcomes for both (Buckley, 2015). Common birth practices have the ability to support or disrupt these processes, and there is a call to respect the Golden Hour after birth to allow privacy and time for critical bonding to take place. One example of the reciprocity of systems is oxytocin release. Skin-to-skin newborn contact stimulates oxytocin, which benefits the mother by causing uterine contractions that control blood loss, inducing calming effects via actions on the central nervous system, and facilitating infant warming through the vasodilation of the maternal chest. The newborn benefits from the second stage surge of oxytocin, which manifests in stress reduction, and a quiet alert state that is inherently attractive to its caregivers. Pleasure centers are activated, and a positive start to life's most important relationships has begun.

Intergenerational attachments patterns are being studied with newer understandings of the influence of genetics on behavioral patterns and epigenetic theories (Liu, 2019). Epigenetics is the study of mechanisms that can activate or deactivate the expression of genes. The changes in the body's biochemical milieu surrounding cells and their genetic material can impact DNA protein replication (Bludau et al., 2019). The social environment can moderate the genetic expression of adaptive behavior as well as pathologic behavior. An example of this process is the epigenome of monozygotic twins who begin life with the same epigenome, but it diverges across their life spans due to differing life circumstances. This area of attachment is just being explored and will evolve understandings of attachment processes in the future.

Long-Term Effects of Disorganized Attachment

Early attachment relationships are prioritized as children begin to make sense of their world. Children are more likely to create beliefs that something is wrong with them rather than their mother or primary caretaker when the primary care provider does not respond to their needs in a timely or sensitive manner. **Disorganized attachment** is relational trauma, a form of complex post-traumatic stress syndrome, when connection and affection between the primary caretaker and the child do not take place. As an infant makes its needs known through limited capacities, responses from the mother or caretaker shape the sense of the environment as friendly and caring or threatening and indifferent (Petri et al., 2018). Biologically, neural pathways are laid down early in life, which embed these formative experiences into the psyche. As the child matures, foundational beliefs, such as concepts of self-worth and belonging, are built from early and prolonged exposures to attentive or neglectful parenting. While the effects of disorganized attachment can be addressed and ameliorated through therapy, it is preferable to take a preventive approach. The prenatal healthcare provider can assess and facilitate attachment and can offer referral to professionals in psychology, psychiatry, and social work when disturbances in attachment are identified.

Maternal Role Development

Rubin

The theories of Reva Rubin, a nurse researcher, have been seminal in the area of maternal **role** development and maternal attachment (Mercer, 1985, 1995, 2010; Rubin, 1984). The maternal role is developed over time as the mother learns to love, respond to, and care for her infant (see Figure 23.1). The role is attained when the woman has developed confidence in herself as a mother, feels competent in care-giving tasks, and expresses gratification and satisfaction with her role (Meighan, 2017). Current prenatal care focuses on biomedical changes and markers, but people are well served by healthcare providers who recognize, appreciate, facilitate, and support the pivotal personal and family dynamic changes that occur during the

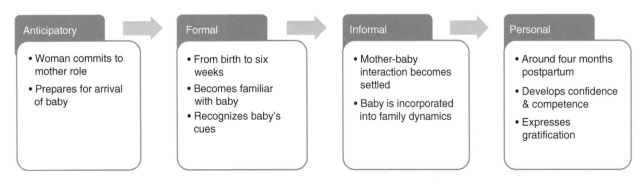

Figure 23.1 Stages of maternal role development. Adapted from Mercer and Walker (2006).

Table 23.1   Indicators for Maternal Role Development

Positive development	Impaired development
Robust fantasies about baby and motherhood	Persistent unrealistic or negative fantasies
Can identify positive maternal role models	No positive maternal role models in one's life
Awareness of fetal/newborn capabilities	Knowledge deficit regarding fetal/newborn capabilities
Wearing clothes that accommodate the pregnant body	Wearing clothes that constrict or hide the pregnant body
Acceptance of bodily changes of pregnancy	Negative response to bodily changes of pregnancy
Seeking care, support, and advice from professionals and family	Dismissing care, support, and advice by professionals and family
Engaging in health-promoting practices	Engaging in practices that are harmful to health
Enriching and empathetic social environment	Impoverished or abusive social environment

Source: Rubin (1984), Mercer and Walker (2006), and Meighan (2017).

childbearing year. Becoming a mother involves changing emotions, attitudes, and behaviors as the child grows.

Rubin conceptualized a series of maternal tasks that were achieved through specific cognitive processes. Her work has been extended, revised, and critiqued over time by herself and by other researchers (Meighan, 2017; Mercer, 1995; Mercer, 2010; Mercer & Walker, 2006; Rubin, 1984). Her theories are still influential in modern conceptions of maternal role development (Cabrera, 2018; Shrestha et al., 2019). Rubin's four tasks of maternal role development arise from a lifetime of social learning that becomes internalized within the individual mother. These tasks include (a) safe passage; (b) acceptance by others; (c) binding-in to the child; and (d) giving of oneself. See Table 23.1 for indicators of positive or impaired development of maternal role attainment.

Tasks of Maternal Role Development

The maternal task of *safe passage* is defined as seeking the means to assure a secure and healthy pregnancy and childbirth for herself and her fetus/newborn. Early in pregnancy, the woman is self-aware and has not yet differentiated the fetus as an individual. She experiences early bodily changes and pregnancy discomforts, such as breast tenderness and enlargement, and nausea and vomiting; her concerns for safety are initially focused on her own health and physical changes. However, safety concerns expand to include embryonic/fetal health and well-being as the fetus becomes psychologically differentiated as an individual for the pregnant woman. This differentiation is used to fully actualize with quickening, but with

the advent of first-trimester ultrasound images of the baby, it can occur with an early ultrasound. The woman becomes aware of the intertwined fates of herself and her baby. Danger for one constitutes danger for the other. Labor and birth are seen as particularly risky events to navigate. Successful attainment of "seeking safe passage" is achieved through acquiring knowledge and skills to help her successfully manage pregnancy and childbirth and through arrangement of tangible aid and social support by family, friends, and professionals.

Pregnancy signals impending changes in the nature of social relationships for the woman, her baby, and her family. This requires letting go of old ways of being to make way for the newer ways of being. To achieve the task of *acceptance by others* for herself as a mother and for her baby as a new family member, the pregnant woman reflects on her current life, her past relationships, and role models with respect to parenting and on her current relationships and aspirations for mothering. She will need to give up certain behaviors of her prepregnancy lifestyle and may want acknowledgment for these changes. If she has more babies in the future, acceptance of the new baby by the siblings will be an important milestone. The ages and developmental stages of the siblings will dictate how she will approach them in gaining this acceptance for her new baby. Her success in navigating this task will largely depend on the quality of her relationships with her partner, her mother, and other important members of her kinship and friendship networks.

The task of *binding-in* to the child is one of establishing a direct form of experience between the mother and her fetus/infant. This entails moving the abstraction of the baby-to-be into a real relationship. An awareness of a separate being, not just being pregnant, is facilitated by ultrasound images, listening to the fetal heartbeat, and recognizing its separate rhythm from her own, and the quintessential experience in differentiating the idea of the baby as a separate being—quickening. The sensation of fetal movement begins an internal awareness of the fetus and its activity patterns for the pregnant woman. Early fetal movements are felt only by the mother and, as such, can be a very special period in gestation. Later in gestation, fetal movements can be palpated externally by others. Mothers-to-be may engage in conversations with their babies about their movements as pregnancy goes along. A dimension of relatedness to the fetus is added to the pregnancy and marks the onset of maternal–infant attachment.

The fourth task of maternal role attainment is "giving of oneself" and is felt by Rubin to be the most complex and demanding task of childbearing. Physical, emotional, and social changes of pregnancy progressively require more and more modifications in the woman's lifestyle and choices. And yet, she must embrace these changes willingly and see their purpose in giving to her child for the child's benefit and well-being. This state of "giving-to" creates a sense of vulnerability, dependence, and a need to be "given-to" in return. "Mothering the mother" is a phrase that symbolizes ways in which family and professionals can support the pregnant woman by assuring her that she will have tangible aid and emotional support that will see her through vulnerable moments.

Cognitive Processes for Maternal Role Development

Rubin articulated three cognitive processes through which the four tasks of maternal role attainment are achieved: replication, fantasy, and dedifferentiation. *Replication* is the active search by the woman for elements of the maternal role that she wishes to incorporate into her interpretation of becoming mother and that she believes are valued by society. Mimicry is an imitation of simple behaviors or practices she has seen other mothers execute. Role-playing is an interactive form of replication and requires a partner in the role-play situation. The woman will closely observe signals from the role-playing partner to see if she is receiving positive or negative feedback from her early mothering behaviors or ideas. She will evolve her role accordingly. Rubin refers to this as "binding-in" to a **maternal identity**.

Cognitive processes in maternal role development

- Replication—seeking elements of mothering that are valued to incorporate into her vision of mothering
- Fantasy—trying on different aspects of mothering through mental contemplation
- Dedifferentiation—synthesizing elements of replication and fantasy work into a single role of mother

---

Fantasy is an essential cognitive component of maternal role taking. It is not to be confused with a stream of consciousness daydream but is rather a series of mental operations that help the pregnant woman accept the pregnancy and the baby, try on various aspects of the mother role mentally, and deal with the hopes and fears she has for her new life ahead. Grief work is another aspect of fantasy work that refers to the gradual disengagement with aspects of the pregnant woman's prior life, no longer useful in the new imagined life. Moving through the grief work allows her to adjust to her new maternal role.

Dedifferentiation is the third cognitive process by which a woman assumes the maternal role. This is an exploration of the goodness of fit of prior fantasy work with the woman's current self-image. The determination of congruence of the fantasized behaviors, **attitudes**, and interactions examined in replication and fantasy work are then assimilated into the woman's formulation of the maternal role.

What can prenatal care providers incorporate into their care practices from an understanding of maternal role development? Providers should inquire about relationships and behaviors important to the woman's attachment to the fetus and her attainment of the maternal role. Clear communication can be encouraged within her primary relationships and can be role-modeled by the prenatal provider. Descriptions of the wide range of normal social and emotional changes she faces can be reassuring to the pregnant woman. Asking about fantasy work and dreams are a chance to engage in discussions that can lead to exploration of her hopes and fears regarding impending childbirth and motherhood. Providing information to enhance the woman's knowledge of her changing needs throughout the course of pregnancy and early postpartum, and of newborn characteristics and behaviors is an essential service. For women who are struggling with serious relationship issues, strategies to assist her include clarifying the problem situation, reviewing steps to conflict resolution, and providing her with appropriate referrals for her psychosocial issues.

Lederman

Dimensions of Psychosocial Adaptation in Pregnancy

Another important theorist in psychosocial concerns in pregnancy is Regina Lederman (Lederman & Weis, 2009), a nurse researcher, who described seven dimensions of maternal development for women from her work examining psychophysiological correlates among pregnancy and childbirth variables. She looked at variables such as maternal **anxiety**, **coping** and safety, labor progress indices, and biochemical markers of **stress**—epinephrine, norepinephrine, and cortisol. Her seven dimensions of psychosocial adaptation include the following areas:

1. Acceptance of pregnancy
2. Identification with a motherhood role
3. Relationship with the mother
4. Relationship with the partner
5. Preparation for labor
6. Fear of loss of control in labor
7. Fear of loss of **self-esteem** in labor.

Her work offers additional important insights to the development of the maternal role, is compatible with Rubin's theories, and will be discussed here.

Acceptance of pregnancy is the adaptive response by the woman to the pregnancy and all that it means in her life. A common feature a woman works toward accepting her pregnancy is ambivalence toward being pregnant. Ambivalence is holding opposing positive and negative thoughts, attitudes, and emotions simultaneously for the same event. Ambivalence is expected to occur in women with an unintended pregnancy as they take in the fact that they are pregnant and consider the implications and choices they have ahead, but it also occurs in women who have planned to be pregnant. Women who are pregnant for the first time face a number of adaptations and limitations with pregnancy and may need to work through both positive and negative emotions (Soltani et al., 2017). The feeling of ambivalence is a normal reaction to the diagnosis of pregnancy and is largely resolved in the early months of pregnancy, but it may recur as the enormity of the life changes are felt by the woman. In Lederman's research (Lederman & Weis, 2009), acceptance of the pregnancy was found to be

Assessment of maternal attachment and adaptation

1. How do you feel about being pregnant?
2. Was this a planned pregnancy or was it unintended? Did both you and your partner agree about the plan?
3. How was pregnancy achieved? Easily? With difficulty? Through assisted reproductive technologies?
4. How do others in your life feel about your pregnancy? Your partner? Your children? Your parents? Your friends?
5. Do you have tangible and emotional support from your partner, family, and friends during pregnancy and beyond?
6. What was your relationship with your mother or primary caretakers like? What were their birth experiences like?
7. How has your relationship with your partner changed during the pregnancy?
8. What bodily changes are you experiencing? How do you feel about these changes?
9. What dreams or fantasies about the baby or about your transition to motherhood do you have?
10. What are you doing differently now that you are pregnant to avoid harm and maintain your health and your baby's health? Changes in habits, such as diet, exercise, rest? Avoidance of smoking, alcohol, drugs?
11. What are you doing to prepare for the baby? Car seat? A room or sleeping space? Clothing, diapers, and other items?
12. Do you talk to your baby in utero? Have a name or nickname for the baby?
13. Are you aware of the baby's movements and position? How would you describe your baby's activities?
14. Are you planning to breastfeed your baby?
15. What are your plans and preferences for labor and birth?

Source: Adapted from Lederman and Weis (2009).

related to a woman's identification with a motherhood role, her relationship with her own mother, and her level of preparation for labor. Additional factors found to be important were the woman's reaction to her bodily changes and whether these reactions manifested in any discomforts of pregnancy. While there are anatomical and physiological explanations for the multitude of common discomforts of pregnancy, the astute care provider will also consider whether these discomforts are a psychosomatic expression of ambivalence, anxiety, stress, or personality issues.

The transition from woman-without-child to woman-as-mother is a process that, when navigated successfully, will end with the *identification with a motherhood role* (Lederman & Weiss, 2009). The extent to which a woman is identifying with a motherhood role can be assessed by exploring the motivation and preparation she has for such a life event. The motivations leading to pregnancy are as varied as are the life stories of the women seen. Some variants on the circumstances surrounding a pregnancy and its meaning can include a planned pregnancy accomplished without difficulty in a committed couple relationship, pregnancy achieved with the use of assisted reproductive technologies amid financial concerns, complicated therapeutic procedures and side effects, a pregnancy in a single woman with several sexual partners in the time frame of conception, and an adolescent who feels social pressure to become pregnant for confirmation that she is desirable and healthy. In some **cultures**, pregnancy will tie a man to a woman in a provider role while the baby is young. This is particularly true in areas of extreme poverty where outsiders view pregnancy as detrimental to the woman's circumstance, and yet her reality may be that a pregnancy and new baby keep the baby's father in a provider role and will help her feed herself and her children for the next several years. These varied pregnancy circumstances lead to varied identification with the

motherhood role and different time frames and emotional journeys in developing the maternal role.

Maternal detachment as a protective mechanism

Women who live with conditions of chronic scarcity and daily struggles to survive, as is seen in impoverished areas of the world, often delay forming attachments to their infants. Maternal attachment is muted and protectively distanced when one's frame of reference is a high fertility rate combined with a high infant mortality rate (Scheper-Hughes, 1985), as is seen in areas such as Haiti, Ethiopia, South Sudan, and remote rural Brazil. Clinicians serving immigrant women from areas with abject poverty or clinicians traveling to provide prenatal care in these areas may note maternal indifference that is in marked contrast to expectations of maternal joy in the United States. Such flat affect is often a reflection of the difficult life path and history of losses experienced in the woman's own precarious efforts to survive. The delay in attachment does not preclude the eventual formation of a secure attachment between mother and child and should be understood in its cultural context.

The desire to be pregnant can be separate from the desire to bear and raise a child. Concerns are raised if the mother-to-be is not preparing for the baby through gathering of supplies and cognitive preparation. However, some cultures do not include preparation for the baby during pregnancy due to the belief that such preparation may invite bad luck. The sensitive care provider will recognize cultural variation in the meaning and expectations ascribed to preparatory activities during pregnancy and will consider maternal behavior in this context. Congruent with Rubin's cognitive processes, Lederman (Lederman & Weis, 2009) found that fantasizing and dreaming were important mental strategies in trying on various maternal behaviors and styles of parenting. These mental operations allowed the woman to envision herself as a mother with characteristics that she desires to develop in that role and to anticipate future life changes as a result of becoming a mother. Her own childhood is reconsidered from a new perspective, including mothering behaviors she experienced that she plans to incorporate or eliminate in her repertoire of mothering behaviors. Role conflicts are anticipated, including the common concerns of job or career demands, childcare arrangements, and concomitant financial implications. Positive identification with the motherhood role involves the clarification of the woman's self-image as mother and the progressive development of confidence in her abilities to successfully complete the tasks of mothering. Women who struggle with low self-esteem, excessive narcissism, lack of good role models, and work–family life balance can experience anxiety related to role adaptations. The psychophysiological influences of these conflicts manifested in this study as prolonged labors and difficult births for a disproportionate number of these women.

It is difficult to generalize theories of maternal role attainment to experiences of Black women because so much of the research has been done on White women (Fouquier, 2013). Black women in the United States experience gendered racism, the intersection of sexism and racism, in their pregnancies (Mehra et al., 2020). While developing their own maternal identities, they are subject to microaggressions and the effects of chronic racism over the life course. Stereotypes combining sexist, racist, and classist images such as mammies (faithful, domestically servile), matriarchs (aggressive, unfeminine), welfare mothers (low-income, unwed), and Jezebels (sexually aggressive) are ascribed to Black mothers (Mehra et al., 2020). In a qualitative study of Black pregnant women, these microaggressions were manifested in assumptions such as Black mothers are on welfare and have too many children. One participant stated "I do think pregnancy is harder for Black, African-American women. We get the most judgement" (Mehra et al., 2020, p. 6). Coping responses to these judgments were to find interconnectedness with friends and family; employ prayer and spiritual beliefs, use problem-solving strategies, and to disengage from the situation. The more active forms of coping acted as a stress buffer and enhanced self-esteem.

The pregnant woman's *relationship with her own mother* is an important line of inquiry for the prenatal clinician to discuss. Intergenerational parenting patterns, while not destiny, are foundations that serve as reference for the development of the maternal role. The love and support present or lacking in her own childhood may shape the pregnant woman's approach to mothering. Inquire about the pregnant woman's relationship with her mother or primary caretaker. This can give rise to discussions about her experiences of being mothered. The grandmother's reaction to the pregnancy and acknowledgment of her daughter as a mother can be influential. Within positive family dynamics, the grandmother-to-be may enjoy sharing memories and reminiscing about her childbearing and childrearing experiences with her pregnant daughter. Their relationship can take on new dimensions as the pregnant woman empathizes with her mother from a new perspective and the grandmother sees her daughter as a mature autonomous adult.

The *relationship with the woman's partner* is a vital element in her adjustment to the mother role. How the pregnant woman perceives the response of her partner to the pregnancy is key and may consist of the partner's empathy toward her, the ability to cooperate under changing conditions, availability for communication and sharing, and reliability in being present to her in both a physical and emotional sense.

The pregnant woman may have concerns about the partner's adjustment to the parenting role; this is something the prenatal care provider can inquire about and provide suggestions and support as appropriate. The nature of the relationship will be important to understand—an interdependent relationship with give and take by both parties can set the stage for success for both parents in assuming their impending parental duties. Mutual caretaking activities during pregnancy are positive signs for the partners' relationship and support for each other as parents. Pregnancy may enhance dependency needs in both partners as they face the restructuring of life as they know it; however, excessive dependency is counterproductive and associated with low autonomy and low self-esteem (Lederman & Weiss, 2009). Partner support during pregnancy has been shown to have a positive effect on selected outcomes such as reducing prenatal anxiety and depression, and supporting smoking cessation (Cheng et al., 2016).

Sexuality may change over the course of pregnancy and early parenting; this can be characterized as a normal evolution of this life phase for a couple. Sexual activities tend to decrease during the first trimester and will gradually be reestablished by six months postpartum (Yeniel & Petri, 2014). Strategies for fostering ongoing closeness and intimacy, such as designating daily time for communication, affection, and connection, can be suggested. Role conflicts that are common for couples can be presented for discussion and consideration. For example, if both partners work, childcare issues are something to begin to sort out during the pregnancy. Who will arrange childcare, transport the child, pack the diaper bag, and so forth? Some places of employment offer parental leaves that support either or both partners during their transition to parenthood; these work policies are important to investigate during the pregnancy. The partner relationship can contribute significantly to adaptation to pregnancy, breastfeeding, and parenthood and will undergo changes that provide the framework for family patterns that extend far into the future.

Preparation for labor is a dimension of psychosocial adaptation to pregnancy that has elements of practical preparation and imagined rehearsal. Preparation can be formal through structured classes or informal through friends, family, and social media. It is important to know the types of childbirth education classes that are available locally and to consider the influence that the classes chosen and taken will have on the pregnant person's knowledge and attitudes toward the childbirth interventions and processes and how this will shape their expectations and hopes for childbirth.

Much of the preparatory activity for pregnancy, labor, and birth is through accessing secondary sources; therefore, knowledge and decision-making about labor and birth today is highly influenced by these sources, such as friends and family's oral histories, books, Internet sources, smartphone apps, television, video, and movie depictions (Johnson, 2014; Luce et al., 2016). Symbolic depictions of others' birth experiences, such as stories of friends' births and television portrayals of labor and birth, are pervasive and almost unavoidable in contemporary culture. Negative experiences tend to be related more frequently and can have an undermining effect on confidence for childbirth. Direct observation of another's birth experience presents a unique learning opportunity. Under the liberal visiting policies in hospitals today or in community birth settings, it is not unusual for a person to have attended the birth of a friend or a family member. Birth has its own special sights, sounds, smells, and sensations, thus creating a multisensory barrage of information for those present. Birth is not experienced directly, but vicariously and within a particular social context. From their **perceptions** of both symbolic and witnessed birth, the observer gives meaning to these events, relevance to their life experience, and incorporates these perceptions into their feelings and beliefs about their abilities to labor and give birth.

Considering choices in labor and birth management and planning for labor and birth is done by pregnant people and encouraged by clinicians. An inherent problem with planning for birth is that there are multiple possibilities of unforeseen situations that may alter birth plans slightly or drastically, calling into play one or many of the labor and birth procedures that had previously been chosen or rejected. Birth satisfaction is positively related to having requests on a birth plan fulfilled and negatively related to the number of birth requests (Mei et al., 2016). Prenatal healthcare providers can assist by reviewing birth plans to foster realistic expectations and the need for flexibility as the labor unfolds in real time. Extensive birth plans should be viewed as an expression of fear and apprehension and an opportunity to discuss emotions and perceptions further. Some clients will avoid thinking about the upcoming labor and birth. This may represent a dysfunctional state or a coping strategy for the individual and should be investigated further.

From a psychological perspective, preparing for labor is also preparing for separation from the fetus. This separation begins with the onset of labor. Contractions and **pain** in labor are a phenomenon toward which much thought and anticipation are invested on the part of the pregnant person. The concept of contractions can be difficult for nulliparous pregnant individuals to imagine, particularly those who do not have prior pain experiences. Multigravid persons can have increased fear because they have

authentic experience to inform their expectations. The prenatal care provider can help clients understand that each labor and birth can be different from previous experiences. A sense of the work, pain, risks, and benefits of labor that are balanced and based on a healthy sense of realistic possibilities is the best place from which to anticipate labor for the pregnant individual.

The final dimension of psychosocial adaptation is related to dealing with significant fears for many childbearing people: *fear of loss of control in labor* and the *fear of loss of self-esteem in labor*. Fear is a powerful emotion with psychological and physical components. These fears are largely centered on the anticipated pain of childbirth and the ability to maintain control over her own physical reactions and emotional responses while in labor. There were also concerns of maintaining social control in terms of interpersonal interactions of respect and mutuality with the staff in the birth setting. Disrespectful and abusive care in childbirth facilities is a global problem, recognized by the World Health Organization as contributing to poor maternal and infant outcomes. In the United States, one in every six laboring women will experience one or more types of maltreatment, including loss of autonomy, being shouted at, scolded, or threatened, and being ignored, refused, or receiving no response to requests for help (Vedam et al., 2019). This problem is magnified for women of color. Respect, dignity, emotional support, and a systemic commitment to a patient-led, informed decision-making are quality care standards that optimize birth outcomes.

The fear of loss of self-esteem in labor is related to how well the woman feels she is able to maintain the level of control she has set for herself. However, a woman's underlying general sense of self-esteem is important as well. In Lederman's analysis (Lederman & Weis, 2009), childbearing women who held themselves in high self-esteem were tolerant with their own imperfections, persistent in working toward their goals, and were able to set boundaries with others who did not value their goals. Women with low self-esteem struggled with a pessimistic attitude toward events in their lives and were less likely to assert their abilities to influence the process and outcomes of their labor and birth experiences.

Fear of childbirth (FOC) is a feature of the complex and dynamic emotional response to the childbearing experience. For most, this fear is moderated by psychological defense mechanisms, such as rationalization and denial, as well as cognitive processes, such as self-esteem and self-efficacy. However, severe fear in childbirth is an issue that is often undetected and, therefore, unexplored in clinical practice. Severe fear in childbirth is called **tokophobia** and falls under the diagnostic category of Specific Phobia as an anxiety disorder. It is estimated that 18–31% of women have moderate levels of FOC, and 5–11% of women have severe levels of FOC (O'Connell et al., 2017). Prenatally, women with high levels of FOC have increased levels of daily stress, prepartum depression, and sleep deprivation that can significantly impair daily functioning and lead to poorer perinatal outcomes. Some pregnant

individuals will try to manage their fears by requesting an elective cesarean birth. A request for an elective cesarean section should trigger a discussion about fears, not simply risks and benefits of the procedure. Predisposing variables to extreme childbirth fear include prior traumatizing birth or medical experiences, low self-esteem, high numbers of daily stressors, and lack of social support (O'Connell et al., 2017).

Consistently over the last several years, about 40% of childbearing people in the United States are pregnant for the first time, while 60% are having repeat pregnancies. This has implications for the individual's expectations, psychological concerns, and family structure adjustments. Multigravidas have an authentic reference point from which to anticipate their impending labor, and while this is highly predictive, it also not a given. Some women will have to be encouraged to open their expectations to other possible trajectories for their labors. The maternal role has been developed to varying degrees of success and satisfaction in multigravid women; now, it is expanded to include another child. Concerns of multigravid women are practical and range from the financial concerns of an additional child to the work of a newborn added to the care and needs of older children (Lederman & Weis, 2009). Additionally, reactions from her partner and extended family may help or hinder her adjustment to becoming mother again.

Body Image

Body image is a subjective awareness and attitude toward one's body and its parts that may or may not correspond to objective measures. Many people have a love–hate relationship with aspects of their body, and this varies over time. Pregnancy is a time in life when body changes are normal, occur gradually over nine months, then resolve rapidly after birth. At few other times of life does a person gain and lose such significant amounts of weight in such a short time frame. Body image is an important psychological concept that influences other psychological processes internal to the individual, as well as behaviors and social relationships. Levels of satisfaction with one's pregnant body change over the course of gestation and have been linked to eating behaviors, gestational weight gain, anxiety disorders, depressive symptoms, exercise behaviors, and duration of breastfeeding (Brown et al., 2015; Inanir et al., 2015; Kiani-Sheikhabadi et al., 2019; Rauff & Downs, 2011).

There is an element of individual assessment of body image that is dynamic and varies over time, but there is also an element of social comparison. Ideals of youthful slender bodies in contemporary culture in the United States are not achievable by most women but are internalized nonetheless. Changes in body image during pregnancy are predicated on cultural norms and can be modified by partner response (Watson et al., 2016). Advanced pregnancy is readily discerned by the public. Public response to the pregnant body can surprise many individuals—for example, well-meaning strangers may approach in a public venue and touch their pregnant abdomen and make comments.

Social media posts can offer appearance ideals or realistic images of bodies in pregnancy and postpartum. Exposure to body positive social media images were found to have a positive effect on body image, with an inverse effect found with idealized body images (Becker et al., 2022). Pregnant people use the Internet for varied reasons including connecting with other pregnant people as a form of support and finding answers to questions about pregnancy and parenting (Baker & Yang, 2018). Because social media use is a significant and ubiquitous aspect of modern life, influences on self-image and mood can be expected.

The simple routine measure of obtaining weight during prenatal care has an emotionally charged meaning to many. Weight stigma is prevalent and can contribute to negative outcomes for pregnant and postpartum individuals (Rodriguez et al., 2019). A person's weight factors into their body image. This single numeric objective measure can elicit an emotional response. Weighing typically occurs at each client visit, despite having limited clinical value (Oken, 2015; Steer, 2015). Some clinicians will forgo weighing when it causes distress. People who enter pregnancy already dissatisfied with their body are more likely to gain outside the recommended weight gain guidelines (Bagheri et al., 2012; Mehta et al., 2010). Beyond the physical health consequences of weight, weight has a powerful link to body image and self-worth that the insightful prenatal care provider will recognize. Little is known about the experience of weight stigma in pregnancy and its effect on body image for trans, nonbinary, and gender-diverse individuals.

Body awareness in pregnancy focuses on the obvious areas of breast and abdominal growth and other physiologic changes. Some of these changes are received positively; others cause dismay. The prenatal care provider can help by providing anticipatory guidance and explanation of the physical changes that can occur. The pregnant body has been celebrated in art since ancient times and is considered beautiful by many people. This fact can be shared with the pregnant person as inspiration and positive affirmation. Pregnant transgender men may react to the bodily changes of pregnancy in various ways. Some view it a functional sacrifice to achieve the goal of having children, with the body changes tolerated or even embraced as part of the process (Charter et al., 2018). For others, the reaction can range from distasteful to dysphoric. Detaching one's self from the pregnant body and creating cognitive distance is a protective coping mechanism used to adapt to pregnancy changes by some transgender men (Charter et al., 2018).

The pregnant body acts as a protective container for the baby. For the individual who accepts and embraces the pregnancy, the body changes may be tangible evidence that the baby is healthy and growing well. However, many people are unprepared for the body changes in early postpartum and the time it can take to return to a nonpregnant body shape (Hodgkinson et al., 2014). Few will regain their prepregnant body shape, although many will approximate it within a few weeks postpartum. This is an area of anticipatory guidance by the prenatal care provider for education, healthy lifestyle promotion, and support.

Clothing can be an extension of the body image. Besides the practical nature of clothing for skin protection and temperature regulation, choice of clothing can communicate identity and project a statement or an image. Additionally, maternity clothing must be functional to accommodate rapid body changes. The change from regular clothing to pregnancy clothes usually occurs of necessity by the 20th week for pregnant nulliparas and by the 16th to 18th week for multiparas. In the past, maternity clothing was used to camouflage pregnancies; however, the newest generation of maternity clothing design highlights and celebrates the wearer's pregnancy (Sohn & Bye, 2015; Weigle & McAndrews, 2021). Maternity clothing that accentuates rather than hides the pregnant body is now being made for a range of activities, from work attire to athletic wear to lingerie.

Body art has moved from a practice of selected subcultures to a practice embraced by many in the mainstream (VanHoover et al., 2017). Some pregnant individuals may have body modification done as part of their identity and body image. It is important to communicate openness and respect for the meaning and motivation of each individual's body art choices. Tattoos may be visually affected by pregnancy if they are in areas of the skin that stretch as the body grows. Tattoos do not cause particular concern during pregnancy. Body piercing may need to be addressed depending on the site of the piercing. Jewelry worn in piercings of the breasts, nipples, abdomen, and genitalia may migrate, extrude through areas of thinning skin, or tear during the changes wrought by pregnancy and birth. It is recommended that pregnant individuals remove jewelry from these sites during advanced pregnancy and childbirth. Breast and nipple jewelry should not be worn while breastfeeding as the jewelry can cause poor latch, choking, and trauma to the infant's oral structures. People planning pregnancy are advised to delay body piercing or acquisition of new tattoos in the months prior to pregnancy due to healing time and potential for infection. It is important to recognize that body modification may be part of the person's self-image. Discussions about body art should be conducted in a supportive and nonjudgmental manner.

Body art adaptations in pregnancy

- Tattoos may be visually affected by pregnancy changes.
- Low back tattoos may affect whether and how epidurals are given; discuss options with anesthesiology professionals.
- Jewelry in pierced areas stretched by the pregnancy may be extruded.
- Remove all jewelry before childbirth to avoid injury.
- Remove nipple jewelry before nursing.
- Avoid acquiring new tattoos or piercings during pregnancy or lactation.

By paying attention to bodily changes, the pregnant person has a unique knowledge of their bodily processes and the life of the fetus. The movements of the fetus and the contractions of the uterus are felt with immediacy and certainty. Technologies in prenatal care, such as ultrasound imaging, fetal heart rate monitors, and screening tests for Down syndrome, are often given more credence in technologically dependent societies. The prenatal care provider needs to honor the information provided by the individual and to carefully balance the information obtained by machine. Although machine-generated information is typically considered more objective than human-generated information, it can create as much uncertainty as it reduces (Lawson & Turriff-Janasson, 2006; Sandelowski, 1993). Additionally, medically controlled information can create a distance between the pregnant person and their organic experience of pregnancy. Just as we encourage people to listen to their bodies, so too are we obligated to listen and respond to their accounts of their body awareness and body knowledge.

Sibling Preparation

Sibling relationships are a dynamic force within the family; children and their parents exert mutual influence on each other in their interactions. Often the new baby is an object of great interest to younger and older siblings alike, though responses vary based on the child's age, personality, and what developmental milestones are being mastered. Toddlers in particular may temporarily demonstrate regressed behaviors, such as increases in pacifier use or clinging to the parent or aggression toward the newborn. An estimated 80% of children will grow up with siblings, so this is a common adjustment in family structure (Volling, 2012).

Preparation of siblings for a new baby may be a parental concern. Sometimes, siblings accompany their mother or pregnant parent to prenatal visits and can be asked about their feelings and expectations for the new baby directly in an age-appropriate manner. If children are not present at prenatal visits, selected questions can be asked of the pregnant individual in regard to the children. Formal sibling preparation classes have not been found to make a significant difference in sibling behavior toward the newborn (Beyers-Carlson & Volling, 2017); however, they can be a rich learning opportunity for the family and can offer parents some coping strategies to deal with sibling concerns. For the prenatal care provider, the most appropriate focus is in assessment, education, and support of the family as they adjust their familial structure and roles to include another child.

Sibling presence at birth can be a positive and meaningful life event for the children and the parents. A recent literature review of sibling-attended birth reported that in home birth, 34% of older siblings were present for labor and 23% attended the birth (Naber et al., 2018). However, the research is this area was primarily done in the 1970s–1980s with few recent contributions. Some hospitals

---

Assessment of sibling preparation

1. What are the ages of the siblings?
2. What have they been told about the pregnancy? How have they responded?
3. What is their understanding of pregnancy, birth, and becoming a big sibling?
4. What is their understanding of the needs of newborns? Of the new demands on their parents' time and energy?
5. What are their expressed feelings about the pregnancy and baby? Are there any notable changes in sibling behavior that coincide with the news of the pregnancy?
6. How are siblings to be included in prenatal visits? In labor and birth?
7. What is the nature of the maternal relationship with each sibling? Partner relationship with each sibling? The sibling-to-sibling relationship? Grandparent relationships with each sibling? Relationship of each sibling with friends or other family?
8. Are the basic needs of the siblings—food, shelter, clothing, developmentally appropriate activities, positive emotional climate, and appropriate supervision and guidance of behavior—provided for by responsible adults? Are there plans in place for the additional resources needed for the new baby?

---

and most birth centers permit siblings at birth, often with the proviso that the child has their own support person available to step out of the intensity of the birth area if this becomes necessary. Midwives are frequently champions of this option as they encourage family-centered care and have witnessed the powerful emotional connections made during sibling-attended birth.

Partner Adaptation and Attachment

Pregnant individuals may or may not have partners in a committed social and legal relationship. Forty percent of births today are to unmarried cisgender women although the nature of unmarried status is changing with more couples choosing informal cohabiting unions (Martin et al., 2017). Lesbian couples may choose to have babies through a pregnancy of one or both of the partners, and gestational surrogates may carry pregnancies for gay and infertile couples. Trans individuals may consider similar reproductive options. Some people choose to proceed with pregnancy without a partner, availing themselves of assisted reproduction technologies to achieve pregnancy. Others are abandoned by their partners after the diagnosis of an unplanned pregnancy. Still others are not certain of paternity, having multiple partners during the time frame of conception. A partner relationship must not be assumed; it must be assessed.

The pregnant person bears the onus of responsibility for nurturing the growing fetus; this may lead to heightened vulnerability and dependency needs that will influence all relationships, but most particularly their relationship with their partner. New roles are forged as the pregnancy progresses in anticipation of the baby. Emotional support and tangible assistance between the pregnant person and their partner are critical elements for positive parental and partner role development requiring clear communication and ongoing effort at this time. Sound information and sensitive guidance by the prenatal care provider can facilitate these changes.

Assessment of partner attachment and adaptation

1. What is the nature of the partner relationship with the pregnant person?
2. Was this a planned pregnancy with partner involvement?
3. What is partner perception of the pregnancy—positive, negative?
4. Does the partner have other children?
5. What past and current experience with parenting does the partner have?
6. Does the partner exhibit bonding behaviors toward the fetus, such as talking to the fetus, patting the pregnant abdomen, protective behavior toward the pregnant person?
7. Is the partner involved in the provision of food, shelter, clothing, and positive emotional climate for the pregnant person? Are there plans in place for the additional resources needed for the new baby?

Partners of the Pregnant Person

Partners of the pregnant person are addressed in this section. Much of the research in this area has been done on cisgender males; for information on partners of other genders, see Chapter 25, *Preconception, Pregnancy, and Postpartum Care of LGBTQ+ Individuals*. The experience of becoming a father is an important milestone in male adult development. Historically, the father has been characterized as a remote figure, busy with the work involved in maintaining financial security for the family. However, men today are rejecting exaggerated definitions of masculinity and are redefining their **paternal identity** to include hands-on involvement and a nurturing component in their relationship with their partner and their children (Gage & Kirk, 2016).

Tradition delegated the father to minor roles in the childbearing experience; however, as access to hospital birth rooms opened to include fathers and others, male partners are now playing a greater role in providing labor comfort and support measures to the laboring person, although there are some cultures that prohibit or discourage this practice. At the birth, some couples want the father to catch the baby or to cut the umbilical cord in an effort to create powerful emotional bonds and family legacy memories.

Couvade, a French verb meaning to brood or to hatch, is a term applied to fatherhood rituals across various historical eras and cultural groups. These rituals serve several purposes for the father and the new family, including warding off evil spirits, publicly acknowledging the new baby as his own, and strengthening the emotional bond between father and child (Devi & Chanu, 2015). Examples of these rituals include avoidance of certain foods, adornment with the pregnant person's clothing, and confinement to a hut for the length of his mate's labor and birth.

While ritual couvade is practiced only in indigenous cultures today, the couvade syndrome is a common condition in which the male partner of a pregnant person experiences physical and emotional symptoms of pregnancy. Estimates of the occurrence of couvade syndrome range from 11% to 80% of male partners, although symptoms may not be recognized as a psychogenic manifestation of the partner's pregnancy (Chase et al., 2021; Navas et al., 2017). Expectant fathers may have one or more signs and symptoms of pregnancy, including nausea, vomiting, weight gain, breast tenderness, food cravings, headaches, abdominal cramps, and sleep disturbances. The couvade syndrome is thought to be a psychosomatic manifestation of the changes in social roles, a reflection of either an overidentification with or an envy reaction to his partner's pregnancy. It is not considered a mental health disorder. Most men will appreciate a simple explanation of the couvade syndrome along with the reassurance that this common male experience will abate with time.

While paternal attachment appears to go through processes similar to maternal attachment, the timing is different (Arghavanian et al., 2018; Vreeswijk et al., 2014). The pregnancy and the baby remain abstractions for the man during early pregnancy; for the woman, the reality of the pregnancy is evident in physical changes. For the man, the changes in his pregnant partner can inform his experience and elicit his response and involvement in the pregnancy. His experience of the pregnancy is through those embodied experiences of his partner that can be shared. Notable events include procuring a home pregnancy test kit, sharing the results, announcing the pregnancy to family and friends, feeling the baby's movements, viewing an ultrasound, supporting the pregnant person through bodily changes, and participating in childbirth classes, prenatal visits, labor, and birth.

The partner relationship may be altered by the experience of pregnancy. Sexual relations may become less frequent in the first trimester due to fatigue, malaise, and nausea experienced by the pregnant person, or in the third trimester due to the discomforts of the enlarging uterus. The male partner may be reluctant to engage in sexual relations for fear of hurting the baby or he may not find the pregnant body arousing. The couple can be reassured that a new normal will be reestablished as they move through a period of fluctuating needs and desires for sexual intimacy (see Chapter 21, *Sexuality*).

The male partner can be encouraged to develop his nurturing father skills throughout pregnancy. He can play a role in buffering some of the stress that the pregnant person undergoes during transitions. Committed partners, whether married, cohabiting, or dating, are found to be a positive influence for the mother's role enactment and stress (Nomaguchi et al., 2012). For mothers no longer linked with the baby's father, the status of relationship with a current partner is the crucial element. Mother–father relationships may be varied and complex.

Role stress and conflict can occur as men adjust their self-image to include the role of father and as they incorporate this new facet of their development into their current social roles and obligations. A recent study showed that men who were invested in the pregnancy and accompanied their partners to hospital were motivated to make at least one positive behavior change in support of family health, such as reducing smoking, alcohol, or improving their diet (Shawe et al., 2019). Another study suggested that expectations to become a father develop relatively early in life and are predictive of paternal involvement throughout their children's lives (Trahan, 2018). Positive fatherhood involvement is related to child emotional self-regulation, child behavior, child literacy, and language outcomes and child educational attainment. Relationship satisfaction and co-parenting alliance can moderate father involvement, but personal confidence for fathering was found to be more meaningful (Trahan, 2018).

Participation in pregnancy, labor, and birth can be interesting and rewarding experiences for partners. The role of the male partner/father includes expressive and nurturant aspects. Direct physical care of very young children and continued open, warm emotional support of his partner and children are among the expectations of the continuous process of learning to negotiate the challenges of fatherhood. Changing societal expectations are based on several assumptions gaining widespread acceptance: (a) the burdens of childrearing are too great to be under the exclusive domain of mothers; (b) the joys of childrearing are too great to be under the exclusive domain of mothers; and (c) children are the responsibility of both parents.

Summary

The prenatal care provider is privileged to see a pregnant person over time and at a key transitional point in their lives. The relationship between an individual and their prenatal care provider begins with a conversation starter as simple as "Tell me about yourself." The process of assessing psychosocial adaptation to pregnancy brings to consciousness and dialogue important concerns that cover a broad range of life experiences, social circumstances, and personality characteristics.

In dealing with psychosocial issues in pregnancy, the primary therapeutic strategy for the prenatal care provider is **active and empathetic listening**. Information, support, and affirmations are provided to assist the individual in gaining insight into their situation. Pregnancy adds another dimension to an already full life that can enhance or overwhelm the ability to cope and function. When coping mechanisms are overwhelmed or mental health concerns are raised, the care provider can refer to local social service agencies and mental health professionals as well as provide empathetic care.

Psychosocial and physiological health outcomes for the pregnant person and the baby are linked to prenatal processes. Attending to the psychosocial adaptations throughout pregnancy is a preventive aspect of prenatal care and includes assessments and interventions to enhance psychosocial wellness and to reduce psychosocial risk. It is important to appreciate the psychosocial background of the pregnant individual in order to best serve their needs and to assist in realizing their goals and optimum health outcomes.

Resources for Clients and Their Families

Body Image and Pregnancy: https://www.womenshealth.gov/mental-health/body-image-and-mental-health/pregnancy-and-body-image

Childbirth Connection. Evidence based childbirth practice to empower childbearing women: https://national-partnership.org/childbirthconnection/

New baby sibling: Helping your older child (or children) adjust: http://www.med.umich.edu/yourchild/topics/newbaby.htm

Resources for Healthcare Providers

Childbirth Connection. Resources for professionals: https://nationalpartnership.org/childbirthconnection/

America's children: Key national indicators of well-being: http://childstats.gov

References

Arghavanian, F. E., Roudsari, R. L., Heydari, A., Dokht, N., & Bahmani, M. (2018). Men's confrontation with pregnancy from women's point of view: An ethno-phenomenological approach. *Journal of Caring Sciences*, 8(4), 231–239. https://doi.org/10.15171/jcs.2019.033

Bagheri, M., Dorosty, A., Sadrzadeh-Yegneh, H., Eshraghian, M., Amirir, E., & Khamoush-Cheshm, N. (2012). Pre-pregnancy body size dissatisfaction and excessive gestational weight gain. *Maternal and Child Health Journal*, 17(4), 1–9. https://doi.org/10.1007/s10995-012-1051-6

Baker, B., & Yang, I. (2018). Social media as social support in pregnancy and the postpartum. *Sexual & Reproductive Healthcare*, 17, 31–34. https://doi.org/10.1016/j.srhc.2018.05.003

Becker, E., Rodgers, R. F., & Zimmerman, E. (2022). # Body goals or# Bopo? Exposure to pregnancy and post-partum related social media images: Effects on the body image and mood of women in the peri-pregnancy period. *Body Image*, 42, 1–10. https://doi.org/10.1016/j.bodyim.2022.04.010

Bergman, J., & Bergman, N. (2013). Whose choice? Advocating birthing practices according to baby's biological needs. *The Journal of Perinatal Education*, 22(1), 8. DOI: 10.1891/1058-1243.22.1.8

Beyers-Carlson, E. E., & Volling, B. L. (2017). Efficacy of sibling preparation classes. *Journal of Obstetric, Gynecologic & Neonatal Nursing*, 46(4), 521–531. https://doi.org/10.1016/j.jogn.2017.03.005

Bjelica, A., Cetkovic, N., Trninic-Pjevic, A., & Mladenovic-Segedi, L. (2018). The phenomenon of pregnancy—A psychological view. *Ginekologia Polska*, 89(2), 102–106. https://doi.org/10.5603/GP.a2018.0017

Blackburn, S. T. (2018). *Maternal, fetal and neonatal physiology* (5th ed.). Saunders Elsevier.

Bludau, A., Royer, M., Meister, G., Neumann, I. D., & Menon, R. (2019). Epigenetic regulation of the social brain. *Trends in Neurosciences*, 42(7), 471–484. https://doi.org/10.1016/j.tins.2019.04.001

Bowlby, J. (1978). *A secure base: Clinical applications of attachment theory*. Routledge.

Brazelton, T. B. (1973). *Neonatal behavioral assessment scale*. J. B. Lippincott Co.

Brown, A., Rance, J., & Warren, L. (2015). Body image concerns during pregnancy are associated with a shorter breastfeeding duration. *Midwifery*, 31(1), 80–89. https://doi.org/10.1016/j.midw.2014.06.003

Buckley, S. J. (2015). Executive summary of hormonal physiology of childbearing: Evidence and implications for women, babies, and maternity care. *The Journal of Perinatal Education*, 24(3), 145–153. https://doi.org/10.1891/1058-1243.24.3.145

Cabrera, J. P. (2018). Maternal role attainment theory: Promoting maternal identity and family health. *International Journal of Childbirth Education*, 33(2), 21–23.

Charter, R., Ussher, J. M., Perz, J., & Robinson, K. (2018). The transgender parent: Experiences and constructions of pregnancy and parenthood for transgender men in Australia. *International Journal of Transgenderism*, 19(1), 64–77. https://doi.org/10.1080/15532739.2017.1399496

Chase, T., Fusick, A., & Pauli, J. M. (2021). Couvade syndrome: More than a toothache. *Journal of Psychosomatic Obstetrics and Gynecology*, 42(2), 168–172. https://doi.org/10.1080/0167482X.2019.1693539

Cheng, E. R., Rifas-Shiman, S. L., Perkins, M. E., Rich-Edwards, J. W., Gillman, M. W., Wright, R., & Taveras, E. M. (2016). The influence of antenatal partner support on pregnancy outcomes. *Journal of Women's Health*, 25(7), 672–679. https://doi.org/10.1089/jwh.2015.5462

Devi, A. M., & Chanu, M. P. (2015). Couvade syndrome. *International Journal of Nursing Education and Research*, 3(3), 109–111. DOI: 10.5958/2454-2660.2015.00017.4

Dubber, S., Reck, C., Müller, M., & Gawlik, S. (2015). Postpartum bonding: The role of perinatal depression, anxiety and maternal-fetal bonding during pregnancy. *Archives of Women's Mental Health*, 18(2), 187–195. https://doi.org/10.1007/s00737-014-0445-4

Eick, S. M., Barrett, E. S., van't Erve, T. J., Nguyen, R., Bush, N. R., Milne, G., Swan, S. H., & Ferguson, K. K. (2018). Association between prenatal psychological stress and oxidative stress during pregnancy. *Paediatric and Perinatal Epidemiology*, 32(4), 318–326. https://doi.org/10.1111/ppe.12465

Fouquier, K. F. (2013). State of the science: Does the theory of maternal role attainment apply to African American motherhood? *Journal of Midwifery & Women's Health*, 58(2), 203–210. https://doi.org/10.1111/j.1542-2011.2012.00206.x

Gage, J. D., & Kirk, R. (2016). First-time fathers: Perceptions of preparedness for fatherhood. *Canadian Journal of Nursing Research Archive*, 34(4A), 15–24.

Hodgkinson, E. L., Smith, D. M., & Wittkowski, A. (2014). Women's experiences of their pregnancy and postpartum body image: A systematic review and meta-synthesis. *BMC Pregnancy and Childbirth*, 14(1), 330. https://doi.org/10.1186/1471-2393-14-330

Hornor, G. (2019). Attachment disorders. *Journal of Pediatric Health Care*, 33(5), 612–622. https://doi.org/10.1016/j.pedhc.2019.04.017

Inanir, S., Cakmak, B., Nacar, M. C., Guler, A. E., & Inanir, A. (2015). Body image perception and self-esteem during pregnancy. *International Journal of Women's Health and Reproduction Science*, 3(4), 196–200. https://doi.org/10.15296/ijwhr.2015.41

Johnson, S. A. (2014). "Maternal devices", social media and the self-management of pregnancy, mothering and child health. *Societies*, 4(2), 330–350. https://doi.org/10.3390/soc4020330

Kennell, M. H., & Klaus, J. H. (1976). *Maternal-infant bonding*. The C. V. Mosby Company.

Kiani-Sheikhabadi, M., Beigi, M., & Mohebbi-Dehnavi, Z. (2019). The relationship between perfectionism and body image with eating disorder in pregnancy. *Journal of Education and Health Promotion*, 8, 242. https://doi.org/10.4103/jehp.jehp_58_19

Klaus, M. H., Kennell, J. H., & Klaus, P. H. (1995). *Bonding: Building the foundations of secure attachment and independence*. Da Capo Press.

Lawson, K. L., & Turriff-Janasson, S. I. (2006). Maternal serum screening and psychosocial attachment to pregnancy. *Journal of Psychosomatic Research*, 60, 371–378. https://doi.org/10.1016/j.jpsychores.2006.01.010

Lederman, R. P., & Weis, K. (2009). *Psychosocial adaptation in pregnancy* (3rd ed.). Springer Publishing Company.

Liu, M. (2019, July). The development of attachment theory: introduction and orientation. In *2019 Scientific Conference on Management, Education and Psychology* (Vol. 1, pp. 122–130). The Academy of Engineering and Education. https://aeescience.org/uploads/ppapers/2019070801SCMEP2019/EMP70326.pdf

Luce, A., Cash, M., Hundley, V., Cheyne, H., Van Teijlingen, E., & Angell, C. (2016). "Is it realistic?" the portrayal of pregnancy and childbirth in the media. *BMC Pregnancy and Childbirth*, 16(1), 40. https://doi.org/10.1186/s12884-016-0827-x

Martin, J. A., Hamilton, B. E., Osterman, M. J., Driscoll, A. K., & Mathews, T. J. (2017). Births: Final data for 2015. National vital statistics reports: from the Centers for Disease Control and Prevention, National Center for Health Statistics. *National Vital Statistics System*, 66(1), 1.

Mehra, R., Boyd, L. M., Magriples, U., Kershaw, T. S., Ickovics, J. R., & Keene, D. E. (2020). Black pregnant women "get the most judgment": A qualitative study of the experiences of black women at the intersection of race, gender, and pregnancy. *Women's Health Issues*, 30(6), 484–492. https://doi.org/10.1016/j.whi.2020.08.001

Mehta, U. J., Siega-Riz, A. M., & Herring, A. H. (2010). Effect of body image on pregnancy weight gain. *Maternal and Child Health Journal*, 15(3), 324–332. https://doi.org/10.1007/s10995-010-0578-7

Mei, J. Y., Afshar, Y., Gregory, K. D., Kilpatrick, S. J., & Esakoff, T. F. (2016). Birth plans: What matters for birth experience satisfaction. *Birth*, 43(2), 144–150. https://doi.org/10.1111/birt.12226

Meighan, M. (2017). *Maternal role attainment—Becoming a mother* (pp. 432). Nursing Theorists and Their Work-E-Book. https://nursekey.com/maternal-role-attainment-becoming-a-mother/

Mercer, R. T. (1985). Relationship of the birth experience to later mothering behaviors. *Journal of Nurse-Midwifery*, 30(4), 204–211. https://doi.org/10.1016/0091-2182(85)90144-2

Mercer, R. T. (1995). A tribute to Reva Rubin. *MCN. The American Journal of Maternal Child Nursing*, 20(4), 184.

Mercer, R. T. (2010). Becoming a mother versus maternal role attainment. In A. I. Meleis (Ed.), *Transitions theory: Middle-range and situation-specific theories in nursing research and practice*. Springer Publishing Company.

Mercer, R. T., & Walker, L. O. (2006). A review of nursing interventions to foster becoming a mother. *Journal of Obstetric, Gynecologic, & Neonatal Nursing*, 35(5), 568–582. https://doi.org/10.1111/j.1552-6909.2006.00080.x

Naber, N. L., Miller, S., & Baddock, S. A. (2018). What do we know about sibling attended birth? An integrative literature review. *Midwifery*, 63, 24–32. https://doi.org/10.1016/j.midw.2018.04.025

Navas, M., Albea, J. G., & Garcia-Parajua, P. (2017). Pregnancy in men: Couvade syndrome. *European Psychiatry*, 41, S415. https://doi.org/10.1016/j.eurpsy.2017.01.362

Neal, Z., & Neal, J. W. (2022). Prevalence, age of decision, and interpersonal warmth judgements of childfree adults. *Scientific Reports*, 12(1), 1–7. https://doi.org/10.1038/s41598-022-15728-z

Nishikawa, M., & Sakakibara, H. (2013). Effect of nursing intervention program using abdominal palpation of Leopold's maneuvers on maternal-fetal attachment. *Reproductive Health*, 10(1), 12. https://doi.org/10.1186/1742-4755-10-12

Nomaguchi, K. M., Brown, S. L., & Leyman, T. M. (2012). *Father involvement and mothers' parenting stress: The role of relationship status*. https://fragilefamilies.princeton.edu/sites/g/files/toruqf2001/files/wp12-07-ff.pdf

O'Connell, M. A., Leahy-Warren, P., Khashan, A. S., Kenny, L. C., & O'Neill, S. M. (2017). Worldwide prevalence of tocophobia in pregnant women: Systematic review and meta-analysis. *Acta Obstetricia et Gynecologica Scandinavica*, 96(8), 907–920. https://doi.org/10.1111/aogs.13138

Oken, E. (2015). Routine weighing of women during pregnancy is of limited value and should be abandoned: AGAINST: Routine weighing in pregnancy is the first step to preventing adverse birth outcomes. *BJOG: An International Journal of Obstetrics & Gynaecology*, 122(8), 1101. DOI: 10.1111/1471-0528.13408

Pallini, S., Baiocco, R., Schneider, B. H., Madigan, S., & Atkinson, L. (2014). Early child-parent attachment and peer relations: A meta-analysis of recent research. *Journal of Family Psychology*, 28(1), 118–123. https://doi.org/10.1037/a0035736

Petri, E., Palagini, L., Bacci, O., Borri, C., Teristi, V., Corezzi, C., Cargioli, C., Banti, S., Perugi, G., & Mauri, M. (2018). Maternal-foetal attachment independently predicts the quality of maternal-infant bonding and post-partum psychopathology. *The Journal of Maternal-Fetal & Neonatal Medicine*, 31(23), 3153–3159. https://doi.org/10.1080/14767058.2017.1365130

Pingeton, B. C., Goodman, S. H., & Monk, C. (2021). Prenatal origins of temperament: Fetal cardiac development & infant surgency, negative affectivity, and regulation/orienting. *Infant Behavior and Development*, 65, 101643. https://doi.org/10.1016/j.infbeh.2021.101643

Pisoni, C., Garofoli, F., Tzialla, C., Orcesi, S., Spinillo, A., Politi, P., Ballottin, U., Manzoni, P., & Stronati, M. (2014). Risk and protective factors in maternal-fetal attachment development. *Early Human Development*, 90, S45–S46. https://doi.org/10.1016/S0378-3782(14)50012-6

Rauff, E. L., & Downs, S. D. (2011). Mediating effects of body image satisfaction on exercise behavior, depressive symptoms, and gestational weight gain in pregnancy. *Annals of Behavioral Medicine*, 42(3), 381–390. https://doi.org/10.1007/s12160-011-9300-2

Robakis, T. K., Williams, K. E., Crowe, S., Lin, K. W., Gannon, J., & Rasgon, N. L. (2016). Maternal attachment insecurity is a potent predictor of depressive symptoms in the early postnatal period. *Journal of Affective Disorders*, 190, 623–631. https://doi.org/10.1016/j.jad.2015.09.067

Rodriguez, A. C. I., Schetter, C. D., Brewis, A., & Tomiyama, A. J. (2019). The psychological burden of baby weight: Pregnancy, weight stigma, and maternal health. *Social Science & Medicine*, 235, 112401. https://doi.org/10.1016/j.socscimed.2019.112401

Rubin, R. (1984). *Maternal identity and the maternal experience*. Springer Publishing Co.

Sahin, B. (2022). Predicting maternal attachment: The role of emotion regulation and resilience during pregnancy. *Journal of Basic and Clinical. Health Sciences*, 6(1), 105–115. https://doi.org/10.30621/jbachs.994182

Sandelowski, M. (1993). Toward a theory of technology dependency. *Nursing Outlook*, 41(1), 36–42.

Scheper-Hughes, N. (1985). Culture, scarcity and maternal thinking: Maternal detachment and infant survival in a Brazilian shantytown. *Ethos*, 13(4), 291–317. https://www.jstor.org/stable/640147

Shawe, J., Patel, D., Joy, M., Howden, B., Barrett, G., & Stephenson, J. (2019). Preparation for fatherhood: A survey of men's preconception health knowledge and behaviour in England. *PLoS One*, 14(3), e0213897. https://doi.org/10.1371/journal.pone.0213897

Shrestha, S., Adachi, K., A Petrini, M., & Shrestha, S. (2019). Maternal role: A concept analysis. *Journal of Midwifery and Reproductive Health*, 7(3), 1732–1741. http://eprints.mums.ac.ir/id/eprint/11770

Sohn, M., & Bye, E. (2015). Pregnancy and body image: Analysis of clothing functions of maternity wear. *Clothing and Textiles Research Journal*, 33(1), 64–78. https://doi.org/10.1177/0887302X14557

Soltani, F., Maleki, A., Shobeiri, F., Shamsaei, F., Ahmadi, F., & Roshanaei, G. (2017). The limbo of motherhood: Women's experiences of major challenges to cope with the first pregnancy. *Midwifery*, 55, 38–44. https://doi.org/10.1016/j.midw.2017.08.009

Steer, P. J. (2015). Routine weighing of women during pregnancy is of limited value and should be abandoned: FOR: Routine weighing does not solve the problem of obesity in pregnancy. *BJOG: An International Journal of Obstetrics & Gynaecology*, 122(8), 1101. https://doi.org/10.1111/1471-0528.13406

Trahan, M. H. (2018). Paternal self-efficacy and father involvement: A bi-directional relationship. *Psychology of Men & Masculinity*, *19*(4), 624. https://doi.org/10.1037/men0000130

Van Rosmalen, L., van der Horst, F. C., & Van der Veer, R. (2016). From secure dependency to attachment: Mary Ainsworth's integration of Blatz's security theory into Bowlby's attachment theory. *History of Psychology*, *19*(1), 22–39. https://doi.org/10.1037/hop0000015

VanHoover, C., Rademeyer, C. A., & Farley, C. L. (2017). Body piercing: Motivations and implications for health. *Journal of Midwifery & Women's Health*, *62*(5), 521–530. https://doi.org/10.1111/jmwh.12630

Vedam, S., Stoll, K., Taiwo, T. K., Rubashkin, N., Cheyney, M., Strauss, N., McLemore, M., Cadena, M., Nethery, E., Rushton, E., Schummers, L., Declercq, E., & the GVtM-US Steering Council. (2019). The giving voice to mothers study: Inequity and mistreatment during pregnancy and childbirth in the United States. *Reproductive Health*, *16*(1), 1–18. https://doi.org/10.1186/s12978-019-0729-2

Volling, B. L. (2012). Family transitions following the birth of a sibling: An empirical review of changes in the firstborn's adjustment. *Psychological Bulletin*, *138*(3), 497. https://doi.org/10.1037/a0026921

Vreeswijk, C. M. J. M., Maas, A. J. B. M., Rijk, C. H. A. M., & van Bakel, H. J. A. (2014). Fathers' experiences during pregnancy: Paternal prenatal attachment and representations of the fetus. *Psychology of Men & Masculinity*, *15*(2), 129–137. https://doi.org/10.1037/a0033070

Watson, B., Broadbent, J., Skouteris, H., & Fuller-Tyszkiewicz, M. (2016). A qualitative exploration of body image experiences of women progressing through pregnancy. *Women and Birth*, *29*(1), 72–79. https://doi.org/10.1016/j.wombi.2015.08.007

Weigle, E. A., & McAndrews, L. (2021). The future of maternity wear: Generation Z's expectations of dressing for pregnancy. *Journal of Fashion Marketing and Management: An International Journal*, *26*(3), 534–549. https://doi.org/10.1108/JFMM-11-2020-0244

Yeniel, A. O., & Petri, E. (2014). Pregnancy, childbirth, and sexual function: Perceptions and facts. *International Urogynecology Journal*, *25*(1), 5–14. https://doi.org/10.1007/s00192-013-2118-7

Zosuls, K. M., Miller, C. F., Ruble, D. N., Martin, C. L., & Fabes, R. A. (2011). Gender development research in sex roles: Historical trends and future directions. *Sex Roles*, *64*(11–12), 826–842. https://doi.org/10.1007/s11199-010-9902-3

24

Health Education during Pregnancy

Kathlyn Albert, Lisa Hanson, and Emily Malloy

The editors gratefully acknowledge Lisa Hanson, Karen Robinson, Leona VandeVusse, and Kathryn Harrod, who were co-authors of the previous edition of this chapter.

Relevant Terms

Birth plan—a written plan that guides birth attendants as to what the birthing family would like for their labor and birth
Childbirth education—a method of preparing pregnant people and their support person(s) for the experience of labor and birth, typically including in-depth information about coping skills, physiology of labor and birth, emotional aspects, and childbirth options
Health literacy—an individual's ability to read, understand, and use healthcare information to make decisions and follow instructions for treatment
Internatal care—a system of care that begins with the birth of a child and extends through the birth of the next

---

Health equity bullet points

- Providers of prenatal health education need to be aware of disparities in pregnancy outcomes that exist for certain groups, especially Black, Indigenous, and other people of color, and offer information and strategies to decrease disparities, such as use of a doula.
- Health literacy disparities parallel health outcome disparities. Therefore, there is a need to find ways to increase health literacy for pregnant clients, such as evaluating the reading level of written materials and using plain language.
- Trauma-informed care as a universal approach may be especially helpful for special populations of pregnant people, including veterans, LGBTQ+ parents, birthing people with higher body mass index (BMI), persons with disabilities, and those with a history of sexual trauma.
- Social Determinants of Health (SDOH) are the environmental conditions in which a person lives, including housing, transportation, access to healthy food and clean water, education, and jobs. Although SDOH are not necessarily modifiable, referrals to community resources can lessen their burden. Prenatal care and education may provide an opportunity to reduce modifiable risk factors.

Introduction

Pregnancy is an ideal time for health education. People are often particularly receptive to learning and using new health information during pregnancy, and many want pregnancy information and want to use it to participate in shared decision-making with a trusted healthcare provider (Avery et al., 2014). Research has also demonstrated that providing health information to pregnant people positively impacts the health of the entire family (Lu et al., 2006). Well-planned health education interactions during pregnancy provide opportunities for healthcare providers to initiate and establish an ongoing healthcare relationship and form the foundation for continued, comprehensive care after pregnancy.

Since all systems of prenatal care involve multiple visits with the healthcare provider, health education during pregnancy can be strategically planned to optimize its impact on the health of pregnant people and their families. This chapter summarizes the specific components of health education that should be addressed before and during pregnancy, suggests the optimal timing for when specific topics should be addressed, and reviews several broad topics related to prenatal education.

Preconception care is ideal, but few people make appointments with providers for that specific purpose. Therefore, providers who care for people of childbearing age should include preconception care in all encounters. For example, planning for a future pregnancy can occur during both annual and interval appointments (Farahi & Zolotor, 2013). Lu et al. (2006) described **internatal care** as a unique type of prenatal care where people of childbearing age (including their families) receive tailored care between pregnancies.

Prenatal and Postnatal Care: A Person-Centered Approach, Third Edition. Edited by Karen Trister Grace, Cindy L. Farley, Noelene K. Jeffers, and Tanya Tringali.
© 2024 John Wiley & Sons Ltd. Published 2024 by John Wiley & Sons Ltd.
Companion website: www.wiley.com/go/grace/prenatal

The goal of preconception care is to enhance perinatal health and reduce risks. The prenatal health education topics to be included in preconception care appear in the 0–12 column of Table 24.5. Preconception care is discussed in detail in Chapter 7, *Preconception Care*.

Sources and Quality of Consumer Childbirth Education

Surprisingly, high-quality scientific evidence is lacking for both individual and group prenatal health education (Gagnon & Sandall, 2007). Published research is criticized for underrepresentation of economically, educationally, and socially disadvantaged participants, and existing research is often based on educators' priorities versus attendees' stated or unstated educational needs (Gagnon & Sandall, 2007).

In the past, it was commonplace for pregnant people and their support person(s) to attend formal **childbirth education** classes beginning at approximately 28 weeks of gestation. The purpose of these classes is to educate about labor and birth, and to prepare them with coping strategies such as breathing, relaxation, movement, and massage as well as how to prepare for unexpected emergencies. The basis of childbirth education is that knowledge lessens fear, which leads to less tension and, consequently, less pain (Dick-Read, 2013). Researchers found that an eight-week series of third-trimester prenatal education classes resulted in reduced fear of childbirth and increased childbirth self-efficacy compared with a control of prenatal care only (Serçekuş & Başkale, 2016). Although individual studies show positive impacts on outcomes, the evidence for effectiveness of childbirth education is overall inconclusive. This may be because childbirth education is viewed as a "single uniform intervention" (Nolan, 2000) rather than in the context of the broader influences on participants, such as self-care, health promotion, quality of life, and outcomes beyond childbirth (Humenick, 2000).

The two most common forms of formal childbirth education available in use today are the Bradley method (American Academy of Husband-Coached Childbirth, 2022) and Lamaze (Lamaze International, 2022). Both of these childbirth education methods have a unique philosophy that provides the basis for the structure and content of classes (Table 24.1).

Hypnobirthing® is a childbirth preparation method that is growing in popularity. This method aims to have expectant people view birth in a positive manner with the belief that childbirth does not have to be painful. It focuses on teaching the skills of deep relaxation, visualization, and self-hypnosis to release fears that can fuel the perception that labor is painful. A study of Australian women using hypnobirthing found that women had fewer interventions, shorter labors, and less pain, and reported feeling more confident, relaxed, less fearful, focused, and more in control compared to those not using this method (Phillips-Moore, 2012). Catsaros and Wendland (2020) conducted a systematic review of nine studies evaluating the effect of hypnosis on childbirth and found that it improved the experience of giving birth. There are no

Table 24.1 Childbirth Education: Comparison of Bradley and Lamaze Approaches

	Bradley	Lamaze
Philosophy	Teaches families how to have natural births. Techniques are based on how the human body works in labor	Originally based on the Pavlovian theory of conditioned behavioral responses through preparation and training (in dogs). Contemporary Lamaze is based on six healthy birth practices that are supported by research
Content	What to expect and how to avoid pain in labor, focusing on a healthy pregnancy and the relationships between the pregnant person and their support people	The six healthy birth practices: 1. Let labor begin on its own 2. Move around and change positions 3. Have continuous support 4. Avoid interventions 5. Avoid being on your back 6. Keep birthing parent and baby together
Structure	12 classes that follow a workbook with a certified Bradley instructor	6 weeks of classes taught by a Lamaze Certified Childbirth Educator

Source: American Academy of Husband-Coached Childbirth (2022) and Lamaze International (2022).

well-controlled studies comparing outcomes using the Lamaze, Bradley, or hypnobirthing methods. Therefore, a shared decision-making approach is recommended to select a childbirth preparation method. Many pregnant people also attend hospital-based classes, which have been criticized for bias toward interventions and practices that are commonplace at the particular facility (Walker et al., 2009). Despite these critiques, some people favor these classes because they are convenient and provide reassurance and familiarity with the birth setting. Compared to online formats, most pregnant patients prefer in person or face-to-face classes (Kovala et al., 2016), and many pregnant people attend classes for the socialization aspect, as a way to connect with others experiencing a similar life event and gain support (Downer et al., 2020). The COVID-19 pandemic, of course, necessitated a pivot toward online format (Inversetti et al., 2021; Pasadino et al., 2020). Prenatal healthcare providers are advised to become aware of the different types of childbirth education classes available to pregnant people in the local area, especially those that may specialize in working with specific populations, such as people from diverse cultures, those who are disabled, expectant parents of multiples, single people, LGBTQ+ people, people in larger bodies, and people with a history of sexual abuse or trauma.

The findings of the national survey *Listening to Mothers (LTM) III* found that 34% of pregnant women received health information in formal classes, and most viewed the information provided as very valuable, second only to the information from their prenatal provider (DeClercq et al., 2013). Although prenatal providers were the most trusted source of health information, a number of perceived barriers to communication with healthcare providers were identified, such as time constraints on visits, fear of bothering the provider, and not understanding medical terminology used (DeClercq et al., 2013).

Pregnant people are increasingly using the Internet as a resource of pregnancy-related information. The LTM III survey identified that over 80% of women searched the Internet on a weekly basis seeking pregnancy health information (DeClercq et al., 2013). The results of a small Canadian survey identified that pregnant women spent an average of 4–6 hours weekly on the Internet searching for health information (Da Costa et al., 2015). Many Internet sites provide communication resources for individuals to discuss pregnancy-related topics, for informal sources of information. Unfortunately, research shows that most pregnant women do not discuss their electronic search findings with their healthcare providers (Daniels & Wedler, 2015; Sayakhot & Carolan-Olah, 2016). The risk of receiving misinformation is high and accuracy can be difficult to assess, making it important for providers to follow up with their clients about their sources of information outside of office visits. It is helpful to develop a list of recommended resources that the provider has evaluated using established criteria. Recommendations for evaluating websites are summarized below, and a list of suggested web resources is provided at the end of this chapter.

A number of additional technologic sources of information have been used to enhance prenatal education including social media, smartphone and device technology, text messaging, personal health records, and electronic health records. Healthcare providers' knowledge of electronic resources of prenatal health information can facilitate open discussions and educational exchanges during prenatal visits.

Mobile device applications ("apps") are commonly available and frequently used by pregnant people to access health information. Many apps allow the user to customize use for their pregnancy and set up health reminders. However, many apps do not have complete or accurate information, cite reliable evidence, or have a search field to access specific topics (Frid et al., 2021).

Reality television shows are common, yet controversial, sources of information for pregnant people and their families. These shows tend to emphasize urgent medical intervention during birth and to underrepresent the diversity of pregnant people and their family structures (Morris & McInerney, 2010).

Public libraries continue to be good sources of free reading material. Some pregnancy books are available for use in digital formats for loan through libraries or for purchase through online bookstores. The ever-expanding options of free or low-cost sources of internet-accessible materials add both opportunity and complexity for pregnant people and their families. Pregnant people can be directed to the most optimal sources for reading material by keeping current with the materials that are available. Developing a recommended reading list or a lending library within the office or clinic setting based on the principles outlined in this chapter can be useful in guiding pregnant people and their partners to quality learning resources. The reading list can be individualized to the philosophy of normal physiologic birth, as well as the culture, language, and age of the population served. Books chosen for inclusion should be reviewed for content, accuracy, health literacy level, and currency.

Delivery of Health Education

A major component of prenatal education takes place during individual prenatal visits and formal prenatal classes. Since a minority of pregnant people attend childbirth education classes, there is an increased emphasis on education during prenatal visits. Clinicians are increasingly pressured to see higher volumes of prenatal clients, making efficient use of time during prenatal visits essential. Health professionals can systematically evaluate the information contained in websites based on components and quality to provide additional resources to clients (Table 24.2).

Table 24.2 Guide to Health Information Website Evaluation

Website component	Evidence of quality
Sources of information	• Appropriate citations are used • References made to accepted health authority, organization, agency and/or scientific evidence • Ability to contact the developer/webmaster
Quality of content	• Reference to an editorial board and/or review • Appropriate use of scientific language • Realistic recommendations • Agreement with findings in other sources and website • Absence of overly dramatic claims that go beyond available evidence • Understandable language used for consumer site; appropriate health literacy level
Currency of information	• Website and/or content contains a date • Embedded web-links are functional
Absence of bias	• Indication of sponsoring organization or funding agency • Absence of funding from commercial sources that hold a financial interest in the content • Advertisements clearly labeled as such
Protection of privacy	• Policy posted that clearly indicates what information is collected and that privacy is assured • If there is a registration process, the privacy policy should indicate what is done with information collected

Another option for delivery of childbirth education is group prenatal care (introduced in Chapter 8, *Prenatal Care*), a system of care that allows more time to be spent on health education. Group prenatal care includes pregnant people of similar gestational ages sharing concerns and questions with each other while receiving prenatal care. At least one group member is a health professional who contributes to and facilitates the discussions. The most well-known form of group prenatal care is CenteringPregnancy, which involves following a specific curriculum plan so that information covered is comprehensive and relevant (Centering Healthcare Institute, 2022). In the LTM III survey, 22% of pregnant women reported participating in group prenatal care (DeClercq et al., 2013). Participants report receiving information that is valuable, current, and individualized (McNeil et al., 2012). Group prenatal care involves multiple directions of information exchange, with the group participants viewed as equals and important sources of information and experience.

Developmental Considerations

Adolescent Education Principles

The rate of adolescent pregnancy and births has recently declined to the lowest rate in four decades (Maddow-Zimet & Kost, 2021). Pregnant teens require special consideration regarding prenatal health education because their cognitive abilities are not yet fully developed. The completion of adolescence is independent of age and is characterized by the person's ability to solve abstract problems and compare plausible explanations for phenomena (Friedman, 2006). Because pregnancy has been associated with regression to earlier cognitive states, assessing the predominant cognitive features of individual adolescents can aid in developing, implementing, and evaluating an appropriate plan of prenatal health education (Friedman, 2006; Maehr & Felice, 2006a, 2006b). Strategies for optimal communication with adolescents include: (a) be succinct; (b) use open-ended questions that are nonthreatening; (c) promote exploration of topics with phrases such as "tell me more"; (d) provide adequate time and opportunity for adolescents to speak; (e) listen more than you speak; (f) reflect the adolescent's mood during interactions (except when it is hostile); (g) model rational decision-making; and (h) raise multiple perspectives during prenatal visits. Because retention of knowledge provided to pregnant teens may be suboptimal, "booster" educational sessions may be necessary to increase long-term retention (Logsdon et al., 2015). An understanding of the cognitive features of early, middle, and late adolescence can guide the prenatal care provider in tailoring communication strategies with teens (Table 24.3).

Adult Education Principles

Knowles (1988) outlined the principles of adult education. Adult learners share a goal: to enrich their knowledge. Applying the principles of adult education creates an environment of mutual exchange of information that is

Table 24.3 Adolescent Cognitive Development

Time frame	Cognitive features
Early teen 11–14 years	• Concrete thinking predominates • Mainly present oriented • Planning is vague, unrealistic • Limited ability to be introspective and to reason abstractly • Commonly reasons by trial and error • Learns and retains information but sometimes unable to apply it • Often exclusive identification of a "best friend" • Concerns about conformity to peers
Middle teen 15–17 years	• Egocentric • Rebellious • Mostly reason by trial and error • Abstract reasoning and introspection becoming more common • Present oriented with limited future planning abilities • Magical thinking leads to risk taking and impulsive behavior • Short term relationships may become sexual
Late teen 18–20 years	• Identity developed, along with "other orientation" • Can apply and use information • Engages in abstract reasoning • Sexual relationships become more interpersonal • Able to plan for the future • Sets goals and takes steps to meet them • Transitioning into adult roles in society (work and family)

relevant to the pregnant person and their family. Adult learning principles include respecting the knowledge the adult already has and building beyond it.

People may enter pregnancy with preconceived thoughts, feelings, and motivation to change while learning more about bodily changes, pregnancy, lactation, and childcare (Table 24.4).

Special Populations

It is important to be aware of certain groups that may need specialized care or education, which should adapt to the individual needs of the client and family situation. Pregnant people from a number of special populations may be marginalized and underserved. Awareness of the impact of SDOH is essential in addressing the educational needs of people from historically underserved and marginalized populations. SDOH are "conditions in the environments where people are born, live, work play, worship and age that affect a wide range of health and functioning and the quality-of-life outcomes and risks" (US Department of Health and Human Services, n.d.-b). The SDOH are categorized into five domains: (a) economic stability; (b) educational access and quality; (c) healthcare access and

Table 24.4 Principles of Adult Education as Applied to Prenatal Education

Principle	Example of incorporation into prenatal education
Autonomous and self-directed	"What would you like to talk about today?"
Need to connect new learning to prior knowledge	"Tell me how what you have learned about discomforts of pregnancy compares to your experiences."
Goal and relevancy oriented	"You are in your third trimester, let's talk about some things that you may experience in the coming weeks."
Practical	"Since you are 36 weeks today, it would be a good idea to finalize your birth plan and discuss the signs and symptoms of labor."
Treat with respect in order to learn effectively	"Good afternoon Ms. Jones. Would it be okay if we discussed postpartum contraceptive options today?"

quality; (d) neighborhood and built environment; and (e) social and community context. A sensitive approach may promote uncovering unique educational needs.

Trauma-informed care as a universal practice is recommended when caring for all pregnant people (Hollander et al., 2017). This approach involves acknowledging the scope of the traumatic experience, recognizing the signs and symptoms of trauma, integrating the knowledge about trauma into the setting/practice, and avoiding retraumatization (Center for Health Care Strategies, 2021). This approach is discussed further in Chapter 26, *Violence and Trauma in the Perinatal Period*.

Pregnant people identifying as LGBTQ+ can experience barriers to care in any healthcare setting, including during pregnancy. Barriers include heteronormative assumptions and implicit and explicit biases. Beginning health encounters with discussing the pronouns used by the provider and patient and continued use of inclusive language can build trust. It is important to provide holistic care to LGBTQ+ individuals, including but not limited to awareness of health disparities, reflection on provider bias, use of gender inclusive terms such as "parent" and "support person," and avoidance of gendered role terminology. See Chapter 25, *Preconception, Pregnancy and Postpartum Care of LGBTQ+ Individuals*.

Veterans

Pregnant people in the military or with a military background have unique needs including but not limited to exposure to violence and trauma, potential PTSD, and exposure to hazardous chemicals and materials (US Department of Veterans Affairs, 2022). Veterans may have a risk of depression and unmet educational needs related to intrapartum care and partner involvement (Sheahan et al., 2022). Health education needs to reflect the awareness of these special circumstances.

Pregnancies at ≥35 Years of Age

Pregnancies at ≥35 years of age continue to remain high due to a national trend in delayed childbearing, as well as the availability of assisted reproductive technologies (Martin et al., 2021). Pregnancies at or after age 35 increase the risk of complications, including increased incidence of chronic conditions, gestational hypertension, preeclampsia, preterm labor, and genetic anomalies. It is critical that persons contemplating pregnancy at or after 35 years of age stabilize chronic illness prior to conception to improve health outcomes. Health education helps modify risks, while also maximizing health.

People with Disabilities

For pregnant people with disabilities, additional or specialized information and support regarding pregnancy, the labor or birth process, as well as adjustment to the postpartum period might be required. This often necessitates understanding the specific condition in order to provide the best care possible and, at times, might require collaboration with a specialist. It is important to understand that the term "disability" can equate to many things, including mobility, cognition, hearing, vision, self-care, and independent living.

People with Higher BMIs

Weight stigma or bias against pregnant people in larger bodies is pervasive in healthcare (Bradford et al., 2020). Nearly 40% of the world's population is overweight or obese (World Health Organization, 2022), which can increase pregnancy risk. People in larger bodies may experience discrimination, discomfort, and safety issues if standard equipment does not fit their body. Bradford et al. (2020) note that weight stigma is sometimes considered an "acceptable" form of discrimination. Respectful treatment of pregnant people of size can decrease barriers to care. Health education that focuses on weight gain guidelines appropriate to prepregnancy BMI and encouraging 30 minutes of vigorous exercise daily can promote health during pregnancy.

People with a History of Sexual Violence or Trauma

Sexual violence and trauma in childhood as well as adulthood is common (see Chapter 26, *Violence and Trauma in the Perinatal Period*). While some people have a conscious awareness of their history of sexual abuse, for others, these experiences remain in the subconscious. Therefore, while asking about a history of sexual abuse is important, it will not universally capture the lived experiences of all individuals. Additionally, because of the nature of pregnancy and birth, including exposure, intimate exams and procedures, and lack of control, the experience may be particularly difficult or trigger flashbacks in people with this history (Simkin & Ancheta, 2017). Prenatal education can help, by offering coping strategies, anticipatory guidance, and encouraging the pregnant person to share their needs with their prenatal provider, or support person.

Issues Integral to Prenatal Education

Literacy, Health Literacy, Written Materials, and Reading Level

Literacy refers to the ability to read, gain knowledge, write coherently, and think critically about what the individual has read. However, even highly literate and educated people may not be *health literate*. **Health literacy** is defined by the US Department of Health and Human Services, Health Resources and Services Administration (2019) as "the degree to which individuals have the capacity to obtain, process and understand basic health information needed to make appropriate health decisions and services needed to prevent or treat illness." The National Assessment of Adult Literacy identified that 16% of women can understand only basic health information and 12% fall below that level (Kutner et al., 2006). Low health literacy is associated with less use of preventive care strategies and poor perinatal outcomes (Hussey et al., 2016) and presents a barrier for correctly interpreting health information related to pregnancy. Additionally, there are few strategies aimed at improving health literacy for pregnant people (Nawabi et al., 2021). Since health literacy is linked to patient safety, the Partnership for Clear Health Communication at the National Patient Safety Foundation (Institute for Healthcare Improvement, 2022) has launched the "Ask me 3" program. This program promotes three simple questions that all patients are encouraged to ask of their providers at every healthcare interaction: "(1) What is my main problem? (2) What do I need to do? and (3) Why is it important for me to do this?" Healthcare providers should use these questions to frame prenatal education in a clear and understandable manner, especially if the person develops a complication during pregnancy.

Plain language is language used in clear, simple terms that is easy to understand. The goal of the "plain language movement" is an effort to bridge the health literacy gap. A basic principle of this movement is that written materials and teaching methods should be understandable to anyone. An example of a plain language method is the "Hey Mama" prenatal education book developed by midwives and successfully used with a diverse population of pregnant women in Boston (Mottl-Santiago et al., 2013). An app is available for patient use.

Written health information materials can be used to supplement individual or group prenatal education. Using written health information at the fourth- to sixth-grade reading level can improve accessibility of information (National Library of Medicine, n.d.). Various tools are available to assess the reading level of a document. For example, the Flesch reading ease test formula is available online and uses the number of words, sentences, and syllables to determine a reading level estimate of inserted text (Readable, 2022; National Library of Medicine, n.d.). It is recommended that written patient education materials be subjected to a reading level test before they are introduced to patients for use. Presenting complex information in simple and understandable terms in written materials will improve their utility and impact. Additionally, the selective use of graphics may convey important information using fewer words in a more memorable manner for some learners.

Functions of Prenatal Communication

Delaney and Singleton (2020) conducted a qualitative study including 21 cisgender, heterosexual women who had recently given birth. They analyzed the communication between women and their healthcare providers. Two major themes with subthemes emerged (Table 24.5). The researchers found that patient communication with antenatal care providers served two interdependent purposes. It allows for both information exchange and the development and maintenance of patient relationships. The authors concluded that more attention to patient centered communication and improved provider patient interactions during pregnancy are necessary. Patient centered communication may be associated with improved outcomes because of the trust building relationship between provider and patient (Delaney & Singleton, 2020).

Guidelines for using plain language in health education material

1. Use words with fewer than three syllables
2. Avoid medical terminology
3. Use general terms of quantity (most or many) instead of statistics
4. Use active voice and friendly terms such as "you"
5. Use bullets of 15 words or less rather than complete sentences
6. Use headings and subheading, 12-point font and plenty of white space
7. Illustrations should be age and culturally appropriate
8. Illustrations should focus on only one idea

Source: Adapted from Mottl-Santiago et al. (2013).

Table 24.5 Information and Relationship Functions of Antenatal Communication between Pregnant People and Providers

Themes	Subthemes
Information functions	• Monitoring pregnancy • Seeking information • Offering information • Normalizing
Relationship functions	• Personalization care • Navigating emotions • Communicating • Power • Self-advocacy

Source: Adapted from Delaney and Singleton (2020).

Prioritizing Prenatal Education Needs

Health professionals are encouraged to develop a comprehensive approach for prenatal health education that can be individualized to meet the needs and priorities of their clients (Hanson et al., 2009). Roberts (1976) identified four priorities in prenatal education in her classic work. In order of importance these were: (a) responding to specific questions; (b) addressing essential health and safety issues; (c) providing anticipatory guidance about pregnancy changes, birth, and infant care; and (d) adding explanations on upcoming topics or policies beyond the immediate needs at the visit. The information is organized by gestation, and the prenatal education plan can be refined as pregnancy progresses. This approach is consistent with principles of adult learning—specifically, the desire for practical information that is relevant and meets their needs. Each of these priorities can be adapted for individual and group prenatal care.

Responding to Questions

Responding to questions of a pregnant person and their partner may seem like a simple task. However, in a busy prenatal office setting, the challenge becomes immediately apparent. Prenatal visits are often scheduled for a brief (or even overbooked) time frame. While patients can ask questions during a prenatal visit at any time, some may be unable to remember their questions if they perceive that the provider is rushing. Taking time to sit and talk to each patient (and their significant other) before or at the end of the appointment will provide the opportunity to answer questions and provide needed education.

Discussing Health and Safety Issues

Issues of safety include environmental health, diet, supplements, and food safety, psychosocial and physical assessments, laboratory testing, and plans to modify risk factors. A careful chart review either before entering the room or with the pregnant person will ensure that vital signs and laboratory findings are carefully addressed.

The issue of food safety is especially significant before and during pregnancy because certain food products and/or contaminants can pose a risk for the developing fetus. The US government has a section of the Food Safety website devoted to preconception and prenatal food safety (US Department of Health and Human Services, 2020) that includes risks of mercury levels in certain types of seafood, unpasteurized milk products, undercooked meats, and certain deli products.

A substantial amount of prenatal health education time is devoted to discussing and reviewing the ever-increasing number of laboratory and diagnostic tests incorporated into the accepted standard of prenatal care. At the same time, as more prenatal tests are added, the expectations for productivity are also increasing (Hanson et al., 2009); however, attention to other important aspects of education may help refocus prenatal visits on wellness.

Anticipatory Guidance

Anticipatory guidance refers to a specific form of health education in which healthcare providers prepare patients for likely pregnancy experiences including physical and emotional symptoms, events, and sensations. The person may be growing and developing into a new role during pregnancy and may be experiencing a unique connection between mind and body. The emotional and physiologic changes that are occurring may be viewed as welcome and exciting, frightening and strange, or for some people, they may not be noticeable. Discussions about what to expect can help reframe the normal discomforts of pregnancy and target education to developing needs.

A clear understanding of pregnant people's experiences during each trimester will help guide the development of a plan of anticipatory guidance. For example, during the first trimester, pregnant people may focus on their profound physiologic changes including nausea, fatigue, urinary frequency, and breast tenderness. Education aimed at coping with these changes will be more effective than attempting to address issues further from the physical and emotional experience. It is also important to maintain a balance between the time spent on the many genetic tests that are offered during early pregnancy and the person's needs to know about the physical and emotional changes occurring.

During the second trimester, relative comfort is accompanied by quickening and a greater awareness of the individuality of the fetus. Therefore, prenatal educational topics can be broadened during this time to include issues of breastfeeding, infant care, and parenting.

During the final trimester, individuals may become increasingly ready to discuss and ultimately experience the process of labor and birth. Tapping into this emotional readiness allows for meaningful dialogues about labor and birth, including fears and hopes for the experience.

Providing Additional Information for Future Use

Providing information about other topics or policies beyond the person's immediate needs is the final priority the provider can address. An example is development of a written **birth plan** for the last trimester. A pragmatic approach to begin a birth plan discussion is sharing features of the birth environment and the processes of care with the pregnant person and the family. This will allow the individual to develop a birth plan that is realistic and useful to guide care during labor and birth.

Trimester-Based Approaches to Prenatal Education

Depending on the structure of the prenatal care environment (individual versus group), pregnant people may experience up to a dozen or more prenatal visits. Considering the priorities of prenatal education and the relative predictability of the emotional and physical changes of pregnancy, education can be efficiently structured by trimester. Table 24.6 contains a detailed teaching

Table 24.6 Prenatal Education Topics with Suggested Timing

Prenatal health education topics	Gestational weeks[a]				
	0[b]–12	12–24	24–32	32–36	36+
Birth setting choices/tour	X				X
Cessation of harmful substances[c]:					
• Alcohol	X				
• Drugs	X				
• Teratogens	X				
• Tobacco	X				
Depression screening	X	X			
Dental care	X				
Employment or school plans	X		X		X
Exercise/activity	X	X	X	X	X
Family planning/Contraception			X	X	X
Fetal growth and status	X	X	X	X	X
Fetal heart tone explanation	X	X	X	X	X
Fetal movement/quickening		X	X	X	X
Fetal presentation			X	X	X
Fundal height measurement	X	X	X	X	X
Hair treatment use	X				
Hot tub/sauna use	X				
Hypertensive disorder screening	X	X	X	X	X
Intimate partner violence	X	X	X	X	X
Option of cervical examination to evaluate for readiness					X
Orientation to provider/practice/prenatal care processes	X				
Over the counter medications	X				
Postterm management					X
Rest and sleep needs	X		X		X
Review laboratory results with patient	X	X	X	X	X
RhoGAM/antepartum			X		
Risk identification/assessment	X	X	X	X	X
Safety/seatbelts	X				
Sexuality	X		X		X
Shared decision-making	X	X	X	X	X
Stripping of membranes >38 weeks					X
Travel	X			X	X
Tubal ligation authorization			X		
Urinary frequency	X				
Vaccines:					
• COVID-19	X	X	X	X	X
• TDaP			X		
• Influenza	X	X	X	X	X
Vaginal discharge		X		X	
VBAC informed consent and support	X			X	X
Warning signs to call provider	X	X	X	X	X

Table 24.6   (*Continued*)

Prenatal health education topics	Gestational weeks[a]				
	0[b]–12	12–24	24–32	32–36	36+
Infant feeding:					
• Breastfeeding education	X	X	X	X	X
• Infant feeding options: breast feeding, breast pumping, formula feeding, or combination	X	X	X	X	X
Labor preparation:					
• Analgesia and anesthesia choices				X	X
• Birth planning/preparation			X	X	X
• Childbirth class attendance		X		X	X
• Involvement of significant other		X			X
• Labor signs/symptoms/when to call provider				X	X
• Methods to facilitate labor coping				X	X
• Plan for care of other children				X	
• Preterm labor		X	X	X	X
Nutrition:					
• Diet and eating patterns	X	X	X	X	X
• Body mass index calculation	X				
• Folic acid	X				
• Food safety	X				
• Supplements such as iron	X		X		
• Weight gain	X	X	X	X	X
Physiologic changes/discomforts:	X	X	X	X	X
• Back pain		X	X	X	X
• Body mechanics		X	X	X	
• Breast care and supportive bra		X	X		
• Breast fullness/tenderness	X				
• Comfortable clothing		X	X		
• Constipation		X		X	
• Contractions (Braxton-Hicks)			X	X	
• Dyspnea/shortness of breath			X	X	
• Emotional changes/fears			X		X
• Fatigue	X			X	
• Heartburn		X	X	X	
• Hemorrhoids		X			
• Leg ache/cramping/varicosities			X	X	X
• Nausea and vomiting	X				
• Round ligament pain		X	X	X	
• Sciatica				X	X
• Supine hypotension		X			
Postterm management					X
Preconception care	X				

(*Continued*)

Table 24.6   (*Continued*)

Prenatal health education topics	Gestational weeks[a]				
	0[b]–12	12–24	24–32	32–36	36+
Preparation for baby:					
Circumcision decision-making					X
Household assistance			X		X
Supplies			X		X
Pediatric provider selection			X		X
Genetic screening:					
• Disease specific (e.g., cystic fibrosis, Tay Sachs)	X				
• Nuchal translucency screen	X	X			
• Serum Screen (NIPT, Quad/AFP)	X	X			
• Anatomy screen ultrasound option (16–20 weeks)		X			
Selective testing as indicated:					
• NST, BPP, Doppler flow			X	X	X
• Ultrasound for fetal growth			X	X	X
• Ultrasound for cervical length		X	X	X	

Source: Adapted from Hanson et al. (2009).
BPP = biophysical profile; EDB = Estimated date of birth; NST = nonstress test; VBAC = vaginal birth after cesarean.
[a] Several prenatal visits can occur within each time frame specified, allowing multiple opportunities and chances to revisit topics as needed.
[b] Zero weeks refers to possible preconception care topics.
[c] Follow-up positives with discussion at each subsequent visit including cessation plan.

plan that includes specific prenatal education topics such as laboratory testing, based on the priorities for prenatal education, and corresponding with timing recommendations based on gestational age. No plan for prenatal health education is complete without making sure that it is individualized. Further, the careful planning of education topics may help to avoid information overload at any single prenatal visit. Prenatal care providers are encouraged to adapt the teaching plans presented in this chapter to the needs of their clients, their practice settings, and the most up-to-date components of prenatal care.

Cultural Considerations

A person's cultural background may affect the manner in which they prepare for and perceive childbirth. Cultural background is an important consideration in preparing an education plan for each pregnant person. Written prenatal educational materials should be culturally relevant whenever possible. Educational materials depicting pregnant people from diverse cultures are available at no cost from several government-sponsored websites, and many of these materials are available in several languages (see *Resources for Healthcare Providers*). The predominantly government-sponsored websites are intended to better serve diverse communities as well as conserve healthcare resources for translation of health information. Several of these websites also contain portals to government and community resources for the care of patients who are refugees.

Health Disparities

Pregnant people comprise a population specifically targeted for improved health outcomes in *Healthy People 2030* (US Department of Health and Human Services, n.d.-a). Health disparities are evident in the poorer perinatal outcomes of many ethnic and racial groups. There is evidence that prenatal health education can make a positive impact on some of these outcomes (Vonderheid et al., 2007), but barriers to receipt of health education can stand in the way. Sperlich et al. (2019) identified that pregnant people who were Black, possessed public insurance, had a lower level of education, or lived in a neighborhood with higher levels of crime were less likely to receive childbirth education. The investigators also found that among the women in the study who attended childbirth classes, there were no meaningful differences in completion rates by race, suggesting that barriers to accessing classes may play a role in childbirth education receipt. Barriers to attending childbirth education classes include lack of transportation, lack of childcare, and cost (Berman, 2006). Doula care has been suggested as an approach to enhance perinatal outcomes for people of color. There is growing evidence to support that doula care can enhance patient decision-making, perinatal outcomes, and access (Attanasio et al., 2021; Thomas et al., 2017). However, based on focus groups of prenatal care recipients, doula care programs may need to be adapted to meet the needs of specific communities (e.g., adolescents). (Attanasio et al., 2021). The accessibility of prenatal and childbirth education could be enhanced by including provisions for transportation, childcare, language, and cultural needs.

The etiology of perinatal health disparities is multifactorial, reflecting a combination of racism, social disadvantage, policy issues, access to care, and historical trauma leading to medical mistrust (Alhusen et al., 2017). McLemore et al. (2018) conducted a secondary analysis of focus group data from a larger community-engaged study of premature birth. The experiences of 54 women of color who were recipients of prenatal care were analyzed. Participants described their prenatal care experiences as both stressful and disrespectful, leaving them with unmet learning needs. Participants made suggestions for improvement including better communication with more careful listening, as well as more attention to birth plans. Altman et al. (2019) conducted a qualitative (grounded theory) interviews with a purposeful sample of 22 women of color who had risk factors for premature birth. Participants described the receipt of incomplete and/or biased information that was "packaged" (p. 3) to benefit the provider rather than the prenatal care recipient. They also described that providers suppressed information or provided misleading or incomplete information that was based on erroneous assumptions about the pregnant person's ability to make sound decisions. The researchers identified two features that influenced the perception of information received from their providers: (a) development of the patient-provider relationship, and (b) the acknowledgment of how the concepts of privilege and marginalization affect prenatal interactions. Urgent attention needs to be given to discrimination, racism, and disrespectful prenatal healthcare encounters to reduce perinatal health disparities.

Documentation of Teaching

Prenatal health education needs to be carefully documented in the prenatal record to assure that all relevant and needed topics are covered. Documenting that the appropriate topics have been covered facilitates continuity, especially when different clinicians are involved in care. Although many of the standardized prenatal health records include a minimal checklist for such documentation, prenatal health education should also be documented in progress notes. Some electronic health record systems include triggers or reminders for health education and timing of laboratory testing. In the absence of these reminders, careful attention to both the timing and documentation of prenatal health and safety information is important. Teaching documentation should include that the patient verbalized understanding of the health education, that they report knowing how and when to contact the healthcare provider, and also that they had no further questions. Such documentation is especially important for topics such as the danger signs of pregnancy complications and the onset of labor. The effectiveness of health teaching can be evaluated at the subsequent visit when the person is asked if they have any questions or concerns about what was discussed at the last visit.

Summary

Prenatal care visits provide opportunities for education that can impact the health of the pregnant person, the fetus, and the entire family. Special consideration of culture, chronologic age, cognitive skills, access and use of health resources, and health literacy all impact the delivery and receipt of prenatal education. Education incorporated into prenatal visits by prioritizing the person's learning needs allows for the individualization of information and opportunities to maximize comprehension, retention, and usage of the information. A well-planned approach with careful documentation is essential to meet the extensive informational needs of pregnant people. Prenatal healthcare providers play an essential role in providing evidence-based and person-centered health education throughout the prenatal period.

Resources	Pregnancy	Labor/Birth	Scientific Evidence
Resources for Clients and Families			
• The American College of Obstetricians and Gynecologists https://www.acog.org/womens-health/pregnancy	X	X	X
• The American Pregnancy Association https://americanpregnancy.org	X	X	
• Bradley Method www.bradleybirth.com		X	
• Centers for Disease Control and Prevention (CDC) https://www.cdc.gov/pregnancy	X		
• Childbirth Connections www.childbirthconnection.org	X	X	
• Evidence-Based Birth https://evidencebasedbirth.com		X	X
• Hey Mama (App) https://www.bmc.org/heymama	X		
• Hypnobirthing method https://us.hypnobirthing.com		X	

Resources	Pregnancy	Labor/Birth	Scientific Evidence
• Lamaze Method www.lamazeinternational.org		X	
• March of Dimes www.marchofdimes.com	X		
• Spinning Babies www.spinningbabies.com.	X	X	
• Text4Baby Initiative (App and texting service) https://www.acf.hhs.gov/text4baby	X		
• US Department of Health and Human Services, Office on Women's Health. Pregnancy http://www.womenshealth.gov/pregnancy	X	X	
Resources for Healthcare Providers			
• American College of Nurse-Midwives https://onlinelibrary.wiley.com/page/journal/15422011/homepage/share-with-women	X	X	X
• The American College of Obstetricians and Gynecologists https://www.acog.org/clinical	X	X	X
• Centers for Disease Control and Prevention (CDC). Plain Language https://www.cdc.gov/healthliteracy/developmaterials/plainlanguage.html	X	X	X
• National Library of Medicine (NLM). MedlinePlus: Pregnancy https://medlineplus.gov/pregnancy.html	X		X

References

Alhusen, J. L., Bower, K., Epstein, E., & Sharps, P. (2017). Racial discrimination and adverse birth outcomes: An integrative review. *Journal of Midwifery & Women's Health*, *61*(6), 707–720. https://doi.org/10.1111/jmwh.12490

Altman, M. R., Oseguera, T., McLemore, M. R., Kantrowitz-Gordon, I., Franck, L. S., & Lyndon, A. (2019). Information and power: Women of color's experiences interacting with health care providers in pregnancy and birth. *Social Science & Medicine*, *238*, N.PAG. https://doi.org/10.1016/j.socscimed.2019.112491

American Academy of Husband-Coached Childbirth. (2022). *The Bradley method of husband-coached natural childbirth*. http://www.bradleybirth.com

Attanasio, L. B., DaCosta, M., Kleppel, R., Govantes, T., Sankey, H. Z., & Goff, S. L. (2021). Community perspectives on the creation of a hospital-based doula program. *Health Equity*, *5*(1), 545–553. https://doi.org/10.1089/heq.2020.0096

Avery, M. D., Saftner, M. A., Larson, B., & Weinfurter, E. V. (2014). A systematic review of maternal confidence for physiologic birth: Characteristics of prenatal care and confidence measurement. *Journal of Midwifery & Women's Health*, *59*, 586–595. https://doi.org/10.1111/jmwh.12269

Berman, R. O. (2006). Perceived learning needs of minority expectant women and barriers to prenatal education. *Journal of Perinatal Education*, *15*(2), 36–42. https://doi.org/10.1624/105812406X107807

Bradford, H., DePalma, K., Mole, K., & Olsen, S. (2020, May 30 – June 1). Weight stigma and fatphobia in healthcare. Are we practicing evidence-based care? [Conference Presentation]. ACNM 65th Annual Meeting & Exhibition, Virtual.

Catsaros, S., & Wendland, J. (2020). Hypnosis-based interventions during pregnancy and childbirth and their impact on women's childbirth experience: A systematic review. *Midwifery*, *84*, 102666. https://doi.org/10.1016/j.midw.2020.102666

Center for Health Care Strategies. (2021). *Trauma-informed care implementation resource center*. https://www.traumainformedcare.chcs.org

Centering Healthcare Institute. (2022). *CenteringPregnancy*. https://centeringhealthcare.org/what-we-do/centering-pregnancy

Da Costa, D., Zelkowitz, P., Bailey, K., Cruz, R., Bernard, J.-C., Dasgupta, K., Lowensteyn, I., & Khalife, S. (2015). Results of a needs assessment to guide the development of a website to enhance emotional wellness and healthy behaviors during pregnancy. *Journal of Perinatal Education*, *24*(4), 213–224. https://doi.org/10.1891/1058-1243.24.4.213

Daniels, M., & Wedler, J. A. (2015). Enhancing childbirth education through technology. *International Journal of Childbirth Education*, *30*(3), 28–32.

Declercq, E. R., Sakala, C., Corry, M. P., Applebaum, S., & Herrlich, A. (2013). *Listening to mothers III: New mothers speak out*. Childbirth Connection. https://www.nationalpartnership.org/our-work/resources/health-care/maternity/listening-to-mothers-iii-pregnancy-and-birth-2013.pdf

Delaney, A. L., & Singleton, G. (2020). Information and relationship functions of communication between pregnant women and their health care providers. *Communication Studies*, *71*(5), 800–822. https://doi.org/10.1080/10510974.2020.1807376

Dick-Read, G. (2013). *Childbirth without fear: The principles and practice of natural childbirth*. Pinter and Martin Ltd.

Downer, T., McMurray, A., & Young, J. (2020). The role of antenatal education in promoting maternal and family health literacy. *International Journal of Childbirth*, *10*(1), 52–64. https://doi.org/10.1891/IJCBIRTH-D-20-00012

Farahi, N., & Zolotor, A. (2013). Recommendations for preconception counseling and care. *American Family Physician*, *88*(8), 499–506.

Frid, G., Bogaert, K., & Chen, K. T. (2021). Mobile health apps for pregnant women: Systematic search, evaluation, and analysis of features. *Journal of Medical Internet Research*, *23*(10), e25667. https://doi.org/10.2196/25667

Friedman, L. S. (2006). Seventeen to twenty-one years: Transition to adulthood. In S. D. Dixon & M. T. Stein (Eds.), *Encounters with children: Pediatric behavior and development* (4th ed., pp. 601–620). Mosby Elsevier.

Gagnon, A. J., & Sandall, J. (2007). Individual or group antenatal education for childbirth or parenthood, or both. *Cochrane Database of Systematic Reviews*, *3*, CD002869.

Hanson, L., VandeVusse, L., Roberts, J., & Forristal, A. (2009). A critical appraisal of guidelines for antenatal care: Components of care and priorities in prenatal education. *Journal of Midwifery & Women's Health*, *54*, 458–468. https://doi.org/10.1016/j.jmwh.2009.08.002

Hollander, M. H., van Hastenberg, E., van Dillen, J., van Pampus, M. G., de Miranda, E., & Stramrood, C. (2017). Preventing traumatic childbirth experiences: 2192 women's perceptions and views.

Archives of Women's Mental Health, 20(4), 515–523. https://doi.org/10.1007/s00737-017-0729-6ItS

Humenick, S. S. (2000). Program evaluation. In F. H. Nichols & S. S. Humenick (Eds.), *Childbirth education: Practice, research, and theory* (2nd ed., pp. 593–608). Saunders.

Hussey, L. C., Frazer, C., & Kopulos, M. I. (2016). Impact of health literacy levels in educating pregnant millennial women. *International Journal of Childbirth Education, 31*(3), 13–18.

Institute for Healthcare Improvement. (2022). *Ask me 3: Good questions for your good health.* http://www.ihi.org/resources/Pages/Tools/Ask-Me-3-Good-Questions-for-Your-Good-Health.aspx

Inversetti, A., Fumagalli, S., Nespoli, A., Antolini, L., Mussi, S., Ferrari, D., & Locatelli, A. (2021). Childbirth experience and practice changing during COVID-19 pandemic: A cross-sectional study. *Nursing Open, 8*(6), 3627–3634. https://doi.org./10.1002/nop2.913

Knowles, M. S. (1988). *The modern practice of adult education: From pedagogy to androgogy.* Prentice Hall/Cambridge.

Kovala, S., Cramp, A. G., & Xia, L. (2016). Prenatal education: Program content and preferred delivery method from the perspective of the expectant parents. *The Journal of Perinatal Education, 25*(4), 232–241. https://doi.org/10.1891/1058-1243.25.4.232

Kutner, M., Greenberg, E., Jin, Y., & Paulsen, C. (2006). *The health literacy of America's adults: Results from the 2003 National Assessment of Adult Literacy (NCES 2006–483).* US Department of Education, National Center for Educational Statistics. https://nces.ed.gov/pubs2006/2006483.pdf

Lamaze International. (2022). *Healthy birth practices.* https://www.lamaze.org/childbirth-practices

Logsdon, M. C., Davis, D. W., Stikes, R., Ratterman, R., Ryan, L., & Myers, J. (2015). Acceptability and initial efficacy of education for teen mothers. *MCN: American Journal of Maternal/Child Nursing, 40*(3), 186–192. https://doi.org/10.1097/NMC.0000000000000126

Lu, M. C., Kotelchuck, M., Culhane, J. F., Hobel, C. J., Klerman, L. V., & Thorp, J. M. (2006). Preconception care between pregnancies: The content of internatal care. *Maternal Child Health Journal, 10*(5), S107–S122. https://doi.org/10.1007/s10995-006-0118-7

Maddow-Zimet, I. & Kost, K. (2021). *Pregnancies, Births and Abortions in the United States, 1973–2017: National and State Trends by Age.* Guttmacher Institute. https://www.guttmacher.org/report/pregnancies-births-abortions-in-united-states-1973-2017

Maehr, J., & Felice, M. E. (2006a). Eleven to fourteen years: Early adolescence: Age of rapid changes. In S. D. Dixon & M. T. Stein (Eds.), *Encounters with children: Pediatric behavior and development* (4th ed., pp. 535–562). Mosby Elsevier.

Maehr, J., & Felice, M. E. (2006b). Fifteen to seventeen years: Mid-adolescence: Redefining self. In S. D. Dixon & M. T. Stein (Eds.), *Encounters with children: Pediatric behavior and development* (4th ed., pp. 565–598). Mosby Elsevier.

Martin, J. A., Hamilton, B. E., Osterman, M., & Driscoll, A. K. (2021). Births: Final data for 2019. *National Vital Statistics Reports, 70*(2), 1–51.

McLemore, M. R., Altman, M. R., Cooper, N., Williams, S., Rand, L., & Franck, L. (2018). Health care experiences of pregnant, birthing and postnatal women of color at risk for preterm birth. *Social Science & Medicine, 201*, 127–135.

McNeil, D. A., Vekved, M., Dolan, S. M., Siever, J., Horn, S., & Tough, S. C. (2012). Getting more than they realized they needed: A qualitative study of women's experience of group prenatal care. *BMC Pregnancy & Childbirth, 12*(17). https://doi.org/10.1186/1471-2393-12-17

Morris, T., & McInerney, K. (2010). Media representations of pregnancy and childbirth: An analysis of reality television programs in the United States. *Birth, 37*(2), 134–140. https://doi.org/10.1111/j.1523-536X.2010.00393.x

Mottl-Santiago, J., Fox, C. S., Pecci, C. C., & Iverson, R. (2013). Multidisciplinary collaborative development of a plain-language prenatal education book. *Journal of Midwifery & Women's Health, 58*, 271–277. https://doi.org/10.1111/jmwh.12059

National Library of Medicine. (n.d.). *Easy-to-read health information.* MedlinePlus. Retrieved April 4, 2022 from https://medlineplus.gov/all_easytoread.html

Nawabi, F., Krebs, F., Vennedey, V., Shukri, A., Lorenz, L., & Stock, S. (2021). Health literacy in pregnant women: A systematic review. *International Journal of Environmental Research and Public Health, 18*(7), 3847. https://doi.org/10.3390/ijerph18073847

Nolan, M. (2000). The influence of antenatal classes on pain relief in labour: A review of the literature. *The Practising Midwife, 3*(5), 23–26.

Pasadino, F., DeMarco, K., & Lampert, E. (2020). Connecting with families through virtual perinatal education during the COVID-19 pandemic. *MCN. The American Journal of Maternal Child Nursing, 45*(6), 364–370. https://doi.org/10.1097/NMC.0000000000000665

Phillips-Moore, J. (2012). Birthing outcomes from an Australian HypnoBirthing programme. *British Journal of Midwifery, 20*(8). https://doi.org/10.12968/bjom.2012.20.8.558

Readable. (2022). *Flesch reading ease and the Flesch Kincaid grade level.* https://readable.com/readability/flesch-reading-ease-flesch-kincaid-grade-level

Roberts, J. E. (1976). Priorities in prenatal education. *Journal of Obstetrical, Gynecological & Neonatal Nursing, 5*(3), 17–20. https://doi.org/10.1111/j.1552-6909.1976.tb02302.x

Sayakhot, P., & Carolan-Olah, M. (2016). Internet use by pregnant women seeking pregnancy-related information: A systematic review. *BMC Pregnancy and Childbirth, 16*, 65. https://doi.org/10.1186/s12884-016-0856-5

Serçekuş, P., & Başkale, H. (2016). Effects of antenatal education on fear of childbirth, maternal self-efficacy and parental attachment. *Midwifery, 34*, 166–172. https://doi.org/10.1016/j.midw.2015.11.016

Sheahan, K. L., Kroll-Derosiers, A., Goldstein, K. M., Sheahan, M. M., Oumarou, A., & Mattocks, K. (2022). Sufficiency of health information during pregnancy: What's missing and for whom? A cross-sectional analysis among veterans. *Journal of Women's Health.* https://doi.org/10.1089/jwh.2021.0462

Simkin, P., & Ancheta, R. (2017). Normal labor and labor dystocia: General considerations. In P. Simkin, L. Hanson, & R. Ancheta (Eds.), *The labor progress handbook: Early interventions to prevent and treat dystocia* (4th ed., pp. 9–48). Wiley Blackwell.

Sperlich, M., Gabriel, C., & St Vil, N. M. (2019). Preference, knowledge and utilization of midwives, childbirth education classes and doulas among U.S. black and white women: Implications for pregnancy and childbirth outcomes. *Social Work in Health Care, 58*(10), 988–1001. https://doi.org/10.1080/00981389.2019.1686679

Thomas, M. P., Ammann, G., Brazier, E., Noyes, P., & Maybank, A. (2017). Doula services within a healthy start program: Increasing access for an underserved population. *Maternal and Child Health Journal, 21*(1), 59–64. https://doi.org/10.1007/s10995-017-2402-0

US Department of Health & Human Services. (2020, September 25). *People at risk: Pregnant women.* https://www.foodsafety.gov/people-at-risk/pregnant-women

US Department of Health and Human Services, Health Resources and Services Administration. (2019, August). *Health literacy.* https://www.hrsa.gov/about/organization/bureaus/ohe/health-literacy/index.html

US Department of Health and Human Services, Office of Disease Prevention and Health Promotion. (n.d.-a). *Maternal, infant, and child health workgroup.* Healthy People 2030. https://health.gov/healthypeople/about/workgroups/maternal-infant-and-child-health-workgroup

US Department of Health and Human Services, Office of Disease Prevention and Health Promotion. (n.d.-b). *Social determinants of health.* Healthy People 2030. https://health.gov/healthypeople/objectives-and-data/social-determinants-health

US Department of Veterans Affairs. (2022, August 18). *Exposure to hazardous chemicals and materials.* https://www.va.gov/disability/eligibility/hazardous-materials-exposure

Vonderheid, S. C., Norr, K. F., & Handler, A. S. (2007). Prenatal health promotion content and behaviors. *Western Journal of Nursing Research, 27*(3), 258–276. https://doi.org/10.1177/0193945906296568

Walker, D. S., Visger, J. M., & Rossie, D. (2009). Contemporary childbirth education models. *Journal of Midwifery & Women's Health, 54*(6), 469–476. https://doi.org/10.1016/j.jmwh.2009.02.013

World Health Organization. (2022). *Obesity.* https://www.who.int/health-topics/obesity#tab=tab_1

25

Preconception, Pregnancy, and Postpartum Care of LGBTQ+ Individuals

Signey Olson and Katie DePalma

"It's easy to fictionalize an issue when you're not aware of the many ways in which you are privileged by it."
—Kate Bornstein & S. Bear Bergman, *Gender Outlaws: The Next Generation* (2010)

Relevant Terms—Sexuality

Asexual—the experience of having little to no sexual attraction or feelings. This accounts for approximately 3% of the population and is not the same as experiencing a low libido. Asexual individuals often still engage in consensual sex for many reasons and are often partnered with partners who are not asexual

Ally—someone who challenges homophobia, biphobia, and transphobia and is actively engaged in advocacy and breaking down their own bias and the biases of those around them. Many LGBTQ+ individuals do not consider the "A" to truly be part of the LGBTQQIA2PA+ acronym because allies themselves do not hold a socially oppressed identity related to gender or sexuality

Bisexual—romantic and/or sexual attraction to more than one gender. Traditionally used in reference to attraction to men and women, though it may also be defined as romantic or sexual attraction to people of any sex or gender identity

Gay—traditionally used to refer to men who are attracted to other men (this includes cis and trans men). This term has also evolved within the LGBTQ+ community to encompass a wider range of same-gender-loving people

Heterosexual—attraction to individuals of the opposite sex or perceived opposite sex

Heteronormativity—a world view that promotes heterosexuality as the normal or preferred sexual orientation

Lesbian—women who are attracted to other women (this includes cis and trans women)

LGBTQQIA2PA+—acronym for Lesbian, Gay, Bisexual, Transgender, Queer, Questioning, Intersex, Asexual, Two-Spirit, Pansexual, Ally, + (often shortened to **LGBTQ+**)

Queer—historically used as a derogatory slur, this word has been reclaimed by the LGBTQ+ community. It encompasses the idea that sexuality and/or gender does not fit neatly into a specific label and instead places the emphasis on fluidity

Questioning—individuals who are unsure of their sexual orientation and/or gender identity and are currently examining and exploring possible aspects of their identity

Sexuality—a broad term encompassing how people experience and express themselves as sexual beings

Sexual orientation—an emotional, romantic, or sexual attraction to other people or no people

Pansexual—attraction to people of all genders

Two-spirit—in some Indigenous cultures, a "third gender" that embodies physical and nonphysical attributes of masculine and feminine. Commonly thought to be the result of supernatural intervention, many two-spirit individuals hold high-level roles as shamans, healers, and ceremonial leaders. Sometimes abbreviated "2" in the LGBTQIA2P+ acronym

---

Relevant Terms—Gender and Sex

Cisgender—the word used to describe an individual who identifies as the same gender as the sex they were assigned at birth, typically either male or female. Often shortened to "cis"

Cisnormativity—a world view that promotes cisgender as the normal or preferred gender identity

Family—a group of people related by blood, legal document, or choice, traditionally with the primary function of raising

---

Prenatal and Postnatal Care: A Person-Centered Approach, Third Edition. Edited by Karen Trister Grace, Cindy L. Farley, Noelene K. Jeffers, and Tanya Tringali.
© 2024 John Wiley & Sons Ltd. Published 2024 by John Wiley & Sons Ltd.
Companion website: www.wiley.com/go/grace/prenatal

children to the age of maturity; variations in family composition and structure exist

Gender—the socially constructed aspects of a person's biological sex or personal identity; may not match categorization of sex assigned at birth

Gender binary—a socially incomplete concept referring to the existence of only two gender categories, male and female

Gender dysphoria—persistent or intermittent feelings of identification with a gender that does not match one's assigned sex at birth, and discomfort with one's assigned gender resulting in distress and impairment

Gender euphoria—persistent or intermittent feelings of embodied joy, comfort, and/or peace when thinking about personal gender and gender expression; generally considered the opposite of gender dysphoria. Pursuing gender euphoria may result in a person opting to change their appearance, name, and documentation, and sometimes medical forms of transitioning

Gender expression (also called gender presentation)—the ways in which a person expresses their gender externally. This may be through clothing, hair, makeup and other appearance-based choices

Gender identity—the ways in which a person experiences their gender internally

Gender nonconforming—relating to a person whose behavior or appearance does not conform to prevailing cultural and social expectations about their gender

Intersex—individuals who possess a variation of hormones, chromosomes, reproductive organs, and secondary sex characteristics which do not neatly fall into the categories of "male" and "female." This term refers to physical characteristics of a person's biology and does not refer to a person's identity

Nonbinary—an umbrella term used to describe someone who does not identify as fully male or fully female. Sometimes also referred to as gender nonbinary

Passing—refers to times when a transgender person is perceived by others to be cisgender instead of the sex they were assigned at birth

Sex—biological classification as female, male, or intersex based on chromosomes, genitalia, and reproductive organs

Sex assigned at birth—the label assigned to a person when they are born, usually based on the external genitalia a person appears to have at birth and it is typically assigned into one of two categories (male and female). There is typically a corresponding assumption that their gender matches their assigned sex—either male or female

Sex binary—a scientifically incomplete concept referring to the existence of only two sex categories, male and female

Stealth—when a trans person consistently passes as a cis individual and intentionally chooses not to disclose their transgender identity. Most people who know them are unaware that they are transgender. Some individuals may choose to be stealth in some areas of their lives are not in others

Transgender—the word used to describe an individual whose internal sense of gender and the sex they were assigned at birth do not match. This term is often shortened to "trans"

Transition—the process that some transgender or nonbinary patients people undergo in which they begin to live in congruence with their gender identity, rather than the gender they were assigned at birth

Introduction

Diversity and fluidity in **gender** and **sexuality** has existed across all cultures for the entirety of human existence. However, cultural understanding of sexual orientation and gender identity differs between communities and is ever-evolving. All clinicians will encounter **LGBTQ+** clients in the clinical setting, regardless of whether the clinician is aware of their client's gender or sexual orientation. Therefore, perinatal healthcare providers must engage in ongoing learning regarding respectful clinical care, inclusive language, and the existence of persistent health disparities in the LGBTQ+ population. A foundational understanding of these concepts will improve the therapeutic relationship with LGBTQ+ patients (Jaffee et al., 2016; Rossi & Lopez, 2017).

Health equity key points

- Gender and sex are distinctly different, and neither are binary.
- Gender-neutral language can be a powerful tool to promote an inclusive environment.
- Care of gender-diverse individuals is not inherently complex and is within the scope of APRNs.
- Focusing on the organs a person has can be a helpful way to determine potential clinical needs.

Why Language Matters

Language is a powerful tool that can be used both to empower and oppress marginalized groups. Recognizing this power, the clinician should utilize language to improve the patient–provider relationship and positively affect clinical outcomes (Rossi & Lopez, 2017). Understanding the importance of language in the LGBTQ+ community is vital to providing culturally humble care. These identities have always existed, though the terms and language we use to describe them have expanded and evolved over time. Finding language to describe a person's experience does not necessarily equate to a new identity, but often represents the relief of affirmation for an individual. Some clinicians may find this evolution and nuance in language confusing as they learn more about this community (Chang et al., 2018). Grounding oneself in shared values of respect, compassion, and openness can help during this process.

While this chapter reviews the most commonly used terms and definitions that are current at the time this book goes to press, there are likely to be instances where clients in the LGBTQ+ community use different languages to describe themselves or their lived experiences. The terminology a person uses may be specific to their age, race, ethnicity, class, native language, and geographic location. When a client shares a part of their identity, such as their sexual orientation or gender identity, it is helpful to have a general understanding of the concept, though the person may experience their identity in a unique way. Therefore, in the clinical setting, it is often best to reflect the language that the patient uses for themselves; while identity labels are important and valid, respectful follow-up clinical questions and clarification are also appropriate (Rossi & Lopez, 2017). A common example illustrating this importance is of a **cisgender** woman who self-identifies as a **lesbian**. This individual may use this term to mean that they are only attracted to and have sex with cisgender women and, therefore, would not have a risk of pregnancy. However, many trans women self-identify as lesbian and do produce sperm, making their lesbian partners at the risk of pregnancy.

Sexual orientation most commonly refers to a person's sexual attraction to others and how they describe that attraction, though not all individuals experience sexual attraction. Sexual orientations include *asexual, lesbian, gay, bisexual, pansexual, queer,* and more (PFLAG, 2022). The majority of societies and cultures have a **heteronormative** perspective. That is, heterosexuality is assumed to be the default sexual orientation. However, it is common for individuals to shift, add, or change their perception of their sexual orientation and the language they use to describe themselves over time. **Questioning** may encompass a state of feeling curious or in flux between various gender identities and/or sexual orientations. While the terms gay and *queer* are not always interchangeable, many individuals who use these terms view them as broad, umbrella terms rather than a reference to a specific type of person to whom they are attracted. Of note, the term queer has historically been used in a derogatory manner and has undergone reclamation by individuals within the LGBTQ+ community. The term lesbian typically describes attraction to women by other women and is inclusive of **transgender** women. In Latin, the term *pan* means "all," and as such, the term pansexual refers to potential attraction to any **gender**. It is important to note that this does not mean a pansexual person experiences attraction to every individual they encounter, but rather they experience attraction to people across the gender constellation.

There are numerous misconceptions about bisexuality, and understanding these can help clinicians avoid unintentional assumptions (Manzer et al., 2018). This term has evolved over time. Bisexual individuals have romantic and/or sexual attraction to more than one gender. Bisexuality is explicitly not a phase or temporary period of experimentation. Men and women are equally likely to be bisexual and engage in romantic and sexual activities with other genders. Attraction to men, women, and non-binary individuals may not be equal, and an individual can be bisexual and have never engaged in sexual activities with more than one sex. Bisexual individuals are not more likely than their nonbisexual peers to have multiple sexual partners or to leave their partner for someone of another gender. Bisexual erasure, or bi erasure, refers to a phenomenon in which bisexual identity is dismissed or delegitimized. An example of this would be to assume that two cisgender women in a relationship are lesbian, without

considering that one or both may be bisexual. This can feel isolating, as identity affirmation is important to many individuals. This may also occur in a couple where one partner **transitions** and changes appearance in such a way that the couple may now be perceived differently in public.

Two-spirit is an Indigenous reference to a third gender or gender expansiveness and often holds specific cultural understanding and role significance within the community. This term is only appropriately used by Indigenous individuals.

Some individuals do not experience sexual attraction, and this is most commonly referred to as **asexuality** (Brunning & McKeever, 2021). There are many misconceptions about this identity, and this experience is distinctly separate from those who experience suboptimal sexual drive or arousal. Asexual individuals may engage in enjoyable, consensual sex, though typically without feeling a strong sexual drive.

It is important to understand the differences between **sex** and gender and not to use this language interchangeably. Sex is a biological construct that refers to inherent physical traits that a person is born with. Sex is most commonly used in reference to the chromosomes that individuals are born with, typically XX or XY (Zemenick et al., 2022). However, while a **sex binary** of these two options is often presumed, there are numerous chromosomal patterns (sexes) that exist both in humans and other species (Grilo & Rosa, 2017; Mastromonaco et al., 2012; Pastorinho et al., 2009; Štrkalj & Pather, 2021). The term **sex assigned at birth** helps to capture the idea that while individuals are often assigned a sex of male or female, that designation is usually only based on the guess of the birth attendant and the appearance of the genitalia. Sometimes the sex is assigned even before birth, based on sonography and some genetic screens and tests. When used, this phrase is typically written as "assigned female at birth" (AFAB) and "assigned male at birth" (AMAB). If an infant appears to have physical characteristics and/or genitalia that does not align with the expected characteristics of male or female, the infant would be documented as **intersex** (Intersex Society of North America, 2019). About 1–2% of the population is intersex. These variations may or may not be obvious at birth. Many countries and organizations deem it unethical to perform nonmedically necessary surgery on infants to align their reproductive organs with male or female sex and recommend waiting until the child is older to allow them to express their own experience of gender. An example could be an infant who is born with one ovary, one testis, and a small phallus. While variations in external genitalia may be noted, intersex characteristics may not be visible externally; thus, the prevalence of intersex individuals is likely higher than recognized.

Gender is a socially constructed idea related to society's roles, norms, and expectations; it is not biological or based on anatomy. Gender is often assumed based on a person's assigned sex (PFLAG, 2022). **Gender identity** refers to an internal sense of one's gender, which cannot be known by external appearance. All individuals, including cisgender, nonbinary, and transgender individuals, have a **gender expression or presentation** (PFLAG, 2022). Even though many people make assumptions about a person's gender or sex assigned at birth based on a person's appearance, there is no way to know a person's identity or anatomy by simply looking at someone. Often, individuals may describe their own appearance or the appearances of others as "masculine" or "feminine," though these concepts are also socially constructed and can have a wide array of meaning across communities and cultures.

Cisgender refers to someone who identifies as the same sex and gender they were assigned at birth. Cisgender men are typically individuals AMAB who experience their gender as male. Cisgender women are typically individuals AFAB who experience their gender as female. **Transgender men** are typically AFAB individuals who experience their gender as male. The term "trans masculine" may also be used to describe someone AFAB who is on the masculine spectrum of gender but may or may not identify fully as male. **Transgender women** are typically AMAB individuals who experience their gender as female. The term "trans feminine" may also be used to describe someone AMAB who is on the feminine spectrum of gender but may or may not identify fully as female. It is important to note that the word **transgender** or **trans** are adjectives and not a noun or verb. The word *trans* should always be used as a separate adjective prior to the word "man" or "woman." It is not correct to write "transman" or "transwoman." It would also not be appropriate to say "a transgender" or "a transgendered person."

The term **nonbinary** may be used to describe AMAB, AFAB, or intersex individuals who do not describe themselves or their genders as falling into the binary categories of male or female (PFLAG, 2022). Because this is related to gender and not sex, it is not based on the anatomy a person has. Some people may use other terms instead of, or in addition to, nonbinary, such as genderfluid, gender expansive, **gender nonconforming**, genderqueer, or other terms.

Trans individuals may also identify as straight/heterosexual, as gender identity is entirely separate from a person's sexual orientation. Gender identities are always valid and do not require a person to have undergone any medical care or procedures in order to hold that identity. For example, a transgender man does not have to have taken testosterone or had any surgeries in order to identify as a transgender man. Many transgender and nonbinary (TGNB) individuals experience **gender dysphoria** surrounding the fact that their internal identities do not match the bodies they were born with (Austin et al., 2022). This is both a DSM-5 diagnosis and an experience that some people who are trans or nonbinary have. It describes an experience of "clinically significant distress or impairment related to a strong desire to be of another gender, which may include desire to change primary and/or secondary sex characteristics." However, it is essential to understand that the experience of gender dysphoria is not required in order to identify as TGNB; many TGNB individuals do not feel acute distress surrounding their bodies, given that outside of socially constructed concepts, anatomical body parts are not inherently gendered (Garg & Marwaha, 2020). Finding ways to experience **gender euphoria** is typically the goal of TGNB individuals, which may include aspects of gender transition (Austin et al., 2022).

Gender transition can look differently depending on what a person's goals are—it could include social, nonmedical appearance changes, or medical approaches. While not all transgender people transition, a great many do at some point in their lives. Because there is no one specific thing that "makes someone trans," many individuals consider their gender transition to be ongoing and, therefore, avoid the term "transitioned" as it implies a completed task. **Passing** occurs when a TGNB person is presumed to be their affirmed gender, typically in a social or public space (Anderson et al., 2020; Billard, 2019). Transgender individuals who live **stealth** typically do not share the fact that they are trans with most or all of the individuals in their lives, though many individuals only live stealth in one area of life, most commonly in the workplace (Anderson et al., 2020). For example, this could occur when a trans man has a masculine gender expression and is presumed to be a cisgender man when interacting with people who do not know he is trans. While passing in public spaces may decrease a person's experience of harassment, discrimination, and violence, an individual's gender is no less valid if they do not pass as cisgender and passing is not always the goal of TGNB individuals (Billard, 2019).

Gender- and Sexuality-Related Biases

Most societies hold norms and biases regarding culturally appropriate roles for each gender. In most cultures, the accepted default of gender is only one of two options, upholding a **gender binary** (Chang et al., 2018). Many transgender individuals still exist within this binary, either identifying as fully male or fully female; however, many genders do not fit into this binary concept. Because of **cisnormativity** and gendered expectations, people are socialized from childhood to label certain traits, appearances, and behaviors as masculine and feminine. Individuals typically recognize their own gender by childhood, often as young as age 3 (Fausto-Sterling, 2021). Gender identity is considered to be an intertwining of social and biological influences. It is important to note that ideas regarding masculinity and femininity are not congruent across all cultures, and the expectation to adhere to these roles may also vary.

Within the context of the United States, identities that hold higher social power and privilege include **heterosexual** and cisgender. LGBTQ+ individuals face discrimination and health disparities, but gender norms and expectations can be harmful to all individuals. Providers should always take care not to assume gender or sexual orientation of patients as well as colleagues.

In order to integrate cultural humility into the health-care setting, clinicians should take time to examine their beliefs regarding gender, sex, and sexuality, many of which may be subconscious (Chang et al., 2018). This may include personal reflection regarding one's appearance, behavior, language, and speaking as well as reflection on how those choices were influenced by their environment. Identifying these beliefs allows an individual to recognize how their bias may affect clinical outcomes and decision-making. Additionally, clinicians should reflect on any assumptions or biases they hold toward the LGBTQ+ community, including any aspects of care they may feel uncomfortable or awkward providing. This is true even if the clinician is a member of the LGBTQ+ community, as their lived experiences may differ greatly from another community member (Chang et al., 2018).

Intersecting identities of power and privilege may change how care is received by clients who hold marginalized identities (Ogungbe et al., 2019). For cisgender clinicians, it is important to recognize that the lived experience of a TGNB person is not something cisgender individuals are able to fully understand. Similarly, straight/heterosexual people are not able to fully understand the experience of an individual who is gay, lesbian, queer, or bisexual. This does not mean that individuals outside these communities should not provide care to LGBTQ+ patients, but rather that this care must be done with intention and humility. Cultural congruence, care provided by clinicians with similar identities or backgrounds to their patients, often increases a feeling of trust and safety for the patient in addition to improving health outcomes (Anakwe et al., 2021). Advocate for patients to be given the option of cultural congruence through seeking diverse candidate pools, diverse and fair hiring committees, and building an inclusive office culture through listening to marginalized voices. While many providers view themselves and their clinic setting as inclusive and supportive to marginalized communities, it is up to members of those communities to make that determination. Demonstrating humility through language, consent, and shared decision-making is foundational to building trust in historically oppressed communities.

Discrimination

Cultural gender norms, beliefs, and expectations can create potentially dangerous environments for individuals to be visibly "out" and openly express their identities, resulting in both overt and subtle discrimination (Center for American Progress [CAP], 2018). **Heteronormativity** and cisnormativity contribute to hostile environments, perpetuating the assumption that heterosexuality and cisgender identity are the preferred sexual orientation and gender identity, respectively (CAP, 2018). These norms can bolster discrimination in all areas of society through media misrepresentation and generational stigma, for example. Some TGNB individuals attribute the severity of their gender dysphoria to the level of anti-trans bias they are subject to and not to their own perception of their

body. Therefore, it is possible that decreased bias may in turn decrease overall gender dysphoria for some people. TGNB individuals may also experience internalized gender bias, which may increase a person's desire to adhere to cultural norms even given their trans identity. The desire to belong and the fear of being excluded through social stigma could likely contribute to individuals choosing not to express their gender externally, which, in turn, may lead to increased high rates of gender dysphoria.

LGBTQ+ youth are particularly vulnerable and often without social or legal protections. **Family** support, which is largely linked to society support, has been shown to be the strongest protective measure against LGBTQ+ youth homelessness and poor health outcomes, including mental health (The Trevor Project, 2022). Access to gender-affirming care, regardless of utilization, has also been shown to be a strong protective factor. In a 2022 national survey of LGBTQ+ youth, fewer than one in three LGBTQ+ youth described their home as LGBTQ+-affirming and more than half of transgender youth said they contemplated suicide within the past year (The Trevor Project, 2022). However, when strong social support was present from family members, TGNB youth attempted suicide less than half as often as those who did not have familial support. TGNB youth who were able to change their name and/or gender marker on legal documents, such as driver's licenses and birth certificates, also reported lower rates of attempting suicide: 11% compared to 25% who were not able to make those changes (The Trevor Project, 2021).

Members of the LGBTQ+ community may also hold multiple, marginalized, intersecting identities. The term *intersectionality* was coined in 1989 by professor Kimberlé Crenshaw to describe the ways in which a person's social identities such as gender, race, class, and other characteristics "intersect" with one another and overlap, resulting in an individual experience and perspective in relation to discrimination and oppression (Crenshaw, 1989). For example, this term assists in presenting ways in which the lived experience of a white, cisgender, lesbian woman from a lower-income background will be inherently different from the experience of a Black, transgender man from an upper-income background because various social identities will result in varied forms of discrimination based on social power (Crenshaw, 2019).

Microaggressions refer to more subtle behaviors, comments, and attitudes, which convey a person's underlying bias. Historically oppressed communities such as the LGBTQ+ community often experience microaggressions on a daily or near daily basis (Miller et al., 2021). While these behaviors may be less apparent to those with more privileged identities, marginalized individuals may be acutely aware of these actions and behaviors. Long-term exposure to microaggressions can increase a person's allostatic load and result in worsening health outcomes (Miller et al., 2021). Coined in the 1980s by social worker Virginia Brooks, the Sexual Minority Stress Theory offers that LGBTQ+ health disparities are caused by environmental stressors such as living in a society with anti-LGBTQ+ bias, which exposes individuals to discrimination, violence, harassment, and social stigmatization (Malmquist et al., 2019). It also posits that even controlling for all other factors, a person's marginalized identity or status can be associated with poor outcomes.

Learning point: Marginalized identities are not health risk factors themself—the true underlying health risk factors are the existing social, political, and cultural biases present. This means a person's transgender identity is not what puts them at risk; society's anti-trans bias is what increases risk.

Sources of discrimination in the clinical setting include:

- Exclusion of diverse gender identities and sexual orientations in health-related data collection and research
- Gendered office environments (decor, signage, photos, brochures, and displayed language)
- Lack of inclusive language on forms
- Lack of staff competency regarding inclusive verbal interactions
- Name discrepancies on documentation including insurance
- Unwanted disclosure of their gender identity and/or sexual orientation to clinicians and clinical staff

Source: Center for American Progress (2018), Hahn, et al. (2019), and Manzer et al. (2018).

Violence

While LGBTQ+ awareness and visibility are increasing globally, this does not always result in increased safety. LGBTQ+ acceptance varies significantly between countries, regions, families, and individuals (Dowd, 2021). Acceptance also varies between identities within the LGBTQ+ community, with TGNB individuals experiencing higher rates of discrimination and violence than their cisgender peers. A 2015 US report from the Center for American Progress (CAP) detailed the experience of transgender people and demonstrated an overall higher rate of violence and mistreatment. Notably, 46% of individuals reported verbal harassment, 9% reported being physically attacked by a stranger because of being transgender, and 10% of respondents were sexually assaulted. Undocumented individuals reported an increased risk for violence, with 24% of respondents reporting being physically attacked. Another survey showed that 50% of transgender people surveyed suffered physical abuse by a romantic partner after coming out as transgender (CAP, 2018).

Medical Trauma

Anti-LGBTQ+ bias exists in all settings and healthcare is no exception. Difficulties in accessing necessary medical care is well documented among all LGBTQ+ demographics but is particularly challenging for TGNB individuals. Detailed below, it is not uncommon for TGNB individuals to experience harmful interactions

with the medical system, sometimes veiled as medical curiosity (Quinn et al., 2015).

LGBTQ+ individuals are more likely to experience discrimination, harassment, and abuse within the healthcare system. A 2017 national survey of LGBTQ+ individuals showed that in the lesbian, gay, and bisexual community:

- 8% said at least one provider refused to see them
- 9% said at least one provider used abusive/harsh language toward them

In the transgender community:

- 29% said at least one provider refused to see them
- 21% said at least one provider used abusive/harsh language toward them
- 23% said at least one provider intentionally misgendered them or used the wrong name
- 29% said they experienced unwanted physical contact from their provider

After experiencing poor, traumatic, or abusive behavior, LGBTQ+ individuals may be advised to find another provider, but this is not always possible.

- 41% of LGBTQ+ patients said it would be difficult or impossible to find services elsewhere (outside a metropolitan area).
- Multiple studies show a high percentage of patients who had poor experiences report they have not seen another provider in over a year due to that poor interaction.

Source: Adapted from CAP (2018).

Health Disparities

Influenced by both historical discrimination and generational community trauma, health disparities are well documented in LGBTQ+ populations. These have multiple etiologies, including previous negative interactions with the healthcare system result in LGBTQ+ patients delaying or forgoing both acute and preventive care including essential screenings and prompt treatment of more serious conditions (Wingo et al., 2018). While access to healthcare and adequate health insurance is a major cause of inequity, research suggests that disparities for LGBTQ+ people persist regardless of access and insurance (Bosworth et al., 2021; CAP, 2018). In order to tackle existing health disparities, clinicians must recognize and advocate for institutional and systemic changes (Yingling et al., 2017). While individualized actions and learning can be foundational and necessary, long-term cultural shifts to decrease anti-LGBTQ+ bias requires accountability by larger systems, including educational institutions responsible for disseminating clinical knowledge and recommendations. At minimum, national professional organizations should include supportive position statements and internal action plans regarding their commitment to including LGBTQ+ affirming care in their education programs. Most importantly, when developing policies and future plans, LGBTQ+ voices must be represented in both leadership and supportive positions.

Health disparities among LGBTQ+ populations

- Mental health disorders
  - LGBTQ+ identities are not mental health disorders themselves, though the experience of discrimination, microaggressions, and social stigma can result in depression, hopelessness, anxiety, and suicidality
- Suicide, attempted suicide, and self-harm
- Cancers, frequently types which are preventable and treatable when diagnosed early
- Chronic conditions such as hypertension, diabetes, cardiovascular disease
  - Increased rates of discrimination, microaggressions, weathering, and generational trauma often result in inflammation which may cause chronic conditions
- Substance use and substance use disorder, often secondary to decreased coping related to discrimination
- Identity-related violence
- Eating disorders, chronic dieting, poor body image
- Homelessness

Source: Bosworth et al. (2021), CAP (2018), and Williams Institute (2019).

Institutional and structural contributors to health disparities among LGBTQ+ populations

- Shortage of knowledgeable, safe, and LGBTQ+-inclusive medical and mental health professionals
- Legal forms of discrimination such as:
  - Employment laws and policies preventing disclosure of identity
  - Exclusionary hiring practices, reduced employment opportunities related to bias and stigma
  - Denial of health insurance, medication, procedures, fertility treatment based on identity
  - Decreased access to equal rights regarding marriage, adoption, retirement benefits, and family building
  - Absence of anti-bullying laws in schools or workplaces

Source: Estevez et al. (2020), Kattari et al. (2020), and National Center for Transgender Equality (2016).

Resiliency

A foundational understanding of the historical context of LGBTQ+ health disparities helps frame these disparities as systemic rather than individual failings and supports a strength-based approach to care. Throughout history and still today, the LGBTQ+ community has continued to discover resourceful and resilient ways to both survive and thrive despite broad cultural discrimination (Elm et al., 2016; Follins et al., 2014). Close-knit, nonbiological community members are often referred to as "chosen family," given that many biological families are unsupportive (Furstenberg et al., 2020). Accepting potential danger by being visibly "out" means that trying to identify other LGBTQ+ community members can be difficult. Stressful and unsupportive family relationships result in significant emotional trauma,

and frequently, it is only through chosen family that individuals find the acceptance and courage to continue living.

Gender-Affirming Practices

Names and Pronouns

Addressing clients with the correct name and pronouns is a critical component of gender-affirming clinical care (Chang et al., 2018). Pronouns are words that refer to a person's gender identity. Although pronouns are often assumed based on a person's perceived gender, this is not always correct. When meeting someone new, it is best practice to ask individuals what pronouns they use and reflect those pronouns when referring to that person, whether they are present or not. During this conversation, it is best to avoid the phrase "preferred pronouns," as an individual's pronouns are not a preference, but an inherent part of their identity. In the event that a person's pronouns are not known, it is better to use gender-neutral pronouns until learning. The most common sets of pronouns include "he/him/his," "she/her/hers," and "they/them/theirs." Many, but not all, nonbinary individuals use "they/them/theirs," which is an example of a gender-neutral pronoun. While this concept may be new for some clinicians, consider that most people will naturally use gender-neutral pronouns as the default when referring to a person you do not know and cannot see or hear. For example, "Oh no, it looks like someone dropped their cell phone on the ground."

Neopronouns are a new category of pronouns that do not identify gender and are used less frequently but still valid. Neopronouns may include pronouns such as "ze/zim/zir" or "xe/xem/xyr." Some individuals may use more than one set of pronouns and the pronouns a person uses may shift over time. Other individuals may want to be referred to without any personal pronouns at all, using their name only. When discussing a person who is transitioning and using a new set of pronouns, always refer to them using their current chosen name and pronouns, even when referring to a past event. Additionally, use correct language even when a person is not present to center respectfulness and practice their new name and/or pronouns.

Pronoun exercise: practice along

Instructions:

Speaking out loud to yourself, tell a theoretical story about a person using "they/them" pronouns. Pretend you are a well-known midwife or nurse practitioner who is going to meet a reporter for an interview to talk about your most recent publication and research. As you are getting ready and talking to a friend on the phone, discuss possible aspects of this encounter. What topics do you think they will find most interesting? What questions will they ask you? What will they use as a headline?

While it may be hard to remain in character, engaging in this type of exercise can help individuals get into the habit of using gender-neutral pronouns as a default and then learning to adjust once you know more about a person's gender identity and pronouns used.

Incorrect name and pronoun experiences are common for TGNB individuals. Misgendering is calling someone by their previously used pronouns. Deadnaming is calling someone by their previously used name. Though both misgendering and deadnaming may not be intentional or always noticed, they can lead to emotional or physical safety concerns, particularly if done in a public place. For example, if a patient who is perceived to be a woman is called from a waiting room using a traditionally masculine name, this may be noticed by other patients who hold strong anti-trans bias and may become aggressive toward the patient as they are exiting the building.

Using correct and respectful language when interacting with TGNB individuals is foundational in providing a safer environment (Hahn et al., 2019; Schreuder, 2019). Dedicating time to practicing language outside of a patient interaction can increase confidence and decrease accidental misgendering. This type of practice and continued education minimizes harm both in the healthcare setting and general public (Diamond-Smith et al., 2018; Sahmoud et al., 2022). Preparing for how to respond when mistakes do happen can help increase a person's comfort and confidence in culturally humble language. When mistakes regarding names and pronouns occur, many individuals feel immediate embarrassment. Recognizing and acknowledging the mistake by simply correcting oneself in the moment is the preferred way to address this type of slip. Defensiveness and extended apologies for using incorrect language commonly results in more discomfort for the person who was misgendered and/or deadnamed. Privately, it can be helpful to engage in personal reflection regarding one's own conscious or subconscious assumptions about gender and/or sexuality. If a scenario or question arises in which clarification or discussion would be helpful, employ intentionality regarding who those questions are brought to. Those with marginalized identities are often flooded with requests for emotional labor regarding their identity and lived experience. It is always best to ask for consent to talk about a person's identity before diving into conversation or questions, especially ones that can feel invasive. When possible, it is also best to compensate individuals for their willingness to teach. Allies without marginalized identities may also be willing to shoulder these conversations.

Inclusive Language

Because language is so important in establishing trust, clinicians should review inclusive terminology and practice integrating these terms into clinical conversations. In particular, learning to utilize gender-neutral language as the default will help clinicians to minimize unintentional harm. This can be challenging, but understanding the fluidity and evolving nature of language helps to maintain cultural humility (Rossi & Lopez, 2017).

When clients arrive for care, there are many potential interactions that can impact a LGBTQ+ client, including with administrative staff and schedulers, other clients in common areas, the medical assistant or nurse performing intake, healthcare clinician, and phlebotomist or other lab personnel. In each of these interactions, there is potential for a positive and affirming experience or a negative, harmful, or traumatic experience. The amount of emotional energy it can take an LGBTQ+ client to schedule and attend an appointment is often immense.

Strategies for respectful interviewing in the clinical setting

- Ask clients what they would like to be called and ensure it is written down in the relevant places for other staff.
- Ask what pronouns someone uses and ask for consent to document that in their record.
- Ask clients if they would like to share their sexual orientation or gender identity. Some clients may decline to share, and others may feel it is important for their care team to know.
- Ask clients what words or language a person uses for their anatomy.
  - This may apply to discussions during the health history-taking process and during any physical exam that may involve evaluation of the chest/breast tissue and/or pelvic area.
- Obtain a sexual health history in an inclusive manner that does not make assumptions about partners, relationships, or practices.

Source: Benyounes (2020) and Fuzzell et al. (2016).

Clinical Care

While LGBTQ+ patients often have cultural considerations that the clinician must take into account, nearly all clinical recommendations remain the same for LGBTQ+ patients as for non-LGBTQ+ patients. In practice, a person's identity may influence language and approach to pregnancy planning, but should not dictate what medical guidance is followed.

When discussing clinical care that may be related to sexual practices and intimacy, clinicians should examine their own personal beliefs, biases, and expectations regarding these topics. It is common for LGBTQ+ individuals to encounter clinicians who inquire about unnecessary aspects of their lives, particularly as it pertains to sexual health. Consider what is clinically relevant and explain to the patient why questions are relevant to keep the conversation respectful.

Family Building and Preconception

When caring for LGBTQ+ individuals across the lifespan, clinicians should not make assumptions about a person's family building goals. While the path to LGBTQ+ parenthood is often costly and may involve additional steps or considerations, LGBTQ+ individuals have similar rates of desire for parenthood when compared to their non-LGBTQ+ peers (Estevez et al., 2020; Family Equality, 2019). Desire for and against parenthood exists across all genders and gender expressions. While some transmasculine individuals may opt for surgical removal of reproductive organs, others may carry a strong desire to become pregnant (Hoffkling et al., 2017).

In caring for LGBTQ+ clients and families, the gender-neutral but clinically accurate term gestational parent is often used to refer to a parent who plans to become or is pregnant. Nongestational parents refer to partners and/or co-parents who are not carrying the pregnancy. Nongestational parents may or may not have contributed genetic material (sperm or eggs) to the pregnancy (Kali, 2022).

LGBTQ+ people can achieve pregnancy in a variety of ways and depends on the preferences of the clients, the biological material and organs present, presence or absence of fertility concerns, and access to safe and affirming care (Table 25.1). Options for conception depend on the patient's partner(s) and may involve biological material from a donor such as sperm, egg, or embryo, any of which could be obtained from an anonymous donor or person known to the patient(s) (Kali, 2022). For clients and their partner who do not have the ability to create or carry a pregnancy, having a child can present costs that are significant and, in some cases, may be prohibitive.

Insurance coverage for fertility treatment is an area of inequity for LGBTQ+ individuals (Estevez et al., 2020). It is not uncommon for insurances to require a patient to meet the medical criteria of infertility—that is, 12 months of trying to conceive without pregnancy—before fertility treatment coverage begins. For many LGBTQ+ individuals, conception within the context of their current relationship is not biologically possible; thus, this criterion cannot be met. Insurances may also contain language that excludes treatment coverage when a procedure utilizes donor biological material like sperm or eggs. Some insurances may require proof of a marriage certificate before approving treatment coverage.

For transgender individuals who wish to have a pregnancy, evidence suggests that gender-affirming hormones do not cause long-term fertility challenges (Ellis et al., 2014). Clients taking gender-affirming hormones should be counseled regarding the timing of discontinuation in order to conceive. Transgender men who discontinue testosterone use in order to conceive are likely to resume their menses in one to three months (University of California, San Francisco Center of Excellence for Transgender Health, 2016). However, while testosterone

Table 25.1 Pathways to Pregnancy

Type of conception	Egg source	Sperm source
Intercourse with an AMAB partner	AFAB client	AMAB partner
Intravaginal insemination (at home or clinic)	AFAB client	AMAB partner (fresh or frozen specimen) Or Known donor (fresh or frozen specimen) Or Anonymous donor (frozen specimen)
Intrauterine insemination (IUI)	AFAB client	AMAB partner (fresh/washed or frozen specimen) Or Known donor (frozen specimen) Or Anonymous donor (frozen specimen)
In-vitro fertilization (IVF)	AFAB client Or Known donor Or Anonymous donor	AMAB partner (fresh or frozen specimen) Or Known donor (frozen specimen) Or Anonymous donor (frozen specimen)
IVF using an AFAB gestational carrier	AFAB client Or Known donor Or Anonymous donor Or Gestational carrier's egg (uncommon)	AMAB partner (fresh or frozen specimen) Or Known donor (fresh or frozen specimen) Or Anonymous donor (frozen specimen)

Source: Ellis et al. (2014), García-Acosta (2019), Kali (2022).

does not cause polycystic ovarian syndrome (PCOS) to develop, some research suggests higher incidence of PCOS in transmasculine individuals, which may necessitate intervention to address oligo- or amenorrhea (Chan et al., 2018; Gezer et al., 2021). Data suggest that most AFAB clients who discontinue testosterone therapy in order to conceive will go on to have healthy pregnancies (Ellis et al., 2014; Light et al., 2014). Additionally, egg or sperm freezing may have been pursued by some clients prior to the initiation of hormones, and clinicians can explore if the client prefers to use cryopreserved gametes or not (Kali, 2022).

Prenatal Care

LGBTQ+ clients entering prenatal care may have some considerations that differ from cisgender and/or heterosexual clients (Ellis et al., 2014; Table 25.2). Depending on the type of conception, family or partner structure, and health history, clients may have difficulty accessing safe and competent care. Though the care is not inherently complicated, lack of cultural competency at the institutional level (i.e., insurance companies, hospital systems, and ambulatory clinics) down to the individual level (i.e., clinicians, nurses, and front desk staff) can cause harm to

Table 25.2   Considerations Important in Prenatal Care of LGBTQ+ Clients

Confirmation of pregnancy	As with all pregnant clients, LGBTQ+ clients may experience planned, unplanned, desired, and undesired pregnancy. Clients may conceive spontaneously or with fertility treatments.
	Clients who conceive via fertility treatments such as induced cycles, IUI, or IVF will likely have had their pregnancy confirmed with their fertility provider.
	Transgender men or nonbinary AFAB clients who do not experience regular menstrual cycles may become aware of pregnancy at later gestational ages. They could then experience further delays in care if they cannot access or find a trans-inclusive clinician. Clinicians should avoid shaming language when discussing the timing of prenatal care.
	Unbiased and affirming counseling about pregnancy options and goals is necessary to create trust between clients and clinicians. It is important to ask only clinically relevant questions related to conception and care. For example, it may be important to know if a pregnancy was conceived using donor egg or sperm, but it is not typically necessary to know *who* the donor is, only if any relevant health history is known.
Finding a clinician	Access to care that is culturally competent, inclusive, and congruent is not only affirming, but can improve health outcomes for clients with marginalized or historically oppressed identities. For clients with intersectional identities that are not adequately represented in healthcare, finding this type of clinician may be challenging at best and impossible at worst. Access to appropriate care can be further challenged by situations like rural settings, citizenship or migration status, health literacy, past medical trauma, and insurance coverage.
Scheduling a visit	For clients who have changed their name or gender on legal documentation, issues may arise if: • Scheduling staff inappropriately question a man who attempts to schedule a gynecological or prenatal visit for himself. • Insurance companies reject a diagnostic or medical billing code typically used for a different sex than that of the client (e.g., a transvaginal ultrasound for a male client).
Abortion care	Access to safe and unrestricted abortion care is necessary for all clients. LGBTQ+ clients are more likely to have experienced delays and/or limited access to other types of care and, thus, may need abortion services at later gestational periods than clients without access issues.

First prenatal visit	This visit should focus on:
	• Establishing a trusting relationship with an emphasis on client autonomy and shared decision-making
	• Ensuring correct names and pronouns are in the records
	• Discussing clients' priorities and goals
	• Taking an inclusive history, including sexual health and history of gender-affirming treatments
	  ○ If a client conceived while using gender-affirming hormones and desires to continue the pregnancy, counseling should include the recommendation for immediate cessation of hormones and the risks and benefits.
	  ○ If a client has had gender-affirming procedures, discuss how pregnancy and birth could impact them, if applicable.
	• Ordering applicable labs and/or imaging

Subsequent routine prenatal visits	Common priorities: • Provide ongoing competent and affirming care. • Confirm accurate documentation so potentially sensitive information does not need to be discussed repeatedly. • Discuss what fosters resilience for individual clients and families and focus care on thriving, not only prevention of harm. • Refer to specialists who are competent and affirming when possible. If it is not known whether a referral is competent and affirming or not, disclose that to clients.
Educational materials	Obtaining affirming pregnancy education can be challenging for LGBTQ+ clients. This can include: printed information or flyers, advertisements, websites, books and magazines, and childbirth education classes. Clinicians should learn local and virtual educational options that can affirm clients and minimize erasure. Within their own facilities, clinicians can advocate for or create inclusive and affirming literature and spaces.

Table 25.2   (*Continued*)

Plans for lactation	Methods of feeding a newborn should be discussed early in a pregnancy so that clients can be well-informed and supported. Depending on their feeding preferences, queer and/or transgender clients can work with their clinician to find affirming lactation support for lactation well before the time of birth. This may include referral to a trans-inclusive lactation consultant.
	Access to inclusive and competent lactational support should be discussed and planned for prior to birth. Some LGBTQ+ individuals may desire chest/breastfeeding and others may not. Yet others may feel obligated to chest/breastfeed but find it emotionally challenging in relation to their sexuality and/or gender identity.
	The experience of transmasculine individuals who opt to breast/chestfeed can vary widely; some may find it challenging to chestfeed with gender dysphoria. With the goal of chest/breastfeeding, it is not uncommon for nonbinary or transmasculine individuals to delay pursuing "top surgery" (bilateral mastectomy) until after the postpartum period.
	For AFAB individuals with a history of bilateral mastectomy, there is frequently a concern regarding regrowth of chest tissue during pregnancy. While this may occur to a small degree, it is often transient and likely to resolve spontaneously after weaning.
	For AFAB individuals without a history of top surgery, chest binding may be desired in the postpartum period.
	If the gestational parent has a partner interested in inducing lactation, protocols such as the Mount Sinai/Zil Goldstein method or Newman method should be considered and discussed early in the pregnancy so as to allow time to fully prepare, as they can take several months to establish. Induced lactation is possible for both trans masculine and trans feminine individuals and the protocol or method will take into account an individual's health background. For AFAB or AMAB nongestational parents, the ability to chest/breastfeed can be an experience that fosters inclusion and connection within a family.
Doula support	Doulas provide important support and advocacy to LGBTQ+ patients, especially if the patient is navigating a healthcare system that does not have queer-inclusive policies.
	Developing and documenting labor and birth preferences that communicate how a team can best support a client and their partner(s) can help optimize a birth experience. Reviewing this information antenatally can give the team time to coordinate and advocate for clients (i.e., trained staff and preadmission forms). This also allows clients to become aware of conditions in which their preferences cannot be supported with enough time to change settings, if desired. For example, visitor policies may necessitate a queer client with two partners to choose between having their doula present or both partners.
Planned birth location	When choosing a setting in which to give birth, LGBTQ+ individuals and families may seek additional information about the policies and practices of the organization (e.g., the presence of staff familiar with LGBTQ+ clients, use of inclusive language on signage and documentation, and policies for induced lactation). For polyamorous families or families with multiple parents, it can be important to proactively discuss the number of people able to be present in the birth room.
	Some individuals who experience gender dysphoria may desire a planned cesarean birth if the experience of vaginal birth presents as a possible triggering event. Other individuals may prefer to plan for an out-of-hospital birth with the intention of minimizing potentially harmful or triggering interactions with hospital employees.
Legal birth documents	Federal and state documents may not accurately reflect the names or roles of parents and families. This may include using legal instead of chosen names or not allowing a legal parent's name on the birth certificate if their gametes were not involved in the pregnancy. Birth certificate data collection policies are state-specific and navigating these policies may present an emotional and/or legal challenge. LGBTQ+ clients should be referred to LGTBQ+ inclusive resources and/or legal advice when necessary. Additionally, for polyamorous families or families with multiple parents, it can be important to proactively discuss the names of the people planned to be on the birth certificate. In some cases, a state may allow three parents' names on a birth certificate, such as when three separate individuals contribute egg, sperm, and gestational carrying capacity.

Source: Follins et al., (2014), García-Acosta et al. (2019), Kerrigan and Cushing (2022), and Trautner et al. (2020).

clients who have marginalized identities. Otherwise, perinatal care recommendations are the same for those who are LGBTQ+ and those who are not.

Postpartum Care

The postpartum period is a time of transition for all new parents. While physical adjustments for LGBTQ+ parents may be similar to non-LGBTQ+ parents, psychological adjustments may vary widely due to familial and peer support, discrimination, geographical location, and social stigma (Manley et al., 2018; Siegel et al., 2022). Specific challenges as well as the ability to thrive in the postpartum period are based on the individual's health and resiliency as well as clinical, community, and societal support (Table 25.3).

Table 25.3   Considerations Important in Postpartum Care of LGBTQ+ Clients

Physiological changes	Some clients may experience unpleasant or dysphoric feelings related to breast/chest changes or engorgement in the perinatal or postpartum period. Clients who use approaches such as chest binding or who wish to suppress lactation should be counseled on the safest ways to do so.
	Genital pain, swelling, trauma, and/or pelvic weakness could be present. Additionally, bleeding and lochia can persist for weeks. If a client experiences discomfort or dysphoria about their genitals, attention to that anatomy during this period may exacerbate that experience. It may be challenging to access hygiene and care products that are not overtly feminine.
	Vaginal/vulvar atrophic changes are common in the postpartum period for all individuals and may persist while breast/chestfeeding. Topical estrogen can help with unpleasant symptoms related to atrophy without interfering with previous or planned gender-affirming therapies such as exogenous testosterone.
Psychosocial changes	Strong community support fosters resiliency and can help families cope during the postpartum period. LGBTQ+ clients experience rejection by their family of origin at higher rates than other groups and this may impact their support system.
	Gender and parental stereotypes and expectations may create feelings of erasure in some LGBTQ+ families who do not ascribe to those views. This can lead to identity and/or role adjustments for new parents who do not see themselves accurately represented in their community or in mainstream society.
	Organized gatherings such as parent/infant play groups or support groups can help combat feelings of isolation that are common in the postpartum period. However, inclusive and affirming spaces for LGBTQ+ families can be difficult to find or may not exist in some regions.
Initiating or Re-initiating hormone therapy	For individuals previously using gender-affirming hormone therapy, the timing of restarting these medications may depend on plans for chest/breastfeeding. While some patients may receive gender-affirming hormone care from their primary care provider or an endocrinologist, prescribing gender-affirming hormones is within the scope of most gynecological providers' practice. This type of care is not medically complex and is similar in approach to managing hormonal contraceptives or postmenopausal hormones, something most gynecological providers commonly provide. Clinician resources and guidelines for gender-affirming hormone therapy are listed at the end of this chapter.
Chest/ breastfeeding	For clients who plan to use testosterone for gender-affirming hormone therapy after pregnancy and who plan to chest/breastfeed, discussion of the timing of starting or restarting testosterone is important. Due to limited data on safety of testosterone therapy in lactation and the likelihood that testosterone will suppress lactation, many clients will delay hormones until they are finished chest/breastfeeding.
Contraceptive needs	Clinicians should revisit any ongoing needs for contraception in the postpartum period. If there is potential for conception, gender-affirming hormone therapy alone is not a reliable method to prevent pregnancy.
	For clients who experience dysphoria related to their menstrual cycles, clinicians should counsel on methods that have the potential for cycle suppression.
Pelvic floor physical therapy	Pelvic floor physical therapy can potentially aid in regaining pelvic floor strength in the postpartum period, though some LGBTQ+ patients may initially avoid this care if they are experiencing dysphoria. Providing a referral to a queer-inclusive pelvic floor physical therapist should be a priority.
Resuming routine gynecological care	Routine care of the LGBTQ+ client is the same as for other groups. Clinical care and routine screenings should be recommended based on the client's anatomy and risk factors and relevant clinical guidelines.
	For LGBTQ+ clients who find it emotionally distressing to pursue reproductive care and/or pelvic exams but need and elect for that care, clinicians should counsel regarding options (pharmacological and nonpharmacological) to help with coping. Some examples include: • Inviting a support person • Allotting extra time for a visit • Starting with a discussion visit without a physical exam • Self-insertion of a speculum • Self-collection of specimens ○ For pap smears, this could include pap sampling without the use of a speculum or HPV-only testing, depending on client age, history, and an informed consent conversation. • Oral anxiolytics • Vaginal or rectal medication (like lorazepam) to reduce pelvic floor hypertonicity during internal exam • Exams or procedures under IV sedation (this depends on cost and availability)
	For TGNB clients who use testosterone and are having pap smears collected, atrophic changes associated with testosterone use increase the rates of insufficient cervical cytology sampling. Offer topical estrogen cream to be used for two weeks prior to pap collection; this improves the rates of adequate sampling and does not interfere with systemic testosterone effects.

Source: Atkins (2020), Furstenberg et al. (2020), Rydström (2020), and Trautner et al. (2020).

Contraception

Clinicians should identify and understand the potential role of contraceptives in the LGBTQ+ community. As sexual practices and partners can vary, determine whether a client is having types of sex that could result in pregnancy, whether intended or unintended (Light et al., 2018; Wingo et al., 2018). Eliciting information regarding partner anatomy and sex practices is critical to determine the potential for pregnancy.

It is also important for clinicians and clients to recognize that gender-affirming hormones (i.e., testosterone, estrogen, estrogen blockers, progestins, and gonadotropin-releasing hormone agonists) are not contraceptives. While testosterone and estrogen blockers may cause menstrual suppression and/or decrease ovarian estrogen production, these effects are not reliable or consistent enough to use as effective contraception (Light et al., 2018; National Institutes of Health, 2022). TGNB AFAB individuals taking testosterone may conceive on this medication, even if they are amenorrheic. Similarly, TGNB AMAB individuals on estrogen may still produce sperm. Misinformation regarding hormone therapy is pervasive, and clients taking gender-affirming hormones may not always be aware of their pregnancy risks.

Counseling regarding contraceptive options for LGBTQ+ clients is similar to counseling cisgender clients (Light, et al., 2018). Risks and benefits should be discussed based on the individual's situation and history. For AFAB clients with dysphoria related to their menstrual cycles, counseling should include contraceptive options that can suppress menstruation and/or other uncomfortable symptoms. TGNB AFAB clients who use testosterone for gender affirmation may still use hormonal forms of contraception like pills, implants, injectables, and intrauterine contraceptive systems with little to no impact on the therapeutic effect of the testosterone (Light et al., 2018).

Summary

Understanding the historical context and current roles that gender and sexuality play in society helps to build inclusive environments for LGBTQ+ individuals. Though clinicians may be initially unacquainted with the logistics of providing clinical care through a gender-neutral lens, practicing the principles discussed above is likely to improve care for all people. Clinicians and health systems should seek out and embrace client feedback, even when challenging, in pursuit of a more just experience for historically marginalized clients. For individuals and groups with more privilege, ongoing learning regarding the LGBTQ+ population, and the intersectionality within this group, is essential in establishing trust, repair, and commitment to center community voices.

Resources for Clients and Their Families

Rainbow Families. *A community-based organization that provides education, resources, and support services for LGBTQ+ parents, families, and parents-to-be.*: https://rainbowfamilies.org

Childbirth Connection. *Evidence based childbirth practice resources to empower childbearing individuals*: https://nationalpartnership.org/childbirthconnection/

La leche league. *Breastfeeding without giving birth*: https://www.llli.org/breastfeeding-without-giving-birth-2

Tagg Magazine. *Queer Fertility 101*: https://taggmagazine.com/queer-fertility

The Lactation Network. *Breastfeeding for Trans and Nonbinary Parents*: https://lactationnetwork.com/blog/breastfeeding-faq-for-trans-and-non-binary-parents

Queer Conception: The Complete Fertility Guide for Queer and Trans Parents-to-Be, by Kristin Liam Kali (2022). https://maiamidwifery.com/book/

Baby Making for Everybody: *Family Building and Fertility for LGBTQ+ and Solo Parents*, by Marea Goodman & Ray Rachlin (2023). https://www.babymakingforeverybody.com/

Resources for Healthcare Providers

Academy of Breastfeeding Medicine: https://www.bfmed.org

Cedar River Clinic Guidelines. *Transgender Health Care Toolkit (led by Simon Adriane Ellis, CNM)*: http://www.cedarriverclinics.org/transtoolkit

Center of Excellence for Transgender Health, University of California, San Francisco, Department of Family and Community Medicine. *Guidelines for the Primary and Gender-Affirming Care of Transgender and Gender Nonbinary People*: https://transcare.ucsf.edu/guidelines

Family Equality Council: www.familyequality.org

GLBT Health Access Project. *Community Standards of Practice for the Provision of Quality Health Care Services to Lesbian, Gay, Bisexual, and Transgender Clients*: http://www.glbthealth.org/CommunityStandardsofPractice.htm

World Professional Association for Transgender Health: https://www.wpath.org

References

Anakwe, A., Green, J., & BeLue, R. (2021). Perceptions of cultural competence and utilization of advanced practice providers. *Journal of Allied Health, 50*(1), 54–62.

Anderson, A. D., Irwin, J. A., Brown, A. M., & Grala, C. L. (2020). "Your picture looks the same as my picture": An examination of passing in transgender communities. *Gender Issues, 37*(1), 44–60. https://doi.org/10.1007/s12147-019-09239-x

Atkins, C. (2020, January 11). *For transgender men, pain of menstruation is more than just physical*. NBC News. https://www.nbcnews.com/feature/nbc-out/transgender-men-pain-menstruation-more-just-physical-n1113961

Austin, A., Papciak, R., & Lovins, L. (2022). Gender euphoria: A grounded theory exploration of experiencing gender affirmation. *Psychology & Sexuality*, 1–21. https://doi.org/10.1080/19419899.2022.2049632

Benyounes, J. (2020). Sexuality education for current and future healthcare providers. In J. Wadley (Ed.), *Handbook of sexuality leadership* (pp. 54–78). Routledge.

Billard, T. J. (2019). "Passing" and the politics of deception: Transgender bodies, cisgender aesthetics, and the policing of inconspicuous marginal identities. In *The Palgrave handbook of deceptive communication* (pp. 463–477). Springer International Publishing. https://doi.org/10.1007/978-3-319-96334-1_24

Bornstein, K., & Bear Bergman, S. (2010). *Gender outlaws: The next generation*. Seal Press.

Bosworth, A., Turrini, G., Pyda, S., Strickland, K., Chappel, A., De Lew, N., and Sommers, B. (2021). *Health insurance coverage and access to care for LGBTQ+ individuals (issue brief No. HP-2021-14)*. Office of the Assistant Secretary for Planning and Evaluation, U.S. Department of Health and Human Services. https://aspe.hhs.gov/sites/default/files/2021-07/lgbt-health-ib.pdf

Brunning, L., & McKeever, N. (2021). Asexuality. *Journal of Applied Philosophy, 38*(3), 497–517. https://doi.org/10.1111/japp.12472

Center for American Progress. (2018, January 18). *Discrimination prevents LGBTQ people from accessing health care*. Center for American Progress. https://www.americanprogress.org/issues/lgbt/news/2018/01/18/445130/discrimination-prevents-lgbtq-people-accessing-health-care

Chan, K., Liang, J., Jolly, D., Weinand, J., & Safer, J. (2018). Exogenous testosterone does not induce or exacerbate the metabolic features associated with PCOS among transgender men. *Endocrine Practice, 24*(6), 565–572. https://doi.org/10.4158/EP-2017-0247

Chang, S. C., Singh, A. A., & Dickey, L. M. (2018). *A clinician's guide to gender-affirming care*. New Harbinger Publications.

Crenshaw, K. (1989). Demarginalizing the intersection of race and sex: A black feminist critique of antidiscrimination doctrine, feminist theory and antiracist politics. *University of Chicago Legal Forum, 1989*(1), 8. https://chicagounbound.uchicago.edu/cgi/viewcontent.cgi?article=1052&context=uclf

Crenshaw, K. (2019). The marginalization of Harriet's daughters: Perpetual crisis, misdirected blame, and the enduring urgency of intersectionality. *Kalfou, 6*(1), 7–23. https://doi.org/10.15367/kf.v6i1.226

Diamond-Smith, N., Warnock, R., & Sudhinaraset, M. (2018). Interventions to improve the person-centered quality of family planning services: A narrative review. *Reproductive Health, 15*. https://doi.org/10.1186/s12978-018-0592-6

Dowd, R. (2021, March 23). *Transgender people over four times more likely than cisgender people to be victims of violent crime*. The Williams Institute. https://williamsinstitute.law.ucla.edu/press/ncvs-trans-press-release

Ellis, S. A., Wojnar, D. M., & Pettinato, M. (2014). Conception, pregnancy, and birth experiences of male and gender variant gestational parents: It's how we could have a family. *Journal of Midwifery & Women's Health, 60*(1), 62–69. https://doi.org/10.1111/jmwh.12213

Elm, J. H. L., Lewis, J. P., Walters, K. L., & Self, J. M. (2016). "I'm in this world for a reason": Resilience and recovery among American Indian and Alaska native two-spirit women. *Journal of Lesbian Studies, 20*(3–4), 352–371. https://doi.org/10.1080/10894160.2016.1152813

Estevez, S. L., Ghofranian, A., Brownridge, S. R., Abittan, B., & Goldman, R. H. (2020). Insurance coverage for LGBTQ patients seeking infertility care. *Fertility and Sterility, 113*(4), e44. https://doi.org/10.1016/j.fertnstert.2020.02.095

Family Equality. (2019) *LGBTQ family building survey*. Family Equality. https://www.familyequality.org/fbs.

Fausto-Sterling, A. (2021). A dynamic systems framework for gender/sex development: From sensory input in infancy to subjective certainty in toddlerhood. *Frontiers in Human Neuroscience, 15*, 613789–613789. https://doi.org/10.3389/fnhum.2021.613789

Follins, L. D., Walker, J. J., & Lewis, M. K. (2014). Resilience in Black lesbian, gay, bisexual, and transgender individuals: A critical review of the literature. *Journal of Gay & Lesbian Mental Health, 18*(2), 190–212. https://doi.org/10.1080/19359705.2013.828343

Furstenberg, F. F., Harris, L. E., Pesando, L. M., & Reed, M. N. (2020). Kinship practices among alternative family forms in western industrialized societies. *Journal of Marriage and Family, 82*(5), 1403–1430. https://doi.org/10.1111/jomf.12712

Fuzzell, L., Fedesco, H. N., Alexander, S. C., Fortenberry, J. D., & Shields, C. G. (2016). "I just think that doctors need to ask more questions": Sexual minority and majority adolescents' experiences talking about sexuality with healthcare providers. *Patient Education and Counseling, 99*(9), 1467–1472. https://doi.org/10.1016/j.pec.2016.06.004

García-Acosta, J. M., San Juan-Valdivia, R. M., Fernández-Martínez, A. D., Lorenzo-Rocha, N. D., & Castro-Peraza, M. E. (2019). Trans* pregnancy and lactation: A literature review from a nursing perspective. *International Journal of Environmental Research and Public Health, 17*(1). https://doi.org/10.3390/ijerph17010044

Garg, G., & Marwaha, R. (2020). *Gender dysphoria (Sexual identity disorders)*. PubMed; StatPearls Publishing. https://www.ncbi.nlm.nih.gov/books/NBK532313

Gezer, E., Piro, B., Cantuerk, Z., Cetinarslan, B., Soezen, M., Selek, A., Polat Isik, A., & Seal, L. J. (2021). The comparison of gender dysphoria, body image satisfaction and quality of life between treatment-naive transgender males with and without polycystic ovary syndrome. *Transgender Health*. https://doi.org/10.1089/trgh.2021.0061

Grilo, T. F., & Rosa, R. (2017). Intersexuality in aquatic invertebrates: Prevalence and causes. *The Science of the Total Environment, 592*, 714–728. https://doi.org/10.1016/j.scitotenv.2017.02.099

Hahn, M., Sheran, N., Weber, S., Cohan, D., & Obedin-Maliver, J. (2019). Providing patient-centered perinatal care for transgender men and gender-diverse individuals: A collaborative multidisciplinary team approach. *Obstetrics and Gynecology, 134*(5), 959–963. https://doi.org/10.1097/AOG.0000000000003506

Hoffkling, A., Obedin-Maliver, J., & Sevelius, J. (2017). From erasure to opportunity: A qualitative study of the experiences of transgender men around pregnancy and recommendations for providers. *BMC Pregnancy and Childbirth, 17*(S2). https://doi.org/10.1186/s12884-017-1491-5

Intersex Society of North America. (2019). *What is intersex? | Intersex Society of North America*. https://isna.org/faq/what_is_intersex

Jaffee, K. D., Shires, D. A., & Stroumsa, D. (2016). Discrimination and delayed health care among transgender women and men. *Medical Care, 54*(11), 1010–1016. https://doi.org/10.1097/mlr.0000000000000583

Kali, K. L. (2022). *Queer conception: The complete fertility guide for queer and trans parents-to-be*. Sasquatch Books.

Kattari, S. K., Bakko, M., Hecht, H. K., & Kinney, M. K. (2020). Intersecting experiences of healthcare denials among transgender and nonbinary patients. *American Journal of Preventive Medicine, 58*(4), 506–513. https://doi.org/10.1016/j.amepre.2019.11.014

Kerrigan, P., & Cushing, A. (2022). "Our story with the state": Birth certificates, data structures and gay and lesbian families. *Sexualities, 136346072211069*. https://doi.org/10.1177/13634607221106913

Light, A., Wang, L.-F., Zeymo, A., & Gomez-Lobo, V. (2018). Family planning and contraception use in transgender men. *Contraception, 98*(4), 266–269. https://doi.org/10.1016/j.contraception.2018.06.006

Light, A. D., Obedin-Maliver, J., Sevelius, J. M., & Kerns, J. L. (2014). Transgender men who experienced pregnancy after female-to-male gender transitioning. *Obstetrics & Gynecology, 124*(6), 1120–1127. https://doi.org/10.1097/aog.0000000000000540

Malmquist, A., Jonsson, L., Wikström, J., & Nieminen, K. (2019). Minority stress adds an additional layer to fear of childbirth in lesbian and bisexual women, and transgender people. *Midwifery, 79*, 102551. https://doi.org/10.1016/j.midw.2019.102551

Manley, M. H., Goldberg, A. E., & Ross, L. E. (2018). Invisibility and involvement: LGBTQ community connections among plurisexual women during pregnancy and postpartum. *Psychology of Sexual Orientation and Gender Diversity, 5*(2), 169–181. https://doi.org/10.1037/sgd0000285

Manzer, D., O'Sullivan, L. F., & Doucet, S. (2018). Myths, misunderstandings, and missing information: Experiences of nurse practitioners providing primary care to lesbian, gay, bisexual, and transgender patients. *The Canadian Journal of Human Sexuality, 27*(2), 157–170. https://doi.org/10.3138/cjhs.2018-0017

Mastromonaco, G. F., Houck, M. L., & Bergfelt, D. R. (2012). Disorders of sexual development in wild and captive exotic animals. *Sexual Development: Genetics, Molecular Biology, Evolution, Endocrinology, Embryology, and Pathology of Sex Determination and Differentiation, 6*(1–3), 84–95. https://doi.org/10.1159/000332203

Miller, H. N., LaFave, S., Marineau, L., Stephens, J., & Thorpe, R. J., Jr. (2021). The impact of discrimination on allostatic load in adults: An integrative review of literature. *Journal of Psychosomatic Research, 146*, 110434. https://doi.org/10.1016/j.jpsychores.2021.110434

National Center for Transgender Equality. (2016). *The report of the 2015 transgender survey.* https://transequality.org/sites/default/files/docs/usts/USTS-Full-Report-Dec17.pdf

National Institutes of Health. (2022). *Testosterone.* Drugs and Lactation Database (LactMed). http://www.ncbi.nlm.nih.gov/books/NBK501721

Ogungbe, O., Mitra, A. K., & Roberts, J. K. (2019). A systematic review of implicit bias in health care: A call for intersectionality. *IMC Journal of Medical Science,* 13(1), 1–16. https://doi.org/10.3329/imcjms.v13i1.42050

Pastorinho, M. R., Telfer, T. C., & Soares, A. M. (2009). Amphipod intersex, metals and latitude: A perspective. *Marine Pollution Bulletin,* 58(6), 812–817. https://doi.org/10.1016/j.marpolbul.2009.02.001

PFLAG. (2022). *National glossary of terms.* PFLAG. https://pflag.org/glossary

Quinn, G. P., Sutton, S. K., Winfield, B., Breen, S., Canales, J., Shetty, G., Sehovic, I., Green, B. L., & Schabath, M. B. (2015). Lesbian, gay, bisexual, transgender, queer/questioning (LGBTQ) perceptions and health care experiences. *Journal of Gay & Lesbian Social Services,* 27(2), 246–261. https://doi.org/10.1080/10538720.2015.1022273

Rossi, A. L., & Lopez, E. J. (2017). Contextualizing competence: Language and LGBT-based competency in health care. *Journal of Homosexuality,* 64(10), 1330–1349. https://doi.org/10.1080/009183 69.2017.1321361

Rydström, K. (2020). Degendering menstruation: Making trans menstruators matter. In C. Bobel, I. T. Winkler, B. Fahs, K. A. Hasson, E. A. Kissling, & T.-A. Roberts (Eds.), *The Palgrave handbook of critical menstruation studies.* Palgrave Macmillan. https://www.ncbi.nlm.nih.gov/books/NBK565621

Sahmoud, A., Hamilton, D., & Pope, R. (2022). A trauma-informed and gender-inclusive medical nomenclature. *Obstetrics & Gynecology,* 140(1), 115–120. https://doi.org/10.1097/aog.0000000000004803

Schreuder, M. C. (2019). Safe spaces, agency, and resistance: A meta-synthesis of LGBTQ language use. *Journal of LGBT Youth,* 18(3), 256–272. https://10.1080/19361653.2019.1706685

Siegel, M., Legler, M., Neziraj, F., Goldberg, A. E., & Zemp, M. (2022). Minority stress and positive identity aspects in members of LGBTQ+ parent families: Literature review and a study protocol for a mixed-methods evidence synthesis. *Children (Basel),* 9(9), 1364. https://doi.org/10.3390/children9091364

Štrkalj, G., & Pather, N. (2021). Beyond the sex binary: Toward the inclusive anatomical sciences education. *Anatomical Sciences Education,* 14(4), 513–518. https://doi.org/10.1002/ase.2002

The Trevor Project. (2021). *2021 national survey on LGBTQ youth mental health.* The Trevor Project. https://www.thetrevorproject.org/survey-2021/?section=SupportingTransgenderNonbinaryYouth

The Trevor Project. (2022). *2022 national survey on LGBTQ youth mental health.* The Trevor Project. https://www.thetrevorproject.org/survey-2022

Trautner, E., McCool-Myers, M., & Joyner, A. B. (2020). Knowledge and practice of induction of lactation in trans women among professionals working in trans health. *International Breastfeeding Journal,* 15(1), 63. https://doi.org/10.1186/s13006-020-00308-6

University of California, San Francisco Center of Excellence for Transgender Health. (2016). *Guidelines for the primary and gender-affirming care of transgender and gender nonbinary people* (2nd ed.). UCSF Transgender Care. https://transcare.ucsf.edu/guidelines

Williams Institute. (2019). *Suicide thoughts and attempts among transgender adults: Findings from the 2015 U.S. transgender survey 2019,* 1-35. https://escholarship.org/content/qt1812g3hm/qt1812g3 hm.pdf

Wingo, E., Ingraham, N., & Roberts, S. C. M. (2018). Reproductive health care priorities and barriers to effective care for LGBTQ people assigned female at birth: A qualitative study. *Women's Health Issues,* 28(4), 350–357. https://doi.org/10.1016/j.whi.2018.03.002

Yingling, C. T., Cotler, K., & Hughes, T. L. (2017). Building nurses' capacity to address health inequities: Incorporating lesbian, gay, bisexual and transgender health content in a family nurse practitioner programme. *Journal of Clinical Nursing,* 26(17–18), 2807–2817.

Zemenick, A. T., Turney, S., Webster, A. J., Jones, S. C., & Weber, M. G. (2022). Six principles for embracing gender and sexual diversity in postsecondary biology classrooms. *Bioscience,* 72(5), 481–492. https://doi.org/10.1093/biosci/biac013

26

Violence and Trauma in the Perinatal Period

Karen Trister Grace

The editors gratefully acknowledge Amy R. Chavez and Nena R. Harris, who authored portions of this chapter in the previous edition.

Relevant Terms

Childhood sexual abuse (CSA)—includes sexual harassment, contact or attempted sexual contact with a child, exposing a child to sexual activity or content, owning or producing child pornography, and other behaviors

Human trafficking—obtaining labor or sex from a person through force or coercion

Intimate partner violence—abusive or violent behavior experienced in the context of a dating, romantic, or sexual relationship

Reproductive coercion—controlling behaviors by a partner or family member that interfere with autonomous reproductive decisions by a person capable of pregnancy

Trauma-informed care—healthcare that recognizes the ubiquity of experiences of trauma and brings that awareness to all patient interactions

---

Health equity key points

- Studies of Black survivors of IPV reveal the complexity of deciding to notify the police whose involvement may contribute to further harm and alienate the survivor from their community.
- There is a need for alternative forms of justice and protection that do not further traumatize IPV survivors or expose partners and communities to a biased legal system.
- Homicide is the leading cause of death during the perinatal period in the United States, especially among young people (under age 25) and people of color.
- There are common factors that result in certain groups being more vulnerable to victimization by human traffickers, including people who were abused as children or who may have run away from chaotic homes, immigrants, members of sexual and gender minority groups, and people who are economically disadvantaged.

Introduction

The experience of traumatic events in childhood or at any point in a person's lifetime can impact their health in myriad ways. Traumatic events may range from physical assault and rape to poor treatment by a healthcare provider, and responses to these events may vary just as widely; some people are able to mobilize strong systems of support, strength, and resilience and exhibit few symptoms of trauma, while others, even with support, may experience difficulty coping. Poor health outcomes, both acute and chronic, may result from trauma experiences. Providing care that recognizes the ubiquity of the experience of trauma and that responds appropriately without retraumatizing the patient is an essential skill, especially in perinatal care, which can be an especially vulnerable time for many people. Screening for **intimate partner violence (IPV)**, **reproductive coercion**, **human trafficking**, and **childhood sexual abuse** (CSA) are critical components of healthcare.

Trauma-Informed Care

Trauma-informed care describes an approach to care in which the healthcare provider enters every care relationship with the knowledge that trauma exists in many people and in many forms. People may experience trauma as a result of violence, abuse, terrorism, environmental disasters, combat, war, incarceration, and structural and interpersonal racism, among other harmful or potentially harmful experiences. The experience of trauma is linked to numerous acute and chronic health problems, including during pregnancy and birth (Gerber, 2019). Because trauma is often not disclosed until the establishment of a trusting relationship, if it is disclosed at all, the tools of trauma-informed care are brought to every care encounter. Each patient should be approached with recognition of the power dynamics inherent in a provider–client relationship and of the

Prenatal and Postnatal Care: A Person-Centered Approach, Third Edition. Edited by Karen Trister Grace, Cindy L. Farley, Noelene K. Jeffers, and Tanya Tringali.
© 2024 John Wiley & Sons Ltd. Published 2024 by John Wiley & Sons Ltd.
Companion website: www.wiley.com/go/grace/prenatal

vulnerability of being pregnant, examined, and evaluated on intimate physical characteristics and lifestyle choices. Powerful emotions can be evoked in the prenatal care encounter. Trauma-informed care emphasizes emotional safety and recognizes the implications of a sense of safety on physiology and behavior.

Trauma-informed practice suggestions are fundamental and implemented in a mindful manner. In the initial introduction to the patient, time is taken to check in and make a warm, nonthreatening physical connection, such as shaking hands. Explanations are given of how the care encounter is structured, and the patient is assured that their choices will be respected through every step. Loss of choice can lead to a feeling of losing one's personal power that can be coupled with a neurophysiologic dysregulation; the body can go into one of the classic physical responses when danger is perceived: fight, flight, freeze, or collapse. The effects of this stress can give rise to somatic and emotional reactions during the exam that range from depersonalization/dissociation to hypervigilant overcontrol or passive surrender. The healthcare provider that practices trauma-informed care helps reduce the stress response and set the stage for a trusting relationship that can be healing. With every opportunity to acknowledge a patient's active participation and choice, trauma-informed care is practiced (Table 26.1).

For the patient who dissociates from their body during an exam due to past trauma, particularly with pelvic or breast exams, it is helpful to slow down time in a way that the person can come into the moment. They can be assisted to connect to their body and not dissociate by asking questions like, "Can you describe physical and emotional sensations you feel going on right now?" or "What do you need to feel safe right now?" It is important to understand that defensive behaviors are protective psychological mechanisms. It is essential to stop any exam or procedure when asked so as not to create conditions that can retraumatize (Reeves, 2015; Seng et al., 2014). The practice of empathetic compassion is the antidote to negative emotions that can dissolve trust in the therapeutic relationship or interfere with the care process. Protective factors that increase resilience among people experiencing or who have experienced trauma include social support, safe and stable relationships, just societal policies, health, housing, faith, and cultural traditions, among others (Kimberg & Wheeler, 2019).

Tools for trauma-informed care

Contain—set safe boundaries with respect to physical and emotional space
Care/Compassion—empathetically accept experience as perceived by the individual, and emphasize self-care for yourself and the patient
Calm—remain calm and breathe, to promote a calming atmosphere
Cope—emphasize coping skills, resilience, and strengths

Source: Adapted from ACOG (2021).

Table 26.1 Trauma-Informed Principles and Practice Suggestions for Prenatal and Postnatal Care

Trauma-informed principle	Practice suggestions
Safety	Obtain fully informed consent for all procedures Allow support people to be present for visits Be mindful of triggering language, especially during pelvic exams Agree to stop any exam at any time if the patient asks or appears uncomfortable or distressed, or dissociates Balance the need for education of student providers with the requirement to avoid retraumatization of patients Position at eye level when talking to patient
Trustworthiness and transparency	Keep patients fully informed and practice shared decision-making Create visible signals that the practice welcomes disclosure, such as resource cards and informational flyers about what will happen if a disclosure is made Implement universal screening and education of all patients, framed as "Because traumatic events are so common, I ask all my patients this. . ." Create transparent systems and policies so that patients and staff feel safe
Peer support	Offer group prenatal care Offer parenting support groups
Collaboration and mutuality	Shared decision-making Provide flexibility in scheduling appointments and avoid punitive policies for lateness/missed visits Ensure clear communication between providers when continuity of care is not possible
Empowerment	Avoid stigmatizing, focus on resilience, and provide resources on self-care Shared decision-making Always obtain consent for all procedures
Awareness of cultural, historical, racial and gender issues	Use language interpreters Address and prevent biased care/practices by providers, staff and the health system Recognize our role as providers in perpetuating trauma and work to reduce harm

Source: Adapted from Gerber (2019), Owens (2021), Sperlich et al. (2017), and ACOG (2021).

Also essential to trauma-informed care is self-care on the part of the healthcare provider. Hearing about past experiences of trauma and supporting patients as they process them and witnessing traumatic events such as bad outcomes during pregnancy can cause secondary or vicarious traumatic stress in providers, especially when the provider has experienced trauma themselves. Many healthcare systems offer mental health services for providers and staff. Engaging in mindful self-care practices can support resiliency and longevity in a career of service.

Intimate Partner Violence during Pregnancy and Postpartum

IPV is defined as physical or emotional injury caused by someone with whom the violence survivor has a close personal relationship. The violence can consist of pushing, slapping, hitting, kicking, biting, repetitive emotional abuse, punching, rape, controlling behavior, stalking, and cyber-abuse, among other behaviors. The person using violence can use verbal threats or physical force to overcome the survivor and commit the act of abuse. According to the Centers for Disease Control and Prevention, one of every four women will experience violence, stalking, or sexual assault from an intimate partner in their lifetime (Smith et al., 2018). Prevalence rates of IPV during pregnancy range from approximately 3% to 9% (Alhusen et al., 2015). However, these are likely low estimates due to underreporting and decreased prenatal care utilization among people experiencing abuse (Jamieson, 2020). Various risk factors are associated with experiencing IPV, including alcohol abuse, cohabitation, young age, experiencing abuse as a child, unemployment, and immigrant status (Abramsky et al., 2011; Sanz-Barbero et al., 2019). There is also significantly elevated risk for experiencing violence among people who identify as sexual and gender minorities (McKay et al., 2019; Swiatlo et al., 2020).

No one pattern characterizes the experience of violence in pregnancy. Pregnancy may be a trigger for violence in a previously nonviolent partner or may be a protective factor for some pregnant people whose violent partners fear harming the fetus. A preexisting pattern of IPV might escalate in episodes and severity during pregnancy. Healthcare providers encounter many people who are experiencing or have experienced abuse who may or may not decide to disclose the abuse to the provider.

Survivors of IPV are more likely to experience both chronic and acute health conditions. Conditions associated with IPV include asthma, irritable bowel syndrome, diabetes, high blood pressure, and headaches, chronic pain, difficulty sleeping, disability, and fair or poor overall health and mental health (Gilbert et al., 2022), as well as decreased use of contraception (Bergmann & Stockman, 2015). Recent research has revealed the profound impacts of one type of IPV, nonfatal strangulation, which can result in traumatic brain injury. A person who has experienced strangulation may present in an

atypical fashion, without obvious signs of injury, but may develop cognitive dysfunction, post-traumatic stress disorder (PTSD) and depression over time (Campbell et al., 2018; Kwako et al., 2011; Zilkens et al., 2016). During pregnancy, IPV poses risks to both the pregnant person and the fetus; IPV in pregnancy is associated with significantly higher risk for inadequate prenatal care, inadequate weight gain, poor nutrition, mental health disorders, substance use, postpartum hemorrhage, preterm birth, low birth weight, small for gestational age, neonatal ICU admission, and maternal and neonatal death (Alhusen et al., 2015; Auger et al., 2021). Adolescents are especially vulnerable to IPV and require targeted intervention since experiencing IPV during adolescence is a risk factor for victimization in adulthood (ACOG, 2012). Children born into abusive home environments are at risk for early sexual initiation, discontinuing education in high school, and early childbearing (Adhia et al., 2019), as well as experiencing and perpetrating various forms of abuse. Additional outcomes can manifest as difficult temperaments, poor health outcomes, poor school performance, and anxiety and depression (Chambliss, 2008; Kimber et al., 2018; McMahon et al., 2011). Some states require mandatory reporting of IPV that occurs in homes with children, regardless of whether it is known that a child is or is not being directly abused. See *Resources for Healthcare Providers* for resources summarizing specific state laws.

IPV often follows a characteristic cycle of building tension, violence, and attempts at reconciliation. The third phase of attempting to convince the survivor that the behavior will change is often effective in keeping the survivor in the relationship and can prolong the abusive relationship for months or years. The decision to remain in an abusive relationship may be impacted by an array of factors, including financial or immigration concerns, impacts on children, lack of alternative housing, lack of social support, and hope that the violence will stop. Further, threats of severe physical harm, homicide, suicide, or violence against children or pets create an overwhelming fear that may lead to a choice of injury over possible death by staying in the relationship.

Cycle of abuse

1. **Building tension**—Arguments, verbal threats, and low-level assaults (pushing), victim tends to appease the abuser in an effort to avoid abuse escalation.
2. **Violent event**—Direct physical harm occurs such as slapping, punching, or rape.
3. **Attempts at reconciliation**—Sometimes called *honeymoon phase*, this often occurs immediately after violence, characterized by the abuser's display of overly affectionate, remorseful, and apologetic behavior.
4. **Calm**—The violent event is not mentioned, and a relative peace ensues. The cycle repeats as difficulties in life circumstances or the relationship leads to tension building.

Homicide is the leading cause of death during the perinatal period in the United States, especially among people under age 25 and people of color (Wallace et al., 2021). Additionally, the majority of perpetrators of perinatal homicide are intimate partners (Campbell et al., 2021). For a person in an abusive relationship, the most dangerous time is when they leave or attempt to leave. However, many people are able to successfully and permanently leave abusive relationships when given the appropriate support. This is the survivor's decision to make. They are the experts on their own lives and on staying safe in their relationships. Appreciation for the context of a person's choice to remain in or leave an abusive relationship is important to express to the individual. There is no place for judgmental reactions to a choice with which the provider may disagree. Empathy for the enormity of the decision at hand aids in compassion and minimizing judgment. Instead, provide information and resources for such time that the person may be ready to leave.

Research demonstrates that a survivor's legal action in the form of a court order of protection against the abuser results in decreased abuse; however, other studies have found that incidences of IPV increase after a court order of protection (McFarlane et al., 2004). Furthermore, there is evidence that temporary court orders for protection might increase psychological abuse, while permanent court orders are more effective in decreasing physical abuse (Holt et al., 2002; Kratochvil, 2010). Obtaining a legal protection order may play a role in decreased depression and PTSD symptoms for some survivors, as well as fewer instance of some types of reabuse (Wright & Johnson, 2012). Studies of Black IPV survivors reveal the complexity of deciding to involve the police who may unjustly cause harm to the partner and alienate the survivor from their community. There is a need for alternative forms of justice and protection in communities traumatized by police inaction or brutality (Decker et al., 2019). In light of these inconsistent findings and the inherent limitations in such studies, individuals in abusive relationships should be made aware of the potential for such action to exacerbate violence and assisted in taking the steps necessary to ensure safety for themselves and any children. The healthcare provider should never force a survivor to take such action if they are not ready or comfortable with the potential consequences. Strategies to enhance safety, self-worth, and empowerment may provide them with the resolve to take legal action should they feel ready to do so in the future.

Screening for IPV is recommended at regular intervals throughout prenatal care; survivors might find it hard to disclose the abuse until they have developed a trusting relationship with the healthcare provider (ACNM, 2002; Anderson et al., 2002; Chang et al., 2012). Regular screening with an openness to hearing the response reminds patients that the clinic is a safe place to seek help when needed. Table 26.2 contains some general principles to follow when assessing for IPV and planning interventions to assist survivors in accessing appropriate resources.

Table 26.2   Intimate Partner Violence: Assessment and Planning

1. Assess for IPV using a formal screening tool or informal questions. Preface with a statement that normalizes universal screening for all patients. Assess for the following:
   - Emotional abuse, humiliation, intimidation, use of threats
   - Physical abuse, including hitting, biting, kicking, slapping, pushing, punching
   - Sexual abuse or rape

   All patients should be assessed for IPV at the initial prenatal visit and regularly throughout the remainder of the pregnancy, at least once per trimester.

2. Assess frequency of abuse and history of injuries and trips to the ER. If there are current injuries, document them in the record with specific descriptions and drawings. Photograph them if a camera is available. If injuries are consistent with abuse but the patient does not disclose abuse, carefully document objective information about the injury.

3. Assess perception of imminent danger. Ask about guns or other weapons in the home. Inquire about suicidal ideations from patient and/or partner. Consider using a tool such as the Danger Assessment (see *Resources for Healthcare Providers*) to assess the risk of homicide.

4. Ask about perceptions of the future of the relationship. Avoid judgment if they have no intention of ending the relationship. Ask sensitive questions to understand the factors that are preventing them from leaving.

5. If there are suspicions of abuse and the partner is always with the patient, use strategies to separate them such as asking for a urine sample and leading the patient to the bathroom, or establish and post universal policies about always speaking to the patient alone for at least a portion of the visit.

6. Assess support network, including sources of financial help, housing, and transportation.

7. Provide contact information for local shelters for abuse survivors and local social services for housing, financial, and medical assistance. Place posters and flyers in bathrooms. Advise the patient on places to keep the numbers hidden, such as under the insert of her shoe or inside the lining of a purse.

8. If the patient wants to obtain a court order of protection, provide information for local agencies that are equipped to provide legal assistance. Do not call agencies or law enforcement on the patient's behalf without permission. If reporting requirements for IPV are state-mandated, inform the patient.

9. Validate the person's experience, choices, and fears and reinforce their self-worth. Withhold judgment and engage in active and supportive listening.

Reproductive Coercion

Reproductive coercion is a type of IPV that can occur with or without concurrent physical abuse. It consists of controlling behaviors by a partner or even a family member that interfere with autonomous reproductive decisions in a person capable of pregnancy. Examples of such behaviors may include preventing someone from accessing contraception, tampering with condoms, coercing a partner to have unprotected sex, threatening to leave a person if they do not get pregnant or do not end a pregnancy, using physical violence in attempts to cause a spontaneous abortion, or using pressure and coercion to encourage pregnancy. Reproductive coercion is strongly associated with IPV and with unintended pregnancy (Miller et al., 2010). As with IPV, providers are recommended to screen for reproductive coercion at multiple points in pregnancy (American College of Obstetricians & Gynecologists [ACOG], 2013). Pregnant people who experienced pregnancy coercion may be interested in a patient-controlled and less detectable method of contraception postpartum, such as intrauterine, injectable, or implanted methods.

Institutional and Provider-Level Coercion

History reveals numerous attempts by government entities to control reproductive decisions by people capable of pregnancy, especially people of color, people with disabilities, poor people, and other marginalized groups. Providers have an ethical responsibility to ensure fully informed consent for any procedure or prescription provided to a patient, and in the area of sexual and reproductive health and contraception, this is especially important. See Chapter 32, *Contraception in the Postnatal Period*, for additional information on avoiding coercive practices in the provision of and counseling for contraception.

Human Trafficking

Healthcare providers may encounter a victim of trafficking upon their entry into prenatal care. Awareness about **human trafficking** has increased in recent years, although there is much more to learn about the role of healthcare providers in the identification of potential survivors and in the facilitation of intervention. Defined as a form of modern-day slavery, human trafficking affects children and adults of various racial/ethnic, socioeconomic, and educational backgrounds (ACOG, 2019; US Department of Homeland Security, 2022). It comprises a broad category of commercial services, including labor and sexual acts involving force, fraud, or coercion. Although no one characteristic confers immunity from trafficking, there are common factors that result in certain groups being more vulnerable to victimization. People who were abused as children or who may have run away from chaotic homes are at particularly high risk for victimization by trafficking, as well as immigrants, members of sexual and gender minority groups, and people who are economically disadvantaged (ACOG, 2019; Geynisman-Tan et al., 2017). In the United States, the majority of people who are trafficked were born in the United States, Honduras, and Mexico; are cisgender female; and of young age (Moukaddam et al., 2021).

Sex trafficking specifically involves the use of coercion, fraud, or force in the provision of commercial sex acts.

Minors under the age of 18 years are not required to be under the influence of force, coercion, or fraud to be considered trafficked. Different from prostitution or sex work, a sex-trafficking victim typically does not have a say about with whom they have sex, does not get paid, may be moved to different locations to maintain secrecy, and has a pimp or trafficker dictating their activities (Dovydaitis, 2010). It is estimated that 40 million people are trafficked globally, and 14,000–17,000 per year are in the United States (Moukaddam et al., 2021).

Victims of sex trafficking may exhibit subtle signs of trauma that may go unnoticed by the unaware healthcare provider. Vague or inconsistent answers to questions about medical and social history, lack of identification, not being in control of or not being paid wages, poor eye contact, tattoos or other types of branding, or elusive response to questions about friends and family members may indicate that a patient is a victim of trafficking (ACOG, 2019; Dovydaitis, 2010; Geynisman-Tan et al., 2017). More noticeable indicators may include reports of multiple recent sexual partners, recurrent sexually transmitted infections, signs of physical or sexual trauma, signs of PTSD, or substance use (ACOG, 2019). Tattoos, such as a dollar sign or a crown, can denote ownership by the enslavers and can be a visible clue to identify victims (Farley et al., 2019). See *Resources for Healthcare Providers* for suggested human trafficking screening questions and for tattoo removal or reconstruction services for survivors of sex trafficking.

Careful and attentive assessment that considers possible indicators of trafficking may mean the difference between a patient's last day as a victim of trafficking and their continued exposure to trauma and violence at the hand of a trafficker. Expedient, collaborative interventions are essential for improving sexual and reproductive health and perinatal and infant outcomes and facilitating short and long-term safety and well-being (Table 26.3).

Table 26.3 Considerations for Providing Care for Potential Victims of Trafficking

- Build a rapport by offering emotional and material support.
- Obtain the person's permission before any contact with law enforcement. Maintain as much confidentiality as possible and be honest about any limitations.
- Be sensitive to the potential impact of immigration issues.
- Be prepared with resources for legal, material, and psychosocial assistance.
- Be aware of the potential security concerns involved in helping trafficking victims, since many traffickers are involved in organized crime, gang activity, drug cartels, or other dangerous activities.
- Consider safety measures for the clinic setting such as limited after-hours access, improved parking lot lighting, electronic locks, security cameras, and emergency notification protocols.

Source: ACOG (2019) and National Human Trafficking Training and Technical Assistance Center (NHTTAC, 2018).

Pregnancy and a History of Childhood Sexual Abuse

CSA is a global public health issue that has affected as many as 37% of pregnant people (Brunton & Dryer, 2021). Pregnancy can trigger feelings of terror and shame for many due to the changes in the pregnant body, the feelings of vulnerability that pregnancy naturally brings, and office procedures such as digital vaginal exams, which can recall the trauma for the individual. This can take the form of flashbacks of previously repressed memories, nightmares, increased anxiety, and behavior changes. For some, pregnancy is the event that brings to consciousness the repressed memories of CSA for the first time in many years, especially among those abused at younger ages. People who have survived CSA have an increase in perinatal complications such as hyperemesis, preterm labor and birth, operative delivery, prolonged labor, cervical insufficiency, fear of childbirth, postpartum depression, and hospitalizations during pregnancy (Brunton & Dryer, 2021; Kendall-Tackett, 2007; Leeners et al., 2010; Lukasse et al., 2010). The psychological burden of processing memories of CSA can directly affect mental health in areas such as fear of childbirth and postpartum mood and anxiety disorders. Connections with other complications, such as preterm birth and prolonged labor, are less clear; it is believed that these complications are in part related to higher levels of catecholamines and stress hormones found in people with prior CSA (Brunton & Dryer, 2021; DeBellis et al., 1994).

Assessing for Childhood Sexual Abuse

All pregnant patients should be asked about a prior history of CSA during the prenatal intake interview. While some people may share their history of CSA and express a preference for being screened, some will not, and they may not disclose until they feel ready to share or until they can judge that the provider "gets it" and is competent at addressing these issues (LoGiudice & Beck, 2016; Sperlich & Seng, 2008). The healthcare provider must be alert to physical, psychological, and behavioral clues that may indicate CSA (Table 26.4).

Providing Care

An acute need for control can motivate behavior that may be exhibited by people who have experienced CSA, stemming from the loss of control endured during their abuse. Certain behaviors may help manage feelings of extreme anxiety and fear that emerge during pregnancy. Some people may seek to learn everything about pregnancy and birth in order to prepare for every possible scenario that might happen to them. This may be manifested as attending multiple childbirth preparation class series, gathering numerous accounts of childbirth experiences, reading many books, and researching childbirth on the Internet (Hobbins, 2004). Some patients may develop very detailed and lengthy birth plans in an effort to control events covering a variety of birth scenarios. This overload of information may contribute to confusion and further anxiety

Table 26.4 Possible Signs and Symptoms of Prior CSA

Physical signs and symptoms	Psychological signs and symptoms	Behavioral signs and symptoms
Prior history of multiple somatic illnesses: • Dizziness and fainting • Chronic pain and fatigue • Severe obesity • Gastrointestinal disorders • Migraine headaches Symptoms related to reproductive health: • Sexual dysfunction • Breast symptoms • Chronic menstrual problems • Chronic urinary tract infection (UTI) • Premenstrual syndrome • History of multiple sexually transmitted infections (STIs) • Multiple unplanned pregnancies • Scars from self-mutilation	• Post-traumatic stress disorder • Compulsive disorders • Dissociative disorders • Panic attacks • Low self-esteem • Depression • Negative reaction to pregnancy • Denial of pregnancy • Poor maternal attachment	• Anorexia or bulimia • Substance abuse • Seeks female healthcare providers • Little or no prenatal care • Frequent healthcare visits for somatic symptoms

or may increase their sense of control over the situation. Some people may exhibit hypervigilance in interpreting their body changes and sensations during pregnancy. This can manifest as frequent telephone contacts with healthcare providers and multiple office visits with problems and many questions (Hobbins, 2004). A history of CSA is associated with increased reports of common discomforts and symptoms of pregnancy during the antepartum period (Lukasse et al., 2009).

Healthcare providers should introduce themselves and talk with patients before they are asked to undress for a physical examination. The initial health interview and history can be incorporated into this time. Once the patient has changed into an examination gown and is ready, providers should knock on the door prior to entering the examination space. During the exam, the healthcare provider explains each physical assessment being done before beginning and obtains fully informed consent from the patient (Tillman, 2020). Since many people have an unknown history of CSA, these should all be routine practice habits. When abuse is disclosed, a calm, nonjudgmental, and empathetic response is essential.

It is of the utmost importance to avoid the use of traumatizing or paternalistic language when providing care to all patients. Some statements that should be strictly avoided are phrases like "just open your legs a little bit wider," "lift your bottom up for me," and "just relax." Not only are these phrases infantilizing to patients, they can also reintroduce traumatizing memories and cause extreme anxiety to CSA survivors (Squire, 2017; Tillman, 2020).

When providing prenatal care, it is essential to understand that survivors of CSA are likely to have strong need for a safe, trusting relationship with their healthcare provider in addition to control over what happens to their bodies. While developing trust is a vital aspect of obtaining quality prenatal care, this can be a difficult task for CSA survivors. To facilitate this process, recognizing and verbalizing understanding of their concerns is important. For example, "I know it may take some time to feel that I am trustworthy. So here are some things about me you can count on. I will keep your confidentiality. I'll try to remember to ask permission to touch you, and I will keep you informed of your condition" (Sperlich & Seng, 2008, p. 68).

Almost half of CSA survivors experience memories of their abuse when undergoing a vaginal exam (Leeners, 2007). They need to be in control of when the exams are done and when they can be stopped for any reason, without penalty. For people who have disclosed CSA and for anyone showing distress during a pelvic exam, it is essential to say, "I see that this is stressful for you. I am going to stop now. Are you okay? Let me know if I may continue." Throughout the perinatal period, vaginal examinations should only be done when absolutely indicated, and the patient should be involved in making the plan of care with a strategy of shared decision-making. Any procedure or examination should be explained prior to being done, and again during every step of the process. This will help the patient anticipate what is being done and gives them the opportunity to accept or decline. Having control over physical exams and invasive procedures is important in reducing retraumatization during pregnancy care.

Summary

Recognizing, responding to, and screening for lifetime and current experiences of trauma are essential components of perinatal care. In some cases, the healthcare provider must operate as a case manager in the beginning stages of the relationship until other professionals with expertise in social services can take over. A familiarity with local community, state, and federal agencies that exist to provide aid to individuals in vulnerable circumstances is essential. Trauma-informed care principles provide a framework to develop relationship-based care that supports survivors as well as providers in promoting health and resilience.

Resources for Pregnant People and Their Families

For adult survivors of child sexual abuse: https://www.rainn.org/articles/adult-survivors-child-sexual-abuse

National Domestic Violence Hotline: https://www.thehotline.org
National Human Trafficking Hotline: https://humantraffickinghotline.org

Resources for Healthcare Providers

Danger Assessment: https://www.dangerassessment.org/
IPV: https://www.ahrq.gov/ncepcr/tools/healthier-pregnancy/fact-sheets/partner-violence.html
IPV resources for healthcare providers (including state reporting laws): https://www.futureswithoutviolence.org/health
Child sexual abuse: https://www.acog.org/clinical/clinical-guidance/committee-opinion/articles/2011/08/adult-manifestations-of-childhood-sexual-abuse
CDC resources on child sexual abuse: https://www.cdc.gov/violenceprevention/childsexualabuse/fastfact.html
Human Trafficking: Human trafficking screening questions and additional resources: National Human Trafficking Training and Technical Assistance Center (NHTTAC). (2018). Adult human trafficking screening tool and guide. https://www.acf.hhs.gov/sites/default/files/documents/otip/adult_human_trafficking_screening_tool_and_guide.pdf
National Human Trafficking Hotline: https://humantraffickinghotline.org
Survivor's Ink: Aids survivors of human trafficking overcome reminders of their past by offering cover-up tattoos or removal services for tattoos they received while being trafficked. http://www.survivorsink.org
Trauma-informed care: https://store.samhsa.gov/product/SAMHSA-s-Concept-of-Trauma-and-Guidance-for-a-Trauma-Informed-Approach/SMA14-4884
Trauma Informed Care Implementation Resource Center: https://www.traumainformedcare.chcs.org

References

Abramsky, T., Watts, C. H., Garcia-Moreno, C., Devries, K., Kiss, L., Ellsberg, M., Jansen, H. A., & Heise, L. (2011). What factors are associated with recent intimate partner violence? Findings from the WHO multi-country study on women's health and domestic violence. *BMC Public Health*, 11(1), 109. https://doi.org/10.1186/1471-2458-11-109

Adhia, A., Drolette, L. M., Vander Stoep, A., Valencia, E. J., & Kernic, M. A. (2019). The impact of exposure to parental intimate partner violence on adolescent precocious transitions to adulthood. *Journal of Adolescence*, 77(August), 179–187. https://doi.org/10.1016/j.adolescence.2019.11.001

Alhusen, J. L., Ray, E., Sharps, P., & Bullock, L. (2015). Intimate partner violence during pregnancy: Maternal and neonatal outcomes. *Journal of Women's Health*, 24(1), 100–106. https://doi.org/10.1089/jwh.2014.4872

American College of Nurse Midwives (ACNM). (2002). Assessment for intimate partner violence in clinical practice. *Journal of Midwifery & Women's Health*, 47(5), 386–390.

American College of Obstetricians & Gynecologists (ACOG). (2012). Intimate partner violence. Committee opinion no. 518 (reaffirmed 2022). *Obstetrics & Gynecology*, 119, 412–417.

American College of Obstetricians & Gynecologists (ACOG). (2013). Reproductive and sexual coercion. Committee opinion no. 554. *Obstetrics & Gynecology*, 121(2), 411–415.

American College of Obstetricians & Gynecologists (ACOG). (2019). Human trafficking. Committee opinion 787. *Obstetrics & Gynecology*, 134(3), e90–e95.

American College of Obstetricians & Gynecologists (ACOG). (2021). Caring for patients who have experienced trauma. Committee opinion no. 825. *Obstetrics & Gynecology, 137*(4), e94–e99. https://doi.org/10.1097/AOG.0000000000004326

Anderson, B. A., Marshak, H. H., & Hebbeler, D. L. (2002). Identifying intimate partner violence at entry to prenatal care: Clustering routine clinical information. *Journal of Midwifery & Women's Health, 47*, 353–359.

Auger, N., Low, N., Lee, G. E., Ayoub, A., & Luu, T. M. (2021). Pregnancy outcomes of women hospitalized for physical assault, sexual assault, and intimate partner violence. *Journal of Interpersonal Violence, 37*(13–14), NP11135–NP11135. https://doi.org/10.1177/0886260520985496

Bergmann, J. N., & Stockman, J. K. (2015). How does intimate partner violence affect condom and oral contraceptive use in the United States? A systematic review of the literature. *Contraception, 91*(6), 438–455. https://doi.org/10.1016/j.contraception.2015.02.009

Brunton, R., & Dryer, R. (2021). Child sexual abuse and pregnancy: A systematic review of the literature. *Child Abuse and Neglect, 111*, 104802. https://doi.org/10.1016/j.chiabu.2020.104802

Campbell, J., Matoff-Stepp, S., Velez, M. L., Cox, H. H., & Laughon, K. (2021). Pregnancy-associated deaths from homicide, suicide, and drug overdose: Review of research and the intersection with intimate partner violence. *Journal of Women's Health, 30*(2), 236–244. https://doi.org/10.1089/jwh.2020.8875

Campbell, J. C., Anderson, J. C., McFadgion, A., Gill, J., Zink, E., Patch, M., Callwood, G., & Campbell, D. (2018). The effects of intimate partner violence and probable traumatic brain injury on central nervous system symptoms. *Journal of Women's Health, 27*(6), 761–767. https://doi.org/10.1089/jwh.2016.6311

Chambliss, L. R. (2008). Intimate partner violence and its implication for pregnancy. *Clinical Obstetrics and Gynecology, 51*(2), 385–397.

Chang, J. C., Dado, D., Schussler, S., Hawker, L., Holland, C. L., Burke, J. G., & Cluss, P. A. (2012). In person versus computer screening for intimate partner violence among pregnant patients. *Patient Education and Counseling, 88*(3), 443–448. https://doi.org/10.1016/j.pec.2012.06.021

DeBellis, M., Lefter, L., Trickett, P. K., & Putnam, F. W. (1994). Urinary catecholamine excretion in sexually abused girls. *Journal of the American Academy of Child and Adolescent Psychiatry, 33*(3), 320–327.

Decker, M. R., Holliday, C. N., Hameeduddin, Z., Shah, R., Miller, J., Dantzler, J., & Goodmark, L. (2019). "You do not think of me as a human being": Race and gender inequities intersect to discourage police reporting of violence against women. *Journal of Urban Health*, 772–783. https://doi.org/10.1007/s11524-019-00359-z

Dovydaitis, T. (2010). Human trafficking: The role of the health care provider. *Journal of Midwifery & Women's Health, 55*, 462–467.

Farley, C. L., Van Hoover, C., & Rademeyer, C. A. (2019). Women and tattoos: Fashion, meaning, and implications for health. *Journal of Midwifery & Women's Health, 64*(2), 154–169. https://doi.org/10.1111/jmwh.12932

Gerber, M. R. (2019). Trauma-informed maternity care. In M. R. Gerber (Ed.), *Trauma-informed healthcare approaches* (pp. 145–155). Springer. https://doi.org/10.1007/978-3-030-04342-1

Geynisman-Tan, J. M., Taylor, J. S., Edersheim, T., & Taubel, D. (2017). All the darkness we don't see. *American Journal of Obstetrics & Gynecology, 216*(2), 135.e1–135.e5. https://doi.org.frontier.idm.oclc.org/10.1016/j.ajog.2016.09.088

Gilbert, L. K., Zhang, X., Basile, K. C., Breiding, M., & Kresnow, M. (2022). Intimate partner violence and health conditions among U.S. adults—National Intimate Partner Violence Survey, 2010–2012. *Journal of Interpersonal Violence*, 1–25. https://doi.org/10.1177/08862605221080147

Hobbins, D. (2004). Survivors of childhood sexual abuse: Implications for perinatal nursing care. *Journal of Obstetric, Gynecologic, & Neonatal Nursing, 33*(4), 485–497.

Holt, V. L., Kernic, M. A., Lumley, T., Wolf, M. E., & Rivara, F. P. (2002). Civil protection order and risk of subsequent police-reported violence. *JAMA: The Journal of the American Medical Association, 288*(5), 589–594.

Jamieson, B. (2020). Exposure to interpersonal violence during pregnancy and its association with women's prenatal care utilization: A meta-analytic review. *Trauma, Violence, and Abuse, 21*(5), 904–921. https://doi.org/10.1177/1524838018806511

Kendall-Tackett, K. (2007). Violence against women and perinatal period: The impact of lifetime violence and abuse on pregnancy postpartum and breastfeeding. *Trauma, Violence and Abuse, 8*(3), 344–353.

Kimber, M., Adham, S., Gill, S., McTavish, J., & MacMillan, H. L. (2018). The association between child exposure to intimate partner violence (IPV) and perpetration of IPV in adulthood—A systematic review. *Child Abuse and Neglect, 76*, 273–286. https://doi.org/10.1016/j.chiabu.2017.11.007

Kimberg, L., & Wheeler, M. (2019). Trauma and trauma-informed care. In M. R. Gerber (Ed.), *Trauma-informed healthcare approaches* (pp. 25–56). Springer. https://doi.org/10.1007/978-3-030-04342-1

Kratochvil, R. (2010). Intimate partner violence during pregnancy: Exploring the efficacy of a mandatory reporting statute. *Houston Journal of Health Law and Policy, 10*, 63–113.

Kwako, L. E., Glass, N., Campbell, J., Melvin, K. C., Barr, T., & Gill, J. M. (2011). Traumatic brain injury in intimate partner violence: A critical review of outcomes and mechanisms. *Trauma, Violence, and Abuse, 12*(3), 115–126. https://doi.org/10.1177/1524838011404251

Leeners, B. (2007). Effect of childhood sexual abuse on gynecological care as an adult. *Psychosomatics, 48*, 385–393.

Leeners, B., Stiller, R., Block, E., Gorres, G., & Rath, W. (2010). Pregnancy complications in women with childhood sexual abuse experiences. *Journal of Psychosomatic Research, 69*(5), 503–510.

LoGiudice, J. A., & Beck, C. T. (2016). The lived experience of childbearing from survivors of sexual abuse: "It was the best of times, it was the worst of times". *Journal of Midwifery & Women's Health, 61*(4), 474–481. https://doi.org/10.1111/jmwh.12421

Lukasse, M., Schei, B., Vangen, S., & Øian, P. (2009). Childhood abuse and common complaints in pregnancy. *Birth, 36*, 190–199.

Lukasse, M., Vangen, S., Øian, P., Kumle, M., Ryding, E. L., Schei, B., on behalf of the Bidens Study Group. (2010). Childhood abuse and fear of childbirth—A population-based study. *Birth, 37*, 267–274.

McFarlane, J., Malecha, A., Gist, J., Watson, K., Batten, E., Hall, I., & Smith, S. (2004). Protection orders and intimate partner violence: An 18-month study of 150 Black, Hispanic, and White women. *American Journal of Public Health, 94*(4), 613–618.

McKay, T., Lindquist, C. H., & Misra, S. (2019). Understanding (and acting on) 20 years of research on violence and LGBTQ + communities. *Trauma, Violence, and Abuse, 20*(5), 665–678. https://doi.org/10.1177/1524838017728708

McMahon, S., Huang, C.-C., Boxer, P., & Postmus, J. L. (2011). The impact of emotional and physical violence during pregnancy on maternal and child health at one year postpartum. *Children and Youth Services Review, 33*, 2103–2111.

Miller, E., Decker, M. R., McCauley, H. L., Tancredi, D. J., Levenson, R. R., Waldman, J., Schoenwald, P., & Silverman, J. G. (2010). Pregnancy coercion, intimate partner violence and unintended pregnancy. *Contraception, 81*(4), 316–322. https://doi.org/10.1016/j.contraception.2009.12.004

Moukaddam, N., Torres, M., Vujanovic, A. A., Saunders, J., Le, H., & Shah, A. A. (2021). Epidemiology of human trafficking. *Psychiatric Annals, 51*(8), 359–363. https://doi.org/10.3928/00485713-20210702-02

National Human Trafficking Training and Technical Assistance Center (NHTTAC). (2018). *Adult human trafficking screening tool and guide.* https://www.acf.hhs.gov/sites/default/files/documents/otip/adult_human_trafficking_screening_tool_and_guide.pdf

Owens, L., Terrell, S., Low, L. K., Loder, C., Rhizal, D., Scheiman, L., & Seng, J. (2021). Universal precautions: The case for consistently trauma-informed reproductive healthcare. *American Journal of Obstetrics and Gynecology, 226*(5), 671–677. https://doi.org/10.1016/j.ajog.2021.08.012

Reeves, E. (2015). A synthesis of the literature on trauma-informed care. *Issues in Mental Health Nursing, 36*(9), 698–709.

Sanz-Barbero, B., Barón, N., & Vives-Cases, C. (2019). Prevalence, associated factors and health impact of intimate partner violence against women in different life stages. *PLoS One, 14*(10), e0221049. https://doi.org/10.1371/journal.pone.0221049

Seng, J. S., D'Andrea, W., & Ford, J. D. (2014). Complex mental health sequelae of psychological trauma among women in prenatal care. *Psychological Trauma: Theory, Research, Practice, and Policy, 6*(1), 41–49.

Smith, S. G., Zhang, X., Basile, K. C., Merrick, M. T., Wang, J., Kresnow, M., & Chen, J. (2018). *National Intimate Partner and Sexual Violence Survey: 2015 Data brief - updated release.* https://www.cdc.gov/violenceprevention/pdf/2015data-brief508.pdf

Sperlich, M., & Seng, J. (2008). *Survivor moms: Women's stories of birthing, mothering and healing after sexual abuse.* Motherbaby Press.

Sperlich, M., Seng, J. S., Li, Y., Taylor, J., & Bradbury-Jones, C. (2017). Integrating trauma-informed care into maternity care practice: Conceptual and practical issues. *Journal of Midwifery and Women's Health, 62*(6), 661–672. https://doi.org/10.1111/jmwh.12674

Squire, C. (2017). Childbirth and sexual abuse during childhood. In C. Squire (Ed.), *The social context of birth* (pp. 229–250). Routledge.

Swiatlo, A. D., Kahn, N. F., & Halpern, C. T. (2020). Intimate partner violence perpetration and victimization among young adult sexual minorities. *Perspectives on Sexual and Reproductive Health, 52*(2), 97–105. https://doi.org/10.1363/psrh.12138

Tillman, S. (2020). Consent in pelvic care. *Journal of Midwifery & Women's Health, 65*(6), 749–758. https://doi.org/10.1111/jmwh.13189

US Department of Homeland Security. (2022, June 3). *What is human trafficking?* Blue Campaign. https://www.dhs.gov/blue-campaign/what-human-trafficking

Wallace, M., Gillispie-Bell, V., Cruz, K., Davis, K., & Vilda, D. (2021). Homicide during pregnancy and the postpartum period in the United States, 2018–2019. *Obstetrics & Gynecology, 138*(5), 762–769. https://doi.org/10.1097/aog.0000000000004567

Wright, C. V., & Johnson, D. M. (2012). Encouraging legal help seeking for victims of intimate partner violence: The therapeutic effects of the civil protection order. *Journal of Traumatic Stress, 25*, 675–681.

Zilkens, R. R., Phillips, M. A., Kelly, M. C., Mukhtar, S. A., Semmens, J. B., & Smith, D. A. (2016). Non-fatal strangulation in sexual assault: A study of clinical and assault characteristics highlighting the role of intimate partner violence. *Journal of Forensic and Legal Medicine, 43*, 1–7. https://doi.org/10.1016/j.jflm.2016.06.005

27

Planning for Physiologic Birth

Carrie E. Neerland and Melissa D. Avery

The editors gratefully acknowledge Melissa A. Saftner, who coauthored the previous edition of this chapter.

Relevant Terms

Confidence for physiologic birth—a person's belief that physiologic birth can be achieved based on their view of birth as a normal process and belief in their body's innate ability to give birth; supported by the social support, knowledge, and information founded in a trusted relationship with a provider in an environment where the person feels safe

Physiologic birth—birth that is powered by the innate human capacity of the birthing person and fetus

Self-efficacy—one's belief in their ability to perform a specific behavior or set of behaviors required to produce an outcome

Tocophobia—extreme fear of childbirth

Introduction

Supporting a physiologic approach to pregnancy, labor, and birth and avoiding the use of unnecessary medical interventions is a critical component of the solution to improving birth outcomes while at the same time reducing cost. The term *physiologic* is used throughout this chapter to highlight an approach to care that supports the body's expected physiologic processes during pregnancy and birth where possible. It includes a person-centered approach to pregnancy where pregnant and birthing people's values and preferences are respected and are part of a reciprocal care process. A physiologic approach is applied where appropriate for individuals at low risk for complications as well as for those with more complex pregnancies. This involves allowing sufficient time for the normal processes to occur and requires an orientation to pregnancy and birth as healthy life events for most people.

It is well recognized and documented that the United States spends more money on healthcare than any other country worldwide, yet it has among the poorest maternal and neonatal outcomes of high-resource nations. Nearly 20% of the US gross domestic product goes to healthcare (Centers for Medicaid & Medicare Services, 2023); childbirth is the most common reason for hospitalization, representing 10% of hospital stays in 2018 (Healthcare Cost and Utilization Project [HCUP], 2022). Newborn and neonatal care represents 61% of all pediatric hospitalizations in 2016 (Moore et al., 2019). Maternal mortality has been increasing in the United States for more than a decade (Douthard et al., 2021) and is higher than other high-resource countries (Tikkanen et al., 2020). Infant mortality is also higher in the United States than similar countries despite declining in recent years (Chen et al., 2016; Mathews & Driscoll, 2017). These data include unacceptable disparities for people of color (Hoyert, 2022).

Most birthing people desire minimal intervention in labor unless medically necessary (Sakala et al., 2018). However, medical interventions that are intended to be used only when indicated have become a routine part of maternity care in the United States. The cesarean birth rate, while slightly declining in recent years, is 32% (Osterman et al., 2022). Approximately 31% of women experienced labor inductions in 2020 (Osterman et al., 2022) and 73% had neuraxial analgesia (Butwick et al., 2018). *Healthy People 2030* includes recommendations for reducing cesarean rates and maternal and infant mortality (Healthy People 2030, n.d.). While many people utilize various childbirth interventions to help them through labor and birth, such as an epidural, this chapter is relevant to facilitating childbearing confidence in all pregnant people during the prenatal period, especially those who desire physiologic birth. However, instilling confidence for birth is relevant to all pregnant and birthing people regardless of their birth preferences and choices.

Prenatal and Postnatal Care: A Person-Centered Approach, Third Edition. Edited by Karen Trister Grace, Cindy L. Farley, Noelene K. Jeffers, and Tanya Tringali.
© 2024 John Wiley & Sons Ltd. Published 2024 by John Wiley & Sons Ltd.
Companion website: www.wiley.com/go/grace/prenatal

Health equity key points

- Increasing the racial and ethnic diversity of the perinatal healthcare workforce is critical to improving equity in childbirth.
- Greater integration of midwifery care in health systems has the potential to improve outcomes and reduce perinatal healthcare disparities.
- Culturally centered care, respectful communication, and shared decision-making may improve client confidence and care outcomes.

Benefits of physiologic birth

- Reduced perinatal infection
- Reduced complications from anesthesia
- Reduced risk of injury or harm from interventions such as induction of labor or operative vaginal birth
- Increased rates of breastfeeding and the potential for
  - improved maternal health (i.e., reduced rates of breast and ovarian cancer, diabetes, hypertension, hyperlipidemia, obesity, and myocardial infarction)
  - improved neonatal and childhood health: (i.e., necrotizing enterocolitis, obesity, sudden infant death syndrome, leukemia, inflammatory bowel disease, and pneumonia)
- Lower out-of-pocket costs for perinatal services
- Increased satisfaction with the childbirth experience
- Lower risk of complications with future birth

Source: Bartick et al. (2017), Bohren et al. (2017), Cragin and Kennedy (2006), Goer et al. (2012), Gregory et al. (2012), Hodnett (2002), Hyde et al. (2012), Johantgen et al. (2012), Moore et al. (2016), Sandall et al. (2018), Schwarz and Nothnagle (2015), and Truven Health Analytics (2013).

What Is Physiologic Birth?

The World Health Organization defined *normal birth* in 1996 as low-risk, vertex fetus between 37 and 42 weeks of gestation, spontaneous in labor onset and progression through the birth of the infant, and both mother and infant in good condition postpartum (WHO, 1996). A similar definition, and adding the nonuse of medical and pharmacologic interventions, was published by the International Confederation of Midwives (ICM, 2014). The American College of Nurse-Midwives, the Midwives Alliance of North America, and the National Association of Certified Professional Midwives partnered on the development of a definition of **physiologic birth** stated more simply as ". . . one that is powered by the innate human capacity of the woman and fetus" (ACNM, MANA, NACPM, 2012, p. 2). More specifically, this definition encompasses spontaneous onset and progression of labor, an environment that supports the biological and psychological processes of labor, vaginal birth and physiologic blood loss, optimal transition of the newborn using skin-to-skin contact, and early breastfeeding initiation (ACNM, MANA, NACPM, 2012).

In addition to formal definitions, nursing and medical societies document support for physiologic approaches to labor and birth. The Association of Women's Health, Obstetric and Neonatal Nurses (AWHONN) has issued multiple position statements advocating for physiologic labor and birth including discouraging nonmedically indicated induction and augmentation of labor (AWHONN, 2014), advocating for fetal monitoring that supports the physiologic labor and birth process (AWHONN, 2015), and shared decision-making as the standard of care (AWHONN, 2011). Reaffirmed in 2021, the American College of Obstetricians and Gynecologists (ACOG) published an opinion in support of limiting medical interventions and utilizing care practices that support physiologic birth (ACOG, 2017).

Benefits of Physiologic Birth

The physical, emotional, and financial benefits of physiologic birth for birthing people and infants are well established. There are no known harms of physiologic birth.

Fear of Childbirth

Some level of fear, worry, or anxiety about birth is normal, given that childbirth can be a person's first experience with a significant amount of pain and first extended experience with the healthcare system. **Tocophobia**, or an extreme fear of childbirth, is reported in varying levels of severity. A systematic review and meta-analysis including 27 studies from around the world found that the prevalence of tocophobia was around 14% (Sanjari et al., 2022); however, tocophobia varies by culture, country, and population. It is unknown how many people in the United States experience tocophobia, but Lowe (2000) found a relationship between decreased **self-efficacy** and fear of childbirth. The greater a person's confidence in their ability to labor and birth, the lower their fear. The increased medicalization of birth likely leads to increased fear for some pregnant and birthing people. More positive opinions about the medicalization of birth are associated with a greater fear of birth (Benyamini et al., 2017). As monitoring and interventions become more routine, interactions with healthcare providers and the broader healthcare system may result in reduced self-efficacy and limit a person's ability to develop confidence (Roosevelt & Low, 2016).

Confidence for Physiologic Birth

Confidence for physiologic birth is a complex concept and can be influenced by numerous factors, including culture, past experiences, social support, as well as psychological and physiologic aspects of health. The term *confidence*, as it relates to labor and birth, has been used in numerous areas including childbirth education methods and courses, consumer literature, birth-related websites, blogs, podcasts, and research literature. Dr. Grantly Dick-Read, often considered the father of the natural childbirth movement, was one of the first to write about confidence for birth in his groundbreaking 1942 publication *Childbirth without Fear* (Dick-Read, 2013). Organizations such as Lamaze International encouraged confident birthing through childbirth preparation in the 1960s and 1970s. A "climate of confidence" was described in the landmark publication, *Our Bodies Ourselves: Pregnancy and Birth,* as an environment that centers on a belief in people's ability to give birth and supports strengths and abilities, while minimizing fear (Boston Women's Health Book Collective, 2008). This is created through providing accurate information, quality prenatal care, encouragement, and love from support persons, and skilled compassionate care from healthcare providers (Boston Women's Health Book Collective, 2008).

In the research literature, the term *confidence for birth* has often been used in association with the term *self-efficacy*. Albert Bandura, a social scientist and psychologist, defines self-efficacy as "one's belief in one's ability to perform a specific behavior or set of behaviors required to produce an outcome" (1977). Bandura's self-efficacy theory has widely been used in the research literature related to childbirth confidence. Lowe defined confidence for childbirth based on Bandura's social learning theory (1993) and developed the most extensively utilized instrument to measure self-efficacy in childbirth, the Childbirth Self-Efficacy Inventory (CBSEI). Lowe's definition of confidence for labor is the woman's belief that she can use specific coping behaviors during labor that will lead to her desired outcome of birth (1993). The CBSEI has been validated in many countries and translated into several languages.

The term *confidence,* however, is used more often by pregnant and birthing people and perinatal healthcare providers and is more easily understood; therefore, confidence may be considered the more person-centered term. In addition, confidence is more applicable to the clinical environment, which is where prenatal healthcare providers can use approaches to improve pregnant and birthing people's confidence for physiologic birth.

Confidence for physiologic birth has more recently been defined as:

> the belief that physiologic birth can be achieved, based on the view of birth as a normal process and belief in the body's innate ability to birth, which is supported by social support, knowledge, and information founded on a trusted relationship with a maternity care provider in an environment where the person feels safe.
> (Neerland, 2018, p. 431)

Confidence for physiologic birth is characterized by four primary attributes or features:

1. Belief in labor and childbirth as a normal process
2. Confidence in people's innate ability to birth

3. Past experiences (e.g., giving birth or being with others during birth)
4. Knowledge/information (Neerland, 2018)

People who express confidence for physiologic birth tend to also hold the belief that childbirth is a normal physiologic process (Attanasio et al., 2014, Avery et al., 2019). Additionally, confidence for physiologic birth is associated with an acceptance of labor pain as a normal part of the process and faith in one's own body to give birth and one's own ability to manage the pain of labor (Stoll & Hall, 2013; Tilden et al., 2016). Previous experience with birth—either first-hand or vicarious experience—is an important characteristic that can shape confidence for physiologic birth (Avery et al., 2014; Grigg et al., 2015; Tilden et al., 2016). People who have previously experienced physiologic birth often express that they feel capable of doing it again (Catling-Paull et al., 2011; Neerland, 2018). Finally, knowledge and information about the childbearing process are defining characteristics. Taking on the responsibility to gain knowledge in pregnancy and using that knowledge toward shared decision-making with a prenatal care provider increases confidence for physiologic childbirth (Avery et al., 2014; Grigg et al., 2015; Neerland, 2018).

Life events, circumstances, and resources that set the stage for the development of confidence for physiologic birth include arising uncertainties, sources of information and preparation, social support, shared birth stories, feeling prepared/equipped for childbirth, continuity of prenatal care, confidence in the system or place of birth, and a trusted relationship with a maternity care provider, including quality, respectful communication, and shared decision-making. Arising uncertainties, although sometimes a hindrance, can also lead to increased confidence.

Pregnancy can be accompanied by many uncertainties for pregnant and birthing people, including uncertainty about the pregnancy diagnosis, fetal growth and development, and the process of labor and birth. Uncertainty can prompt individuals to seek new knowledge and information, which has the potential to enhance childbirth confidence (Borrelli et al., 2018; Luyben & Fleming, 2005). Many sources of information are used to gain confidence for birth, including books, the Internet, prenatal education classes, healthcare providers, and friends (Catling-Paull et al., 2011; Sanders & Crozier, 2018). Previous experiences are an important source of information as well as friends and relatives (Edmonds et al., 2015; Stoll & Hall, 2013). Social support including understanding, caring, and information-giving from partners, midwives, and other perinatal care providers increases one's sense of control and security (Howarth et al., 2010).

The physical labor environment can enhance or diminish confidence and anxiety. Most laboring patients prefer a private, calm, relaxing environment with attendants who maintain a calm atmosphere in the room (Attanasio et al., 2014; Catling-Paull et al., 2011; Neerland & Skalisky, 2022). People gain confidence when they have confidence in the system or the birth setting of their choice (Attanasio et al., 2014; Catling-Paull et al., 2011; Grigg et al., 2015). A trusted relationship with a perinatal care provider is important in increasing confidence for birth (Grigg et al., 2015; Catling-Paull et al., 2011, Saftner et al., 2017). People with confidence for birth at home or a birth center describe a trusting relationship with their midwives that included respect, closeness, expertise, information sharing, and a positive approach to birth (Grigg et al., 2015; Leap et al., 2010; Neerland & Skalisky, 2022) and may search for a provider who will provide information, choices, shared decision-making, and encouragement (Luyben & Fleming, 2005). Those who receive care within a culturally centered birth center model have higher levels of autonomy and feel more respect from the care team, with less variance in experience for Black, Indigenous, and people of color (BIPOC) individuals, suggesting that this model may offer enhanced childbirth experiences (Almanza et al., 2022).

Taking the responsibility to gain knowledge in pregnancy and using that knowledge toward shared decision-making with a prenatal care provider increases confidence for physiologic childbirth (Avery et al., 2014; Grigg et al., 2015). When pregnant and birthing people feel confident about childbirth, they have a belief in themselves that they can achieve a physiologic birth, manage labor pain and discomfort, have a decreased fear of childbirth, and have a high level of satisfaction with the childbirth experience.

Evidence Related to Prenatal Confidence for Physiologic Birth

Pregnant people prepare for labor and birth in a variety of ways. Childbirth education courses have been a mainstay recommendation made by perinatal healthcare providers over many decades. These courses often include a series of weekly classes that typically occur later in pregnancy to provide pregnant people and support persons with information about labor and birth, the postpartum period, and newborn care. One goal of childbirth education is to provide information that fosters a person's ability to reduce fears surrounding childbirth and to cope with childbirth pain. Some studies suggest that antenatal classes can reduce fear of pregnancy (Gökçe İsbir et al., 2016) and postpartum stress, increase confidence to handle labor and birth (Brixval et al., 2016), and decrease interventions such as epidural use and cesarean birth (Hong et al., 2021), yet benefits of childbirth education classes vary by the curriculum offered and remain largely unexplored.

There is scarce research related to specific actions prenatal care providers can take to help pregnant people feel confident about physiologic labor and birth during the prenatal period (Avery et al., 2014). Qualitative explorations of prenatal care experiences and how those helped during labor and birth suggest that patients are more confident or able to act on their own behalf when they experience a respectful relationship with their provider in which information is provided to them (Avery et al., 2019; Brown, 1998; Coughlan & Jung, 2005; Leap et al., 2010) and where they can participate in decisions about their care (Coughlan & Jung, 2005; Leap et al., 2010). Connections with other pregnant people are also perceived as increasing confidence for labor and birth (Leap et al., 2010). Confidence increases among nulliparas as pregnancy progresses and birth approaches, most likely due to increased knowledge of a variety of coping methods (Kish, 2003).

Discussions about a person's risk for certain conditions or situations can decrease confidence in pregnancy in general. Prenatal care providers want to share evidence related to risk for certain conditions yet struggle to balance that information without overstating dangers during pregnancy and increasing fear. Prenatal care providers feel office time is too limited to thoroughly discuss all pregnancy risks; that using words other than "risk" and acknowledging the limits of applying research results to individual people can help reduce fears and help balance the information; and that balance is needed to avoid unnecessary technology use (Van Wagner, 2016). Information is often provided to patients without a concomitant message that pregnancy is safer than ever. Prenatal care providers need to be cautious about presenting pregnancy as inherently risky and help pregnant people and their support persons build their confidence in the physiologic process of pregnancy and birth (Bisits, 2016). Providers can communicate their own confidence in the normalcy of pregnancy, labor, and birth, which contributes to confidence for birth and feeling on the "same page" with the care team (Avery et al., 2019).

Examining approaches to home and birth center birth care can provide some understanding about childbirth confidence because home and birth center birth by its very nature represents a low intervention type of childbearing experience for individuals at low risk of complications. Preparation and planning for labor and birth during pregnancy in partnership with support persons and providers increase confidence for an out-of-hospital labor and birth (Lothian, 2010). In one study, women who chose a midwife-led freestanding birth center expressed confidence in their choice of birth environment, their ability to give birth, and the birth process (Grigg et al., 2015). Further, women who birthed in birth centers identified that the calm homelike environment, longer unrushed visits, and respectful care in birth centers led to feelings of confidence for physiologic birth (Neerland & Skalisky, 2022). Planning for physiologic birth is a major focus of prenatal care for people who choose to give birth in a birth center or at home because the options available to cope with labor are nonpharmacologic, physiologic approaches because labor induction and augmentation, and epidural analgesia are not available in these environments. Therefore, careful planning and discussions with the healthcare team, including nutrition, physical activity, sleep, attention to emotional health, and support systems, are critical so that pregnant people are in the best health possible when labor begins. In addition, careful planning for labor includes discussions about an individual's preferences for labor support techniques, the makeup of their labor support team, plans for transport in emergent situations, and conditions that may necessitate a change in birth environment.

Enhancing Confidence for Physiologic Birth

Prenatal care practices to enhance confidence for physiologic birth are organized into those that can occur within the broader healthcare system, those that can occur during prenatal care visits, and variable strategies and supports based on individual preferences.

Healthcare System Supports

Healthcare system supports that may enhance confidence for physiologic birth include examining payment and other financial and social incentives to focus on increasing vaginal births and decreasing unnecessary labor and birth interventions with their attendant risks, such as elective labor inductions and elective cesareans. Labor unit staff can examine their processes to ensure that when a birthing person plans a physiologic approach to their labor and birth, comfort measures in labor are provided and staff are experienced with their use. These include adequate nurse staffing to allow for continuous labor support, the use of intermittent auscultation for fetal heart rate monitoring, hydrotherapy, and other nonpharmacologic measures that promote comfort and physiologic processes. Clinics and hospitals can also ensure that their clinical environments and communications include images, positive messaging, and educational materials that support a physiologic approach.

Administrative and multidisciplinary support for promoting physiologic labor and birth when appropriate and consistent with patients' wishes is critical for this philosophy to be consistently implemented. Support for full-scope, integrated midwifery practice within health systems is also important, given the consistency between midwifery practice, physiologic birth, and improved outcomes including the potential to reduce healthcare disparities for Black birthing people (Vedam et al., 2018). Critically important to improving equity in childbirth is increasing the diversity of the perinatal care workforce. Representative and culturally congruent care may lead to increased quality care (Kozhimannil et al., 2021).

Prenatal Care Strategies

Potential enhancements to prenatal care include group prenatal care, periodic group sessions for pregnant people organized by providers, and longer individual, education-focused visits at certain points in pregnancy. These variations compared to the more common individual 10–15 minute visits could be used to discuss integrative therapies, provide yoga or other integrative classes, meet additional providers in the practice who may attend the person's birth, and discuss preparation for physiologic birth including support and coping measures for labor and planning for assembling a labor support team.

Sessions dedicated to providing information on the benefits of physiologic birth and labor-coping strategies can increase confidence in an individual's ability to give birth (Ip et al., 2009). Initiating prenatal care with a discussion about hopes and plans for pregnancy and birth, recording important items in the health record to aid care continuity, and making time to address those topics throughout the pregnancy can be helpful. Providers can start each visit by identifying the most important topics to the client and focusing on those first, then completing required assessments and using purposeful supportive language about their strength and providing appropriate positive responses to their self-care. Members of group practices can develop plans for supporting physiologic birth consistently as a group to provide pregnant people with the continuity they desire and that providers wish to offer. Finally, group strategies to improve consistency across care providers, such as group chart reviews and effective use of the electronic health record, can enhance the client's experience of feeling that the care team is "on the same page."

Individual Strategies

Talking with pregnant people about their level of confidence regarding childbirth with a focus on providing information and developing a trusting relationship can facilitate the development of childbirth confidence. Providers can offer guidance about how to respond to negative birth stories and any other communication in the person's environment that may cause concern. Specific recommendations for resources of interest to each person such as integrative therapies like mindfulness, relaxation techniques, yoga, aromatherapy, acupressure or acupuncture, breastfeeding resources in the health system, and links to community resources for additional support outside the health system are valuable. Purposeful focus on family and friends that are part of the person's support team and including them in the prenatal care process will be beneficial as they prepare for labor and birth. Helping a person decide who they would like to be present for birth, what roles support people might play, and inviting those individuals to attend a prenatal visit or special sessions offered by a health system to discuss and demonstrate labor support techniques is an important strategy to foster the inclusion of the family. Doulas are also a valuable source of information and support, leading to confidence for birth (Avery et al., 2019). Including doulas as part of the labor support team and providing community resources to assist clients in accessing doulas should be discussed prenatally. Comfort measures, such as the use of birth and peanut balls, ambulation, water immersion, massage, aromatherapy, and music, can be offered during labor and birth. Birth and peanut balls are large inflatable balls that can be used for upright mobility or for positioning in bed for comfort and to aid labor progress. Tangible help and practical strategies can enhance confidence.

All persons, whether they specifically request a low intervention or physiologic labor and birth, deserve care that is respectful of their values and preferences and focuses on enhancing their confidence for their birth experience. While 59% of women agree or strongly agree that birth should not be interfered with unless necessary, 73% reported using epidural analgesia (Butwick et al., 2018). An approach aimed at promoting confidence prenatally may result in some persons choosing to labor physiologically, while others will choose an epidural in advance or find it a helpful intervention in certain labors. Many of these strategies can be used with all pregnant and laboring people to improve their childbirth experience regardless of individual childbirth choices.

Summary

Pregnancy, labor, and birth are physiologic processes that can proceed in most cases with support, monitoring, and education from perinatal care providers and a broader network, with minimal medical intervention. Preparation during pregnancy for those who prefer a physiologic approach to labor and birth should be included in prenatal care visits, individualizing as appropriate for each person. Taking time to understand each individual's values, hopes for their pregnancy and birth, and supporting them in ways that increase their confidence for labor and birth can be incorporated into care, while research is conducted to provide additional evidence for this approach to care. Perinatal care providers and pregnant people and their families can advocate for system and policy changes to provide individualized and equitable prenatal care, focused on supporting a physiologic approach to care.

Resources for Clients and Their Families

Six Care Practices that Support Healthy Birth: http://www.lamaze.org/HealthyBirthPractices
Evidence Based Birth: https://evidencebasedbirth.com

Resources for Healthcare Providers

America College of Nurse-Midwives. Healthy birth initiative: http://www.midwife.org/ACNM-Healthy-Birth-Initiative
America College of Nurse-Midwives, Share with women handout: Writing a birth plan: https://onlinelibrary.wiley.com/doi/10.1111/jmwh.12192
ACOG. (2019). Committee Opinion No. 766: Approaches to limit intervention during labor and birth. *Obstetrics & Gynecology, 33(2)*, e164–173.
Adams, E. D., Stark, M. A., & Low, L. K. (2016). A nurse's guide to supporting physiologic birth. *Nursing for Women's Health, 20*(1), 76–86.

Strategies to enhance confidence for physiologic birth

System-Level Supports

- High-level administrative support for physiologic birth
- Payment and rewards aligned with outcomes over volume
- Staff education to routinely support physiologic labor and birth for people choosing that approach
- Staff education on care practices that support physiologic labor and birth (e.g., ambulation, labor support, use of intermittent auscultation, and equipment such as birth balls)
- Clinic messaging and environment that support people's ability to birth including artwork and educational materials
- Administrative support for time for extended prenatal visits and group sessions
- Cultural respect and humility as the norm throughout the health system
- Recruit and retain diverse multidisciplinary workforce
- Support for full-scope midwifery services

Prenatal Care Strategies

- Group prenatal care to optimize social support
- Group classes to discuss labor and birth and to provide specific labor-coping techniques
- Longer prenatal visits to discuss birth preparation, support team, comfort measures, and tools to support coping and physiologic birth
- Encourage the use of a doula or continuous labor support person

Individual Care Strategies

- Assess individual level of confidence for physiologic birth
- Assess and promote optimal social support, birth team support
- Provide information on the benefits of physiologic birth
- Discuss any concerns or fears, previous birth experiences, and positive and negative birth stories
- Encourage reading or listening to podcasts about positive birth stories
- Allow adequate time for discussing labor and birth processes and individual birth preferences
- Specific individualized options provided such as books/videos/other resources supporting physiologic birth, specific classes such as yoga, hypnobirthing, and mindfulness

References

Almanza, J. I., Karbeah, J., Tessier, K. M., Neerland, C., Stoll, K., Hardeman, R. R., & Vedam, S. (2022). The impact of culturally-centered care on peripartum experiences of autonomy and respect in community birth centers: A comparative study. *Maternal & Child Health Journal, 26*, 895–904. https://doi.org/10.1007/s10995-021-03245-w

American College of Nurse-Midwives (ACNM); Midwives Alliance of North America (MANA); National Association of Certified Professional Midwives (NACPM). (2012). Supporting healthy and normal physiologic childbirth: A consensus statement by the American College of Nurse-Midwives, Midwives Alliance of North America, and the National Association of Certified Professional Midwives. *Journal of Midwifery & Women's Health, 57*(5), 529–532.

American College of Obstetricians and Gynecologists (ACOG). (2017, reaffirmed 2021). Committee opinion no. 766: Approaches to limit intervention during labor and birth. *Obstetrics & Gynecology, 133*(2), e164–e173.

Association of Women's Health, Obstetric and Neonatal Nurses (AWHONN). (2011). Quality patient care in labor and delivery: A call to action. *Journal of Midwifery & Women's Health, 41*, 151–153.

Association of Women's Health, Obstetric and Neonatal Nurses (AWHONN). (2014). Non-medically indicated induction and augmentation of labor. *Journal of Obstetric, Gynecologic & Neonatal Nursing, 43*(5), 678–681.

Association of Women's Health, Obstetric and Neonatal Nurses (AWHONN). (2015). Fetal heart monitoring. *Journal of Obstetric, Gynecologic, & Neonatal Nursing, 44*, 683–686.

Attanasio, L. B., McPherson, M. E., & Kozhimannil, K. B. (2014). Positive childbirth experiences in US hospitals: A mixed methods analysis. *Maternal and Child Health Journal, 18*(5), 1280–1290.

Avery, M. D., Neerland, C. E., & Saftner, M. A. (2019). Women's perceptions of prenatal influences on maternal confidence for physiologic birth. *Journal of Midwifery & Women's Health, 64*(2), 201–208. https://doi.org/10.1111/jmwh.12897

Avery, M. D., Saftner, M. A., Larson, B., & Weinfurter, E. V. (2014). A systematic review of maternal confidence for physiologic birth: Characteristics of prenatal care and confidence measurement. *Journal of Midwifery & Women's Health, 59*(6), 586–595.

Bandura, A. (1977). Self-efficacy: Toward a unifying theory of behavioral change. *Psychological Review, 84*(2), 191–215.

Bartick, M. C., Schwarz, E. B., Green, B. D., Jegier, B. J., Reinhold, A. G., Colaizy, T. T., Bogen, D. L., Schaefer, A. J., & Stuebe, A. M. (2017). Suboptimal breastfeeding in the United States: Maternal and pediatric health outcomes and costs. *Maternal & Child Nutrition, 13*(1), e12366. https://doi.org/10.1111/mcn.12366

Benyamini, Y., Molcho, M. L., Dan, U., Gozlan, M., & Preis, H. (2017). Women's attitudes towards the medicalization of childbirth and their associations with planned and actual modes of birth. *Women and Birth, 30*(5), 424–430.

Bisits, A. (2016). Risk in obstetrics—Perspectives and reflections. *Midwifery, 38*(2016), 12–13.

Bohren, M. A., Hofmeyr, G. J., Sakala, C., Fukuzawa, R. K., & Cuthbert, A. (2017). Continuous support for women during childbirth. *Cochrane Database of Systematic Reviews, 7*, CD003766.pub6. https://doi.org/10.1002/14651858.CD003766.pub6

Borrelli, S. E., Walsh, D., & Spiby, H. (2018). First-time mothers' expectations of the unknown territory of childbirth: Uncertainties, coping strategies and 'going with the flow'. *Midwifery, 63*, 39–45. https://doi.org/10.1016/j.midw.2018.04.022

Boston Women's Health Book Collective. (2008). *Our bodies, ourselves: Pregnancy and birth.* Simon & Schuster.

Brixval, C. S., Axelsen, S. F., Thygesen, L. C., Due, P., & Koushede, V. (2016). Antenatal education in small classes may increase childbirth self-efficacy: Results from a Danish randomised trial. *Sexual & Reproductive Healthcare, 10*, 32–34.

Brown, C. E. (1998). Women and their care providers: An exploration of knowledge, confidence, and relationships in the context of childbearing and childbirth. *Birth Issues, 7*(3), 95–100.

Butwick, A. J., Bentley, J., Wong, C. A., Snowden, J. M., Sun, E., & Guo, N. (2018). United States state-level variation in the use of neuraxial analgesia during labor for pregnant women. *JAMA Network Open, 1*(8), e186567. https://doi.org/10.1001/jamanetworkopen.2018.6567

Catling-Paull, C., Dahlen, H., & Homer, C. C. (2011). Multiparous women's confidence to have a publicly funded homebirth: A qualitative study. *Women and Birth, 24*(3), 122–128.

Centers for Medicaid & Medicare Services. (2023). *National health expenditure fact sheet.* https://www.cms.gov/research-statistics-data-and-systems/statistics-trends-and-reports/nationalhealthexpenddata/nhe-fact-sheet

Chen, A., Oster, E., & Williams, H. (2016). Why is infant mortality higher in the United States than in Europe? *American Economic Journal. Economic Policy, 8*(2), 89–124. https://doi.org/10.1257/pol.20140224

Coughlan, R., & Jung, K. E. (2005). New mothers' experiences of agency during prenatal and delivery care: Clinical practice, communication and embodiment. *Journal of Prenatal & Perinatal Psychology & Health, 20*(2), 99.

Cragin, L., & Kennedy, H. P. (2006). Linking obstetric and midwifery practice with optimal outcomes. *Journal of Obstetric, Gynecologic & Neonatal Nursing, 35*(6), 779–785.

Dick-Read, G. (2013). *Childbirth without fear: The principles and practice of natural childbirth.* Pinter & Martin.

Douthard, R. A., Martin, I. K., Chapple-McGruder, T., Langer, A., & Chang, S. (2021). U.S. maternal mortality within a global context: Historical trends, current state, and future directions. *Journal of Women's Health, 30*(2), 168–177. https://doi.org/10.1089/jwh.2020.8863

Edmonds, J. K., Cwiertniewicz, T., & Stoll, K. (2015). Childbirth education prior to pregnancy? Survey findings of childbirth preferences and attitudes among young women. *Journal Perinatal Education, 24*(2), 93–101.

Goer, H., Romano, A., & Sakala, C. (2012). *Vaginal or cesarean birth: What is at stake for women and babies? A best evidence review.* Childbirth Connection.

Gregory, K., Jackson, S., Korst, L., & Fridman, M. (2012). Cesarean versus vaginal delivery: Whose risks? Whose benefits? *American Journal of Perinatology, 29*(01), 7–18.

Grigg, C. P., Tracy, S. K., Schmied, V., Daellenbach, R., & Kensington, M. (2015). Women's birthplace decision-making, the role of confidence: Part of the evaluating maternity units study, New Zealand. *Midwifery, 31*(6), 597–605.

Healthcare Cost and Utilization Project (HCUP). (2022). *Healthcare cost and utilization project.* https://www.hcup-us.ahrq.gov

HealthyPeople 2030. (n.d.). *Pregnancy and childbirth.* https://health.gov/healthypeople/objectives-and-data/browse-objectives/pregnancy-and-childbirth

Hodnett, E. (2002). Pain and women's satisfaction with the experience of childbirth: A systematic review. *American Journal of Obstetrics & Gynecology, 186*(5), S160–S172.

Hong, K., Hwang, H., Han, H., Chae, J., Choi, J., Jeong, Y., Lee, J., & Lee, K. J. (2021). Perspectives on antenatal education associated with pregnancy outcomes: Systematic review and meta-analysis. *Women and Birth: Journal of the Australian College of Midwives, 34*(3), 219–230. https://doi.org/10.1016/j.wombi.2020.04.002

Howarth, A., Swain, N., & Treharne, G. (2010). A review of psychosocial predictors of outcome in labour and childbirth. *New Zealand College of Midwives, 42*, 17–20.

Hoyert, D. L. (2022). *Maternal mortality rates in the United States, 2020.* National Center for Health Statistics Health E-Stats. https://doi.org/10.15620/cdc:113967

Hyde, M. J., Mostyn, A., Modi, N., & Kemp, P. R. (2012). The health implications of birth by caesarean section. *Biological Reviews, 87*(1), 229–243.

ICM Position Statements. (2014). *Keeping birth normal.* https://internationalmidwives.org/assets/files/statement-files/2018/04/keeping-birth-normal-eng.pdf

Ip, W. Y., Tang, C. S., & Goggins, W. B. (2009). An educational intervention to improve women's ability to cope with childbirth. *Journal of Clinical Nursing, 18*(15), 2125–2135.

Isbir, G. G., Inci, F., Onal, H., & Yildiz, P. D. (2016). The effects of antenatal education on fear of childbirth, maternal self-efficacy and post-traumatic stress disorder (PTSD) symptoms following childbirth: An experimental study. *Applied Nursing Research, 32*, 227–232. https://doi.org/10.1016/j.apnr.2016.07.013

Johantgen, M., Fountain, L., Zangaro, G., Newhouse, R., Stanik-Hutt, J., & White, K. (2012). Comparison of labor and delivery care provided by certified nurse-midwives and physicians: A systematic review, 1990 to 2008. *Women's Health Issues, 22*(1), E73–E81.

Kish, J.A. (2003). *The development of maternal confidence for labor among nulliparous pregnant women.* [Doctoral dissertation, University of Maryland]. Digital Repository at the University of Maryland.

https://drum.lib.umd.edu/bitstream/handle/1903/275/dissertation.pdf?sequence=1

Kozhimannil, K. B., Almanza, J., Hardeman, R., & Karbeah, J. (2021). Racial and ethnic diversity in the nursing workforce: A focus on maternity care. *Policy, Politics, & Nursing Practice, 22*(3), 170–179. https://doi.org/10.1177/15271544211005719

Leap, N., Sandall, J., Buckland, S., & Huber, U. (2010). Journey to confidence: Women's experiences of pain in labour and relational continuity of care. *Journal of Midwifery & Women's Health, 55*(3), 234–242.

Lothian, J. A. (2010). How do women who plan homebirth prepare for childbirth? *The Journal of Perinatal Education, 19*(3), 62–67.

Lowe, N. K. (1993). Maternal confidence for labor: Development of the Childbirth Self-Efficacy Inventory. *Research in Nursing & Health, 16*(2), 141–149.

Lowe, N. K. (2000). Self-efficacy for labor and childbirth fears in nulliparous pregnant women. *Journal of Psychosomatic Obstetrics and Gynecology, 21*(4), 219–224.

Luyben, A. G., & Fleming, V. E. (2005). Women's needs from antenatal care in three European countries. *Midwifery, 21*(3), 212–223.

Mathews, T. J., Driscoll, A. K. (2017). *Trends in infant mortality in the United States, 2005–2014.* National Center for Health Statistics (U.S.). *NCHS Data Brief* no. 279, 2017–1209 https://stacks.cdc.gov/view/cdc/45082

Moore, B. J., Freeman, W. J., & Jiang, H. J. (2019). Costs of pediatric hospital stays, 2016. *HCUP Statistical Brief, 250,* 1–12. https://www.ncbi.nlm.nih.gov/books/NBK547762/

Moore, E. R., Bergman, N., Anderson, G. C., & Medley, N. (2016). Early skin-to-skin contact for mothers and their healthy newborn infants. *Cochrane Database of Systematic Reviews, 11,* CD003519. https://doi.org/10.1002/14651858.CD003519.pub4

Neerland, C. (2018). Maternal confidence for physiologic birth: A concept analysis. *Journal of Midwifery & Women's Health, 63*(4), 425–435. https://doi-org.ezp3.lib.umn.edu/10.1111/jmwh.12719

Neerland, C. E., & Skalisky, A. E. (2022). A qualitative study of US women's perspectives on confidence in the birth center model of prenatal care. *Journal of Midwifery & Women's Health, 67*(4), 435–441. https://doi.org/10.1111/jmwh.13349

Osterman, M. J. K., Hamilton, B. E., Martin, J. A., Driscoll, A. K., & Valenzuela, C. P. (2022). Births: Final data for 2020. *National Vital Statistics Reports, 70*(17). https://doi.org/10.15620/cdc:112078

Roosevelt, L., & Low, L. K. (2016). Exploring fear of childbirth in the United States through a qualitative assessment of the Wijma Delivery Expectancy Questionnaire. *Journal of Obstetric, Gynecologic & Neonatal Nursing, 45*(1), 28–38.

Saftner, M. A., Neerland, C., & Avery, M. D. (2017). Enhancing women's confidence for physiologic birth: Maternity care providers' perspectives. *Midwifery, 53,* 28–34.

Sakala, C., Declercq, E., Turon, J., & Corry, M. (2018). *Listening to mothers in California: A population-based survey of women's childbearing experiences, full survey report.* National Partnership for Women & Families. https://www.chcf.org/wp-content/uploads/2018/09/ListeningMothersCAFullSurveyReport2018.pdf

Sandall, J., Tribe, R. M., Avery, L., Mola, G., Visser, G. H., Homer, C. S., Gibbons, D., Kelly, N. M., Kennedy, H. P., Kidanto, H., Taylor, P., & Temmerman, M. (2018). Short-term and long-term effects of caesarean section on the health of women and children. *Lancet, 392*(10155), 1349–1357. https://doi.org/10.1016/S0140-6736(18)31930-5

Sanders, R. A., & Crozier, K. (2018). How do informal information sources influence women's decision-making for birth? A meta-synthesis of qualitative studies. *BMC Pregnancy and Childbirth, 18,* 21. https://doi.org/10.1186/s12884-017-1648-2

Sanjari, S., Chaman, R., Salehin, S., Goli, S., & Keramat, A. (2022). Update on the global prevalence of severe fear of childbirth in low-risk pregnant women: A systematic review and meta-analysis. *International Journal of Women's Health and Reproduction Sciences, 10*(1), 3–10. https://doi.org/10.15296/ijwhr.2022.02

Schwarz, E. B., & Nothnagle, M. (2015). The maternal health benefits of breastfeeding. *American Family Physician, 91*(9), 603–604.

Stoll, K., & Hall, W. (2013). Vicarious birth experiences and childbirth fear: Does it matter how young Canadian women learn about birth? *The Journal of Perinatal Education, 22*(4), 226–233.

Tikkanen, R. Gunja, M.Z., FitzGerald, M. & Zephyrin, L. (2020). *Maternal mortality and maternity care in the United States compared to 10 other developed countries.* Commonwealth Fund. https://www.commonwealthfund.org/publications/issue-briefs/2020/nov/maternal-mortality-maternity-care-us-compared-10-countries

Tilden, E. L., Caughey, A. B., Lee, C. S., & Emeis, C. (2016). The effect of childbirth self-efficacy on perinatal outcomes. *Journal of Obstetric, Gynecologic & Neonatal Nursing, 45*(4), 465–480.

Truven Health Analytics. (2013). *The cost of having a baby in the United States.* Truven Health Analytics.

Van Wagner, V. (2016). Risk talk: Using evidence without increasing fear. *Midwifery, 38,* 21–28.

Vedam, S., Stoll, K., MacDorman, M., Declercq, E., Cramer, R., Cheyney, M., Fisher, T., Butt, E., Yang, Y. T., & Kennedy, H. P. (2018). Mapping integration of midwives across the United States: Impact on access, equity, and outcomes. *PLoS One, 13*(2), e0192523. http://doi.org/10.1371/journal.pone.0192523

World Health Organization (WHO). (1996). *Care in normal birth: A practical guide.* Department of Reproductive Health and Research. World Health Organisation.

28

Triage during Pregnancy

Catherine Ruhl

Relevant Terms

Acuity—seriousness of a person's condition
Acuity index—tool to classify acuity
Disposition—outcome of triage and evaluation in terms of the decision for either admission or discharge
Emergency Medical Treatment and Labor Act—federal law enacted in 1986, assures access to emergency healthcare regardless of the ability to pay
Emergency Severity Index (ESI)—a five-level acuity classification system for triage, can be applied to adults and children, used in emergency departments
Evaluation—the healthcare provider's clinical assessment of a person's condition after assignment of acuity
Maternal Fetal Triage Index (MFTI)—a five-level acuity classification system for triage that can be applied to the pregnant person and fetus(es)
Medical screening examination (MSE)—a medical exam done to determine if there is an emergency condition
Triage in pregnancy—systematic, brief maternal and fetal assessments which determine a pregnant person's acuity and priority for full evaluation
Qualified medical person (QMP)—the provider who performs the medical screening exam. The QMP may be a physician, a midwife (CNM/CM), nurse practitioner (NP), physician assistant (PA) or a registered nurse (RN) who meets criteria set out by the hospital's credentialing committee.
Throughput—moving clients through processes of care
Triage—the process of assigning the level of urgency of a person's condition and their need for evaluation, treatment and healthcare resources

Introduction

Triage is a process first described in the early 1800s on the battlefields in France, used to decide priorities for the care of injured soldiers (Robertson-Steel, 2006). The concepts of triage are still applied to battlefields, mass casualties and disasters, and in hospital emergency settings to prioritize care and resources based on acuity. Since the beginning of the twenty-first century, separate and distinct pregnancy triage and evaluation units have become more common within hospital settings, and there has been a focus on defining the purposes of these units and improving triage care. The need for pregnancy triage units was spurred by a need to better utilize hospital resources and decrease the amount of client turnover in labor units, decrease unneeded admissions to labor units, minimize wait times, concentrate on appropriate and timely maternal and fetal assessment, and promote more rapid response when people arrive with pregnancy emergencies (Angelini, 2013). The Institute of Medicine's (2001) report "Crossing the Quality Chasm: A New Health System for the 21st Century" lists six goals for healthcare that are aptly applied to triage and evaluation in maternity care. These goals are to provide healthcare that is safe, effective, patient-centered, timely, efficient, and equitable.

Health equity key points

- Triage unit clients often feel vulnerable when they are experiencing emergent healthcare needs; those who identify as belonging to marginalized groups may feel especially vulnerable.
- Acuity classification tools, also called **acuity indexes**, have potential to reduce bias in decision-making about care priority.

Objectives and Goals of Triage Care and Evaluation

The initial minutes and hours of care in triage settings serving pregnant and postpartum people provide opportunities for healthcare providers to positively influence subsequent interactions, care, and outcomes. These opportunities include:

- Efficient initial assessment of a person's presenting condition and classification of their **acuity**, so appropriate resources and treatment can be provided in a timely manner.

Prenatal and Postnatal Care: A Person-Centered Approach, Third Edition. Edited by Karen Trister Grace, Cindy L. Farley, Noelene K. Jeffers, and Tanya Tringali.
© 2024 John Wiley & Sons Ltd. Published 2024 by John Wiley & Sons Ltd.
Companion website: www.wiley.com/go/grace/prenatal

- Nonbiased application of triage acuity tools to equitably prioritize care across groups and populations.
- Identification of a person's needs and strengths, including coping and family dynamics.
- Identification of perinatal risk factors.
- Setting a person on a path of care (especially important for a person with comorbidities).
- Positively influencing a person's subsequent care in the facility if care in the triage unit is perceived as safe and welcoming.
- Providing sensitive and nonbiased care. Triage unit clients often feel vulnerable when they are experiencing urgent or emergent healthcare needs; those who identify as belonging to marginalized groups may feel especially vulnerable.
- Setting the stage for physiologic labor and birth by helping people understand early labor processes and coping strategies.

Prenatal and Postpartum Triage in the Hospital Setting

Most prenatal and postpartum triage occurs within a hospital setting, either in the main emergency department (ED), the labor and birth suite, or in a dedicated triage and **evaluation** area of a hospital maternity unit. Regardless of triage location, the need for timely and efficient person-focused care is the same.

Triage in hospital settings involves collecting relevant patient information needed to assign acuity and determine which patients cannot wait for full medical evaluation (ACOG, 2016; Emergency Nurses Association, 2023). Typical triage protocols guide the initial assessment and decisions about the priority level for clinical evaluation. This initial assessment may be conducted by a registered nurse (RN), midwife, nurse practitioner (NP), physician assistant (PA), or physician depending on the institution's model of care. The healthcare team member performing triage typically assigns the person's acuity during the first encounter. **Triage in pregnancy** is followed by the complete evaluation of the person and the fetus by a healthcare provider with appropriate skills and training for evaluating the pertinent issues identified during triage. Within perinatal care units, an RN often performs the initial assessment in the triage area. The Association of Women's Health, Obstetric and Neonatal Nurses (AWHONN) defines triage in perinatal settings as the initial assessment of the person and fetus(es) by the RN consistent with the term triage in main ED settings, meaning, RNs perform the initial assessment and assign acuity (Ruhl et al., 2015a). This distinguishes triage from a full evaluation and plan for management by the maternity provider. There are maternity units where nurses are credentialed to perform both triage and the full evaluation, depending on the person's clinical condition, and then consult the provider about management and **disposition**. This arrangement is more likely when providers are not on site or nearby and are not able to provide expeditious evaluation and management.

Primary Responsibilities of Professionals during Triage and Evaluation

- **Registered nurse**: Initial assessment and assignment of priority for evaluation based on acuity (triage), and possible need for a higher level of care than the setting provides; reassessing at regular intervals until disposition is decided and assisting with evaluation as directed by the provider.
- **Healthcare provider**: Responding in an appropriate time frame to evaluate people as indicated by prioritization, carry out evaluation, make decisions about observation, admission or discharge, and plan follow-up care.
- **All team members:** Assessing people's needs and strengths and involving them as much as possible throughout triage and evaluation, including in decisions about admission or discharge, ensuring the person and their support people understand and agree with the plan of care during and after triage and evaluation.

Common Reasons People Seek Urgent/Emergent Care during Pregnancy

Pregnant people are often seen in triage and evaluation settings during pregnancy when they have symptoms of labor, either at term or preterm. Other common reasons people seek urgent healthcare during pregnancy include vaginal bleeding, dysuria, abdominal pain, nausea/vomiting, falls, minor motor vehicle accidents, headaches, decreased fetal movement, and vaginal discharge (ACOG, 2016; Kodama et al., 2021). Signs and symptoms of preeclampsia, preterm premature rupture of membranes, and acute abdominal pain are also reported frequently in triage units. Acute and critical conditions, such as motor vehicle collision injury, placental abruption, or seizure, are less common, but they demand immediate attention and management. People presenting for triage who lack access to prenatal care or do not have maternity care insurance coverage present providers with opportunities to connect them with the prenatal care system. Providers can assess critical history components and presence of any chronic medical conditions and can initiate referrals for social services or care for the management of medical conditions. Two categories of common conditions evaluated in obstetric triage that present unique challenges within a triage unit are discussed below. Other conditions commonly evaluated within triage units are covered in more detail in separate chapters.

Threatened or actual miscarriage is a common presenting condition for people seeking urgent care. People experiencing early pregnancy loss need appropriate psychological and physical care. When they are cared for in EDs, the staff may not be prepared to provide the holistic care needed for clients and families. ED professionals may not recognize the grief associated with early pregnancy loss or may not be able to support clients and families in early stages of bereavement (Bacidore et al., 2009; Merrigan, 2018; Punches et al., 2019). An approach informed by a framework for fetal loss that prioritizes the person's need for prompt evaluation, supportive comfort care, compassionate sharing of the news of pregnancy loss, and encouragement for the person and their family to express their feelings, along with coordination of follow-up care can positively affect how they recover from and process miscarriage (Bacidore et al., 2009; National Perinatal Association, 2017).

Postpartum clients are often seen in EDs for conditions that may be a result of childbirth complications but could be overlooked by healthcare providers unfamiliar with perinatal care. Appropriate and timely recognition, assessment, and management of postpartum complications, including preeclampsia, postpartum mood and anxiety disorders, pulmonary embolus or venous thromboembolism, delayed postpartum hemorrhage, cardiac disease, and infection are essential to providing high-quality postpartum triage and care (Chagolla et al., 2013; Glazer et al., 2022). Such recognition and assessment become more critical if a person is taken to a hospital without perinatal services, or if they do not alert the ED staff that they have had a recent childbirth. When a postpartum person who is breastfeeding presents to triage with a complication, appropriate clinical support for the breastfeeding dyad can be lacking in triage and EDs, and infants may not be allowed to remain with the breastfeeding parent. Policies that support the unique needs of postpartum parents and their newborns can enhance quality care.

Collaboration between Perinatal and Emergency Departments

Providing optimal care for clients experiencing complications during both early gestation and postpartum requires collaboration and close communication between emergency and perinatal departments (ACOG, 2016; Chagolla et al., 2013). Institutional policies and algorithms that specify the unit where pregnant and postpartum clients will be evaluated based on clinical condition, appropriate care practices, and guidelines for interdepartmental collaboration have potential to improve client safety and outcomes (Chagolla et al., 2013). When pregnant clients have medical or surgical conditions that have pregnancy implications, they should be evaluated by a perinatal healthcare provider (AAP & ACOG, 2017). Institutions should also have policies addressing interdepartmental collaboration in the care of pregnant clients with highly transmissible infectious diseases (ACOG, 2016).

Obstetric Triage Unit Organization

Pregnancy triage and evaluation units can differ in the model of care. Elements that vary are healthcare provider team, scope of services provided, and types of conditions evaluated.

Examples of obstetric triage unit models

- Hospitalist-staffed units with a mix of providers including physicians, certified nurse-midwives/certified midwives (CNMs/CMs), nurse practitioners (NPs), and PAs
- CNM/CM/NP-led units
- Units in hospitals that have no in-house perinatal providers. RNs triage, evaluate, report findings to providers by phone unless there's an urgent need for a bedside provider, and carry out decisions on disposition as directed by the provider
- Units that include antenatal testing capabilities
- Units that accommodate pregnant clients of all gestations, or only pregnant clients over 16- or 20-week gestation

Perinatal triage and evaluation units are optimal settings for clients and professionals to benefit from collaborative, interprofessional models of care. Midwives have increasingly been utilized in hospital-based pregnancy triage units in the United States in the past 20 years (Angelini & Howard, 2014). Greater client satisfaction and significantly shorter triage unit stays have been demonstrated when midwives managed triage care (Paul et al., 2013). A recent analysis showed that clients admitted in labor by midwives working in a perinatal triage unit were less likely to have oxytocin augmentation, epidural anesthesia for labor, or cesarean births (Breman et al., 2021).

Elements of Triage

If a person reports labor contractions, their discomfort and coping can be assessed via the Coping with Labor Algorithm, version 2, rather than a pain rating of 0–10 (Roberts et al., 2010). This algorithm was developed by nurses and midwives at the University of Utah to provide a pain assessment tool more appropriate for labor than the standard 0–10 pain scale and assess a laboring person as either coping with their labor pain or not coping. The initial triage assessment of the pregnant person includes the following elements (AAP & ACOG, 2017; Ruhl et al., 2015a; Ruhl, 2019).

- The person's reason for presenting for care
- Estimated gestational age
- Status of fetal movement
- Reports of pain: source and pain rating
- Mental status
- Maternal vital signs and SpO_2 by pulse oximetry
- Fetal heart rate, and if contractions present, measured before, during, and after contractions
- Frequency, intensity, and length of contractions
- Coping
- Status of amniotic membranes
- Vaginal bleeding
- Vaginal discharge
- Prenatal care course
- Past pregnancy, gynecologic, medical, and surgical histories
- Social history and substance use
- Allergies

Elements of Healthcare Provider Evaluation

In addition to the initial assessments, provider evaluation elements can include (Ruhl, 2019):

- Review of electronic medical record for past medical and surgical histories, past pregnancy and gynecologic histories, and review of prenatal course
- Interval history to include review of systems, recent sleep and rest, recent food, and fluids
- Allergies
- Medication use
- Recent substance use (nicotine, marijuana, opioids, other drugs, and alcohol)
- Social history
- Presence or absence of support people
- Assessment of coping, anxiety, educational needs
- Discussion of pregnancy complications
- **For clients with symptoms of labor:**
  - Method used to establish gestational age
  - Pelvic exam: cervical dilation, effacement, position, and consistency, assessment of adequacy of pelvis, fetal presentation, and station of the presenting part (unless contraindicated)
  - Confirmation of status of amniotic membranes
  - Abdominal exam: findings of Leopold's maneuvers, including estimated fetal weight and presentation
  - Confirmation of presence or absence of vaginal bleeding
  - Exam of lower extremities for edema and reflexes

Best Practices in Triage Units

Triage Acuity Tools

Prioritizing clients based on acuity and anticipated need for resources is key to promoting efficient, high-quality, and timely care for clients and appropriate use of staff and resources such as lab, imaging, and other ancillary services (ENA, 2023). Using a standardized triage classification tool improves the quality of care (ACEP, 2017).

Classifying a pregnant person's acuity when they present for care is valuable for several reasons that go beyond deciding which clients should be seen first by the provider. It is acknowledged that assigning a priority level for evaluation may be less necessary in a low-volume setting. All settings, regardless of size, can benefit from implementing an acuity tool to standardize the process of triage, enhance communication between nurses and providers, more efficiently mobilize resources for higher acuity clients or their fetus(es), identify potential need for transport in a timely manner, and track acuity trends over time to inform staffing plans.

Acuity classification tools are an objective means of determining priority for evaluation. The value of pregnancy triage tools in reducing biased decision-making about care priority compared to not using a tool has not yet been established. Equitable application of these tools across populations of pregnant clients is another area needing study. Racial disparities have been found in the application of triage tools in pediatric and adult populations (Dennis, 2021, Vigil et al., 2016).

The Maternal Fetal Triage Index

A commonly used tool for triage classification of emergent hospital visits is the **Emergency Severity Index** (ESI), which contains limited pregnancy content (Emergency Nurses Association, 2023). An acuity classification instrument, the **Maternal Fetal Triage Index** (MFTI), was developed specifically for triaging pregnant clients and their fetus(es) in the hospital setting (Ruhl et al., 2015b). The MFTI is the only pregnancy triage acuity classification tool developed for use in the United States with a national panel of multidisciplinary content validators and reliability testers—physicians, midwives, and nurses with expertise in pregnancy triage (Ruhl et al., 2015a). The validity of the MFTI in appropriately prioritizing people with urgent needs so that they can be evaluated expeditiously was demonstrated by Kodama et al. (2021); clients in their study assigned higher priority levels had shorter lengths of triage evaluations. The MFTI is organized as an algorithm (Figure 28.1). Questions on the left for each level of acuity are associated with corresponding exemplary clinical conditions on the right. Vital signs are a key parameter for levels 1, 2, and 3. The initial vital-sign values are used to make the priority level assignment, not subsequently obtained values. Although the MFTI has not been tested for use with postpartum clients, the emphasis on vital signs, elevated blood pressure with or without symptoms of preeclampsia, bleeding, and pain make it relevant to the triage of this population. The MFTI provides common examples of conditions but cannot address all the conditions clients may have. Clinicians must apply critical thinking and clinical judgment for proper use.

Assessment of Pain and Coping in the MFTI

The MFTI assessment of pain is with the 0–10 pain rating scale for nonlabor pain and the Coping with Labor Algorithm, version 2, for the assessment of labor pain (Roberts et al., 2010). This is important because it allows the clinician to distinguish pain not related to labor from that associated with contractions. When people report symptoms such as headaches and epigastric pain, specifying the sources and the pain rating can help the clinician focus on the person's overall condition and potentially prevent missing the diagnosis of emergent conditions. Using the Coping with Labor Algorithm, version 2, for labor pain assessment allows clients and clinicians to understand the multifaceted context of the labor process. This algorithm reinforces a person's coping ability and provides helpful suggestions for clients, their families, and clinicians when a person needs additional support (Roberts et al., 2010).

Relevance of the MFTI for Providers

The nurse, not the healthcare provider, generally assigns client acuity level. Healthcare providers will benefit from knowing if their institutions use an acuity tool,

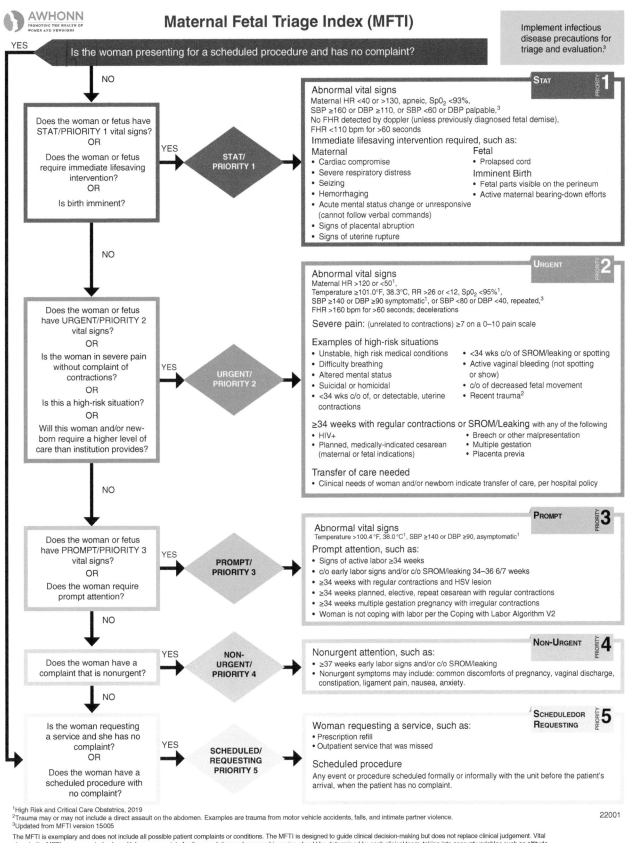

Figure 28.1   The Maternal Fetal Triage Index classification algorithm. AWHONN Maternal Fetal Triage Index (2022). Reprinted with permission from the Association of Women's Health, Obstetric and Neonatal Nurses (AWHONN) (www.awhonn.org).

understanding how a tool works, and the specific conditions and vital-sign parameters for each level. The attention to abnormal vital signs in levels 1, 2, and 3 in the MFTI guides healthcare providers to focus on early warning signs of maternal or fetal distress. The blood pressure parameters in level 2 are consistent with those identified in the American College of Obstetricians and Gynecologists' (2020) practice bulletin on hypertension and preeclampsia in pregnancy. The Alliance for Innovation on Maternal Health (2022) safety bundle on severe hypertension in pregnancy calls for all facilities in the United States where pregnant and postpartum clients may present for care to implement facility-wide processes for timely triage and evaluation of hypertension. The implementation of a pregnancy acuity tool such as the MFTI supports these goals.

Clinical Decision Tools for Triage and Evaluation

Screening tools, decision algorithms, and practice protocols for triage and evaluation can improve documentation, assessment, and overall quality of care, and improve client flow through the unit (Angelini & Howard, 2014; Smithson et al., 2013). The implementation of the MFTI in one hospital reduced time from presentation to the nurse's assignment of acuity from an average of 33 minutes to an average of 6 minutes, and provider response time was reduced on average from 78 to 13 minutes (Ruhl et al., 2020). Triage using decision aids when evaluating clients with preeclampsia and hemorrhage during pregnancy has improved triage assessment and documentation of those conditions (McCarthy et al., 2013). Management protocols for many common presenting conditions in pregnancy triage will be helpful to healthcare providers working in such settings and are found in textbooks devoted to the topic.

Emergency Medical Treatment and Labor Act

The **Emergency Medical Treatment and Labor Act** (EMTALA) is a federal law enacted in 1986 to ensure that patients presenting to emergency care settings are not turned away because of their inability to pay for services. EMTALA applied to pregnant clients requires a **medical screening examination** (MSE) by a **qualified medical person** (QMP), which may be a healthcare provider or RN who meets requirements set by each hospital, to determine whether the person or fetus has an emergency medical condition (Centers for Medicaid and Medicare Services, 2021). The EMTALA requires that the hospital stabilize the person and/or fetus and arrange for transfer to another facility if indicated, if benefits of transfer outweigh risks (Wilson-Griffin, 2021).

Violations of EMTALA regulations can result in penalties for hospitals. Typical violations can include not performing the MSE, or not consulting, treating, or stabilizing and transporting appropriately. A lack of timely response from consultants or a lack of urgency communicated to consultants can also result in penalties (Angelini & Howard, 2014).

Liability Issues in Pregnancy Triage and Evaluation

Key areas of liability concern in triage and evaluation include lack of timeliness in assessments and consultations, sending a person home without establishing fetal well-being, and not diagnosing active labor (Angelini & Howard, 2014). Delays in initial triage can result in critical treatment delays for clients with higher acuity because of conditions like active preterm labor, hemorrhage, or severe hypertension. The time a person arrives to the triage unit and the time a perinatal provider is notified of their status should be documented for every person (AAP & ACOG, 2017). Delays in provider response and not communicating appropriate urgency to providers are critically important areas of liability especially when providers are not on site (Angelini & Mahlmeister, 2005). Other common sources of liability include not identifying or failing to follow up on a nonreassuring fetal heart rate pattern and lack of policies detailing what conditions mandate bedside evaluation by a perinatal provider and discharging clients whose condition is unstable (Angelini & Mahlmeister, 2005; Simpson, 2014).

The triage and evaluation process was the second-most common source of alleged professional liability in obstetrics in a 25-year review by Muraskas et al. (2012), who found that 21% of cases were attributed to failure to triage a pregnant person appropriately. In that review, "triage" referred to the entire process of triage, evaluation, and decisions about disposition. Case examples included misdiagnosis, inaccurate presentation of the case by a triage nurse or house staff when reporting to an attending obstetrician, missing abruption or HELLP syndrome (hemolysis, elevated liver enzymes, and low platelets), not correctly diagnosing ruptured membranes, and sending clients in active labor home. The fourth-most common reason for liability, accounting for 11% of cases, involved delays in transporting a person to a tertiary care center when it was indicated because of extreme prematurity, triplets or higher-order multiples, complicated twin pregnancies, congenital anomalies, and expected difficult births with high-risk neonates.

Clinicians should be aware that clear communication is key to minimizing errors and liability risks throughout the triage and evaluation process, but especially during clinical hand-offs (Angelini & Howard, 2014). All clinicians evaluating clients should be aware of their facility's triage policies on wait times, transports, mobilizing extra staff when needed for emergent clinical cases or excess volume, and timing and extent of the reassessment of clients who present with lower acuity and are awaiting full evaluation.

Quality Measures in Triage

Quality measures addressing **throughput** in EDs focus on median time from arrival to departure from the ED and median time from the decision to admit a client until departure from the ED (AHRQ, 2020). The AWHONN published a draft perinatal quality measure aimed at increasing the percentage of clients who are triaged within 10 minutes of arrival to the unit (AWHONN, 2022). Other relevant measures of timeliness for pregnancy triage and evaluation that individual units may desire to track are time from arrival to disposition, time from completion of triage to disposition, and time from disposition to departure of the client from the triage and evaluation unit.

Anticipatory Guidance about Triage during Prenatal Care

Clients benefit from education during prenatal care on what to expect if they are asked to go to perinatal triage units, and on common reasons why that may be necessary before labor. Clients should know that care is not necessarily provided first come, first served, but that clients with more serious conditions or urgency for care will be given priority. Practical advice such as bringing beverages and snacks and planning for the possibility of waiting and being aware that the triage and evaluation process could take several hours will allow for reasonable expectations. Clients should be advised that it is optimal to discuss the decision to go to the triage unit with their prenatal care providers before arriving. Pregnant and postpartum clients should expect timely triage care and that clinicians will respond to their concerns, support their physical and emotional well-being, appropriately inform them of each step of the process, ensure their comfort with a plan for admission or discharge, and make sure they understand discharge teaching and plans for referrals and follow-up.

Summary

Triage is a process; a triage unit is a place. Pregnancy triage and evaluation units in the twenty-first century are better defined than in the past, and the goals of care are clearer. Clients who receive care in these units deserve the same standards as are maintained in EDs, including acuity-prioritized care in a system that values timely throughput and equitable and efficient use of resources. Pregnancy triage and evaluation units provide midwives, NPs, and other advanced healthcare providers with opportunities to lead interdisciplinary quality initiatives to promote nonbiased care, streamline processes, and partner with clients to improve their satisfaction with care in this critically important area.

Resources for Clients and Their Families

American Federation of Teachers: The Importance of Respectful Maternity Care for Women of Color: https://www.aft.org/hc/spring2021/taylor

New York City Standards for Respectful Care at Birth: https://www1.nyc.gov/assets/doh/downloads/pdf/ms/respectful-care-birth-brochure.pdf

Why is my provider sending me to the hospital birth unit? AWHONN consumer article: https://www.health4mom.org/provider-sending-hospital-birth-unit

Resources for Healthcare Providers

ACOG Committee Opinion 667: *Hospital-based Triage of Obstetric Patients:* https://www.acog.org/clinical/clinical-guidance/committee-opinion/articles/2016/07/hospital-based-triage-of-obstetric-patients

AWHONN Maternal Fetal Triage Index video: https://www.youtube.com/watch?v=apzgT1zpHzg

Emergency Nurses Association. (2023). Emergency Severity Index Handbook 5th Edition. https://enau.ena.org/Listing/e9af283e-444a-43c3-9b1f-70b25b901482

National Perinatal Association: *Interdisciplinary Guidelines for Care of Women Presenting to the Emergency Department with Pregnancy Loss (2017)*: http://www.nationalperinatal.org/interdisciplinary-guidelines

Reinforcement of EMTALA Obligations specific to Patients who are Pregnant or are Experiencing Pregnancy Loss (2022): https://www.cms.gov/medicareprovider-enrollment-and-certificationsurveycertificationgeninfopolicy-and-memos-states-and/reinforcement-emtala-obligations-specific-patients-who-are-pregnant-or-are-experiencing-pregnancy

References

Agency for Healthcare Research and Quality (AHRQ). (2020). *Improving patient flow and reducing emergency department crowding: A guide for hospitals.* https://www.ahrq.gov/research/findings/final-reports/ptflow/section3.html

Alliance for Innovation on Maternal Health. (2022). *Severe hypertension in pregnancy.* https://saferbirth.org/psbs/severe-hypertension-in-pregnancy/

American Academy of Pediatrics (AAP) & American College of Obstetricians and Gynecologists (ACOG). (2017). *Guidelines for perinatal care* (8th ed.). American Academy of Pediatrics (AAP) & American College of Obstetricians and Gynecologists (ACOG).

American College of Emergency Physicians. (2017). *ACEP policy statements: Triage scale standardization.* American College of Emergency Physicians. https://www.acep.org/patient-care/policy-statements/triage-scale-standardization

American College of Obstetricians and Gynecologists (ACOG). (2016). Hospital-based triage of obstetric patients. Committee opinion no. 667. *Obstetrics & Gynecology, 128,* e16–e19.

American College of Obstetricians and Gynecologists (ACOG). (2020). Gestational hypertension and preeclampsia. ACOG practice bulletin no. 222. *Obstetrics & Gynecology, 135,* e237–e260.

Angelini, D., & Howard, E. (2014). Obstetric triage: A systematic review of the past fifteen years: 1998–2013. *MCN: The American Journal of Maternal/Child Nursing, 39*(5), 284–297.

Angelini, D. J. (2013). Overview of obstetric triage and potential pitfalls. In D. Angelini & D. LaFontaine (Eds.), *Obstetric triage and emergency care protocols* (pp. 1–9). Springer Publishing.

Angelini, D. J., & Mahlmeister, L. R. (2005). Liability in triage: Management of EMTALA regulations and common obstetric risks. *Journal of Midwifery & Women's Health, 50*(6), 472–478.

Association of Women's Health, Obstetric and Neonatal Nurses (AWHONN). (2022). *Maternal Fetal Triage Index (MFTI).* AWHONN. www.awhonn.org

Bacidore, V., Warren, N., Chaput, C., & Keough, V. A. (2009). A collaborative framework for managing pregnancy loss in the emergency department. *Journal of Obstetric, Gynecologic, & Neonatal Nursing, 38*(6), 730–738.

Breman, R. B., Phillippi, J. C., Tilden, E., Paul, J., Barr, E., & Carlson, N. (2021). Challenges in the triage care of low-risk laboring patients: A comparison of 2 models of practice. *The Journal of Perinatal & Neonatal Nursing, 35*(2), 123–131.

Centers for Medicaid and Medicare Services. (2021). Emergency Medical Treatment & Labor Act (EMTALA). http://www.cms.gov/regulations-and-guidance/legislation/emtala

Chagolla, B. A., Keats, J. P., & Fulton, J. M. (2013). The importance of interdepartmental collaboration and safe triage for pregnant women in the emergency department. *Journal of Obstetric, Gynecologic, & Neonatal Nursing, 42*(5), 595–605.

Dennis, J. A. (2021). Racial/ethnic disparities in triage scores among pediatric emergency department fever patients. *Pediatric Emergency Care, 37*(12), e1457–e1461.

Emergency Nurses Association. (2023). *Emergency severity index handbook* (5th Ed.). ENA University. https://enau.ena.org/Listing/e9af283e-444a-43c3-9b1f-70b25b901482

Glazer, K. B., Harrell, T., Balbierz, A., & Howell, E. A. (2022). Postpartum hospital readmissions and emergency department visits among high-risk, Medicaid-insured women in new York City. *Journal of Women's Health*. Advance online publication. https://doi.org/10.1089/jwh.2021.0338

Institute of Medicine. (2001). *Crossing the quality chasm: A new health system for the 21st century*. National Academy Press.

Kodama, S., Mokhtari, N. B., Iqbal, S. N., & Kawakita, T. (2021). Evaluation of the maternal-fetal triage index in a tertiary care labor and delivery unit. *American Journal of Obstetrics & Gynecology MFM, 3*(4), 100351.

McCarthy, M., McDonald, S., & Pollock, W. (2013). Triage of pregnant women in the emergency department: Evaluation of a triage decision aid. *Emergency Medicine Journal, 30*(2), 117–122.

Merrigan, J. L. (2018). Educating emergency department nurses about miscarriage. *MCN: The American Journal of Maternal/Child Nursing, 43*(1), 26–31.

Muraskas, J., Ellsworth, L., Culp, E., Garbe, G., & Morrison, J. (2012). Risk management in obstetrics and neonatal-perinatal medicine. In O. Ozdemir (Ed.), *Complementary pediatrics* (pp. 269–286). IntechOpen Ltd.

National Perinatal Association. (2017). *Interdisciplinary guidelines for care of women presenting to the emergency department with pregnancy loss*. https://www.nationalperinatal.org/interdisciplinary-guidelines

Paul, J., Jordan, R., Duty, S., & Engstrom, J. L. (2013). Improving satisfaction with care and reducing length of stay in an obstetric triage unit using a nurse-midwife-managed model of care. *Journal of Midwifery & Women's Health, 58*(2), 175–181.

Punches, B. E., Johnson, K. D., Acquavita, S. P., Felblinger, D. M., & Gillespie, G. L. (2019). Patient perspectives of pregnancy loss in the emergency department. *International Emergency Nursing, 43*, 61–66.

Roberts, L., Gulliver, B., Fisher, J., & Cloves, K. G. (2010). The coping with labor algorithm: An alternate pain assessment tool for the laboring woman. *Journal of Midwifery & Women's Health, 55*(2), 107–116.

Robertson-Steel, I. (2006). Evolution of triage systems. *Emergency Medicine Journal, 23*(2), 154–155.

Ruhl, C. (2019). Obstetric triage tools. In N. H. Troiano, P. M. Witcher, & A. M. Baird (Eds.), *High-risk & critical care obstetrics* (4th ed., pp. 196–197). Wolters Kluwer.

Ruhl, C., Garpiel, S. J., Priddy, P., & Bozeman, L. L. (2020). Obstetric and fetal triage. *Seminars in Perinatology, 44*(4), 151240.

Ruhl, C., Scheich, B., Onokpise, B., & Bingham, D. (2015a). Content validity testing of the maternal fetal triage index. *Journal of Obstetric, Gynecologic, & Neonatal Nursing, 44*(6), 701–709.

Ruhl, C., Scheich, B., Onokpise, B., & Bingham, D. (2015b). Interrater reliability testing of the Maternal Fetal Triage Index. *Journal of Obstetric, Gynecologic, & Neonatal Nursing, 44*(6), 710–716.

Simpson, K. R. (2014). Perinatal patient safety and professional liability issues. In K. R. Simpson & P. A. Creehan (Eds.), *Perinatal nursing* (4th ed., pp. 1–40). Lippincott Williams & Wilkins.

Smithson, D. S., Twohey, R., Rice, T., Watts, N., Fernandes, C. M., & Gratton, R. J. (2013). Implementing an obstetric triage acuity scale: Interrater reliability and patient flow analysis. *American Journal of Obstetrics & Gynecology, 209*(4), 287–293.

Vigil, J. M., Coulombe, P., Alcock, J., Kruger, E., Stith, S. S., Strenth, C., Parshall, M., & Cichowski, S. B. (2016). Patient ethnicity affects triage assessments and patient prioritization in US Department of Veterans Affairs emergency departments. *Medicine, 95*(14), 1–7.

Wilson-Griffin, J. (2021). Maternal-fetal transport. In K. R. Simpson & P. A. Creehan (Eds.), *Perinatal nursing* (5th ed., pp. 316). Lippincott Williams & Wilkins.

29

Assessment and Care at the Onset of Labor

Amy Marowitz

Relevant Terms

Active labor—the phase of labor during which contractions are strong and regular and rapid cervical dilation occurs

Braxton Hicks contractions—the uterine activity of pregnancy, perceived as painless by many people, so named after John Braxton Hicks, who wrote about this phenomenon in 1871

Continuous labor support—the presence of a supportive companion throughout the labor process

Contractions—periodic tightening and relaxing of the uterine muscle (myometrium)

Dilation—the diameter of the opening of the cervix, measured in centimeters

Early labor—the preparatory phase of labor during which contractions become more regular and stronger, and the cervix slowly effaces and dilates; different terms are used to denote this part of labor, for example, latent labor, prelabor, and prodromal labor

Effacement—thinning of the cervix that occurs during labor, measured as a percentage

Ketonuria—the presence of ketones in the urine resulting from inadequate caloric intake

Labor—a function of the birthing person by which the infant is expelled from the uterus through the vagina into the outside world

Oxytocin—a hormone that stimulates contractions of the smooth muscle of uterus

Prostaglandins—a group of hormones that stimulate contractions of the smooth muscle of the uterus and aid in cervical ripening, in part by causing collagen breakdown

Station—the location of the presenting part of the fetus relative to the ischial spines of the pregnant person's pelvis, measured in centimeters above or below the spines; presenting part at the spines is zero station

Therapeutic rest—administration of medication to relieve discomfort to enable sleep during the early part of labor

---

Introduction

Although the onset of **labor** is often portrayed in popular media as an abrupt and dramatic event, the signs and symptoms of early labor are often subtle or indistinguishable from uterine activity and other discomforts associated with late pregnancy. The onset of labor is a retrospective diagnosis, making this a challenging time for pregnant persons, their families, and healthcare providers. This chapter reviews issues related to diagnosing labor onset, teaching, and anticipatory guidance regarding the onset of labor, components of an evaluation for labor, and ways to provide support during the early phases of labor.

Health equity key points

- Providers should reflect on their own implicit and/or unconscious bias in the provision of care at the onset of labor; providers' perceptions of the ability of persons to make decisions sometimes impact the information given.
- Systemic racism, negative social determinants of health, and health inequality increase the risk of poor birth outcomes for some pregnant persons. The knowledge of a possible increased risk of poor outcomes may increase psychological discomfort regarding remaining at home during early labor.
- Trauma-informed care practices should be considered in care of pregnant persons during early labor.

Determining the Onset of Labor

It has long been recognized that uterine activity in the form of **contractions** occurs throughout much of pregnancy (Reynolds, 1968). Over the course of pregnancy, contractions gradually increase in strength and frequency and eventually result in labor. The hormonal milieu to initiate and support labor evolves during this time as well. Increasing secretion of **prostaglandins,** estrogen, and **oxytocin** causes remodeling of the connective tissue of the cervix and gradually more coordinated and frequent uterine contractions.

Initiation of labor is triggered by a complex cascade of events with maternal, placental, and fetal components. This includes maternal, fetal, and placental hormone production and excretion; structural changes in the uterus,

Prenatal and Postnatal Care: A Person-Centered Approach, Third Edition. Edited by Karen Trister Grace, Cindy L. Farley, Noelene K. Jeffers, and Tanya Tringali.
© 2024 John Wiley & Sons Ltd. Published 2024 by John Wiley & Sons Ltd.
Companion website: www.wiley.com/go/grace/prenatal

cervix, and membranes; and inflammatory processes in the cervix, placenta, membranes, and fetus. No single component brings about labor. Though the process is not fully understood, it is thought that several interrelated feedback loops are responsible for the onset of labor.

The complexity of the process and the ongoing contractions throughout pregnancy explain why it can be difficult to precisely define when labor begins. Adding to the uncertain nature of diagnosing labor onset is the significant variation in how individuals experience the uterine activity leading up to established labor. Some pregnant persons are unaware of these contractions, and others find them to be very mild and have little difficulty continuing their activities of daily living when they occur. In contrast, some pregnant persons experience considerable discomfort for hours, days, or longer, resulting in life disruption, lost sleep, and several trips to the healthcare provider for evaluation. In addition, periods of regular, painful contractions that appear to be labor but then stop for hours, days, or weeks are common.

There is no consensus among clinicians and researchers on how to define the onset of labor (Hanley, et al., 2016). Various criteria are used in different combinations including cervical change, bloody show, ruptured membranes, and characteristics of the contractions such as regularity, frequency, and strength (Friedman, 1978; O'Driscoll et al., 1973; Simkin et al., 2017). Pregnant people themselves may define it differently, noting not only contractions, bloody show, and leaking fluid but also emotional changes, sleep alterations, and gastrointestinal symptoms as heralding the onset of labor (Gross et al., 2003).

Timing of Admission to the Birth Setting

One of the most challenging decisions for pregnant persons and their healthcare providers is when to seek admission to the planned birth site. It is generally accepted that it is best to delay admission until the period of relatively rapid cervical **dilation** commonly known as **active labor** has begun. This recommendation is based on three considerations. First, a number of studies have found that rates of cesarean birth and other interventions, such as the use of epidural analgesia and oxytocin augmentation, are higher in pregnant persons admitted prior to the active phase of labor (Davey et al., 2013; Kauffman et al., 2016; Lundgren et al., 2013; Miller et al., 2020; Neal, et al., 2014, 2017; Rota et al., 2018; Rahnama et al., 2006). A systematic review found that those admitted to the labor unit in active labor have shorter labor unit stays, feel in more control of their experience, and use fewer drugs to progress labor or for pain relief (Lauzon & Hodnett, 2009). Second, care provided in the hospital or birth center prior to active labor increases healthcare costs by requiring more staffing, equipment, and space. Finally, there is a longstanding assumption that pregnant persons will be more comfortable at home during this early part of labor.

The assumption that home is the most comfortable place for pregnant and birthing people has been challenged by research on the experience of **early labor**. This research demonstrates tension between clinicians trying to delay admission and pregnant persons who want to be admitted to the birth setting (Eri et al., 2011; Nyman et al., 2011; Spiby et al., 2013). Pregnant persons perceive incongruences between what they are told and what they experience. Some are uncertain about when to seek care and are worried about erroneously seeking care too early. Some feel unsupported by care providers who may not appreciate the difficulty of this part of labor. Family members are also uncomfortable with the responsibility of caring for the person in early labor, and both pregnant persons and families may want to "hand over" responsibility to healthcare professionals. Some birth sites have strict policies requiring delay of admission until the onset of active labor. This is a dilemma for pregnant persons who do not feel safe or comfortable being at home in early labor. An option for individuals needing support to remain at the birth site in such situations is ideal. When this is not possible, frequent phone contact between the provider and pregnant person may be helpful.

Reframing "False Labor"

When a pregnant person experiences contractions that later stop, this is often referred to as "false" labor. True labor contractions are said to steadily increase in strength and frequency and increase with activity. False labor contractions, sometimes called **Braxton Hicks contractions**, are said to be irregular, not increase in strength or frequency, and stop or decrease with maternal activity. Although these distinctions between true and false labor are widely accepted, they are not evidence based. The quantification of uterine activity based on intrauterine pressure catheters shows a gradual increase in contraction strength and frequency from late gestation to active labor (Caldeyro-Barcia & Poseiro, 1960). This evidence refutes the concept of dividing uterine activity prior to active labor into distinct phases.

Numerous studies have documented the negative impact on pregnant persons when they are sent home after a labor evaluation during which they are told they are experiencing false labor and have come to the birth setting too soon (Barnett et al., 2008; Eri et al., 2011). Those in this situation report feeling anxious, confused, and unsupported and uncertain about how to recognize "true" labor. The term "false labor" is problematic. It is physiologically inaccurate and invalidates the pregnant person's experience. A better approach is to reframe this phenomenon by describing early labor as an essential phase of preparatory activity by the body in advance of active labor.

Periods of contractions that appear to be labor but then stop are very common. The normalcy of this should be communicated, and reassurance given that these contractions help prepare the cervix for labor. Accurate anticipatory guidance during prenatal visits on the realities of the onset of labor and early labor is important.

Determining Active Labor

Mid-twentieth-century obstetrician Emanuel Friedman defined the onset of active labor as the time when the rate of cervical dilation sharply increases (1978). This definition is considered the most accurate but can be difficult to recognize in real time. Historically, the criteria of regular contractions and a cervical dilation of 3 or 4 cm have been used to define active labor. However, current evidence indicates that many pregnant persons are not in active labor until a cervical dilation of about 6 cm (Neal et al., 2010; Neal & Lowe, 2012; Zhang et al., 2010a, 2010b). An accurate diagnosis is important because once active labor is thought to have begun, there are often specific cultural and institutional time expectations regarding labor progression. If a pregnant person is mistakenly diagnosed as being in active labor when they are not, interventions such as oxytocin augmentation and cesarean births for slow **labor** may be used unnecessarily (Gifford, 2000; Neal & Lowe, 2012; Neal et al., 2010).

Accuracy of an active labor diagnosis increases if multiple factors are considered. These factors include cervical **effacement** and dilation, contraction frequency, intensity, and pattern development over time. Affect should be considered also, as most pregnant persons are unable to converse during contractions and become more internally focused once active labor begins. Healthcare providers tend to rely on serial digital vaginal exams for labor diagnosis. This procedure can seem safe, but it inoculates the cervix with vaginal bacteria, even when performed aseptically, and multiple exams are associated with higher rates of chorioamnionitis (Gluck et al., 2020). Additionally, digital vaginal exams are invasive and range from uncomfortable to painful. The procedure itself can retraumatize those with a history of physical or sexual abuse. Vaginal exams are to be used judiciously, with explanation regarding the rationale for the exam, and with consent of the pregnant person. It should be performed gently, and the care provider should be responsive to feedback during the exam, altering the pressure or position of the examining hand or ending the exam altogether. The astute clinician will rely on multiple assessments to arrive at a diagnosis of labor.

Anticipatory Guidance during the Prenatal Period

Accurate anticipatory guidance during the prenatal period can help pregnant persons prepare more effectively for the onset of labor. Adequate time should be spent during late pregnancy prenatal visits to provide information on the process of labor onset and self-care in early labor. Specific instructions on when and how to contact the healthcare provider can guide the pregnant person and their family in decision-making when labor starts.

Anticipatory guidance emphasizes that labor onset is a gradual process, and it is often difficult to distinguish from the contractions and common discomforts of late pregnancy. The variability in individual experience of labor onset should be explained. The normalcy of a lengthy preparatory phase and common experience of contractions that stop and start over days and weeks should also be discussed. Finally, anticipatory guidance includes an explanation of the reasons to delay admission to the birth site until active labor begins.

Commonly, pregnant persons are told to contact their healthcare provider or go to the planned birth site when they have contractions that are 5 minutes apart or closer and painful for at least 1 hour, if they think their membranes have ruptured, or if they have heavy bleeding. These are reasonable guidelines, but it is essential to explain that not everyone is in active labor when these events occur, and that returning home may be suggested if active labor has not yet started at the time of the evaluation. Acknowledging the challenging nature of determining the onset of active labor for both the pregnant person and healthcare provider may decrease negative feelings about going home following a labor evaluation. Finally, pregnant people are encouraged to contact the healthcare provider with any questions or if they experience difficulty coping with early labor.

Other important topics to cover during prenatal teaching about labor are the importance of adequate food, fluids, and rest. Coping strategies and comfort measures for early labor should also be addressed. The benefits of **continuous labor support** during early labor should be emphasized. See Chapter 27, *Planning for Physiologic Birth*, for information on labor support. Pregnant persons should be encouraged to identify support persons before labor begins, seeking those who are knowledgeable about and comfortable with birth who can provide a calming presence. Including support persons during prenatal visits is a good way to make sure that these individuals are prepared to provide support and comfort measures during early labor.

Assessment of the Pregnant Person with Report of Labor Onset

An encounter with a patient regarding the possible onset of labor can occur by telephone or in person in the office, birth center, or triage area of the labor and birth unit. For birth care providers offering home birth, the initial assessment may occur in the person's home. Any such encounter must begin with the necessary collection of data. These include information on the pregnant person, the fetus, and the labor. Questions should be tailored to the individual and the circumstances. Begin with determining the pregnant person's due date and whether they have had any health concerns preceding or during this pregnancy.

Subjective Data

Uterine Contractions

The presence of contractions may or may not be the primary symptom leading the pregnant person to contact you. If they are having contractions, when did they start? What has the contraction pattern been since starting? What is the current frequency, length, and strength of the contractions? Do they need to stop what they are doing when they occur, or can they continue their activities? Can they sleep through them? Where do they feel them? What are they doing to cope with contractions? Do they have any other pain?

Other Signs and Symptoms of Possible Labor

Is there any vaginal bleeding or spotting, bloody show, or leaking fluid?

Fetal Status

Is the fetus moving? Is fetal movement the same or has it changed?

Fatigue

Recent sleep history: If it is night, have they slept? If it is day, how much sleep did they have last night? Recent history regarding rest and activity: Their degree of fatigue will be different if they have been walking for hours trying to get labor going or working all day, as compared to relaxing. How tired do they feel? How is their energy? If it is night, do they feel like they could sleep?

Hydration/Nutrition

Have they been eating and drinking normally? What is their recent food/fluid intake? How is their appetite? Do they have any nausea or vomiting? Are they urinating with usual frequency and a normal amount? Is their urine a light-yellow color or dark and concentrated in appearance?

Environment, Transportation, and Support

What is the time of day and the weather? How far away from the birth site does the pregnant person live? Do they have access to transportation? Is home a quiet place where they can rest if needed?

Coping

What is their affect? If the contact is by telephone, how do they sound? Do they stop talking during contractions? Do they sound anxious, relaxed, energetic, exhausted? If this is a face-to-face visit, what is their general appearance? How do they seem to be coping? How do they feel they are coping? What have they been doing?

Other Information

Ask about any signs or symptoms of a urinary tract infection such as burning or pain with urination or increased frequency of urine. Urinary tract infections can stimulate contractions.

Have they had recent sexual intercourse or a recent digital vaginal examination? Both of these can stimulate contractions and a small amount of bleeding or spotting.

Objective Data for a Face-to-Face Labor Onset Assessment

Additional physical assessments are included when the pregnant person presents for evaluation of labor onset and include:

- Vital signs
- Fetal heart rate assessment
- Urine dipstick for proteinuria and **ketonuria**, assess specific gravity as needed
- Leopold's maneuvers to determine fetal lie, presentation, position, and estimated fetal weight
- Abdominal palpation for uterine tone and contraction frequency

A digital vaginal exam for cervical dilation, effacement, position, and consistency, fetal **station**, and to confirm presentation should be performed by a healthcare provider skilled in this type of assessment. If there is a possibility of ruptured membranes, a digital vaginal exam should be deferred and a sterile speculum exam performed to assess pooling of fluid and to obtain samples for laboratory or microscopic confirmation of the presence of amniotic fluid. The assessment of cervical effacement is an important aspect of the evaluation since the cervix usually effaces considerably before more rapid dilation can occur, particularly in **nulliparous** persons. It is important to note that often some cervical effacement and dilation occurs prior to the onset of labor. For this reason, one digital vaginal exam might not be definitive in determining if a pregnant person is in labor. When the diagnosis is not clear, serial cervical examinations showing cervical change may be a more accurate indication of labor.

Plan of Care

At the onset of an encounter with a pregnant person for labor evaluation, the need for immediate admission to the planned birth site must be determined. Reasons for immediate admission include, but are not limited to, active labor, vaginal bleeding heavier than normal bloody show, or concerns about patient or fetal status. Institutional policies and individual healthcare provider practices regarding the timing of admission vary greatly for pregnant persons with ruptured membranes in the absence of labor. If immediate admission is necessary, assessment by phone or in the office is limited and the pregnant person is directed to the planned birth site. In this situation, the provider will notify personnel at the birth setting that the pregnant person should arrive in the birth unit shortly.

If there is no indication of a need for immediate admission and early labor is occurring, the plan of care should be tailored to meet the individual's needs. Thus, it is essential to include the pregnant person in the decision-making. For example, if the encounter is by telephone, it is helpful to ask the pregnant person if they want to be evaluated in person. If the pregnant person is comfortable remaining at home, management is centered on self-care, coping strategies, social support, and timing of admission. If active labor does not ensue, remind them to keep their next scheduled prenatal appointment. Shared decision-making and autonomy in healthcare decisions are critical components of care at the onset of labor. Providers should reflect on their own implicit and/or unconscious bias in the provision of care at the onset of labor. Research reveals that providers' perceptions of the ability of persons to make decisions sometimes impact the information given (Altman et al., 2019).

Structural racism, negative social determinants of health, and health inequality increase the risk of poor birth outcomes for some pregnant persons. The knowledge of a possible increased risk of poor outcomes may increase psychological discomfort regarding remaining at home during early labor. Trauma-informed care practices should be considered in the care of pregnant persons during early labor (see Chapter 26, *Violence and Trauma in the Perinatal Period*; Reissig et al., 2021).

The following discussion on self-care and coping should be read with the understanding that little to no research has been conducted on optimal strategies for early labor. Common recommendations come from conventional wisdom, empirical data, and general nursing and midwifery principles.

Self-Care

Self-care in early labor primarily involves hydration, nutrition, and rest. Close attention to these issues is needed during longer periods of early labor. There are several reasons why pregnant persons may not keep themselves hydrated and nourished in early labor. Some believe that they should not eat or drink once labor begins. This common misconception should be corrected and the importance of continued intake of fluids and calories in early labor emphasized during prenatal education about labor. Most pregnant persons do not feel well if they are dehydrated, and dehydration may make the uterus irritable, resulting in increased discomfort and inefficient contractions. Once significant dehydration occurs, it can be difficult to correct with oral fluids. Thus, many clinicians recommend the consumption of at least 8 oz of fluid per hour when awake. Pregnant persons can easily monitor their own hydration status by drinking when thirsty and by observing the color of their urine, which should be light yellow. Continued caloric intake is also important during early labor. The goal is for the pregnant person to remain well hydrated and nourished with adequate caloric reserves for the physical exertion of labor. Eating normally during early labor is ideal, although frequent light snacks and caloric beverages can be an adequate source of nutrition and calories.

Some pregnant persons experience nausea and/or vomiting in early labor, making it more difficult to stay adequately hydrated and nourished. With mild nausea, it is often possible to continue to sip fluids and eat small amounts of easily digestible food such as refined carbohydrates or fruits. With significant nausea or vomiting, admission for intravenous fluids and possibly antiemetic medication may be needed.

Sleep and Rest

Sufficient rest and sleep are important with long periods of early labor. Coping with early labor and subsequent active labor is much more difficult with significant sleep deprivation and fatigue. As with hydration and nourishment, adequate rest and sleep help a pregnant person manage the physical exertion of active labor. There are several reasons why pregnant persons may experience fatigue in early labor. Many individuals have difficulty sleeping in advanced pregnancy and may start labor with a sleep deficit. For some, the excitement and/or anxiety experienced with the onset of labor make it difficult to sleep. Some pregnant persons believe they should be physically active once early labor begins in order to speed labor progress. Finally, some individuals cannot sleep due to the pain of early labor contractions.

Advising pregnant persons on the importance of adequate rest and sleep in early labor should start during prenatal visits and be emphasized during any encounter related to possible labor. Suggestions for preventing fatigue include napping frequently in the last weeks of pregnancy, trying to sleep between the contractions if it is night, and conserving energy by alternating periods of rest and activity during the day. If the pregnant person cannot sleep through contractions, dozing in between is helpful. Various relaxation measures can also help the pregnant person sleep. Examples include a warm bath, chamomile tea, massage, aromatherapy, guided imagery, or meditation, and listening to relaxing music. A small amount of alcohol to promote sleep, such as a half glass of wine, has been a time-honored recommendation to support rest in early labor. Alcohol also inhibits contractions and, in fact, was used as a tocolytic in the 1960s. Though some consider any alcohol consumption in pregnancy to be inappropriate, it can be argued that it has the same fetal effects as opioids, a class of drug often used to promote rest in early labor (Greulich & Tarrant, 2007).

When a pregnant person cannot sleep during a period of early labor and becomes fatigued or exhausted, medication can be a useful tool. Medications that can be provided to take at home include antihistamines such as Benadryl® (diphenhydramine) available over the counter, and Vistaril® (hydroxyzine), and other nonbenzodiazepine sedative-hypnotics such as Ambien® (zolpidem) by prescription. Barbiturate sedative-hypnotics such as Seconal® (secobarbital) were commonly used in this circumstance in the past; however, these drugs have prolonged depressant effects in the newborn and are now considered contraindicated for use in early labor (Greulich & Tarrant, 2007; King & Brucker, 2017). Importantly, none of the sedative-hypnotics have analgesic properties, and they are not helpful in promoting rest when painful contractions prevent sleep. If a pregnant person is extremely fatigued and cannot sleep due to painful contractions, admission to the planned birth site for **therapeutic rest** with an opioid analgesic such as morphine sulfate should be considered.

Coping Strategies and Comfort Measures for Early Labor

An important strategy for coping in early labor is distraction. Distracting activities help pass the time and may decrease the pregnant person's focus on contractions.

Suggestions include continuing a normal routine as much as possible or engaging in diverting activities such as watching a movie, playing cards, preparing food, or working on a project. Nesting behaviors, such as preparing the home environment for the baby, increase as pregnancy draws to a close and may be a positive distraction during early labor.

The degree of discomfort experienced in early labor varies greatly. Generally, recommendations for comfort and nonpharmacological pain relief in early labor are similar to those suggested for active labor. Measures such as water immersion, superficial application of heat and cold, position changes and other movements, touch, and massage are effective in active labor (ACOG, 2017) and may be helpful in managing the discomforts of early labor.

Continuous support during labor has well-established benefits (Hodnett et al., 2013), and there is some evidence of its benefits in early stages of labor (Simkin & Bolding, 2004). The evidence shows the greatest benefit when support is provided by a person who is experienced and trained and is not part of the patient's social network (Hodnett et al., 2013); however, it is most commonly provided by a partner, family member, or friend in early labor. The support pregnant persons receive during this time affects their experience and ability to cope and sets the stage for improved coping in later labor.

Ambulation in Early Labor

Unrestricted movement in **active labor** is associated with greater satisfaction with the birth experience, decreased pain, and possibly shorter labor (ACOG, 2017). Though no studies have examined the benefits of unrestricted movement in early labor, common sense dictates that pregnant persons should be encouraged to move around as desired during this time. Some pregnant persons and clinicians believe that ambulation hastens the transition from early to active labor. Pregnant persons may be advised that continued walking helps determine if their contractions are "real" labor because of the belief that activity diminishes the contractions of "false" labor and stimulates the contractions of true labor. Neither of these rationales is evidence-based. The common practice of instructing pregnant persons in early labor to walk for an hour or two to assess the effect on the contraction pattern should be critically evaluated. This practice contributes to fatigue and is unlikely to be beneficial. Pregnant persons should be advised to move about and rest during early labor as comfort dictates.

Summary

Progression from late pregnancy to established labor is a process that, for many, unfolds over days or weeks. Identifying the onset of labor and coping with the early phases of labor can be challenging. An understanding of the psychophysiological nature of these events is needed to provide appropriate teaching to pregnant persons and to support them during this unique period of time.

Resources for Clients and Their Families

Stages of labor and birth from Mayo Clinic: https://www.mayoclinic.org/healthy-lifestyle/labor-and-delivery/in-depth/stages-of-labor/art-20046545

"Ask the Midwife" about what starts labor: https://wsnm.org/midwife-natural-hormones-labor/#:~:text=Even%20when%20birth%20is%20scheduled,brain%20produces%20it%20in%20waves

Getting through early labor at home: www.babycentre.co.uk/x1037973/how-can-i-get-through-early-labour-at-home

Resources for Healthcare Providers

ACOG's Committee Opinion: Approaches to Limit Intervention During Labor and Birth: https://www.acog.org/clinical/clinical-guidance/committee-opinion/articles/2019/02/approaches-to-limit-intervention-during-labor-and-birth

References

Altman, M. R., Oseguera, T., McLemore, M. R., Kantrowitz-Gordon, I., Franck, L. S., & Lyndon, A. (2019). Information and power: Women of color's experiences interacting with health care providers in pregnancy and birth. *Social Science & Medicine*, 238, 112491. https://doi.org/10.1016/j.socscimed.2019.112491

American College of Obstetricians & Gynecologists (ACOG). (2017). Approaches to limit interventions during labor and birth. Committee opinion no. 687. *Obstetrics & Gynecology*, 129(2), e20–e28.

Barnett, C., Hundley, V., Cheyne, H., & Kane, F. (2008). 'Not in labour': Impact of sending women home in the latent phase. *British Journal of Midwifery*, 16(3), 144–148.

Caldeyro-Barcia, R., & Poseiro, J. J. (1960). Physiology of the uterine contraction. *Clinical Obstetrics and Gynecology*, 3(2), 386–410.

Davey, M., McLachlan, H., Forster, D., & Flood, M. (2013). Influence of timing of admission in labour and management of labour on method of birth: Results from a randomised controlled trial of caseload midwifery (COSMOS trial). *Midwifery*, 29, 1297–1302.

Eri, T., Blystaf, A., Gjengedal, E., & Blaaka, G. (2011). 'Stay home for as long as possible': Midwives' priorities and strategies in communicating with first-time mothers in early labour. *Midwifery*, 27, e286–e292.

Friedman, E. (1978). *Labor: Clinical evaluation and management* (2nd ed.). Appleton.

Gifford, D. (2000). Lack of progress in labor as a reason for cesarean. *Obstetrics & Gynecology*, 94(4), 589–595.

Gluck, O., Mizrachi, Y., Ganer Herman, H., Bar, J., Kovo, M., & Weiner, E. (2020). The correlation between the number of vaginal examinations during active labor and febrile morbidity, a retrospective cohort study. *BMC Pregnancy and Childbirth*, 20(1), 246. https://doi.org/10.1186/s12884-020-02925-9

Greulich, B., & Tarrant, B. (2007). The latent phase of labor: Diagnosis and management. *Journal of Midwifery & Women's Health*, 52(3), 190–198.

Gross, M. M., Haunschild, T., Stoexen, T., Methner, V., & Guenter, H. (2003). Women's recognition of the spontaneous onset of labor. *Birth*, 30(4), 267–271.

Hanley, G. E., Munro, S., Greyson, D., Gross, M. M., Hundley, V., Spiby, H., & Janssen, P. A. (2016). Diagnosing onset of labor: A systematic review of definitions in the research literature. *BMC Pregnancy and Childbirth*, 16, 71. https://doi.org/10.1186/s12884-016-0857-4

Hodnett, E. D., Gates, S., Hofmeyr, G. J., & Sakala, C. (2013). Continuous support for women during childbirth. *Cochrane Database of Systematic Reviews*, (7), CD003766.

Kauffman, E., Souter, V., Katon, J., & Sitcov, K. (2016). Cervical dilation on admission in term spontaneous labor and maternal and newborn outcomes. *Obstetrics & Gynecology*, 127(3), 481–488.

King, T. L., & Brucker, M. C. (2017). *Pharmacology for women's health* (2nd ed.). Jones and Bartlett.

Lauzon, L., & Hodnett, E. D. (2009). Labour assessment programs to delay admission to labour wards. *Cochrane Database of Systematic Reviews*, (1), CD000936.

Lundgren, I., Andren, K., Nissen, E., & Berg, M. (2013). Care seeking during the latent phase of labour—Frequencies and birth outcomes in two delivery wards in Sweden. *Sexual & Reproductive Healthcare*, 4(4), 141–146.

Miller, Y. D., Armanasco, A. A., McCosker, L., & Thompson, R. (2020). Variations in outcomes for women admitted to hospital in early versus active labour: An observational study. *BMC Pregnancy and Childbirth*, 20(1), 469. https://doi.org/10.1186/s12884-020-03149-7

Neal, J., Lamp, J., Buck, J., Lowe, N., Gillespie, S., & Ryan, S. (2014). Outcomes of nulliparous women with spontaneous labor onset admitted to hospitals in preactive versus active labor. *Journal of Midwifery & Women's Health*, 59(1), 28–34.

Neal, J., Lowe, N., Phillipi, J., Ryan, S., Knupp, A., Dietrich, M., & Thung, S. (2017). Likelihood of cesarean delivery after applying leading active labor diagnostic guidelines. *Birth*, 44(2), 1–9.

Neal, J., Lowe, N. K., Patrick, T. E., Cabbage, L. A., & Corwin, E. J. (2010). What is the slowest-yet-normal cervical dilation rate among nulliparous women with spontaneous labor onset? *Journal of Obstetric, Gynecologic, & Neonatal Nursing*, 39(4), 361–369.

Neal, J. L., & Lowe, N. K. (2012). Physiologic partograph to improve birth safety and outcomes among low-risk, nulliparous women with spontaneous labor onset. *Medical Hypotheses*, 78(2), 319–325.

Nyman, V., Downe, S., & Berg, M. (2011). Waiting for permission to enter the labour ward world: First time parents' experiences of the first encounter on a labour ward. *Sexual & Reproductive Healthcare*, 2(3), 129–134.

O'Driscoll, K., Stronge, J. M., & Minogue, M. (1973). Active management of labour. *British Medical Journal*, 3(5872), 135–137.

Rahnama, P., Ziaei, S., & Faghihzadeh, S. (2006). Impact of early admission in labor on method of delivery. *International Journal of Gynaecology and Obstetrics*, 92(3), 217–220.

Reissig, M., Fair, C., Houpt, B., & Latham, V. (2021). An exploratory study of the role of birth stories in shaping expectations for childbirth among nulliparous Black women: Everybody is different (but I'm scared). *Journal of Midwifery & Women's Health*, 66(5), 597–603. https://doi.org/10.1111/jmwh.13282

Reynolds, S. R. (1968). The uses of Braxton Hicks contractions. *Obstetrics & Gynecology*, 32(1), 134–140.

Rota, A., Antolini, L., Colciago, E., Nespoli, A., Borrelli, S. E., & Fumagalli, S. (2018). Timing of hospital admission in labour: Latent versus active phase, mode of birth and intrapartum interventions. A correlational study. *Women & Birth*, 31(4), 313–318. https://doi.org/10.1016/j.wombi.2017.10.001

Simkin, P., & Bolding, A. (2004). Update on nonpharmacologic approaches to relieve labor pain and prevent suffering. *Journal of Midwifery & Women's Health*, 49(6), 489–504.

Simkin, P., Hanson, L., & Ancheta, R. (2017). *The labor progress handbook: Early interventions to prevent and treat dystocia* (4th ed.). Wiley Blackwell.

Spiby, H., Walsh, D., Green, J., Crompton, A., & Bugg, G. (2013). Midwives' beliefs and concerns about telephone conversations with women in early labour. *Midwifery*, 30(9), 1036–1042.

Zhang, J., Landy, H. J., Ware Branch, D., Burkman, R., Haberman, S., Gregory, K. D., Hatjis, C. G., Ramirez, M. M., Bailit, J. L., Gonzalez-Quintero, V. H., Hibbard, J. U., Hoffman, M. K., Kominiarek, M., Learman, L. A., Van Veldhuisen, P., Troendle, J., Reddy, U. M., & Consortium on Safe Labor. (2010a). Contemporary patterns of spontaneous labor with normal neonatal outcomes. *Obstetrics and Gynecology*, 116(6), 1281–1287.

Zhang, J., Troendle, J., Mikolajczyk, R., Sundaram, R., Beaver, J., & Fraser, W. (2010b). The natural history of the normal first stage of labor. *Obstetrics & Gynecology*, 115(4), 705–710.

30

Components of Postnatal Care

Tia P. Andrighetti and Judith M. Butler

Relevant Terms

Ankyloglossia—commonly referred to as tongue-tie; an unusually short frenulum that can decrease tongue mobility, can interfere with newborn attaining adequate latch for breastfeeding, varies in severity

Boggy—when referring to the uterus, it means soft and not fully contracted

Diastasis recti—a midline separation of the rectus abdominis muscles at the linea alba

Eschar—area in the uterus where the placenta was attached; at about 10 days postpartum, this "scab" will be released; bright red bleeding for 1–2 hours is normal, then back to previous lochia color and amount

First-degree laceration—tear of the perineum, labia, or vagina involving the superficial layers of tissue

Fourth-degree laceration—tear that lacerates the external and internal anal sphincter and rectovaginal septum

Fourth trimester—time from birth of the placenta lasting for approximately three months postpartum

Fundus—the topmost part of the uterus; felt during abdominal evaluation of the uterus

Involution—normal process the body undergoes after birth; when referred to the uterus, the shrinking back of the uterus to an almost nonpregnant size

Kegel exercises—tightening and lifting, holding, then releasing pelvic floor muscles to improve muscle tone

Lochia—vaginal blood, tissue, and mucus loss after birth; lasting up to six to eight weeks postpartum

Matrescence—the physical, emotional, hormonal, and social transition to becoming a mother

Pelvic organ prolapse—descent of pelvic viscera, often due to a weakness, in the supporting structures of the pelvic floor

Second-degree laceration—tear involving the fascia and perineal muscle

Third-degree laceration—tear involving the perineal muscle as well as the external anal sphincter

---

Introduction

Postnatal care begins with the onset of the postpartum period; it is also referred to as the puerperium. It has been generally defined as a six- to eight-week period beginning with the delivery of the placenta. Despite this long-standing definition, the postpartum period actually lasts for several months, into the first year and beyond, and is a neglected aspect of modern healthcare. Literature is sparse on the **puerperium**, but what does exist deals primarily with abnormal **involution** and pathology. Respecting and supporting the length of restoration in the postpartum client has long been the belief and practice in most other developed and developing countries but continues to be overlooked in the United States.

There are many adaptations and adjustments that need to be made by the birthing person and family to accommodate the new family member into an already established structure. Quality healthcare during this time offers support, education, surveillance, and interaction. The focus is on supporting families through this adjustment and providing education, consultation, collaboration, and referral when indicated.

Health equity key points

- Thirty-six percent of maternal deaths occur in the first postpartum week and another 33% occur between one week and one year after birth with Black and American Indian/Alaskan natives three times as likely to die from pregnancy-related causes.
- Rooted in the false narrative that there are physiologic differences in the way people of various races and ethnicities experience pain, Black people are less likely to have their pain assessed and treated in the postpartum period, contributing to the inequities in outcomes.
- To prevent erroneous assumptions and harm to those who are not heteronormative, always ask about sexual practices before recommending contraception.

Discharge home from the birth facility comes at a time when most clients are being bombarded by the sensory overload that accompanies rapid physical and psychological changes after birth. Sleep deprivation is common as well. The ability to integrate new information during this time is often diminished and challenges clinicians to find

Prenatal and Postnatal Care: A Person-Centered Approach, Third Edition. Edited by Karen Trister Grace, Cindy L. Farley, Noelene K. Jeffers, and Tanya Tringali.
© 2024 John Wiley & Sons Ltd. Published 2024 by John Wiley & Sons Ltd.
Companion website: www.wiley.com/go/grace/prenatal

teachable moments. Therefore, postpartum teaching ideally begins during pregnancy and continues throughout postpartum and includes the client and family members. Because information is often passed down through family members, the inclusion of family during teaching sessions can reduce confusion or correct inaccurate information.

The degree of postpartum discomfort, adjustment of the birthing person to baby and baby to the birthing person, and the amount of support received all affect recovery and adaptation to their new role. It is important for healthcare providers to facilitate planning for postpartum recovery and newborn care, identify social and tangible support, and optimize psychological resiliency and physical and mental health, all important components for optimal health in the puerperium. Anticipatory guidance is approached in a realistic manner. Teaching includes the expected physiological and psychological tasks that client's face during this time.

Fourth-trimester tasks

- Physical restoration
- Psychological adaptation to a new role
- Development of knowledge and skills to care for a dependent infant
- Establishment of bond with the baby
- Adjustments to lifestyle issues and relationship changes to accommodate a new family member

---

The primary concerns of a person who has recently given birth include learning about infant behavior and care, physical recovery, and juggling demands of employment or other obligations, including household duties, relationships, and other children. A client is able to adapt to their new role faster when the concerns for their own recovery are met. If the changes the birthing person is experiencing are normal, reassurance can help the client focus on meeting their own needs as well as those of the infant.

Immediate Postpartum Care

Postpartum care in the first few days after birth can be delivered by a variety of healthcare providers. In-hospital postpartum care requires the provider to have hospital privileges. Innovative methods of assessing the birthing person's needs in the first one to two days after birth include client-centered collaborative rounds where the healthcare provider, nurse, case manager, lactation consultant, and social worker make rounds together. This model can improve interprofessional communication and enhance care and planning for each birthing person's postpartum needs (Segel et al., 2010). Patient navigation programs, which are used in other healthcare specialties, may also be beneficial to help meet client needs during this time, especially for low-income women (Ruderman et al., 2021). If the birth occurred in a birth center or home birth setting, the provider usually stays for a specified

period of time, followed by birth assistants assessing the client for a specified number of hours after birth. Births that occur in these settings are usually followed by a series of home visits or visits for the birthing person and newborn to their provider's office the day after birth and again in a few subsequent days. Components of postpartum care remain the same regardless of where the birth occurred.

An assessment of client and family adjustment during this immediate postpartum time is crucial. A review of the birth event with the birthing person helps them process the experience. If the provider making rounds did not attend the birth, a review of the birth record is essential prior to beginning the discussion. It is important to keep in mind that the client will have their own perceptions of their labor and birth process that may differ from information derived from reading the chart. Support a wide range of emotional responses when asking the individual to share their birth story. The general areas to address during the immediate postpartum period are noted below and are discussed in depth throughout the rest of this chapter.

Postpartum care considerations

- Homeostasis
- Involution
- Bladder function
- Vital signs
- Comfort and report of symptoms
- Initiation of lactation, if breastfeeding
- Suppression of lactation, if not breastfeeding
- Review of birth experience
- Client family bonding
- Infant care-taking
- Preparation for home care and assistance

Later Postpartum Care

After initial postpartum care following childbirth, many clients are not seen by a healthcare provider until a postpartum visit six to eight weeks later. Opportunities to assess physical and psychosocial adjustment are missed with this length of time between clinical visits and can delay interventions for adjustment concerns or complications. A two-week postpartum visit is recommended; however, adding a single visit to standard postpartum care will not be enough. Recently, some practices have been tailoring the time frames of visits to client needs, seeing patients at one and five weeks, for example. There is no set time frame in which visits should be done but are best tailored to every situation, with the first visit in the first 3 weeks and the last visit before 12 weeks after birth (ACOG, 2018a). Tables 30.1 and 30.2 reflect suggested assessment and care components covered at each of the one- to two- and five- to six-week visits. The one- to two-week visit is done to assure that postpartum involution is proceeding normally, noting psychological

Table 30.1 One- to Two-Week Postpartum Visit

Subjective assessment to consider	• Physical and emotional adjustment • Birth experience • Family adaptation • Infant feeding • Exercise/activity • Rest/sleep • Diet/fluids • Lochia • Afterbirth pains • Perineal comfort • Diuresis/diaphoresis • Constipation/hemorrhoids • Sexuality/resumption of intercourse • Family planning • Warning signs and symptoms of complications (i.e., postpartum preeclampsia or infection)
Objective assessment to consider *Consideration of some components is based upon the information gathered in the subjective assessment*	Vital signs Weight Heart/lungs Breasts Uterus-abdominal assessment Costovertebral angle tenderness Perineum/bleeding prn Extremities/edema Postpartum mood disorders Intimate partner violence screening

Plan to consider	• Teaching
	  ○ Family adaptation
	  ○ Matrescence
	  ○ Infant feeding (frequency, duration, latch)
	  ○ Normal involution
	  ○ Exercise/activity
	  ○ Rest/sleep
	  ○ Diet/fluids
	  ○ Family planning
	  ○ Review warning signs and symptoms of potential complications
	• Follow-up at six weeks and prn
	• Consult, collaborate, refer prn

Table 30.2 Five- to Six-Week Postpartum Visit

Subjective assessment to consider	• Physical and emotional adjustment • Birth experience • Family adaptation • Infant feeding • Exercise/activity • Rest/sleep • Diet/fluids • Lochia • Perineal comfort • Constipation/hemorrhoids • Sexuality/resumption of intercourse • Family planning • Chronic Conditions
Objective assessment to consider	Vital signs Weight Heart/lungs Breasts Abdomen Uterus Costovertebral angle tenderness Extremities Perineum and vagina Hemorrhoids Postpartum mood disorders and intimate partner violence screening

Plan to consider	• Teaching
	  ○ Family adaptation
	  ○ Matrescence
	  ○ Normal involution
	  ○ Infant feeding
	  ○ Exercise/activity
	  ○ Rest/sleep
	  ○ Diet/fluids
	  ○ Resumption of menses and ovulation
	  ○ Family planning
	  ○ Returning to work
	  ○ Review warning signs of postpartum mood and anxiety disorders
	  ○ Chronic disease management
	  ○ Health maintenance
	• Lab testing as dictated by history (i.e., GCT, thyroid function tests, etc.)
	• Follow-up at annual exam or prn
	• Consult, collaborate, refer prn

adjustment, and determining any maladaptations either physically or emotionally. The five- to six-week visit is focused on assessing that postpartum involution is more complete, that the psychological adjustment of the family is continuing, and that family planning has been addressed. Any indicated follow-up laboratory testing is done at this time.

Postpartum care in the United States is considered woefully inadequate by many experts, and a restructuring of current practices is urgently needed (ACOG, 2018a; Cornell et al., 2016). Thirty-six percent of maternal deaths occur in the first postpartum week (usually due to bleeding, infection, and high blood pressure) and another 33% occur between one week and one year (usually due to cardiomyopathy) after birth, with Black and American Indian/Alaskan Natives three times as likely to die from pregnancy-related causes than White people (CDC, 2019). Postpartum care is limited in scope and typically completed after the first six weeks. The six weeks historically may be due to the confinement or resting period seen in many cultures for the first 40 days following a birth (ACOG, 2018a). Better education and tangible support during this time would help clients while also lessening the use of emergency departments and acute care treatment facilities (Brousseau et al., 2018). Hospital stays after birth are quite short for most birthing people, even those undergoing a surgical birth. Office visits require time and travel for the birthing person with a new baby and are not always seen as essential, leading to high no-show rates for these appointments. Some studies have found that up to 50% of clients do not attend the postpartum visit (Geissler et al., 2020). The highest rate of nonattendance is seen in clients with limited resources and real and perceived discrimination during hospital care (Attanasio & Kozhimannil, 2017). These health inequities are due to institutional and internalized racism and classism and need to be addressed. Current postpartum care does not offer the support required to help birthing people and families adjust to their new roles and responsibilities and, more importantly, to assist in their recoveries from and adjustments to the anatomic, physiological, and psychological changes after childbirth.

Home visits, postpartum group care, postpartum doula care, caring for the birthing person-baby dyad, and connection through various social media platforms are some innovative strategies that are being explored to fill this gap in care (Baker & Yang, 2018). Experts have proposed moving from a disease-screening approach to an integrated health promotion approach that encompasses four life skills that have documented influence on health: (a) mobilization of social and tangible support; (b) positive coping skills; (c) self-efficacy; and (d) realistic expectations (Fahey & Shenassa, 2013). The CenteringPregnancy™ model of care is a program that has successfully implemented this health promotion approach during the prenatal and postpartum period, incorporating all four of the life skills in its process of care. Some of the positive postpartum health outcomes attributed to CenteringPregnancy include reduced postpartum weight retention, reduced rates of postpartum depression (PPD), higher rates of attending postpartum healthcare appointments, increased use of postpartum contraception, and higher confidence levels (DeCesare et al., 2017; Magriples et al., 2015; Robertson et al., 2009). CenteringParenting is a continuation model in the postpartum year that recognizes that the health of the client is tied to the health of the infant and that assessment and interventions are more appropriate and efficient when done in a dyad context (Connor et al., 2018).

The increased use of telehealth has opened another venue for seeing clients postnatally. This may be attractive to clients with transportation issues, other children, restrictive work schedules, or many of the myriad other challenges faced by people during this time. This modality has the possibility of improving the poor rates of attendance for postpartum visits. Virtual office visits via videoconferencing have been trialed in several populations of postpartum people and have been found to be effective (Ackerman et al., 2021; Pflugeisen et al., 2016; Saad et al., 2021; Zhao et al., 2021). This method has the advantage of reducing the number of office visits and travel and allows individuals more opportunities to consult health staff from their own home. Also, the client's environment is visible in the background during the videoconference and can highlight important clues that add to a more complete picture of their physical and emotional

state. Healthcare providers should also consider potential barriers to the use of telehealth. At a minimum, clients must have access to a phone or the internet with a connection speed capable of video streaming. Not all clients are able to speak freely in their homes, and providers should remember that they cannot see who or what is outside the view of the camera.

Placental Encapsulation

Placental consumption, or placentophagia, is not a new phenomenon; there is information on placental consumption by humans dating back to biblical times (Joseph et al., 2016). There is little that is known about the benefits of placental consumption in humans. Some common beliefs about the benefits of placentophagia in humans include enhanced lactation, improved bonding, increased vitamin and nutritional value, as well as the ability to prevent some postpartum complications such as depression and anemia (Hayes, 2016; Joseph et al., 2016; Stanley et al., 2019). Theoretical risks of placentophagia include infection, thromboembolic events, and ingestion of toxins accumulated in the placenta (Hayes, 2016). The Centers for Disease Control and Prevention (CDC; 2017) recommend not ingesting encapsulated placentas due to an isolated case of a newborn being exposed to Group B strep (GBS) after its mother ingested encapsulated placenta. While the cause of the neonatal infection could not be definitively determined, one possible mechanism is that the placenta may not have been heated to the appropriate temperature. Clinicians should inquire about placental ingestion in cases of late onset GBS (Association of Placenta Preparation Arts [APPA], 2021b; Buser et al., 2017).

There are no state or federal regulations or standards on placental encapsulation; however, the APPA (2021a) has guidelines and standards for encapsulation, as well as a search engine to locate trained specialists. The placenta must remain refrigerated until it is dried by the encapsulator. For clients who express interest in placental encapsulation, clinicians should provide education about current evidence and facilitate placenta collection and storage after birth.

Assessment of Physical and Emotional Adjustment

A birthing person's emotional status and physical recovery are evaluated during postpartum visits. Some clients may not feel comfortable sharing intimate feelings or how their family is adjusting, unless specifically asked. The provider's ability to use shared decision-making and integrate client preferences and values into care is vital to ensuring open and respectful dialogue. Communication can be facilitated by asking open-ended questions and by giving time to answer, without unduly hurrying on to the physical exam part of the visit. The healthcare provider can start by asking the client to describe their life with the new baby. Follow-up questions and probes can be targeted to areas for a fuller picture of the experience.

Attaining a realistic life balance is one of the major tasks of the childbearing year. The new parent needs to care for their infant, provide continued attention to siblings, help siblings adjust to a new baby's presence, and maintain relationships separate from the children. Additionally, there may be concerns regarding finances, employment, and the maintenance of daily tasks and household management. It is important to the client's overall health to participate in outside activities and continue to maintain contact with others; however, this is challenging particularly in the early postpartum weeks. Prioritizing and asking for help are key. Give the birthing person permission to let some tasks go at home while prioritizing what is most important to them. For a client who is struggling with this concept, write a script noting that their job in the early postpartum period is to care for their own needs, the baby, and other children. Postpartum doulas are another resource to consider for the early postpartum adjustment. They offer a range of services, from breastfeeding support to light housekeeping and meal preparation. Family and friends are often willing to help, and the new parent should be encouraged to graciously accept these offers of help from their extended social network. Encourage the client to keep a list of chores, so that when someone offers, an immediate need is fulfilled. Paternity or partner leave is an important employment benefit for some; these should be explored and arranged in the prenatal period.

Assessing mood in the early postpartum period is vital since 30–80% of clients experience postpartum blues (Iwanowiscz-Palus et al., 2021). This wide range reflects differing criteria for diagnosing postpartum blues. The etiology of postpartum blues is unknown, but many common postpartum aspects such as fatigue, decreased support, hormonal fluctuation, social isolation, and marital or relationship conflict can contribute. It is not unusual for a birthing person to cry for unexplained reasons, experience anxiety, feel overly fatigued, have trouble sleeping, an increased appetite or none at all, and mixed feelings regarding the birth experience. Symptoms that are severe or last more than two weeks warrant evaluation for postpartum mood and anxiety disorders. It is important to understand that the onset of postpartum mood and anxiety disorders can be weeks or months after the birth. Chapter 43, *Common Complications during the Postnatal Period*, contains more detail on postpartum mood and anxiety disorders.

Healthcare providers can help clients experiencing the postpartum blues in a variety of ways. Active listening can be very therapeutic. Individuals need to be reassured that their feelings do not make them a bad parent but are a normal response to expected physiologic and emotional changes during this adjustment period. Suggest increased help at home by enlisting family and friends to cook, clean, watch other children, and help care for the baby. Encourage the birthing person to take some time for themselves such as reading a book, taking a bath, visiting with friends, or getting out of the house for a walk. Encourage them to sleep when the baby sleeps and take every opportunity to rest, as caring for a newborn is a 24-hour-a-day job. By trying a variety of tactics, the client can find what coping measures work best for them.

Review of Birth Experience

The individual who gave birth needs to integrate and accept the reality of their own birth and newborn experience while reconciling expectations and fantasies that may have been unmet. The actual birth experience can vary from the way it was imagined. Encouraging clients to discuss their birth can facilitate the task of integrating their imagined birth with reality. Failure to complete this process can interfere with their ability to become comfortable with their new identity. The psychological task of fitting the pieces of the birth experience into their own narrative can generate a positive perspective on the experience. Birth is an intense event; its memory may reflect focused and selected aspects of the experience. They may need help in understanding how and why their own birth varied from their hopes and expectations. This review can help them to make sense of the experience, to express their emotions, and incorporate this transformative event into their identity. How a person feels about their birth experience can also affect their attachment process with the baby.

Family Adaptation

Family structure affects individual function. Understanding the structure of the client's family as they define it will help clinicians provide culturally sensitive and realistic information and care. Family structure has evolved to include a wider variety of configurations over the last half century. Families can be almost any configuration of people imaginable and extended family may or may not be involved. More than 35% of birthing people are unmarried (DePaulo, 2017). Do not assume family structure. Ask directly whom they include in their family. Regardless of family structure, adjustments will be made to accommodate a new family member, and bonding with the new baby will remain an essential feature of this adjustment.

Bonding is the emotional tie that the childbearing person develops with their unborn baby and later with their newborn (see Chapter 23, *Psychosocial Adaptations in Pregnancy*). Bonding can occur between other important members of the family and the newborn, such as father or partner, grandparents, and siblings. This process develops over time and provides a powerful source of motivation for ongoing care-taking activities. The capabilities of parents to recognize their baby's behavioral cues and respond appropriately are influenced by numerous factors and can have lasting effects on parent–child bonding (Kerstis et al., 2016). Strong parent–child bonds can persist throughout a lifetime, despite separation of time and distance.

The stage is set immediately after birth for attachment to begin. A cascade of hormones is generated during the labor and birth process. Endorphins promote an exhilarated sense of achievement about the birth, while prolactin and oxytocin facilitate a peaceful and deepening love for the neonate. However, routine interventions done without medical indication, such as induction of labor, cesarean section, or epidural anesthesia, can mute the hormonal response and influence the bonding process.

A healthy newborn should not be separated from the birthing person after birth if not medically necessary. Becoming acquainted with the newly born baby immediately after birth typically proceeds in a progressive journey using gaze, proximity, fingertips, palms, voice, embrace, and movement. The en face position allows optimal eye contact, so the birthing person and neonate can fixate on the other's features. Birthing people may communicate with a high-pitched voice suited to the newborn's hearing range, while babies imitate with mouth and tongue movement (Kennell & Klaus, 1998). This process requires close physical contact and should not be interrupted by hospital procedures, all of which can be done at a later time for a healthy newborn.

Many factors can affect bonding. Client's perceptions of their own abilities and skills to care for their newborn can shape their interactions with the baby and each other. Parents are influenced by the way they were parented, both consciously and unconsciously. Parents who are made more aware of their baby's competencies and abilities can optimize opportunities for bonding and mutuality. Past experiences with infants influence their expectations and motivation to parent and shape their efforts to nurture, love, and provide for their baby. The personality of the baby and any special needs the baby has can also play a part. Some factors that influence parental behaviors are important to appreciate; these include the baby's sex, birth order, weight, interfamilial and cultural background, and child-rearing practices they experienced from their own parents. Healthcare providers can positively influence modifiable factors, such as parenting knowledge and confidence, by providing education, supportive care, and affirming the abilities of both baby and parents. Access to racially concordant care for the postpartum person is emerging as an important step in improving health disparities and has been shown to improve satisfaction, trust, and adherence (Karbeah et al., 2019).

Each parent tends to interact differently with their babies. Traditionally, fathers were removed from the daily work of caring for the infant and provided discipline or playtime as the child grew, while mothers assumed primary care of the baby. As family structure has evolved and many more birth parents work, the roles of child-rearing vary from family to family. There are many factors that influence men's roles with their children including their relationship with their own father, culture, personality, infants' health, and employment status (Shorey & Ang, 2019). Many fathers in contemporary society want to be involved with the daily aspects of newborn care and are creating the space in their lives to do so (Shorey & Ang, 2019; Singley, 2015).

Sibling Adjustment

Sibling adjustment is an important part of family adaptation. Gender, personality, and interests of the older sibling can influence adjustment. The family's culture, size, setting, and support system also influence this relationship. Parental factors such as well-being, sense of competence, relationship with each other, and personality also have an effect on sibling adjustment (Coleman Smith, 2013; Volling, 2012). Parents may be confident about their care-taking abilities for the new infant but may be more concerned with how to manage two or more children adequately.

Changes in sibling behavior are common with the addition of a new family member. A child's response involves a whole multitude of factors, many of which are only a small part of having a new sibling. A person's relationship with their firstborn may feel disrupted, and their relationship with their partner may change, all of which can influence sibling adjustment. Resorting to more immature behaviors such as mimicry or imitation can occur as the older child attempts to get parental attention. Younger children may have behaviors such as increases in pacifier use, toileting accidents, difficulty being left with a sitter, following parents around the house, or aggression to the newborn. Older children can find it hard to play well with other children, have communication difficulties, and may spend more time lying around the house (Coleman Smith, 2013; Stewart et al., 1987; Volling, 2012). The addition of a new sibling can also be a period of rapid maturation for the older child (Stewart et al., 1987). And often, siblings enjoy interacting and caring for the new baby in ways that are appropriate to their age and abilities. Many of these behaviors will depend on what developmental milestones are occurring when the new sibling is introduced.

Anticipatory guidance can help families navigate these sibling adjustments. Sibling prenatal preparation should be tailored to their age and development. Some examples of preparation strategies are allowing participation during antepartum visits by using the tape measure and listening to fetal heart tones, helping with newborn preparations, and talking about "our" baby and what the sibling can expect the baby to do when born in realistic terms, not as a playmate. Attendance at sibling preparation classes has shown no difference in older sibling adjustment over time (Beyers-Carlson & Volling, 2017).

Adjustment can be facilitated by encouraging the belief that this is a time of acclimation versus a time of rivalry. Parents should not scold regressive behavior, but instead offer special time and attention to the older siblings. Visitors should be encouraged to spend time with older siblings when coming to visit the newborn. Parents can keep small gifts on hand for older siblings to decrease jealousy when visitors bring gifts for the newborn. Older siblings should have opportunities to interact with the newborn with supervision. Children can help with baby care as desired and age appropriate. It is important to encourage parents to spend some alone time with each sibling each day. Finally, it is good to remind parents that open communication and expression of frustration can help prevent aggressive behaviors during this time of sleep and schedule adjustments for the whole family (Coleman Smith, 2013; Volling, 2005).

Sibling adjustment can have a huge impact on the family as a whole (Volling, 2012). Relationship conflict and parental frustration can arise due to sibling maladjustment, which has also been found to increase postpartum mood and anxiety disorders, behavior issues, and substance abuse in siblings later in life (Dirks et al., 2015; Gallagher et al. 2018; Volling, 2005; Waid et al., 2020). Facilitating the adjustment of the whole family to the new baby is a health-promoting practice.

Matrescence

Maternal role attainment is a historical concept used to describe the process a mother goes through in taking on this new role (Rubin, 1967). The role attainment process may be influenced by culture, personal experiences with being parented, physical condition, socioeconomic status, preparation for this life event, and attitudes about parenting. While birth people begin this journey during pregnancy, continuous changes and honing of the concept of self will occur through transition to the first child and subsequent children. Matrescence is not a static one-time event but the beginning of a lifelong transformation that is being continually reevaluated and altered. Mercer and Walker have built on Rubin's and others work to develop the Becoming a Mother mid-range theory (Meighan, 2017). This newer theory takes into consideration the environmental factors and personal familiar characteristics that affect role development.

There are many things that can be done to help clients as they evolve their role. The healthcare provider can encourage clients to prepare in advance, trust their instincts about their child, offer suggestions and advice at postpartum and well-child visits, and demonstrate childcare practices (Mercer, 2004). Praise them for all that they are doing, while also emphasizing realistic expectations; encourage the client to use their support system and what has effectively worked for them in the past (Fahey & Shenassa, 2013). Ultimately, this is an important life process for the birthing person and will influence their self-esteem and satisfaction with their family, as well as set the stage for a nurturing environment for the child where infant development is enhanced.

Infant Feeding

The chosen infant feeding method will dictate how to approach this topic during postpartum visits. For those clients choosing formula-feeding, a discussion on specifics related to formula should occur. Education includes timing, frequency, and amount of feeding. Newborns should formula-feed every 2–3 hours for the first two weeks of life and then every 3–4 hours thereafter. Longer periods between feeds at night are fine as long as the infant is gaining weight. After the first 48 hours, the amount of formula taken will increase over the first month to at least 24 oz/day (American Academy of Pediatrics, 2018). Bottle care and formula storage should be discussed. Discard any infant formula that is left in bottles after feedings as the combination of formula and saliva can cause bacterial growth (CDC, 2022). Bottles can be washed by hand or in the dishwasher. Sterilization is not necessary.

Breast assessment is important in the client who is formula-feeding. These clients should be encouraged to wear a form-fitting bra around the clock and have minimal stimulation of the breasts. Nonsteroidal anti-inflammatory drugs (NSAIDs) can be beneficial for the discomfort experienced during this time. Breast engorgement, its resolution, and continuing leakage of milk should be determined. By the six-week visit, milk production has typically ceased and the breasts have returned to a non-pregnant state.

For those individuals choosing breastfeeding, the timing, frequency, and duration of feedings should be assessed, as well as the client's adjustment to feeding demands and the neonate's acceptance of breastfeeding. Breastfed babies typically eat 8–12 times in a 24-hour period for the first 2 weeks. Feeding on demand is encouraged. Both breasts are used for feeding, but at any given feeding, the baby can get enough supply from one breast.

Clients who are breastfeeding should also be taught to assess their nipples after each feeding. This can help determine early signs of nipple breakdown. A crease on the nipple after it is removed from the infant's mouth may signify poor latch. A reddened area or pain with latch may denote malpositioning, **ankyloglossia**, or a plugged duct. An exam of the breasts by inspection and palpation may be done based on history or any noted masses as needed. A visual inspection of the nipples can verify reports of nipple integrity or nipple problems. Chapter 31, *Lactation and Breastfeeding*, contains more detailed information.

Activity and Exercise

Postpartum fatigue and sleep deprivation are of significant concern because of their overall impact on parental health, as well as the ability to function and care for the newborn. It is difficult in the early postpartum days to recognize differences between what is normal or what is an early manifestation of an impending problem. Fatigue will impact everything the birthing person does during this time. They will need to prioritize rest and make time for themself and the other children. Encourage acceptance of help from family and friends. Household chores should be delegated to others. Encourage the birthing person to nap when the baby naps, as this will bolster strength for nighttime infant care and feedings.

All birthing people should be up and moving relatively soon after birth, even those who gave birth by cesarean section. Altered clotting factors increase the risk for thrombosis at this time; activity is a preventive practice. Advancement of activity beyond normal walking or home

Kegel exercises can begin shortly after birth and can help restore vaginal muscle tone as well as maintain urinary continence. Data suggest a link between pelvic floor muscle training and reduced incidence of urinary incontinence (Dong et al., 2021). During the vaginal exam at the six-week examination, ask the birthing person to perform a Kegel exercise around the examiner's gloved finger if during shared decision making this was agreed upon; muscle tone can be assessed and advice given accordingly.

Abdominal musculature has been stretched with the pregnancy and will take time to return to its nonpregnant state. Clients can begin abdominal strengthening exercises any time after an uncomplicated vaginal birth. These exercises can begin with the client lying flat on their backs on the floor with their knees bent pulling their abdomen toward the floor. If the individual had a cesarean birth, then abdominal exercises should be delayed until the incision has healed.

Walking can begin early in the postpartum period. Going outside in the fresh air benefits the whole family. Encourage clients to start slowly and build back to their normal routine. By monitoring lochial discharge, clients can gauge how their body is tolerating the increase in exercise. Heavier or brighter red lochia means they are doing too much too soon and need to slow down.

Safe limits for vigorous exercise during the early postpartum period have not been determined, so recommendations should be supportive but cautious. Encourage clients to listen to their bodies and remind them of the physiologic changes occurring that may necessitate altering their typical exercise patterns for a brief amount of time. However, in the absence of any complications, the resumption of exercise by starting slow and building back to regular routines can be beneficial and has not demonstrated harm (ACOG, 2020). Clients should be cautioned to stop exercising if they experience bright red vaginal bleeding, increased pain, shortness of breath, or lightheadedness. If symptoms do not improve with rest, they should seek care (see Chapter 20, *Physical Activity and Exercise in the Perinatal Period*).

Diet and Nutrition

The individual recovering from childbirth needs a high-quality, well-balanced diet. After assessing food security, clients can follow the MyPlate guidelines and should not calorie-restrict early in the postpartum period (US Department of Agriculture, n.d.; see Chapter 9, *Nutrition during Pregnancy*). Encouraging food choices with high nutritional value while minimizing empty calorie foods is important for their health. When breastfeeding, the average person needs approximately 500 calories more than what was needed prepregnancy. It is common to advise clients to continue the daily prenatal vitamin supplementation postpartum and through the duration of breastfeeding, with additional iron for clients who are anemic.

A calorie-restricted diet to intentionally lose weight should be avoided until lactation has been well established. Normal diet alone often results in weight loss after birth (McKinley et al., 2018). Over the first few weeks postpartum, weight loss will naturally occur through diuresis and diaphoresis of the excess fluid retained during pregnancy. It is important to encourage clients to drink when thirsty to maintain hydration. Encouraging water is best for hydration. Soda, fruit juices, and other high sugar drinks should be limited.

Weight Loss

Many clients are very concerned about returning to their prepregnant weight. It is important for clients to attain a healthy weight in the first several months postpartum to prevent obesity in subsequent pregnancies and later in life (ACOG, 2021; McKinley et al., 2018). Adequate time should be planned during the postpartum visit to assess diet, lifestyle, nutrition, and health risk factors. Reminding clients that they put on pregnancy weight over several months can help them realize that it may take several months for the weight to come off. A realistic time frame is to achieve prepregnancy weight by 6–12 months after birth (ACOG, 2021). Though many clients are motivated to lose excess weight, they are also adjusting to the demands of a new infant. Clients experiencing a difficult postpartum transition are less likely to engage in weight self-management behaviors in the 12 weeks following their baby's birth (McKinley et al., 2018). Evidence suggests that exercise can improve mood in the postpartum period (Poyatos-Leon et al., 2017). Exercise as an intentional therapy should be prescribed in the postpartum period to improve mood and facilitate weight loss. Individualized and realistic goals for weight loss are key.

Lochia

Lochia is the vaginal blood, tissue, and mucus loss occurring after birth and often lasting up to six or eight weeks postpartum. Lochia flow progresses through three predictable stages, but timing can vary. This bleeding contains erythrocytes, decidua, bacteria, and epithelial cells and is initially sterile until three to four days postpartum. Lochia rubra begins after birth and lasts for the first few days postpartum. Patterns of lochia flow vary in amount and duration between people and pregnancies (Table 30.3).

Each day, the amount of bleeding should be less and the color lighter. An exception to this rule is **eschar** bleeding

Table 30.3 Patterns of Lochial Flow

Lochial flow	Time frame
Lochia rubra	Lasts 1–4 days postpartum
Lochia serosa	After rubra—up to about 9 days postpartum
Lochia alba	After serosa—up to 5 weeks postpartum

Source: Adapted from Chauhan and Tadi (2020).

that occurs at about 10 days postpartum. At approximately 10 days, this "scab" over the placental site in the uterus will be released. Some may experience heavier, brighter red bleeding, which should only last for a few hours. If it persists beyond that time frame, they should be evaluated. It is important to note when postpartum lochia bleeding stopped. This helps determine whether bleeding at a future date is a return of menses or the continuation of lochial flow.

Afterbirth Pain

Afterbirth pains are caused by uterine contractions, and although the uterus does not return to its prepregnant size, it does return to a nonpregnant state. This process may be less intense in first-time clients as the uterus stays well contracted after birth. However, in multiparas or those with uterine overdistension, the uterus has to work harder to maintain muscle tone and return to a nonpregnant state. Thus, they often experience more severe cramping. Other factors increasing the frequency and strength of the afterbirth pains are breastfeeding and a full bladder. The act of breastfeeding leads to the release of endogenous oxytocin, which stimulates the uterus to contract. The bladder fills quickly due to postpartum diuresis and a full bladder can displace the uterus resulting in uterine atony. Both the endogenous oxytocin and emptying of a full bladder facilitates uterine contractions and may cause more intense afterbirth pains.

There are several recommendations to alleviate the discomfort. First, help the client understand that the sensation of cramping is the uterus working to contract and ligate the uterine vessels to diminish bleeding. This may give a different perspective to the afterpains. Second, physically helping the uterus to stay contracted may decrease the intensity of the afterpains. This can be accomplished by emptying the bladder regularly, gently massaging the **fundus** periodically, or lying prone with a pillow under the fundus. NSAIDs are the medication of choice. Ibuprofen 600 mg po Q6h prn is a common choice. If that does not suffice, then alternate acetaminophen 500 mg po q4h with the NSAIDs (Berens, 2022). Finally, stronger medications such as narcotics may be needed to control pain in the first hours or days after birth, particularly in multiparous women, and can be added to the NSAID regimen. Severe afterpains that last longer than two to three days should be evaluated to determine if there is a pathological cause of the pain (Deussen et al., 2020).

Perineal Discomfort

Some women will not sustain a perineal injury during childbirth. Intact perineum rates vary with providers. Midwives often use warm compresses, perineal massage in second stage, left lateral maternal position, and positions other than lithotomy, which can decrease the laceration rate. These methods have been shown to increase the rate of intact perineums and reduce the rate of third- and

fourth-degree lacerations (Magoda et al., 2019). Even with an intact perineum, the vaginal and perineal tissues may be bruised, edematous, and tender for several days after birth. The type of **laceration** or episiotomy will guide the assessment and management of the perineum. Some lacerations require minimal, if any, suturing, while others may need extensive suturing. By three weeks postpartum, most repairs should be well healed, and the sutures should have resorbed, except for the external knot. The knot will eventually be released when the suture underneath has been resorbed which may take four to five weeks.

Each day postpartum, the perineal area should evidence more healing, reflected in increasing comfort in the area. If there is increasing irritation or pain, then an examination is recommended. Diagnoses that are considered include perineal infection, hematoma, and dehiscence of the repair. Inquire about activities that could potentially irritate the area, such as intercourse or overexertion. For some people, it can take several months for the perineum to feel fully comfortable again.

For treatment to be effective, pain must first be diagnosed. Diagnosis of pain relies primarily on patient self-report, although there can be behavioral cues indicating pain. White clients have their pain assessed, diagnosed, and treated more frequently than Hispanic and non-Hispanic Black women. Black and Hispanic women are not only evaluated less frequently, they often have higher pain scores that are undertreated. This may result in negative effects on bonding, healing, breastfeeding, sexuality, and mood disorders (Johnson et al., 2019).

Options to relieve immediate postpartum perineal discomfort

- Ice packs: 20 min applications, especially in the first 2–24 hours after childbirth
- Cool or warm water bath
- Kegel exercises
- Topical anesthetics—benzocaine spray such as Dermoplast
- Herbal compresses—witch hazel, comfrey, and lavender oil
- Aromatherapy

Source: Adapted from Rezaie-Keikhaie et al. (2019).

Diuresis and Diaphoresis

The body's removal of excess water accumulated during pregnancy begins soon after birth. This usually occurs on days 2–5 but may start as early as 12 hours postpartum and lasts into the second week, especially if large amounts of intravenous (IV) fluids were used in labor.

Diuresis of about 3000 mL/day is common. A single void can be 500 mL or more (Blackburn, 2018). Remind clients of the importance of keeping the bladder empty and the uterus contracted and reassure them that the loss of this extra fluid is a natural part of the postpartum recovery process. This process should be completed by three weeks postpartum.

Diaphoresis is another route for shedding the excess extracellular fluid retained during pregnancy. Remind clients of its normalcy and discuss comfort measures. Encourage frequent showering or bathing, wearing natural fibers, and dressing in layers. Keep fluids at the bedside and drink to thirst. Explain that weight loss of 5–6 pounds of fluid during this time can be expected. Breastfeeding clients may experience diaphoresis during breastfeeding.

Constipation and Hemorrhoids

For many people, resumption of regular bowel habits can take up to a week in part because many will have had limited intake during labor. Some will push out stool during birth but may be unaware they have done so. This should be shared with clients to relieve some of the anxiety surrounding the lack of a bowel movement the first few days after birth. Fear of disrupting sutures or causing more pain to an already sensitive area may cause clients to withhold bowel movements. Medications such as iron supplementation or narcotics, which have the side effect of constipation, can also make this more of an issue postpartum. Constipation often leads to straining, which can cause hemorrhoids or worsen ones that developed during pregnancy or were exacerbated during birth.

Constipation and hemorrhoid treatment often overlap. Constipation treatments include increasing fluids, high-fiber foods such as raw fruits, vegetables and whole grains, and moderate activity such as walking. Over-the-counter stool softeners such as Docusate Sodium can relieve some of the fear associated with a bowel movement and adding a mild laxative for those with a third- or fourth-degree laceration is common practice. Clients often fear that having a bowel movement may disrupt their sutures. Reassure them that this is rarely the case. Relief measures for hemorrhoids are aimed at reducing the size, discomfort, and itching with over-the-counter Tucks or witch hazel compresses, Preparation H ointment, and anesthetic sprays. Warm perineal baths and preventive behaviors such as avoiding prolonged sitting on the toilet or straining during bowel movements are also beneficial. Finally, remind clients that preventing constipation may prevent hemorrhoids as well.

Sleep

The postpartum period is characterized by a significant lack of sleep for most new parents. Sleep disturbance can include both sleep deprivation and sleep fragmentation that disrupts the integrity of the sleep cycle. Despite extreme fatigue, insomnia can increase for some people and further reduce sleep time. Cumulative lack of sleep and sleep fragmentation increasingly worsen up to three months postpartum and can significantly affect daytime functioning and mood (Gueron-Sela et al., 2021; Ladyman et al., 2021). Lower sleep quality at three months postpartum is associated with worse symptomatology for

perinatal mood and anxiety disorders and parenting stress. This can lead to a vicious cycle of sleep disturbances, mood disorders, parenting stress, and poor infant outcomes including poor growth, disturbed infant bonding, and later developmental delays (Gueron-Sela et al., 2021; Slomian et al., 2019). The assessment of the family's sleep duration and quality is essential during postpartum visits. Areas to assess include employment, household assistance, use of medications, alcohol and herbal preparations, sleep duration and quality, and number of nighttime awakenings. Some parents feel that co-sleeping improves the quality of their sleep since they can feed without getting out of bed. However, some research has shown that the opposite may also be true (Volkovich et al., 2015). This is an opportunity for active listening and shared decision-making between families and healthcare providers.

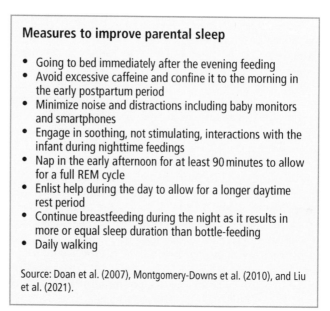

Measures to improve parental sleep

- Going to bed immediately after the evening feeding
- Avoid excessive caffeine and confine it to the morning in the early postpartum period
- Minimize noise and distractions including baby monitors and smartphones
- Engage in soothing, not stimulating, interactions with the infant during nighttime feedings
- Nap in the early afternoon for at least 90 minutes to allow for a full REM cycle
- Enlist help during the day to allow for a longer daytime rest period
- Continue breastfeeding during the night as it results in more or equal sleep duration than bottle-feeding
- Daily walking

Source: Doan et al. (2007), Montgomery-Downs et al. (2010), and Liu et al. (2021).

Sleep deprivation and insomnia are significantly associated with maternal mental health disorders (Da Costa et al., 2021; Hutchens & Likis, 2019). If clients continue to have difficulty falling asleep or returning to sleep for more than two to four weeks, screening for perinatal depression and anxiety should be done and referral to a sleep clinic considered.

Sexuality

Resuming intimacy in the postpartum period is an important but often overlooked or avoided subject. In order to provide holistic care, it is critical to understand that resuming sexual practice is not a medical decision and there is no evidence to support six weeks as the time to resume intercourse. Some couples will have resumed sexual relations before the six-week visit. Physically, perineal discomfort, vaginal bleeding or discharge, dyspareunia, fatigue, insufficient lubrication, leaking or tender breasts, fear of waking the infant, fear of injury, fear of pregnancy, or a decreased sense of attractiveness may be experienced and typically these have been the focus of discussion (Ollivier et al., 2020). Psychologically, the birth experience, relationship issues, body image, and role conflict (Khajehei & Doherty, 2017) can also affect the resumption of intimacy. Social support, understanding, and empathy from partners is a critical element to postpartum healing and positive well-being in relation to sexuality and sexual identity (Ollivier et al., 2020).

Healthcare providers may need to help couples redefine intimacy. Sometimes intimacy does not involve the resumption of sexual practices, particularly penetrative sex, but intimacy needs may be fulfilled in various ways such as holding, touching, and caressing. Expressing goodwill and humor, creating time and space to be together, feeling nurtured, and getting adequate sleep can strengthen relationships during this transitional time and can lead to enhanced sexual desire.

When penetrative sex is desired, vaginal lubrication may be reduced, especially if the person is breastfeeding. Extended foreplay and use of lubricants can improve sexual experiences for postpartum clients. Lubricants such as Astroglide and K-Y Jelly are water soluble and safe to use with latex condoms. Silicone-based lubricants last longer and can also be used with latex condoms but not with toys or tools made of silicone. Natural oils, such as mineral oil and olive oil, can be used but can weaken the integrity of latex condoms.

Providing open communication and creation of a safe space will facilitate the client's self-definition of what is important to them and how they want to define their sexual health. This will help prevent further harm to those who are not heteronormative and provide space for clients to be the experts in their own sexual health. Allow room for sexual health to look and feel different, not as a problem, but as one point along the continuum (Handelzalts et al., 2018; Ollivier et al., 2020; see Chapter 21, *Sexuality*).

Resumption of Menses and Ovulation

In order to help birthing people anticipate the resumption of menses and ovulation in the postpartum period, it is important to take a thorough history including gender identity, sexual orientation, values, and fertility goals. Knowing the client's lochial flow pattern can help determine if bleeding or spotting is a resumption of lochia or menses. Note their infant feeding method, including frequency and amounts of supplementation with pumped milk and formula. Clients who breastfeed, even for a short amount of time, may have a delayed resumption of menses due to the hormonal shifts that occur to sustain lactation.

There is no certainty as to when menses and ovulation will begin. Understanding that fertility can return before menses resumes is essential contraceptive teaching. Clients who formula-feed their baby can anticipate a return of menses within four to six weeks postpartum (Makins & Cameron, 2020). Generally, when exclusively

breastfeeding, high prolactin levels delay the resumption of ovulation and menses. However, this varies between 2 and 18 months postpartum. Emphasis should be placed on the unknown nature of the return of ovulation and the ability for ovulation to precede menses, especially for those who want to prevent further or closely spaced pregnancies.

Contraception

Discussions about family planning should ideally begin in the prenatal period. For those who want contraception, many will choose to resume the method previously used. Method of infant feeding, sexual history, types of contraception, ease of use, success with prior use, lifestyle, partner responsibilities, and reproductive life plans are important components of this discussion.

Combined hormonal contraceptive (CHC) methods are contraindicated before 21 days postpartum due to the heightened risk of venous thromboembolism (VTE; CDC, 2016). Clients with risk factors for VTE should be evaluated between days 21 and 42 and included in a risk/benefit analysis regarding contraception decisions; however, the risk of using CHCs must be balanced against the risk of pregnancy. Other methods may be more appropriate for these individuals. After 42 days postpartum, standard criteria for eligibility for CHC are used (CDC, 2016).

Progestin-only pills are the most commonly recommended choice for clients who breastfeed and desire oral contraceptives. Some prefer to limit newborn exposure to exogenous hormones during this time, as progesterone and estrogen can be found in the milk supply (Kennedy & Goldsmith, 2018). While there are concerns about infant exposure to progestins, there is no evidence of harm.

Breastfeeding influences contraception in several ways. Most exclusively breastfeeding people will experience lactational amenorrhea, which is considered a reliable birth control method for three to six months postpartum (Kennedy & Goldsmith, 2018; Van der Wijden & Manion, 2015). For this to be a reliable method of contraception, clients must breastfeed frequently around the clock with minimal supplementation and have not resumed menses or given their infant other food sources. For more detailed information on postnatal contraception, see Chapter 32, *Contraception in the Postnatal Period*.

Postpartum Physical Examination

Breast Exam

For clients who choose to breastfeed, a visual inspection of the breasts and nipples for any areas of breakdown or redness is done. Observation of a feeding can assist in the assessment for signs of poor latch. Infant malpositioning and poor latch can lead to nipple breakdown. Educate clients to evaluate their breasts on a regular basis; this can help identify early signs of tissue breakdown. Excessive redness, a break in the skin, or a compressed nipple right after feeding may be signs of poor latch or an infant with ankyloglossia. While inspecting the breast, assess for warm or reddened areas as well as breast discomfort. Such areas can indicate mastitis; this is discussed in more detail in Chapter 44, *Common Lactation and Breastfeeding Problems.*

Clients who choose not to breastfeed may experience breast engorgement on days 2–4 postpartum. They should be encouraged to refrain from stimulating the breasts in any way. A form-fitting bra should be worn, even to sleep at night. Cold compresses and NSAIDs can be used as needed. Lack of breast stimulation will decrease the levels of prolactin and milk production will decline and then cease. Milk production may take several days to decrease and several weeks to stop.

Palpation of lactating or nonlactating breasts should be done in a standard and thorough manner. Compress the nipple at the end of the exam and observe any discharge. Follow-up and collaboration or referral should be undertaken for any abnormal breast changes or persistent areas of concern.

A breast exam is typically performed at the six-week postpartum visit. Historically, it was thought that palpation of the lactating breast would not yield relevant information due to the inherent physical changes. Approximately 7% of all breast cancers in clients under 45 are diagnosed during pregnancy or the first year postpartum, and incidence is on the rise (Case, 2016). Clients who have breast cancer detected postpartum have a worse prognosis than breast cancer detected at any other life stage (Hartman & Eslick, 2016; Lefrere, et al., 2021). The hormonal influences during pregnancy, delays in evaluation and diagnosis during pregnancy and lactation, and the increasing incidence of women initiating pregnancy at a later age can contribute to a poorer prognosis (Case, 2016; Hartman & Eslick, 2016, Lefrere et al., 2021). However, childbearing is associated with long-term risk reductions in breast cancer—a reduction of 4.3% for every 12 months of breastfeeding and up to 33% for clients who breastfeed for up to 2 years. The negative effect is that there is a transient increased risk immediately postpartum that can last up to 10 years (Lefrere et al., 2021). Clients should be instructed to report concerning changes. Follow-up should be initiated without delay for any persistent lump. While clogged ducts are likely, the healthcare provider should maintain a high index of suspicion for malignancies.

Abdominal Exam

Involution of the uterus is assessed by the location of the fundus compared to either the umbilicus or symphysis pubis as landmarks. Involution of the uterus follows a typical pattern approximating one fingerbreadth of descent per day from the umbilicus to the pubis symphysis. During the first few days after birth, the uterus should be at or below the umbilicus. If the uterus is above or displaced to the side of the umbilicus, the bladder may be full. Ask the client to empty their bladder and reassess. On day 3 postpartum, the fundus should be about three fingerbreadths below the

umbilicus; day 4, four fingerbreadths (see Figure 6.2 in Chapter 6, *Physiologic Alternations during the Postnatal Period*). The fundus of the uterus should only be palpable abdominally for up to two weeks, after which time, the involuted uterus sits below the symphysis pubis and is a pelvic organ once again. If the fundus is not located where anticipated, and the client's bladder is empty, further evaluation is needed. At the six-week exam, the uterus is evaluated on pelvic exam, as it is no longer felt abdominally.

The consistency of the fundus is also noted. A firm consistency means the myometrial fibers are contracting and there is less blood loss. A soft or **boggy** uterus means the fibers are relaxed, which can result in heavier bleeding. The fundus is massaged and any clots expelled, which allows the fundus to contract and maintain a firm consistency.

The route of birth will determine expectations and extent of the abdominal examination. Abdominal inspection after cesarean birth includes assessing for signs of infection (warmth, redness, and drainage) and wound dehiscence. Incision staples are usually removed around day 4 postpartum. Sutures will dissolve on their own. If there is concern for wound dehiscence, then staples may remain in situ for a week or more postpartum. An office visit for a one- to two-week incision check is a standard practice.

To assess the degree of **diastasis recti**, the client should lie in a supine position with knees bent. Place examining fingers midline on the abdomen. Palpate using just the fingertips angled toward the floor from the xiphoid process to the pubic symphysis noting width and depth. Repeat after having the client bring their chin to their chest to engage the rectus muscles. A separation may be noted anywhere along the midline between these two sheaths. Ideally, the separation will narrow with the engagement of the rectus muscles. Estimate this space in fingerbreadths. Knowing the degree of diastasis can be a motivating factor to help clients resume exercise and regain muscle tone. It can also help to identify people who could benefit from working with a physical therapist to further assist with this aspect of postpartum recovery. This is discussed in greater detail in Chapter 20, *Physical Activity and Exercise in the Perinatal Period*.

Costovertebral Angle Tenderness

Consider assessing for costovertebral angle tenderness (CVAT) during any postpartum encounter. There is an increased risk for urinary tract infection (UTI) in the postpartum period due to events and interventions that can occur during labor and birth. Urinary stasis, overdistention of the bladder, and vulvar trauma all increase the risk of UTI.

Perineal Exam

A thorough birth history noting second-stage events will facilitate what to expect when performing a perineal assessment. If the client had an episiotomy or a laceration, then the inspection of the area can be done during postpartum care in the birth facility or home visit and at the 6–12-week postpartum visit. Assessment of the perineum is individualized unless there are specific perineal concerns.

Superficial perineal tissues should be healed by two to three weeks postpartum, but it can take up to a few months to be completely healed if extensive tearing occurred or an episiotomy was performed. Removal of the last knot of suture may be warranted based on complaints and observation. If all remaining repaired tissue is healed, then it is safe to remove the last suture. Areas noted as pink, granular tissue from chronic inflammation can be very tender and friable. The use of silver nitrate to cauterize the area and reset the wound healing process may offer the client relief. A faint pinkish line should be noted where the tissues have approximated and healed. If there is redness, edema, purulent exudate, or a fever, then a perineal infection should be suspected, and appropriate management initiated.

Vaginal and Uterine Exam

After birth, the vagina can be bruised, lacerated, and edematous. Over the first few days postpartum, increased vaginal tone will be noted as the edema subsides. A vaginal exam is not necessary at the two-week visit unless the client is reporting symptoms indicative of excessive postpartum bleeding or endometritis. If the uterus is larger than anticipated for two weeks postpartum, then subinvolution is suspected and the cause investigated. If the individual is saturating more than one pad per hour, a speculum and bimanual pelvic exam is performed to determine the cause of postpartum hemorrhage. The management will depend on symptoms and findings.

Rugae return at approximately three to four weeks postpartum. However, the vagina never fully returns to its prepregnant state. Hymenal tag remnants can be observed, as well as scars from lacerations and repairs.

At six weeks postpartum, a speculum exam is considered for cultures, a Pap smear if indicated, and for the visual inspection of internal tissues. A digital vaginal exam is considered to assess uterine size, shape and tenderness, palpate ovaries, and assess vaginal muscle tone. The uterus is approximately the size of a nonpregnant uterus by six weeks postpartum. Before removing examining fingers from the client's vagina, ask them to perform a Kegel exercise to assess vaginal tone. See Chapter 2, *Ethics in Perinatal Care*, for more discussion on informed consent and shared decision-making.

Assessment for pelvic organ prolapse (POP) may also be indicated at this time. Symptoms commonly reported include a lump or bulge in the genital area, pressure or heaviness, or the feeling that something is falling out (i.e., a tampon or one's uterus). It is important for providers to note that symptoms do not correlate well to the degree of prolapse. Referral to a pelvic floor physical therapist should be offered to anyone reporting symptoms, regardless of severity.

Rectal Exam

Some clients have preexisting hemorrhoids and others will develop these during pregnancy and childbirth. In many cases, these will resolve in the early postpartum period with time and comfort measures, such as topical ointments and Sitz baths. Symptomatic hemorrhoids are evaluated to guide further treatment. Occasionally, referral to a proctologist will be indicated.

A rectal exam may be indicated after a third- or fourth-degree laceration to assess the healing, integrity, and tonus of the internal and external anal sphincters. Any report of fecal incontinence warrants an assessment of the rectovaginal wall. Occult tears of the anal sphincter during childbirth are emerging as a high-risk litigation area. While rectal exams are used sparingly, it is important to note appropriate healing of all areas traumatized during childbirth. There is debate in the literature on whether a client with a third- or fourth-degree laceration should have a vaginal birth or cesarean section with a subsequent birth. There is a lack of robust evidence on whether and under what conditions to recommend an elective cesarean birth but an expected birth weight of >4000 g and a duration of second stage >30 m are statistically significant risk factors for recurrence of obstetric anal sphincter injury. Mediolateral episiotomy is associated with significantly lower rates of sphincter injury in both spontaneous vaginal and operative vaginal deliveries (Van Bavel et al., 2020). However, they are also associated with more acute pain and are more difficult to repair. There are some who advocate that cesarean birth should be offered in subsequent pregnancies to individuals who have had a fourth-degree laceration with shared decision-making including risks, benefits, and harms, and then the client's decision should be honored (Yogev et al., 2014).

Leg Exam

Evaluation of the lower extremities is done in the days following birth and should be considered at the two- and six-week visit. Some people will develop varicosities during pregnancy; postpartum assessment can direct further management. An evaluation of any leg pain or tenderness should be done to assess potential deep or superficial venous thrombosis. If a cord-like vessel is noted, or the patient has warmth over an area, edema, or reports pain or tenderness, consultation and testing may be indicated. Homan's sign is not highly predictive and may or may not be positive in the presence of venous thrombosis. Normal pregnancy edema of the legs has usually dissipated by two weeks postpartum.

Postpartum Mental Health Disorders

The incidence of postpartum depression (PPD) and postpartum anxiety (PPA) is increasing. They are treatable yet underdiagnosed conditions with significant adverse health effects for postpartum clients, newborns, and the families (McKee et al., 2020). As many as 85% of postpartum clients experience the transitory *baby blues*.

Women in developed countries experience PPD with the highest rates being in the United States (Slomian et al., 2019; United States Preventive Services Task Force, 2019) and 20% experience anxiety (Nakić Radoš et al., 2018).

A Healthy People 2030 goal and the American Association of Pediatrics recommendation is to screen for depression during every postpartum encounter: routine postpartum visits, problem visits, and well-child checks. Anxiety has a 75% comorbidity rate alongside depression (Nakić Radoš et al., 2018), and therefore, the American College of Obstetricians and Gynecologists (ACOG) also recommends anxiety screening during the postpartum visits. Validated screening tools such as the Edinburgh Postnatal Depression Scale (EPDS) and Generalized Anxiety Disorder-7 (GAD-7) should be used (ACOG, 2018a). Some postpartum clients may be stigmatized, distrustful of the healthcare system, and fearful that their children could be taken from them. Some people may not screen positively on the EPDS but may show somatic symptoms such as high blood pressure, unexplained body aches, and nausea. These symptoms should be seen as potential warning signs. In this case, there are other screening tools such as the Centers for Epidemiologic Studies Depression Scale (CES-D), Beck Depression Inventory-II (BDI-II), or the International Depression Symptom Scale (IDSS; Haroz et al., 2017). These screening tools can be given to clients in the waiting area or as they enter the exam room, allowing privacy to complete the tool while waiting to be seen. If the early postpartum visit is taking place via telehealth, the screening can be done verbally or electronically. Clinicians can then score responses and talk to them about their answers. Some individuals may be ashamed about their feelings or feel they should be happy since they just had a baby and may not want to share their negative feelings. Self-report screening tools, in conjunction with further evaluation, may be helpful for clients who are reluctant to self-disclose. If a diagnosis of PPD/PPA is made, then collaboration with mental health practitioners is warranted. It has been shown that anticipatory guidance before discharge from the hospital, birth center, or before the provider leaves the home followed by a phone call at two weeks reduces symptoms of PPD and increases breastfeeding duration through six months postpartum among African Americans and Hispanic clients (ACOG, 2018b). Postpartum mood and anxiety disorders are discussed in detail in Chapter 43, *Common Complications during the Postnatal Period*, and Chapter 47, *Mood and Anxiety Disorders*.

Intimate Partner Violence Screening

All postpartum clients should be screened at every encounter to determine if they are safe in their home from intimate partner violence (IPV; ACOG, 2012) as one in three clients experiences physical violence over their lifetime. Almost half of Black, American Indian, and Alaskan Native women report physical violence, sexual violence, and/or stalking by an intimate partner in their lifetime (National Partnership for Women & Families, 2021). Questioning about IPV may occur many times before a client is comfortable sharing this information. Make IPV questioning a routine part of all encounters, so that clients know they can choose to share this information. If they report abuse and are ready to make a change, community resources can be activated. For many clients, pregnancy and childbirth can be a vulnerable time when abuse escalates. PPD/PPA and IPV often coexist. People who experience recurrent past or current IPV are at significantly higher risk for postpartum mood and anxiety disorders (Velonis et al., 2017). Clients can be motivated to seek care due to concerns about the safety of their baby (CDC, 2021a). See Chapter 26, *Violence and Trauma in the Perinatal Period*, for a more detailed discussion on IPV.

Postpartum Warning Signs

According to the CDC, 36% of maternal deaths occur during birth and up to the first week postpartum and another 33% occur between one week and one year postpartum (CDC, 2019). Signs and symptoms can appear during the postpartum period and are linked to various differential diagnoses and should be considered (Table 30.4). Sharing this information with the birthing person and their support system is key to decreasing maternal mortality.

Cultural Considerations

Cultural traditions and practices are common during childbirth and the postpartum period. Clients often look to family members or community for support and guidance. Postpartum rituals can act to support clients and affirm their sense of family and community. However, if cultural beliefs or practice are not supported by the healthcare team, the client can feel isolated and belittled, which can influence one's risk of PPD (Abdollahi et al., 2016). Therefore, every client should be given the opportunity to discuss their desire to incorporate family and cultural practices into their care.

Cultural traditions are assessed during the prenatal period, and practices should be honored without interference and encouraged unless safety is a concern. Healthcare providers should not make assumptions based on ethnicity. Determine individual needs and facilitate meeting these needs. By gaining a basic understanding of the common cultures in the local community, the practitioner can better care for clients during the postpartum period.

Many cultures value postpartum as a time of healing for the postpartum person and specify a period when the client and baby will remain relatively secluded and cared for by female relatives (Kim-Godwin, 2003). This practice contrasts with many Western cultures, where clients are often expected to resume normal activities relatively soon after birth. Some cultures specify that sexual intercourse cannot resume until all bleeding has stopped or a specified period has elapsed, such as Orthodox Jews. Many cultures

Table 30.4 Postpartum Warning Signs

Symptom	Differential diagnoses
Saturating maxi pad in <1 hour × 1–2 hours And/or Passing golf ball-sized clots, more than 1	Postpartum hemorrhage, endometritis, or retained products of conception
A return of bright red bleeding after that phase of lochia has passed	Eschar bleeding, delayed postpartum hemorrhage, overexertion, or endometritis
Temperature > 101 °F (38 °C)	Endometritis, mastitis, viral infection, or UTI
Severe headache Visual disturbances GI upset (pain, nausea, and vomiting)	Postpartum preeclampsia or postepidural headache
Seizure	Postpartum eclampsia
Lump and/or warmth on breast	Plugged duct, mastitis, or malignancy
Chest pain and difficulty breathing	Pulmonary emboli
Warm area, pain, or edema in calf	Deep vein thrombosis or superficial thrombophlebitis
Difficulty or pain with urination	Urinary retention, UTI, or periurethral laceration
Pus, redness, and foul odor at cesarean section scar	Incision infection, wound dehiscence, or granulation tissue
Pus, redness, or foul odor of perineum	Endometritis, perineal infection, or granulation tissue
Hopelessness, despair, anger, or fear of harming self, infant, or other children	Postpartum depression, anxiety, psychosis, or postpartum thyroiditis
Worsening of any symptoms is cause for more in-depth evaluation and usually face-to-face evaluation	

view postpartum as a cold period and encourage particular foods, at certain temperatures or with certain food characteristics that are considered hot, in order to help restore balance and help prevent ailments later in life (Leung, 2017). For example, the standard hospital pitcher of ice water on the bedside table will be ignored by those who hold these beliefs, whereas tepid water will be accepted. By helping facilitate cultural traditions and practices, healthcare providers communicate respect for this heritage. See Chapter 19, *Culture and Community*, for further discussion of this topic.

Health Disparities and Vulnerable Populations

Health disparities are a national travesty in populations that are marginalized in the United States. Postpartum clients of color, immigrants or refugees, uninsured or underinsured, homeless, adolescents, LGBTQIA+, and those who suffer abuse will all need additional considerations during postpartum follow-up. Some clients may simultaneously fall into several vulnerable categories, putting them at added risk for problems.

A growing body of literature confirms that people of color experience racism and racial biases throughout their healthcare experiences. Women of color have reported that their experience of pregnancy and birth care were negatively impacted by providers who withheld or present biased and incomplete information (Altman, et al., 2019). They felt that the "packaging" of information was intended to influence their decision-making (Altman et al., 2019).

Additionally, Black people who experience pain are less likely to be assessed and treated in the postpartum period, contributing to the inequities in outcomes. This is rooted in the false narrative that there are physiologic differences in the way people of various races and ethnicities experience pain (Hoffman et al., 2016).

Immigrant or refugee clients may not speak the language, understand rites or customs, or be able to negotiate everyday systems such as taking a bus or finding their clinic within a hospital. Food, shelter, and healthcare can be daunting tasks. Taking time during visits to assess available resources, and supplementing where appropriate, can facilitate optimal health for the whole family. Clients struggle to care for themselves and their newborns if they are worried about how to eat or maintain shelter.

The uninsured and underinsured in the United States have many barriers including healthcare costs. Healthcare practices are often influenced by reimbursement, and lack of reimbursement is one reason why many practices do not offer additional postpartum services in spite of need. Most insurance payers only reimburse for one postpartum visit, which is often part of the global fee. However, if clients can be screened earlier, and problems averted, then less healthcare dollars will be spent to rectify ailments after the fact (Luca et al., 2019). Since 2018, ACOG's Optimizing Postpartum Care has recommended an initial assessment within the first 3 weeks postpartum, either by phone or in person, and then a comprehensive postpartum visit no later than 12 weeks after birth guided by the health concerns present after the birth. Incorporating this flexibility into the visits provides space to be patient-centric versus provider-centric.

Adolescents face numerous challenges during the postpartum period. While teen pregnancy rates are down overall, some groups, such as teens living in southern or northwestern states, continue to have higher rates with Hispanic and non-Hispanic Black teens two times the rate of non-Hispanic White teens. American Indian/Alaska Natives had the highest teen pregnancy rate among all races and ethnicities (CDC, 2021b). Teenage clients are challenged in the development of a parental role, as they are going through their own adolescent growth and development at the same time. Self-esteem can be an important factor in the developing relationship between teen parent and child. Teenage clients face social and economic disadvantages. Healthcare providers play important roles in education and support. Health education and advice should be tailored to appropriate developmental levels. Authentic praise and compassionate support can go a long way in facilitating positive behaviors. Role modeling of appropriate care and parenting behaviors can also be helpful. About a third of teens will experience a repeat pregnancy within a short time interval (McCracken & Loveless, 2014). Postpartum follow-up is essential to help ameliorate this cycle. Discussions about reliable contraception should begin prenatally and continue at each postpartum encounter. Teen clients should be screened for IPV and asked if they feel safe during postpartum visits.

There is a high rate of failure to show for postpartum visits; as many as 40% of clients did not have timely postpartum care (ACOG, 2018b). Some of the most marginalized clients are the least likely to receive postpartum care. Clients who are from ethnic minorities, have Medicaid or no insurance, and are younger than aged 25 are less likely to attend postpartum care visits (The National Committee for Quality Assurance, 2016; Wilcox et al., 2016). Lack of transportation or childcare, fatigue, employment, and a perception that the visit is not essential are barriers to attending postnatal visits (Dibari et al., 2014). Patient-centric interventions prenatally in the form of postpartum care planning to improve attendance rates may include topics such as timing of postpartum visits, choice of telehealth or in person visits, who the care team is and how to reach them, as well as what is to be accomplished at each visit (Fowler et al., 2016). Helping clients learn about care for themselves, their baby, and family can be very challenging when access to information is limited, and other daily living needs take precedence. The identification of barriers to care, health teaching, and communicating the purpose for postpartum follow-up visits are important aspects of care before discharge following childbirth.

Incorporating home visits and the creative use of social media for monitoring, education, and support has been shown to be effective and to enhance and expand postpartum care during the COVID-19 pandemic. However, many marginalized populations have shown decreased completed telehealth visits and decreased video visits, which reveal that there is a potential to increase health disparities in these populations (Eberly et al., 2020), which must be addressed before this can become part of the normative healthcare routine. Not everyone has the ability to afford smartphones, computers, and internet access. A reexamination and restructuring of postpartum care as currently offered is considered essential to increasing utilization and improving health in the childbearing year.

Interprofessional Care

Consultation, collaboration, and referral can occur with physicians, therapists, social workers, lactation consultants, as well as other providers. Bringing in the expertise of other professionals with different knowledge and skill sets to serve the client's needs is an important clinical decision point that can promote optimal health.

There are varying levels of involvement of other providers. Consultation refers to talking with another provider about the care of a client. This person may have more expertise in a particular area, or a consultation may be warranted based on protocols or practicing at the boundaries of scope of practice. An example in postnatal care is when a client has recurrent plugged ducts while breastfeeding. A lactation consultant can be contacted for a more detailed assessment and treatment plan to ameliorate this problem and prevent mastitis.

Collaboration occurs when each practitioner assumes part of the care for the client. A client having a cesarean birth is an example of collaborative care. A physician performs the cesarean birth, and the original provider may be involved in inpatient postsurgical care and ongoing postpartum care.

Referral is necessary when patient condition dictates that another provider would better serve the client. Referral is warranted when a client presents with a high fever, abdominal tenderness, foul-smelling lochia, abnormal bleeding, or subinvolution. One clinician may begin the workup, obtaining cultures or blood work, and a physician will assume care of this client and treat the severe endometritis requiring hospitalization.

Employment Considerations

The United States ranks last among industrialized countries in providing paid maternity or parental leave. As of 2019, the United States and New Guinea are the only two countries worldwide that do not guarantee paid maternity leave and of the countries that offer paid leave over half also offer paternity leave. The International Labour Organization, a United Nations agency, recommends at least 18 weeks of maternity leave (Rubin, 2016). In many Scandinavian and European countries, maternity leave is subsidized for 10 months to 3 years (Fisher et al., 2016). Canada provides a year or more of paid parental leave with 55% of pay replaced. Currently, only eight states have paid maternity leave (World Population Review, 2021).

During postpartum, the Family and Medical Leave Act (FMLA) entitles eligible employees of covered employers to take unpaid, job-protected leaves for specified family and medical reasons with the continuation of group health insurance coverage under the same terms and conditions as if the employee had not taken leave. The company must have at least 50 employees, and an employee must have worked there for 1 year to be eligible. The FMLA allows up to 12 work weeks of unpaid leave in a 12-month period for childbirth and care of the newborn within 1 year of birth (United States Department of Labor, n.d.). Many employers require documentation of a six-week postpartum exam before returning to work. More than 40% of US workers do not meet all of FMLA's requirements, and even if they do, many cannot afford to take unpaid leave (US Department of Labor, 2018). Clients of lower socioeconomic status and who are younger and unmarried are less likely to be able to utilize the benefits, as there is no income to offset the time.

There are multiple benefits of paid parental leave for the newborn, client, and family. Increased breastfeeding initiation and duration has been found with paid leave (Mirkovic et al., 2016; Van Niel et al., 2020). Breastfeeding, in turn, helps decrease Sudden Infant Death Syndrome, obesity, asthma, and necrotizing enterocolitis rates in children, while helping decrease breast and ovarian cancer in birthing people (Mirkovic et al., 2016). Paid leave of a minimum of six months improves mental and physical health (Aitken et al., 2015), results in higher rates of well-baby physical examinations and immunization uptake, and decreases infant morbidity and mortality (Van Niel et al., 2020). Long-term benefits of paid leave include reduced high school dropout rate and higher income in adulthood (Carneiro et al., 2015). Postpartum is a time of physical recovery from pregnancy and birth, and of psychosocial adjustment in family structure and relationships. All of this can place a strain on families and can lead to maladaptation. Postpartum mood and anxiety disorders are a significant health challenge not only for the client but also for the family and employers. Even 12 weeks of leave might not be enough time for all of these adaptations to occur (Dagher et al., 2014). The American Academy of Pediatrics and Pediatric Policy Council both recommend 12 weeks paid leave (Dodson & Talib, 2020). UNICEF recommends six months (Chzhen et al., 2019). Advocacy efforts at the legislative level are needed to help make this change.

Healthcare providers must become politically active and advocate for a change to the current system. Paid maternity leave should be the rule, rather than the exception. Partners should be allowed paid time to help support the recovering postpartum person, to bond with the infant, and to support the establishment of breastfeeding. This will take political will and advocacy from a broad range of constituents to bring the United States in line with other countries, but it will reap financial and health benefits for the nation in the long run.

Summary

The postpartum period follows one of the most significant life-changing experiences and is a critical phase in the individual's and the family's life. Half of maternal deaths occur postnatally, and the United States was one of only two countries to report a significant increase in its overall mortality ratio. Even worse, Black clients die at rates 2.5 times higher than White clients and 3 times higher than Hispanic clients (Declercq & Zephyrin, 2020). During pregnancy, it is natural to focus on one's current needs and the preparation for childbirth; however, little emphasis is placed on anticipatory guidance for postpartum. Warning signs for postpartum physical and mental health abnormalities must be shared. Families need to feel they are in a safe partnership with the healthcare team. Many of the physical and emotional problems that clients suffer after childbirth can be prevented or ameliorated with good postpartum care. A postpartum care plan initiated in the prenatal period and incorporated into the client's medical record is one step toward this goal. An increase in the attention and support clients receive during this time can positively affect their long-term well-being, as well as the health and well-being of their infant and their family (Bartel et al., 2019).

Resources for Clients and Families

Websites/Hotlines

Domestic violence Hotline: 1-800-799-SAFE, Multilingual

March of Dimes, Postpartum Care Plan: https://www.marchofdimes.org/pregnancy/your-postpartum-checkups.aspx

Nutrition, exercise, weight loss: https://www.myplate.gov/life-stages/pregnancy-and-breastfeeding

Perinatal mood and anxiety disorders: Postpartum Support International: www.postpartum.net; 1-800-944-4PPD (Assistance available in Spanish).

Placental encapsulation: Association of Placenta Preparation Arts, http://placentaassociation.com

Resources for Healthcare Providers

Edinburgh Postnatal Depression Scale: https://perinatology.com/calculators/Edinburgh%20Depression%20Scale.htm

Nutrition, exercise, weight loss: https://www.myplate.gov/professionals

Patient Safety Bundles: https://saferbirth.org/patient-safety-bundles/

AHRQ Toolkit for Improving Perinatal Safety: https://www.ahrq.gov/hai/tools/perinatal-care/index.html

ACOG Safe Motherhood Initiative: https://www.acog.org/community/districts-and-sections/district-ii/programs-and-resources/safe-motherhood-initiative

References

Abdollahi, P., Etemadinezhad, S., & Lye, M. (2016). Postpartum mental health in relation to sociocultural practices. *Taiwanese Journal of Obstetrics & Gynecology*, 55, 76–80.

Ackerman, M., Greenwald, E., Noulas, P., & Ahn, C. (2021). Patient satisfaction with and use of telemental health services in the perinatal period; a survey study. *The Psychiatric Quarterly*, 92(3), 925–933.

Aitken, Z., Garrett, C. C., Hewitt, B., Keogh, L., Hocking, J. S., & Kavanagh, A. M. (2015). The maternal health outcomes of paid maternity leave: A systematic review. *Social Science & Medicine*, 130, 32–41.

Altman, M., Oseguera, T., McLemore, M., Kantrowitz-Gordon, K., Franck, L., & Lyndon, A. (2019). Information and power: Women of color's experiences interacting with healthcare providers in pregnancy and birth. *Social Science & Medicine, 238*. https://doi.org/10.1016/j.socscimed.2019.112491

American Academy of Pediatrics, (2018). Amount and schedule of formula feedings. https://www.healthychildren.org/English/ages-stages/baby/formula-feeding/Pages/Amount-and-Schedule-of-Formula-Feedings.aspx

American College of Obstetricians and Gynecologists. (2018a). Optimizing postpartum care. ACOG Committee Opinion 736. *Obstetrics & Gynecology, 131*(5), e140–e150.

American College of Obstetricians and Gynecologists. (2018b, 2018). Screening for perinatal depression. ACOG Committee opinion number 757. *Obstetrics & Gynecology, 132*, e208–e212.

American College of Obstetricians and Gynecologists. (2021). Interpregnancy care. Obstetric care consensus 8. *Obstetrics & Gynecology, 133*(1), 251–272.

American College of Obstetricians and Gynecologists (ACOG). (2012, reaffirmed 2022). Committee opinion no. 518. *Obstetrics & Gynecology, 119*, 412–417.

American College of Obstetricians and Gynecologists (ACOG). (2020). Physical activity and exercise during pregnancy and the postpartum period. ACOG Committee opinion no. 804. *Obstetrics & Gynecology, 135*(4), e178–e188.

Association of Placenta Preparation Arts. (2021a). *Association of Placenta Preparation Arts.* https://placentaassociation.com

Association of Placenta Preparation Arts. (2021b). *Group B strep (GBS) and placenta encapsulation.* Association of Placenta Preparation Arts. https://placentaassociation.com/group-b-strep-placenta-encapsulation

Attanasio, L., & Kozhimannil, K. B. (2017). Health care engagement and follow-up after perceived discriminations in maternity care. *Medical Care, 55*(9), 830–833. https://doi.org/10.1097/MLR.0000000000000773. PMID: 28692572

Baker, B., & Yang, I. (2018). Social media as support in pregnancy and the postpartum. *Sexual & Reproductive Healthcare, 17*, 31–34.

Bartel, A., Kim, S., Nam, J., Rossin-Slater, M., Ruhm, C. & Waldfogel, J. (Jan 2019). *Racial and ethnic disparities in access to and use of paid family and medical leave: evidence from four nationally representative datasets.* US bureau of labor statistics: Monthly labor review. https://www.bls.gov/opub/mlr/2019/article/racial-and-ethnic-disparities-in-access-to-and-use-of-paid-family-and-medical-leave.htm

Berens, P. (2022). *Overview of the postpartum period: Normal physiology and routine maternal care.* https://www.uptodate.com/contents/overview-of-the-postpartum-period-normal-physiology-and-routine-maternal-care?search=afterpains&sectionRank=1&usage_type=default&anchor=H3036838181&source=machineLearning&selectedTitle=1~4&display_rank=1#H3036838181

Beyers-Carlson, E. E. A., & Volling, B. L. (2017). Efficacy of sibling preparation classes. *Journal of Obstetrics, Gynaecologic and Neonatal Nursing, 46*(4), 521–531.

Blackburn, S. (2018). *Maternal, fetal & neonatal physiology; a clinical perspective* (5th ed.). Elsevier Science.

Brousseau, E. C., Danilack, V., Cai, F., & Matteson, K. A. (2018). Emergency department visits for postpartum complications. *Journal of Women's Health, 27*, 253–257.

Buser, G., Mató, S., Zhang, A., Metcalf, B., Beall, B., & Thomas, A. (2017). Notes from the field: Late onset infant group B streptococcus infection associated with maternal consumption of capsules containing dehydrated placenta, Oregon, 2016. *Morbidity and Mortality Weekly Report, 66*(25), 677–678. https://www.ncbi.nlm.nih.gov/pmc/articles/PMC5687501

Carneiro, P., Loken, K. V., & Salvanes, K. G. (2015). A flying start? Maternity leave benefits and long-run outcomes of children. *Journal of Political Economy, 123*(2), 365–412.

Case, A. S. (2016). Pregnancy-associated breast cancer. *Clinical Obstetrics and Gynecology, 59*, 779–788.

Centers for Disease Control and Prevention. (2016). US medical eligibility criteria for contraceptive use, 2016. *MMWR Morbidity and Mortality Weekly Report, 65*, 1–105.

Centers for Disease Control and Prevention. (2017). Notes form the field; late-onset group B streptococcus infection associated with

maternal consumption of capsules containing dehydrated placenta. *Morbidity and Mortality Weekly Report, 66*(25), 677–678.

Centers for Disease Control and Prevention. (2019). *Pregnancy-related deaths.* https://www.cdc.gov/vitalsigns/maternal-deaths

Centers for Disease Control and Prevention. (2021a). *Preventing intimate partner violence.* https://www.cdc.gov/violenceprevention/intimatepartnerviolence/fastfact.html

Centers for Disease Control and Prevention. (2021b). *Reproductive health: teen pregnancy.* https://www.cdc.gov/violenceprevention/intimatepartnerviolence/fastfact.html

Centers for Disease Control and Prevention. (2022). *Infant formula preparation and storage.* https://www.cdc.gov/nutrition/infantand-toddlernutrition/formula-feeding/infant-formula-preparation-and-storage.html#:~:text=Throw%20out%20any%20infant%20formula,can%20cause%20bacteria%20to%20grow

Chauhan, G., & Tadi, P. (2020, 2021). Physiology, postpartum changes. In *StatPearls*. StatPearls Publishing. https://www.ncbi.nlm.nih.gov/books/NBK555904

Chzhen, Y., Gromada, A. & Rees, G. (2019). *Are the world's richest countries family friendly?* http://www.unicef-irc.org/family-friendly

Coleman Smith, V. (2013). Preparing a child for the birth of a sibling. *International Journal of Childbirth Education, 28*, 20–24.

Connor, K. A., Duran, G., Faiz-Nassar, M., Mmari, K., & Minkovitz, C. S. (2018). Feasibility of implementing group well baby/well woman dyad care at federally qualified health centers. *Academic Paediatrics, 18*(5), 510–515.

Cornell, A., McCoy, C., Stampfel, C., Bonzon, E., & Verbiest, S. (2016). Creating new strategies to enhance postpartum health and wellness. *Maternal and Child Health Journal, 20*(1), 39–42.

Da Costa, D., Lai, J. K., & Zelkowitz, P. (2021). A prospective study on the course of sleep disturbances in first-time fathers during the transition to parenthood. *Infant Mental Health Journal, 42*(2), 222–232. https://doi.org/10.1002/imhj.21911

Dagher, R. K., McGovern, P. M., & Dowd, B. E. (2014). Maternity leave duration and postpartum mental and physical health: Implications for leave policies. *Journal of Health Politics, Policy and Law, 39*(2), 369–416.

DeCesare, J. Z., Hannah, D., & Amin, R. (2017). Postpartum contraception use rates of patients participating in the centering pregnancy model of care versus traditional obstetric care. *The Journal of Reproductive Medicine, 62*(1–2), 45–49.

Declercq, E., & Zephyrin, L. (2020). *Maternal mortality in the United States: A primer.* https://www.commonwealthfund.org/publications/issue-brief-report/2020/dec/maternal-mortality-united-states-primer

DePaulo, B. (2017). *Reminder: marriage is no longer the mode.* Council on Contemporary Families. https://sites.utexas.edu/contemporary-families/2017/09/12/singles2017factsheet

Deussen, A. R., Ashwood, P., Martis, R., Stewart, F., & Grzeskowiak, L. E. (2020). Relief of pain due to uterine cramping/involution after birth. [John Wiley & Sons, Ltd]. *Cochrane Database of Systematic Reviews,* (10), CD004908. https://doi.org/10.1002/14651858.CD004908.pub3

Dibari, J. N., Yu, S. M., Chao, S. M., & Lu, M. (2014). Use of postpartum care predictors and barriers. *Journal of Pregnancy, 2014*, 530769.

Dirks, M. A., Persram, R., Recchia, H. E., & Howe, N. (2015). Sibling relationships as sources of risk and resilience in the development and maintenance of internalizing and externalizing problems during childhood and adolescence. *Clinical Psychology Review, 42*, 145–155.

Doan, T., Gardiner, A., Gay, C. L., & Lee, K. A. (2007). Breast-feeding increases sleep duration of new parents. *The Journal of Perinatal & Neonatal Nursing, 21*(3), 200–206.

Dodson, N. & Talib, H. (2020). *Paid parental leave for mothers and fathers can improve physician wellness.* AAP News. https://publications.aap.org/aapnews/news/12432, https://doi.org/10.1007/s00737-018-0932-0.

Dong, Y., Obmerga, F., & Garcia, R. (2021). Comparative study on the quality of life of postpartum mothers with urinary incontinence undergoing biofeedback therapy and Kegel exercises. *International Journal of Research and Analytical Reviews, 8*(2), 48–52.

Eberly, L. A., Kallan, M. J., Julien, H. M., Haynes, N., Sameed Ahmed, M. K., Ashwin, S. N., Snider, C., Chokshi, N. P., Eneanya, N. D.,

Takvorian, S. U., Anastos-Wallen, R., Chaiyachati, K., Ambrose, M., O'Quinn, R., Seigerman, M., Goldberg, L. R., Leri, D., Choi, K., Gitelman, Y., . . . Adusumalli, S. (2020). Patient characteristics associated with telemedicine access for primary and specialty ambulatory care during the COVID-19 pandemic. *JAMA Network Open, 3*(12), e2031640. https://doi.org/10.1001/jamanetworkopen.2020.31640

Fahey, J. O., & Shenassa, E. (2013). Understanding and meeting the needs of women in the postpartum period: The perinatal maternal health promotion model. *Journal of Midwifery & Women's Health, 58,* 613–621.

Fisher, G. G., Valley, M. A., Toppinen-Tanner, S., & Mattingly, V. P. (2016). Parental leave and return to work. In C. Spitzmueller & R. A. Matthews (Eds.), *Research perspectives on work and the transition to motherhood.* Springer International Publishing.

Fowler, J. D., Varma, V., Siedel, K., Rodriguez, J., & Batra, P. (2016). Improving rates of postpartum visit completion in an urban resident obstetrics clinic. *Obstetrics & Gynecology, 127,* 58S–59S.

Gallagher, A. M., Updegraff, K. A., Padilla, J., & McHale, S. M. (2018). Longitudinal associations between sibling relational aggression and adolescent adjustment. *Journal of Youth and Adolescence, 47,* 2100–2113.

Geissler, K., Ranchoff, B. L., Cooper, M. I., & Attanasio, L. B. (2020). Association of insurance status with provision of recommended services during comprehensive postpartum visits. *JAMA Network Open, 3*(11). https://doi.org/10.1001/jamanetworkopen.2020.25095

Gueron-Sela, N., Shahar, G., Volkovich, E., & Tikotzky, L. (2021). Prenatal maternal sleep and trajectoris of ppstartum depresiosn and anxirty symptoms. *Journal of Sleep Research, 30*(4), e13258.

Handelzalts, J. E., Levy, S., Yadid, L., & Goldzweig, G. (2018). Mode of delivery, childbirth experience and postpartum sexuality. *Archives of Gynecology and Obstetrics, 297*(4), 927–932. https://doi.org/10.1007/s00404-018-4693-9

Haroz, E. E., Bass, J., Lee, C., Oo, S. S., Lin, K., Kohrt, B., Michalopolous, L., Nguyen, A. J., & Bolton, P. (2017). Development and cross-cultural testing of the international depression symptom scale (IDSS): A measurement instrument designed to represent global presentations of depression. *Global Mental Health, 4*(e17). https://doi.org/10.1017/gmh.2017.16

Hartman, E. K., & Eslick, G. D. (2016). The prognosis of women diagnosed with breast cancer before, during and after pregnancy; a meta-analysis. *Breast Cancer Research and Treatment, 160,* 347–360.

Hayes, E. H. (2016). Consumption of the placenta in the postpartum period. *Journal of Obstetric, Gynecologic & Neonatal Nursing, 45*(1), 78–89.

Hoffman, K., Trawalter, S., Axt, J., & Oliver, M. (2016). Racial bias in pain assessment and treatment recommendations, and false beliefs about biological differences between blacks and whites. *Proceedings of the National Academy of Sciences of the United States of America, 19*(113). https://doi.org/10.1073/pnas.1516047113. Epub 2016 Apr 4. PMID: 27044069; PMCID: PMC4843483

Hutchens, B. F., & Likis, F. E. (2019). A mental health acronym that must be stopped: PMAD. *Archives Womens Mental Health, 22,* 709. https://doi.org/10.1007/s00737-018-0932-0

Iwanowiscz-Palus, G., Marcewicz, A., & Bien, A. (2021). Analysis of determinants of postpartum emotional disorders. *BMC Pregnancy and Childbirth, 21*(1), 517.

Johnson, J. D., Asiodu, I. V., McKenzie, C. P., Tucker, C., Tully, K. P., Bryant, K., Verbiest, S., & Stuebe, A. M. (2019). Racial and ethnic inequities in postpartum pain evaluation and management. *Obstetrics and Gynecology, 134*(6), 1155–1162. https://doi.org/10.1097/AOG.0000000000003505

Joseph, R., Giovinazzo, M., & Brown, M. (2016). A literature review of the practice of placentophagia. *Nursing for Women's Health, 20,* 476–483.

Karbeah, J. M., Hardeman, R., Almanza, J., & Kozhimannil, K. B. (2019). Identifying the key elements of racially concordant care in a freestanding birth center. *Journal of Midwifery & Women's Health, 64*(5), 592–597. https://doi.org/10.1111/jmwh.13018

Kennedy, K. I., & Goldsmith, C. (2018). Contraception after pregnancy. In R. A. Hatcher, A. L. Nelson, J. Trussell, C. Cwiak, P. Cason, M. S. Policar, A. Edelman, A. R. A. Aiken, J. Marrazzo, & D. Kowal (Eds.), *Contraceptive technology* (21st ed., pp. 511–541). Ayer Company Publishers.

Kennell, J., & Klaus, M. (1998). Bonding: Recent observations that alter perinatal care. *Pediatrics in Review, 19*(1), 4–12.

Kerstis, B., Aarts, C., Tillman, C., Persson, H., Engstrom, G., Edlund, B., Öhrvik, J., Sylvén, S., & Skalkidou, A. (2016). Association between parental depressive symptoms and impaired bonding in the infant. *Archives of Women's Mental Health, 19,* 87–94.

Khajehei, M., & Doherty, M. (2017). Exploring postnatal depression, sexual dysfunction, and relationship dissatisfaction in Australian women. *The British Journal of Midwifery, 25,* 162. https://doi.org/10.12968/BJOM.2017.25.3.162

Kim-Godwin, Y. S. (2003). Postpartum beliefs & practices among non-Western cultures. *The American Journal of Maternal/Child Nursing, 28,* 75–80.

Ladyman, C., Gander, P., Huthwaite, M., Sweeney, B., & Signal, T. L. (2021). Sleep HAPi: A feasibility and descriptive analysis of an early and longitudinal sleep education intervention for pregnant women. *Behavioral Sleep Medicine, 19*(4), 427–444. https://doi.org/10.1080/15402002.2020.1772265

Lefrere, H., Lenaerts, L., Borges, V. F., Schedin, P., Neven, P., & Amant, F. (2021). Postpartum breast cancer: Mechanisms underlying its worse prognosis, treatment implications, and fertility preservation. *International Journal of Gynecological Cancer: Official Journal of the International Gyencological Cancer Society, 31*(3), 412–425. https://doi.org/10.1136/ijgc-2020-002072

Leung, G. (2017). Cultural considerations in postnatal dietary and infant feeding practices among Chinese mothers in London. *British Journal of Midwifery, 25*(1), 18–24.

Liu, Y., Chang, C., Hung, H., & Chen, C. (2021). Outcomes of a walking exercise intervention in postpartum women with disordered sleep. *The Journal of Obstetrics and Gynaecology Research, 47*(4), 1380–1387. https://doi.org/10.1111/jog.14672

Luca, D. L., Garlow, N., Staatz, C., Margiotta, C., & Zivin, K. (2019). *Societal costs of perinatal mood and anxiety disorders in the United States.* Mathematica policy research. https://www.mathematica.org/download-media?MediaItemId={E24EE558-B67B-4BF6-80D0-3BC75DB12EB6}

Magoda, G., Saccone, G., Al-Kouatly, H. B., Dahlen, G. H., Thornton, C., Akbarzadeh, M., Ozcan, T., & Berghella, V. (2019). Warm perineal compresses during the second stage of labor for reducing perineal trauma: A meta-analysis. *European Journal of Obstetrics, Gynecology, and Reproductive Biology, 240,* 93–98. https://doi.org/10.1016/j.ejogrb.2019.06.011

Magriples, U., Boynton, M. H., Kershaw, T. S., Lewis, J., Rising, S. S., Tobin, J. N., Epel, E., & Ickovics, J. R. (2015). The impact of group prenatal care on pregnancy and postpartum weight trajectories. *American Journal of Obstetrics & Gynecology, 213*(5), 688–e1.

Makins, A., & Cameron, S. (2020). Post pregnancy contraception. *Best Practice & Research.Clinical Obstetrics & Gynaecology, 66,* 41–54. https://doi.org/10.1016/j.bpobgyn.2020.01.004

McCracken, K. A., & Loveless, M. (2014). Teen pregnancy; an update. *Current Opinion in Obstetrics & Gynecology, 26,* 355–359.

McKee, K., Admon, L. K., Winkelman, T. N. A., Muzik, M., Hall, S., Dalton, V. K., & Zivin, K. (2020). Perinatal mood and anxiety disorders, serious mental illness, and delivery-related health outcomes, United States, 2006–2015. *BMC Women's Health, 20*(1), 150. https://doi.org/10.1186/s12905-020-00996-6

McKinley, M. C., Allen-Walker, V., McGirr, C., Rooney, C., & Woodside, J. V. (2018). Weight loss after pregnancy: Challenges and opportunities. *Nutrition Research Reviews, 31*(2), 225–238. https://doi.org/10.1017/S0954422418000070

Meighan, M. (2017). Maternal role attainment—Becoming a mother. *Nursing Theorists and Their Work-E-Book, 432.*

Mercer, R. T. (2004). Becoming a mother versus maternal role attainment. *Journal of Nursing Scholarship, 36*(3), 226–232.

Mirkovic, K. R., Perrine, C. G., & Scanlon, K. S. (2016). Paid maternity leave and breastfeeding outcomes. *Birth, 43*(3), 233–239.

Montgomery-Downs, H. E., Clawges, H. M., & Santy, E. E. (2010). Infant feeding methods and maternal sleep and daytime functioning. *Pediatrics, 126*(6), e1562–e1568.

Nakić Rados, S., Tadinac, M., & Herman, R. (2018). Anxiety during pregnancy and postpartum: Course, predictors and comorbidity with postpartum depression. *Acta Clinica Croatica*, *57*(1), 39–51. https://doi.org/10.20471/acc.2018.57.01.05

National Committee for Quality Assurance. (2016). *The state of health care quality report*. National Committee for Healthcare Quality Assurance. http://www.ncqa.org/report-cards/health-plans/state-of-health-care-quality

National Partnership for Women & Families. (2021). *Intimate partner violence endangers pregnant people and their infants*. https://www.nationalpartnership.org/our-work/health/moms-and-babies/intimate-partner-violence.html

Ollivier, R., Aston, M., & Price, S. (2020). Exploring postpartum sexual health: A feminist poststructural analysis. *Health Care for Women International*, *41*(10), 1081. https://doi.org/10.1080/07399332.2019.1638923

Pflugeisen, B. M., McCarren, C., Poore, S., Carlile, M., & Schroeder, R. (2016). Virtual visits: Managing prenatal care with modern technology. *MCN: The American Journal of Maternal/Child Nursing*, *41*(1), 24–30.

Poyatos-Leon, R., Garcia-Hermoso, A., Sanabria-Martinez, C., Alvarez-Bueno, C., Cavero-Redondo, I., & Martinez-Vizcaino, V. (2017). Effects of exercise-based interventions on postpartum depression; a meta-analysis of randomized controlled trials. *Birth*, *44*(3), 200–208.

Rezaie-Keikhaie, K., Hastings-Tolsma, M., Bouya, S., Shad, F. S., Sari, M., Shoorvazi, M., . . . Balouchi, A. (2019). Effect of aromatherapy on post-partum complications: A systematic review. *Complementary Therapies in Clinical Practice*, *35*, 290–295. https://doi.org/10.1016/j.ctcp.2019.03.010

Robertson, B., Aycock, D. M., & Darnell, L. A. (2009). Comparison of CenteringPregnancy to traditional care in Hispanic mothers. *Maternal and Child Health Journal*, *13*(3), 407–414.

Rubin, R. (1967). Attainment of the maternal role. Part 1. Processes. *Nursing Research*, *16*, 237–245.

Rubin, R. (2016). Despite potential health benefits of maternity leave, US lags behind other industrialized countries. *JAMA*, *315*(7), 643–645.

Ruderman, R. S., Dahl, E. C., Williams, B. R., Feinglass, J. M., Kominiarek, M. A., Grobman, W. A., & Yee, L. M. (2021). Obstetric provider perspectives on postpartum patient navigation for low-income patients. *Health Education & Behaviour*. https://doi.org/10.1177/10901981211043117

Saad, M., Chan, S., Nguyen, L., Srivastava, S., & Appiredy, R. (2021). Patient perceptions of the benefits and barriers of virtual postnatal care; a qualitative study. *BioMed Central Pregnancy and Childbirth*, *21*(1), 543.

Segel, S., Hashima, J., Gregory, W. T., Edelman, A., Li, H., & Guise, J. M. (2010). A new approach to postpartum rounds: Patient-centered collaborative care improves efficiency. *Journal of Graduate Medical Education*, *2*(1), 67–72.

Shorey, S., & Ang, L. (2019). Experiences, needs and perceptions of parentl involvement during the first year after their infant's birth: A meta analysis. *PLoS One*, *14*(1). https://doi.org/10.1371/journal.pone.0210388

Singley, D. B. (2015). Men's perinatal mental health in the transition to fatherhood. *Professional Psychology: Research and Practice*, *46*, 309–316.

Slomian, J., Honvo, G., Emonts, P., Reginster, J. Y., & Bruyère, O. (2019). Consequences of maternal postpartum depression: A systematic review of maternal and infant outcomes. *Women's Health (London, England)*, *15*, 1745506519844044. https://doi.org/10.1177/1745506519844044

Stanley, C., Baillargeon, A., & Selk, A. (2019). Understanding placentophagy. *Journal of Obstetric, Gynaecologic and Neonatal Nursing*, *48*(1), 37–49.

Stewart, R. B., Mobley, L. A., Van Tuyl, S. S., & Salvador, M. A. (1987). The firstborn's adjustment to the birth of a sibling: A longitudinal assessment. *Child Development*, *58*, 341–355.

United Sstates Preventive Services Task Force. (2019). Interventions to prevent perinatal depression: US preventive services task force recommendation statement. *Journal of American Medical Association*, *321*(6), 580. https://doi.org/10.1001/jama.2019.0007

US Department of Agriculture. (n.d.). *Pregnancy and breastfeeding*. https://www.myplate.gov/life-stages/pregnancy-and-breastfeeding.

US Department of Labor. (2018). *2018 Family and Medical Leave Act surveys*. https://www.dol.gov/agencies/oasp/evaluation/fmla2018

US Department of Labor. (n.d.). *Family and medical leave*. https://www.dol.gov/agencies/whd/fmla#:~:text=The%20FMLA%20entitles%20eligible%20employees,employee%20had%20not%20taken%20leave.

Van Bavel, J., Ravelli, A., Abu-Hanna, A., Roovers, J., Mol, B. W., & de Leeuw, J. W. (2020). Risk factors for the recurrence of obstetrical anal sphincter injury and the role of a mediolateral episiotomy: An analysis of a national registry. *BJOG: An International Journal of Obstetrics and Gynaecology*, *127*(8), 951–956. https://doi.org/10.1111/1471-0528.16263

Van der Wijden, C., & Manion, C. (2015). Lactational amenorrhoea method for family planning. *Cochrane Database of Systematic Reviews*, *10*, CD001329. https://doi.org/10.1002/14651858.CD001329.pub2

Van Niel, M. S., Bhatia, R., Riano, N. S., de Faria, L., Catapano-Friedman, L., Ravven, S., Weissman, B., Nzodom, C., Alexander, A., Budde, K., & Mangurian, C. (2020). The impact of paid maternity leave on the mental and physical health of mothers and children: A review of the literature and policy implications. *Harvard Review of Psychiatry*, *3/4*(28), 113. https://doi.org/10.1097/HRP.0000000000000246

Velonis, A. J., O'Campo, P., Kaufman-Shriqui, V., Kenny, K., Schafer, P., Vance, M., Dunkel Schetter, C., Hillemeier, M., Lanzi, R. & Chinchilli, V. M. (2017). The impact of prenatal and postpartum partner violence on maternal mental health: Results from the community child health network. *Journal of Women's Health*, *26*(10), 1153. https://doi.org/10.1089/jwh.2016.6129

Volkovich, E., Ben-Zion, H., Karny, D., Meiri, G., & Tikotzky, L. (2015). Sleep patterns of co-sleeping and solitary sleeping infants and mothers: A longitudinal study. *Sleep Medicine*, *16*(11), 1305–1312.

Volling, B. L. (2005). The transition to siblinghood: A developmental ecological systems perspective and direction for future research. *Journal of Family Psychology*, *19*, 542–549.

Volling, B. L. (2012). Family transitions following the birth of a sibling: An empirical review of changes in the firstborn's adjustment. *Psychological Bulletin*, *138*, 497–528.

Waid, J. D., Tanana, M. J., Vanderloo, M. J., Voit, R., & Kothari, B. H. (2020). The role of siblings in the development of externalizing behaviours during childhood and adolescence: As coping review. *The Journal of Family Social Work*, *23*(4), 318–337.

Wilcox, A., Levi, E. E., & Garrett, J. M. (2016). Predictors of nonattendance to the postpartum follow-up visit. *Maternal and Child Health Journal*, *20*(1), 22–27.

World Population Review. (2021). *Maternity leave by country*. https://worldpopulationreview.com/country-rankings/maternity-leave-by-country

Yogev, Y., Hiersch, L., Maresky, L., Wasserberg, N., Wiznitzer, A., & Melamed, N. (2014). Third and fourth degree perineal tears-the risk of recurrence in subsequent pregnancy. *The Journal of Maternal-Fetal & Neonatal Medicine*, *27*, 177–181.

Zhao, L., Chen, J., Lan, L., Deng, N., Liao, Y., Yue, L., Chen, I., Wen, S. W., & Xie, R. H. (2021). Effectiveness of telehealth interventions for women with postpartum depression: Systemic review and meta-analysis. *JMIR mHealth and uHealth*, *9*(10), e32544.

31

Lactation and Breastfeeding

Marsha Walker

Note about language: While this chapter occasionally includes some gendered language such as "mother" and "maternal" to reflect commonly used terms in the field of lactation and breastfeeding, the author and editors reiterate our acknowledgment that people of all genders get pregnant, give birth, and also breastfeed and parent. We further acknowledge that some patients may prefer terms like "chestfeeding" or "human milk feeding." Providers should inquire about language preferences of their patients, to support a respectful and inclusive patient/provider relationship and to avoid miscommunication and alienation.

Introduction

Lactation is an ancient and robust process that provides both nutrition and immunologic protection to infants and young children. Infants who are not fed breastmilk have an increased risk of acute and chronic diseases such as otitis media, lower respiratory tract infections, gastrointestinal (GI) infections, necrotizing enterocolitis, sudden infant death syndrome (SIDS), obesity, types 1 and 2 diabetes, and childhood leukemia (Table 31.1). The lactation process is also important to the mother and to a lactating parent's health. Women who do not breastfeed have an increased risk of premenopausal breast cancer, ovarian cancer, endometrial cancer, type II diabetes, hypertension, hyperlipidemia, obesity, metabolic syndrome, myocardial infarction (MI), and cardiovascular disease (Louis-Jacques & Stuebe, 2018). These diseases are costly. If 90% of US families were to feed breastmilk exclusively for six months, the United States would save $13 billion per year and prevent over 900 infant deaths annually (Bartick & Reinhold, 2010). For every 597 women who optimally breastfeed, one maternal or child death is prevented (Bartick et al., 2017a). Breastfeeding is a public health issue and forms the foundation for lifelong health outcomes.

Health equity key points

- Specific culturally relevant interventions are needed among populations and facilities with lower prevalence.
- Healthcare providers should avoid delivering care to Black families based on stereotypes or assumptions that Black people prefer formula or do not wish to breastfeed.

- "Chestfeeding" is a term preferred by some gender nonconforming individuals to acknowledge their gender identity and to avoid gender dysphoria.
- White women have the longest breastfeeding duration when they are not working, whereas Black women have the longest breastfeeding duration when they are working in professional/managerial positions. Individuals working in service/labor jobs have the shortest breastfeeding duration when compared to other professional/managerial positions or those who do not work.

Central to successful breastfeeding is the support of knowledgeable and skilled healthcare providers (US Preventive Services Task Force, 2016). However, many healthcare providers receive little training in the provision of evidence-based lactation care in their academic preparation or through continuing education programs. This chapter provides an overview of breastfeeding as a public health issue, the unique properties of human milk, related anatomy and physiology, the role of the healthcare provider in promoting and supporting breastfeeding, and the basics of support and assessment. The management of common breastfeeding problems is addressed in Chapter 44, *Common Lactation and Breastfeeding Problems.*

Breastfeeding contributes to improved health outcomes for both the mother and the infant through the lifespan. It programs the infant's immune system and contributes to optimal brain growth and development. Lactation provides metabolic and cancer-preventing advantages to the lactating parent. In a study conducted to quantify the excess cases of pediatric and maternal disease, death, and costs attributable to suboptimal breastfeeding rates in the United States, it was found that annual excess deaths totaled 3340, 78% of which were maternal deaths due to MI, breast cancer, and diabetes. Excess pediatric deaths totaled 721, mostly due to SIDS and necrotizing enterocolitis. Medical costs totaled $3.0 billion, 79% of which were for care given to the birthing person. Costs of premature death total $14.2 billion (Bartick et al., 2017a).

All major health organizations recommend breastfeeding. The American Academy of Pediatrics (AAP) recommends exclusive breastfeeding for six months, followed by the introduction of appropriate complementary foods and continued breastfeeding for two years or as long as is desired by the dyad (Meek et al., 2022). This recommendation is the standard of care. It is the goal toward which efforts should be directed to achieve optimal health outcomes.

Table 31.1 Health outcomes related to breastfeeding

Maternal	Infant/child
Reduced:	Reduced:
• Postpartum blood loss	• Neonatal death
• Breast cancer	• Sudden infant death syndrome
• Ovarian cancer	• Necrotizing enterocolitis
• Type 2 diabetes	• Otitis media
• Hypertension	• Eczema
• Cardiovascular disease	• Asthma
• Hyperlipidemia	• Childhood leukemia
• Metabolic syndrome	• Allergies
Increased:	• Mortality, hospitalization, outpatient visits
• Rapid uterine involution	• Gastrointestinal disease (inflammatory bowel disease, rotavirus, and celiac disease)
• Response to infant cues	• Respiratory tract infections (pneumonia and respiratory syncytial virus)
• Dyad bonding behaviors	• Oral malocclusion (from the use of artificial nipples)
	• Type 1 diabetes
	• Urinary tract infection
	• Sepsis
	• Obesity
	• Occurrence of genes associated with antibiotic resistance in the gut
Increased:	Increased:
• Cognitive function	• Cognitive development

Source: Adapted from Binns et al. (2016), Krawczyk et al. (2016), Victora et al. (2016), Meek (2021), Fox et al. (2021), and Pärnänen et al. (2021).

Breastfeeding as a Public Health Issue

Increasing the rate of breastfeeding in the United States has been a public health priority for more than a century. The US Department of Health and Human Services (HHS) has promulgated breastfeeding objectives for the nation through the Healthy People initiative, which provides science-based, 10-year national objectives for improving the health of all Americans (Table 31.2).

Breastfeeding rates are tracked by the Centers for Disease Control and Prevention (CDC). For infants born in 2018 in the United States, 83.9% initiated breastfeeding, 56.7% were breastfeeding at six months, and 35.0% were breastfeeding at 12 months. Exclusive breastfeeding through three months was 46%, through six months was 25.8%, and breastfed infants receiving formula before two days of age was 19.4% (Centers for Disease Control and Prevention, 2021a). However, there is a rapid drop in exclusive breastfeeding rates over the first two weeks (Table 31.3), emphasizing the need for increased monitoring and appropriate interventions in the early postpartum period.

While breastfeeding rates for those who have ever breastfed have increased from 26.5% in 1970 to 83.9% for infants born in 2018, this increase has taken a concerted effort by federal and state health agencies, breastfeeding and professional health organizations, breastfeeding initiatives, and lactation personnel such as healthcare providers, lactation consultants, doulas, and breastfeeding educators and counselors. Contributing to the progress in lactation support over the last 25 years has been the increase in employers who provide time and space to express milk at work, the increase in state legislation mandating worksite support for lactating employees, laws protecting the right to breastfeed in public, expansion in lactation education and training opportunities for healthcare providers, the availability of advanced lactation support and services from International Board Certified Lactation Consultants (IBCLCs), and increased research on breastfeeding and lactation.

Even though steady progress has been made, there remain many challenges and gaps in care that prevent people from meeting their breastfeeding goals. Some public policies or lack of policies have a detrimental effect on breastfeeding. For example, the United States still has no

Table 31.3 Decline in exclusive breastfeeding rates

U.S. National Breastfeeding Rates, 2018 Births

Child Age	Breastfeeding (n = 21,428)	Exclusive Breastfeeding (n = 20,760)
At birth	83.9 ± 0.9	
7 days	83.1 ± 0.9	63.3 ± 1.2
14 days	82.4 ± 1.0	61.0 ± 1.2
21 days	80.9 ± 1.0	58.9 ± 1.2
28 days	80.2 ± 1.0	58.2 ± 1.2
1 month	79.9 ± 1.0	57.8 ± 1.2
2 months	75.6 ± 1.0	51.9 ± 1.2
3 months	70.9 ± 1.1	46.3 ± 1.2
4 months	64.5 ± 1.2	39.4 ± 1.2
5 months	59.3 ± 1.2	31.2 ± 1.1
6 months	56.7 ± 1.2	25.8 ± 1.0
7 months	49.1 ± 1.2	
8 months	46.4 ± 1.2	
9 months	42.9 ± 1.2	
10 months	39.5 ± 1.2	
11 months	36.9 ± 1.1	
12 months	35.0 ± 1.1	
18 months	14.8 ± 0.8	

Source: Division of Nutrition, Physical Activity, and Obesity, National Center for Chronic Disease Prevention and Health Promotion/ Public Domain/US Department of Health and Human Services.

Table 31.2 Healthy People 2030 breastfeeding objectives

Objective number	Objective	Baseline (2015 births)	2030 Target
MICH-15	Increase the proportion of infants who are breastfed exclusively through age six months	24.9%	42.5%
MICJ-16	Increase the proportion of infants who are breastfed at one year	35.9%	54.1%

national paid family leave policy, resulting in some people returning to work within a few weeks of giving birth and often before breastfeeding has become well established. Research consistently indicates that those who return to work within several weeks or months after giving birth have lower rates of breastfeeding initiation, success, and duration (Hamner et al., 2021). Occupation and breastfeeding appear to be racially patterned, and it is likely that race moderates the relationships between work and breastfeeding (Whitley et al., 2021). For example, working in a service or labor job was associated with about one month less breastfeeding compared to not being employed at all or working in a professional or management position. Among Black mothers, the longest duration occurred among those in professional or management work, not service or labor jobs. Racial disparities were smaller among those in managerial/professional occupations. Adding to the basic challenge of breastfeeding while employed, Black women are disproportionately employed in low-wage service and minimum and subminimum wage jobs that lack flexibility and accommodations for expressing milk. This adds a substantial burden to employed Black parents' ability to sustain breastfeeding (Entmacher et al., 2014).

Racial Disparities

The consistently lower prevalence of breastfeeding among Black infants warrants increased attention and action (Bartick et al., 2017a). Initiation rates vary by race and ethnicity, ranging from 90.3% among Asian people to 73.6% among Black people. In 26 states, the initiation rates are lowest among infants of Black people (Chiang et al., 2021). Suboptimal breastfeeding is associated with a greater burden of disease among Black infants (Bartick et al., 2017b). This persistent gap in breastfeeding rates between Black people and those of other races indicates that Black people are more likely to encounter unsupportive cultural norms, live in environments that are unsupportive of breastfeeding, lack role models, perceive it as inferior to formula feeding have medical providers who assume that they prefer infant formula, lack partner support, have socioeconomic challenges, or have unsupportive work environments. A study performed in North Carolina assessed whether there were differences in breastfeeding support services available through the Supplemental Nutrition Program for Women, Infants, and Children (WIC) program based on the county-level racial/ethnic composition of the WIC sites. It found that breastfeeding initiation by WIC sites was negatively associated with the percentage of Black clients. They were also less likely to offer clinic-based support services (Evans et al., 2011). There are also racial disparities in access to hospital care practices known to support breastfeeding. Hospitals in zip codes where the percentage of Black residents was >12.2% were less likely than facilities in zip codes where the percentage was ≤12.2% to meet five indicators for recommended practices supportive of breastfeeding (Centers for Disease Control and Prevention, 2014). Specific interventions might be needed among populations and facilities with lower breastfeeding prevalence. A study in the southern United States showed that implementing the Ten Steps to Successful Breastfeeding through the Baby-Friendly Hospital Initiative (BFHI) resulted in reduced disparities among Black infants with substantial increases in initiation and exclusivity (Merewood et al., 2019). Black breastfed newborns are much more likely to be fed formula in the hospital than newborns of White people. If hospital formula supplementation was eliminated, the gap between Whites and Blacks could be reduced by about 1.8 weeks or 20% of the overall difference (McKinney et al., 2016). Clinicians must avoid microaggressions and stereotyping, must listen closely, and pay attention to the feelings, information, plans, and thoughts of Black pregnant and breastfeeding people. They must be empathetic and allow the voices of Black people to be heard and respected (Knox-Kazimierczuk et al., 2021). An app entitled "Irth" (2021) provides prenatal, birthing, postpartum, and pediatric reviews of pregnancy and childbirth care that are entered by Black and Brown people. The "B" is dropped to signify that racism and bias must be eliminated from birth care.

LGBTQIA+ Families

Approximately 5.6% of adults in the United States identify as gay, lesbian, bisexual, or transgender (Jones, 2021). Clinicians should provide informed, inclusive, affirming, and welcoming care by using language that is comfortable for everyone (Duckett & Ruud, 2019). Explore the preferred terms for each family to assure comfort, to employ the use of gender affirming language, and to provide optimal care. LGBTQIA+ families face the unique challenges posed by their individual family dynamics as well as the usual challenges of new parents. A welcoming approach by clinicians should include gender-inclusive language on intake forms, websites, signage, and educational materials, asking for preferred pronouns, and educating themselves regarding co-nursing, induced lactation, nursing after chest reduction (top surgery in transgender men), breast augmentation in transgender women, use of medications specific to transgender individuals (such as testosterone, spironolactone), and gender dysphoria (unease or distress when parts of their body do not match their gender identity; Farrow, 2015).

LGBTQIA+ family dynamics can vary and include:

- Co-nursing and/or co-lactation. Co-nursing involves both partners nursing the baby. Co-nursing may involve inducing lactation in the nongestational parent, the nongestational parent using a tube feeding device to provide expressed breastmilk for feedings but not specifically inducing lactation, or the nongestational parent providing comfort nursing with no expectation of milk production. The birthing parent might exclusively nurse for the first two weeks or so to encourage an abundant milk supply, while the partner may choose to comfort feed or work to induce lactation. The birthing partner may choose to express breastmilk to provide milk for the nonbirthing partner to use when feeding the infant. A helpful co-lactation feeding plan is available from the Academy of Breastfeeding Medicine (Ferri et al., 2020).
- Transgender women (those assigned male at birth) desiring to nurse their infant may wish to induce lactation and establish milk production. They may be taking medications such as estradiol and progesterone as feminizing hormones and spironolactone (Aldactone) to suppress testosterone. Mammary tissue may or may not be well developed. The breast tissue that develops, using standard estrogen hormone therapy, has been described as radiographically (Sonnenblick et al., 2018) and histologically (Kanhai et al., 2000) indistinguishable from that of cisgender women, leading to the presence of galactophores, ducts, lobes, and alveoli. Increasing glandular volume may result in functional milk secretion. A protocol for inducing lactation in transgender women includes pumping several times per day in addition to the hormones, spironolactone, and domperidone (Reisman & Goldstein, 2018). Transgender women may be able to produce some milk but may not be able to supply all of the milk that an infant requires, especially as the growing infant's needs increase. Transgender

women may or may not continue androgen blockade medication during lactation. Supplementation may be necessary using donor human milk or infant formula. Informal milk sharing may occur and should be used with knowledge and caution. Analysis of milk from transgender women is sparse, but older research has shown the presence of lactose, proteins, and electrolytes that are within the range of colostrum and milk obtained from lactating women (Kulski et al., 1981).

- Transgender men (those assigned female at birth) may become pregnant and nurse or not nurse their infant. Some transgender men may have had prior chest contouring surgery, which flattens the chest but does not completely remove all mammary tissue. This is not a mastectomy or breast reduction surgery. The remaining breast tissue may grow under the influence of pregnancy hormones and could be disconcerting to some transmasculine people. Different types of top surgery can be performed, but one procedure that leaves a pedicle of intact tissue under the nipple may be more conducive to milk flow and production. This may present a challenge for infant latching as the chest is flatter and the skin can be quite taut. Techniques such as molding the areolar tissues into a sandwich and application of a nipple shield may aid in latching, while a nursing supplementer device may help deliver milk and stimulate milk production (MacDonald, 2019). Use nursing positions that do not cause the chest tissue to become stretched or tighter such as a clutch hold or cross cradle. Laid-back positioning may tighten the chest tissue. Binding the breasts is sometimes done to reduce gender dysphoria but during lactation may run the risk of causing milk stasis, plugged ducts, reduced milk production, and mastitis (Garcia-Acosta et al., 2019). Sometimes testosterone is taken by transgender men to help reduce feelings of gender dysphoria (MacDonald, 2019), and while testosterone appears safe

for the infant, it can reduce milk production and serum prolactin levels (Drugs and Lactation Database, 2021a). In the past, testosterone was used therapeutically to suppress lactation; therefore, close monitoring of infant weight gain should be exercised with the use of testosterone during lactation establishment. Lactating transgender patients should be taught to recognize engorgement, plugged ducts, and mastitis whether or not they had gender affirming surgery (MacDonald, 2019). Other feeding options can be offered if appropriate (MacLean, 2021) such as finger feeding, inducing lactation in the partner, cup feeding, and running a tube feeding device under a nipple shield. Some flanges may not fit well over the chest contours. Breast pump use following top surgery could be complicated by difficulty finding pump flanges that fit properly over the remolded chest contours. Clinicians may need to help with fitting and the use of specialized flange inserts.

Hospital-Based Care

The lack of knowledge regarding breastfeeding assessment and the consistent lack of assessment during the hospital stay increases the risk for poor outcomes and early weaning. Hospital lactation care and services are critical to the successful initiation and continuation of breastfeeding, yet only 27.96% of US infants are born in Baby-Friendly hospitals (Baby-Friendly USA, 2021). The BFHI was started in 1991 by United Nations International Children's Emergency Fund (UNICEF) and the World Health Organization (WHO) to recognize hospitals with best practices in supporting breastfeeding. To be designated as Baby-Friendly, a hospital must implement the WHO/UNICEF Ten Steps to Successful Breastfeeding (Table 31.4) and comply with the *International Code of Marketing of Breastmilk Substitutes*, which requires

Table 31.4 Ten steps to successful breastfeeding

Critical management procedures
1a. Comply fully with the International Code of Marketing of Breastmilk Substitutes and relevant World Health Assembly resolutions.
1b. Have a written infant feeding policy that is routinely communicated to staff and parents.
1c. Establish ongoing monitoring and data-management systems.
2. Ensure that staff have sufficient knowledge, competence, and skills to support breastfeeding.
Key clinical practices
3. Discuss the importance and management of breastfeeding with pregnant women and their families.
4. Facilitate immediate and uninterrupted skin-to-skin contact and support mothers to initiate breastfeeding as soon as possible after birth.
5. Support mothers to initiate and maintain breastfeeding and manage common difficulties.
6. Do not provide breastfed newborns any food or fluids other than breastmilk, unless medically indicated.
7. Enable mothers and their infants to remain together and to practice rooming-in 24 hours a day.
8. Support mothers to recognize and respond to their infants' cues for feeding.
9. Counsel mothers on the use and risks of feeding bottles, teats, and pacifiers.
10. Coordinate discharge so that parents and their infants have timely access to ongoing support and care.

hospitals to pay fair market value for infant formula and not promote items detrimental to breastfeeding, including discharge bags that contain formula (UNICEF, 2021).

Every two years, the CDC conducts a national survey of hospitals with maternity services called the Maternity Practices in Infant Nutrition and Care (mPINC) survey. It measures the impact of practices and policies on breastfeeding rates. Hospitals receive points for patient and staff education, staff skills, feeding practices, and discharge support. The national score for 2020 was 81% with significant variations in scoring on the various components (Centers for Disease Control and Prevention, 2021b). For example, in some hospitals, up to 75% of breastfeeding newborns are supplemented with infant formula. State-specific reports detail where improvements need to be made in each state's hospitals. The CDC sends a report to every participating hospital showing specific changes they can make to better support breastfeeding mothers.

Hospital-based lactation personnel should be easily available. Specialized lactation services delivered by IBCLCs are important because 71% of people experiencing breastfeeding issues are not able to be deferred to the bedside nurse or nonclinician support person. This is true even when the staff nurses are well trained in basic breastfeeding support (Francis-Clegg & Francis, 2011). Taking acuity of the breastfeeding issue into consideration may improve lactation care. For example, staff nurses can provide care and support for low-acuity situations where no problems have been identified and IBCLCs intervene in high-acuity situations. This model has been shown to improve the quality of patient care, productivity, and increased staff satisfaction (Mannel, 2010). Table 31.5 lists examples of high-acuity situations that should be referred to an IBCLC.

Healthcare providers play an important role in promoting, supporting, and protecting breastfeeding. All healthcare providers should have basic core competencies in providing evidence-based lactation support and services

Table 31.5   High-acuity risk factors for referral to an IBCLC

Infant risk factors	Maternal risk factors
Small for gestation age (SGA)	High BMI (obesity)
Large for gestation age (LGA)	Diabetes
Intrauterine growth retardation (IUGR)	Maternal request
Preterm and late preterm	Pregnancy induced hypertension
Multiples	Cesarean delivery
Infant readmissions	Anxiety, depression
Cardiac, neurologic, metabolic issues	Separation
Oral anomalies	Breast pathology
Congenital anomalies, syndromes	Physically challenged
Signs of insufficient intake (weight loss and jaundice)	Neurodiversity

Table 31.6   United States Breastfeeding Committee Core competencies in breastfeeding care and services for all health professionals

Knowledge

All health professionals should understand:

Basic anatomy and physiology of lactation

How human milk prevents disease and illness

Why exclusive breastfeeding matters

How pregnancy and birth practices influence breastfeeding

Societal and cultural factors influencing breastfeeding

Risks of formula feeding

Contraindications to breastfeeding

When and how to refer for lactation services

Resources for families

Role of formula company marketing

Skills

All health professionals should be able to:

Protect, promote, and support breastfeeding in their practice

Complete a lactation health history and be aware of factors that could influence breastfeeding

Refer and seek assistance from lactation professionals

Protect confidentiality

Use new technologies to ensure evidence-based practice

Attitudes

All health professionals should:

Value human milk/breastfeeding as a public health issue

Recognize and respect cultural differences related to breastfeeding care and support

Respect confidentiality

Remain free of the influence of formula company marketing

Seek collaboration with interdisciplinary lactation care teams

Encourage employers to develop employee lactation programs

Be aware of personal values that could bias care

Support colleagues who are breastfeeding

Support family-centered policies at the local, state, and federal levels

as described by the United States Breastfeeding Committee (2010; Table 31.6).

The BFHI delineates 16 competencies necessary for implementing the Ten Steps to Successful Breastfeeding in their Guidelines and Evaluation Criteria (Table 31.7) for hospitals working to achieve the Baby-Friendly designation.

There are a number of helpful practices that breastfeeding individuals have identified about their interactions with healthcare providers, including prenatal information regarding the realities of breastfeeding, practical help with positioning and latch, provision of effective interventions for early problems, and the receipt of evidence-based

Table 31.7 Competencies necessary for implementing the Ten Steps to Successful Breastfeeding

Use skills for building confidence and giving support whenever engaging in a conversation with a mother
Engage in antenatal conversation about breastfeeding
Implement immediate and uninterrupted skin-to-skin
Facilitate breastfeeding within the first hour, according to cues
Discuss with a mother how breastfeeding works
Assist mother getting her baby to latch
Help a mother respond to feeding cues
Help a mother manage milk expression
Help a mother to breastfeed a low-birth-weight or sick baby
Help a mother whose baby needs fluids other than breastmilk
Help a mother who is not feeding her baby directly at the breast
Help a mother prevent or resolve difficulties with breastfeeding
Ensure seamless transition after discharge

answers to questions such as how long and how often to breastfeed, when to switch sides, and whether nipple shields and supplementing with bottles of formula will undermine their efforts (Graffy & Taylor, 2005). Remaining with clients during early feedings, assuring correct latch, and documenting milk transfer provide the type of assistance that is most valuable, making sure that these tasks are demonstrated but allowing the parent to perform the task themself (Gill, 2001). Individuals wish to receive support from healthcare professionals that are knowledgeable, who listen to their concerns and desires, take their time, and who can offer advice, tools, and solutions other than quickly suggesting formula feeding by bottle (Ranch et al., 2019).

Other care practices that are not helpful have been described by those who breastfeed. These practices include inconsistent advice about techniques, quick intervention with a bottle when feeding difficulties are present, and lack of skilled assistance (McInnes & Chambers, 2008; Mozingo et al., 2000; Nelson, 2007). Rough handling of the breast or infant (such as pushing the breast into the infant's mouth or pushing the baby to the breast), packaged advice that is not tailored to the individual situation, information delivered in a lecture format, and education that consists of literature left at the bedside with no explanation have been identified as unhelpful (Schmied et al., 2011). Healthcare provider neutrality negatively affects initiation and duration (DiGirolamo et al., 2003). People who receive unsatisfactory care from healthcare providers may turn to social media sites for support. While these sites may provide around-the-clock access to support, emotional reassurance, empathy from others who shared similar experiences, and mitigate feelings of isolation, these sites can also promulgate inaccurate information, be judgmental and polarizing, and lack moderation from knowledgeable experts (Regan & Brown, 2019).

Following birth, new parents should be given the opportunity to learn and develop the essential knowledge and skills needed for a positive initiation of breastfeeding (Figure 31.1). An essential knowledge and skills checklist is provided in Figure 31.2.

Birth facility discharge instructions should be provided so that people leave with a clear feeding plan (Figure 31.3).

Once discharged, new parents continue to have questions. They need ongoing guidance and support to prevent premature weaning for problems such as sore nipples, real or perceived insufficient milk supply, latch issues, and return to employment. Healthcare providers can contact their clients the day after discharge to assess progress. While telephone contact can be helpful, two-way text messaging may be a more effective way to perform triage and engage mothers (Martinez-Brockman et al., 2018). Clients should also receive information on how to assess for themselves if feedings are going well, as well as a list of community resources to call with questions or problems.

Composition of Human Milk

Human milk has evolved and adapted over the millennia into a living, dynamic fluid that both nurtures and protects the human infant. In contrast, the composition of infant formula is set by its manufacturer and cannot adjust to meet the changing needs of the infant. Formula lacks the enzymes, hormones, disease-protective factors, and the myriad of other components that combine to program the immune system and promote the brain growth and development observed in human-milk-fed infants.

Colostrum is the first milk that is present in the breasts from 12 to 16 weeks of gestation onward. This milk is thicker than mature milk, and its yellowish color is due to the presence of beta-carotene. Colostrum is higher in protein, sodium, chloride, potassium, magnesium, carotenoids, and fat-soluble vitamins, and lower in sugars, fat, and lactose than mature milk. Colostrum contains abundant amounts of antioxidants, antibodies, and immunoglobulins, with especially high concentrations of secretory IgA (sIgA). Also present is interferon, with its strong antiviral activity, fibronectin that makes certain phagocytes more aggressive, and pancreatic secretory trypsin inhibitor that protects and repairs the delicate intestines of the newborn, preparing this organ to process future foods. The composition of colostrum changes and increases in volume over the first several days as it transitions to mature milk. When **tight junction closure** occurs in the mammary epithelium, the sodium-to-potassium ratio declines and lactose concentration increases. This signals secretory activation, the onset of copious milk production, and the change to transitional milk. This is often referred to as the milk "coming in." Since newborns have very small stomachs and digestive systems, colostrum delivers its nutrients in a very concentrated low-volume form. It has a mild laxative effect, which aids in the passing of meconium. Colostrum has a mean energy value of 18.76 kcal/oz, while mature milk is about 21 kcal/oz but varies widely from person to person. The volume of colostrum ingested by newborns during the first

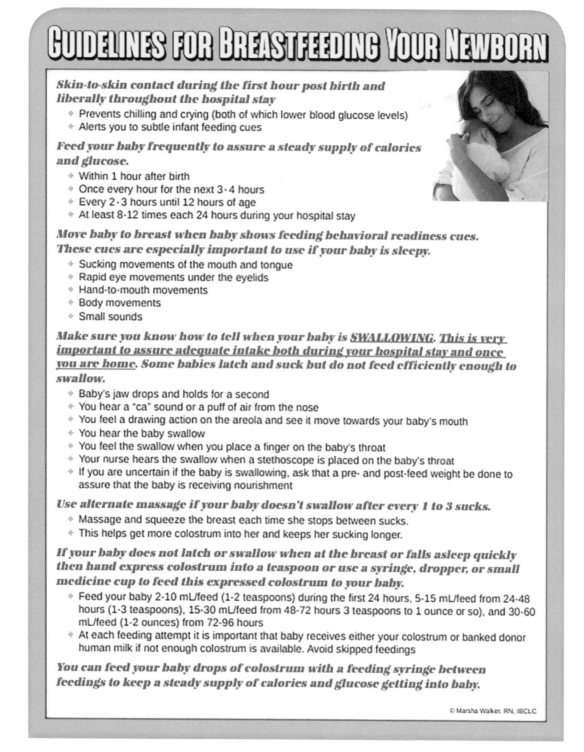

GUIDELINES FOR BREASTFEEDING YOUR NEWBORN

Skin-to-skin contact during the first hour post birth and liberally throughout the hospital stay

- Prevents chilling and crying (both of which lower blood glucose levels)
- Alerts you to subtle infant feeding cues

Feed your baby frequently to assure a steady supply of calories and glucose.

- Within 1 hour after birth
- Once every hour for the next 3-4 hours
- Every 2-3 hours until 12 hours of age
- At least 8-12 times each 24 hours during your hospital stay

Move baby to breast when baby shows feeding behavioral readiness cues. These cues are especially important to use if your baby is sleepy.

- Sucking movements of the mouth and tongue
- Rapid eye movements under the eyelids
- Hand-to-mouth movements
- Body movements
- Small sounds

Make sure you know how to tell when your baby is _SWALLOWING_. This is very important to assure adequate intake both during your hospital stay and once you are home. Some babies latch and suck but do not feed efficiently enough to swallow.

- Baby's jaw drops and holds for a second
- You hear a "ca" sound or a puff of air from the nose
- You feel a drawing action on the areola and see it move towards your baby's mouth
- You hear the baby swallow
- You feel the swallow when you place a finger on the baby's throat
- Your nurse hears the swallow when a stethoscope is placed on the baby's throat
- If you are uncertain if the baby is swallowing, ask that a pre- and post-feed weight be done to assure that the baby is receiving nourishment

Use alternate massage if your baby doesn't swallow after every 1 to 3 sucks.

- Massage and squeeze the breast each time she stops between sucks.
- This helps get more colostrum into her and keeps her sucking longer.

If your baby does not latch or swallow when at the breast or falls asleep quickly then hand express colostrum into a teaspoon or use a syringe, dropper, or small medicine cup to feed this expressed colostrum to your baby.

- Feed your baby 2-10 mL/feed (1-2 teaspoons) during the first 24 hours, 5-15 mL/feed from 24-48 hours (1-3 teaspoons), 15-30 mL/feed from 48-72 hours 3 teaspoons to 1 ounce or so), and 30-60 mL/feed (1-2 ounces) from 72-96 hours
- At each feeding attempt it is important that baby receives either your colostrum or banked donor human milk if not enough colostrum is available. Avoid skipped feedings

You can feed your baby drops of colostrum with a feeding syringe between feedings to keep a steady supply of calories and glucose getting into baby.

© Marsha Walker, RN, IBCLC

Figure 31.1   Hospital breastfeeding instructions. Trendsetter Images/Adobe Stock.

three days of life ranges from 2 to 20 mL per feeding, with about 100 mL of colostrum available during the first 24 hours following birth.

Various factors can affect the composition of colostrum such as:

- Preterm birth whereby colostrum is higher in protein for the first few weeks and is more highly enriched with potent disease-protective factors compared with mature milk from those who give birth at term.
- Colostrum of diabetic people can be lower in some disease-protective factors, making it important to tightly control diabetes to minimize immune property alterations.
- Colostrum of those giving birth by cesarean section has been shown to be lower in antioxidant status (Simsek

MY HOSPITAL DISCHARGE CHECKLIST

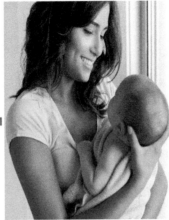

- ❏ I can position my baby correctly on both breasts
- ❏ It does not hurt once the baby starts sucking
- ❏ The baby can latch to each breast
- ❏ I can tell when the baby is swallowing milk
- ❏ I know how many times in 24 hours to feed the baby
- ❏ I know when my milk should come in & who to call if it doesn't by day 3
- ❏ I know how long to feed the baby on each side
- ❏ I know that feedings lasting longer than 30 minutes is a sign of baby not feeding well
- ❏ I know that if baby does not feed well from the breast I should hand express colostrum and/or pump milk and feed the baby as much of that milk as he will take
- ❏ I know when it is time to feed my baby
- ❏ I know the five feeding cues to use if my baby is sleepy
- ❏ I know how many diapers baby should have each day
- ❏ I know how to tell if a disposable diaper is wet
- ❏ I know how much weight baby should gain weekly
- ❏ I know that artificial nipples and pacifiers can confuse my baby and have been shown other ways to feed him if necessary
- ❏ I know I should hand express and pump milk if baby does not feed well
- ❏ I know that persistent, inconsolable crying may be a sign of underfeeding and will feed baby expressed colostrum or pumped milk
- ❏ I know how to tell if my baby is jaundiced
- ❏ Someone will visit me a day or two after I get home, or.... I will see my pediatrician or family doctor in one to two days
- ❏ I know when and who to call for help with nursing if I have any concerns

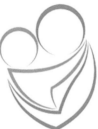

Figure 31.2 Discharge checklist of knowledge and skills. Trendsetter Images/Adobe Stock.

et al., 2015) and contain a higher abundance of microorganisms of environmental origin.

- Colostrum of individuals who smoke during lactation has a significantly lower antioxidant capacity than the colostrum of those who do not smoke (Napierala et al., 2019) as well as significantly lower cytokine (IL-1β and IL-8) levels (Piskin et al., 2012), increasing the newborn's vulnerability to infection.

Bacteria are normal residents in breastmilk, with over 700 species having been identified (Cabrera-Rubio et al., 2012) and 100–10,000 viable bacteria present per milliliter (Fernandez et al., 2013). *Lactobacillus* species and *bifidobacteria* typically dominate the breastfed infant's gut. Bifidobacteria are nourished by oligosaccharides. Human milk oligosaccharides (HMOs) are complex, highly abundant sugars that function as substrates or food for specific microbes, including certain species of *Bifidobacterium*. The microbiomes of newborns and young infants are enriched in genes required for the degradation of those HMOs. The rich diversity of bacterial species in breastmilk imprint the infant gut and influence and select for the bacteria that follow.

Human milk is 87.5% water. All of the other components are either dissolved, dispersed, or in suspension. Infants consuming adequate amounts do not require extra water, even in hot or arid climates (Ashraf et al., 1993). Consuming extra water can depress the infant's appetite and reduces caloric intake, which raises the risk for hyperbilirubinemia and, if given in abundance over a short period of time, can contribute to water intoxication. Supplementation with sterile water or glucose water is contraindicated because it does not provide sufficient nutrition, can lead to weight loss, does not reduce serum bilirubin levels, and can cause hyponatremia (Kellams et al., 2017).

Milk lipids or fats provide about 50% of the energy in human milk. The fat content of milk varies throughout a feeding or pumping session. The early milk or foremilk is

LOOK! LISTEN! ACT!

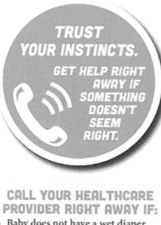

TRUST YOUR INSTINCTS.

GET HELP RIGHT AWAY IF SOMETHING DOESN'T SEEM RIGHT.

CALL YOUR HEALTHCARE PROVIDER RIGHT AWAY IF:

- Baby does not have a wet diaper for longer than 6 hours
- Urine is dark and smells strong
- Baby is lethargic, limp or docile
- Baby has dry mouth and no tears
- Baby is irritable
- Baby has inconsolable crying
- Baby has a sunken fontanel
- Baby is feverish
- Baby has yellow skin
- Skin when pinched remains tented up

WHERE TO FIND HELP

To locate a lactation consultant:
www.USLCA.org

To find a variety of breastfeeding support services:
www.zipmilk.org

App for 24/7 breastfeeding support:
www.pacify.com

Office on Women's Health Helpline:
800-994-9662

My local number for help:

_____

WIC Offices • La Leche League
State Breastfeeding Coalitions • Baby Cafes
Local breastfeeding support organizations

© 2018 Marsha Walker, RN, IBCLC

BREASTFEEDING PROBLEMS CAN HAPPEN!

Know when and where to seek help!

Most breastfeeding mothers find that the early days of nursing a baby is a time of exploring and learning what works best for both mom and baby. With basic instruction and support from your healthcare providers, breastfeeding usually gets off to a good start. However, sometimes mother- nature throws you a curve ball and problems crop up that need attention right away. Learning to recognize these problems and act on them quickly helps you meet your breastfeeding goals and enjoy a satisfying breastfeeding relationship.

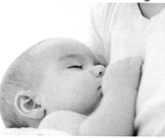

CAUSES FOR CONCERN

Make sure you are working with an IBCLC (International Board Certified Lactation Consultant) and contact your IBCLC or other knowledgeable lactation care provider immediately if:

You
- Are a first time mother
- Had a cesarean delivery
- Have a history of low milk supply
- Are diabetic
- Are obese
- Are hypothyroid
- Have polycystic ovary syndrome
- Have tubular or asymmetric breasts
- Took prenatal SSRI medication
- Have sore nipples
- Think you don't have enough milk

Your Baby
- Is preterm or late preterm
- Small or large for gestational age
- Had vacuum extraction
- Lost more than 7% of birth weight
- Cannot be heard or seen to swallow colostrum or milk
- Is a twin or triplet
- Does not latch to the breast
- Has uric acid crystals after day 2
- Is jaundiced (yellow skin or whites of the eyes)
- Cries all the time/never satisfied after feedings
- Takes more than 30 minutes to feed
- Is extremely sleepy

What I need to know

Feed your baby 8-10 times each 24 hours during the early days.
Put a sleepy baby to breast when you see feeding cues...
- Rapid eye movements under eyelids
- Hand-to-mouth movements
- Small sounds
- Sucking movements of mouth
- Body movements

✳ Massage & compress the breast when baby pauses between sucks.
✳ Have your lactation consultant/nurse verify that baby is swallowing.
✳ Make sure you know when baby is swallowing.
✳ If baby does not latch or nurse well, express your colostrum/milk and feed your baby 2-10 mL/feed (1-2 teaspoons) during the first 24 hours, 5-15 mL/feed from 24-48 hours (1-3 teaspoons), 15-30 mL/feed from 48-72 hours (3 teaspoons to 1 ounce or so), and 30-60 mL/feed (1-2 ounces) from 72-96 hours
✳ Consult your healthcare provider and LC if more supplementation is needed.

Figure 31.3 Discharge information sheet.

more dilute, whereas the milk at the end of a feeding or pumping session has a higher fat content. There are several types of fats in human milk, with triacylglycerols being the most abundant at 98–99% of the total fat. The rest of the fats consist of di- and monoacylglycerols, non-esterified fatty acids, phospholipids, cholesterol, and cholesterol esters. Eighty-five percent of the triacylglycerols are fatty acids, of which there are over 200 different types. Human milk fat contains mostly medium- and long-chain fatty acids, including long-chain polyunsaturated fatty acids (LCPUFAs). The amounts and types of fatty acids are highly dependent on diet and vary from person to person and across cultures. The LCPUFA (particularly docosahexaenoic acid [DHA]) present in human milk is thought to be especially important in the development and maturation of the retina and central nervous system (CNS) and is the most abundant omega-3 fatty acid in the brain and retina.

Oils from fish and algae are usually the main sources of DHA and arachidonic acid (ARA) added to infant formulas—DHA from fermented microalgae (*Crypthecodinium cohnii*) and ARA from soil fungus (*Mortierella alpina*). The fatty acid blends in formulas that contain palm oil and palm olein oil can interfere with calcium and fat absorption (Souza et al., 2017) and may not be suitable for preterm infants. While formula manufacturers have marketed DHA-supplemented formula as a product to enhance cognitive development, full-term babies fed formula milk supplemented with LCPUFA did not have better outcomes than were reported for full-term babies fed formula milk without LCPUFA (Jasani et al., 2017). The DHA in infant formula may have the same chemical formula as the DHA in breastmilk, but it is structurally different than the DHA in breastmilk and is unlikely to function identically to the naturally occurring DHA in breastmilk. A review of the scientific literature that was published by the international research network Cochrane found no clear evidence that DHA-supplemented formula benefits babies' brain development (Jasani et al., 2017).

The maturation of the GI tract is influenced by short- and medium-chain fatty acids. Long-chain fatty acids have antiviral and antiprotozoal effects besides being involved in infant visual and brain development. Among the several classes of sphingolipids and glycolipids are gangliosides, which bind bacterial toxins. Sphingomyelins in the milk fat globule membrane are important in the myelination of the CNS.

Cholesterol is an essential part of all membranes and is required for normal growth and functioning. Serum cholesterol levels are higher in breastfed infants than in formula-fed infants. This difference may have a long-term effect on the ability of the adult to metabolize cholesterol. Cholesterol is part of and necessary for the development of the myelin sheath that is involved in nerve conduction in the brain. Formula contains little to no cholesterol. Adolescents who were exclusively breastfed were shown to have lower low-density lipoprotein, lower total cholesterol levels, and lower levels of triglycerides compared to those who were exclusively formula fed or mixed fed (Hui et al., 2019).

Factors that can influence breastmilk lipid content include maternal age, geographic location, gestational age of the infant, parity, maternal diet during pregnancy and lactation, body mass index (BMI), stage of lactation, time of day, beginning or end of a feeding, smoking, and the number and duration of feedings per day. Breastmilk fat content is lower in the presence of gestational diabetes (Shapira et al., 2019), mastitis (Say et al., 2016), smoking (Baheiraei et al., 2014), and when frozen over time (Orbach et al., 2019). A high BMI increases proin-flammatory fatty acids and decreases anti-inflammatory fatty acids (de la Garza Puentes et al., 2019). Fat rises to the top of refrigerated milk, forming a high-calorie cream layer.

Proteins in human milk have multiple functions that include the enhancement of the immune system, defensive duties against pathogens, and stimulation of the growth and development of the gut. The protein content of human milk is approximately 9 g/L, or 1% on average, and comprising over 400 different proteins within three major groups (casein, whey, and mucins). Caseins constitute about 13% of the total protein and give milk its characteristic white color. Alpha-lactalbumin and lactoferrin are the chief whey fractions, each possessing different antibacterial and immune stimulation activity (Lonnerdal et al., 2017). The protein content in infant formulas ranges from 12 to 19 g/L in standard infant formulas and from 16 to 27 g/L in formulas designed for older infants. The high protein content of infant formula has been implicated in the increased risk for obesity in formula-fed infants (Luque et al., 2015). Protein concentration is highest in the early days, declines to relatively stable levels in mature milk, and is higher in preterm milk during the early weeks than in term milk.

Whey proteins represent about 90% of the total protein in colostrum and 60% of the total protein in mature milk. Whey proteins comprise many different proteins that include major immunological proteins such as lactoferrin, lysozyme, and sIgA, and α-lactalbumin and bile salt-stimulated lipase, which have nutritional roles. Lactoferrin binds to iron and facilitates its uptake into cells. The bacteriostatic effects of lactoferrin act to withhold iron from bacteria that require it for growth. However, lactoferrin needs to be in an environment with a low iron concentration to maintain this bacteriostatic capacity. If exogenous iron is added to breastmilk, the benefits of lactoferrin might be impaired, which could increase the risk of infection in newborns (Chan et al., 2007). One study showed adding human milk fortifier that contained iron to term colostrum reduced the bacteriostatic action of breastmilk against *Escherichia coli* (Campos et al., 2013). Lysozyme lyses the cell walls of most gram-positive bacteria such as *Staphylococcus aureus*. Human milk lysozyme supports the growth of resident commensal bifidobacteria in breastmilk while inhibiting the growth of adult-like strains of bifidobacteria (Minami et al., 2016). Secretory IgA is abundant in human milk. It is highest in colostrum and gradually decreases over time. IgA shields mucosal surfaces from invasion by preventing the adherence of pathogens to the intestinal epithelial surface, while it neutralizes toxins and viruses. α-lactalbumin is a digestible whey protein that makes up 25–35% of the protein in breastmilk. It is involved in lactose synthesis, milk production, and binds zinc, calcium, and iron. Mucins are glycoproteins present in the milk fat globule membrane. Their diverse functions include regulating cell signaling and transcription and modulating the binding of bacteria to the intestinal mucosa epithelium.

Enzymes are proteins that act as catalysts to increase the rate of chemical reactions within cells. Bile salt-stimulated lipase represents about 1–2% of total human milk protein. It is activated by bile salts in the intestine allowing it to hydrolyze or break down fats, separating them into free fatty acids and glycerol to aid in fat digestion and absorption. Amylase is necessary for the infant to digest starch and compensates for immature pancreatic function.

Cytokines are a large group of 80 proteins, peptides, or glycoproteins that are secreted by specific cells of the immune system. Cytokines are a category of signaling molecules that mediate and regulate immunity, inflammation, and hematopoiesis. Milk-derived cytokines affect infant intestinal epithelial proliferation and repair. These duties are essential for maturation and healing of the GI tract as well as inducing oral tolerance and allergy reduction (Dawod & Marshall, 2019).

Growth factors present in human milk have a wide range of effects on the intestinal tract, vasculature, the nervous system, and the endocrine system. Hormones in breastmilk have various functions that permanently shape infant physiologic processes.

Carbohydrates in human milk include lactose, monosaccharides, neutral and acid oligosaccharides, peptide-bound and protein-bound carbohydrates, glucose, galactose, and other complex carbohydrates. Lactose (milk sugar) is the primary carbohydrate in human milk and is a disaccharide composed of galactose and glucose. It is broken down by the enzyme lactase, which is present in the infant by 24 weeks gestation. Lactose is involved in newborn growth; it enhances calcium absorption and is a readily available source of galactose, which is essential to the production of galactolipids such as cerebroside. Galactolipids are essential to CNS development and brain myelinization. Infant formula that has had the lactose removed, such as soy-based formula or lactose-free formulas, cannot provide this important factor to infants. HMOs, biologically active carbohydrates, represent the third largest solid component in human milk after lactose and triglyceride. There are more than 200 neutral and acidic HMOs that differ in composition from those of any other mammal. HMOs are essentially indigestible and are not utilized as a macronutrient, but are delivered to the infant gut intact, where they nourish the infant's gut microbiota acting as the infant's first prebiotic. They serve as decoys in the infant gut through their ability to mimic intestinal cell receptors, preventing bacterial, viral, or protozoan parasite pathogens from attaching to their respective receptors on the infant's intestinal cells. HMOs are a source of sialic acid, which is an essential nutrient for optimal brain development and cognition. Each person has a unique composition and concentration of HMOs in their milk. Some infant formulas are currently supplemented with oligosaccharides. While biotechnological means exist to produce commercially available oligosaccharides, the composition and abundance of HMOs found in human milk have not been artificially reproduced.

Vitamins, both water-soluble and fat-soluble, are fully present in breastmilk. The breast cannot synthesize water-soluble vitamins, so they are derived from the maternal diet. Ascorbic acid (vitamin C) is an important antioxidant in breastmilk and is heat labile and subject to photodegradation. Pasteurized donor human milk may contain lower levels of vitamin C than freshly expressed milk. People who smoke have lower levels of vitamin C in their milk (Dror & Allen, 2018). Vitamin B_{12} is a nutrient critical to an infant's developing nervous system. Vegans may produce milk that is deficient in vitamin B_{12} unless they are supplemented. Symptoms of a B_{12} deficiency in exclusively breastfed infants may be noted between 4 and 10 months of age and include anemia, irritability, infections, hypotonia, microcephaly, refusal to suck, failure to thrive, apathy, anorexia, movement disorders, and gross developmental delay or regression. Infants with these symptoms and the lactating parent should be tested for B_{12} deficiency and offered treatment. Breastfeeding can continue. While breastmilk contains all the nutrients an infant requires, vitamin D may be reduced, as the normal acquisition of vitamin D is dependent on skin exposure to sunshine. People who live in northern latitudes or cold climates, who use sunscreen, have dark skin, or wear clothing that covers large portions of their skin may be deficient in vitamin D themselves. If a breastfeeding individual is vitamin D deficient, the milk may not contain the recommended levels of vitamin D for optimal infant health. While infants can be supplemented with vitamin D drops if necessary, a more reliable way to assure adequate amounts of vitamin D in breastmilk might be to supplement the mother if needed. A randomized controlled trial demonstrated that maternal vitamin D supplementation alone with 6400 IU/day safely supplies breastmilk with adequate amounts of vitamin D to meet the requirements of the infant (Hollis et al., 2015).

Minerals and trace elements are contained in full complements in breastmilk. During pregnancy, breast involution, mastitis, and the first four days postpartum, the junctions between the alveolar cells (milk-making cells) have large gaps that allow sodium and chloride to enter the milk. Thus, under these conditions, milk has greatly increased concentrations of sodium and chloride and decreased concentrations of lactose and potassium. After four days postpartum under usual circumstances, the alveolar cells swell through the influence of prolactin, which closes these gaps. However, during the first few days postpartum, sodium levels can remain high if the infant transfers little colostrum and/or there is a delay in **lactogenesis II**. Sodium concentration in breastmilk during at least the first week postpartum may serve as a biomarker, with high sodium levels representing inadequate infant feeding, insufficient milk removal, a delay in lactogenesis II, and insufficient milk production. Zinc concentration in breastmilk is usually completely adequate for normal infant growth and development, but low levels of zinc can occur. In such cases, the infant may present with persistent perioral, neck, and/or groin rashes, poor weight gain, irritability, poor appetite, slowed growth and development, diarrhea, or immune system deficiencies. Zinc levels can be low even when normal in the maternal serum. Transient neonatal zinc deficiency may be the result of mutations in the maternal SLC30A2 gene, which encodes the ZnT2 transporter—the protein vehicle that imports zinc into the milk-secreting cells in the breast (Golan & Assaraf, 2020). In people lacking this transport mechanism, zinc cannot be effectively secreted into the milk and milk synthesis may be depressed. Zinc supplementation of the infant will restore normal zinc levels, and breastfeeding is recommended to continue.

Defense agents in human milk are composed of an army of components whose interplay is both complex and synergistic. These agents are a compensatory mechanism for the immature immune system of the human newborn with their antimicrobial, anti-inflammatory, and immunoregulatory effects. The antimicrobial proteins in milk include lactoferrin, sIgA, lysozyme, alpha-lactalbumin, lactadherin, defensins, and others. Macrophages and leukocytes are important and abundant cellular components.

Circadian rhythms affect the concentration of a number of breastmilk components. For example, temporal variations exist for cortisol (higher during the day), which promotes alertness, activity, and feeding behaviors and decreases at night. Nighttime milk has high levels of melatonin and tryptophan, which promote sleep. Immune components often exhibit higher activity during the daytime, and the hormonal composition of breastmilk also varies during the 24 hour cycle. The infant circadian clock is not fully functional at birth. The variations in milk components over the day and night may act as environmental cues for the acquisition of infant circadian rhythms. Therefore, some may wish to label expressed milk with the time of day that it was expressed, and select the stored milk that best corresponds with the current time that the infant is being fed (Italianer et al., 2020).

Contraindications to Breastfeeding

There are a few contraindications to breastfeeding. These include classic galactosemia (galactose 1-phosphate uridyltransferase deficiency) in the infant, active untreated maternal tuberculosis, and maternal human T-cell lymphotropic virus (HTLV) type I or II posititivity. People receiving radioactive isotopes or who have had exposure to radioactive materials and those receiving antimetabolites or chemotherapeutic agents or a small number of other medications should not give their milk to their babies until they clear the milk. People using illicit drugs and those with active herpes simplex lesions on a breast should also abstain. However, the infant may feed from the other breast if there are no lesions.

In developed countries such as the United States, people infected with human immunodeficiency virus (HIV) are advised not to breastfeed their infants. However, expressed milk from HIV-positive people can be made safe when it is pasteurized (Israel-Ballard et al., 2007). In developing areas of the world with populations at increased risk of other infectious diseases and nutritional

deficiencies resulting in increased infant death rates, the mortality risks associated with artificial feeding may outweigh the possible risks of acquiring HIV infection. The use of antiretroviral agents by pregnant people is a critical component of the prevention of transmission during antepartum, peripartum, and early postpartum periods. For people with HIV in countries that support breastfeeding with antiretroviral interventions, the WHO recommends exclusive breastfeeding for six months, in combination with antiretroviral therapy for the parent and short-term treatment for infant prophylaxis, to minimize HIV transmission while delivering the health benefits of breastfeeding to the infant (World Health Organization, 2016). However, new recommendations have been issued from the U.S. Department of Health and Human Services (HHS) and the Office of AIDS Research (OAR) regarding medical practice guidelines for infant breastfeeding in the presence of maternal HIV. Individuals with HIV who are on antiretroviral therapy with a sustained undetectable viral load and who choose to breastfeed should be supported in this decision. Clinicians should review the complete guidelines (Panel on Treatment of HIV During Pregnancy and Prevention of Perinatal Transmission, 2023).

Anatomy of the Breast

The breast does not become fully developed and functional until pregnancy and lactation. Breast development occurs in stages during fetal development. By 24 weeks of gestation, the basic framework of the mammary gland has been laid down. In the third trimester of pregnancy, the epidermis in the area where the nipple will eventually appear recedes, forming the mammary pit where the nipple is created from smooth muscle fibers arranged in a circular and longitudinal manner. This depression later elevates forming the protruding nipple. If this pit does not elevate, it can result in a true inverted nipple. The areola surrounds the nipple structure and is formed during the fifth month of gestation. At the end of a full-term pregnancy, 15–20 lobes of glandular tissue have formed within the fetal mammary glands, containing the cells that synthesize milk and that are connected to **lactiferous ducts**. Generally, one pair of breasts form along each milk line, but occasionally accessory or supernumerary nipples and/or breast tissue forms in the axilla or just below the breasts and can swell and secrete milk during lactation. Breasts may be slightly different in size and shape from each other, which is not generally related to their overall milk-producing capacity. However, tuberous, asymmetrical, or cone-shaped breasts may be at risk of producing lower volumes of milk. Such breasts may have large areolas relative to the size of the breast where herniation of breast tissue into the nipple/areolar complex is evident. These breasts may be hypoplastic and point down and sideways. They may show a high location of the submammary folds (lower boundary of the breast where the breast and chest meet), contain dense fibrous rings around the areola, have reduced breast tissue and milk ducts in the lower

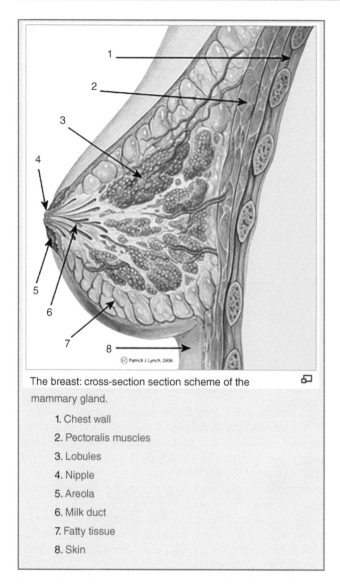

The breast: cross-section section scheme of the mammary gland.

1. Chest wall
2. Pectoralis muscles
3. Lobules
4. Nipple
5. Areola
6. Milk duct
7. Fatty tissue
8. Skin

Figure 31.4   Gross anatomy of the breast. Patrick J. Lynch/Wikimedia Commons/CC BY 3.0.

quadrants, and/or have an intramammary distance of more than 1.5 in (indicating medial breast hypoplasia).

The breast (Figure 31.4) is composed of glandular tissue surrounded by fatty tissue and supported by fibrous tissue and suspensory **Cooper ligaments**. The **tail of Spence**, which projects into the axilla, is connected to the breast's ductal system. Between 5 and 10 main ducts branch and extend from the nipple in a complex and intertwined pattern of 15–25 secretory lobules composed of branching ductules that end in alveolar clusters. The **alveolus** is the milk-secreting unit with lactocytes lining the alveolus and functioning as the milk-synthesizing cells. The alveolus is surrounded by a rich vascular supply and smooth muscle myoepithelial cells. The myoepithelial cells contract under the influence of oxytocin and push the milk down the ductwork to the nipple, an event known as the let-down reflex or **milk ejection reflex**.

The ductal system of the breast is convoluted with peripheral ducts draping over central ducts in a radial

fashion, much like the roots of a tree. Research has shown that not all the milk ducts and connecting lobes make milk at the same time. The first ductal system to be active in lactation was shown to be in the lower-outer quadrant of the breast and, as the baby grew and milk requirements increased, more areas of the breast were recruited to become active. The last area in the breast that was activated to produce milk was the upper-outer quadrant. Controversy exists as to whether there are lactiferous sinuses or dilated sacs beneath the areola. Under ultrasound examination, the absence of any sac-like features in the ductwork under the areola has been reported (Gooding et al., 2010; Ramsay et al., 2005). However, breasts removed by mastectomy were described as having a small antechamber or lactiferous sinus (Love et al., 2015). Nicholson et al. (2009) state, "The collecting ducts that drain each segment, which typically measure about 2 mm in diameter, coalesce in the subareolar region into lactiferous sinuses approximately 5–8 mm in diameter."

The nipple sits in the center of the areola and contains nerve fiber endings, five to nine main milk ducts that open on the nipple tip, smooth muscle fibers, and a rich blood supply. Milk ducts at the base of the nipple are very superficial and easily compressed. Their depth ranges from 0.7 to 7.9 mm. Thus, excessive compression applied incorrectly may occlude these ducts, impeding the flow of milk out of the nipple. Proper latch and sucking are important for clinicians to monitor, as is the fit of the flange on a breast pump and the fit of a nipple shield to avoid excessive pressure on the superficial ductwork of the nipple. Appropriate placement of fingers for hand expression is also important to avoid blocking milk egress. Nipples vary in size and shape. Some nipple variations have the potential for causing a difficult latch such as nipples that are flat, inverted, dimpled, bulbous, bifurcated, or extremely large or mulberry shaped. Prenatal nipple preparation techniques are no longer recommended since they have not been shown to improve nipple protractility or prevent sore nipples.

The areolae enlarge and darken during pregnancy. **Montgomery glands** become prominent during pregnancy and secrete substances such as milk during lactation as well as substances that lubricate and protect the nipple and areola. The ducts of sebaceous glands often empty near or into the ducts of the Montgomery glands. The Montgomery glands have a secretory apparatus, which can become infected, inflamed, or obstructed, presenting a raised bump or fluid-filled blister. They also secrete an odor helping to orient the newborn to the nipple. The nipple and areola should not be washed off as the odor is a chemical attractant to the infant helping babies recognize their own mother's breast. Nipple creams may also mask the olfactory properties of the areola as could full contact nipple shields.

The main sources of blood supply to the breast are the internal thoracic, lateral thoracic, and posterior intercostal arteries. The anterior and lateral cutaneous branches of the second to sixth intercostal nerves innervate the breast and skin. The fourth intercostal nerve supplies the nipple and areola with additional cutaneous branches from the third and fifth nerves. Disruption of the intercostal thoracic nerves T4, T5, or T6 within their respective vertebrae from spinal injury, surgery, or spinal anomalies could inhibit feedback signals to the brain resulting in a diminished release of prolactin and compromised milk production. The lymphatic system of the breast is extensive and functions to collect excess fluid, bacteria, and cast-off cell parts, ridding the breasts of toxins and waste products. The main lymphatic drainage of the breast is to the axilla and the internal mammary nodes, with at least three-quarters of the drainage to the axillary nodes.

Physiology of Lactation

Following the expulsion of the placenta, the abrupt withdrawal of progesterone in the presence of high levels of prolactin initiates lactogenesis II between 36 and 96 hours following birth. Milk ejection is regulated by oxytocin, which acts on myoepithelial cells that surround the lactocytes and propels the milk through the ducts to the nipple. Milk secretion from lactocytes is conducted by a suite of reproductive and metabolic hormones, including glucocorticoids, insulin, insulin-like growth factor 1, growth hormone, and thyroid hormone. Prolactin is the principal lactogenic hormone that regulates mammary gland differentiation, milk production, and the active secretory mechanisms that facilitate milk synthesis. It is synthesized and secreted from the anterior pituitary gland when the infant suckles at the breast. There are three forms of prolactin:

- The monomeric isoform known as "little prolactin" which accounts for 80–95% of the active circulating hormone
- The dimeric isoform known as big prolactin accounts for <10% of the total prolactin
- The polymeric isoform known as big-big prolactin or macroprolactin accounts for a smaller and variable percentage of the total prolactin

The latter two forms have low biologic activity, with macroprolactin unable to cross capillary membranes and stimulate prolactin receptors but still registering as part of the total prolactin level. An imbalance in the types of prolactin should be considered when insufficient milk production is resistant to multiple interventions.

Oxytocin is required for the secretion of prolactin and is synthesized in the hypothalamus and transported to the posterior pituitary, from which it is released into the bloodstream and through a closed system into the brain. Release of oxytocin from infant sucking, mechanical breast pumping, or even thinking about the baby causes contractions of the smooth muscle myoepithelial cells surrounding the mammary alveoli, moving milk into the collecting ducts, dilating the ducts, and propelling the milk toward the nipple resulting in the milk ejection reflex.

The endocrine system is thought to determine maximum milk-producing potential, but local control mechanisms (autocrine) acting in concert actually regulate the short-term synthesis of milk such as:

- The degree of breast fullness and the short-term rate of milk synthesis are inversely related. The emptier the breast, the higher the rate of milk synthesis (Daly et al., 1996; Lai et al., 2010). Clinicians could advise those who need to increase milk production to decrease the time between feeding or pumping sessions.
- Shortened intervals between feedings or milk expression results in higher fat content of the milk (Kent et al., 2006). Shortening the intervals between feedings or milk expression may provide higher fat content milk when an infant is not gaining weight appropriately.
- A factor or factors in the milk termed the feedback inhibitor of lactation (FIL) seem not to be one protein or substance such as serotonin but may be a collection of bioactive factors that concentrate in the breastmilk when breast draining is delayed or abruptly stopped. The increasing concentration of these factors provides negative feedback to the alveoli in a chemical feedback loop, and the process seems reversible with more frequent or thorough draining of the breasts.

Infant Contribution to Breastfeeding

Infants bring their own distinctive anatomical structures to the breastfeeding relationship and must coordinate sucking, swallowing, and breathing to successfully remove milk from the breast. Evaluation of the infant's oral and other structures related to breastfeeding is important when providing guidance or managing problems (Table 31.8).

Sucking at the breast involves a complex and coordinated series of behaviors that have been studied for decades yet remain controversial and somewhat inconclusive (Azarnoosh & Hassanipour, 2020; Mills et al., 2020). Sucking at the breast is a dynamic process with both undulating movements of the tongue and vacuum-generating movements necessary to withdraw an appropriate volume of milk during a feeding (Genna et al., 2021). Infants suck in bursts followed by rests. The less mature the infant, the fewer sucks per burst and the longer the rest periods between sucking bursts. Fewer sucks per burst and longer rest periods can lead to insufficient milk transfer, insufficient milk production, and infant weight gain issues.

Swallowing involves more than two dozen muscles and is initiated when the milk bolus accumulates between the soft palate and epiglottis. Swallowing should be assessed by both the clinician and parents, especially during the early days. Even though an infant's jaw may move up and down resembling sucking and swallowing, jaw movement itself is not a sign of milk transfer. Unless the infant is actually swallowing, little to no milk is ingested. Signs of swallowing include deep jaw excursions, audible swallowing sounds, visualization of the throat during a swallow, a small puff of air from the nose, and a "ca" sound from the throat. If a clinician is uncertain whether an infant is swallowing, cervical auscultation can be performed with a small stethoscope placed to the side of the larynx to listen

Table 31.8 Evaluation of infants' oral structures

Structure	Function	Normal appearance	Alteration
Lips	Seal the oral cavity; stabilize the nipple	Soft, closed, bow-shaped upper lip, well-defined philtrum	Suction blisters can be an indication of ankyloglossia; high or low tone; cleft; asymmetrical; smooth philtrum and thin upper lip can be present with fetal alcohol spectrum; short or flat philtrum may indicate genetic anomalies
Tongue	Seals the oral cavity; changes configuration to compress nipple and propel bolus to back of throat	Soft, well defined, rests in bottom of mouth; actively cups around a finger or nipple forming a central groove	Protruding out of mouth, humped, bunched, or retracted; restricted movement due to ankyloglossia
Jaw	Provides stable base for tongue movement; helps creates negative oral pressure (vacuum) when moved downward	Upper and lower alveolar ridges are aligned	Hanging open or clenched; retracted (micrognathia); wide or excessive jaw excursions; clenching or biting during sucking; asymmetrical or deviating to one side
Cheeks	Provide stability to oral cavity; aid in bolus formation	Fat pads visible	Puckering or dimpled during sucking; drooping to one side
Hard palate	Helps compress the nipple and maintain its position	Intact with rugae	Cleft; high, arched, bubble
Soft palate	Assists in creating posterior oral seal; elevates during swallow	Intact; does not sag to one side	Cleft; bifid uvula; decreased movement; nasal regurgitation of milk
Muscles	Coordinate movement of food and air through the oral cavity; affect lip movement, allow graded jaw movements, influence the shape and action of the tongue and cheeks, elevate the soft palate to seal the nasopharynx, protect the airway, and move and clear a bolus of food	Normal strength and coordination	High or low tone; uncoordinated or ineffective
Nerves	Six cranial nerves overlap in function to enable suck, swallow, and breathe	Gather and channel sensory input from oral structures; motor aspect allows normal movement of oral structures	Damage or ineffective innervation; drooping cheeks and oral structures; failure of proper movements
Reflexes	Secure food in a safe and effective manner without needing to be a learned behavior	When stimulated, all primitive neonatal reflexes are intact	Depressed or absent reflexes such as swallowing, sucking, gag, phasic bite, transverse tongue, rooting

for the pharyngeal swallow (Vice et al., 1995). In special situations, pre- and postfeed weights can be taken to validate the volume of milk ingested by the infant.

Breastfeeding Basics

Proper positioning, latch, suck, and swallow are the foundation for successful breastfeeding. The breastfeeding individual should be helped into a comfortable position, using pillows if necessary, so they can maintain comfort for the entire feeding. While there are several effective breastfeeding positions, it is best to introduce only a few in the beginning. Prior to discharge, they should be able to demonstrate at least one position comfortably, be able to position the infant without assistance, assure proper

latch and milk transfer, state when the infant is swallowing, and not experience nipple pain.

Positioning during Feedings

In the cradle position, the infant is held in their parent's arm, completely facing them and slightly angled so that the head is higher than the hips, but the head, neck, and trunk are all in alignment (Figure 31.5). This position should place the infant's nose at the level of the nipple and the lower lip and chin slightly below the nipple. This is the most common breastfeeding position but may be a little awkward at first.

The cross-cradle position (Figure 31.5) uses the same alignment as the cradle position, but the infant is held with the opposite arm with a hand behind the infant's

Breastfeeding positions

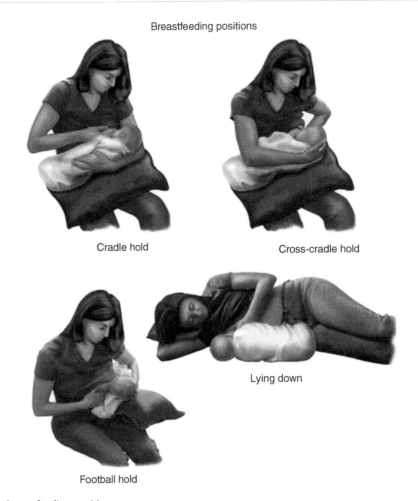

Cradle hold   Cross-cradle hold

Lying down

Football hold

Figure 31.5 Common breastfeeding positions.

head. This position is often useful for early feeding sessions and is also appropriate for feeding preterm and small infants, or any time better head control is needed.

In the football or clutch position, the infant is placed to the side of the parent on a pillow and turned slightly sideways or in a more upright sitting position (Figure 31.5). Care should be taken not to place a heavy breast directly on top of the infant's chest. This is an easy position to learn and can be useful for small or preterm infants. It provides good control of the infant's head and excellent visualization of the nipple and areola.

A restful way to feed an infant is with the parent lying on their side and the infant also on their side completely facing the breast (Figure 31.5). The infant's body can be supported by the parent's arm or a rolled towel or blanket. This position can be helpful following cesarean births.

The ventral or laid-back position places the infant in a prone position on the parent who is reclining at about a 30° angle (Figure 31.6). This position is frequently used for positioning sick or preterm infants, late preterm infants, infants with upper airway anomalies, tongue-tied infants, infants having difficulty handling a fast flow of milk, or infants having difficulty feeding in other positions.

There are many options for positioning twins. The football or clutch hold for both infants, one infant in a

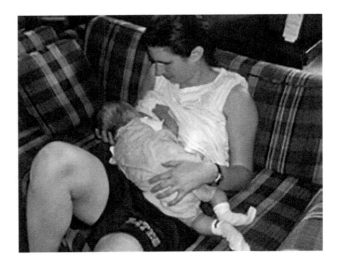

Figure 31.6 Laid-back or ventral position.

cradle hold and one in a clutch hold, infants crisscrossed in cradle holds, or both infants in a prone position (Figure 31.7). Many will start out feeding one infant at a time, so they can learn each infant's manner of feeding and then feed both simultaneously as a time-saving method as they build confidence.

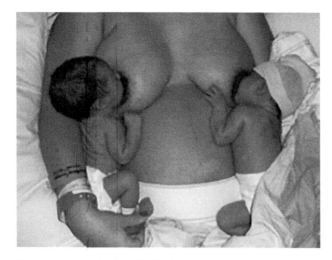

Figure 31.7 Twins in a laid-back or prone position. Courtesy of Lucia Jenkins.

Hand Positions

Many will find it helpful to support the breast during the feeding by using the "C" hold. The thumb is placed above the areola and the index finger below the areola, well away from the nipple. This technique allows the weight of the breast to be supported by the hand rather than the infant's jaw.

The "U" hold or "dancer" hand position is the "C" hold rotated 90° such that the infant's chin rests on the space between the thumb and index finger, while the palm of the hand supports the breast. This hand position is often used with preterm infants, infants with a weak suck, or infants with muscular or neurological challenges that keep them from securely latching to the breast.

Latch

Once positioned correctly, the infant is brought to the breast without leaning down or pushing the breast to the baby. The infant's nose should be at the level of the nipple and the chin contacting the breast as the mouth opens wide and grasps the nipple/areola (Figure 31.8).

Characteristics of a correct latch include the infant's mouth opened wide enough so that the angle at the corner of the mouth is about 160° (Figure 31.9). The nipple and at least one-fourth to one-half of an inch of the areola should be drawn into the infant's mouth and remain in place during sucking; the infant should not pop on and off the breast during feeding. The nipple should not be flattened or distorted when the baby comes off the breast, nor should it be blanched, creased, flattened, or demonstrate blisters, fissures, or cracks.

Correcting the latch may require a position change for the parent and assuring that the infant is in close contact with their body without an arm tucked in between their chest and the breast. The ventral position may be a reasonable choice. If the infant's mouth is not wide open enough or the infant cannot open wide, the parent can use their index finger to gently draw the mouth open, as illustrated in Figure 31.10.

Getting your baby to latch:

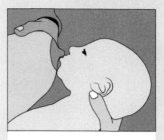

Tickle the baby's lips to encourage him or her to open wide.

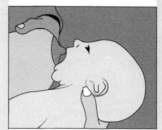

Pull your baby close so that the chin and lower jaw move into your breast first.

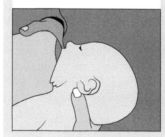

Watch the lower lip and aim it as far from the base of the nipple as possible, so the baby takes a large mouthful of breast.

Figure 31.8 Latch sequence. US Department of Health & Human Services last accessed November 30, 2022/Public Domain/ Department of Health and Human Services.

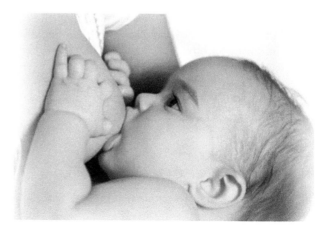

Figure 31.9 Mouth configuration for correct latch. Office on Women's Health, US Department of Health and Human Services (2018).

Parents and helpers should avoid pushing on the back of the infant's head to achieve latch-on. This does not hasten or improve the latch and can cause the infant to extend

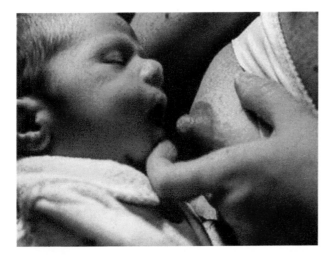

Figure 31.10 Index finger gently draws the mouth open for a better latch.

the head, bite the nipple, or detach from the breast. Healthcare providers should avoid grabbing the breast or manipulating it roughly as people resent this type of handling. A correct latch ensures uniform drainage of all the mammary lobes, avoids nipple discomfort or damage, does not occlude the superficial milk ducts, allows free flow of milk, and ensures maximum milk intake. Proper latch should be checked prior to birth facility discharge, especially if there is a report of sore or damaged nipples, if there is infant weight loss beyond 5–7% of the birth weight, or if the infant appears consistently unsettled following feedings.

Swallowing should be either heard or seen and should be documented in the maternal or infant record. Both the upper and lower lips should be flared out, not rolled or tucked under, although many infants with a correct latch may appear to have the upper lip in a neutral position rather than flanged out (Mills et al., 2020). The lips should form a complete seal with no leakage of milk at the corners of the mouth. The cheeks should not be dimpled or drawn in during sucking, and the cheek line should be a smooth arc. There should be no smacking or clicking sounds during sucking. This indicates that the tongue is losing contact with the nipple/areola. To remedy this, the parent can place their index finger in the soft area under the infant's chin where the tongue attaches and gently push up to provide support.

Breastmilk Production

Lactogenesis I denotes secretory initiation and takes place during the second half of pregnancy. Lactogenesis II, the onset of copious milk production, varies widely but is most commonly seen between 36 and 96 hours postpartum (median 66 hours). The rapid drop in maternal progesterone levels following the expulsion of the placenta combines with the secretion of prolactin and other permissive hormones such as cortisol and insulin to trigger lactogenesis II. Delayed onset of lactogenesis refers to the maternal perception of lactogenesis occurring after

72 hours postpartum and the transfer of less than 9.2 g of milk per feeding (Chapman & Perez-Escamilla, 2000). This is discussed in detail in Chapter 44, *Common Lactation and Breastfeeding Problems.*

During the first three days postpartum, milk synthesis will occur, even in the absence of a suckling infant or expressing milk. The composition of colostrum is similar in breastfeeding and nonbreastfeeding people over the first three days postpartum. However, when milk is not removed from the breast, milk reverts to the composition of colostrum rather than continuing to change to its more mature composition and increase in volume. Thus, efficient milk removal is necessary for continued lactation.

Milk production varies widely, with small volumes of colostrum available during the first one to three days (7–123 mL/day) until lactogenesis II occurs and the volume of milk increases rapidly to an average of 408 mL on day 3, 625 mL on day 4, and 576 mL on day 7. Milk volume continues to increase (750 mL/day at four weeks to 800 mL/day at six months) until it levels off around six months. During the first one to three days, the volume of colostrum may seem small relative to the amount of formula an infant can be persuaded to consume from a bottle. This is in keeping with the physiologic needs and nutrient stores of a newborn infant. The newborn infant's stomach capacity is small, and the stomach itself is somewhat noncompliant during the early hours following birth. Over the next three days, the stomach becomes more compliant and able to handle larger amounts of milk. The average volume per feeding on day 1 ranges from 5 to 10 mL or more depending on the size of the infant and increases to approximately 10–20 mL on day 2, 38 mL on day 3, 58 mL on day 4, 65 mL on day 7, and 94 mL at four weeks. Clinicians should avoid unnecessary or routine supplementation with infant formula as human milk is rapidly digested, and breastfed infants can show hunger signs sooner than 2 or 3 hours after a feeding, especially in the early days after birth. Formula supplementation in the early days can alter the infant gut microbiome (Forbes et al., 2018; Pannaraj et al., 2017) disrupting the programming of the immune system.

Milk production is a continuous process and is influenced by several control mechanisms. The endocrine system is thought to set an individual's maximum potential for milk production, but local control mechanisms regulate the short-term synthesis of milk (Hartmann et al., 1998; Table 31.9).

Breastfeeding Patterns

Breastfed infants usually nurse between 8 and 12 times each 24 hours (Holmes et al., 2013). However, this varies depending on the actual age and gestational age of the infant, their condition, the birth experience, and the culture into which the infant is born. They may even show a diurnal pattern. Frequent feedings during the early days are important to reduce the occurrence of hyperbilirubinemia and excessive weight loss (Hassan & Zakerihamidi, 2018).

Table 31.9 Local factors regulating milk production

Degree of fullness of the breast	Computerized breast measurements have shown that the emptier the breast, the higher the rate of milk synthesis (Daly et al., 1992). Each breast controls its own rate of milk synthesis so one breast may produce more milk than the other (Kent et al., 2006).
Infant's demand for milk	The milk supply adjusts to the infant's appetite. Some infants may feed more frequently as their need increases or they may simply consume more milk per feeding.
Storage capacity of the breasts	The size of the breast does not determine the amount of milk that can be produced but larger breasts may be able to store more milk. People whose breasts have a smaller storage capacity make similar amounts of milk in a 24-hours period, but their infant may feed more frequently.
Feedback inhibitor of lactation (FIL)	A collection of bioactive factors that inhibit milk secretion as milk accumulates in the alveoli. The longer milk remains in the breast, the higher the concentration of FIL, which downregulates milk production.

The average length of breastfeeding sessions decreases over time, and feedings become shorter throughout the first year. Feedings lasting less than 10 minutes are rare in the first month (Shealy et al., 2008). However, total milk intake during feedings between one and three months increases (Kent et al., 2013). Infants may cluster or bunch their feedings toward the end of the day and during the early evening, where intervals between feedings are very short. This is normal and not an indication of insufficient milk or that formula supplementation is necessary. New parents often ask questions such as how long to feed on each side, when to switch sides, or how to know when the infant is done on the first side. Rather than using time limits, better indicators of when the infant is done or should switch sides are either when the infant comes off the breast on their own or when the infant will no longer suck and swallow when the breast is massaged and compressed. Infants may feed on one breast per feeding in the early days and do not always take both breasts at each feeding. After lactogenesis II and after the first few days, infants will usually take both sides at most feedings.

Assessing Intake

There are several tools that have been developed to assess the feeding effectiveness of the breastfed infant. These tools vary in their purpose and usefulness, as some are designed to organize the assessment of the actual feeding, while others are more predictive of those infants who need follow-up and referral (Walker, 2023). Most of the feeding assessment tools are used to identify feeding problems in neonates, and a tool such as the LATCH tool (Jensen et al., 1994) provides a mechanism for clinicians to be consistent when evaluating feeding sessions (Table 31.10).

Table 31.10 The LATCH Tool

L: Latch, i.e., How well the baby latches on
A: Audible swallowing
T: Type, i.e., nipple type
C: Comfort
H: Help, i.e., how much help is needed to hold the baby at the breast

Source: Adapted from Jensen et al. (1994).

Measuring the actual intake of breastmilk in a healthy, full-term normal infant is not necessary. Sufficient milk intake is generally verified by diaper output and weight gain. Adequately breastfed infants typically lose about 5–7% of their birth weight during the birth facility stay and/or by day 4 after birth (Martens & Romphf, 2007; Mulder et al., 2010). However, some adequately breastfed infants will lose more than 5–7% of their birth weight due to the normal diuresis of excess fluid from the maternal fluid load (Mulder et al., 2010) and stooling. The timing and amounts of maternal intravenous (IV) fluids during labor are correlated with neonatal output and newborn weight loss. Neonates appear to experience diuresis and correct their fluid status in the first 24 hours after birth (Noel-Weiss et al., 2011). Intrapartum fluid administration can cause fetal volume expansion and greater fluid loss after birth that is reflected in rapid weight loss following delivery (Chantry et al., 2011). This needs to be accounted for when evaluating weight, feeding parameters, and adequacy of intake.

Breastfed infants generally void a median of two times on days 1 and 2, three times on day 3, five times on day 4, six times on day 5, and seven times on days 6 and 7 (Nommsen-Rivers et al., 2008). The median number of stools are three on days 1–3, four on days 4 and 5, five on day 5, and six on days 6 and 7 (Nommsen-Rivers et al., 2008).

Breastfed infants who do not have three to five stools per day by five to seven days of age, stools not having transitioned to yellow by day 7 following birth, or who demonstrate uric acid crystals in the diaper after day three should be assessed for hydration, adequate weight gain, and breastfeeding difficulties (Mulder et al., 2010; Shrago et al., 2006). Producing less than four stools on day 4 or the delay of lactogenesis II beyond 72 hours postpartum suggests difficulty in establishing breastfeeding. The nursing couplet in this situation should be seen by a healthcare provider and an IBCLC. While wet diapers are an indication of hydration, stool output indicates sufficient caloric intake. Assessing that swallowing is taking place at the breast for most of the feeding is also an important observation in assessing that adequate breastfeeding is occurring.

After the initial weight loss during the early days following birth, most breastfed infants regain their birth weight by two weeks. From two to six weeks of age, the average breastfed female infant is expected to gain approximately 34 g/day and the male breastfed infant gains about 40 g/day, with a minimum gain of 20 g/day for both male and female infants. A general rule of thumb places weight gain of 4–7 oz (112–200 g) a week during the first month, an average of 1–2 lb (0.5–1 kg)/month for the first six months, and an average of 1 lb (0.5 kg)/month from six months to one year. Infants usually grow in length by about an inch a month (2.5 cm) during the first six months, and around 0.5 in/month from six months to one year. However, these numbers are quite variable.

Nutrition for Optimal Lactation

Lactation is a normal physiologic process. While it places an extra requirement on the body, humans adapt without major adjustments in diet or starting a new or special diet. Breastmilk has a relatively constant composition across cultures although some components can be altered through diet or supplementation such as DHA and other fatty acids (Ueno et al., 2020). The Dietary Reference Intake (DRI) Calculator for Healthcare Professionals can be used to estimate calorie needs based on sex, age, height, weight, activity level, pregnancy, and lactation status (US Department of Agriculture, 2021). Iodine and choline requirements increase during lactation, but not all people need to take a multivitamin supplement unless there are identified dietary deficiencies. Lower-mercury-containing fish is recommended. Vegans and some vegetarians need to supplement vitamin B_{12} to avoid infant deficiency. Dietary supplements may also be necessary for those who have had bariatric-type surgery. There is no need to make feeding difficult by providing lists of foods to avoid or imposing strict dietary requirements. People should not hesitate to feed their babies breastmilk even if their diet is of lower quality, since most key nutrients will be available in their milk. The effects of postpartum weight loss and exercise on lactation are discussed in Chapter 20, *Physical Activity and Exercise in the Perinatal Period.*

Smoking and Vaping

Despite public health messages to the contrary, many people of childbearing age continue to smoke. Nicotine is secreted into breastmilk and is approximately three times higher than the amount in maternal circulation (Napierala et al., 2016). Nicotine and other compounds in cigarettes have several effects on the infant. For example, nicotine, when found in breastmilk, can decrease heart rate variability in some infants in a dose-dependent manner, altering their autonomic cardiovascular control (Dahlstrom et al., 2008). Nicotine can alter the taste of milk. Smoking causes adverse changes to breastmilk composition, reducing its protective properties, and decreasing supply (Napierala et al., 2016). Smoking is associated with a lower content of lipids, calories, and proteins, decreased antioxidant properties, and an altered immune status (Macchi et al., 2021). It also affects infant behavior and sleep patterns causing some to spend significantly less time sleeping during the hours immediately after the breastfeeding individual smokes, with less time spent in active sleep as

the nicotine dose increases (Mennella et al., 2007). This particular side effect might serve as an incentive to help with smoking cessation or reduction. Infant tobacco smoke exposure has well-documented negative consequences on infant growth, increased episodes of otitis media, upper and lower respiratory infections, as well as an increased risk for SIDS.

Smoking has the potential to decrease milk supply as prolactin levels are lower in those who smoke (Bahadori et al., 2013). Nicotine has been shown to directly inhibit α- and β-casein secretion in lactating mammary epithelial cells and induce mammary epithelial cell apoptosis, reducing milk production (Kobayashi et al., 2020). Nicotine raises circulating adrenaline significantly, which modulates the release of oxytocin. This may result in a reduction of oxytocin and interfere with milk ejection in those who smoke (Napierala et al., 2017). Parents who give birth to preterm infants may produce significantly lower amounts of milk at two weeks postpartum, 514 mL/day in nonsmokers compared with 406 mL/day in smoking mothers (Hopkinson et al., 1992). Smokers should be encouraged to feed more frequently to help offset potential milk supply problems, and infants of smokers should be weighed more frequently to assure that adequate growth is taking place. Smokers are at risk for short feeding duration, possibly because of the infant behaviors that are exacerbated by smoking, such as crying or disturbed sleep patterns, or by a dose-dependent adverse effect on milk supply (Banderali et al., 2015).

While smoking should always be discouraged, if individuals find it impossible to quit, breastfeeding should still be encouraged to help protect the infant against a number of diseases and conditions, including SIDS. Nicotine replacement methods to achieve smoking cessation (e.g., the nicotine patch, gum, and inhaler) can be safely used. It has been shown that the absolute dose of nicotine and its metabolite continues to decrease by about 70% from when cigarettes are smoked or use of the 21-mg patch to when they use the 7-mg patch. The lower-dose patch showed no significant impact on milk intake and seems a safer option than continued smoking (Ilett et al., 2003) or high dose transdermal patches.

Vaping is the use of electronic cigarettes (e-cigarettes), which are battery-operated cigarettes that turn chemicals, including nicotine, into a vapor, which is then inhaled. E-cigarettes can also contain other substances that are harmful to both the pregnant person and the developing fetus, like heavy metals, flavorings, and cancer-causing chemicals. A study in mice showed that nicotine exposure was associated with craniosynostosis (premature fusing of cranial sutures), raising concerns regarding teratogenicity (Mohi et al., 2020).

Alcohol

While avoidance of alcohol use is recommended during pregnancy, its use is ubiquitous in society and pregnant people may ask about alcohol intake during lactation. Alcohol easily passes into human milk, and its concentration is equal to or greater than the concentration of alcohol in blood. Milk alcohol levels peak about 30–60 minutes after consumption, but peak levels can be delayed by an hour when alcohol is consumed with food. If an infant consumes milk during the time of maximum alcohol concentration, the amount of alcohol the infant consumes is estimated to be about 5–6% of the weight-adjusted intake (Pepino & Mennella, 2004). Alcohol test strips are commercially available for use to detect the presence of alcohol in breastmilk, but does not indicate the level of inebriation in the lactating individual, a concern for any infant caretaker. A nomogram is probably more reliable for determining when breastmilk is free of alcohol (Ho et al., 2001). Expressing and discarding milk after alcohol consumption is not necessary and will not hasten its elimination. Contrary to cultural beliefs, alcohol is not a galactogogue; it delays the milk ejection reflex and can reduce consumption in the hours following beer consumption. Alcohol blocks the release of oxytocin, which delays the milk ejection reflex and reduces milk yield to the infant. Infants consume an average of 20% less milk in the 3–4 hours following the maternal intake of alcohol (Mennella & Garcia-Gomez, 2001).

People who breastfeed should be encouraged to continue, even if they plan to have an occasional alcoholic drink, as recommending abstinence may serve as a deterrent to breastfeeding. The number of alcoholic beverages should ideally be limited to one drink per day or less during lactation, and binge drinking should be avoided. Adverse effects from occasional and moderate drinking can be minimized if recommendations are given to limit the amount of alcohol consumed and to wait 2 hours after ingesting alcohol before feeding or expressing milk. Parents can minimize their infants' exposure by feeding or expressing milk just prior to alcohol consumption (Crowe & Wright, 2021).

Cannabis sativa (Marijuana)

As this goes to press, recreational marijuana use is legal in 18 states, while medical marijuana use is legal in 36 states. Marijuana use is rising in the general population and is of particular concern for lactating people. In a population of WIC clients in one of the largest health departments in Colorado, of those who reported any history of marijuana use (past, ever, or current), 35.8% reported having used marijuana at some point in their pregnancy, and 18% report having used it while breastfeeding (Ryan, 2018). Cannabinoids, such as phytocannabinoid tetrahydrocannabinol (THC), are transferred to breastmilk. Levels remain relatively low after 4 hours following inhaled marijuana use and are largely determined by how much and how often the parent smokes. The oral absorption of THC following feeding an infant is relatively low, about 1–5% of the human milk dose (Baker et al., 2018). The AAP recommends the avoidance of marijuana use during pregnancy and lactation (Ryan et al., 2018). Health professionals' opinions on the acceptability of breastfeeding by cannabis-using parents vary because of insufficient

long-term data on the outcome of infants exposed to cannabis via milk (Drugs and Lactation Database, 2021b). Parents can be advised to avoid feeding at times of peak drug concentrations (the first four hours post use). If parents cannot abstain from marijuana use during lactation, then it is recommended to use marijuana after feedings and before the infant's longest sleep period.

Substance Use Disorders

Substance use disorder (SUD) remains a significant problem among people of childbearing age. The Academy of Breastfeeding Medicine has a clinical protocol that outlines recommendations for drug-dependent people, specifying those who should be discouraged from breastfeeding, those who should be supported in their decision to continue, and those whose situations require more careful evaluation (Reece-Stremtan et al., 2015). People with an SUD who have begun or wish to initiate breastfeeding should be closely monitored along with their infant. Ongoing substance abuse treatment, postpartum care, psychiatric care when warranted, and pediatric care are recommended for those with SUDs. Lactation support is particularly important for infants experiencing neonatal abstinence syndrome (NAS) and their parents. Breastmilk may help lessen the severity of neonatal drug withdrawal and the need for pharmacologic treatment of the infant. Those with SUDs (including those receiving medication assisted treatment with methadone or buprenorphine) with no other medical contraindication should be encouraged to continue unless the risks of substance use clearly outweigh the medical, psychosocial, and financial benefits of breastfeeding (Northern New England Perinatal Quality Improvement Network, 2017). People using alcohol or drugs should be advised, educated, and supported to avoid or cease alcohol or drug use due to risks of harm to infants. When lactating parents continue substance use with significant risk to the infant and refuse treatment, clinicians can recommend against breastfeeding.

Prescription Medications

Most medications are compatible with breastfeeding, but there are a few medications that are contraindicated or that should be used with caution. For example, discontinuing breastfeeding for hours or days may be necessary with some medications such as radioactive compounds. Breastfeeding should almost always be recommended, as the risk of not breastfeeding is usually higher than the risk from most medications. Reliance on medication package inserts is an inaccurate source of information regarding the use of drugs while breastfeeding. Because data on drug effects in lactation are often limited, healthcare providers need to understand the principles underlying the transfer of drugs into breastmilk, as well as have an awareness of the potential adverse effects on the infant.

All medications transfer into breastmilk to some degree, and for many drugs, the amount transferred is less than 1% of the adult dose. Medications penetrate more during the colostral phase of milk production and less after the milk matures. Herbal preparations and supplements are also biologically active and should be used with caution. The purity and dosage of herbal preparations varies widely. Preterm or unstable infants should be evaluated carefully in terms of their ability to handle even small amounts of medication. For those who have been taking medications during pregnancy, the dose of medication in breastfed infants is a fraction of that received by the fetus in utero. Both over-the-counter medications and prescribed medications should be evaluated for the absolute dose received by the infant so that abandonment of breastfeeding is not suggested due to anxiety or lack of knowledge on the part of the clinician (Hale, 2021). See the resources section of this chapter for sources of drug safety during lactation.

Employment and Lactation

Six in ten new lactating individuals return to the workforce, many of them within four to six weeks of giving birth. Employment can have a profound effect on feeding choices, as those returning to employment are more likely to stop breastfeeding than those who are not employed. Many forgo breastfeeding altogether because they feel that it is incompatible with employment, and they cannot imagine how they will be able to combine the two. Many challenges have been identified by those returning to the workplace that include issues of unpaid leave, stress, cost of a pump, finding childcare, unsupportive supervisors and coworkers, lack of a place and time to express milk at work, inflexible working hours, lack of sufficient break time, embarrassment, and irregular work hours with long or rotating shifts. Those with longer leaves and those who anticipate working part-time are more likely to initiate breastfeeding and do so for longer than those who plan to return early to work and work full-time.

Until the 2010 Patient Protection and Affordable Care Act (ACA) was passed, breastfeeding employees had little in the way of worksite protection or accommodations for expressing milk. Under this law, employers are required to provide "reasonable break time for an employee to express milk for her nursing child for one year after the child's birth each time such employee has need to express the milk." Employers are also required to provide "a place, other than a bathroom, that is shielded from view and free from intrusion from coworkers and the public, which may be used by an employee to express breastmilk." This law applies only to nonexempt employees (hourly workers who receive payment for overtime work). The requirement for break time to express breastmilk does not preempt state laws that provide greater protections to employees. Thirty states currently have laws related to breastfeeding in the workplace (National Conference of State Legislatures, 2021).

Clinicians can provide practical information and resources to help parents continue providing breastmilk after their return to work by assuring that feedings get off to a good start before the parent returns to work. Planning helps reduce many challenges. Clinicians can help by assessing the type and extent of support available for their client's particular situation. New parents should inform their employer that they will be expressing milk when they return to work and should be aware of any worksite protection laws that apply to them. A place to pump should be arranged for as well as breaks of sufficient length to accommodate pumping. Childcare arrangements should be made before the infant is born. Some employers allow parents to bring young infants to work or have onsite childcare. To maximize efficiency and supply, parents should obtain a multiuser, double-electric pump. Some individuals are able to work from home and feed their baby directly when needed. Having another caregiver available may be helpful to manage work commitments and breastfeeding.

Supporting parents with a short maternity leave is different than for those with a longer leave. Dwindling milk production and/or insufficient milk supply are often pressing problems when returning to work soon after giving birth. These parents can use a similar approach to avoiding insufficient milk supply that is used to initiate and maintain abundant milk production in preterm births. This model promotes a high milk production by 10–14 days postpartum, such that the parent is producing 50% more milk than what the infant actually needs (Hill et al., 1999). This strategy increases production quickly and serves as a reserve to compensate for any volume decreases that may occur when the parent returns to work or school. This excess milk is frozen for use on the first day back to work or school and anytime a fluctuation occurs in the amount of milk pumped while separated from the infant.

To produce more milk than the baby requires, parents will need to hand express and/or pump milk several times each day in addition to directly feeding the baby. Combining hand expression with electric pumping during the first days after birth increases milk production in parents of preterm infants (Morton et al., 2009). Time-saving ideas for pumping at work are provided in Table 31.11.

Summary

Breastfeeding is widely recognized as the optimal way to nourish the newborn. The health benefits of breastmilk are related to its unique nutritional composition, which is ideally suited to the needs of the human infant. Moreover, breastmilk contains several other important components, including immunoprotectants, anti-inflammatory agents, and growth factors. Infants that are breastfed have improved health outcomes and improved cognitive function compared to formula-fed infants. Close physical contact of the nursing dyad during feeding contributes to attachment and influences infant neurodevelopment. Women also derive long-lasting health benefits from including protection from breast and ovarian cancers as

Table 31.11 Time-saving ideas for pumping at work

- Learn how to hand express as a back-up to pumping and for use while pumping.
- Use of a hands-free bra allows for continued working while pumping.
- Hands-free pumps might also be suggested for some people.
- Have two or three pump collection kits for use at work; these can be brought home for cleaning instead of having to wash pump collection parts after each use at work.
- Those with access to refrigeration can place the pump collection parts in a sealed, clean plastic bag in a refrigerator between uses and then clean them at home.
- Those without access to refrigeration can use a cooler with "blue" ice to keep expressed milk cold.
- Use sanitizing wipes to quickly clean pump parts if they do not have access to running water.
- Pump directly into the bottles that will be used the next day. This eliminates having to transfer milk into other containers.
- Keep nursing pads at work to avoid stains on clothing, especially if the parent is in long meetings or has a long duty assignment. Keep a change of clothing at work, just in case.
- Listen to the baby's sounds while pumping. The sounds can be recorded and played back during pumping or made into a slide show with photos and sounds that can be played back on smartphones or other electronic devices with earbuds. This provides a relaxed atmosphere and a mechanism to condition the let-down reflex.

Source: Adapted from Walker (2011) and Roche-Paull (2016).

well as a reduced risk of cardiovascular disease and diabetes. Healthcare professionals have a responsibility to promote breastfeeding and to develop the knowledge and skills needed to help initiate and maintain breastfeeding, and cope with common feeding problems.

Resources for Healthcare Providers

Books

Genna C.W. (2017). *Supporting sucking skills in breastfeeding infants*, 3rd ed. Jones & Bartlett Learning.

Hale, T.W. (2021). *Medications and mothers' milk*, 19th ed. Springer Publishing Company.

Lauwers, J., & Swisher, A. (2021). *Counseling the nursing mother: A lactation consultant's guide*. 7th ed. Jones & Bartlett Learning.

Lawrence, R.A., & Lawrence, R.M. (2022). *Breastfeeding: A guide for the medical profession*, 9th ed. Elsevier.

Walker, M. (2023). *Breastfeeding management for the clinician: Using the evidence*, 5th ed. Jones & Bartlett Learning.

Wambach K., & Spencer, B. (2021). *Breastfeeding and human lactation*, 6th ed. Jones & Bartlett Learning.

Wilson-Clay B., & Hoover, K. (2022). The breastfeeding atlas, 7th ed. LactNews Press, LLC.

Web Resources

The Melanated Mammary Atlas (2021). Searchable directory of various breast-related conditions on brown and black skin. https://www.mmatlas.com

Getting started with breastfeeding. Stanford Medicine, Newborn Nursery at Lucile Packard Children's Hospital. https://med.stanford.edu/newborns/professional-education/breastfeeding.html

Apps

Breastfeeding Management 2. Helps the clinician identify, triage, and manage common breastfeeding problems in the first weeks of life. Includes five calculators, including two feeding calculators and a weight loss calculator. Massachusetts Breastfeeding Coalition. https://apps.apple.com/us/app/breastfeeding-management-2/id366578339

InfantRisk for healthcare professionals. (n.d.). Gives health care providers access to up-to-date and evidence-based information about prescription and nonprescription medications and their safety during pregnancy and breastfeeding. Infant Risk Center at Texas Tech University Health Sciences Center. https://www.infantrisk.com/infantrisk-center-resources

BiliTool. (2021). Designed to help clinicians assess the risks toward the development of hyperbilirubinemia or "jaundice" in newborns over 35 weeks gestational age. https://bilitool.org/?page_id=46

Newborn Weight Loss Tool (NEWT). (2021). Allows pediatric healthcare providers and parents to see how a newborn's weight during the first days and weeks following childbirth compares with a large sample of newborns, which can help with early identification of weight loss and weight gain issues. https://www.newbornweight.org/#:~:text=What%20is%20it%3F,gain%20issues.%22%20Ian%20M

Organizations and Agencies

Academy of Breastfeeding Medicine. https://www.bfmed.org

American Academy of Pediatrics. https://www.aap.org

Baby Friendly USA. www.babyfriendlyusa.org/

California Perinatal Quality Care Collaborative. https://www.cpqcc.org

Centers for Disease Control and Prevention. https://www.cdc.gov

Human Milk Banking Association of North America. https://www.hmbana.org

International Lactation Consultant Association. www.ilca.org

La Leche League International. https://www.llli.org

National Lactation Consultant Alliance. https://nlca.us

Office of Women's Health, US Department of Health and Human Services. https://www.womenshealth.gov

United States Breastfeeding Committee. http://www.usbreastfeeding.org

Women, Infants, and Children (WIC) Program US Department of Agriculture, Food and Nutrition Service. https://www.fns.usda.gov/wic

United States Lactation Consultant Association. www.uslca.org

Medications and Breastfeeding

Briggs, G.G., Towers, C.V., & Forinash, A.B. (2022). *Briggs drugs in pregnancy and lactation*, 12th ed. Wolters Kluwer.

Hale, T.W. (2021). *Medications and mothers' milk*, 19th ed. Springer Publishing Company.

Drugs and Lactation Database (LactMed). Searchable database for drug safety use during lactation. National Library of Medicine. https://www.ncbi.nlm.nih.gov/books/NBK501922

InfantRisk for healthcare professionals. Gives health care providers access to up-to-date and evidence-based information about prescription and nonprescription medications and their safety during pregnancy and breastfeeding. Infant Risk Center at Texas Tech University Health Sciences Center. https://www.infantrisk.com/infantrisk-center-resources

Nice, F. (2011). *Nonprescription drugs for the breastfeeding mother.* Praeclarus Press.

Nice, F.J., Luo, A.C., & Harrow, C.A. (2016). *Recreational drugs and drugs used to treat addicted mothers: Impact on pregnancy and breastfeeding.* Nice Breastfeeding LLC.

Employment and Breastfeeding

Business case for breastfeeding. Office on Women's Health. https://www.womenshealth.gov/breastfeeding/breastfeeding-home-work-and-public/breastfeeding-and-going-back-work/business-case

Break time for nursing mothers. US Department of Labor, Wage and Hour Division. https://www.dol.gov/agencies/whd/nursing-mothers

Breastfeeding state laws. National Conference of State Legislatures. https://www.ncsl.org/research/health/breastfeeding-state-laws.aspx https://www.ncsl.org/health/breastfeeding-state-laws

Patient Protection and Affordable Care Act. https://www.healthcare.gov/where-can-i-read-the-affordable-care-act/

Resources for Clients and Families

Apps

Anya. https://anya.health/?fbclid=IwAR0z88quR4LShbE38f7rF6gatkXSUb0sdhDI6TFMHCMRuIEG81q7z_ZJOZ0

MommyMeds for Moms. Provides drug safety and ingredients information for safe use of prescription and over-the counter medications. https://apps.apple.com/us/app/mommymeds-pregnancy-safety/id669222544?ls=1

Breastfeeding Solutions. Guide for overcoming breastfeeding problems. https://apps.apple.com/us/app/breastfeeding-solutions/id720156246?ls=1

Irth. Provides prenatal, birthing, postpartum, and pediatric reviews of care for Black and brown women. https://apps.apple.com/us/app/irth-birth-without-bias/id1537466974

Pacify Health. Connects parents to a nationwide network of lactation consultants and registered nurses. https://apps.apple.com/us/app/pacify-spiepr DHYPhelping-spiepr DHYPnew-spiepr DHYPparents/id981698864

Books

Marasco & West. (2019). *Making more milk*, 2nd ed. McGraw-Hill Education.

Mohrbacher & Kendall-Tackett. (2010). *Breastfeeding made simple*, 2nd ed. New Harbinger Publications.

Spangler. (2021). *Breastfeeding: A parent's guide.* Baby GooRoo https://babygooroo.com/books

Spangler. (2019). *Breastfeeding: Keep it simple.* Baby GooRoo https://babygooroo.com/store/product/breastfeeding-keep-it-simple

Wiessinger et al. (2010). *The womanly art of breastfeeding*, 8th ed. Random House Publishing group.

Where to Find Help

US Lactation Consultant Association. To find a lactation consultant. https://uslca.org/resources/find-an-ibclc

ZipMilk. To find lactation care and support. https://www.zipmilk.org/

WIC. Local WIC agencies. https://www.fns.usda.gov/wic/program-contacts

Baby Café. Drop-in informal breastfeeding support groups. https://www.babycafeusa.org

La Leche League International. Mother-to-mother support. https://www.llli.org

Mahmee. Provides care managers for personalized breastfeeding support. https://www.mahmee.com

References

Ashraf, R. N., Jalil, F., Aperia, A., & Lindblad, B. F. (1993). Additional water is not needed for healthy breastfed babies in a hot climate. *Acta Paediatrica Scandinavica*, 82(12), 1007–1011. https://doi.org/10.1111/j.1651-2227.1993.tb12799.x

Azarnoosh, J., & Hassanipour, F. (2020). Fluid–structure interaction modeling of lactating breast. *Journal of Biomechanics*, 103, 109640. https://doi.org/10.1016/j.jbiomech.2020.109640

Baby Friendly USA. (2021). *Baby friendly USA.* https://www.babyfriendlyusa.org

Bahadori, B., Riediger, N. D., Farrell, S. M., Uitz, E., & Moghadasian, M. F. (2013). Hypothesis: Smoking decreases breast feeding duration by suppressing prolactin secretion. *Medical Hypotheses*, 81(4), 582–658. https://doi.org/10.1016/j.mehy.2013.07.007

Baheiraei, A., Shamsi, A., Khaghani, S., Shams, S., Chamari, M., Boushehri, H., & Khedri, A. (2014). The effects of maternal passive smoking on maternal milk lipid. *Acta Medica Iranica*, 52(4), 280–285.

Baker, T., Datta, P., Rewers-Felkins, K., Thompson, H., Kallem, R. R., & Hale, T. W. (2018). Transfer of inhaled cannabis into human breast milk. *Obstetrics and Gynecology, 131*(5), 783–788. https://doi.org/10.1097/AOG.0000000000002575

Banderali, G., Martelli, A., Landi, M., Moretti, F., Betti, F., Radaelli, G., Lassandro, C. & Verduci, E. (2015). Short and long term health effects of parental tobacco smoking during pregnancy and lactation: A descriptive review. *Journal of Translational Medicine, 13*(1), 327.

Bartick, M., & Reinhold, A. (2010). The burden of suboptimal breastfeeding in the United States: A pediatric cost analysis. *Pediatrics, 125*, e1048–e1056.

Bartick, M. C., Jegier, B. J., Green, B. D., Schwarz, E. B., Reinhold, A. G., & Stuebe, A. M. (2017b). Disparities in breastfeeding: Impact on maternal and child health outcomes and costs. *Journal of Pediatrics, 181*, 49–55.

Bartick, M. C., Schwarz, E. B., Green, B. D., Jegier, B. J., Reinhold, A. G., Colaizy, T. T., Bogen, D. L., Schaefer, A. J., & Stuebe, A. M. (2017a). Suboptimal breastfeeding in the United States: Maternal and pediatric health outcomes and costs. *Maternal Child Nutrition, 13*, e12366.

Binns, C., Lee, M., & Low, W. Y. (2016). The long-term public health benefits of breastfeeding. *Asia Pacific Journal of Public Health, 28*, 7–14.

Cabrera-Rubio, R., Collado, M. C., Laitinen, K., Salminen, S., & Isolauri, E. (2012). The human milk microbiome changes over lactation and is shaped by maternal weight and mode of delivery. *American Journal of Clinical Nutrition, 96*, 544–551.

Campos, L. F., Repka, J. C., & Falcão, M. C. (2013). Effects of human milk fortifier with iron on the bacteriostatic properties of breast milk. *Journal of Pediatrics, 89*(4), 394–399. https://doi.org/10.1016/j.jped.2012.12.003

Centers for Disease Control and Prevention. (2014). Racial disparities in access to maternity care practices that support breastfeeding – United States, 2011. *Morbidity and Mortality Weekly Report, 63*, 725–728.

Centers for Disease Control and Prevention. (2021a). *Results: Breastfeeding rates. National Immunization Survey.* US Dept. of Health and Human Services. https://www.cdc.gov/breastfeeding/data/nis_data/results.html

Centers for Disease Control and Prevention. (2021b). *2020 National Results Report.* CDC Survey of Maternity Care Practices in Infant Nutrition and Care. https://www.cdc.gov/breastfeeding/data/mpinc/national-report.html

Chan, G. M., Lee, M. L., & Rechtman, D. J. (2007). Effects of a human milk derived human milk fortifier on the antibacterial actions of human milk. *Breastfeeding Medicine, 2*, 205–208.

Chantry, C. J., Nommsen-Rivers, L. A., Peerson, J. M., Cohen, R. J., & Dewey, K. G. (2011). Excess weight loss in first-born breastfed newborns relates to maternal intrapartum fluid balance. *Pediatrics, 127*, e171–e179.

Chapman, D. J., & Perez-Escamilla, R. (2000). Lactogenesis stage II: Hormonal regulation, determinants, and public health consequences. *Recent Research Developments in Nutrition, 3*, 43–63.

Chiang, K. V., Li, R., Anstey, E. H., & Perrine, C. G. (2021). Racial and ethnic disparities in breastfeeding initiation – United States, 2019. *Morbidity and Mortality Weekly Reports, 70*, 769–774.

Crowe, S., & Wright, T. (2021). Breastfeeding dilemma: What are the impacts of alcohol use during lactation? *Contemporary OB/GYN Journal, 66*, 16–20.

Dahlstrom, A., Ebersjo, C., & Lundell, B. (2008). Nicotine in breast milk influences heart rate variability in the infant. *Acta Paediatrica, 97*, 1075–1079.

Daly, S. E., Kent, J. C., Owens, R. A., & Hartmann, P. E. (1996). Frequency and degree of milk removal and the short-term control of human milk synthesis. *Experimental Physiology, 81*, 861–875.

Daly, S. E. J., Kent, J. C., Huynh, D. Q., Owens, R. A., & Hartmann, P. E. (1992). The determination of short-term breast volume changes and the rate of synthesis of human milk using computerized breast measurement. *Experimental Physiology, 77*, 79–87.

Dawod, B., & Marshall, J. S. (2019). Cytokines and soluble receptors in breast milk as enhancers of oral tolerance development. *Frontiers in Immunology, 10*, 16. https://doi.org/10.3389/fimmu.2019.00016

de la Garza Puentes, A., Martí Alemany, A., Chisaguano, A. M., Montes Goyanes, R., Castellote, A. I., Torres-Espínola, F. J., García-Valdés, L., Escudero-Marín, M., Segura, M. T., Campoy, C., & López-Sabater, M. C. (2019). The effect of maternal obesity on breast milk fatty acids and its association with infant growth and cognition – The PREOBE follow-up. *Nutrients, 11*(9), 2154. https://doi.org/10.3390/nu11092154

DiGirolamo, A. M., Grummer-Strawn, L. M., & Fein, S. B. (2003). Do perceived attitudes of physicians and hospital staff affect breastfeeding decisions? *Birth, 30*, 94–100.

Dror, D. K., & Allen, L. H. (2018). Overview of nutrients in human milk. *Advances in Nutrition, 9*(Suppl 1), 278S–294S.

Drugs and Lactation Database. (2021a). *Testosterone.* https://www.ncbi.nlm.nih.gov/books/NBK501721

Drugs and Lactation Database. (2021b). *Cannabis.* https://www.ncbi.nlm.nih.gov/books/NBK501587

Duckett, L. J., & Ruud, M. (2019). Affirming language use when providing health care for and writing about childbearing families who identify as LGBTQI. *Journal of Human Lactation, 35*, 227–232.

Entmacher, J., Frolich, L., Robbins, K. G., Martin, E., & Watson, L. (2014). *Underpaid & overloaded: Women in low-wage jobs.* National Women's Law Center. https://nwlc.org/wp-content/uploads/2015/08/final_nwlc_lowwagereport2014.pdf

Evans, K., Labbok, M., & Abrahams, S. W. (2011). WIC and breastfeeding support services: Does the mix of services offered vary with race and ethnicity? *Breastfeeding Medicine, 6*, 401–406.

Farrow, A. (2015). Lactation support and the LGBTQI community. *Journal of Human Lactation, 31*, 26–28.

Fernandez, L., Langa, S., Martin, V., Maldonado, A., Jimenez, E., Martin, R., & Rodriguez, J. M. (2013). The human milk microbiota: Origin and potential roles in health and disease. *Pharmacological Research, 69*, 1–10.

Ferri, R. L., Rosen-Carole, C. B., Jackson, J., Carreno-Rijo, E., Greenberg, K. B., & Academy of Breastfeeding Medicine. (2020). ABM clinical protocol #33: Lactation care for lesbian, gay, bisexual, transgender, queer, questioning, plus patients. *Breastfeeding Medicine, 15*, 284–293.

Forbes, J. D., Azad, M. B., Vehling, L., Tun, H. M., Konya, T. B., Guttman, D. S., Field, C. J., Lefebvre, D., Sears, M. R., Becker, A. B., Mandhane, P. J., Turvey, S. E., Moraes, T. J., Subbarao, P., Scott, J. A., Kozyrskyj, A. L., & Canadian Healthy Infant Longitudinal Development (CHILD) Study Investigators. (2018). Association of exposure to formula in the hospital and subsequent infant feeding practices with gut microbiota and risk of overweight in the first year of life. *JAMA Pediatrics, 172*, e181161.

Fox, M., Siddarth, P., Oughli, H. A., Nguyen, S. A., Milillo, M. M., Aguilar, Y., Ercoli, L., & Lavretsky, H. (2021). Women who breastfeed exhibit cognitive benefits after age 50. *Evolution, Medicine, and Public Health, 9*, 322–331.

Francis-Clegg, S., & Francis, D. T. (2011). Improving the "bottom-line": Financial justification for the hospital-based lactation consultant role. *Clinical Lactation, 2*, 19–25.

García-Acosta, J. M., San Juan-Valdivia, R. M., Fernández-Martínez, A. D., Lorenzo-Rocha, N. D., & Castro-Peraza, M. E. (2019). Trans* pregnancy and lactation: A literature review from a nursing perspective. *International Journal of Environmental Research and Public Health, 17*(1), 44. https://doi.org/10.3390/ijerph17010044

Genna, C. W., Saperstein, Y., Siegel, S. A., Laine, A. F., & Elad, D. (2021). Quantitative imaging of tongue kinematics during infant feeding and adult swallowing reveals highly conserved patterns. *Physiological Reports, 9*(3), e14685.

Gill, S. L. (2001). The little things: Perceptions of breastfeeding support. *Journal of Obstetric, Gynecologic, & Neonatal Nursing, 30*, 401–409.

Golan, Y., & Assaraf, Y. G. (2020). Genetic and physiological factors affecting human milk production and composition. *Nutrients, 12*(5), 1500. https://doi.org/10.3390/nu12051500

Gooding, M. J., Finlay, J., Shipley, J. A., Halliwell, M., & Duck, F. A. (2010). Three-dimensional ultrasound imaging of mammary ducts in lactating women. *Journal of Ultrasound in Medicine, 29*, 95–103.

Graffy, J., & Taylor, J. (2005). What information, advice, and support do women want with breastfeeding? *Birth, 32*, 179–186.

Hale, T. W. (2021). *Medications and mothers' milk* (19th ed.). Springer Publishing Company.

Hamner, H. C., Chiang, K. V., & Li, R. (2021). Returning to work and breastfeeding duration at 12 months, WIC infants and toddler feeding practices Study-2. *Breastfeeding Medicine: the Official Journal of the Academy of Breastfeeding Medicine*, 16(12), 956–964. https://doi.org/10.1089/bfm.2021.0081

Hartmann, P. E., Sherriff, J. L., & Mitoulas, L. R. (1998). Homeostatic mechanisms that regulate lactation during energetic stress. *Journal of Nutrition*, 128, 394S–399S.

Hassan, B., & Zakerihamidi, M. (2018). The correlation between frequency and duration of breastfeeding and the severity of neonatal hyperbilirubinemia. *Journal of Maternal, Fetal, and Neonatal Medicine*, 31, 457–463.

Hill, P. D., Aldag, J. C., & Chatterton, R. T. (1999). Effects of pumping style on milk production in mothers of non-nursing preterm infants. *Journal of Human Lactation*, 15, 209–216.

Ho, E., Collantes, A., Kapur, B. M., Moretti, M., & Koren, G. (2001). Alcohol and breastfeeding: Calculation of time to zero level in milk. *Biology of the Neonate*, 80, 219–222.

Hollis, B. W., Wagner, C. L., Howard, C. R., Ebeling, M., Shary, J. R., Smith, P. G., Taylor, S. N., Morella, K., Lawrence, R. A., & Hulsey, T. C. (2015). Maternal versus infant vitamin D supplementation during lactation: A randomized controlled trial. *Pediatrics*, 136, 625–634.

Holmes, A. V., McLeod, A. Y., & Bunik, M. (2013). ABM clinical protocol #5: Peripartum breastfeeding management for the healthy mother and infant at term, revision 2013. *Breastfeeding Medicine*, 8(6), 469–473. https://doi.org/10.1089/bfm.2013.9979

Hopkinson, J. M., Schanler, R. J., & Garza, C. (1992). Milk production by mothers of premature infants. Influence of cigarette smoking. *Pediatrics*, 90, 934–938.

Hui, L. L., Kwok, M. K., Nelson, E. A. S., Lee, S. L., Leung, G. M., & Schooling, C. M. (2019). Breastfeeding in infancy and lipid profile in adolescence. *Pediatrics*, 143(5), e20183075. https://doi.org/10.1542/peds.2018-3075

Ilett, K. F., Hale, T. W., Page-Sharp, M., Kristensen, J. H., Kohan, R., & Hackett, L. P. (2003). Use of nicotine patches in breastfeeding mothers: Transfer of nicotine and cotinine into human milk. *Clinical Pharmacology and Therapeutics*, 74, 516–524.

IRTH. (2021, November 23). *Irth*. Retrieved March 23, 2022, from https://irthapp.com

Israel-Ballard, K., Donovan, R., Chantry, C., Coutsoudis, A., Sheppard, H., Sibeko, L., & Abrams, B. (2007). Flash-heat inactivation of HIV-1 in human milk: A potential method to reduce postnatal transmission in developing countries. *Journal of Acquired Immune Deficiency Syndromes*, 45, 318–323.

Italianer, M. F., Naninck, E., Roelants, J. A., van der Horst, G., Reiss, I., Goudoever, J., Joosten, K., Chaves, I., & Vermeulen, M. J. (2020). Circadian variation in human milk composition, a systematic review. *Nutrients*, 12(8), 2328. https://doi.org/10.3390/nu12082328

Jasani, B., Simmer, K., Patole, S. K., & Rao, S. C. (2017). Long chain polyunsaturated fatty acid supplementation in infants born at term. *Cochrane Database of Systematic Reviews*, 3(3), CD000376. https://doi.org/10.1002/14651858.CD000376.pub4

Jensen, D., Wallace, S., & Kelsay, P. (1994). LATCH: A breastfeeding charting system and documentation tool. *Journal of Obstetric, Gynecologic, & Neonatal Nursing*, 23, 27–32.

Jones, J.M. (2021). *LGBT identification rises to 5.6% in latest U.S. estimate.* Gallup Poll Social Series. https://news.gallup.com/poll/329708/lgbt-identification-rises-latest-estimate.aspx.

Kanhai, R. C., Hage, J. J., van Diest, P. J., Bloemena, E., & Mulder, J. W. (2000). Short-term and long-term histologic effects of castration and estrogen treatment on breast tissue of 14 male-to-female transsexuals in comparison with two chemically castrated men. *American Journal of Surgical Pathology*, 24, 74–80.

Kellams, A., Harrel, C., Omage, S., Gregory, C., Rosen-Carole, C., & Academy of Breastfeeding Medicine. (2017). ABM clinical protocol #3: Supplementary feedings in the healthy term breastfed neonate, revised 2017. *Breastfeeding Medicine*, 12, 188–198.

Kent, J., Hepworth, A., Sherriff, J. L., Cox, D. B., Mitoulas, L., & Hartmann, P. (2013). Longitudinal changes in breastfeeding patterns from 1 to 6 months of lactation. *Breastfeeding Medicine*, 8(4), 401–407.

Kent, J. C., Mitoulas, L. R., Cregan, M. D., Ramsay, D. T., Doherty, D. A., & Hartmann, P. E. (2006). Volume and frequency of breastfeeds and fat content of breastmilk throughout the day. *Pediatrics*, 117, e387–e395.

Knox-Kazimierczuk, F. A., Nommsen-Rivers, L., Ware, J., Graham, C., & Conner, N. (2021). Exploring the breastfeeding experiences of African American mothers through a critical race theory lens. *Breastfeeding Medicine*, 16(6), 487–492. https://doi.org/10.1089/bfm.2020.0328

Kobayashi, K., Tsugami, Y., Suzuki, N., Suzuki, T., & Nishimura, T. (2020). Nicotine directly affects milk production in lactating mammary epithelial cells concurrently with inactivation of STAT5 and glucocorticoid receptor in vitro. *Toxicology In Vitro*, 63, 104741. https://doi.org/10.1016/j.tiv.2019.104741

Krawczyk, A., Lewis, M. G., Venkatesh, B. T., & Nair, S. N. (2016). Effect of exclusive breastfeeding on rotavirus infection among children. *Indian Journal of Pediatrics*, 83, 220–225.

Kulski, J. K., Hartmann, P. E., & Gutteridge, D. H. (1981). Composition of breast fluid of a man with galactorrhea and hyperprolactinaemia. *Journal of Clinical Endocrinology and Metabolism*, 52, 581–582.

Lai, C. T., Hale, T. W., Simmer, K., & Hartmann, P. E. (2010). Measuring milk synthesis in breastfeeding mothers. *Breastfeeding Medicine*, 5, 103–107.

Lönnerdal, B., Erdmann, P., Thakkar, S. K., & Sauser, J. (2017). Longitudinal evolution of true protein, amino acids and bioactive proteins in breast milk: A developmental perspective. *Journal of Nutritional Biochemistry*, 41, 1–11.

Louis-Jacques, A., & Stuebe, A. (2018). Long-term maternal benefits of breastfeeding. *Contemporary OB/GYN*, 64, 26–29.

Love, S. M., Lindsey, K., & Love, E. (2015). *Dr. Susan Love's breast book* (6th ed.). Da Capo Press.

Luque, V., Closa-Monasterolo, R., Escribano, J., & Ferre, N. (2015). Early programming by protein intake: The effect of protein on adiposity development and the growth and functionality of vital organs. *Nutrition and Metabolic Insights*, 8, 49–56.

Macchi, M., Bambini, L., Franceschini, S., Alexa, I. D., & Agostoni, C. (2021). The effect of tobacco smoking during pregnancy and breastfeeding on human milk composition—A systematic review. *European Journal of Clinical Nutrition*, 75, 736–747.

MacDonald, T. K. (2019). Lactation care for transgender and nonbinary patients: Empowering clients and avoiding aversives. *Journal of Human Lactation*, 35, 223–226.

MacLean, L. R. (2021). Preconception, pregnancy, birthing, and lactation needs of transgender men. *Nursing for Women's Health*, 25, 129–138.

Mannel, R. (2010). Lactation rounds: A system to improve hospital productivity. *Journal of Human Lactation*, 26, 393–398.

Martens, P. J., & Romphf, L. (2007). Factors associated with newborn in-hospital weight loss: Comparisons by feeding method, demographics, and birthing procedures. *Journal of Human Lactation*, 23, 233–241.

Martinez-Brockman, J. L., Harari, N., & Pérez-Escamilla, R. (2018). Lactation advice through texting can help: An analysis of intensity of engagement via two-way text messaging. *Journal of Health Communication*, 23, 40–51.

McInnes, R. J., & Chambers, J. A. (2008). Supporting breastfeeding mothers: Qualitative synthesis. *Journal of Advanced Nursing*, 62, 407–427.

McKinney, C. O., Hahn-Holbrook, J., Chase-Lansdale, P. L., Ramey, S. L., Krohn, J., Reed-Vance, M., Raju, T. N. K., Shalowitz, M. U., & on behalf of the Community Child Health Research Network. (2016). Racial and ethnic differences in breastfeeding. *Pediatrics*, 138(2), e20152388. https://doi.org/10.1542/peds.2015-2388

Meek, J. Y. (2021). Infant benefits of breastfeeding. In A. G. Hoppin (Ed.), *Up to date*. UptoDate. https://www.uptodate.com/contents/infant-benefits-of-breastfeeding

Meek, J. Y., Noble, L., & The Section on Breastfeeding. (2022). Policy statement: Breastfeeding and the use of human milk. *Pediatrics*, 150(1). https://doi.org/10.1542/peds.2022-057988

Mennella, J. A., & Garcia-Gomez, P. L. (2001). Sleep disturbances after acute exposure to alcohol in mothers' milk. *Alcohol*, 25, 153–158.

Mennella, J. A., Yourshaw, L. M., & Morgan, L. K. (2007). Breastfeeding and smoking: Short-term effects on infant feeding and sleep. *Pediatrics*, 120, 497–502.

Merewood, A., Bugg, K., Burnham, L., Krane, K., Nickel, N., Broom, S., Edwards, R., & Feldman-Winter, L. (2019). Addressing racial inequities in breastfeeding in the southern United States. *Pediatrics, 143*(2), e20181897. https://doi.org/10.1542/peds.2018-1897.

Mills, N., Lydon, A. M., Davies-Payne, D., Keesing, M., Geddes, D. T., & Mirjalili, S. A. (2020). Imaging the breastfeeding swallow: Pilot study utilizing real-time MRI. *Laryngoscope Investigative Otolaryngology, 5*, 572–579.

Minami, J., Odamaki, T., Hashikura, N., Abe, F., & Xiao, J. Z. (2016). Lysozyme in breast milk is a selection factor for bifidobacterial colonisation in the infant intestine. *Beneficial Microbes, 7*, 53–60.

Mohi, A., Kishinchand, R., Durham, E., & Cray, J. (2020). Maternal nicotine exposure during lactation alters craniofacial development. *The FASEB Journal, 34*, 1–1. https://doi.org/10.1096/fasebj.2020.34.s1.02917

Morton, J., Hall, J. Y., Wong, R. J., Thairu, L., Benitz, W. E., & Rhine, W. D. (2009). Combining hand techniques with electric pumping increases milk production in mothers of preterm infants. *Journal of Perinatology, 29*, 757–764.

Mozingo, J. N., Davis, M. W., Droppleman, P. G., & Merideth, A. (2000). "It wasn't working": Women's experiences with short-term breast-feeding. *MCN The American Journal of Maternal Child Nursing, 25*, 120–126.

Mulder, P. J., Johnson, T. S., & Baker, L. C. (2010). Excessive weight loss in breastfed infants during the postpartum hospitalization. *Journal of Obstetric, Gynecologic, & Neonatal Nursing, 39*, 15–26.

Napierala, M., Mazela, J., Merritt, T. A., & Florek, E. (2016). Tobacco smoking and breastfeeding: Effect on the lactation process, breast milk composition and infant development. A critical review. *Environmental Research, 151*, 321–338.

Napierala, M., Merritt, T. A., Mazela, J., Jablecka, K., Miechowicz, I., Marszalek, A., & Florek, E. (2017). The effect of tobacco smoke on oxytocin concentrations and selected oxidative stress parameters in plasma during pregnancy and post-partum—An experimental model. *Human & Experimental Toxicology, 36*, 135–145.

Napierala, M., Merritt, T. A., Miechowicz, I., Mielnik, K., Mazela, J., & Florek, E. (2019). The effect of maternal tobacco smoking and second-hand tobacco smoke exposure on human milk oxidant-antioxidant status. *Environmental Research, 170*, 110–121.

National Conference of State Legislatures. (2021). *Breastfeeding state laws.* https://www.ncsl.org/research/health/breastfeeding-state-laws.aspx

Nelson, A. M. (2007). Maternal-newborn nurses' experiences of inconsistent professional breastfeeding support. *Journal of Advanced Nursing, 60*, 29–38.

Nicholson, B. T., Harvey, J. A., & Cohen, M. A. (2009). Nipple-areolar complex: Normal anatomy and benign and malignant processes. *Radiographics, 29*, 509–523.

Noel-Weiss, J., Woodend, A. K., Peterson, W. E., Gibb, W., & Groll, D. L. (2011). An observational study of associations among maternal fluids during parturition, neonatal output, and breastfed newborn weight loss. *International Breastfeeding Journal, 6*, 9. https://doi.org/10.1186/1746-4358-6-9

Nommsen-Rivers, L. A., Heinig, M. J., Cohen, R. J., & Dewey, K. G. (2008). Newborn wet and soiled diaper counts and timing of onset of lactation as indicators of breastfeeding inadequacy. *Journal of Human Lactation, 24*, 27–33.

Northern New England Perinatal Quality Improvement Network. (2017). *Breastfeeding guidelines for women with a substance use disorder.* https://ilpqc.org/wp-content/docs/toolkits/MNO-OB/Breastfeeding-Guidelines-for-Women-with-SUD.pdf

Orbach, R., Mandel, D., Mangel, L., Marom, R., & Lubetzky, R. (2019). The effect of deep freezing on human milk macronutrients content. *Breastfeeding Medicine, 14*, 172–176.

Panel on Treatment of HIV During Pregnancy and Prevention of Perinatal Transmission. (2023). *Recommendations for the Use of Antiretroviral Drugs During Pregnancy and Interventions to Reduce Perinatal HIV Transmission in the United States.* Department of Health and Human Services. https://clinicalinfo.hiv.gov/sites/default/files/guidelines/documents/perinatal-hiv/guidelines-perinatal.pdf

Pannaraj, P. S., Li, F., Cerini, C., Bender, J. M., Yang, S., Rollie, A., Adisetiyo, H., Zabih, S., Lincez, P. J., Bittinger, K., Bailey, A., Bushman, F. D., Sleasman, J. W., & Aldrovandi, G. M. (2017). Association between breast milk bacterial communities and establishment and development of the infant gut microbiome. *JAMA Pediatrics, 17*, 647–654.

Pärnänen, K. M. M., Hultman, J., Markkanen, M., Satokari, R., Rautava, S., Lamendella, R., Wright, J., McLimans, C. J., Kelleher, S. L., & Virta, M. P. (2021). Early-life formula feeding is associated with infant gut microbiota alterations and an increased antibiotic resistance load. *American Journal of Clinical Nutrition, 115*(2), 407–421. https://doi.org/10.1093/ajcn/nqab353

Pepino, M. Y., & Mennella, J. A. (2004). Advice given to women in Argentina about breast-feeding and the use of alcohol. *Revista Panamericana de Salud Publica, 16*, 408–414.

Piskin, I. E., Karavar, H. N., Arasli, M., & Ermis, B. (2012). Effect of maternal smoking on colostrum and breastmilk cytokines. *European Cytokine Network, 23*, 187–190.

Ramsay, D., Kent, J., Hartmann, R., & Hartmann, P. (2005). Anatomy of the lactating human breast redefined with ultrasound imaging. *Journal of Anatomy, 206*, 525–534.

Ranch, M. M., Jämtén, S., Thorstensson, S., & Ekström-Bergström, A. C. (2019). First-time mothers have a desire to be offered professional breastfeeding support by pediatric nurses: An evaluation of the mother-perceived-professional support scale. *Nursing Research and Practice, 8731705.* https://doi.org/10.1155/2019/8731705

Reece-Stremtan, S., Marinelli, K. A., & The Academy of Breastfeeding Medicine. (2015). ABM clinical protocol #21: Guidelines for breast-feeding and substance use or substance use disorder, revised 2015. *Breastfeeding Medicine, 10*, 135–141.

Regan, S., & Brown, A. (2019). Experiences of online breastfeeding support: Support and reassurance versus judgement and misinformation. *Maternal & Child Nutrition, 15*(4), e12874. https://doi.org/10.1111/mcn.12874

Reisman, T., & Goldstein, Z. (2018). Case report: Induced lactation in a transgender woman. *Transgender Health, 3*, 24–26.

Roche-Paull, R. (2016). *Breastfeeding in combat boots: A survival guide to successful breastfeeding while serving in the military.* CreateSpace Independent Publishing Platform.

Ryan, S. A. (2018). A modern conundrum for the pediatrician: The safety of breast milk and the cannabis-using mother. *Pediatrics, 142*, e20181921.

Ryan, S. A., Ammerman, S. D., O'Connor, M. E., Committee on Substance Use And Prevention, Section on Breastfeeding, Gonzalez, L., Patrick, S. W., Quigley, J., Walker, L. R., Meek, J. Y., Johnston, M., Stellwagen, L., Thomas, J., & Ware, J. (2018). Marijuana use during pregnancy and breastfeeding: Implications for neonatal and childhood outcomes. *Pediatrics, 142*(3), e20181889. https://doi.org/10.1542/peds.2018-1921

Say, B., Dizdar, E. A., Degirmencioglu, H., Uras, N., Sari, F. N., Oguz, S., & Canpolat, F. E. (2016). The effect of lactational mastitis on the macronutrient content of breast milk. *Early Human Development, 98*, 7–9.

Schmied, V., Beake, S., Sheehan, A., McCourt, C., & Dykes, F. (2011). Women's perceptions and experiences of breastfeeding support: A metasynthesis. *Birth, 38*, 49–60.

Shapira, D., Mandel, D., Mimouni, F. B., Moran-Lev, H., Marom, R., Mangel, L., & Lubetzky, R. (2019). The effect of gestational diabetes mellitus on human milk macronutrients content. *Journal of Perinatology, 39*, 820–823.

Shealy, K. R., Scanlon, K. S., Labiner-Wolfe, J., Fein, S. B., & Grummer-Strawn, L. M. (2008). Characteristics of breastfeeding practices among US mothers. *Pediatrics, 122*(Suppl. 2), S50–S55.

Shrago, L. C., Reifsnider, E., & Insel, K. (2006). The neonatal bowel output study: Indicators of adequate breast milk intake in neonates. *Pediatric Nursing, 32*, 195–201.

Simsek, Y., Karabiyik, P., Polat, K., Duran, Z., & Polat, A. (2015). Mode of delivery changes oxidative and antioxidative properties of human milk: A prospective controlled clinical investigation. *Journal of Maternal Fetal and Neonatal Medicine, 28*, 734–738.

Sonnenblick, E. B., Shah, A. D., Goldstein, Z., & Reisman, T. (2018). Breast imaging of transgender individuals: A review. *Current Radiology Reports, 6*(1), 1. https://doi.org/10.1007/s40134-018-0260-1

Souza, C. O., Leite, M. E. Q., Lasekan, J., Baggs, G., Pinho, L. S., Druzian, J. I., Ribeiro, T. C. M., Mattos, A. P., Menezes-Filho, J. A., & Costa-Ribeiro, H. (2017). Milk protein-based formulas containing different oils affect fatty acids balance in term infants: A, randomized blinded crossover clinical trial. *Lipids in Health and Disease, 16*(1), 78. https://doi.org/10.1186/s12944-017-0457-y

Ueno, H. M., Higurashi, S., Shimomura, Y., Wakui, R., Matsuura, H., Shiota, M., Kubouchi, H., Yamamura, J. I., Toba, Y., & Kobayashi, T. (2020). Association of DHA concentration in human breast milk with maternal diet and use of supplements: A cross-sectional analysis of data from the Japanese Human Milk Study Cohort. *Current Developments in Nutrition, 4*(7), nzaa105. https://doi.org/10.1093/cdn/nzaa105

UNICEF. (2021). *Baby-Friendly Hospital Initiative.* https://www.unicef.org/documents/baby-friendly-hospital-initiative

United States Breastfeeding Committee. (2010). *Core Competencies in Breastfeeding Care and Services for All Health Professionals.* Rev ed. Washington, DC.

US Department of Agriculture, National Agricultural Library. (2021). *DRI calculator for healthcare professionals.* https://www.nal.usda.gov/legacy/fnic/dri-calculator

US Preventive Services Task Force. (2016). Primary care interventions to support breastfeeding: U.S. preventive services task force recommendation statement. *Journal of the American Medical Association, 316,* 1688–1693.

Vice, F. L., Bamford, O., Heinz, J. M., & Bosma, J. F. (1995). Correlation of cervical auscultation with physiological recording during suckle-feeding in newborn infants. *Developmental Medicine and Child Neurology, 37,* 167–179.

Victora, C. G., Bahl, R., Barros, A. J., Franca, G. V., Horton, S., Krasevec, J., Murch, S., Sankar, M. J., Walker, N., Rollins, N. C., & Lancet Breastfeeding Series Group. (2016). Breastfeeding in the 21st century: Epidemiology, mechanisms, and lifelong effect. *The Lancet, 387*(10017), 475–490.

Walker, M. (2011). *Breastfeeding and employment: Making it work.* Praeclarus Press.

Walker, M. (2023). *Breastfeeding management for the clinician: Using the evidence* (5th ed.). Jones and Bartlett Learning.

Whitley, M. D., Ro, A., & Palma, & A. (2021). Work, race and breastfeeding outcomes for mothers in the United States. *PLoS One, 16*(5), e0251125. https://doi.org/10.1371/journal.pone.0251125

World Health Organization. (2016). *Consolidated guidelines on the use of antiretroviral drugs for treating and preventing HIV infection* (2nd ed.). https://apps.who.int/iris/bitstream/handle/10665/208825/9789241549684_eng.pdf?sequence=1&isAllowed=y

32

Contraception in the Postnatal Period

Katie Daily

The editors are grateful to Patricia Aikins Murphy and Leah Torres, who coauthored this chapter in the prior editions.

Relevant Terms

Behind the counter—drugs stocked behind the pharmacy counter and dispensed by a pharmacist without needing a healthcare provider's prescription or other form of compliance

Combined hormonal contraceptives—hormonal contraceptives that contain both estrogen and progestin

Emergency contraception—any contraceptive method used after sexual intercourse to prevent pregnancy; hormonal-based methods are commonly used, but the copper intrauterine device can also be used

Fertility awareness-based methods—a variety of methods that use the menstrual cycle and signs of ovulation to determine the fertile period and avoid intercourse during that time; also known as "natural family planning"

Intrauterine contraception—small device placed in the uterus to prevent pregnancy

Lactational amenorrhea method—temporary contraceptive that can be used during the first months after birth in people who are exclusively breastfeeding and meet selected other criteria

Long-acting reversible contraceptive methods—reversible contraceptive method that provides long-acting protection without requiring the user to do anything on a daily, weekly, or monthly basis; examples include intrauterine devices and contraceptive implants

Medical eligibility criteria—evidence-based guidelines about the use of contraceptives in the presence of medical conditions and risk factors for complications, as well as in normal health states such as postpartum and breastfeeding

Morning-after pill—emergency contraception containing progestin; inhibits or delays ovulation

Progestin-only pills—hormonal oral contraceptive pills that contain only progestin; also known as the "minipill"

Sterilization—permanent contraceptive method; not intended to be reversible; involves surgical alteration of the fallopian tubes or the vas deferens

Introduction

Postpartum contraception is important because the adequate spacing of pregnancies is a critical factor in improving maternal and infant health outcomes in future pregnancies. It is an opportunity to assist people in achieving their reproductive life goals and provide choices that meet their needs.

The greatest risk for low birth weight and preterm births in future pregnancies occurs when there is less than six months between birth and the next pregnancy (American College of Obstetricians and Gynecologists [ACOG], 2018). Ideally, pregnancy spacing should be 18 months for optimal maternal and child health (ACOG, 2018). A meta-analysis of adverse outcomes associated with short interpregnancy intervals showed that intervals shorter than 6 months are associated with a 30–60% increased risk of preterm birth, low birth weight, and small-for-gestational-age infants, and intervals of 18 months or less were associated with a smaller but still significant increase in the risk of adverse perinatal outcomes (Conde-Agudelo et al., 2006). An 18-month interval is particularly important for people who gave birth by cesarean section, for best outcomes and opportunities for a trial of labor after cesarean.

For those with contraceptive needs, counseling and decision-making ideally begin during early pregnancy and continue throughout prenatal care into the early postpartum period. Qualitative evidence supports frequent sessions of contraceptive counseling throughout the prenatal period, with reinforcement of counseling and family planning decisions after birth (Yee & Simon, 2011). Contraceptive choices may be influenced by method effectiveness, access, availability, convenience, cost, side effects, previous experience, partner approval, and societal norms (Dam et al., 2021). Counseling should follow the principals of

Prenatal and Postnatal Care: A Person-Centered Approach, Third Edition. Edited by Karen Trister Grace, Cindy L. Farley, Noelene K. Jeffers, and Tanya Tringali.
© 2024 John Wiley & Sons Ltd. Published 2024 by John Wiley & Sons Ltd.
Companion website: www.wiley.com/go/grace/prenatal

reproductive justice as defined by the advocacy group SisterSong as, "the human right to maintain personal bodily autonomy, have children, not have children, and parent the children we have in safe and sustainable communities" (SisterSong, n.d.). Clinicians can honor and respect individuals' choices in their reproductive health by utilizing the principles of shared decision-making and person-centered care. Autonomous decision-making in contraceptive care is paramount. Coercion may be well intentioned when providers believe the most effective method of contraception is the best method for that person, but it is essential to remember that the patient's own values, preferences, and comfort level are what determine the best contraceptive method for that person.

Values and preferences that guide contraceptive decision-making are dynamic and may change over time from immediately postpartum, to three months, six months, and onward. Prior experiences with various methods, future fertility plans, and health concerns also impact preferences (Dam et al., 2021). People who desire more children may prefer short acting methods, and people who are satisfied with their family size may prefer long-acting reversible contraception (Carr et al., 2018; Dam et al., 2021; DeSisto et al., 2018). Immediate postpartum insertion of **long-acting reversible contraceptive (LARC) methods** may be preferred by some people for convenience (Dam et al., 2021), but this factor must be balanced within a framework of reproductive justice to prevent coercion by providers (Dam et al., 2021; Harper et al., 2020). Some patients who are able to easily access LARCs in the birth setting may not have the same access to care when they are ready for removal.

Evidence-based tools and trainings are available for providers to assist in counseling families on their choices. These include the client-centered PATH questions focused on **P**arenting/pregnancy **A**ttitudes, **T**iming, and **H**ow important delaying pregnancy is for that individual. This tool covers key questions to ask, including: Do you think you want more children, when, and how important is pregnancy prevention? (Geist et al., 2019). Other tools for use in the clinical setting include the "one key question" that encourages providers to simply ask at each healthcare encounter, "Would you like to become pregnant in the next year?" (Power to Decide, 2022). The client's response guides the provider to offer preconception care, contraception, or other resources to match their needs. This simple tool allows primary care providers to address many unmet needs for families.

Transgender and nonbinary individuals who are at risk for pregnancy need access to evidence-based contraceptive counseling (Light et al., 2018). There are no contraindications for the use of contraception for those on testosterone therapy (Boudreau & Mukerjee, 2019). Providers should provide guidance to those choosing an intrauterine device (IUD) on the anticipated pelvic exams, cramping, and menses changes, as they may cause physical or psychological distress and influence one's choice in method (Boudreau & Mukerjee, 2019). Research on postpartum contraceptive methods in transgender and nonbinary people is lacking.

Health equity key points

- Access to postpartum contraception may be limited for birthing families who rely on Medicaid services to cover the cost of their care. Strategies to address these barriers include expansion of Medicaid until one-year postpartum, immediate postpartum LARC insertion, telehealth, and optimizing postpartum care with an initial visit within the first three weeks postpartum.
- Contraceptive counseling should be person-centered and follow principles of reproductive justice.
- Providers must be aware of their own biases and internalized racism when counseling clients.
- Fully informed consent for sterilization is essential; a shameful history of racist and eugenicist practices such as forced sterilization and sterilization procedures performed without consent, generally performed on groups deemed undesirable to reproduce, is documented throughout the world.

Postpartum Care and Return to Fertility after Childbirth

Optimal postpartum care is an ongoing process that includes multiple care visits tailored to each individual's need, with the first visit recommended to occur by three weeks postpartum (ACOG, 2018). This allows for ample opportunity to meet contraceptive needs according to each individual's preferences and to educate on the rationale for pregnancy spacing. The challenge is that many postpartum people do not attend their routine care visits. As many as 40% of postpartum people receive no care at all (Bennett et al., 2014). Many people (40–57%) will have resumed sexual activity, usually without utilizing a method of contraception, by the time of the traditional six-week visit, placing them at risk for an unintended and closely spaced pregnancy (ACOG, 2016b).

A common misconception of postpartum people is that they are not at risk of ovulation and unintended pregnancy in the first weeks or months after birth. The average time of return to ovulation in nonbreastfeeding people is about 6 weeks after birth, with an average mean of 45–94 days postpartum; 20–71% of first menses are preceded by ovulation (Jackson & Glasier, 2011). For those not exclusively breastfeeding, it is unpredictable when ovulation and menstruation will return. Although a certain proportion of first bleeding episodes after childbirth are anovulatory and luteal phase abnormalities occur in some early ovulatory cycles, it is not possible to predict which of the first postpartum cycles will be ovulatory and potentially fertile. Thus, healthcare providers must consider that all people who are not exclusively breastfeeding are at risk of unintended pregnancy as early as three to four weeks postpartum.

For breastfeeding people, the return of ovulation is also variable (Wang & Fraser, 1994); feeding patterns and supplementation with formula, fluids, or foods determines the risk of ovulation. It is not possible to predict when fertility and the risk of pregnancy will resume. The **lactational amenorrhea method (LAM)** of family planning is based on the contraceptive effects of breastfeeding. People who exclusively breastfeed and remain amenorrheic have a very small risk of becoming pregnant in the first six months after giving birth (Van der Wijden & Manion, 2015). Once breastfeeding is discontinued, prolactin levels decline, and ovulation can return within 14–30 days (King, 2007).

Although the return to ovulation is delayed in breastfeeding people, who on average ovulate between five and six months postpartum, variability in feeding practices means that some will ovulate earlier than five months. Therefore, contraceptive methods should be initiated earlier to provide adequate protection from an unintended pregnancy. LAM should be considered as a transitional method, best used by those who plan to exclusively breastfeed for the first six months, with plans in place to initiate additional contraception for those who desire to avoid pregnancy at that time, or if menses return or additional supplementation is started (King, 2007).

Access to Postpartum Contraception

Although studies show most postpartum women desire to avoid pregnancy in the first two years postpartum, about 70% of those women are not using contraception (Dam et al., 2021). Ambivalence toward pregnancy can lead to lower uses of contraception (LaCross et al., 2019), but this gap between stated preferences and actual use can also be attributed to multiple other factors, including issues of health equity and access to care.

For the many birthing people who rely on Medicaid services for perinatal care, access to contraceptive services in the postpartum period is limited (Rodriguez et al., 2022; Sakowicz et al., 2021; Steenland et al., 2021). Traditional Medicaid coverage lasts until 60 days postpartum, while emergency Medicaid covers only the cost of the birth. In 2020, Medicaid covered 42% of births (Kaiser Family Foundation [KFF], 2022b). A portion of the American Rescue Plan Act of 2021 allowed states the option to expand their postpartum coverage for up to one year (KFF, 2022a). This would greatly expand access to key medical services and address underlying health inequities. When barriers to access are removed, as demonstrated in the Contraceptive CHOICE Project that offered participants easy and free access to the method of their choice, LARC methods were most often selected and rates of unintended pregnancies decreased (McNicholas et al., 2014).

Another mechanism to expand access to postpartum contraception is the use of telehealth. This innovative method of providing healthcare via audio or video visits can provide opportunities for contraceptive counseling and prescribing hormonal contraceptive method for ongoing use or as a bridge to a patient's preferred placement of a LARC device. Prior to the COVID-19 pandemic, both provider-driven telehealth and nurse- or other support staff-driven telehealth interventions were shown to improve perinatal care (DeNicola et al., 2020). Since the start of the pandemic, telehealth has been widely used in the provision of postpartum care, for dispensing contraception, counseling clients to prepare for LARC insertion, and counseling prior to a nurse-led clinic visit to start depot medroxyprogesterone acetate (DMPA).

The need to initiate or refill a prescription through a provider appointment is often a barrier for patients to access their chosen method. There is a strong advocacy movement within healthcare organizations to promote over-the-counter access to benefit patients and in recognition of the general low risks of hormonal contraceptive methods (ACOG, 2019). The emergency contraceptive pill is already available without a prescription to meet this need.

The stress of new parenthood, whether for a first-time parent or a parent with other children, is well documented (Vernon et al., 2010). Lack of time, the responsibilities of caregiving, household tasks and work, lack of childcare, and other factors all contribute to challenges in remembering to take oral contraceptives on time, getting to the pharmacy for refills, and scheduling appointments with a provider for initiation of contraception.

Breastfeeding and Contraception

The choice of contraceptive method should not interfere with a person's ability to breastfeed. Breastfeeding is the optimal feeding method for infants, and it confers significant health benefits for both the lactating person and infant. Lactogenesis II, the process by which a person begins to produce copious amounts of milk, is initiated in part by the withdrawal of progesterone that occurs when the placenta is delivered. There are theoretical concerns that the early administration of hormonal, especially progestin-containing, contraceptives may impact lactogenesis II. Some clinicians may feel it is prudent to delay the administration of a large progesterone bolus (such as an injection of DMPA or the insertion of the progestin implant) until copious milk production occurs (Hatcher et al., 2018). Most research shows that the initiation of progestin-only methods in the early postpartum period does not have a negative effect on lactation, but this theoretical concern leads some clinicians and patients to choose to delay the start until six weeks postpartum, when breastfeeding is well established.

In most cases, progestin-only contraceptives can be administered in the immediate postpartum period without adverse effects on lactation and may even increase milk volume (King, 2007). Initiating **combined hormonal contraceptives (CHCs)** after six weeks postpartum has few adverse effects on lactation (Kapp & Curtis, 2010). Although some CHCs have been shown to reduce the duration of breastfeeding and diminish the quantity of milk, the evidence is limited. No adverse effects on infant growth or development have been described in children breastfed by parents taking CHCs (Tepper et al., 2016), though the theoretical risks of hormonal transfer to infants lead some to choose nonhormonal methods.

Physiologic Postpartum Changes

Contraceptive method choice must also be tailored to the normal expected physiologic changes of the puerperium. For example, the increased risk of venous thromboembolism (VTE) associated with pregnancy continues until its peak at 3 weeks postpartum and then gradually declines before returning to a prepregnancy baseline level of risk around 12 weeks postpartum (Tepper et al., 2014). Estrogen-containing contraceptives are, therefore, contraindicated for at least three weeks after birth or longer, depending on the postpartum person's risk factors for VTE (Curtis, et al., 2016).

People who have had certain perinatal complications need to be carefully evaluated prior to initiating a contraceptive method. For example, the physiological and biochemical changes associated with preeclampsia may persist for several weeks and even months postpartum (Firoz & Melnik, 2011). There are also several health conditions associated with an increased risk for adverse events as a result of unintended pregnancy for those who live with these conditions, including diabetes, hypertension, and heart disease (Curtis, et al., 2016).

Immediate Postpartum LARC Insertion

One solution to broaden access to contraception for postpartum people is to offer LARC insertion in the early postpartum period. Options for this include placing an IUD right after placental delivery (*postplacental*) or placing an IUD or implant device prior to hospital discharge (*immediate*; ACOG, 2016b; 2017; Escobar & Shearin, 2019). A recent systematic review on immediate postpartum implant placement revealed higher rates of contraception use in the early postpartum period, with a higher number of days of abnormal bleeding in the first six weeks postpartum (Sothornwit et al., 2017). Postplacental IUD insertion can be accomplished with either a manual technique after vaginal or cesarean birth or with the assistance of ring forceps after a vaginal birth; placement within ten minutes of placental delivery is ideal (ACOG, 2016b; Lopez et al., 2015b). This technique requires specialized training, which may be accessed through ACOG's Postpartum Contraceptive Access Initiative (PCAI; see *Resources for Clients and Healthcare Providers* for more information). In addition to standard IUD contraindications, early postpartum IUD insertion is also contraindicated in cases of hemorrhage, intraamniotic infection, endometritis, and sepsis (ACOG, 2016b). Postplacental insertion is associated with higher rates of expulsion compared to delayed insertion (four or more weeks after childbirth), ranging from 10% to 27% (ACOG, 2016b). One study of the levonorgestrel device showed a 24% expulsion rate in the postplacental insertion group, compared to 4.4% in the delayed insertion group (Chen et al., 2010). It is important to note that delay in placing the device, though having a reduced risk of expulsion, may impose an additional barrier to the person having it placed at all.

People are at a higher risk of not receiving the device when asked to return for delayed placement. The social circumstances of a new parent must, therefore, be considered, and the risks and benefits of early versus delayed insertion must be discussed. Thorough counseling and shared decision-making are required in determining the most appropriate insertion timing for each individual.

The benefits of immediate LARC insertion include higher rates of contraceptive continuation, decreased rates of short birth intervals, provision of contraception to those who lose access to healthcare in the early postpartum period, and cost effectiveness (ACOG, 2016b; Escobar & Shearin, 2019). Counseling should begin during prenatal care to review the risks and benefits of immediate insertion. Barriers to immediate insertion include lack of provider training and reimbursement challenges. Additionally, providers must recognize their own potential biases that may lead them to give coercive counseling to people of color, encouraging them to use a LARC method that may not fit their personal preferences or values (Escobar & Shearin, 2019).

Medical eligibility criteria (MEC) for contraceptive use have been developed by the World Health Organization (WHO) and are periodically updated by expert groups. The criteria were established to assist individual countries in the development of guidelines specific to their populations and health systems. The Centers for Disease Control and Prevention (CDC) developed recommendations for US healthcare providers to base contraceptive management on the best available evidence and to reduce medical barriers to contraceptive use. All of the contraceptive methods reviewed in the document include recommendations for postpartum and breastfeeding people as well as an extensive array of health conditions. The document can be used to determine whether a particular contraceptive can be used by a person with a medical condition such as diabetes or a health behavior such as smoking. The recommendations for contraceptive use are grouped into four categories known as the MEC categories. These categories are described in Table 32.1.

Healthcare providers need to be aware of all contraceptive methods and the recommendations for their use in the postpartum period in order to assist people in making appropriate reproductive health choices.

Contraceptive Methods

Counseling on contraceptive methods includes starting with the most effective methods and moving down to the least effective with the caveat that contraceptive effectiveness will depend on the ability of the person to use the method correctly and consistently, their preferences, and other influences. Autonomous contraceptive decision-making is paramount (Senderowicz, 2020). The effectiveness of contemporary contraceptive methods is usually described by reporting the percentage of people who will experience a pregnancy during the first year of "perfect" or "typical" use. Perfect use refers to correct and

Table 32.1   MEC Categories for Contraceptive Use

Category	Overall recommendation	Recommendation for a specific medical condition or health behavior
1	Use method in any circumstance	No restriction
2	Generally use the method	Advantages generally outweigh the theoretical or proven risks
3	Use of method not recommended unless more appropriate methods are not available or acceptable	Theoretical or proven risks usually outweigh advantages
4	Do not use method	Unacceptable health risk

Source: Adapted from Curtis et al. (2016).

Table 32.2   Contraceptive Methods Grouped by Level of Effectiveness

Level	Effectiveness	Contraceptive methods
Tier 1	Most effective methods; failure rates are less than 1 pregnancy per 100 people per year	Sterilization Intrauterine contraception Implant contraception
Tier 2	Very effective methods; failure rates are 6–12 pregnancies per 100 people per year	Injectable contraception Contraceptive patch Contraceptive ring Contraceptive pills
Tier 3	Less effective methods; failure rates are 12 or more pregnancies per 100 people per year	External condom Diaphragm Internal condom Fertility awareness-based methods Withdrawal Spermicides

Source: Adapted from Hatcher et al. (2018).

consistent contraceptive use at all times; typical use refers to actual use that includes incorrect and inconsistent use of a method. Typical use effectiveness rates have more relevance to actual risk of unintended pregnancy. Methods are grouped according to their estimated effectiveness in preventing pregnancy, from less effective (about 30 pregnancies per 100 people per year) to most effective (less than 1 pregnancy per 100 people per year) (see Table 32.2).

Providers may consider using patient-friendly education tools to assist counseling that categorize methods by effectiveness. One easy-to-use tool is included here and is available in multiple languages (Figure 32.1).

Tier 1 Methods

Tier 1 contraceptives are the most effective methods for preventing pregnancy. Failure rates are typically much less than 1 pregnancy per 100 people per year. The methods in this tier are less susceptible to user error, and once initiated, they provide contraceptive protection for long periods of time without the need for daily maintenance. You can "set it and forget it" in the words of marketing personality and inventor Ron Popeil (Gladwell, 2000, p. 65).

Long-term coverage without daily maintenance may be useful for those in the early postpartum period with multiple demands from family, missed sleep, and returning to work. An additional benefit, with the exception of vasectomy, is that the use of tier 1 methods is not partner-dependent, and they are also less detectable by partners. This may be an advantage for people with abusive or coercive partners who may seek to interfere with contraceptive methods (see Chapter 26, *Violence and Trauma in the Perinatal Period*).

Long-Acting Reversible Contraceptive Methods

LARC methods are as effective as permanent **sterilization** in preventing pregnancy. An advantage of LARC methods is that once placed, the methods require little attention: there are no frequent provider visits or prescription refills to manage, the method is not coitus dependent, and the user does not need to remember daily, weekly, or monthly ingestion, insertion, or reapplication. Fertility returns rapidly once the device is removed. There are both non-hormonal and hormonal options. LARCs can be used in the early postpartum period and do not interfere with breastfeeding. The disadvantages include lack of autonomy to remove the device when desired, discomfort during placement, and potential complications during placement or removal. Some devices also cause bleeding pattern changes, which may increase or decrease acceptability.

Intrauterine contraception (IUC) involves the placement of a small T-shaped device in the uterus to prevent pregnancy. There are two types of IUDs available in the United States. The nonhormonal Copper T 380A (brand name ParaGard`) and the hormonal levonorgestrel intrauterine systems (LNG IUS, brand names Mirena®, Kyleena™, Skyla®, Liletta®). A healthcare provider inserts an IUD during an office visit, providing the additional advantage of avoiding the risks and costs of surgery. Each type of IUD has a string that passes from the uterus and protrudes through the cervix to facilitate removal as well as provide a palpable and visible clue that the device is still in the uterus.

The *copper IUD* is approved for 10 years of contraceptive use, although research suggests it may be effective for 12 years or longer, and some providers counsel patients about the option of prolonged use (Bahamondes

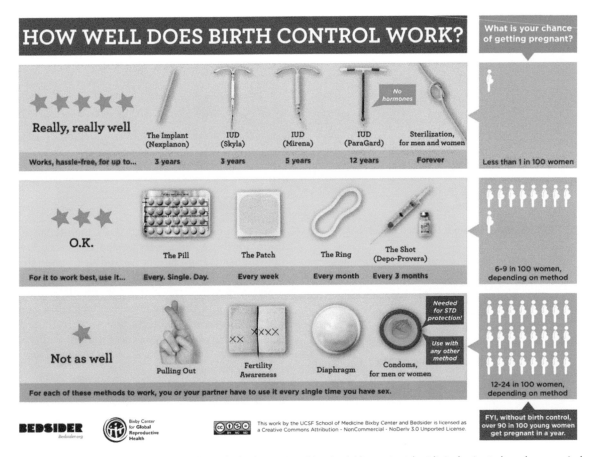

Figure 32.1 How well does birth control work? Bedsider https://providers.bedsider.org/articles/clinical-minute-how-long-are-iuds-and-implants-effective.

et al., 2005; Sivin, 2007). Once placed, the device produces a sterile inflammatory response within the uterus that creates a hostile environment for sperm, preventing the fertilization of the egg. The copper device is effective almost immediately after insertion: indeed, it is used for **emergency contraception (EC)** up to five days after unprotected intercourse and has a failure rate between 0.5% and 1% in the first year (Kulier et al., 2007; Meirik et al., 2009). Cumulative pregnancy rates at 7 years and 8–12 years are 1.4–1.6% and 2.2%, respectively (Hatcher et al., 2018). The copper device is associated with an increased amount and duration of bleeding during menses (up to 55%), as well as increased dysmenorrhea during the first several menstrual cycles (Hatcher et al., 2018). These are the most common reasons for the removal of the device in the first year. However, these symptoms are often relieved with the use of nonsteroidal anti-inflammatory drugs (NSAIDs), and the heavier menses rarely leads to anemia. People using this method should be counseled regarding these potential side effects.

The *levonorgestrel IUDs* are equally effective for pregnancy prevention, but differ in their mechanism of action, length of use, and side effects from the nonhormonal IUD. Once placed, the device releases a small amount of levonorgestrel into the uterus, producing a thickening of cervical mucus that inhibits sperm motility and function. The steady local hormone effect also produces

endometrial atrophy and tubal immobility that prevents transport of the ovum through the tube. Due to the steady systemic absorption of levonorgestrel, ovulation is often inhibited as well. These combined mechanisms effectively prevent fertilization. The levonorgestrel device is presumed to be effective approximately seven days after placement. Currently, there is insufficient evidence to support its use for EC; however, new evidence is emerging supporting its use (Turok et al., 2021). The failure rate of the Mirena in the first year of use is between 0.1% and 0.2%, while at five years of continuous use, the cumulative pregnancy rate is 0.5–1.1% (Hatcher et al., 2018). The failure rate does not appear to increase at seven years of use (Hatcher et al., 2018). In contrast to the increased bleeding that can occur with the copper IUD, the levonorgestrel device is associated with a marked decrease in menstrual blood flow as it thins the lining of the uterus. An additional benefit of these devices, though the mechanism is unclear, is the treatment of endometriosis (Gibbons et al., 2021; Tanmahasamut et al., 2012).

Both the Mirena and Liletta have a 52-mg LNG drug reservoir within a T-shaped polyethylene frame to provide slow and gradual hormonal release. Mirena is US Food and Drug Administration (FDA) approved for up to seven years of use for contraception, and five years for control of heavy menses, while Liletta is approved for up to six years for contraception (Actavis & Medicines360, 2019; Bayer

HealthCare Pharmaceuticals, 2021). The Liletta device is a lower cost hormonal IUD created by nonprofit Medicines360 in 2015 to expand access and is available to public health clinics at approximately one third of the price of the Mirena device (Actavis & Medicines360, 2019). While Liletta is not yet FDA approved for heavy menses, it has been used in clinical practice with success, and the device is in clinical trials to gain FDA approval for its use for this noncontraceptive benefit (Creinin & Uhm, 2020). Kyleena offers a lower dose of LNG (19.5 mg) for use up to five years, while the Skyla offers a smaller size and lower hormonal dose (13.5 mg) for use up to three years and is marketed for use in nulliparous people and adolescents (Teal & Edelman, 2021).

There are few absolute contraindications to the use of IUCs: active pelvic infection, cervical or endometrial cancer, and current breast cancer for the levonorgestrel devices, anomalies of the reproductive tract, gestational trophoblastic disease, pelvic tuberculosis, and copper allergy or Wilson's disease for the copper device. Nulliparity, infection with human immunodeficiency virus (HIV), immunocompromise, and adolescent age are *not* contraindications to the use of IUC and are, arguably, characteristics of populations that may have greater interest in effective methods to prevent unplanned pregnancy. The CDC supports the insertion of IUDs with screening for sexually transmitted infections (STIs) at the time of insertion, and if positive, patients are able to continue their IUC with proper STI treatment (Curtis et al., 2016).

There are some preexisting medical conditions that warrant caution with the use of IUC (MEC category 3), but the more common cautions and complications involve the risks of infection, expulsion, and uterine perforation. These complications are uncommon but warrant attention, particularly for postpartum people. The infection risk associated with IUC is low, primarily associated with insertion, and is often due to an undetected STI at the time of insertion. A postpartum person who has had puerperal sepsis or endometritis after childbirth should not have the device inserted until the infection is completely resolved. Once inserted, the device does not have to be removed should an infection develop, unless the infection is unresponsive to therapy.

Expulsion of the device is uncommon (2–10% within the first year) but can occur and is more common when inserted shortly after childbirth (ACOG, 2016a). Perforation of the uterus is uncommon with IUD insertion, occurring in 1 per 1000 insertions or less (Hatcher et al., 2018). Concerns that perforations are increased in postpartum breastfeeding people are not supported by data, and the MEC categories for insertion of an IUD are the same regardless of breastfeeding status (Curtis et al., 2016).

There are no known adverse effects of IUC on breastfeeding in users of either the copper or the levonorgestrel devices. There is no evidence of increased copper concentration in the human milk of users of copper devices. Transfer of progestin from milk to the infant is low among those who use a levonorgestrel contraceptive system (Hatcher et al., 2018). Common side effects of increased cramping and irregular menses may be managed expectantly or with a short-term trial of NSAIDs (ACOG, 2016a). If there is ongoing cramping or heavy bleeding more than three months after placement, consider evaluation for IUD expulsion, malposition, pregnancy, or cervical dysplasia.

The IUC device itself and the cost of a provider visit for insertion is covered by third-party insurance due to federal policy mandate of the Affordable Care Act. Over time, IUCs are one of the least expensive methods because of the potential length of contraceptive protection. However, the entire cost is paid at the initiation of the method, and for those without healthcare coverage, it may be prohibitive. Fortunately, there are many federally qualified health centers and Title X funded clinics that offer these methods on a sliding fee scale for those without insurance.

Implant contraception involves the placement of a subdermal capsule on the inner side of the nondominant upper arm. Once placed, the device can be palpated but is usually not visible. Nexplanon° is currently the only implant available in the United States. It is a single flexible rod about 4 cm in length and 2 mm in diameter that releases etonogestrel, a synthetic progestin, at a steady rate. Prior implant devices included multiple rods, and providers may still encounter these devices, particularly in patients who immigrated to the United States who desire removals.

The steady release of etonogestrel from the implant suppresses ovulation and provides effective contraception for at least three years. Some providers now recommend off-label use up to five years due to recent clinical research showing effectiveness for prolonged use (Ali et al., 2016; McNicholas et al., 2017; Thaxton & Lavelanet, 2018). Formal clinical trials for FDA approval for this five-year interval are still in progress (Ali et al., 2016; McNicholas et al., 2017). The implant must be inserted and removed by a trained healthcare provider, which can limit access. The method is effective immediately after insertion if inserted within the first five days of their menstrual cycle. The failure rate is less than 1 per 1000, and fertility returns rapidly after discontinuation.

Menstrual cycle irregularities are the most commonly reported side effects of the implant method. Irregular bleeding is a primary reason for discontinuing the method. Management can be expectant by providing education on common bleeding patterns and reminding patients that improvements are expected after several months of use, or in some cases, with the addition of low-dose combined oral contraceptives (COCs) or a trial of Ibuprofen 400–800 mg three times a day for 5–10 days to control breakthrough bleeding (ACOG, 2016a). There are no clinically significant metabolic changes noted in users of the device.

Because the implant only contains progestin, it is a good choice for people who cannot use estrogen. It should not be placed in people experiencing unexplained abnormal uterine bleeding. The only absolute contraindication to implant use is current breast cancer. It is considered MEC category 3 for initiation in people with multiple cardiovascular risk factors and chronic medical conditions such as liver disease.

Like other tier 1 contraceptive methods, the implant requires little attention, an advantage in the stressful, even chaotic, postpartum adjustment period. The changes in menstrual bleeding may be more or less acceptable to some people. The device and the cost of a provider visit for insertion may or may not be covered by third-party insurance. The implant can also be one of the least expensive contraceptive choices because of the potential length of time that contraceptive protection lasts, but as with IUCs, the entire cost is paid at the initiation of the method and, thus, may be prohibitive for some people without private insurance or access to low-cost federally funded contraception.

Permanent Methods

Sterilization is the most commonly used contraceptive method in the world. It is intended to be permanent (despite occasional failures) and not reversible (despite the existence of a reversal procedure). Thus, counseling about the permanency of sterilization is critical to ensuring that the actual sterilization procedure is well understood and that people who choose this method have no further pregnancy plans. Individuals or couples who are not sure whether they have completed their families may prefer the option of using LARCs that are as effective as sterilization, and more accessible to most people through provision at Title X funded and other sites.

Tubal sterilization involves the excision or occlusion of the fallopian tubes. For most procedures, it is effective immediately, and failure rates in the first year after sterilization are less than 1%. Failures do occur, though, and are related to the procedure type, the skill of the surgeon, and the anatomical characteristics of the person being sterilized. Over a 10-year period, the cumulative failure rate for tubal sterilization is about 1.85%, ranging from less than 1% when performed as a postpartum tubal excision to over 2% when bipolar coagulation methods are used. People who experience failure of a tubal sterilization and become pregnant are more likely to have an ectopic pregnancy. Healthcare providers must be aware of this risk in any person presenting with pregnancy who has previously undergone tubal sterilization.

Tubal occlusion can be accomplished abdominally by laparotomy and laparoscopy or transcervically. Procedures include electrosurgical methods (which coagulate the tube), use of clips or rings, sclerosing agents to mechanically occlude the tube, or the surgical excision of portions of the tube. Transcervical insertion of metal coils into the fallopian tubes was previously available, but the device used in this procedure has been discontinued. Surgeons will recommend a method based on patient physical factors and with shared decision-making with the patient.

Tubal sterilization can be accomplished immediately after a cesarean or a vaginal birth (before leaving the hospital), or as an interval procedure after the postpartum recovery period. There is no evidence of associated major risk or adverse effects on postpartum recovery or lactation from having the procedure performed shortly after birth, other than the usual risks associated with anesthesia and surgery.

The younger a person is when they undergo permanent sterilization, the more likely they are to regret the decision later (Danvers & Evans, 2022). Yet contraceptive autonomy is important for people of all reproductive ages, and sterilization should not be withheld based on a person's age. Surgical reanastamosis of the tubes to reverse the procedure can be attempted, but its success is dependent on the type of procedure and the amount of tube that has been damaged. Counseling should address these issues in addition to those surrounding the risks and benefits of the procedure. Cost is also an important consideration since third-party insurers may not cover this procedure, interval outpatient procedures may be less expensive than in-hospital procedures, some procedures require additional follow-up testing that is costly (e.g., hysterosalpingogram for transcervical procedures), and there may be varying access to publicly funded or subsidized procedures for people without insurance or financial means.

Some types of coverage (particularly federally supported insurance programs) have strict rules about the timing of consent and counseling that must be followed for coverage to be secured. Typically, consent must be signed and dated at least 30 days prior to the procedure and readily available for review while the patient is in the hospital. The importance of fully informed consent for sterilization cannot be overstated. A shameful history of racist and eugenicist practices such as forced sterilization and sterilization procedures performed without consent, generally performed on groups deemed undesirable to reproduce, is documented throughout the world (Patel, 2017).

Vasectomy is also an option some couples consider. Vasectomy involves the ligation/excision or cautery of the vas deferens and is considered a permanent sterilization method. It is associated with lower risk, lower cost, and a lower failure rate than tubal sterilization methods (Jamieson et al., 2004; Sokal & Labrecque, 2009). The outpatient procedure commonly uses a "no scalpel" technique that is associated with relatively minor discomfort and bruising. The use of another form of contraception is essential until the person has a negative sperm count, which takes at least three months (Sokal & Labrecque, 2009).

Tier 2 Methods

Methods in this category are very effective in preventing pregnancy, are patient-controlled (as opposed to partner-controlled), but are more susceptible to user error in typical use. Typical use accounts for human error such as forgetting to take a daily pill, forgetting to replace a contraceptive patch or ring, missing an appointment for a repeat injection, or not closely following the criteria for effective use of the LAM. These errors can be common in

Turok, D. K., Gero, A., Simmons, R. G., Kaiser, J. E., Stoddard, G. J., Sexsmith, C. D., Gawron, L. M., & Sanders, J. N. (2021). Levonorgestrel vs. copper intrauterine devices for emergency contraception. *New England Journal of Medicine*, *384*(4), 335–344. https://doi.org/10.1056/nejmoa2022141

Upadhyay, U. D., Zlidar, V. M., & Foster, D. G. (2016). Interest in self-administration of subcutaneous depot medroxyprogesterone acetate in the United States. *Contraception*, *94*(4), 303–313.

Van der Wijden, C., & Manion, C. (2015). Lactational amenorrhoea method for family planning. *Cochrane Database of Systematic Reviews*, (10), CD001329. https://www.cochranelibrary.com/cdsr/doi/10.1002/14651858.CD001329.pub2/full

Vernon, M. M., Young-Hyman, D., & Looney, S. W. (2010). Maternal stress, physical activity, and body mass index during new mothers' first year postpartum. *Women & Health*, *50*(6), 544–562.

Wang, I. Y., & Fraser, I. S. (1994). Reproductive function and contraception in the postpartum period. *Obstetrical & Gynecological Survey*, *49*(1), 56–63.

World Health Organization. (2007). *Technical consultation on the effects of hormonal contraception on bone health*. http://whqlibdoc.who.int/hq/2007/WHO_RHR_07.08_eng.pdf?ua=1.

Yee, L., & Simon, M. (2011). Urban minority women's perceptions of and preferences for postpartum contraceptive counseling. *Journal of Midwifery & Women's Health*, *56*(1), 54–60.

Zapata, L. B., Steenland, M. W., Brahmi, D., Marchbanks, P. A., & Curtis, K. M. (2013). Effect of missed combined hormonal contraceptives on contraceptive effectiveness: A systematic review. *Contraception*, *87*, 685–700.

Part III

Complex Prenatal and Postnatal Conditions

33

Bleeding during Pregnancy

Sascha James-Conterelli

The editors gratefully acknowledge Robin G. Jordan, who authored the previous edition of this chapter.

Relevant Terms

Biochemical pregnancy—fertilization of egg and sperm that produces measurable human chorionic gonadotropin but does not develop far enough to be visualized by ultrasound

Cervical motion tenderness—an unpleasant sensation elicited by moving the cervix side to side with gloved examining fingers; a possible sign of ectopic pregnancy

Choriocarcinoma—a malignant form of gestational trophoblastic disease

Couvelaire uterus—a condition in which blood invades the uterine musculature; can occur with placental abruption

Early pregnancy loss—loss of an intrauterine pregnancy in the first trimester of pregnancy; also called miscarriage or spontaneous abortion

Ectopic pregnancy—a fertilized ovum that has implanted outside of the uterine endometrium

Gestational trophoblastic disease (GTD)—a spectrum of rare disease conditions in which placental trophoblasts develop into tumors, ranging from benign to malignant

Hydatidiform mole—a condition of varying degrees of abnormal trophoblastic proliferation of tissue with an absent embryo (complete mole) or some fetal or embryonic tissue (partial mole)

Kleihauer–Betke test—a maternal blood test that measures the amount of fetal hemoglobin transferred from the fetus to the maternal bloodstream to quantify fetal-maternal hemorrhage

Leiomyoma—benign uterine tumor, also known as fibroid

Luteal phase deficiency—a clinical diagnosis associated with an abnormal luteal phase length of ≤10 days (alternate acceptable definitions include ≤11 or ≤9 days); a potential cause of infertility that may be caused by low progesterone or endometrium not responding adequately to progesterone to support fertilized ovum

Pelvic rest—a general term denoting avoidance of sexual activity (intercourse, orgasm, and vaginal penetration with finger or object), tampons, and douching.

Placental abruption—premature separation of the placenta from the uterine wall prior to birth

Placenta accreta—pathologic placental attachment to the myometrium due to trophoblastic invasion beyond the decidua basalis

Placenta increta—deep myometrial invasion of the trophoblastic villi

Placenta percreta—deepest myometrial invasion of the trophoblastic villi through the myometrium, uterine serosa, and possibly internal organs

Placenta previa—a placenta implanted at the margin of or over the cervical os

Placental-site trophoblastic tumor—arising from cells that form the placenta, rare, slow growing benign for GTD

Recurrent pregnancy loss—two or more pregnancy losses prior to 20 weeks of gestation

Subchorionic hemorrhage—separation of the chorion from uterine lining resulting in a collection of blood between the uterine wall and the chorionic membrane

Succenturiate lobed placenta—placenta with one or more accessory lobes located at a distance from the edge of the main lobe, usually much smaller than the largest lobe, often with of infarcts or atrophy

Trophotropism—the phenomenon of dynamic placental migration at its insertion throughout gestation

Vasa previa—a placental condition in which the fetal vessels run through the amniotic membranes and over the cervix, unprotected by the umbilical cord or placental tissue

Prenatal and Postnatal Care: A Person-Centered Approach, Third Edition. Edited by Karen Trister Grace, Cindy L. Farley, Noelene K. Jeffers, and Tanya Tringali.
© 2024 John Wiley & Sons Ltd. Published 2024 by John Wiley & Sons Ltd.
Companion website: www.wiley.com/go/grace/prenatal

Introduction

Approximately 14–20% of pregnant people will experience vaginal bleeding at some time during pregnancy (Liu et al., 2021). This can range from mild without serious consequences to severe and can result in morbidity and mortality. Regardless of severity, vaginal bleeding during pregnancy can be very frightening to the individual and family and should be carefully and thoroughly evaluated. This chapter will explore the etiologies, presentation, assessment, and treatments of vaginal bleeding throughout the course of pregnancy and is organized by time period in pregnancy when they usually occur. Vaginal bleeding outside of pregnancy is beyond the scope of this text.

Health equity key points

- Uterine fibroids are more common in Black women; the intersectionality of racism and gender oppression may be contributing factors.
- Women with disabilities experience higher odds of experiencing miscarriage than women without disabilities. Additional research is necessary to understand this disparity, but potential contributors might include life stressors, exposure to discrimination and adversity across the life course, and increased exposure to preconception risk factors.

Early Pregnancy Bleeding

Bleeding during the first trimester of pregnancy occurs in approximately 15–25% of pregnant people (American College of Obstetricians and Gynecologists [ACOG], 2021c; Hendriks et al., 2019). The etiology is often unknown, and the diagnostic process is one of exclusion, with the completion of a thorough history and physical examination. Bleeding without cramping that occurs after intercourse or around the time of the first missed menses can usually be attributed to physiologic causes such as implantation (Table 33.1; Pontius & Vieth, 2019). Light bleeding episodes, especially those without pain and lasting only a day or two, do not increase the risk of an **early pregnancy loss** above the baseline risk of 15% for all pregnancies (Quenby et al., 2021). The bleeding from nonpathological etiologies typically is of small volume and subsides within hours (Pontius & Vieth, 2019). Some people will experience significant bleeding in early pregnancy. The most common

pathologic reasons for bleeding in the first half of pregnancy are early pregnancy loss and **ectopic pregnancy** (Hendriks et al., 2019).

Differential Diagnosis for Bleeding in the First Half of Pregnancy

Ectopic pregnancy is the most concerning cause of early pregnancy bleeding and must be considered as a differential diagnosis. An empty uterus found on ultrasound examination may signal a **biochemical pregnancy** or complete early pregnancy loss, but this diagnosis is not definitive until ectopic pregnancy is excluded.

Potential etiologies of bleeding in the first half of pregnancy

Ectopic pregnancy
Implantation bleeding
Spontaneous pregnancy loss
Leiomyomas
Molar pregnancy
Subchorionic hemorrhage
Vaginal trauma
Infection

Evaluation

Timing, amount of vaginal bleeding, and visualization of the cervix are essential data to discriminate between normal and abnormal etiology. It is critical to recognize an early ectopic pregnancy before tubal rupture occurs. A systematic approach to evaluating the source of the vaginal bleeding allows for the development of an appropriate and efficient management plan.

Essential data to gather when assessing a client with early pregnancy vaginal bleeding

- Is the client hemodynamically stable?
- Is fever present?
- Is the bleeding intrauterine or extrauterine?
- Is the pregnancy intrauterine or ectopic?
- Is the pregnancy viable?

Table 33.1 Benign Causes of Bleeding in Early Pregnancy

Potential etiologie	Physiology	Comments
Implantation spotting	Blastocyst implants into the endometrium 6–11 days after conception.	Lasts one to several days, small amount, bright red to darker in color.
Cervical polyps	Benign tumor on the surface of the cervical canal, bleeding caused by inflammation or vasocongestion.	More common in parous people, dark or bright red color. Often intermittent spotting.
Postcoital spotting	Increase in pelvic blood flow causes cervix to become engorged and friable or can be attributed to infection.	Bleeding may also occur after pelvic exam or Pap smear.

Focused History

A detailed menstrual, gynecologic, and obstetric history is key in evaluating a client presenting with vaginal bleeding during pregnancy. It is also important to assess the person's desired plan for the current pregnancy. The date of the last known menstrual period is ascertained to estimate gestational age along with data from any ultrasounds done for pregnancy dating. Ask about bleeding severity, amount, location, and severity of pain or cramping to assess acuity. The client may be able to quantify the number of sanitary pads used over a specified time and the amount that each pad is soaked. This estimate can be helpful as soaking a pad in less than an hour suggests significant bleeding that requires prompt attention. The presence of clots can also indicate heavy bleeding. Associated symptoms such as shoulder pain, feeling faint, and vomiting are also important to assess. History is reviewed for risk factors for various etiologies of pregnancy bleeding such as previous ectopic or molar pregnancy, prior early pregnancy loss, history of vaginal infections (such as *Chlamydia trachomatis,* human papilloma virus, and *Neisseria gonorrhoeae*), uterine fibroids, or current use of an intrauterine device.

The present pregnancy history is obtained, including the presence and onset of early pregnancy signs such as breast tenderness, date of pregnancy diagnosis, any illness, fever, or substance exposures since pregnancy. When inquiring about personal habits, sexual history, medication use, substance use, and environmental exposures, sensitivity in tone and demeanor is essential. Some clients experiencing a spontaneous pregnancy loss search their past actions diligently to find an explanation and may experience needless guilt over causing the loss (Kendig et al., 2017).

Physical Exam

Vital signs including blood pressure, pulse, and temperature are obtained. The abdomen is palpated for adnexal masses or tenderness. Auscultation of fetal heart tones by Doppler is attempted if the last normal menses was at least 10 weeks prior. During the speculum examination, external tissues are observed for nonobstetric causes of bleeding such as trauma, infection, and nonvaginal bleeding from external or internal hemorrhoids. The cervix is examined for signs of infection, discharge, polyps, friability, active bleeding, tissue at the os, and dilation. Any tissue found in the vaginal vault or removed from the cervical os can be sent to pathology to determine the presence of chorionic villi, which verifies an intrauterine pregnancy. Bimanual pelvic examination is done to assess uterine size, shape, and **cervical motion tenderness**. Pain or discomfort during this procedure can be significant with an ectopic pregnancy. Assessment of the adnexa is made for masses and tenderness.

Laboratory Evaluation

The determination of serial beta-human chorionic gonadotropin (ßhCG) can augment interpretation of ultrasound findings and differentiate between normal and abnormal pregnancy conditions. Serial ßhCG is obtained in a suspected ectopic pregnancy or if viability of the fetus is in question. The level of ßhCG in a normally progressing pregnancy doubles every 2–3 days from the time of blastocyst formation, peaks at 8–10 weeks, and then declines starting at 10–12 weeks of gestation to a nadir at 16 weeks of gestation (Table 33.2). For clients who are experiencing more than minimal bleeding, a complete blood count (CBC) with differential, and blood type and screen with possible crossmatch is also done.

Diagnostic Testing

The rapid availability of ultrasonography has allowed for more individualized management of first-trimester bleeding. A combination of transabdominal and transvaginal ultrasound may be used.

Subchorionic Hemorrhage

Subchorionic hemorrhage (also called subchorionic hematoma) is defined as bleeding due to the separation of the chorion from the uterine lining. This results in a collection of blood between the uterine wall and the chorionic membrane (retroplacental clot). Painless spotting or bleeding is a common sign of subchorionic hemorrhage; however, many are detected as an incidental

Table 33.2 Discriminatory Levels for Beta-human Chorionic Gonadotropin

Parameter	Ultrasound detection[a] (approximate weeks of gestation)	Quantitative ßhCG (mIU/mL)
Gestational sac detection	Detectable at 4.5 weeks when mean diameter is 2–3 mm	Detectable on TVUS at 1000 mIU/mL, detectable on abdominal ultrasound at 1800 mIU/mL
Yolk sac identification	5 weeks at 5–6 mm	1000–7200
Fetal pole identification	5–7 weeks	7200–10800
Cardiac activity detection	6–7 weeks	>10,800

Source: Adapted from Hendriks et al. (2019).
TVUS: transvaginal ultrasound.
[a] Individual institutions may have varying guidelines for ultrasound parameters.

finding during a routine ultrasound without any signs or symptoms noted by the pregnant person.

When there is evidence on ultrasound of a subchorionic hemorrhage, the outcome depends on the size of the hemorrhage and fetal gestational age. Pregnancy outcomes are typically favorable when bleeding is earlier in pregnancy since the hemorrhage usually regresses and is often small in size. Most subchorionic hemorrhages resolve on their own by 20 weeks of gestation via reabsorption. Prognosis tends to be poorer when bleeding occurs late first trimester or early second trimester as the amount of bleeding and the size of the retroplacental clot is generally larger. Subchorionic hemorrhage may cause intermittent bleeding periodically throughout pregnancy. The typical management of subchorionic hemorrhage is **pelvic rest** for several weeks and reassurance that this condition usually resolves spontaneously.

Leiomyomas

Leiomyomas, commonly called uterine fibroids, are benign smooth muscle tumors that are found in approximately 11% of pregnant people (Coutinho et al., 2021) and can cause vaginal bleeding during pregnancy. These are more common with increasing age and in people of color, specifically Black people (Mukherjee et al., 2013). Black women are three times more likely to have uterine fibroids than White women (Henshaw et al., 2022). Also, uterine fibroids tend to have faster growth rates in Black women than White women (Henshaw et al., 2022). As race is a social rather than biological construct, genetics are not a contributing factor to the increased prevalence of leiomyomas in Black people; however, the underlying cause remains unclear. The intersectionality of racism and gender oppression as contributing factors to physiologic changes and gene expression may provide more insight (Zota & VanNoy, 2021). Fibroids can grow under the influence of pregnancy hormones, or they may decrease in size or remain unchanged. There are several types of fibroids, classified by location within the myometrium (Figure 33.1). Most pregnant people with fibroids will be asymptomatic, but bleeding can occur when an intramural fibroid twists on its stalk or the placenta implants over a fibroid. Pregnant persons with uterine fibroids have an increased risk of spontaneous pregnancy loss compared to those without fibroids (Coutinho et al., 2021).

Spontaneous Pregnancy Loss

Spontaneous pregnancy loss is the most common early pregnancy complication and is defined in several ways. According to the ACOG, early pregnancy loss is an intrauterine sac that contains a nonviable embryo or fetus prior to 12 6/7 weeks gestation (ACOG, 2021c). Several terms are used to describe early spontaneous pregnancy loss: *miscarriage* is the commonly used lay term and *spontaneous abortion* is the medical term for early pregnancy loss. There is no consensus on terminology for pregnancy loss prior to viability in the literature. The European Society of Human Reproduction and

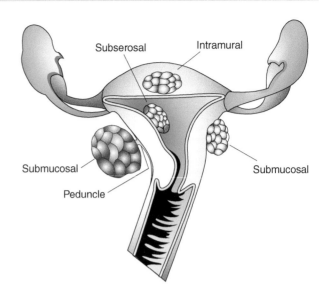

Figure 33.1 Leiomyomas: Intramural—most common, develop within the uterine wall; subserosal—develop on the outside wall of the uterus and grow outward; submucosal—least common, develop on the inside wall of the uterine cavity and grow inward. Source: Adapted from http://www.nichd.nih.gov/health/topics/uterine/conditioninfo/Pages/default.aspx, National Institute of Child Health and Development.

Embryology (ESHRE) early pregnancy loss interest group has developed recommendations for consistent terminology and definitions by characterizing the pregnancy loss according to the fetal stage of development and clinical findings (Kolte et al., 2014). They recommend using the term *early pregnancy loss* for pregnancy failure up to 10 weeks of gestation at the completion of organogenesis and *fetal miscarriage* for losses after 10 weeks of gestation. In contrast, the ACOG notes a time frame of early pregnancy loss up to 13 weeks of gestation. For the remainder of this chapter, we will use ACOG's recommended term, *early pregnancy loss*. The various types of early pregnancy loss according to characteristics, clinical presentation, and commonly used terms are presented in Table 33.3.

Determining precise incidence is challenging since an early pregnancy loss may occur before a person is aware of the pregnancy. It is often due to a biochemical pregnancy, which can produce enough ßhCG to induce a positive home pregnancy test, yet continues no further than four to five weeks post-last menstrual period (LMP). The resulting vaginal bleeding can easily be interpreted as a late menstrual period. However, it is estimated that approximately 15% of clinically recognized pregnancies end in a loss (Quenby et al., 2021). The peak incidence of early pregnancy loss is between five and eight weeks of gestation with 80% occurring within the first trimester (ACOG, 2021c).

Although the etiology of first-trimester loss can be multifactorial and often unknown, it is estimated that 50% of losses are due to chromosomal abnormalities (ACOG, 2021c). Certain risk factors increase the likelihood of pregnancy loss; advanced age of the pregnant person and the number of prior early pregnancy losses are two independent risk factors.

Table 33.3 Classification of Early Pregnancy Loss

Diagnosis	Characteristics and presentation
Complete pregnancy loss (complete abortion)	Heavy cramping, bleeding, and passage of clots and/or tissue followed by an abrupt decrease in pain and bleeding. Complete passage of products of conception Cervix closed Uterus small May see blood in vaginal vault
Incomplete pregnancy loss (threatened abortion, inevitable abortion)	Cramping may be intense; bleeding may be heavy. Partial passage of products of conception Cervix open or closed
Delayed pregnancy loss (missed/delayed abortion)	Cervix closed The uterus may be small or appropriate for gestational age. Amenorrhea many be the only symptom; often found during routine office visits when fetal heartbeat is not heard at the appropriate time.
Septic pregnancy loss (septic abortion)	Loss accompanied by uterine infection and sepsis Very rare

Table 33.4 Maternal Age and Early Pregnancy Loss Rate

Age	Early pregnancy loss rate (%)
12–19	13
20–24	8–11
24–29	12
30–35	15
35–39	20–25
40–42	35
42–45	51
>45	93

Source: Adapted from Dimitriadis et al. (2020).

The rate of spontaneous pregnancy loss increases with advancing age due to aging oocytes (Table 33.4).

Some groups are more likely to experience early pregnancy loss. Black women experience early pregnancy loss at higher rates than White women with the highest risk between 10 and 20 weeks of gestation (Mukherjee et al., 2013). While limited research has examined explanatory pathways for race-based disparities in early pregnancy loss, the impact of racism on the social determinants of health provides a plausible root cause (Prather et al., 2018). Women with disabilities also experience higher odds of experiencing miscarriage than women without disabilities (Dissanayake et al., 2020). Additional research is necessary to understand this disparity, but potential contributors might include the role of associated comorbidities or life stressors (Dissanayake et al., 2020). Finally, exposure to adversities across the life course is associated with increased risk of early pregnancy loss; stress associated with both acute life events and chronic, long-term exposure to negative circumstances, may play a role in increasing vulnerability to early pregnancy loss (Li & Marren, 2018).

Signs and Symptoms

Bleeding and cramping are the most common presenting symptoms of early pregnancy loss. Some clients report a cessation of previously present pregnancy symptoms such as breast tenderness.

Risk factors for early pregnancy loss

Racism[a]
Prior history of early pregnancy loss
Advanced age (either parent)
Uterine abnormalities
    Leiomyomas
    Bicornuate, unicornuate, septate, or didelphic uterus
Medication use in early pregnancy
    Isotretinoin (Accutane)
    Nonsteroidal anti-inflammatory drugs
Endocrine disorders
    Diabetes mellitus
    Progesterone deficiency and luteal phase deficiency
Smoking
Alcohol use
Caffeine intake of 200 mg/day or more
Malnutrition
Chronic diseases such as factor V Leiden coagulation defect, renal or cardiac disease
Autoimmune disorders such as systemic lupus erythematosus (SLE) or antiphospholipid antibody syndrome.

Source: Adapted from ACOG (2021c) and Quenby et al. (2021).
[a] Due to the effects of racism, Black individuals experience early pregnancy loss at higher rates than White individuals. Black birthing people are at an increased risk of miscarriage due to intersectionality of racism and oppression in the United States, leading to physiologic changes that may impact pregnancy outcomes.

Signs and symptoms of spontaneous early pregnancy loss

- Bleeding that progresses from light to heavy
- Cramps that continue until tissue is passed
- Abdominal pain
- Weakness
- Vomiting
- Back pain

Diagnosis and Management

It is essential to make a definitive diagnosis in order to monitor for complications and to provide accurate information for the parents. This is accomplished through a combination of medical history, physical examination, ultrasound, and serum ß-hCG levels. No single parameter is highly sensitive for predicting an impending loss, although certain clinical and ultrasound findings are suggestive of pregnancies that will not reach viability. Ultrasound may identify an absent or slowing fetal heart rate (<100 BPM at five to seven weeks of gestation), an empty yolk sac, retained products of conception (POCs), subchorionic hemorrhage, or other abnormalities. When found in conjunction with absent cardiac activity, findings of a crown rump length (CRL) of 7 mm or greater and/or mean gestational sac diameter of 25 mm or greater are diagnostic of pregnancy loss (ACOG, 2021c). The most reassuring marker of a healthy pregnancy is the presence of cardiac activity, which should be evident after approximately six weeks of gestation. When cardiac activity is present, the risk of spontaneous loss declines.

There are no effective therapies to interrupt a threatened or inevitable early pregnancy loss. Most first-trimester pregnancy losses occur completely without further need for intervention. Clients who are experiencing an early pregnancy loss are counseled to expect bleeding and cramping until the uterus has emptied. Over-the-counter analgesia such as ibuprofen can be suggested. Although infection and hemorrhage are rare, clients should be advised of signs and symptoms of both and instructed to report them if they occur. A follow-up visit is established to assess for any retained POCs and to review contraceptive and emotional needs.

For those with missed or incomplete early pregnancy loss, options include expectant, medical, and surgical management, and selection is guided by clinical presentation, hemodynamic stability, the presence of infection, and the person's preference. In a nonviable pregnancy without complications, the person's preference should be a primary consideration in management. There is no evidence that any one option produces better long-term outcomes (ACOG, 2021c).

Expectant Management

Expectant management is often the initial treatment choice for spontaneous pregnancy loss and has a success rate of approximately 80% (ACOG, 2021c). If unable to make an immediate decision on management, it is appropriate to give the person time to consider options, as long as the clinical condition remains stable. This method has the greatest variation in presentation, and the client should be informed that in some cases, expectant management can last up to a month. In the absence of hemorrhage or infection, there is no limit to how long it is safe to wait for the process to complete naturally, and the option of changing management strategies remains available. The client should be counseled to report signs of endometritis (fever and uterine tenderness) and heavy bleeding (soaking through two sanitary pads per hour for 2 hours in a row).

Medical Management

The use of the prostaglandin analogue, misoprostol, in a hemodynamically stable person with an incomplete or delayed pregnancy loss and a gestational age less than 13 weeks is an effective and safe alternative to surgical management. Pregnancy expulsion with misoprostol occurs in approximately 80–99% of cases with incomplete or delayed pregnancy loss in the first trimester (ACOG, 2021b). Several protocols for medical management with misoprostol, which vary by route, dose, and dosing interval, can be used (ACOG, 2021b). A common protocol is intravaginal administration of misoprostol with initial dose of 800 mcg, repeating the dose between 3 hours and seven days after administration (ACOG, 2021b). Misoprostol can also be given in doses of 600 mcg orally or 400 mcg sublingually (ACOG, 2021b). This may be preferred if heavy bleeding is present or for the client's convenience. Oral treatment may be repeated twice with a 3-hour interval. A 6- to 12-hour spacing of repeat dosing is often more tolerable for clients experiencing side effects. The addition of mifepristone to enhance the efficacy of uterine contractions is recommended prior to administration of misoprostol when available (ACOG, 2021b; Beaman et al., 2020; Chu et al., 2020). Clients choosing medical management of early pregnancy loss report a greater sense of control and feeling more actively engaged in their treatment plan (Shorter et al., 2019).

Counseling on what to expect with medical management is an important component of care. Nausea, vomiting, fever, and chills are common side effects and can be more significant with oral and sublingual routes. Clients are informed that cramping will increase and bleeding will become heavier with an increased likelihood of visible clots. Pretreatment with a nonsteroidal anti-inflammatory drug (NSAID) before administering the misoprostol is helpful to alleviate side effects. A combination narcotic/acetaminophen can also be prescribed. If a client calls during the miscarriage process, careful questions about the degree of soaking of pads or about the relation of fever to misoprostol use often reveal a normal process. Recommending another dose of an NSAID, with a follow-up call in 1 hour, is often sufficient to assess safety and provide reassurance. Once the gestational tissue is passed, cramping quickly subsides. The bleeding pattern experienced with tissue passage is typically described as heavier than the usual menstrual flow and lasts approximately three or four days. This is followed by a transition to vaginal spotting that may last for a week or longer. Symptoms of retained POC or endometritis include high fever, heavy bleeding, pelvic pain, or feeling ill several days after, and warrant further evaluation. See the *Resources for Clients and Their Families* section for a handout to provide people choosing medical management.

Surgical Management

Immediate surgical management of first-trimester pregnancy loss can be done by electric vacuum aspiration, manual vacuum aspiration, or sharp curette. Cervical ripening agents are often used first to facilitate the evacuation procedure. Surgical management is indicated for clients with severe hemorrhage, signs of infection, significant pain, and failure of medical management. Surgical management may also be a preferred pathway choice. Some states allow midwives, nurses, and physician assistants to perform select surgical aspiration, particularly manual vacuum aspiration, in the office setting (Mainey et al., 2020). Safety and efficacy data for these providers are the same as for physicians (Renner et al., 2013).

Early Pregnancy Loss Follow-Up Care

Any person with vaginal bleeding who is Rhesus (Rh) factor negative and is not sensitized should receive Rh(D) immune globulin within 48–72 hours of the onset of bleeding, regardless of whether the pregnancy ends in a loss or continues. Before 12 weeks of gestation, the dose of Rh(D) immune globulin is 50 mcg, though the more readily available 300 mcg may be used; after 12 weeks of gestation, the dose is 300 mcg.

A follow-up visit is typically scheduled one to two weeks after a pregnancy loss. The physical exam is focused on confirming uterine involution and resolution of pregnancy symptoms. Confirmation of pregnancy expulsion can be done by ultrasound, though serial serum ß-hCG measurement (reaching <5 mlU/mL) can be used where ultrasound services are not readily available. If pregnancy symptoms have resolved and heavy bleeding and cramping have abated, it is reasonable to assume the confirmation of complete tissue passage and forgo confirmatory tests.

It has been common practice to advise one to two weeks of pelvic rest after experiencing a pregnancy loss; however, this is not an evidence-based recommendation. Ovulation may resume as early as day 21 after pregnancy loss and menses typically returns by approximately six weeks postloss. Initiation of contraception, if desired, may be accomplished immediately after completion of early pregnancy loss or at the follow-up visit (ACOG, 2021c). Persons who have experienced an early pregnancy loss often ask about the optimal timing for attempting the next pregnancy. There is no physiologic reason to wait. Subsequent pregnancy timing must take into account a holistic approach including the client's personal and medical factors. It is common practice to advise that it is safe to try for conception when they feel emotionally and physically ready. Most people go on to experience a successful pregnancy after a spontaneous loss, regardless of the interpregnancy interval (Shorter et al., 2019).

Early Pregnancy Loss and Grief

The loss of a desired pregnancy is often a deeply felt event. Emotional attachment to the pregnancy and the developing fetus can begin early in the first trimester, and feelings of loss and grief are often more intense than expected. Emotional healing can take longer than physical healing. One study found that nine months after a pregnancy loss, 18% of clients met the criteria for posttraumatic stress, 17% for moderate or severe anxiety, and 6% for moderate or severe depression (Quenby et al., 2021).

The way in which news of a pregnancy loss is communicated is important. Reassurance about the commonplace nature of pregnancy loss and what does *not* cause early loss to reduce self-blame is important in providing care. Experiences vary, but for many, it is a difficult and vulnerable time and grief reactions should be evaluated. See Chapter 45, *Perinatal Loss and Grief*, for more information.

Recurrent Pregnancy Loss

Recurrent pregnancy loss (RPL) is defined as two or more pregnancy losses prior to 20 weeks of gestation and affects approximately 2.5% of the population trying to conceive (Dimitriadis et al., 2020). The likelihood of a repeat early pregnancy loss increases after each successive loss. Because the risk of subsequent loss is only slightly lower among those who have had two versus three miscarriages, and the probability of finding a treatable etiology is similar among the two groups, most experts agree that there is a role for evaluation after two losses (Li & Marren, 2018). Primary RPL is defined as recurrent losses in a person who has never experienced a live birth. Secondary RPL occurs in people who have previously had a live birth. The causes of RPL include genetic chromosomal abnormalities, uterine structural abnormalities like bicornuate uterus, and immunologic factors such as antiphospholipid antibody syndrome (APS). APS is a thrombophilic condition that is increasingly recognized as a potential etiology of RPL. Tests for antiphospholipid antibodies signaling the presence of APS are increased in women with early pregnancy losses (Zhu et al., 2019). Additional etiologies include endocrine problems such as hypothyroidism, polycystic ovarian syndrome, diabetes mellitus, **luteal phase deficiency**, and infectious causes. Environmental factors including excessive alcohol or caffeine intake are also implicated in RPL. After a thorough evaluation, a cause will be identified for approximately 30–50% of the population experiencing RPL (Li & Marren, 2018).

People who experience RPL should be offered genetic counseling and referred to a fertility specialist for further evaluation and management. Various therapeutic strategies to increase the likelihood of viable pregnancy in this group such as oral, vaginal, and intramuscular progesterone, and intravenous administration of immunoglobulin been evaluated in randomized control trials, but no consistently effective treatment has yet been identified (Dimitriadis et al., 2020). Higher rates of depression and emotional stress are found in this population; thus, screening and treatment for psychological disorders is warranted (Kendig et al., 2017).

Risks for recurrent pregnancy loss

Of note, no risk factors are identified in 50–75% of couples with recurrent pregnancy loss
Client age
Previous number of pregnancy losses
Antiphospholipid syndrome
Congenital uterine malformation (uterine septum)
Acquire uterine malformations (leiomyomas, polyps, or adhesions)
Chronic endometriosis
Overt hypothyroidism
Obesity
Lifestyle factors (stress, smoking, and excessive alcohol consumption)

Ectopic Pregnancy

An **ectopic pregnancy** occurs when a fertilized ovum implants outside of the uterine cavity. Approximately 1–2% of all documented pregnancies are ectopic (Hendriks et al., 2019). Although a rare event, ectopic pregnancy is the leading cause of pregnancy-related maternal death in the first trimester. Ectopic pregnancy can result in loss of a fallopian tube and can reduce fertility.

The incidence of ectopic pregnancy has increased significantly since the early 1970s but has become stable in the last decade. This increase is attributed to the rise of risk factors associated with ectopic pregnancy such as smoking and pelvic inflammatory disease (PID) among people of reproductive age, the growing use of assisted reproductive technology (ART), and improvement in the detection and diagnosis of ectopic pregnancy. Risk factors can be categorized by the strength of association (Table 33.5); however, 50% of ectopic pregnancies occur without risk factors (Hendriks et al., 2019). Ectopic pregnancy most commonly occurs in the fallopian tubes. More rarely, ectopic pregnancy occurs in the ovary, the cervical canal, or the peritoneum.

Table 33.5 Risk Factors for Ectopic Pregnancy

Prior ectopic pregnancy
Previous damage to fallopian tubes
Tubal pathology/surgery
Prior genital tract infection including PID
Assisted reproductive technology
Infertility
Smoking
Intrauterine device (IUD)

Source: Adapted from ACOG (2018) and Hendriks et al. (2019).

Clinical Presentation

Ectopic pregnancy may develop enough to produce symptoms such as bleeding or lower-quadrant pain between six and eight weeks. Many people are asymptomatic when attending the first prenatal visit, and atypical presentation is common. Since ß-hCG is produced, some may have early pregnancy symptoms such as breast tenderness and nausea. Table 33.6 lists signs and symptoms of ectopic pregnancy.

Diagnosis and Management

Ectopic pregnancy may be subacute in early stages; however, it can quickly become an obstetric emergency. Early diagnosis is critical to reducing morbidity and mortality and to outcomes preserving tubal function and fertility. Ectopic pregnancy is included in the differential diagnosis in all people of reproductive age presenting with vaginal bleeding and a positive pregnancy test in the first trimester. Diagnosis of an unruptured ectopic pregnancy is accomplished with serum ßhCG measurements and transvaginal ultrasound. Serial measurement of serum ßhCG values (Table 33.7) can help to distinguish between a potentially viable intrauterine gestation, a resolving spontaneous pregnancy loss, and an ectopic pregnancy.

Diagnosis and Management

The use of discriminatory human chorionic gonadotropin (hCG) levels differs and has been challenged. If discriminatory levels are utilized, the value should be conservatively high to avoid misdiagnosis. Most viable first-trimester intrauterine pregnancies have hCG levels that double every 48 hours. Ectopic pregnancies can present with increasing or decreasing hCG levels, and the rise or decline occurs more slowly than would be expected with an early spontaneous pregnancy loss (ACOG, 2018). Ultrasound findings are correlated with hCG levels to determine diagnosis and appropriate management.

Table 33.6 Signs and Symptoms of Ectopic Pregnancy

Abdominal pain
Amenorrhea, positive pregnancy test
Bleeding often brownish in color
Dizziness, fainting, syncope
May have breast tenderness, nausea, and other pregnancy signs
Physical exam Adnexal mass Acute pain on cervical motion
Signs of rupture include Hypotension Nausea Pallor Shoulder pain (blood irritating diaphragm) Urge to defecate (blood pooling in cul de sac)

Source: ACOG (2018)/The American College of Obstetricians and Gynecologists.

Table 33.7 Criteria for Ectopic Pregnancy Management Options

Expectant management

Candidate should be asymptomatic

Objective evidence of resolution (i.e., a plateau or decrease in hCG levels)

Counseled on potential risks and willing to accept risks (i.e., tubal rupture, hysterectomy, and emergency surgery)

Medical management with methotrexate

Stable vital signs

No medical contraindication for methotrexate therapy

No evidence of tubal rupture

Absence of embryonic cardiac activity

Ectopic mass of 35 mm or less

Starting hCG level less than 1500 IU/mL

Prompt availability of surgery if patient does not respond to treatment

Dosage: single intramuscular dose of 1 mg/kg or 50 mg/m^2

Follow-up: hCG on the fourth and seventh posttreatment days, then weekly until undetectable, which usually takes several weeks

Expected hCG changes: initial slight increase, then 15% decrease between days 4 and 7; if not, repeat dosage or consider surgery

Surgical management

Unstable vital signs or signs indicating rupture

Advanced ectopic pregnancy (high hCG levels, large mass, cardiac activity)

Patient unreliable for follow-up

Contraindications to expectant management or methotrexate

Source: ACOG (2018)/ The American College of Obstetricians and Gynecologists.

The treatment of an ectopic pregnancy can be expectant, surgical, or medical, depending on presentation and preferences (Table 33.7). When hCG values decrease at a rate that is at least as high as that expected in spontaneous pregnancy loss, continued outpatient surveillance and expectant management is warranted until levels are undetectable. Reasons for abandoning expectant management include intractable or significantly increased pain, insufficient decrease of hCG levels, or tubal rupture with hemoperitoneum.

Medical management of ectopic pregnancy with the administration of systemic methotrexate, a folic acid antagonist, is a common, low-cost, and safe alternative to surgery in those who are hemodynamically stable. Multiple-dose and single-dose intramuscular administration regimens are used: the single-dose regimen is most common and carries considerably fewer side effects. Surgical management may involve removing the affected fallopian tube (salpingectomy) or dissecting the ectopic pregnancy with conservation of the tube (salpingotomy).

The risk of recurrence is approximately 10–27% among those with previous ectopic pregnancy, at least 25% among those with two or more previous ectopic pregnancies (Petrini & Spandorfer, 2020) and highest in birthing people experiencing infertility or salpingotomy (Hendriks et al., 2019). Most people who experience ectopic pregnancy can go on to have a healthy pregnancy. The person can still be experiencing the loss of a pregnancy, even though it was not viable, and can experience grieving similar with any other early pregnancy loss.

Gestational Trophoblastic Disease

Gestational trophoblastic disease (GTD) includes a spectrum of premalignant conditions (partial and complete **hydatidiform moles [HM]**) and malignant tumors (**epithelioid trophoblastic tumor (ETT), and placental-site trophoblastic tumor (PSTT**; Table 33.8; Ning et al., 2019). Approximately 80% of GTD falls in the category of HM, a benign neoplastic disease in which a normally fertilized ovum implants into the uterus, but the chorionic villi do not develop properly (Ning et al., 2019). The pregnancy is not viable, and the normal pregnancy process develops into a benign tumor. There are two subtypes of HM: complete HM (CHM) and partial HM (PHM; Table 33.8). The symptoms of CHM tend to be more severe than those of PHM, and there is a difference in histology between the two types. Genetic markers have shown that most HMs are derived entirely from paternal genes. This can happen when the sperm penetrates an ovum that has no nucleus.

HM occurs in approximately 1–2 in 1000 pregnancies (Clark et al., 2021) and is more common at the extremes of reproductive age. People older than 35 years have a twofold increase in risk, and people over the age of 40 have a fivefold to tenfold increase in risk compared to younger people (Clark et al., 2021).

Potential Problems

People who have had a molar pregnancy are at risk for developing one of several malignant trophoblastic conditions. **Choriocarcinoma** involves direct invasion of the myometrium and its blood supply. This is a highly malignant form of GTD that spreads rapidly throughout the body and requires aggressive treatment. Choriocarcinoma is rare, occurring in only 1 of every 20,000–40,000 pregnancies (Ning et al., 2019). Approximately half of all cases of choriocarcinoma are related to a molar pregnancy. The other cases arise from a spontaneous pregnancy loss or a normal pregnancy (Soper, 2021). PHMs are rarely followed by malignant changes, whereas this may occur in approximately 2.5–7.5% of CHMs (Soper, 2021). Malignancy typically occurs within six months of molar evacuation. An invasive mole penetrates the myometrium and can embolize to distant sites such as the parametrial tissues, spinal cord, brain, or lungs. The tumor typically grows rapidly, invading blood vessels and causing local tissue destruction and bleeding at those sites with related complications. PSTT and ETT are rare types of GTD. Diagnosis and treatment of PSTT and ETT are dependent on staging and metastasis (Hancock & Tidy, 2021).

Presentation

The most common classic symptom of GTD is vaginal bleeding, occurring in the majority of cases with this condition. Molar tissue separates from the decidua, causing

Table 33.8   Types of Gestational Trophoblastic Disease

Type	Physiology	Physical findings
Hydatidiform mole		
Partial	Some fetal tissue present One set of maternal haploid genes and two sets of paternal haploid genes	Vaginal bleeding Absence of fetal heart tones Signs and symptoms of incomplete or missed abortion Uterus can be S < D
Complete	No fetal tissue present Duplication of the haploid sperm after fertilization of an empty ovum Increased potential for malignancy	Vaginal bleeding Absence of fetal heart tones Uterus can be S > D
Gestational trophoblastic neoplasms		
Invasive mole	Trophoblastic invasion confined to the myometrium	Continued bleeding Uterine subinvolution
Gestational choriocarcinoma	Rapidly growing trophoblastic cells invade myometrium and blood vessels Extremely malignant	Continued bleeding Uterine subinvolution Asymptomatic
Placental-site trophoblastic tumor	Slow growing form of GTD Very rare	Can present years after pregnancy

Source: Adapted from Hancock and Tidy (2021), Ning et al. (2019), and Soper (2021).

bleeding that can vary from spotting to heavy and be bright red clots or watery brown discharge. The bleeding can persist intermittently for weeks. Uterine growth is often more rapid than is expected for gestational age and can result in a sensation of increased pelvic pressure. No fetal heartbeat is present. Due to extremely high levels of hCG, some may report severe nausea and vomiting. Signs and symptoms of hyperthyroidism can be present, especially with high hCG levels, due to stimulation of the thyroid gland by hCG or by a thyroid-stimulating substance produced by the trophoblasts. People with CHM can develop preeclampsia in the first or second trimester.

Risk factors for gestational trophoblastic disease

Maternal age <20 or >35

Prior molar pregnancy

Prior history of miscarriage

Family history

Poor nutritional status

Source: Adapted from Hancock and Tidy (2021), Ning et al. (2019), and Soper (2021).

Diagnosis and Management

Most molar pregnancies are diagnosed in the first trimester prior to the onset of the classic signs and symptoms due to the common practice of early pregnancy dating with ultrasound. Serum quantitative hCG level greater than expected for gestational age is also an indicator. Complete blood cell count with platelets is obtained as anemia and coagulopathy could occur. Although people with GTD are usually clinically euthyroid, plasma thyroxine is obtained and can be markedly elevated.

Some people present with spontaneous passage of molar tissue. After the expulsion of tissue, it is essential to determine whether a miscarriage is complete. A physical examination and, in some cases, evaluation with ultrasound and serial hCG levels are necessary shortly after or, if symptoms are stable, within a few days of expulsion. For those who do not pass molar tissue spontaneously, treatment is suction curettage under ultrasound guidance, which reduces potential for sequelae. **Pelvic rest** is recommended for two to four weeks after evacuation of the uterus, and the person is instructed not to become pregnant for six months, to avoid confusion about the development of malignant disease once when serum hCG is detected. Some people who have completed childbearing or who have higher risk for malignancy can be offered a hysterectomy to reduce risk for choriocarcinoma. The prognosis for retained fertility is excellent and most people experience a complete cure with standard therapy (Clark et al., 2021).

Because of the small but real potential for the development of malignant disease and because these malignancies are usually very responsive to treatment, the importance of consistent follow-up care is strongly emphasized. Once a molar pregnancy is diagnosed, a baseline chest X-ray is often done, as the lungs are a primary site of metastasis for malignant trophoblastic tumors. Serial hCG levels are commonly monitored weekly until they are within normal limits for three to four weeks and then monthly for six months to one year

(Soper, 2021) to identify the rare patient who develops malignant disease. Levels should consistently drop and should never increase. Normal levels are usually reached within 8–12 weeks after the evacuation of GTD. As long as the hCG levels are falling, intervention is not needed.

The risk of recurrence of HM is 1–2% (Soper, 2021). Pregnant persons with a prior history of GTD should undergo early ultrasound evaluation to rule out repeat molar gestation.

Bleeding during the Second Half of Pregnancy

Bleeding during the late second or third trimester of pregnancy is most often abnormal. The bleeding can range from very mild to extremely brisk and may or may not be accompanied by abdominal pain. The role of the healthcare provider is to move toward diagnosis and to determine the need for direct care and the need for referral or consultation. Additionally, emotional support, especially if the bleeding results in a poor pregnancy outcome, is an important component of competent and compassionate care.

Differential Diagnoses

Cervical bleeding from benign conditions should be considered. Spotting after intercourse or a digital vaginal examination due to cervical friability is common at any gestation in pregnancy.

Potential Etiologies of Bleeding in the Second Half of Pregnancy

Cervical insufficiency
Preterm labor
Placenta previa
Placental abruption
Vasa previa
Vaginal infection
Cervical bleeding relative to:

- Postcoital bleeding
- Cervicitis
- Cervical ectropion
- Polyps

Impact of *Dobbs v. Jackson Women's Health Organization* Supreme Court Decision on Management of Early Pregnancy Loss, Ectopic Pregnancy, and Emergency Termination of Pregnancy

Dobbs v. Jackson Women's Health Organization (2022) was a landmark decision of the US Supreme Court in which the Court held that the Constitution of the United States does not protect the right to abortion. On June 28, 2022, the Court overturned *Roe v. Wade* (1973) and *Planned Parenthood v. Casey* (1992)—prior cases that affirmed the constitutional right to an abortion. The *Dobbs* decision has complicated the management of early pregnancy loss, ectopic pregnancy, and emergency termination of

pregnancy (which may be required for a number of conditions including intrauterine sepsis, hypertensive disorders of pregnancy before fetal viability, and obstetric hemorrhage before fetal viability; MacDonald et al., 2022). In an attempt to address this, the US Department of Health and Human Services issued a mandate on July 11, 2022, indicating that the 1996 Federal legislation Emergency Medical Treatment and Labor Act (EMTALA) applies to patients needing abortion care to treat an emergency medical condition (US Department of Health and Human Services, 2022). However, at the time of publication of this text, legal challenges regarding whether EMTALA takes precedence over state laws are ongoing. Healthcare providers should be aware of local laws and regulations on the elective termination of pregnancy, which may impact their management of early pregnancy loss, ectopic pregnancy, and emergency termination of pregnancy.

Placenta Previa

Placenta previa is a condition where the placenta overlies the cervical os (Jain et al., 2020). Normally, the placenta implants in the muscular upper uterine segment. In placenta previa, the placenta is totally or partially implanted in the lower uterine segment, which is thinner and less vascular. Terminology to describe the condition has been inconsistent. Placenta previa had been commonly classified as complete, partial, or marginal, depending on proximity or coverage of the internal os (Figure 33.2). However, the use of transvaginal ultrasound allows for precise localization of the placental margins and cervical os. Accordingly, newer nomenclature eliminates the use of the terms *marginal* and *partial*. Instead, placenta previa is reclassified into two conditions: true placenta previa where placental tissue covers the cervical os in any degree (includes complete, partial, and marginal previa), and low-lying placenta, where the edge of the placenta is within 2 cm of the cervical os (Jain et al., 2020). The literature continues to reflect a variety of terms to describe the continuum of placental tissue near or over the internal cervical os.

A low-lying placenta is a common finding on second-trimester ultrasonography; however, it is not necessarily pathologic. It is estimated that over 90% of low-lying placentas seen on ultrasound at 20 weeks of gestation will migrate away from the cervix and out of the lower uterine segment (Anderson-Bagga & Sze, 2023). This **trophotropism** occurs as the placenta naturally grows toward the more highly vascularized uterine fundus. The majority of clients with a placenta previa seen on ultrasound in the second trimester will no longer have a placenta previa in the third trimester (Haino et al., 2018).

Placenta previa in the third trimester occurs in approximately 1 in 200 pregnancies at term (Cresswell et al., 2013). The incidence of placenta previa is rising in correlation with the increase in cesarean birth in the United States, which is associated with an increased risk for placenta previa in a subsequent pregnancy with the risk increasing with each cesarean birth (Silver, 2015).

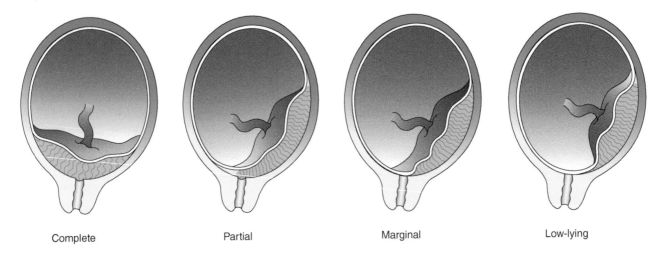

Complete   Partial   Marginal   Low-lying

Figure 33.2 Types of placenta previa.

Risk Factors for Placenta Previa

Maternal age >35
Multiparity
Prior cesarean section or other uterine surgery or curettage
Infertility treatments
Smoking
Unexplained elevated alpha-fetoprotein (AFP)
Multiple gestation
Short interpregnancy interval

Potential Problems

Placenta previa is associated with multiple adverse maternal and fetal/neonatal complications. Many of the maternal sequelae are due to consequences of hemorrhage. Clients with placenta previa are more likely to experience cesarean birth and, thus, are exposed to potential surgical complications. Placenta accrete spectrum disorders, such as **placenta accreta, increta,** or **percreta**, are associated with placenta previa and place the client at risk for emergency hysterectomy. The presence of placenta previa increases risk for thrombophlebitis, blood transfusions, intensive care admission, septicemia, and even death (Anderson-Bagga & Sze, 2023). Active bleeding at any point in pregnancy due to placenta previa increases risk for emergency cesarean birth (Anderson-Bagga & Sze, 2023). Cases of placenta previa in which the placenta is attached anteriorly have a higher rate of significant hemorrhage compared to a posterior placental attachment (Jing et al., 2018). Clients with placenta previa may suffer considerable emotional distress due to recurrent bleeding, hospitalizations, feelings of helplessness, and acute concern for maternal and fetal health. Fetal potential problems relate primarily to preterm birth and an increase in perinatal morbidity and mortality.

Presentation

The classic clinical presentation of placenta previa includes painless bright red vaginal bleeding in the late second or early third trimester of pregnancy. The first episode of bleeding often stops after a few hours. Subsequent episodes of bleeding tend to be worse due to increased development of the lower uterine segment and further detachment of the placenta. The painless bleeding occurs due to stretching of the lower uterine segment and detachment at the placenta. Some may experience associated pain and cramping due to uterine irritability caused by bleeding.

Birth Planning

Vaginal birth is an option with ultrasound evidence that the placental edge is >2 cm from the internal cervical os. Current guidelines recommended that a late-preterm or early-term cesarean birth should be conducted between 36 weeks and 0 days and 37 weeks and 6 days (ACOG, 2021a).

Placental Abruption

Placental abruption is defined as antepartal decidual hemorrhage leading to the premature separation of the placenta. The immediate cause of the premature placental separation is often the rupture of the pregnant person's blood vessels in the decidua basalis, where it comes into contact with the anchoring villi of the placenta. Since the separation lies within the maternal decidua, the bleeding is almost always maternal in origin. Placental abruptions can be concealed or visible (Qiu et al., 2021). Concealed placental abruption most often occurs when a midsection of placenta has separated from the uterine wall and the edges of placenta remain attached (Figure 33.3).

The incidence of placental abruption is estimated at 0.3–4.4% (Qiu et al., 2021). One-third of all cases of third-trimester bleeding are caused by placental abruption, with approximately half of the cases of abruption occurring prior to 37 weeks of gestation (Tikkanen, 2011). The presence of hypertension during pregnancy, whether from chronic hypertension or a pregnancy-related hypertensive disease, significantly increases the risk of placental

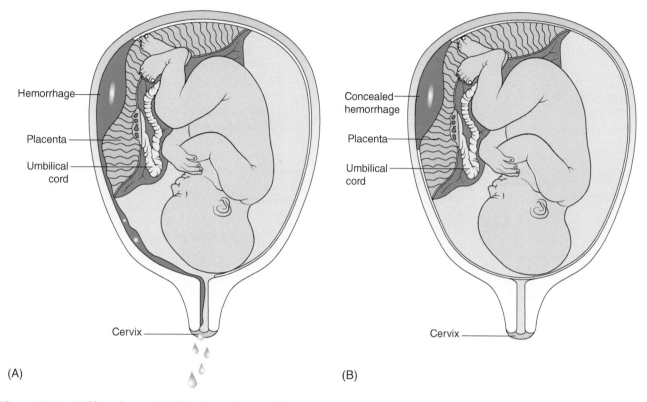

Figure 33.3   Visible and concealed bleeding in placental abruption. Types of abruption: (A) with visible abruption, blood tracks between the membranes and escapes through the vagina and cervix and (B) with concealed abruption, blood collects behind the placenta, with no evidence of vaginal bleeding. Reprinted with permission from Oyelese and Ananth (2006). Illustration by John Yanson.

abruption (Araji et al., 2017). The underlying pathophysiological mechanism is thought to be ischemic placental disease, characterized by chronic reduced blood flow. Smoking is a risk factor with a dose–response relationship between the number of cigarettes smoked and the risk of placental abruption. A likely etiology is chronic placental ischemia resulting in decidual necrosis. Preterm prelabor rupture of membranes is associated with an increase in placental abruption, possibly due to infection and inflammatory processes. Cesarean birth is known to cause lasting damage to the myometrium and endometrium and is associated with a twofold increased risk of placental abruption in subsequent pregnancies (Klar & Michels, 2014; Table 33.9).

Potential Problems

Clients with placental abruption are at higher risk for shock, consumptive coagulopathy, renal failure, and death, all of which are due to the significant blood loss. **Couvelaire uterus**, a rare condition describing blood seeping into the uterine musculature, is associated with placental abruption. Clients who experience placental abruption have a high recurrence rate in subsequent pregnancies. Clients who have had a placental abruption have a twofold to sixfold higher risk for death and long-term morbidity due to cardiovascular disease compared to normal pregnancy (Ananth et al., 2021). Fetal complications include decreased oxygenation resulting in cerebral compromise and stillbirth.

Presentation

The signs and symptoms of placental abruption can vary markedly, making timely diagnosis difficult. In its early stages, there may be no signs or symptoms clinically evident. The only symptoms of a concealed abruption may be cramping, contractions, uterine tenderness, or back pain. The clinical hallmarks of visible placental abruption are vaginal bleeding with abdominal pain. The amount of bleeding correlates with the severity of the placental detachment and with fetal sequelae. These classic symptoms are often accompanied by uterine hypertonicity and tenderness. The client may experience tachycardia and an abnormal fetal heart rate pattern can be present. When the placenta is attached to the posterior wall of the uterus, back pain can accompany placental abruption.

Vasa Previa

Vasa previa occurs when fetal vessels emerging from the placenta extend over the cervical os (Figure 33.4). Vasa previa is often seen in conjunction with a velamentous cord insertion. The exposed vessels often lack Wharton's jelly, making them more vulnerable to compression and tears. It is a rare condition occurring in 1 in 1275–2500 pregnancies; however, it has a high rate of fetal and neonatal morbidity and mortality if not diagnosed prenatally (Ranzini & Oyelese, 2021). If the unprotected fetal vessels rupture, which often occurs at the time of rupture of membranes, the fetus can exsanguinate within minutes.

Table 33.9 Risk Factors for Placental Abruption

Risk factor	Comment
Prior placental abruption	Recurrence risk 5–15%
Hypertension, chronic and pregnancy-related	Fivefold increase in risk
Increasing parity	
Increased age	Due to chronic disease or higher parity
Preterm prelabor rupture of membranes (PPROM)	Occurs in 2–5% of PPROM cases
Smoking	Increases risk 40%
Alcohol use	
Short interpregnancy interval	
Cocaine use in third trimester	Occurs in 10% of pregnant cocaine users
Uterine and factors Leiomyoma Prior cesarean birth	Twofold increase in risk with prior cesarean birth
Rapid uterine decompression Multiple gestation Polyhydramnios	Twin gestation has threefold increase in risk
Maternal diseases Thrombophilia Hypothyroidism Asthma	
Blunt or penetrating trauma	Occurs in 7–13% of abdominal injury
Unexplained abnormally elevated maternal serum AFP	

Source: Adapted from Araji et al. (2017).

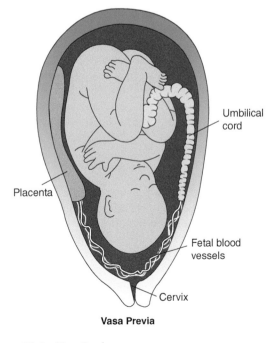

Vasa Previa

Figure 33.4 Vasa Previa.

Most cases of vasa previa are diagnosed prenatally by routine ultrasound, even though screening for vasa previa is not a standard component of the complete ultrasound examination (Ranzini & Oyelese, 2021). Risk-based ultrasound screening is recommended for pregnant people with placenta previa, low-lying placenta, **succenturiate lobed placenta** advanced age, multiple gestation, and in-vitro fertilization. Strategies include administration of antenatal steroids between 30 and 32 weeks of gestation and scheduled delivery at 34 weeks of gestation and possibly as early as 33 weeks of gestation (Melcer et al., 2018).

Diagnosis and Management of Bleeding in the Second Half of Pregnancy

The amount, color, and characteristics of the bleeding, as well as any associated symptoms, are ascertained. Chart review is done for blood type and Rh, risk factors, and placental location noted with any prior ultrasound examination. Abdominal palpation for uterine tone and tenderness and vital sign assessment is performed. A digital pelvic examination in people experiencing second- or third-trimester bleeding is never performed until placental location is identified. Even a gentle digital exam can precipitate severe hemorrhage in the presence of placenta previa.

Sonographic evaluation is required to determine placental location. Transvaginal ultrasound is superior to abdominal ultrasound in diagnosing placenta previa; it allows for the visualization of the internal cervical os and the lower placental edge, and the fetal head does not obscure visualization of the placental edge. Ultrasound may reveal retroplacental clotting, indicating possible placental abruption; however, because the placenta and fresh bleeding have similar appearances on sonography images, negative findings on ultrasound do not exclude the possibility of placental abruption.

A CBC and type and screen are done, and coagulation studies may be helpful. Rh-negative patients receive Rh(D) immune globulin within 48–72 hours of the onset of bleeding. A **Kleihauer–Betke test** should be performed first to determine the appropriate dose of Rh(D) immune globulin.

Hospitalization is appropriate for people with placenta previa during an acute bleeding episode or in the presence of uterine contractions. Conservative expectant management is appropriate when bleeding from documented placenta previa subsides so that birth can occur as close to term is possible. Outpatient management of placenta previa may be appropriate for patients in stable condition with home support, close proximity to a hospital, and ready access to transportation.

The management of placental abruption varies, depending on gestational age and the status of the pregnant person and fetus. Placental abruption can occur early in pregnancy and can be associated with poor placentation, which can lead to fetal growth restriction. Serial ultrasound evaluation of fetal growth may be indicated.

Obstetrical collaboration or referral is warranted since most causes of second- and third-trimester bleeding are abnormal. In the case of placenta previa, consultation or referral is done for possible tocolysis, outpatient or inpatient management decisions, and steroid administration. Placental abruption is an obstetric emergency and physician management is essential.

Pregnant individuals with late pregnancy bleeding may suffer considerable emotional distress due to recurrent bleeding, hospitalizations, feelings of helplessness, and acute concern for maternal and fetal health. Family and other support systems can be crucial to maintaining family function and reducing maternal stress. People with limited support may benefit from social and community services.

Interprofessional Care

Of note, obstetrical consultation is appropriate for clients in stable condition with bleeding of unknown etiology. Uncomplicated early intrauterine pregnancy loss can be managed independently. Referral to physician management is appropriate for any pregnancy bleeding event that is potentially life-threatening.

Resources for Healthcare Providers

American College of Obstetricians & Gynecologists (ACOG) Committee opinion no. 831: Medically indicate late-preterm and early-term deliveries. https://www.acog.org/clinical/clinical-guidance/committee-opinion/articles/2021/07/medically-indicated-late-preterm-and-early-term-deliveries

American College of Obstetricians & Gynecologists (ACOG) Practice bulletin no. 193: Tubal ectopic pregnancy. https://www.acog.org/clinical/clinical-guidance/practice-bulletin/articles/2018/03/tubal-ectopic-pregnancy

American College of Obstetricians & Gynecologists (ACOG). Practice bulletin no. 200: Early pregnancy loss. https://www.acog.org/clinical/clinical-guidance/practice-bulletin/articles/2018/11/early-pregnancy-loss

American College of Obstetricians & Gynecologists (ACOG). Practice bulletin no. 225: Medication abortion up to 70 days of gestation: https://www.acog.org/clinical/clinical-guidance/practice-bulletin/articles/2020/10/medication-abortion-up-to-70-days-of-gestation#:~:text=Combined%20mifepristone%E2%80%93misoprostol%20regimens%20are,regimen%20is%20the%20recommended%20alternative

Resources for Clients and Their Families

Association of Reproductive Health Professionals. Miscarriage resource handouts: https://www.reproductiveaccess.org/miscarriage

Association of Reproductive Health Professionals. Ectopic pregnancy fact sheet: https://www.reproductiveaccess.org/resource/ectopic-pregnancy

Reproductive Health Access Project. Protocols for medication management of early pregnancy loss handout: http://www.reproductiveaccess.org/resource/medication-management-miscarriage-misoprostol-protocol

American College of Obstetricians and Gynecologists. Early pregnancy loss: Frequently asked questions: https://www.acog.org/womens-health/faqs/early-pregnancy-loss

American College of Obstetricians and Gynecologists. Bleeding during pregnancy: Frequently asked questions: https://www.acog.org/womens-health/faqs/bleeding-during-pregnancy

American College of Obstetricians and Gynecologists. Repeated miscarriages (Recurrent pregnant loss): Frequently asked questions: https://www.acog.org/womens-health/faqs/repeated-miscarriages

References

American College of Obstetricians and Gynecologists (ACOG). (2018). Practice bulletin no. 193: Tubal ectopic pregnancy. *Obstetrics & Gynecology*, *131*(3), e91–e103. https://doi.org/10.1097/aog.0000000000002464

American College of Obstetricians and Gynecologists (ACOG). (2021a). Committee opinion no. 831: Medically indicate late-preterm and early-term deliveries. *Obstetrics & Gynecology*, *138*(1), e91–e103. https://doi.org/10.1097/AOG.0000000000004447

American College of Obstetricians and Gynecologists (ACOG). (2021b). Practice bulletin no. 224: Medication abortion up to 70 days of gestational. *Obstetrics & Gynecology*, *132*(5), e197–e207. https://doi.org/10.1097/aog.0000000000002899

American College of Obstetricians and Gynecologists (ACOG). (2021c). Practice bulletin no. 200: Early pregnancy loss. *Obstetrics & Gynecology*, *132*(5), e197–e207. https://doi.org/10.1097/aog.0000000000002899

Ananth, C. V., Patrick, H. S., Ananth, S., Zhang, Y., Kostis, W. J., & Schuster, M. (2021). Maternal cardiovascular and cerebrovascular health after placental abruption: A systematic review and meta-analysis (CHAP-SR). *American Journal of Epidemiology*, *190*(12), 2718–2729. https://doi.org/10.1093/aje/kwab206

Anderson-Bagga, F. M., & Sze, A. (2023). Placenta previa. In *StatPearls [Internet]*. StatPearls Publishing. http://www.ncbi.nlm.nih.gov/books/NBK539818/

Araji, S., Khoury, A., Elkafrawi, D., & Miller, J. (2017). Etiologies and risk factors of placental abruption and neonatal mortality: A retrospective study [6K]. *Obstetrics & Gynecology*, *129*(5), 113S.

Beaman, J., Prifti, C., Schwarz, E. B., & Sobota, M. (2020). Medication to manage abortion and miscarriage. *Journal of General Internal Medicine*, *35*(8), 2398–2405. https://doi.org/10.1007/s11606-020-05836-9

Chu, J. J., Devall, A. J., Beeson, L. E., Hardy, P., Cheed, V., Sun, Y., Roberts, T. E., Ogwulu, C. O., Williams, E., Jones, L. L., Papadopoulos, J. H. L. F., Bender-Atik, R., Brewin, J., Hinshaw, K., Choudhary, M., Ahmed, A., Naftalin, J., Nunes, N., Oliver, A., & Izzat, F. (2020). Mifepristone and misoprostol versus misoprostol alone for the management of missed miscarriage (MifeMiso): A randomised, double-blind, placebo-controlled trial. *The Lancet*, *396*(10253), 770–778. https://doi.org/10.1016/S0140-6736(20)31788-8

Clark, J., Slater, S., & Seckl, M. J. (2021). Treatment of gestational trophoblastic disease in the 2020s. *Current Opinion in Obstetrics & Gynecology*, *33*(1), 7–12. https://doi.org/10.1097/GCO.0000000000000674

Coutinho, L. M., Assis, W. A., Spagnuolo-Souza, A., & Reis, F. M. (2021). Uterine fibroids and pregnancy: How do they affect each other? *Reproductive Sciences*, *29*, 2145–2151. https://doi.org/10.1007/s43032-021-00656-6

Cresswell, J. A., Ronsmans, C., Calvert, C., & Filippi, V. (2013). Prevalence of placenta praevia by world region: A systematic review and meta-analysis. *Tropical Medicine & International Health*, *18*(6), 712–724.

Dimitriadis, E., Menkhorst, E., Saito, S., Kutteh, W. H., & Brosens, J. J. (2020). Recurrent pregnancy loss. *Nature Reviews Disease Primers*, *6*(1), 98. https://doi.org/10.1038/s41572-020-00228-z

Dissanayake, M. V., Darney, B. G., Caughey, A. B., & Horner-Johnson, W. (2020). Miscarriage occurrence and prevention efforts by disability status and type in the United States. *Journal of Women's Health, 29*(3), 345–352. https://doi.org/10.1089/jwh.2019.7880

Haino, K., Ishii, K., Kanda, M., Kanai, A., Hayashi, S., & Mitsuda, N. (2018). Variations of placental migration in patients with early third trimester malposition. *Journal of Medical Ultrasonics, 45*(1), 99–102.

Hancock, B. W., & Tidy, J. (2021). Placental site trophoblastic tumour and epithelioid trophoblastic tumour. *Best Practice & Research Clinical Obstetrics & Gynaecology, 74*, 131–148.

Hendriks, E., MacNaughton, H., & MacKenzie, M. (2019). First trimester bleeding: Evaluation and management. *American Family Physician, 99*(3), 166–174.

Henshaw, C. A., Goreish, M. H., Gornet, M. E., & Cross, C. I. (2022). The impact of uterine fibroids on fertility: How the uncertainty widens the gap in reproductive outcomes in Black women. *Reproductive Sciences, 29*(7), 1–7.

Jain, V., Bos, H., & Bujold, E. (2020). Guideline no. 402: Diagnosis and management of placenta previa. *Journal of Obstetrics and Gynaecology Canada, 42*(7), 906–917.e1. https://doi.org/10.1016/j.jogc.2019.07.019

Jing, L., Wei, G., Mengfan, S., & Yanyan, H. (2018). Effect of site of placentation on pregnancy outcomes in patients with placenta previa. *PLoS One, 13*(7), e0200252. https://doi.org/10.1371/journal.pone.0200252

Kendig, S., Keats, J. P., Hoffman, M. C., Kay, L. B., Miller, E. S., Moore Simas, T. A., Frieder, A., Hackley, B., Indman, P., Raines, C., Semenuk, K., Wisner, K. L., & Lemieux, L. A. (2017). Consensus bundle on maternal mental health: Perinatal depression and anxiety. *Obstetrics & Gynecology, 129*(3), 422–430. https://doi.org/10.1097/AOG.0000000000001902

Klar, M., & Michels, K. B. (2014). Cesarean section and placental disorders in subsequent pregnancies-a meta-analysis. *Journal of Perinatal Medicine, 42*(5), 571–583.

Kolte, A. M., Bernardi, L. A., Christiansen, O. B., Quenby, S., Farquharson, R. G., Goddijn, M., & Stephenson, M. D. (2014). Terminology for pregnancy loss prior to viability: A consensus statement from the ESHRE early pregnancy special interest group. *Human Reproduction, 30*(3), 495–498. https://doi.org/10.1093/humrep/deu299

Li, Y. H., & Marren, A. (2018). Recurrent pregnancy loss: A summary of international evidence-based guidelines and practice. *Australian Journal of General Practice, 47*(7), 432–436. https://doi.org/10.31128/ajgp-01-18-4459

Liu, S., Yu, L., Wu, Q., Cui, H., Lin, X., & Wang, W. (2021). Study on the correlation between vaginal bleeding in first trimester and preterm birth: A birth cohort study in Lanzhou, China. *Journal of Obstetrics and Gynaecology Research, 47*(6), 1997–2004. https://doi.org/10.1111/jog.14750

MacDonald, A., Gershengorn, H. B., & Ashana, D. C. (2022). The challenge of emergency abortion care following the Dobbs ruling. *JAMA, 328*(17), 1691–1692. https://doi.org/10.1001/jama.2022.17197

Mainey, L., O'Mullan, C., Reid-Searl, K., Taylor, A., & Baird, K. (2020). The role of nurses and midwives in the provision of abortion care: A scoping review. *Journal of Clinical Nursing, 29*(9–10), 1513–1526.

Melcer, Y., Maymon, R., & Jauniaux, E. (2018). Vasa previa. *Current Opinion in Obstetrics and Gynecology, 30*(6), 385–391. https://doi.org/10.1097/gco.0000000000000478

Mukherjee, S., Velez Edwards, D. R., Baird, D. D., Savitz, D. A., & Hartmann, K. E. (2013). Risk of miscarriage among Black women and White women in a US prospective cohort study. *American Journal of Epidemiology, 177*(11), 1271–1278. https://doi.org/10.1093/aje/kws393

Ning, F., Hou, H., Morse, A. N., & Lash, G. E. (2019). Understanding and management of gestational trophoblastic disease. *F1000Research, 8*, 1–9. https://doi.org/10.12688/f1000research.14953.1

Oyelese, Y., & Ananth, C. V. (2006). Placental abruption. *Obstetrics & Gynecology, 108*(4), 1005–1016. https://doi.org/10.1097/01.AOG.0000239439.04364.9a

Petrini, A., & Spandorfer, S. (2020). Recurrent ectopic pregnancy: Current perspectives. *International Journal of Women's Health, 12*, 597–600. https://doi.org/10.2147/IJWH.S223909

Pontius, E., & Vieth, J. T. (2019). Complications in early pregnancy. *Emergency Medicine Clinics of North America, 37*(2), 219–237. https://doi.org/10.1016/j.emc.2019.01.004

Prather, C., Fuller, T. R., Jeffries, W. L., IV, Marshall, K. J., Howell, A. V., Belyue-Umole, A., & King, W. (2018). Racism, African American women, and their sexual and reproductive health: A review of historical and contemporary evidence and implications for health equity. *Health Equity, 2*(1), 249–259. https://doi.org/10.1089/heq.2017.0045

Qiu, Y., Wu, L., Xiao, Y., & Zhang, X. (2021). Clinical analysis and classification of placental abruption. *The Journal of Maternal-Fetal & Neonatal Medicine, 34*(18), 1–5. https://doi.org/10.1080/14767058.2019.1675625

Quenby, S., Gallos, I. D., Dhillon-Smith, R. K., Podesek, M., Stephenson, M. D., Fisher, J., Brosens, J. J., Brewin, J., Ramhorst, R., Lucas, E. S., McCoy, R. C., Anderson, R., Daher, S., Regan, L., Al-Memar, M., Bourne, T., MacIntyre, D. A., Rai, R., Christiansen, O. B., & Sugiura-Ogasawara, M. (2021). Miscarriage matters: The epidemiological, physical, psychological, and economic costs of early pregnancy loss. *The Lancet, 397*(10285), 1658–1667. https://doi.org/10.1016/S0140-6736(21)00682-6

Ranzini, A. C., & Oyelese, Y. (2021). How to screen for vasa previa. *Ultrasound in Obstetrics & Gynecology, 57*(5), 720–725.

Renner, R. M., Brahmi, D., & Kapp, N. (2013). Who can provide effective and safe termination of pregnancy care? A systematic review. *BJOG: An International Journal of Obstetrics & Gynaecology, 120*(1), 23–31.

Shorter, J. M., Atrio, J. M., & Schreiber, C. A. (2019). Management of early pregnancy loss, with a focus on patient centered care. *Seminars in Perinatology, 43*(2), 84–94. https://doi.org/10.1053/j.semperi.2018.12.005

Silver, R. M. (2015). Abnormal placentation: Placenta previa, vasa previa, and placenta accreta. *Obstetrics & Gynecology, 126*(3), 654–668.

Soper, J. T. (2021). Gestational trophoblastic disease: Current evaluation and management. *Obstetric Anesthesia Digest, 41*(4), 168–169. https://doi.org/10.1097/01.aoa.0000796088.25096.4b

Tikkanen, M. (2011). Placental abruption: Epidemiology, risk factors and consequences. *Acta Obstetricia et Gynecologica Scandinavica, 90*(2), 140–149.

US Department of Health and Human Services. (2022). *Reinforcement of EMTALA obligations specific to patients who are pregnant or are experiencing pregnancy loss.* https://www.cms.gov/medicareprovider-enrollment-and-certificationsurveycertificationgeninfopolicy-and-memos-states-and/reinforcement-emtala-obligations-specific-patients-who-are-pregnant-or-are-experiencing-pregnancy-0

Zhu, H., Wang, M., Dong, Y., Hu, H., Zhang, Q., Qiao, C., Xie, X., Fan, F., Zeng, J., Jia, Y., Chen, L., Liu, J., Li, L., Zhai, Y., Zhao, Z., Shen, M., & Cao, Z. (2019). Detection of non-criteria autoantibodies in women without apparent causes for pregnancy loss. *Journal of Clinical Laboratory Analysis, 33*(9), e22994. https://doi.org/10.1002/jcla.22994

Zota, A. R., & VanNoy, B. N. (2021). Integrating intersectionality into the exposome paradigm: A novel approach to racial inequities in uterine fibroids. *American Journal of Public Health, 111*(1), 104–109.

34

Amniotic Fluid and Fetal Growth Disorders

Victoria H. Burslem and Cindy L. Farley

Relevant Terms

Amniotic fluid index (AFI)—the largest vertical pocket (LVP) of amniotic fluid visualized by ultrasound without the presence of umbilical cord measured in centimeters in each of the four maternal abdominal quadrants. The AFI is the sum of those four pockets. An AFI between 5 and 24 cm is considered normal

Amniotic fluid volume (AFV)—the total amniotic fluid present in utero

Arterial Doppler flow studies—a measurement of blood flow in the umbilical arteries, fetal aorta, and middle cerebral artery during the diastolic phase to determine downstream vascular resistance; commonly performed on the umbilical artery and expressed as a ratio of systolic to diastolic flow

Biophysical profile (BPP)—assessment of five fetal biophysical activities sensitive to hypoxia, including gross body movements, fetal breathing, fetal tone, AFV, and nonstress test (NST); scoring criteria have a strong correlation to fetal acidemia within one week of the test

Chorioamnionitis—an acute inflammation or infection of the membranes and chorion of the placenta, also referred to as "Triple I" (intrauterine inflammation or infection or both)

Deepest (maximal) vertical pocket (DVP or MVP)—a reliable method for estimating AFV on ultrasound, done by measuring a pocket of maximal depth of amniotic fluid free of umbilical cord and fetal parts; normal range is considered 2–8 cm

Doppler velocimetry—a Doppler flow ultrasonic measurement of the arterial and/or venous vascular beds in the fetus to detect normal or abnormal uteroplacental blood flow patterns

Fern test—a microscopic examination of a fluid sample obtained on a cotton-tipped swab from the posterior fornix of the vagina by sterile speculum exam. If present, amniotic fluid will crystallize on the slide due to its high sodium chloride concentration, seen as a fern pattern

Fetal growth restriction (FGR)—inadequate growth of the fetus in utero, leading to a failure to attain full growth potential; also known as intrauterine growth restriction (IUGR)

Idiopathic—arising spontaneously or occurring without a known cause

Individual growth potential curve—methodology for assessing optimal growth potential in both fetal and newborn weight calculated by computer software that is based on a number of variables, which include fetal sex and the maternal characteristics of height, weight in first trimester, parity, and ethnic origin

Large for gestational age (LGA)—newborn weight greater than or equal to the 90th percentile for gestational age; one range of a method used to classify neonates into risk categories by weight relative to gestational age

Low birth weight (LBW)—newborn weight <2500 g; one range of a method used to classify neonates into risk categories by weight; not categorized in relation to gestational age

Macrosomia—variously defined as birth weight greater than 4000 or 4500 g. Recent literature has described it as 4000 g in a pregnant person with diabetes (of any type, due to increased fetal abdominal circumference) or 4500 g in pregnant person without diabetes; an abdominal circumference of >35 cm identifies >90% of macrosomic infants

Modified biophysical profile (modified BPP)—the combined results of an NST and AFI, two of the BPP components most associated with accurate assessment of current fetal status

Nonstress test (NST)—antenatal assessment of the fetal heart rate (FHR) pattern. A reactive FHR pattern in the normal range of 110–160 beats per minute with variability, two accelerations, and no decelerations over a 20-minute period has a very low likelihood of adverse perinatal outcomes within one week following the test

Oligohydramnios—less than normal AFV; variously defined as ≤200–500 mL, an LVP of <2 cm or an AFI of ≤5 cm

Placental lake—intravillous spaces in the placenta filled with maternal blood found on ultrasound; a few can be normal; multiple lakes can be associated IUGR

Placentation—formation of the placental structure

Polyhydramnios—greater than normal AFV; commonly defined as >2,100 mL, an AFI of ≥25 cm at any gestational age, or a single measurement of any LVP >8 cm

Prenatal and Postnatal Care: A Person-Centered Approach, Third Edition. Edited by Karen Trister Grace, Cindy L. Farley, Noelene K. Jeffers, and Tanya Tringali.
© 2024 John Wiley & Sons Ltd. Published 2024 by John Wiley & Sons Ltd.
Companion website: www.wiley.com/go/grace/prenatal

Ponderal index—the ratio of birth weight to length [(birth weight (g)/crown heel length)³ × 100]

Small for gestational age (SGA)—a weight for gestation below a given threshold; commonly defined as less than or equal to the 10th percentile; may be associated with FGR or may be constitutionally small with a normal growth pattern

Targeted ultrasound—also known as a level II ultrasound; this ultrasound examination is done by a certified technician to look for specific fetal anomalies or conditions

Very small for gestational age (VSGA)—less than the third percentile (>2 SD below normal); associated with a significantly increased risk of poor outcome

Introduction

The gestational intrauterine environment is influenced by multiple factors, each of which has the ability to significantly impact fetal growth and development, positively or negatively. Placental development and functioning, amniotic fluid production and volume, as well as numerous maternal and fetal conditions, all contribute individually and cumulatively to the environmental factors influencing perinatal health outcomes. This chapter provides a review of normal amniotic fluid physiology, normal **placentation**, and patterns of fetal development, along with maternal, fetal, and placental conditions that contribute to abnormal amniotic fluid and fetal growth patterns.

Health equity key points

- Past studies exploring racial and ethnic differences in amniotic fluid and fetal growth patterns demonstrated higher intrauterine inflammatory responses in African Americans and other people of color. There was no or limited consideration of the role of the chronic stress of racism in the genesis of these physiologic responses in this body of evidence.
- Heightened immunomodulatory responses leading to higher rates of amniotic fluid and fetal growth disorders, such as chorioamnionitis and low birth weight neonates, found in African Americans and other people of color are driven primarily by social and economic factors and systemic racism.

Amniotic Fluid Dynamics

The amniotic fluid is a clear, watery liquid that contains several components. The main component is water; within this water, there is a soluble component consisting of carbohydrates, proteins, lipids, electrolytes, and metabolites. The insoluble component contains lanugo, vernix, and cellular elements, such as fetal epithelial cells (Mao et al., 2019). Amniotic fluid is found within the amniotic cavity by six weeks of gestation from the last menstrual period (LMP).

Amniotic fluid surrounds the fetus during intrauterine development and is vital to the well-being of the fetus. Amniotic fluid cushions the fetus from abdominal trauma to the pregnant person, provides a constant temperature, protects the umbilical cord from compression, and provides the necessary fluid, space, and growth factors to allow normal development of the fetal lungs and musculoskeletal and gastrointestinal systems. Amniotic fluid also

contains antibacterial properties that help protect the fetus from infection. Studies of the amniotic fluid through amniocentesis provide fetal genetic karyotyping and information about fetal lung maturity. Given the important functions of amniotic fluid, it is not surprising that abnormalities in **amniotic fluid volume (AFV)** are associated with increased perinatal morbidity and mortality.

Amniotic fluid maintains a balanced volume by constantly being produced and reabsorbed in a dynamic process that increases with gestational age. Early in pregnancy, most amniotic fluid comes from the pregnant person. By the second trimester, the fetus contributes to AFV and composition through the production of lung fluid and, predominantly, through urination. During the first half of pregnancy, AFV correlates with fetal weight and, thus, is fairly predictable. At 10 weeks of gestation, the average volume is 30 mL; at 16 weeks, it is 190 mL.

After 20 weeks of gestation, there is a greater variation in volume of amniotic fluid, with a general increase in total volume up to approximately 33 weeks of gestation. Around this time, the AFV plateaus. Near 38 weeks of gestation, volume starts to decline by an estimated 125 mL/week to an average volume of 800 mL by 40 weeks of gestation (Blackburn, 2018) (Figure 34.1). There is a wide range of normal biological variability to the volume that fluctuates from day to day within the same individual. Changes in AFV tend to occur gradually; however, modest changes can be influenced by hydration and activity of the pregnant person (Lim et al., 2017). After 40 weeks of gestation, it declines at a rate of 8% a week,

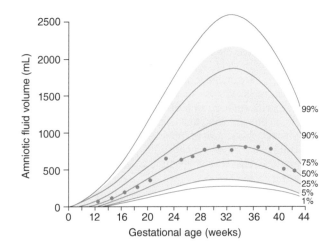

Figure 34.1 Nomogram showing amniotic fluid volume as a function of gestational age. The points indicate the mean for each two-week interval. Brace and Wolf (1989)/with permission of Elsevier.

with an average of 400 mL volume at 42 weeks of gestation (Blackburn, 2018).

The fetus begins to swallow amniotic fluid at 16–18 weeks of gestation. Near term, a fetus swallows from 200 to 500 mL/day, removing 50% of the amniotic fluid produced through fetal urination (Brace & Cheung, 2014). This fluid is absorbed through the fetal gastrointestinal system and is either recycled through the kidneys or is transferred to the tissues of the pregnant person through the placenta. Near term, the turnover of amniotic fluid is approximately 1000 mL/day regardless of the total volume present.

There is recent interest and increased debate about microbial transfer at the feto/neonatal–maternal interface. One study challenged the long-held belief that the amniotic fluid and uterine cavity are sterile environments in normal pregnancies (Collado et al., 2016). These researchers characterized the placenta and membranes as permeable, not impenetrable, barriers and suggested that in-utero seeding of the fetal microbiome begins through oral and vaginal flora transfer via the pregnant person's bloodstream to the placenta. However, studies since that time have confirmed that prior to the onset of uterine contractions and rupture of membranes (ROM), the amniotic fluid is devoid of microbes in uncomplicated term pregnancies (Lim et al., 2018; Rehbinder et al., 2018). Neonatal gut colonization is initiated through the bacteria picked up through the birth process, skin-to-skin contact, and breastfeeding. While the health implications of this finding are not yet fully understood, the maternal microbiota during pregnancy may influence fetal and infant health. The newborn microbial gut colonization process appears to be a physiologic phenomenon with potential to influence short-term and long-term health.

Placentation and Perinatal Outcomes

Fetal development is largely dependent on proper implantation and function of the placenta, beginning with its formation and secure attachment to the uterine wall by day 10 after fertilization (Figure 34.2). The cytotrophoblast, the embryo at seven days after fertilization, forms several types of extravillous trophoblastic tissue, the tissue responsible for the formation of the placenta. By 10–12 weeks of gestation, the trophoblast has eroded the maternal spiral arterioles sufficiently so that blood flows into the intervillous spaces, signaling a properly maturing placenta. The placenta serves a number of functions during pregnancy, including immunologic acceptance of the fetus, transfer of nutrients and gases, heat regulation, and removal of waste products. The placenta also performs as an endocrine organ, secreting over 100 peptides and steroids influencing adaptation to pregnancy and fetal health. Further details of placental formation are found in Chapter 4, *Conception, Implantation, and Embryonic and Fetal Health.*

The placenta is formed by the chorionic villi of the embryo and the decidua basalis of the endometrium of the mother.

A number of pregnancy complications can be related back to the process of trophoblastic invasion. The extent and degree of the placental vascular lesions resulting from defective placentation explains the varied clinical presentations and degree of severity. For example, if the invasive process is defective with only 10% of the spiral arterioles fully penetrated into the endometrium, rather than the 96% penetration seen in a normal pregnancy, the placenta will fail to establish proper maternal circulation and the fetus will die (Osol & Moore, 2014). This defective process of invasion has been definitively associated with spontaneous abortion, preeclampsia, **fetal growth restriction (FGR)**, preterm labor, and fetal death (Knöfler et al., 2019). Conversely, reduced arteriole invasion may actually be the result of a conceptus that is defective as in the case of chromosomal abnormalities. The health of the uterine cavity plays a role in how well placentation proceeds. Pregnant individuals with abnormal endometrial glandular tissue and those with scarring from cesarean sections or other uterine surgeries are at greater risk of developing abnormal placentation and its associated morbidities (Mainigi et al., 2014; Poonia et al., 2017).

Throughout pregnancy, the fetus is in a constant state of rapid growth, in both cellular formation and cellular size. To meet this need, uteroplacental blood flow increases throughout the pregnancy, resulting in a greater than 50-fold increase in uterine blood flow as compared to the nonpregnant person. Placental growth and factors contributing to vasodilation of maternal arteries permit the increased uterine blood flow that result from a blood volume increase of 40% and a doubling of the pregnant person's cardiac output. A disruption to either the placental attachment process or the uterine blood flow will impact fetal growth and development; the greater and longer the disruption, the greater the insult.

Amniotic Fluid Disorders

Oligohydramnios

Oligohydramnios is diagnosed by ultrasound and defined by varying parameters, such as an AFV of <200 mL, a **deepest vertical pocket (DVP)** of <2 cm, or an **amniotic fluid index (AFI)** of <5 cm. The DVP was found to be the best predictor of fetuses at risk for adverse perinatal outcomes in a recent meta-analysis (Kehl et al., 2016; Rabie et al., 2017). Figure 34.3 shows AFI values at various points in gestation.

The exact incidence of oligohydramnios is difficult to determine since varying criteria are used to establish a diagnosis, but the generally accepted rate is between 1% and 3% of all pregnancies. Approximately 20% of pregnancies requiring increased antepartum surveillance for a maternal or fetal condition also have oligohydramnios (Kehl et al., 2016). Amniotic fluid disorders should be suspected whenever there is a clinically significant discrepancy in fundal height measurement, prompting an ultrasound evaluation of fluid status.

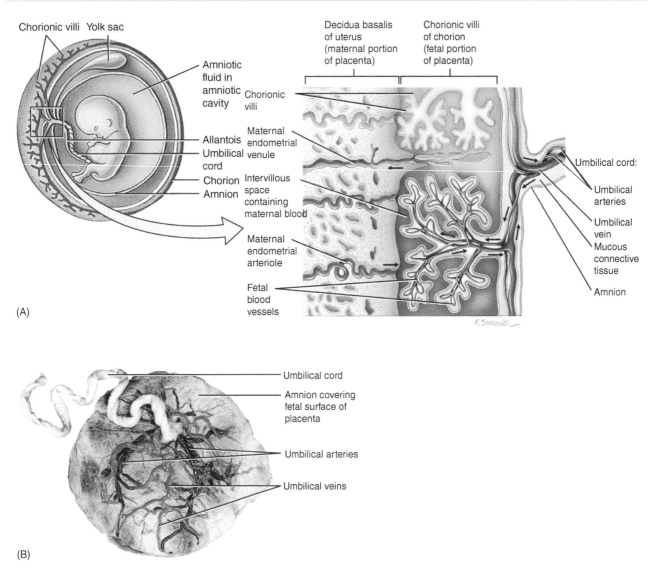

Figure 34.2 Formation of the placenta and umbilical cord. (A) Details of the placenta and umbilical cord. (B) Fetal surface of the placenta. Tortora and Derrickson (2017)/with permission from John Wiley & Sons.

Oligohydramnios is associated with a number of fetal and maternal conditions, including fetal renal abnormalities, placental insufficiency, and abnormalities of the amnion. It also may simply be an isolated, **idiopathic** condition not associated with any underlying pathology. Understanding the timing of onset as well as the cause of oligohydramnios is paramount because implications for perinatal outcomes and, therefore, prenatal management of the condition, vary significantly (Sammour & Sagi, 2019). There is no consensus regarding management of idiopathic oligohydramnios. Early induction is being questioned due to growing evidence of increased neonatal morbidity with late-preterm and early-term inductions.

Oligohydramnios that develops in the second trimester is considered early onset and has a high perinatal mortality rate (PMR) due to the etiologies associated with it (Kehl et al., 2016). Early-onset oligohydramnios is commonly caused by fetal anomalies, such as renal agenesis, dysplasia, or obstructive disorders, where there is either a lack of urine production or the inability to pass urine. Because fetal urine is a necessary component of amniotic fluid that contributes to fetal lung development, some renal anomalies carry a PMR close to 100%. With preterm prelabor rupture of membranes (PPROM), another etiology for midpregnancy oligohydramnios, the PMR will depend on fetal gestational age and the presence of other conditions that may result from PPROM, like chorioamnionitis.

In the third trimester, oligohydramnios is more commonly associated with either uteroplacental insufficiency or postterm pregnancy. However, in the presence of an otherwise normal pregnancy, a significant percentage of third-trimester onset oligohydramnios is idiopathic, resolving spontaneously in three to four days or in response to increased maternal hydration. The clinical management dilemma in the third trimester results from oligohydramnios having an association with poor fetal outcomes. Low AFV should not be the sole indication for an expedited birth (Modi et al., 2016; Sammour & Sagi, 2019). The clinical condition of the pregnant person and their fetus must also be considered for management decisions in a shared

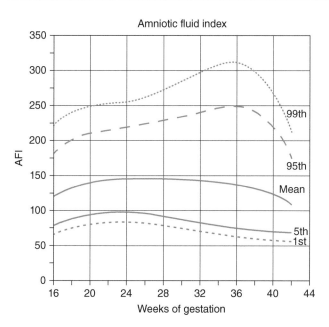

Figure 34.3   Amniotic fluid index (in millimeters) plotted with gestational age (weeks). The solid line denotes the 50th percentile; dashed lines, the 5th and 95th percentiles; and dotted lines, +2 standard deviations (2.5th and 97.5th percentiles). Adapted from Moore and Cayle (1990).

decision-making model. Expectant management is preferred over intervention by induction when the decision is based solely on an isolated low AFI. Neonatal outcomes are similar between the two management options and unwarranted interventions can lead to potential harms for the pregnant individual's short- and long-term health (Sammour & Sagi, 2019). The importance of differentiating idiopathic oligohydramnios from that associated with an abnormal maternal or fetal condition is in the recognition of risks inherent to labor induction with an unfavorable cervix. If all other fetal assessment and surveillance parameters are normal, the risks of cesarean section due to failed induction must be taken into account in the provider's and the patient's clinical decision-making process.

Causes of oligohydramnios

In the Fetus

- Renal agenesis
- Urinary tract obstruction
- Prelabor spontaneous rupture of the membranes
- Abnormal placentation
- Elevated maternal serum alpha-fetoprotein (AFP)
- Postterm pregnancy
- Severe FGR

In the Pregnant Person

- Idiopathic
- Dehydration
- Hypertensive disorders
- Uteroplacental insufficiency
- Antiphospholipid syndrome

Oligohydramnios found in association with hypertensive disorders or FGR carries a high risk of poor perinatal outcomes. The low fluid volume is due to decreased fetal kidney perfusion, a result of the vascular constriction that accompanies hypertension, or placental insufficiency resulting from poor placentation in early gestation. While the PMR of later-onset oligohydramnios is not as high as that associated with early onset, it nonetheless has a strong association with perinatal morbidity and mortality and has been linked to cerebral palsy (CP) and adult-onset cardiovascular disease (Modi et al., 2016). Late pregnancy oligohydramnios is generally the result of a maternal condition requiring close observation and prudent decision-making for the timing of birth. An evaluation of the environment that is best for the fetus, in utero or extrauterine, is determined by close monitoring with tests that assess fetal status.

Postterm pregnancy is another etiology of late-onset oligohydramnios (Murzakanova et al., 2020). Although AFV has a wide range of normal variations, it is known to decrease from an average of 700–800 mL at 40 weeks of gestation to 400 mL by 42 weeks of gestation. Oligohydramnios in a postterm pregnancy is associated with an increased risk of meconium-stained amniotic fluid (MSAF), fetal intolerance of labor, neonatal intensive care unit (NICU) admissions, and poor neonatal outcomes. Meconium aspiration syndrome, with its risk of chemical pneumonitis and neonatal death, is one of the more serious sequelae associated with MSAF in the presence of oligohydramnios.

Diagnosis and Management

Accurate pregnancy dating and serial assessment of fundal height are essential to detecting oligohydramnios. Leopold maneuvers reveal an easily palpated fetus when amniotic fluid is low. If the fundal height is measuring smaller than expected by dates, a screening ultrasound should be obtained to confirm the expected date of birth (EDB) and evaluate fluid volume. The status of the amniotic sac should be evaluated by history and physical exam as indicated. If screening ultrasound for dating has been performed and EDB is confirmed, a **targeted ultrasound** should be scheduled to obtain an anatomy scan and AFV. This will assist in determining if fetal anomalies or signs of aneuploidy are the cause of the oligohydramnios; if these are suspected, genetic counseling and testing are offered. If PPROM is suspected, verification can be done through sterile speculum exam for pooling of amniotic fluid in the posterior vagina, nitrazine test to assess if vaginal pH has changed from acid to neutral, **fern test**, or point-of-care ROM test.

Serial Doppler blood flow studies have advanced to allow evaluation of the fetal renal circulation in addition to umbilical artery and cerebral artery blood flow (Refaat et al., 2021). These studies can provide information on current fetal status with data that support either expectant management or the need to intervene and facilitate birth. If expectant management is chosen, fetal surveillance procedures such as fetal movement counting, **nonstress testing (NST)**, **biophysical profile (BPP)**, or the **modified BPP** are done.

Management of pregnancy with oligohydramnios after 40 weeks of gestation is the source of significant debate in the professional and lay literature, concerning the value and type of antepartum surveillance, the pros and cons of spontaneous labor versus induction of labor, and the decision about if and when to intervene. This is a multifaceted issue, and discussion with a pregnant person includes the findings of current well-designed studies, along with the individual's cultural perspective and personal preferences. Current evidence suggests that the induction of labor at or after 41 weeks of gestation is not associated with an increase in cesarean section compared to expectant management. This finding is reassuring to healthcare providers desiring to minimize the risk of poor neonatal outcomes and to maximize the probability of a vaginal birth. Labor induction at 41 weeks of gestation or beyond may improve perinatal outcome slightly, but if fetal and maternal status are reassuring, either induction or expectant management is a reasonable choice (Murzakanova et al., 2020).

Simple hydration is an effective, evidence-based treatment for oligohydramnios, particularly in cases of idiopathic oligohydramnios (Azarkish et al., 2022). Maternal hydration is safe, easily implemented and tolerated, and inexpensive. Oral or intravenous routes or a combination can be used; hypotonic fluids seem to work best in restoring volume in the amniotic fluid compartment. Extreme oligohydramnios has been treated with transabdominal amnioinfusion in rare cases.

Mild idiopathic oligohydramnios can be managed expectantly while awaiting spontaneous labor. The decision to continue expectant management with monitoring or to schedule an induction is one that is determined in collaboration with the pregnant person and after consultation or referral to a physician colleague, depending on the practice model and setting.

Polyhydramnios

Polyhydramnios, greater than normal amniotic fluid, is defined as a DVP of >8 cm and an AFI of >24 cm at any gestational age (Dashe et al., 2018). The overall incidence of polyhydramnios is 1–3%; the earlier it develops, the longer it persists, and the greater deviation from normal fluid volume, the greater the perinatal morbidity and mortality. Polyhydramnios can develop gradually or rapidly, with or without a cause identified, and may benignly run its course or be associated with poor maternal and/or fetal outcomes. The pathophysiology underlying polyhydramnios is most often related to impaired fetal swallowing or overproduction of fetal urine. These mechanisms disrupt the normal turnover of amniotic fluid, allowing fluid to accumulate.

When no etiology is determined, polyhydramnios is deemed idiopathic, and this represents over half of cases. Mild idiopathic polyhydramnios is generally associated with positive outcomes and managed expectantly (Dashe et al., 2018). However, moderate to severe polyhydramnios is found to be associated with significant fetal and maternal conditions. Congenital fetal anomalies, primarily gastrointestinal, cardiac, and neural tube defects, aneuploidy, preterm birth, multiple gestation, **macrosomia**, fetal intolerance of labor, meconium-stained fluid, emergency cesarean sections, cord pH <7, low 5-minute Apgar scores, and increased NICU admissions all are fetal conditions or outcomes found in conjunction with polyhydramnios. Maternal conditions associated with polyhydramnios are poorly controlled type I or II diabetes and fetal-maternal hemorrhage. Placental abruption and postpartum hemorrhage are serious maternal outcomes that can result from polyhydramnios due to uterine overdistension (Vanda et al., 2022).

Causes of polyhydramnios

In the Fetus

- Gastrointestinal disorders: duodenal atresia, gastroschisis, diaphragmatic hernia
- Central nervous system abnormalities: anencephaly, other neural tube defects
- Cystic hygromas
- Nonimmune hydrops
- Some genetic syndromes
- Congenital infections: toxoplasmosis, rubella, cytomegalovirus (CMV), herpes simplex, parvovirus B19
- Placental abnormalities
- Twin-to-twin transfusion syndrome

In the Pregnant Person

- Idiopathic
- Poorly controlled diabetes mellitus
- Maternal-fetal hemorrhage

Diagnosis and Management

Accurate pregnancy dating and serial assessment of fundal height are essential to detecting polyhydramnios. Fundal height can measure larger than expected for gestational age. Leopold maneuvers may reveal an easily ballotable fetus and an unstable lie may be noted. A fluid thrill can be elicited in polyhydramnios by placing the palm of one hand flat on one side of the uterus, tapping the other side of the uterus, and noting vibrations on the palm of the palpating hand. Medical and family history of diabetes and the results of any screening tests for gestational diabetes mellitus (GDM) should be reviewed. A repeat screen for gestational diabetes can be considered if sudden onset polyhydramnios occurs with a prior high-normal testing result. Serial Doppler blood flow studies are typically obtained for a pregnancy confirmed to have polyhydramnios. Fetal surveillance measures depend on the etiology of polyhydramnios, but include various schedules of fetal movement counting, NSTs, and BPPs or modified BPPs.

While polyhydramnios is associated with few symptoms in the pregnant person, severe forms can lead to respiratory difficulties due to the pressure of the expanded uterus. Treatment of severe polyhydramnios may include administration of a prostaglandin synthetase inhibitor, such as indomethacin, administered to decrease production of fetal urine, increase fluid reabsorption by the fetal lungs, and increase the amount of intermembranous fluid movement from the fetus to the pregnant person (Vanda et al., 2022). AFV has been noted to decrease within 24 hours of the administration. Prostaglandin synthetase inhibitors as a long-term treatment option are limited due to serious maternal and fetal side effects noted with exposure, particularly if given after 32 weeks of gestation.

Removal of fluid by serial amniocentesis reductions may be done in individuals with severe polyhydramnios (Erfani et al., 2019). This is an effective method of removing from 1 to 5 L of amniotic fluid; however, it must be repeated since the amniotic fluid is regenerated in the body every 48–72 hours. Theoretical risks to this procedure are ROM, preterm labor, and placental abruption if the uterine volume is decompressed too rapidly; however, these are uncommon outcomes (Erfani et al., 2019). This management strategy is typically reserved for those suffering from acute cardiopulmonary decompensation due to the polyhydramnios and is most frequently used in twin-to-twin transfusion syndrome.

Postnatal follow-up of infants born after idiopathic polyhydramnios in pregnancy is important. Not all anomalies are visible on prenatal ultrasound. One study found chromosomal or genetic disorders on follow-up in about 13% of neonates with a prenatal diagnosis of polyhydramnios (Boito et al., 2016). The severity of polyhydramnios and maternal perception of reduced fetal movements were independently associated with the presence of such anomalies.

Mild idiopathic polyhydramnios can be managed expectantly while awaiting spontaneous labor. The decision to continue expectant management with monitoring or to schedule an induction is one that is determined in collaboration with the pregnant person and after consultation or referral to a physician colleague, depending on the practice model and setting.

Chorioamnionitis or Triple I

Chorioamnionitis is a polymicrobial ascending infection affecting the fetal membranes—the chorion and amnion—as well as the surrounding fluid. The term "intrauterine inflammation or infection or both" abbreviated as "Triple I" has been suggested by a National Institute of Child Health and Human Development (NICHD) expert panel to replace the term chorioamnionitis to more accurately represent the pathophysiologic processes involved (Higgins et al., 2016). Prevalence estimates are 2–4% of the general population of pregnant people and up to 70% of those who give birth preterm (Peng et al., 2018). Laboratory testing is confirmatory but is often not timely for clinical decision-making, so diagnosis is based on clinical signs and symptoms. The primary clinical marker for chorioamnionitis is maternal fever >38 °C (>100.4 °F) that persists for more than an hour once other potential diagnoses have been investigated, such as dehydration, overheating from hydrotherapy, or epidural-related fever. Clinical markers are nonspecific; look for multiple markers to support a diagnosis of Triple I. Treating all maternal fevers with antibiotics results in overtreatment and can cause harm.

Clinical markers for chorioamnionitis

- Maternal fever >38 °C (>100.4 °F) persisting more than 1 hour
- Maternal white blood cell count >15 000 mm^3
- Maternal tachycardia >100 bpm
- Fetal tachycardia >160 bpm
- Uterine tenderness
- Foul-smelling amniotic fluid or vaginal discharge

Although this infection is often recognized during labor, its origin can be in the prenatal period. Infection and inflammation are strongly associated with preterm birth. Placental lesions indicating chronic or acute chorioamnionitis are commonly found on histological examination with spontaneous preterm birth (Peng et al., 2018). The mechanisms that lead from infection to preterm birth are not fully understood; however, inflammation is believed to play a significant role. Bacterial infection of the amniotic membranes, amniotic fluid, or placenta causes increased prostaglandin production. Prostaglandins are associated with increased uterine activity, cervical softening, and dilation that may ultimately result in preterm labor and birth. However, clinical trials of prophylactic antibiotic treatment in pregnant people at high risk for preterm birth have not consistently demonstrated efficacy, and some clinical trials have suggested harm.

Prompt diagnosis and treatment are essential, as serious sequelae can occur, including complications such as endometritis and sepsis, and neonatal pneumonia, sepsis, and CP. The most common treatment for chorioamnionitis is the combination of ampicillin or penicillin plus gentamicin. These antibiotics specifically target the two organisms most likely to cause neonatal infection—Group B Streptococcus (GBS) and *Escherichia coli*. Clindamycin is used for those who are allergic to penicillin. Acetaminophen can be given for fever.

Prelabor Rupture of Membranes

Prelabor rupture of membranes (PROM) is defined as the ROM before the onset of labor; it occurs in approximately 8–10% of term pregnancies (Marowitz, 2016). The majority of individuals with term PROM will enter labor within 28 hours, up to 95% without intervention (ACNM, 2018; Middleton et al., 2017). The pathophysiologic mechanism leading to PROM is theorized to be local inflammatory processes that weaken the membranes which then yield to biomechanical pressures. PROM is usually first suspected by patient report of leaking vaginal fluid; however, other diagnoses must be considered. Questions to rule out urinary incontinence, recent sexual intercourse, and vaginal discharge should be posed. The diagnosis of PROM can be complicated by a slow or intermittent amniotic fluid leak or blood in vaginal discharge (Ghafoor, 2021).

It is important to verify ROM with a sterile speculum exam and to scrupulously avoid a digital vaginal exam. Digital vaginal exams for membrane and cervical status introduce vaginal microbes into the lower uterus, essentially setting the stage for chorioamnionitis. Individuals with ≥8 cervical exams had 1.7 times the risk of developing chorioamnionitis compared with those with one to three exams (Slagle et al., 2022). Rupture can be verified with visual inspection when copious fluid is coming from the vagina. Color and odor should be noted. When ROM is not obvious, nitrazine, fern tests, or point-of-care ROM tests, such as Amnisure®, can be used. Management options for term PROM can be developed based on verified rupture alone without a digital vaginal exam. Options include expectant management and immediate induction, typically with low-dose oxytocin induction protocols. Expectant management is an important option to offer those with term PROM (ACNM, 2018).

Maternal and fetal/neonatal infection and cord compression are the primary concerns for term PROM; these concerns are raised with the loss of the protection that an intact amniotic sac provides to the laboring person and their baby. Induction of labor at time of term PROM may reduce the risk of infection, but it does not reduce rates of serious morbidity or mortality (ACNM, 2018; Middleton et al., 2017). Expectant management is an option for individuals with term PROM that promotes physiologic birth and decreases the need for intervention. Clients eligible for expectant management include those individuals who are afebrile with a single vertex fetus, reactive NST, clear fluid, GBS negative, or prophylaxis initiated if positive (ACNM, 2018; Marowitz, 2016). Clients can be sent home or admitted to the hospital; instructions or orders include temperature every 4 hours while awake, nothing per vagina, and repeat NST the following day if no labor ensues.

PPROM is ROM that occurs before the pregnancy has reached 37 weeks; management rests on gestational age considerations, underlying infection, and other concomitant conditions. PPROM occurs in approximately 3% of US births (Kuba & Bernstein, 2018). Management options are similar to term PROM—expectant management versus induction of labor. However, gestational age is a key consideration. The patient should be transferred to a facility equipped to care for the preterm infant in the event of spontaneous labor arising and the neonatal team should be notified. Additionally, a course of antenatal corticosteroids is considered to assist in accelerating the maturation of the fetal lungs. Treatment reduces the risk of perinatal death, neonatal death, respiratory distress disease, and intraventricular hemorrhage (McGoldrick et al., 2020). A single course of corticosteroids is recommended for pregnant individuals with ruptured membranes between 24 0/7 weeks and 33 6/7 weeks of gestation who are at risk of preterm birth within 7 days (ACOG, 2017). For those pregnant people between 34 0/7 weeks and 36 6/7 weeks at risk of preterm birth, a single course of betamethasone is recommended if they have not received antenatal corticosteroids previously (ACOG, 2017).

Fetal Growth Disorders

Determination of Growth Disorders

Historically, the terms **small for gestational age** (SGA) and FGR have been used interchangeably. This practice evolved because, prior to the advent of diagnostic fetal ultrasound assessment, research into fetal growth and development was based solely on neonatal outcomes. Earlier twentieth century observers noted that two parameters were associated with newborn outcomes, gestational age, and birth weight, with the distinction between them not yet clear. By the 1960s, newborn birth weight ranges had become standardized, providing an initial frame of reference for weight relative to outcome. These weight classifications are:

- extremely low birth weight (ELBW <1000 g)
- very low birth weight (VLBW <1500 g)
- **low birth weight** (LBW <2500 g)
- macrosomia (>4000 g).

With advancements in the field of neonatology, it was ascertained that a newborn's weight relative to gestational age enabled the prediction of perinatal and neonatal morbidity and mortality. Population-based reference ranges of birth weight relative to gestational age norms were developed, adding significantly to clinicians' ability to assess risks and to determine management strategies. The classifications are:

- **very small for gestational age** (VSGA; less than the 3rd percentile)
- small for gestational age (SGA; less than the 10th percentile)
- appropriate for gestational age (AGA; 10th to the 90th percentile)
- **large for gestational age** (LGA; greater than the 90th percentile; Figure 34.4)

While this methodology brought great improvement in the ability to further identify infants at greater risk, it did not take into account differences inherent to a neonate's anthropometric measurements. Therefore, a newborn could fit by weight in the AGA category but have FGR by characteristics, while an SGA infant by weight could simply be constitutionally small, resulting in false negatives and false positives (Sharma et al., 2016a, 2016b). To address this flaw, the **ponderal index** was developed, defined as the ratio of birth weight to length (crown to heel). This classification was the first methodology that

Gestational age birth weight percentiles

Week of gestation	5th	10th	50th	90th	95th
24	539	567	680	850	988
25	540	584	765	938	997
26	580	637	872	1080	1180
27	650	719	997	1260	1467
28	740	822	1138	1462	1787
29	841	939	1290	1672	2070
30	952	1068	1455	1883	2294
31	1080	1214	1635	2101	2483
32	1232	1380	1833	2331	2664
33	1414	1573	2053	2579	2861
34	1632	1793	2296	2846	3093
35	1871	2030	2549	3119	3345
36	2117	2270	2797	3380	3594
37	2353	2500	3025	3612	3818
38	2564	2706	3219	3799	3995
39	2737	2877	3374	3941	4125
40	2863	3005	3499	4057	4232
41	2934	3082	3600	4167	4340
42	2941	3099	3686	4290	4474

Figure 34.4 Birth weight percentiles throughout gestation. Duryea et al. (2014)/Wolters Kluwer Health, Inc.

appeared to more closely correlate with actual perinatal morbidity and outcomes (Walther & Ramaekers, 1982; Weiner & Robinson, 1989). More recent studies, however, failed to demonstrate that longitudinal growth assessment alone is predictive of adverse outcomes (Figueras et al., 2018).

Coinciding with the advancements in treatment options available to neonatologists, the field of ultrasound technology was growing in its ability to analyze fetal growth patterns prior to birth. A new avenue of research opened, focused on the identification of in-utero patterns of abnormal growth, while exploring fetal assessment modalities and antenatal intervention to improve outcomes. Concern arose as studies began to show that some neonates diagnosed with FGR in utero were being incorrectly identified, leading to unnecessary intervention and iatrogenic prematurity, adding both cost and morbidity without benefit (Figueras et al., 2018). In fact, while the morbidity and mortality risks have been well documented for newborns who weigh less than the 10th percentile for gestational age, 18–22% of newborns in the SGA category are normally developed, small newborns who are not at risk for adverse outcome (SMFM et al., 2020).

Recent research has identified yet another improvement in the ability to correctly identify and classify fetal growth and birth weight: an **individual growth potential curve**. This model assesses a customized growth potential calculated for each fetus in each pregnancy, applying this new standard to fetal weight as well as birth weight. The model is customized for fetal sex in addition to maternal characteristics of height, weight, parity, and ethnic origin (Fay et al., 2021; Gardosi et al., 2018; Sharma et al., 2016a). The optimal birth weight that is calculated is then projected backward for all gestational ages, thus avoiding the standard of preterm neonatal weights, which are skewed by the pathology of many preterm neonates. Research validates that the use of this methodology results in more correct identification of fetuses and newborns previously categorized as SGA by population referencing, as normal size by customized growth potential calculations and not at risk. Additionally, this calculation identifies a substantial number of fetuses greater than the 10th percentile that are actually FGR and at risk (Deter et al., 2018; Gardosi et al., 2018). In this text, FGR will refer to those neonates identified as growth restricted as defined by an estimated fetal weight (EFW) or abdominal circumference (AC) less than the 10th percentile for gestational age and SGA will refer to those neonates constitutionally small, less than the 10th percentile for gestational age, but not growth restricted (American College of Obstetricians and Gynecologists (ACOG) 2021; SMFM et al., 2020).

A stronger association of abnormal Doppler studies, fetal intolerance of labor, need for cesarean birth, NICU admissions, stillbirths, and neonatal deaths has been found with infants identified as having actual FGR by the customized growth potential model (Figueras et al., 2018; Gardosi et al., 2018). Evidence is mounting that validates this approach, with the anticipation that growth potential curves will become the standard tool utilized for antenatal identification of a fetus at risk (Deter et al., 2018; SMFM et al., 2020).

Fetal Growth Restriction

FGR, also known as intrauterine growth restriction (IUGR), is defined as the failure of a fetus to achieve its genetic growth potential in utero as indicated by EFW < 10th percentile and/or AC < 10th percentile for gestational age (SMFM et al., 2020). While the various weight classifications focus primarily on establishing neonatal risk status by birth weight, the focus of FGR is on the impact of the prenatal environment on current fetal well-being. FGR is the second highest cause of perinatal mortality, after prematurity. The negative effects of FGR are well documented and include increased perinatal and neonatal morbidity and mortality, long-term neurologic impairment with developmental delays and disabilities, and in-utero metabolic programming associated with cardiovascular and endocrine diseases (Li et al., 2020). While FGR affects 10% of pregnancies, it is associated with 28–45% of nonanomalous stillbirths and a two- to fivefold increased rate of perinatal deaths in FGR preterm fetuses compared with term infants (Kalpashri & Devaskar, 2019; McCowan et al., 2018; Ortigosa Rocha et al., 2010; SMFM et al., 2020).

The causes of FGR are multifactorial, with approximately one-third due to genetic abnormalities and two-thirds related to the fetal environment. Maternal, placental, fetal, and environmental factors are individually or synergistically potential contributors to this condition. FGR is detected by a slowing growth pattern on serial ultrasounds overall and, in particular, with an AC in the <10th percentile for gestational age.

The literature differentiates FGR by the gestational age of development, with early-onset FGR, typically more severe, diagnosed at <32 weeks' gestation and late-onset FGR, commonly with milder presentation, diagnosed >32 weeks' gestation. These designations are important in helping to determine the most appropriate surveillance and management for prevention of poor outcomes and long-term sequalae (Figueras et al., 2018; SMFM et al., 2020). FGR is also described in relation to its impact on fetal cell development, with symmetric FGR, where the entire fetal body is proportionally small, accounting for 25% of cases and associated with worse outcomes. Asymmetric FGR, where the fetal head and brain are the expected size while the rest of the body is smaller than expected, with 75% of cases, is more commonly diagnosed later in pregnancy and has less risk for adverse perinatal outcomes (Sharma et al., 2016a). While this differentiation was once thought to be predictive of long-term sequalae, more recent studies have shown similar growth and developmental outcomes in symmetric and asymmetric growth-restricted preterm newborns (SMFM et al., 2020).

Symmetric FGR is due to an early alteration in the process of normal cell division that results in the creation of a smaller number and size of cells, commonly caused by genetic, infectious, or teratogenic insults. It can be apparent in early-second-trimester ultrasounds, with uniform diminishment of fetal organs, length, and weight, resulting in an overall proportionately smaller newborn. Symmetric FGR is usually caused by chromosomal or congenital anomalies, but is also associated with infections, such as CMV and rubella, or exposure to other teratogens, such as smoking, alcohol, cocaine, narcotics, or antiseizure medications, such as phenytoin or valproate (Sharma et al., 2016a, 2016b). Because the insult has occurred during the period of hyperplasia, it is less amenable to improvement by prenatal interventions. Management decisions are informed by weighing the risk of prematurity against the risk of an adverse in-utero environment.

Asymmetric FGR is usually the result of uteroplacental insufficiency, which causes chronic fetal hypoxemia and malnutrition in utero, with onset most common in the third trimester (Sharma et al., 2016a). In this case, the insult occurs during the phase of hypertrophy, causing the fetal cell to be smaller in size but normal in number. With this growth pattern, the abdomen and lower body experience a delay with relative sparing of head growth. Asymmetric FGR is associated with maternal hypertensive disorders, including preeclampsia, malnutrition, especially protein and glucose deficiencies, diabetes and other diseases affecting vascularity such as renal disease, abnormal placentation, such as circumvallate placenta or placenta previa, multiple gestation, autoimmune disorders, such as systemic lupus erythematosus, and hemoglobinopathies, such as sickle cell anemia. Additionally, individual behavioral factors, such as moderate alcohol intake, smoking, and use of substances, are associated with development of asymmetric FGR.

Diagnosis and Management

Screening, detection, and collaborative management and/or referral are the focus of primary care management for a pregnant person with suspected FGR. Screening should be done throughout pregnancy for risk factors associated with FGR with follow-up assessment performed as indicated. Universal screening for FGR in the first and second trimesters by Doppler studies, biochemical markers, and maternal factors have been effective in detecting early-onset FGR up to 90% (Figueras et al., 2018). However, there is currently no evidence that routine FGR screening in any trimester improves outcomes and it is not currently recommended (ACOG, 2021; Henrichs et al., 2019).

Numerous studies have evaluated potential strategies with the hope of preventing development of FGR. To date, prescribing bed rest or the prophylactic use of low-dose aspirin, low-molecular-weight heparin, or sildenafil have not been shown effective. In regard to nutritional counseling, while it is always prudent to encourage a healthy diet appropriate to the pregnant person's dietary preferences and requirements, research has failed to demonstrate any specific nutritional or dietary strategies to be effective in FGR prevention. Therefore, other than providing standard pregnancy nutritional counseling, additional nutritional approaches, restrictions, and supplements are not effective and not recommended (ACOG, 2021).

The clinical hallmark for the detection of FGR is a fundal height measurement of at least 3 cm less than dates in an individual with certain pregnancy dating. Experienced clinicians sometimes are able to detect a fetal weight smaller than expected for gestational age through palpation. These physical findings have a low sensitivity in detecting FGR but are often the trigger to initiate further testing (ACOG, 2021; Figueras et al., 2018; Lausman & Kingdom, 2013). While serial fundal height measurements and fetal weight estimation by palpation have been shown to have minimal intrinsic value, the benefit of these primary care screening tools abides more in the opportunity presented by prenatal visits in obtaining a thorough history, careful exploration of a client's perception of fetal growth and movement, and supportive counseling for healthy lifestyle choices (Hargreaves et al., 2011). Precise determination of gestational age is essential to detecting and diagnosing FGR. Ongoing thorough subjective and objective assessments should identify those individuals at risk for the development of FGR and in need of follow-up ultrasound and testing (Table 34.1).

The diagnosis of FGR is made by consecutive ultrasound measurements performed at least two weeks apart (ACOG, 2021; Figueras et al., 2018). If not previously involved in the diagnostic process, the healthcare provider should include a collaborative physician in the ongoing management plan once FGR has been identified by ultrasound. The pregnant person cared for in a rural or community office may need to be referred to a facility equipped to handle the prenatal, perinatal, and neonatal requirements of the pregnancy.

Table 34.1 Risk Factors for Development of FGR

Prepregnancy conditions	• Hypertensive disorders • Diabetes • Renal disease • Cyanotic cardiac disease • Collagen vascular disease • Autoimmune disorders (e.g., systemic lupus erythematosus) • Antiphospholipid antibody syndrome • Thrombophilias • Some hemoglobinopathies • Severe anemia • Prepregnancy BMI <20 or >30 • Use of assisted reproductive technologies
Present pregnancy conditions	• Multiple gestation • Fetal genetic or structural disorders • Hypertensive disorders • Inadequate weight gain, particularly if associated with low protein intake • Placental and umbilical cord abnormalities (circumvallate placenta, placenta accreta, single umbilical artery, partial placental infarction, hemangioma, **placental lakes**, placental abruption, and placenta previa) • Relative hypoglycemia or a "flat response" on a 3-hour glucose tolerance test, reflecting reduced glucose supply to the placenta • Unexplained abnormal serum genetic screening
Prior pregnancy history	• Prior history of FGR infant
Family history	• Family or personal history of infant with chromosomal abnormalities, congenital malformations, or genetic syndromes
Teratogenic exposures	• Smoking • Moderate alcohol use • Substance use • Environmental teratogen exposure • Infection (CMV, Rubella, Toxoplasmosis, Herpes simplex, Syphilis; especially in first trimester)
Social determinants	• Inadequate prenatal care • Systemic and interpersonal racism

Source: Adapted from Sharma et al. (2016a), Nasiri et al. (2020), Gavanier et al. (2021), and ACOG (2021).

Once FGR is diagnosed, targeted ultrasounds are performed to evaluate fetal anatomy and AFV. This will assist in determining if fetal anomalies or signs of aneuploidy are the cause of the FGR, in conjunction with genetic counseling and testing if not previously obtained (Sharma et al., 2016a). There is no single protocol for optimal methods and timing of fetal surveillance for the growth-restricted fetus. Care strategies should be individualized and modified as indicated (ACOG, 2021; SMFM et al., 2020). Serial fetal growth ultrasounds are commonly performed at three- to four-week intervals to assess the fetal growth curve (ACOG, 2021). Measurements of the biparietal diameter (BPD), head circumference (HC)/AC ratio, fetal weight, and AFV should be included. The fetal AC provides the best single measurement to screen for poor growth (Rad et al., 2018). Serial **arterial Doppler flow studies** of the umbilical artery are performed weekly or biweekly to assess for the presence of fetal acidemia. Strong evidence exists that serial Doppler flow studies improve perinatal outcomes and reduce perinatal deaths through identification of fetuses in jeopardy in the intrauterine environment and prompt cesarean birth (ACOG, 2021; Figueras et al., 2018; Sharma et al., 2016a; SMFM et al., 2020). Recent studies indicate that fetal weight below the third percentile combined with abnormal **Doppler velocimetry** of uterine arteries is most strongly associated with poor fetal and neonatal outcomes (Figueras et al., 2018; SMFM et al., 2020; Unterscheider et al., 2013). Serial NSTs performed every three to seven days, depending on the fetal risk status, also provide clinical evidence of fetal acid–base status. The **BPP** or **modified BPP** continues to be a clinical tool used for ongoing surveillance of high-risk pregnancies; however, it has been found to be a late indicator of diminishing placental functioning. The high number of false positive and false negative results has also diminished its efficacy as a tool to assess for fetal well-being (SMFM et al., 2020). An estimate of AFV by itself is poorly correlated with fetal acidemia; however, a declining AFI in the presence of FGR is an indicator of worsening uteroplacental function and warrants umbilical artery Doppler flow studies and a period of prolonged monitoring, and consideration of expedited birth (SMFM et al., 2020; Sharma et al., 2016a; Unterscheider et al., 2013). Daily maternal evaluation of fetal movement is an appropriate adjunct to antepartum fetal surveillance.

The decision to continue expectant management with close monitoring or to schedule an immediate induction is one that is determined in collaboration with or after referral to a physician colleague, depending on the practice model and setting. Of note, induction prior to term solely due to the presence of FGR without indicators of placental deterioration or worsening fetal status has not been found to improve perinatal outcomes, nor is it cost-effective, and potentially increases NICU admissions due to morbidities associated with the delivery of late-preterm and early term neonates (<38 weeks of gestation; Figueras et al., 2018).

Macrosomia

Macrosomia is variously defined as a newborn weight of greater than 4000 g (8 lb 13 oz) to 4500 g (9 lb 14 oz), with the latter parameter more commonly used (Wang et al., 2016). An alternative descriptor of macrosomia is the classification of birth weight relative to gestational age, which defines LGA as birth weight above the 90th percentile for gestational age (Araujo Júnior et al., 2017). Macrosomia is further described by categories with the risk of adverse outcomes increasing with each birth weight category: 4000–4499 g, 4500–4999 g, and >5000 g (ACOG, 2020).

The definition of macrosomia is further differentiated due to its association with maternal diabetes. Because of increased total fetal body fat, larger shoulder and upper-extremity circumferences, and AC that tends to be larger relative to the BPD than in patients without diabetes, the risk of vaginal birth complicated by shoulder dystocia is increased significantly. Thus, macrosomia is considered greater than 4500 g in a person without diabetes, but greater than 4000 g in a person with diabetes (ACOG, 2020; Wang et al., 2016).

Risk factors for fetal macrosomia

- Diabetes (all types, including gestational)
- Abnormal 1-hour glucose screen with a normal 3-hour glucose tolerance test
- Previous birth of an infant >4000 g
- Dyslipidemia
- Maternal prepregnant obesity
- Excessive prenatal weight gain
- Postterm pregnancy
- Tall maternal height
- Male-sex fetus
- High paternal birth weight

Diagnosis and Management

Accurate prenatal identification of a macrosomic fetus is difficult and available assessment methods have poor sensitivity. A fundal height growth pattern >3 cm more than expected for gestation, particularly if performed serially by the same examiner, is an initial indicator of macrosomia. Experienced clinicians sometimes detect a fetal weight larger than expected for gestational age through palpation. As with FGR, gross assessments of fetal size are fraught with inherent variation—multiple provider measurements, changes in fetal station, presentation or position, maternal obesity, or personal bias. Interestingly, a pregnant person's own perception of fetal size has been found to have as good a correlation to actual birth weight as fetal weight estimation by Leopold maneuvers and/or sonographic EFW determination (Ashrafganjooei et al., 2010; Torloni et al., 2008).

The ability of ultrasound to accurately assess fetal weight has been disappointing (ACOG, 2020; Scifres et al., 2015). Late pregnancy ultrasound estimates of fetal weight are notoriously inaccurate and must be considered in conjunction with other findings and the individual's informed decision in developing a plan for birth. Despite the fact that only 50% of shoulder dystocia cases involve macrosomic fetuses, providers may be reluctant to attempt vaginal birth if there is concern about perinatal risks associated with macrosomia, and thus increasingly rely on sonographic EFW measurement in late pregnancy (Dadkhah et al., 2013). The inaccuracy of ultrasound EFW results in early inductions of labor and scheduled

cesarean births, only to discover at birth an infant of normal weight (Chauhan et al., 2005; Scifres et al., 2015). An ultrasound that predicts a macrosomic infant is an independent variable that predisposes a pregnant person to having a cesarean birth, in spite of its known inaccuracy, clearly impacting both the provider and patient (ACOG, 2020).

The assessment of risk factors for the development of macrosomia include a review of the patient's medical, obstetrical, and family history, with focus on any history of diabetes and current GDM screening test results, as well as current physical examination findings.

If an ultrasound for dating has been performed and EDB confirmed, a targeted ultrasound should be scheduled to obtain an anatomy scan and an EFW. This will assist in determining if fetal anomalies or signs of aneuploidy are the cause of the size greater than dates, with genetic counseling and testing made available as indicated. Serial fetal growth ultrasounds at three- to four-week intervals to assess the fetal growth curve should be initiated. Measurements of the BPD, HC/AC ratio, fetal weight, and AFV should be included. A fetal AC of >35 cm identifies more than 90% of macrosomic infants (Dadkhah et al., 2013).

A prudent clinical course is the combination of EFW measurement with Leopold maneuvers by an experienced examiner, sonographic findings, and the individual's own perception of fetal size when having any discussion regarding mode of birth. A question frequently posed by those in this situation is about the possibility of early labor induction in the hope of avoiding continued fetal growth and increased risk of cesarean birth. The evidence is inconsistent on the benefits of induction versus expectant management. Some earlier studies that included pregnant people without diabetes documented an increased risk of cesarean birth with induction prior to 41 weeks, particularly with a Bishop's score of <6; however, waiting the onset of spontaneous labor or delaying induction until >41 weeks of gestation has been associated with a lower rate of cesarean birth, even in the presence of macrosomia (Bailey & Kalu, 2009; Sanchez-Ramos et al., 2002). However, more recent meta-analyses have demonstrated similar cesarean birth rates for inductions compared to expectant management with a lower incidence of shoulder dystocia (Boulvain et al., 2016; Magro-Malosso et al., 2017). Further, pregnant individuals can be counseled that the ACOG recommends that elective cesarean birth be considered for suspected fetal macrosomia with an EFW of *at least 5000 g in those without diabetes* and at least *4500 g in those with diabetes* (ACOG, 2020). This recommendation is based on consensus and expert opinion, not evidence from clinical trials. It is important to note that even with excellent attention to nutritional recommendations, extensive prenatal care, and experienced providers, prebirth estimates of fetal weight are frequently inaccurate. There are risks inherent in attending the vaginal birth of a macrosomic infant. A study of community birth demonstrated adverse outcomes increased incrementally as the size of the macrosomic infants increased, particularly of note in those >4500 g. Negative outcomes that increased on a continuum with larger birth weight included perineal trauma, postpartum hemorrhage, cesarean birth, neonatal birth injury, shoulder dystocia, and neonatal NICU stays of longer than 24 hours (Pillai et al., 2020).

The decision to offer an induction prior to 41 weeks of gestation or a scheduled cesarean birth for macrosomia is one that is guided by the principle of shared decision-making and determined in collaboration with or after referral to a physician colleague, depending on the practice model and setting.

Summary

A careful and systematic approach to the examination of the pregnant abdomen will reveal concerns related to amniotic fluid and fetal growth disturbances. Additionally, listening to the woman or pregnant person as they relate their interval history and their sense of fetal growth and activity will provide clues that assist in differentiating normal variation from conditions requiring further evaluation. Amniotic fluid and fetal growth disturbances are important contributors to perinatal morbidity and mortality with short-term implications regarding timing and route of birth and long-term implications regarding the health and well-being of the birthing person and their baby. Establishment of an accurate due date early in pregnancy, along with the use of customized fetal growth charts, will assist the healthcare provider in identifying the fetus at risk. The provision of evidence-based practice in collaboration with physician colleagues and shared decision-making with the pregnant person are critical components in the development of a management plan that will provide the best outcome for both.

Resources for Clients and Their Families

Amniotic fluid disorders:
https://www.marchofdimes.org/complications/polyhydramnios.aspx
https://www.marchofdimes.org/complications/oligohydramnios.aspx
Intrauterine growth restriction:
https://www.marchofdimes.org/complications/low-birthweight.aspx
https://kidshealth.org/en/parents/iugr.html?ref=search#catpregnancy
https://familydoctor.org/condition/intrauterine-growth-restriction
Low birth weight: https://www.marchofdimes.org/complications/low-birthweight.aspx

Resources for Healthcare Providers

Triple I:
https://www.obgproject.com/2016/10/16/chorioamnionitis-nichd-workshop-terminology-management

Fetal macrosomia:
https://www.acog.org/clinical/clinical-guidance/practicebulletin/articles/2020/01/macrosomia
Intrauterine fetal growth restriction:
http://aium.s3.amazonaws.com/resourceLibrary/SMFM_fetal_Growth_Restriction.pdf
Regimens of fetal surveillance for impaired fetal growth:
https://pubmed.ncbi.nlm.nih.gov/33481528
https://pubmed.ncbi.nlm.nih.gov/33251165
https://pubmed.ncbi.nlm.nih.gov/31615781

References

American College of Nurse-Midwives. (2018). *Position statement: Prelabor rupture of membranes at term.* https://www.midwife.org/acnm/files/ACNMLibraryData/UPLOADFILENAME/000000000233/PS-Prelabor-rupture-of-membranes-FINAL-22-MAR-18.pdf

American College of Obstetricians & Gynecologists (ACOG). (2020). Macrosomia: Practice bulletin, number 216. *Obstetrics & Gynecology*, 135(1), e18–e35. https://doi-org.frontier.idm.oclc.org/10.1097/AOG.0000000000003606

American College of Obstetricians & Gynecologists (ACOG). (2021). Fetal growth restriction. Practice bulletin, number 227. *Obstetrics & Gynecology*, 137(2), e16–e28. https://doi.org/10.1097/AOG.0000000000004251

American College of Obstetricians & Gynecologists (ACOG). Committee on Obstetric Practice. (2017). Committee opinion no. 713: Antenatal corticosteroid therapy for fetal maturation. *Obstetrics & Gynecology*, 130(2), e102–e109.

Araujo Júnior, E., Peixoto, A. B., Zamarian, A. C., Elito Júnior, J., & Tonni, G. (2017). Macrosomia. *Best Practice & Research. Clinical Obstetrics & Gynaecology*, 38, 83–96. https://doi.org/10.1016/j.bpobgyn.2016.08.003

Ashrafganjooei, T., Naderi, T., Eshrati, B., & Babapoor, N. (2010). Accuracy of ultrasound, clinical and maternal estimates of birth weight in term women. *Eastern Mediterranean Health Journal*, 16(3), 313–317.

Azarkish, F., Janghorban, R., Bozorgzadeh, S., Arzani, A., Balouchi, R., & Didehvar, M. (2022). The effect of maternal intravenous hydration on amniotic fluid index in oligohydramnios. *BMC Research Notes*, 15(1), 1–5. https://doi.org/10.1186/s13104-022-05985-6

Bailey, C., & Kalu, E. (2009). Fetal macrosomia in non-diabetic mothers: Antenatal diagnosis and delivery outcome. *Journal of Obstetrics and Gynaecology: The Journal of the Institute of Obstetrics and Gynaecology*, 29(3), 206–208. https://doi.org/10.1080/01443610902743763

Blackburn, S. T. (2018). *Maternal, fetal, and neonatal physiology: A clinical perspective* (5th ed.). Elsevier Saunders.

Boito, S., Crovetto, F., Ischia, B., Crippa, B. L., Fabietti, I., Bedeschi, M. F., Lalatta, F., Colombo, L., Mosca, F., Fedele, L., & Persico, N. (2016). Prenatal ultrasound factors and genetic disorders in pregnancies complicated by polyhydramnios. *Prenatal Diagnosis*, 36(8), 726–730. https://doi.org/10.1002/pd.4851

Boulvain, M., Irion, O., Dowswell, T., & Thornton, J. G. (2016). Induction of labour at or near term for suspected fetal macrosomia. *The Cochrane Database of Systematic Reviews*, 2016(5), CD000938. https://doi.org/10.1002/14651858.CD000938.pub2

Brace, R. A., & Cheung, C. Y. (2014). Regulation of amniotic fluid volume: Evolving concepts. In L. Zhang & C. A. Ducsay (Eds.), *Advances in fetal and neonatal physiology* (pp. 49–68). Springer. https://doi.org/10.1007/978-1-4939-1031-1_5

Brace, R. A., & Wolf, E. J. (1989). Normal amniotic fluid volume changes throughout pregnancy. *American Journal of Obstetrics & Gynecology*, 161, 382–388. https://doi.org/10.1016/0002-9378(89)90527-9

Chauhan, S. P., Grobman, W. A., Gherman, R. A., Chauhan, V. B., Chang, G., Magann, E. F., & Hendrix, N. W. (2005). Suspicion and treatment of the macrosomic fetus: A review. *American Journal of Obstetrics & Gynecology*, 193(2), 332–346. https://doi.org/10.1016/j.ajog.2004.12.020

Collado, M. C., Rautava, S., Aakko, J., Isolauri, E., & Salminen, S. (2016). Human gut colonisation may be initiated in utero by distinct microbial communities in the placenta and amniotic fluid. *Scientific Reports*, 6(1), 1–13. https://doi.org/10.1038/srep23129

Dadkhah, F., Kashanian, M., Bonyad, Z., & Larijani, T. (2013). Predicting neonatal weight of more than 4000 g using fetal abdominal circumference measurement by ultrasound at 38–40 weeks of pregnancy: A study in Iran. *The Journal of Obstetrics and Gynaecology Research*, 39(1), 170–174. https://doi.org/10.1111/j.1447-0756.2012.01918.x

Dashe, J. S., Pressman, E. K., Hibbard, J. U., & Society for Maternal-Fetal Medicine (SMFM). (2018). SMFM consult series# 46: Evaluation and management of polyhydramnios. *American Journal of Obstetrics and Gynecology*, 219(4), B2–B8. https://doi.org/10.1016/j.ajog.2018.07.016

Deter, R. L., Lee, W., Yeo, L., Erez, O., Ramamurthy, U., Naik, M., & Romero, R. (2018). Individualized growth assessment: Conceptual framework and practical implementation for the evaluation of fetal growth and neonatal growth outcome. *American Journal of Obstetrics and Gynecology*, 218(2S), S656–S678. https://doi.org/10.1016/j.ajog.2017.12.210

Duryea, E. L., Hawkins, J. S., McIntire, D. D., Casey, B. M., & Leveno, K. J. (2014). A revised birth weight reference for the United States. *Obstetrics & Gynecology*, 124(1), 16–22. https://doi.org/10.1097/AOG.0000000000000345

Erfani, H., Diaz-Rodriguez, G. E., Aalipour, S., Nassr, A., Rezaei, A., Gandhi, M., Mendez-Figuero, M., Aagard, A. A., & Shamshirsaz, A. A. (2019). Amnioreduction in cases of polyhydramnios: Indications and outcomes in singleton pregnancies without fetal interventions. *European Journal of Obstetrics & Gynecology and Reproductive Biology*, 241, 126–128. https://doi.org/10.1016/j.ejogrb.2019.05.019

Fay, E., Hugh, O., Francis, A., Katz, R., Sitcov, K., Souter, V., & Gardosi, J. (2021). Customized GROW vs INTERGROWTH-21st birthweight standards to identify small for gestational age associated perinatal outcomes at term. *American Journal of Obstetrics & Gynecology MFM*, 4(2), 100545. https://doi.org/10.1016/j.ajogmf.2021.100545

Figueras, F., Caradeux, J., Crispi, F., Eixarch, E., Peguero, A., & Gratacos, E. (2018). Diagnosis and surveillance of late-onset fetal growth restriction. *American Journal of Obstetrics and Gynecology*, 218(2). https://doi.org/10.1016/j.ajog.2017.12.003

Gardosi, J., Francis, A., Turner, S., & Williams, M. (2018). Customized growth charts: Rationale, validation and clinical benefits. *American Journal of Obstetrics and Gynecology*, 218(2), S609–S618. https://doi-org.frontier.idm.oclc.org/10.1016/j.ajog.2017.12.011

Gavanier, D., Berthet, G., Hajri, T., Allias, F., Atallah, A., Massoud, M., Golfier, F., Bolze, P. A., & Massardier, J. (2021). Vesicles or placental lakes in ultrasonography, determining the correct etiology. *Journal of Gynecology Obstetrics and Human Reproduction*, 50(6), 101738. https://doi.org/10.1016/j.jogoh.2020.101738

Ghafoor, S. (2021). Current and emerging strategies for prediction and diagnosis of prelabour rupture of the membranes: A narrative review. *The Malaysian Journal of Medical Sciences: MJMS*, 28(3), 5. https://doi.org/10.21315/mjms2021.28.3.2

Hargreaves, K., Cameron, M., Edwards, H., Gray, R., & Deane, K. (2011). Is the use of symphysis-fundal height measurement and ultrasound examination effective in detecting small or large fetuses? *Journal of Obstetrics and Gynaecology*, 31(5), 380–383. https://doi.org/10.3109/01443615.2011.567343

Henrichs, J., Verfaille, V., Jellema, P., Viester, L., Pajkrt, E., Wilschut, J., van der Horst, H. E., Franx, A., de Jonge, A., & IRIS study group. (2019). Effectiveness of routine third trimester ultrasonography to reduce adverse perinatal outcomes in low risk pregnancy (the IRIS study): Nationwide, pragmatic, multicentre, stepped wedge cluster randomised trial. *BMJ*, 367, l5517. https://doi.org/10.1136/bmj.l5517

Higgins, R. D., Saade, G., Polin, R. A., Grobman, W. A., Buhimschi, I. A., Watterberg, K., Silver, R. M., Raju, T. N., & The Chorioamnionitis Workshop participants. (2016). Evaluation and management of women and newborns with a maternal diagnosis of chorioamnionitis: Summary of a workshop. *Obstetrics and Gynecology*, 127(3), 426. https://doi.org/10.1097/AOG.0000000000001246

Kalpashri, K., & Devaskar, S. U. (2019). Intrauterine growth restriction. *Pediatric Clinics of North America*, 66(2), 403–423. https://doi.org/10.1016/j.pcl.2018.12.009

Kehl, S., Schelkle, A., Thomas, A., Puhl, A., Meqdad, K., Tuschy, B., Berlit, S., Weiss, C., Bayer, C., Heimrich, J., Dammer, U., Raabe, E., Winkler, M., Fashingbauer, F., Beckmann, M. W., & Dammer, U. (2016). Single deepest vertical pocket or amniotic fluid index as evaluation test for predicting adverse pregnancy outcome (SAFE trial): A multicenter, open-label, randomized controlled trial. *Ultrasound in Obstetrics & Gynecology*, 47(6), 674–679. https://doi.org/10.1002/uog.14924

Knöfler, M., Haider, S., Saleh, L., Pollheimer, J., Gamage, T. K., & James, J. (2019). Human placenta and trophoblast development: Key molecular mechanisms and model systems. *Cellular and Molecular Life Sciences*, 76(18), 3479–3496. https://link.springer.com/article/10.1007/s00018-019-03104-6

Kuba, K., & Bernstein, P. S. (2018). ACOG practice bulletin no. 188: Prelabor rupture of membranes. *Obstetrics & Gynecology*, 131(6), 1163–1164. https://doi.org/10.1097/AOG.0000000000002663

Lausman, A., & Kingdom, J. (2013). Intrauterine growth restriction: Screening, diagnosis, and management. *Journal of Obstetrics and Gynaecology Canada*, 35(8), 741–748. https://doi.org/10.1016/S1701-2163(15)30865-3

Li, T., Wang, Y., Miao, Z., Lin, Y., Yu, X., Xie, K., & Ding, H. (2020). Neonatal adverse outcomes of induction and expectant management in fetal growth restriction: A systematic review and meta-analysis. *Frontiers in Pediatrics*, 8, 2296–2360. https://doi.org/10.3389/fped.2020.558000

Lim, E. S., Rodriguez, C., & Holtz, L. R. (2018). Amniotic fluid from healthy term pregnancies does not harbor a detectable microbial community. *Microbiome*, 6(1), 1–8. https://doi.org/10.1186/s40168-018-0475-7

Lim, K. I., Butt, K., Naud, K., & Smithies, M. (2017). Amniotic fluid: Technical update on physiology and measurement. *Journal of Obstetrics and Gynaecology Canada*, 39(1), 52–58. https://doi.org/10.1016/j.jogc.2016.09.012

Magro-Malosso, E. R., Saccone, G., Chen, M., Navathe, R., Di Tommaso, M., & Berghella, V. (2017). Induction of labour for suspected macrosomia at term in non-diabetic women: A systematic review and meta-analysis of randomized controlled trials. *BJOG: An International Journal of Obstetrics and Gynaecology*, 124(3), 414–421. https://doi.org/10.1111/1471-0528.14435

Mainigi, M. A., Olalere, D., Burd, I., Sapienza, C., Bartolomei, M., & Coutifaris, C. (2014). Peri-implantation hormonal milieu: Elucidating mechanisms of abnormal placentation and fetal growth. *Biology of Reproduction*, 90(2), 26. https://doi.org/10.1095/biolreprod.113.110411

Mao, Y., Pierce, J., Singh-Varma, A., Boyer, M., Kohn, J., & Reems, J. A. (2019). Processed human amniotic fluid retains its antibacterial activity. *Journal of Translational Medicine*, 17(1), 1–9. https://doi.org/10.1186/s12967-019-1812-8

Marowitz, A. (2016). Management of prelabor rupture of the membranes at term: Using the evidence (pp. 411–428). In B. A. Anderson & S. E. Stone (Eds.), *Best practices in midwifery: Using the evidence to implement change*. Springer.

McCowan, L. M., Figueras, F., & Anderson, N. H. (2018). Evidence-based national guidelines for the management of suspected fetal growth restriction: Comparison, consensus, and controversy. *American Journal of Obstetrics and Gynecology*, 218(2S), S855–S868. https://doi.org/10.1016/j.ajog.2017.12.004

McGoldrick, E., Stewart, F., Parker, R., & Dalziel, S. R. (2020). Antenatal corticosteroids for accelerating fetal lung maturation for women at risk of preterm birth. *Cochrane Database of Systematic Reviews*, (12), CD004454. https://www.cochranelibrary.com/cdsr/doi/10.1002/14651858.CD004454.pub4/pdf/full

Middleton, P., Shepherd, E., Flenady, V., McBain, R. D., & Crowther, C. A. (2017). Planned early birth versus expectant management (waiting) for prelabour rupture of membranes at term (37 weeks or more). *Cochrane Database of Systematic Reviews*, 2017(1), CD005302. https://doi.org/10.1002/14651858.CD005302.pub3

Modi, J. Y., Patel, R. V., Shah, P. T., & Agrawal, A. G. (2016). Fetomaternal outcome in pregnancy with oligohydramnios. *International Journal of Reproduction, Contraception, Obstetrics and Gynecology*, 5(11), 4037–4040.

Moore, T. R., & Cayle, J. E. (1990). The amniotic fluid index in normal human pregnancy. *American Journal of Obstetrics & Gynecology*, *162*(5), 1168–1173. http://10.0.3.248/0002-9378(90)90009-V

Murzakanova, G., Räisänen, S., Jacobsen, A. F., Sole, K. B., Bjarkø, L., & Laine, K. (2020). Adverse perinatal outcomes in 665,244 term and post-term deliveries—A Norwegian population-based study. *European Journal of Obstetrics & Gynecology and Reproductive Biology*, *247*, 212–218. https://www.theseus.fi/bitstream/handle/10024/345047/Adverse_perinatal_outcomes_in_665244_.pdf?sequence=1

Nasiri, K., Moodie, E., & Abenhaim, H. A. (2020). To what extent is the association between race/ethnicity and fetal growth restriction explained by adequacy of prenatal care? A mediation analysis of a retrospectively selected cohort. *American Journal of Epidemiology*, *189*(11), 1360–1368. https://doi.org/10.1093/aje/kwaa054

Ortigosa Rocha, C., Bittar, R. E., & Zugaib, M. (2010). Neonatal outcomes of late-preterm birth associated or not with intrauterine growth restriction. *Obstetrics and Gynecology International*, *2010*, 231842. https://doi.org/10.1155/2010/231842

Osol, G., & Moore, L. G. (2014). Maternal uterine vascular remodeling during pregnancy. *Microcirculation*, *21*(1), 38–47. https://doi.org/10.1111/micc.12080

Peng, C. C., Chang, J. H., Lin, H. Y., Cheng, P. J., & Su, B. H. (2018). Intrauterine inflammation, infection, or both (Triple I): A new concept for chorioamnionitis. *Pediatrics & Neonatology*, *59*(3), 231–237. https://www.pediatr-neonatol.com/article/S1875-9572(17)30027-X/fulltext

Pillai, S., Cheyney, M., Everson, C. L., & Bovbjerg, M. L. (2020). Fetal macrosomia in home and birth center births in the United States: Maternal, fetal, and newborn outcomes. *Birth*, *47*(4), 409–417. https://doi.org/10.1111/birt.12506

Poonia, S., Satia, M. N., & Bang, N. (2017). Study of placentation and maternal and fetal outcomes in cases of 2 or more caesarean sections. *International Journal of Reproduction, Contraception, Obstetrics and Gynecology*, *5*(7), 2402–2406. https://go.gale.com/ps/i.do?id=GALE%7CA459171330&sid=googleScholar&v=2.1&it=r&linkaccess=abs&issn=23201770&p=HRCA&sw=w&userGroupName=anon%7Ebda6f39a

Rabie, N., Magann, E., Steelman, S., & Ounpraseuth, S. (2017). Oligohydramnios in complicated and uncomplicated pregnancy: A systematic review and meta-analysis. *Ultrasound in Obstetrics & Gynecology*, *49*(4), 442–449. https://doi.org/10.1002/uog.15929

Rad, S., Beauchamp, S., Morales, C., Mirocha, J., & Esakoff, T. F. (2018). Defining fetal growth restriction: Abdominal circumference as an alternative criterion. *Journal of Maternal and Fetal Neonatal Medicine.*, *31*(23), 3089–3094. https://doi.org/10.1080/14767058.2017.1364723

Refaat, M., Khater, H., & Helmy, M. (2021). Value of fetal renal artery doppler indices in idiopathic oligohydramnios and polyhydramnios. *Benha Medical Journal*, e-pub 1–10. https://doi.org/10.21608/bmfj.2021.67624.1397

Rehbinder, E. M., Carlsen, K. C. L., Staff, A. C., Angell, I. L., Landrø, L., Hilde, K., Gaustad, P., & Rudi, K. (2018). Is amniotic fluid of women with uncomplicated term pregnancies free of bacteria? *American Journal of Obstetrics and Gynecology*, *219*(3), 289-e1. https://doi.org/10.1016/j.ajog.2018.05.028

Sammour, R., & Sagi, S. (2019). Isolated oligohydramnios-the dilemma of proper management. *Harefuah*, *158*(11), 728–731. PMID: 31721516

Sanchez-Ramos, L., Bernstein, S., & Kaunitz, A. M. (2002). Expectant management versus labor induction for suspected fetal macrosomia: a systematic review. *Obstetrics & Gynecology*, *100*(5), 997_1002. https://doi.org/10.1016/S0029-7844(02)02321-9

Scifres, C. M., Feghali, M., Dumont, T., Althouse, A. S., Speer, P., Cari-tis, S. N., & Catov, J. M. (2015). Large-for-gestational-age ultrasound diagnosis and risk for cesarean delivery in women with gestational diabetes mellitus. *Obstetrics & Gynecology*, *126*(5), 978–986. https://doi.org/10.1097/AOG.0000000000001097

Sharma, D., Farahbakhsh, N., Shastri, S., & Sharma, P. (2016b). Intrauterine growth restriction—Part 2. *The Journal of Maternal-Fetal & Neonatal Medicine*, *29*(24), 4037–4048. https://doi.org/10.3109/14767058.2016.1154525

Sharma, D., Shastri, S., Farahbakhsh, N., & Sharma, P. (2016a). Intrauterine growth restriction—Part 1. *The Journal of Maternal-Fetal & Neonatal Medicine*, *29*(24), 3977–3987. https://doi.org/10.3109/14767058.2016.1154429

Slagle, H. B. G., Hoffman, M. K., Fonge, Y. N., Caplan, R., & Sciscione, A. C. (2022). Incremental risk of clinical chorioamnionitis associated with cervical examination. *American Journal of Obstetrics & Gynecology MFM*, *4*(1), 100524.

Society for Maternal-Fetal Medicine (SMFM), Martins, J. G., Biggio, J. R., & Abuhamad, A. (2020). Society for Maternal-Fetal Medicine consult series #52: Diagnosis and management of fetal growth restriction. *American Journal of Obstetrics and Gynecology*, *223*(4), B2–B17. https://doi.org/10.1016/j.ajog.2020.05.010

Torloni, M. R., Sass, N., Sato, J. L., Renzi, A. C. P., Fukuyama, M., & Lucca, P. R. D. (2008). Clinical formulas, mother's opinion and ultrasound in predicting birth weight. *Sao Paulo Medical Journal*, *126*(3), 145–149. https://doi.org/10.1590/S1516-31802008000300002

Unterscheider, J., Daly, S., Geary, M. P., Kennelly, M. M., McAuliffe, F. M., O'Donoghue, K., & Malone, D. (2013). Optimizing the definition of intrauterine growth restriction: The multicenter prospective PORTO study. *American Journal of Obstetrics & Gynecology*, *208*(4), 290e1–e6. https://doi.org/10.1016/j.ajog.2013.02.007

Vanda, R., Bazrafkan, M., Rouhani, M., & Bazarganipour, F. (2022). Comparing pregnancy, childbirth, and neonatal outcomes in women with idiopathic polyhydramnios: A prospective cohort study. *BMC Pregnancy and Childbirth*, *22*(1), 1–7. https://doi.org/10.1186/s12884-022-04625-y

Walther, F. J., & Ramaekers, L. H. (1982). The ponderal index as a measure of the nutritional status at birth and its relation to some aspects of neonatal morbidity. *Journal of Perinatal Medicine*, *10*(1), 42–47. https://doi.org/10.1515/jpme.1982.10.1.42

Wang, D., Zhu, L., Zhang, S., Wu, X., Wang, X., Lv, Q., Gan, D., Liu, L., Li, W., Zhou, Q., Lu, J., He, H., Wang, J., Xin, H., Li, Z., & Chen, C. (2016). Predictive macrosomia birthweight thresholds for adverse maternal and neonatal outcomes. *The Journal of Maternal-Fetal & Neonatal Medicine*, *29*(23), 3745–3750. https://doi.org/10.3109/14767058.2016.1147549

Weiner, C. P., & Robinson, D. (1989). Sonographic diagnosis of intrauterine growth retardation using the postnatal ponderal index and the crown-heel length as standards of diagnosis. *American Journal of Perinatology*, *6*(04), 380–383. https://doi.org/10.1055/s-2007-999622

35

Spontaneous Preterm Birth

Esther Ellsworth Bowers

The editors gratefully acknowledge Robin G. Jordan and Nancy Jo Reedy, who were co-authors of the previous edition of this chapter.

Relevant Terms

Age of viability—the stage of development at which a fetus can survive outside of the uterus; occurs sometime between 22 and 26 weeks, usually when fetal weight is greater than 500 g.

Cervical cerclage—a minor prenatal surgical procedure to stitch the cervix closed to prevent preterm birth in persons with short cervix or cervical insufficiency.

Cervical insufficiency—a condition where the cervix is weakened and begins to dilate early in pregnancy, often without clinical symptoms.

Epigenetics—modification of gene expression rather than alteration of the genetic code itself, can occur in offspring either before or after birth and thus program individuals for lifelong health outcomes.

Interpregnancy interval—spacing between a live birth and the beginning of the following pregnancy.

Preterm birth rate—the number of births occurring at less than 37 completed weeks of gestation divided by the total number of live births, multiplied by 100 to be expressed as a percent.

Pessary—an elastic, rigid circular device that is inserted into the vagina to support the uterus.

Stress—demands that tax or exceed the adaptive capacity of an organism and that result in psychological and biological changes.

Tocolytics—drugs that inhibit uterine contractions.

Vaginal microbiome—the bacteria that colonize the vagina, the composition of which has implications for a person's health.

To prevent an early birth, wear a lodestone (magnet) to hold the child within . . .

(Cotton Mather, 1710, in Wertz & Wertz, 1989)

Introduction

Preterm birth (PTB) is defined as a birth after 20 weeks of gestation and prior to 37 completed weeks of gestation. On a global basis, PTB is the leading cause of neonatal morbidity and mortality. The **PTB rate** has substantial significance as a measure of the health and well-being of a nation, and it is tracked by global and national organizations, governments, and policy makers. The United States is the sixth highest in the world for its total number of neonates born preterm and 54th highest out of 184 countries in the world for its rate of PTB (World Health Organization [WHO], 2018). The PTB rate in the United States is one of the highest among developed nations (March of Dimes, 2016), slightly over 10% of all births (Martin et al., 2021).

Although the PTB rate in the United States declined by 15% between 2006 and 2013, it rose again in the years 2014–2019 (Martin & Osterman, 2022). The societal cost of PTB is significant. Prematurity is associated with approximately one-third of all infant deaths in the United States, and it negatively impacts long-term educational attainment and income in adults who were born prematurely (Hall & Greenberg, 2016).

Fetal growth and maturation occur along a continuum throughout pregnancy; therefore, PTB is categorized by gestational age to guide discussion about the impact of PTB on infant morbidity and mortality. (Note that gestational age is never rounded up, so, e.g., 36 weeks and 6 days of gestation is considered 36 weeks and not 37 weeks of gestation.)

- Late preterm: 34–36 weeks of gestation
- Moderate preterm: 32–33 weeks of gestation
- Very preterm: 28–31 weeks of gestation
- Extremely preterm: <28 weeks of gestation

Prenatal and Postnatal Care: A Person-Centered Approach, Third Edition. Edited by Karen Trister Grace, Cindy L. Farley, Noelene K. Jeffers, and Tanya Tringali.
© 2024 John Wiley & Sons Ltd. Published 2024 by John Wiley & Sons Ltd.
Companion website: www.wiley.com/go/grace/prenatal

PTB can be subdivided into iatrogenic (medically indicated, such as for preeclampsia with severe features) versus spontaneous and subdivided again between singleton and multiple gestation pregnancies. The remainder of this chapter will discuss spontaneous PTB (sPTB). Distinctions will be made between singleton and multiple gestation when appropriate.

> ### Health equity key points
>
> - In the United States, non-Hispanic Black individuals face a higher risk of PTB (both spontaneous and iatrogenic) than non-Hispanic White individuals, a disparity that persists even for Black populations with high socioeconomic status.
> - A key mechanism underlying the relationship between race/ethnicity, socioeconomic status, and sPTB is lifetime exposure to stress from racism and negative social determinants of health.
> - Primary prevention strategies for sPTB that have strong research support include: smoking cessation, adequate weight gain, interpregnancy interval >18 months, and use of a midwife-led continuity of care model.

Social and Racial/Ethnic Disparities

Some racial groups and groups with lower socioeconomic status have higher rates of sPTB. Worldwide, rates of sPTB are inversely related to income and education (Brink et al., 2020; Bushnik et al., 2017; Joseph et al., 2014). In the United States, disparities in sPTB rates by socioeconomic status are also well documented (Dunlop et al., 2021). In addition, the United States demonstrates striking disparities in PTB rates (both spontaneous and iatrogenic) by race/ethnicity (Figure 35.1). In the United States, non-Hispanic Black individuals face 65% higher risk of PTB than non-Hispanic White individuals (Martin & Osterman, 2022). These disparities are accentuated for Black individuals

born in the United States, versus those who immigrated as adults (Burris & Hacker, 2017), and disparities persist even for Black populations with high socioeconomic status (Collins et al., 2007, 2011; Johnson et al., 2020). Persistent disparities are of great concern for population health, as PTB is predictive of developmental problems and adverse health outcomes later in life.

Explanations for disparities in the rate of sPTB in the United States have typically focused on access to high-quality healthcare, incidence of malnutrition, exposure to environmental pollution, and prevalence of comorbidities (Burris & Hacker, 2017). Of significance, exposure to interpersonal and institutional racism has also been established as an independent contributor to sPTB disparities (Figure 35.2; Alhusen et al., 2016; Collins et al., 2004; Kim et al., 2020).

One mechanism underlying the relationship between socioeconomic status, race/ethnicity, and sPTB is lifetime exposure to **stress**. Frequent exposure to stress hormones can induce **epigenetic** changes in the hypothalamic–pituitary–adrenal (HPA) axis of a person with childbearing potential (Traylor et al., 2020), resulting in heightened reactivity of their HPA axis. When the person becomes pregnant, this ongoing heightened reactivity results in elevated amounts of cortisol passing into fetal circulation during critical periods of neuroendocrine development (Kramer et al., 2013). This passage has two effects:

1. It leads to premature activation of the fetal HPA axis, one of the key pathways to onset of preterm labor.
2. It contributes to an infant or child developing high stress reactivity later in life, consequently placing individuals assigned female at birth at greater risk for sPTB as an adult.

Examining the fetal/infant/childhood effects of toxic stress (Jiang et al., 2019) helps explain the apparent transmission of sPTB disparity across generations. It also undergirds an urgent call for interventions that can

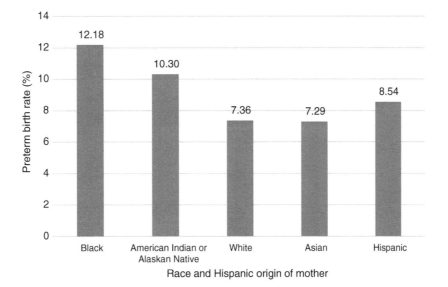

Figure 35.1 Singleton PTB rates, by race and Hispanic origin of mother: United States, 2020. Adapted from Martin and Osterman (2022).

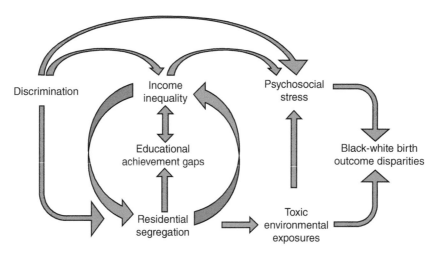

Figure 35.2 Conceptual model of factors in the United States that contribute to racial disparities in birth outcomes. Burris and Hacker (2017)/with permission of Elsevier.

(a) decrease people's exposure to the chronic stress of impoverishment and racism and (b) offer protection and promote healing when chronic stress does occur.

Pathophysiology of Preterm Birth

sPTB is not a single entity but the outcome of a multifactorial, complex process. For sPTB to occur, the cervix undergoes considerable change, including collagen remodeling and altered cellular content, allowing effacement and dilatation. In addition, the myometrium shifts from a quiescent to contractile state, often accompanied by a shift in signaling between anti-inflammatory and proinflammatory pathways. Biophysical pathways leading to these changes can be categorized as three overall processes (Buhimschi et al., 2010; Talati et al., 2017; Waldorf et al., 2015):

1. *Premature activation of the hypothalamus pituitary adrenal axis in the pregnant person or fetus.* This activation leads to a release of prostaglandins and stimulation of placental estrogens, which, in turn, promote cervical remodeling and myometrium activation.
2. *Frequent or ongoing inflammation.* Systemic infection, ascending genital tract infections, and uterine overdistention (as seen in multifetal gestation or polyhydramnios) all stimulate inflammation. An inflammatory response increases prostaglandin production, which, in turn, promotes cervical remodeling, myometrial activation, and breakdown of extracellular matrix in the fetal membranes (increasing risk for preterm premature rupture of membranes).
3. *Decidual hemorrhage.* Decidual bleeding can trigger the release of thrombin, which promotes inflammation in the decidua and fetal membranes, increasing the risk of preterm premature rupture of membranes.

Perinatal Morbidity Related to Prematurity

Premature infants are at greater risk for short- and long-term complications, including disabilities and impediments in growth and mental development (Table 35.1).

Table 35.1 Potential Neonatal Complications of Prematurity

Respiratory distress syndrome
Intraventricular hemorrhage
Feeding difficulties
Hypoglycemia
Difficulty maintaining body temperature
Apnea
Necrotizing enterocolitis
Patent ductus arteriosus
Infection
Jaundice
Hypothermia
Neurobehavioral problems
Retinopathy of prematurity
Anemia
Cerebral palsy
Cognitive and developmental deficits

With each additional week of prematurity, a newborn is at greater risk for medical complications.

Risk Factors for Preterm Birth

There are multiple risk factors for sPTB (Table 35.2), although 50% of persons who give birth prematurely have no clearly delineated risk factor. While most persons with a prior history of sPTB will go on to have a term birth, a prior sPTB is the strongest risk factor for sPTB.

Chronic stress has been associated with sPTB, operating through an epigenetic mechanism (see discussion above regarding socioeconomic and racial/ethnic disparities). Research implicates several of the stress response hormones (e.g., corticotropin releasing hormone, corticotropin, and cortisol) as likely contributors to sPTB

Table 35.2 Risk Factors for Spontaneous Preterm Birth

Prior obstetric/gynecologic history
Prior history of sPTB
Short **interpregnancy interval** (greatest risk if <6 months)
Cervical surgery (cone biopsy, LEEP, etc.)
Multiple cervical dilation and uterine evacuation procedures
Uterine anomalies
Demographics
<17, >35 years of age
Less education (<12 years)
Single marital status
Lower socioeconomic status
Nutritional status/physical activity
Prepregnancy BMI < 19
Low or excessive gestational weight gain
Poor nutritional status
Long working hours (>80 hours/week)
Hard physical labor (including frequent lifting and standing >8 hours)
Current pregnancy characteristics
Assisted reproductive technologies
Multiple gestation
Congenital malformation
Poly- or oligohydramnios
Fetal infection
Chorioamnionitis
Short cervical length <24 weeks of gestation
Positive fetal fibronectin 22–34 weeks of gestation
Medical conditions of the pregnant person
Genetic loci associated with preterm birth
Chronic medical condition (e.g., hypertension, diabetes, thyroid disease, and asthma)
Abdominal surgery during pregnancy
Non-genital tract bacterial infection (e.g., pyelonephritis, appendicitis, pneumonia, and periodontal disease)
Genital tract bacterial infection (e.g., bacterial vaginosis, chlamydia, gonorrhea, and trichomoniasis)
Psychological factors (e.g., stress and depression)
Substance use (e.g., tobacco, marijuana, alcohol, cocaine, and opioids)

(Traylor et al., 2020). While a solid physiological foundation exists for the relationship between stress and sPTB, stress has been a difficult concept to uniformly measure and treat in the clinical setting.

Genetic factors have long been postulated as contributing influences in length of gestation, and especially in sPTB. Current research has confirmed a genetic link and

provided the identity of genes that are associated with the length of gestation. PTB is associated specifically with variants on the human genome at the EBF1, EEFSEC, and AGTR2 loci (Zhang et al., 2017).

Occupational physical activity has been implicated in the etiology of sPTB. A study of work patterns in over 62,000 childbearing-aged women found a dose response relationship between occupational lifting and sPTB, with the strongest associations for sPTB less than 31 weeks of gestation (Runge et al., 2013). The underlying theory linking occupational activity to sPTB centers on sleep deprivation or disrupted circadian rhythms, resulting in neuroendocrine changes that affect the timing of parturition.

Recent studies indicate that exposure to fine particulate matter is a global contributor to sPTB, especially in Southeast Asia where air pollution is significant (Malley et al., 2017). Persons living in large US cities and near industry are also at higher risk for particulate matter inhalation and sPTB. Systemic inflammation is the mechanism linking air pollution with sPTB.

The causal pathway between risk factors and the actual outcome of sPTB continues to be the subject of much research. Current topics under investigation include the role of the **vaginal microbiome** in sPTB risk, and investigations into molecular and epigenetic-based risk assessment.

Predicting Preterm Birth

Efforts to reduce sPTB rates are hampered by both the difficulty of sPTB prediction in an asymptomatic population and the limited availability of targeted intervention for people at high risk of sPTB.

Risk Scoring

Risk-factor-based prenatal scoring systems have been developed in an effort to identify persons who are most likely to experience sPTB; however, they have failed to achieve that goal. More than half of pregnant persons who give birth prematurely are not identified by risk scoring (low sensitivity), and the majority of pregnant persons who screen positive go on to give birth at term (low predictive value) (Davey et al., 2015).

Fetal Fibronectin Testing

Fetal fibronectin (fFN) is a glycoprotein found in high concentrations in the amniotic fluid and in the interface between the decidua and the trophoblast cells. It is thought to play a role in blastocyst implantation, as well as maintenance of the attachment between the uterine decidua and fetal chorion during pregnancy. Although normally found in the cervical and vaginal secretions before 16–20 weeks of gestation, its presence in cervicovaginal secretions after 20 weeks of gestation is abnormal, except as a marker of the imminent onset of labor at term.

The fFN test is used for persons presenting with signs and symptoms of preterm labor. A positive test has limited utility, with only a 12–16% positive predictive value for

PTB occurring within 1–2 weeks (Hologic, 2020). A negative fFN result is strongly predictive that a person will *not* have a PTB in the next two weeks (>99% negative predictive value). Using fFN to confirm risk status can help decrease unnecessary and potentially harmful interventions, but it does not aid in the prevention of sPTB (Berghella & Saccone, 2016).

The fFN test is performed by placing a swab in the posterior fornix of the vagina and rotating it for 10 seconds. The test may produce a false positive result if the pregnant person had sexual intercourse, vaginal bleeding, transvaginal ultrasonography, or a vaginal exam within the previous 24 hours.

Cervical Length Measurement

Transvaginal ultrasound to determine cervical length (CL) is an effective screening tool to predict sPTB. A short CL (<25 mm) in the second trimester has been associated with a marked increased risk of sPTB. The risk of sPTB is inversely proportional to CL; those persons with the shortest CL have the highest risk of sPTB.

CL measurement is best obtained between 16 and 24 weeks of gestation. Before this time, it is more difficult to discern the lower uterine segment from the endocervical canal. After 24 weeks of gestation, the time frame for effective interventions to prevent sPTB has passed.

Persons with a singleton pregnancy and a prior history of sPTB should undergo serial transvaginal CL measurement between 16 and 24 weeks (Berghella et al., 2016). Some experts strongly advocate a one-time screening CL measurement in all pregnancies. The screening is cost-effective and has demonstrated utility in reducing sPTB in clinical trials (Khalifeh & Berghella, 2016; Orzechowski et al., 2014). Currently, however, there is no recommendation for universal CL screening in the United States.

Primary Prevention of Spontaneous Preterm Birth

Given the difficulty of accurately predicting sPTB, prevention efforts should target all persons who are pregnant or wishing to become pregnant, not solely individuals with risk factors. Primary sPTB prevention strategies that have strong research support as effective in preventing sPTB include:

- Smoking and other substance use cessation
- Adequate nutrition and weight gain
- Interpregnancy interval (IPI) >18 months
- Midwife-led continuity of care model

Primary sPTB prevention strategies that have demonstrated some potential for reducing the risk of sPTB include:

- Infection treatment
- Psychological stress reduction
- Normalization of sleep patterns
- Occupational task modification

Smoking and Substance Use Cessation

Smoking cessation is considered one of the most important measures to reduce sPTB and other complications of pregnancy. A higher proportion of women stop smoking in pregnancy than during any other time in their lives (Lumley et al., 2009). Pregnant persons who stop smoking in the first or second trimesters of pregnancy have a decreased risk of sPTB, compared with those who continue smoking; this decrease follows a dose–response curve, demonstrating improved outcomes with both smoking reduction and smoking cessation efforts (Liu et al., 2020; Wallace et al., 2017).

One-to-one counseling using evidence-based interventions can be effective in reducing smoking during pregnancy (American College of Obstetricians and Gynecologists [ACOG], 2020). Appropriate smoking cessation counseling includes providing information on the impacts of tobacco use on fetal/infant safety, such as increased risk for sPTB, low birth weight, fetal growth restriction, and sudden infant death syndrome. For further information on smoking cessation and other substance use during pregnancy, refer to Chapter 18, *Substance Use during Pregnancy*.

Nutrition and Weight Gain

The risk of sPTB is increased for people who begin pregnancy underweight. In addition, across all body mass index (BMI) categories, gestational weight gain that is more or less than recommended is associated with an increase in sPTB risk (Santos et al., 2019). The magnitude of this risk is greatest for people who enter pregnancy underweight (Girsen et al., 2016; Hannaford et al., 2017).

Gaining adequate pregnancy weight can significantly reduce PTB risk. Interestingly, underweight Black persons who reach weight gain goals for pregnancy benefit from a greater reduction in sPTB, compared to underweight White persons (Leonard et al., 2017). This is a potentially promising opportunity for targeted intervention to address disparities in sPTB risk.

Working with individuals to improve diet quality during pregnancy may also have potential to prevent sPTB. Deficiencies in iron, folic acid, B12, zinc, vitamin D, calcium, and omega-3 fatty acids have been associated with sPTB (Dunlop et al., 2011; Kar et al., 2016). However, there is mixed evidence regarding the role of micronutrient supplementation (either preconceptionally or during pregnancy) in reducing the risk of sPTB (Imdad & Bhutta, 2012; Li et al., 2017b; Mozurkewich & Klemens, 2012; Rahman et al., 2016; Rogne et al., 2017). For example, Cantor et al. (2015) discuss that for pregnant persons with anemia, iron supplementation has been shown in some trials to reduce the risk of sPTB, but systematic review has shown no impact of supplementation on sPTB. The role of micronutrients in the pathophysiology of sPTB is complex, and precise mechanisms of action and optimal requirements are not fully known.

Studies also indicate that pregnant persons who do not eat three meals plus two snacks daily have a higher risk of sPTB, compared to those who are able to follow this recommended food intake pattern (Englund-Ogge et al., 2017). It is postulated that the body reacts to missed meals as a stressor, and elevated levels of stress hormones have been implicated in the events leading to sPTB. Counseling regarding this relationship should be individualized and solution-oriented, working with pregnant persons to optimize eating patterns given the particular financial and schedule constraints they face. Counseling should also recognize the multifactorial nature of sPTB and maintain respect for cultural practices such as Ramadan fasting, which in the absence of other risk factors has little relationship with sPTB (Glazier et al., 2018).

Nutritional interventions to reduce sPTB risk

Support all pregnant persons in their efforts to:

- Achieve an appropriate prepregnancy weight.
- Gain an adequate amount of pregnancy weight for BMI.
- Take 200–300 mg of omega-3 fatty acids daily or eat two fish meals a week.
- Take a prenatal multivitamin supplement that includes vitamin D.
- Have a healthy, balanced diet.
- Eat three meals plus two snacks daily; do not routinely miss meals.
- Achieve adequate iron stores.

Interpregnancy Interval

Multiple studies demonstrate a dose–response relationship between an IPI less than 18 months and sPTB (Appareddy et al., 2016; Nerlander et al., 2015). This relationship is stronger for individuals with a history of prior sPTB (Kouallali et al., 2016). One proposed mechanism of action is insufficient time for micronutrient replenishment between pregnancies, particularly folate and iron (Getz et al., 2012). Recommendations for IPI are between a minimum of 18 months and 24 months (ACOG, 2019; WHO, 2005). Advising individuals to wait at least 1.5 years between pregnancies and providing reliable birth control options are appropriate interventions for reducing the risk of sPTB. With >50% of short IPI pregnancies unintended, helping individuals achieve their desired pregnancy spacing through postpartum access to birth control can reduce this share of short IPI pregnancies and reduce sPTB risk (Gemmill & Lindberg, 2013).

Midwife-Led Care

In 2016, the Cochrane Collaboration published evidence that midwifery-led care models, whether using a primary midwife structure or team-based care, are associated with decreased risk of sPTB compared to care programs led by obstetricians or family physicians (Sandall et al., 2016). Researchers suggest this relationship may be based on the following (Sandall et al., 2019):

- Midwifery care often reaches populations underserved by the healthcare system.

- Strong relationships between midwives and pregnant persons may decrease stress as the pregnant person navigates the health system and social programs.
- Strong relationships between midwives and pregnant persons may increase participation in prenatal care, which, in turn, provides opportunities for prevention and early diagnosis of complications.
- Midwifery care can facilitate coordination when referral to obstetric or maternal-fetal medicine (MFM) is necessary.

Infection Treatment

In most cases, the vaginal microbiome is dominated by lactobacilli. During pregnancy, the presence of lactobacilli increases. This physiologic change is thought to have a protective effect to prevent the growth of potentially harmful bacteria (Nelson et al., 2016). In persons whose vaginal microbiota is not lactobacilli-dominant, antibacterial defense mechanisms are reduced. High numbers of pathogenic bacteria and a weakened cervical mucus barrier can allow lower genital tract bacteria to pass into the endometrium and amniotic cavity. Here, ascending bacteria can stimulate the production of chemokines and cytokines and inflammatory mediators, which can eventually trigger preterm uterine muscle activity or weaken the amniotic and chorionic membranes.

Multiple studies have reported an association between sPTB and lower genital tract infections, including group B streptococci, *Chlamydia trachomatis,* bacterial vaginosis (BV), *Neisseria gonorrhoeae,* syphilis, and *Trichomonas vaginalis.* However, a causal association for most of these infections has not been demonstrated, and only one screen-and-treat trial for lower genital tract sexually transmitted infections (STIs) has demonstrated a significant effect on sPTB prevention (Sangkomkamhang et al., 2015). The current recommendation is to test pregnant persons who are symptomatic for lower genital tract infection and to screen persons who are otherwise at risk (Centers for Disease Control and Prevention [CDC], 2021; US Preventive Services Task Force [USPSTF], 2020). If positive, treatment should be per CDC guidelines. Additionally, the therapeutic use of probiotics is under consideration to promote vaginal microbiome health in an effort to reduce sPTB (Yang et al., 2015). Trials to date have been small, with an effect demonstrated only in groups already at high risk of sPTB (Kirihara et al., 2018).

The treatment of asymptomatic bacteriuria (ASB) in pregnancy has long been considered a strategy to reduce sPTB risk. However, more recent meta-analyses have found little support for routine screening and treatment of ASB as an effective intervention for reducing sPTB risk (Angelescu et al., 2016; Smaill & Vazquez, 2019). Additionally, a randomized controlled trial (RCT) involving close to 6000 pregnant persons did not confirm an association between ASB and sPTB (Kazemier et al., 2015). While screening and treating persons with ASB is useful in preventing pyelonephritis (USPSTF, 2019), these findings question routine screen-and-treat protocols for the purpose of preventing sPTB.

Periodontal disease has been associated with a sevenfold increase in sPTB (Boggess & Edelstein, 2006). The theory behind this association lies in the subclinical systemic inflammatory process that accompanies periodontal infections. Known labor mediators, such as cytokines and prostaglandins, are chronically produced in individuals with periodontal infection (Perunovic et al., 2016). However, despite this association, studies conflict regarding the impact of treating periodontal infections in pregnancy. For example, a systematic review of RCTs found that when periodontal treatment is appropriately and adequately administered during the prenatal period, it can reduce the risk of sPTB in some populations (Lopez et al., 2015). Another review indicated there is insufficient evidence to determine if periodontal treatment during pregnancy has an impact on sPTB (Iheozor-Ejiofor et al., 2017). This variation in conclusions is likely due to different definitions, treatment protocols, and study rigor. Given that chronic oral infection is common—it has been estimated that close to 50% of the US population has some degree of periodontal disease (Eke et al., 2015)—it may be beneficial to identify and treat periodontal disease prior to pregnancy or in early gestation, especially for individuals at risk for sPTB.

Prenatal Stress and Depression

Psychological stress and altered mood states during pregnancy are linked with sPTB. Pregnant persons with posttraumatic stress disorder (PTSD) experience a fourfold increase in sPTB (Yonkers et al., 2014). Persons with prenatal depression also have higher rates of sPTB (Mesches et al., 2020). The underlying mechanism is thought to be an increase in stress hormones, which can prematurely activate the fetal HPA axis.

Studies assessing the impact of antidepressant therapy on the prevention of sPTB have had variable outcomes. Early research failed to demonstrate an ability of selective serotonin reuptake inhibitor (SSRI) treatment to reduce sPTB risk, compared to a cohort of pregnant patients with depression and no pharmaceutical treatment (Wisner et al., 2009). However, a more recent study reported decreased rates of sPTB in pregnant patients receiving SSRI therapy (Malm et al., 2015). The different findings between studies may relate to the timing at which treatment began or the amount to which depressive symptoms were reduced (Mesches et al., 2020). At present, it is unclear how much depression treatment using other modalities (such as counseling, meditation, or biofeedback monitoring) can protect against sPTB (Traylor et al., 2020).

Epidemiologic studies have shown inverse correlations between social support and stress biomarkers such as cortisol in pregnant persons (Hoffman et al., 2016; Stewart et al., 2015), suggesting that acute stress during pregnancy may be a target for intervention. However, RCTs of interventions aiming to provide social support for pregnant individuals at high risk of sPTB demonstrate only a slight reduction in sPTB risk (East et al., 2019). Interventions aiming to support relaxation, such as yoga and massage, also only show a slight reduction in sPTB risk (Field et al., 2012).

Group prenatal care, such as CenteringPregnancy, brings individuals of similar gestational ages together into a group setting for ongoing care. This model intentionally facilitates social support among members of the group and holds potential for reducing sPTB in select populations. A systematic review and meta-analysis of 4 RCTs and 10 observational studies comparing group prenatal care to traditional care found that group prenatal care might decrease the risk of PTB for Black pregnant persons. Although the authors note that their results are not statistically significant, they did show that the rate of PTB was 7.9% in group care compared with 9.3% in traditional care (Carter et al., 2016). A plausible explanation for the reduced rate of sPTB in Black persons is increased social support and stress reduction provided within the group prenatal care setting.

Disturbed Sleep and Fatigue

Disturbed sleep appears to play a role in many adverse pregnancy outcomes, including sPTB. Poor sleep quality, occupational fatigue, insomnia, and sleep apnea are associated with a significantly increased risk for PTB (Felder et al., 2017; Li et al., 2017a; Okun et al., 2012). The mechanism underlying these associations is thought to be a proinflammatory response with increased production of cytokines, which are known to promote labor.

Sleep is a potentially modifiable risk factor for sPTB. Assessing individuals' sleep quality and habits during pregnancy, and implementing behavioral interventions accordingly, may be a relatively simple intervention to reduce the risk of sPTB. The Pittsburgh Sleep Quality Index is a self-rated questionnaire that can be used with pregnant persons who report extreme fatigue or disordered sleep. Research indicates that moderate exercise during pregnancy is associated with improved sleep quality and might be a worthwhile adjunct treatment to combat sleep disturbances (Baker et al., 2016). For pregnant persons with sleep apnea, continuous positive airway pressure (CPAP) is a safe and effective intervention to improve sleep quality.

Improving sleep quality and reducing fatigue

Throughout pregnancy:

- Evaluate sleep habits.
- Evaluate sleep quality.
- Evaluate level of fatigue.

Measures to improve sleep quality:

- Exercise regularly.
- Avoid large meals close to bedtime.
- Establish a consistent bedtime and waking time.
- Establish a regular relaxing bedtime routine.
- Associate the bed with sleep; avoid watching TV, reading, or using a computer in bed.
- Use comfortable bedding and a cooler room.
- Block out distracting noise.
- Practice relaxation techniques before bedtime.
- Use CPAP for sleep apnea.

Occupational and Physical Activity

Some individuals are exposed to highly demanding occupational physical activities during pregnancy. Studies on the relationship between occupational activities and sPTB have yielded contradictory results. One systematic review found a strong association between physically demanding work during pregnancy (prolonged standing, heavy lifting, physical exertion, occupational fatigue, and demanding posture) and sPTB (van Beukering et al., 2014). Another review noted only a modest relationship between strenuous work activities and sPTB (Palmer et al., 2013). Currently, no guidelines exist on reduced work or standing hours for the purpose of sPTB risk reduction. It is appropriate to evaluate each pregnant person's occupational tasks and schedule in the context of the person's total health and physical fitness, prior to making recommendations regarding occupational activity.

Individuals with a history of sPTB or at risk for sPTB are often concerned about their physical activity in relation to PTB. In the past, persons with a history of sPTB or those considered at high risk for sPTB were often placed on bedrest or activity restriction during pregnancy. However, bedrest is now understood to be a harmful intervention. Bedrest is associated with blood clots, bone density loss, changes in cardiovascular and muscular conditioning, and stress from changing financial and household responsibilities. In addition, bedrest does not decrease the risk of sPTB (Medley et al., 2018).

Activity restriction does not carry the same physical risks as bedrest, but it can also cause stress for the pregnant person. Because there are minimal data to support activity restriction, it should be framed as an option but not an evidence-based recommendation. Recent research has suggested that regular physical activity and 30-minute exercise daily is safe and does not increase the risk of sPTB, even for pregnant people with a history of a prior sPTB (Satterfield et al., 2016). However, it is recommended that people who have a cerclage in place do not participate in regular exercise, extended standing, or lifting (Satterfield et al., 2016).

Secondary Prevention of Spontaneous Preterm Birth

Secondary prevention measures are recommended for the specific populations of individuals with a history of sPTB or individuals with clinical signs associated with sPTB.

Progesterone Therapy

In a healthy pregnancy, progesterone has the following effects on the uterus and cervix:

- Suppresses production of contractile proteins
- Reduces myometrial response to oxytocin
- Suppresses response to cytokines and prostaglandins
- Prevents the formation of gap junctions

Together, these effects help maintain gestation by suppressing myometrial activity. The natural actions of progesterone have been put to therapeutic use for sPTB prevention.

Vaginal progesterone has been shown to reduce the rate of sPTB in individuals with a short cervix (<25 mm), when initiated before 24 weeks of gestation (Romero et al., 2016). Vaginal progesterone is self-administered daily in doses of 90-mg gel or 200-mg suppository, from diagnosis through 36 weeks of gestation. While the use of vaginal progesterone originally was reserved for individuals diagnosed with a short cervix in mid-second trimester, RCTs have also demonstrated the efficacy of daily vaginal progesterone therapy for sPTB risk reduction in persons with a history of sPTB (Elimian et al., 2016), typically beginning at 16 weeks of gestation. Vaginal progesterone is now accepted as first-line treatment for either persons with a short cervix or persons with a normal-length cervix and a history of sPTB (ACOG, 2021).

In 2011, the US Food and Drug Administration (FDA) approved the administration of 17-hydroxyprogesterone caproate (17-OHPC, brand name Makena®) to reduce the risk of sPTB in persons with singleton pregnancy and a history of at least one sPTB. The usual dose was 250 mg in either an intramuscular or subcutaneous preparation, administered weekly from 16 to 20 weeks of gestation through 36 weeks of gestation. In 2019, results from the PROLONG trial in Europe called into question the effectiveness of 17-OHPC for the reduction of sPTB risk, because study participants receiving 17-OHPC showed no benefit compared to participants receiving placebo. However, the study population in Europe was not reflective of the US population where original trials for 17-OHPC took place, in indices of race/ethnicity, age, socioeconomic status, or marital status (SMFM, 2020). Given these differences, researchers have questioned whether contrasting results between PROLONG and original 17-OHPC trials might reflect 17-OHPC having focal effectiveness in persons who experience chronic stress. That question remains unanswered. In the meantime, professional organizations in the United States have reframed their recommendations to present 17-OHPC as a prevention option for persons with a history of sPTB, alongside the option of daily vaginal progesterone (ACOG, 2021).

The prenatal healthcare provider should be aware that the use of progesterone for sPTB prevention is evolving, and a number of clinical trials are currently ongoing. At the time of publication, FDA approval for use of Makena and generic 17-OHPC had been withdrawn, and professional societies were making decisions about recommendations for practice.

Cerclage

Cervical cerclage is a therapeutic option to reduce sPTB risk in persons with documented short cervix and/or a history of cervical insufficiency (Alfirevic et al., 2013). Cerclage aims to give mechanical support to the cervix to keep it closed (Figure 35.3). It can also reduce the production of local inflammatory cytokines within the cervix, providing a secondary mechanism of action to prevent labor (Monsanto et al., 2017).

Cervical cerclage procedure

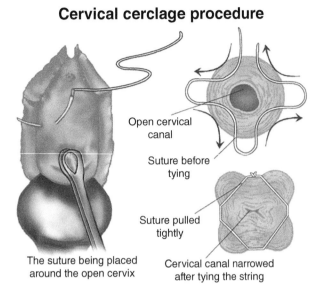

Open cervical canal

Suture before tying

Suture pulled tightly

Cervical canal narrowed after tying the string

The suture being placed around the open cervix

Figure 35.3 Cervical cerclage procedure.

Individuals with cervical insufficiency tend to have progressive shortening of the cervix prior to 24 weeks of gestation and are often either asymptomatic or present with mild symptoms such as pelvic pressure, premenstrual-like cramping or backache, and increased vaginal discharge over several days or weeks. In most cases, the diagnosis of cervical insufficiency is elusive and is only made after several midtrimester pregnancy losses, or after several pregnancies that result in progressively earlier sPTB.

The optimal timing, method, and selection criteria for cerclage depend on whether the procedure is performed due to a person's obstetric history or due to current symptoms and cervical shortening (ACOG, 2014). History-indicated cerclage is generally performed between 12 and 16 weeks of gestation. Cerclage indicated by short cervix on ultrasound or by physical exam findings of cervical dilation and effacement can be performed up to the time of viability (in the United States, typically 24 weeks of gestation). Once placed, the cerclage remains in position until the onset of active labor or 36–37 weeks of gestation.

Pregnant persons who may be candidates for cerclage include those with a history of prior cerclage, cervical trauma such as conization or LEEP, second-trimester pregnancy loss, progressively earlier births, or sPTB <34 weeks. Possible candidates should receive MFM consultation regarding risks and benefits of the procedure (Koullali et al., 2016). Cerclage would then be placed by either an experienced OB/GYN or MFM physician. Pregnancy after cerclage can be comanaged by the specialist who placed the cerclage and a midwife, nurse practitioner, family practice physician, or community OB/GYN.

Pessary

Pessaries have been used for sPTB prevention for over 50 years. The typical **pessary** is a cone-shaped flexible silicon device that is inserted into the upper fornices of the vagina and is designed to support and incline the cervix. Different sizes of pessary are available to allow better adaptation to the pregnant person's individual characteristics. Custom-fit pessaries based on ultrasound measurements can also be created by 3-D printers (Tudela et al., 2016). A pessary is placed before 24 weeks of gestation and removed around 37 weeks of gestation. Pessaries are generally well tolerated, and there are no associated side effects (Falcao et al., 2017).

Unfortunately, current efficacy data do not support pessary use for sPTB prevention. Early RCTs reported that pessary use significantly improved sPTB rates in persons at risk for sPTB (Goya et al., 2012). However, later studies found no improvement (Conde-Agudelo et al., 2020; Nicolaides et al., 2016). The American College of Obstetricians and Gynecologists and the Society for Maternal-Fetal Medicine now recommend against pessary use for the prevention of sPTB (ACOG, 2021).

Prenatal Education on Signs and Symptoms of Preterm Labor and Related Conditions

During the course of prenatal care, all pregnant persons should receive information on the signs and symptoms of preterm labor, preterm prelabor rupture of membranes (PPROM), and cervical insufficiency. When a person recognizes possible preterm labor or these related conditions and has clear instruction about actions to take, they can receive expedited care and potentially delay or prevent sPTB. Additionally, they can receive interventions to improve neonatal outcomes if current conditions progress to PTB.

Signs and symptoms of preterm labor, PPROM, or cervical insufficiency

- Menstrual-like uterine cramps
- Uterine contractions more than four to six times in an hour
- Pressure in the lower abdomen
- Low backache (intermittent back pain and/or a change in the character of back pain)
- Vaginal bleeding
- Increased vaginal discharge of clear, watery, pink, or tan fluid
- Pelvic pressure or a feeling that "something" is in the vagina
- Persistent abdominal cramping with or without nausea, vomiting, or diarrhea

---

Diagnosis and Management of Individuals with Preterm Labor

Preterm labor is defined as contractions of sufficient frequency and intensity to cause progressive effacement and dilation of the cervix prior to 37 completed weeks of pregnancy (37 weeks and 0 days). Although preterm labor is one of the most common reasons for hospitalization during pregnancy, it is challenging to identify those persons with preterm labor who will go on to give birth preterm. Less than 10% of persons diagnosed in preterm labor will give birth within seven days (ACOG, 2016). Approximately 40–50% of persons with suspected preterm labor stop contracting and go on to give birth at term (ACOG, 2016).

When a person presents with signs of preterm labor, a thorough review of the prenatal record and present pregnancy history should be conducted to evaluate risk factors and provide context for current symptoms. Evaluation of fetal well-being should begin, typically through continuous electronic fetal monitoring. A speculum exam is recommended to allow visual examination of the cervix and membranes and to collect cervical-vaginal cultures for STIs, BV, and rapid screen for GBS. Swabs may be collected for fFN and for amniotic fluid in the vaginal secretions, followed by ultrasound to evaluate CL and amniotic fluid volume. Additional testing can include urine culture, as well as urine drug screening with consent from the pregnant person. A digital vaginal examination for cervical dilation and effacement is the last step of evaluation, but digital exam should only be done if membranes are intact and placental location is known (Table 35.3).

When a diagnosis of preterm labor is made, interventions to promote positive neonatal outcomes should be initiated. Exogenous corticosteroids accelerate fetal lung maturity and are indicated for all pregnant persons between 23 weeks of gestation through 33 weeks 6 days who are at risk for PTB (spontaneous or iatrogenic) within the next 7 days (ACOG, 2016). From 34 weeks of gestation through 36 weeks 6 days, corticosteroids can also be administered to pregnant persons at risk for PTB who have not previously received corticosteroid therapy. Both betamethasone and dexamethasone are effective and

acceptable. Studies show that a single course of antenatal corticosteroids is associated with a reduction in serious outcomes related to prematurity, such as perinatal and neonatal death, respiratory distress syndrome, intraventricular hemorrhage, and necrotizing enterocolitis (Roberts et al., 2017).

Magnesium sulfate provides neuroprotection to the very preterm or extremely preterm fetus, decreasing the incidence and severity of cerebral palsy due to prematurity. It should be administered in pregnancies less than 32 weeks of gestation when birth is likely in the next seven days (ACOG, 2016).

Tocolytics, such as indomethacin, nifedipine, and terbutaline, can be effective for delaying birth for two to seven days (ACOG, 2016; Haas et al., 2009). Tocolytics are administered over the course of 48 hours, with a primary goal of prolonging pregnancy to provide time for the administration of corticosteroids and magnesium sulfate. Tocolysis also allows time for transport to another facility as needed. Tocolysis should not be used after 34 weeks of gestation, even if a complete course of corticosteroids has not been administered. Ongoing tocolytic therapy to control preterm contractions, whether administered inpatient or in the home setting, is ineffective in preventing sPTB, is associated with significant side effects for the pregnant person and/or fetus, and should not be used.

Age of viability is a consideration when an individual presents in preterm labor. There is general medical consensus based on outcomes data that treatment for preterm labor should be initiated in pregnancies at or beyond 24 weeks of gestation (Leuthner, 2014). In the peri-viable period (time frames just under 24 weeks of gestation), the preferences of pregnant persons and their families are important considerations in decision-making about intervention for preterm labor.

Diagnosis and Management of Individuals with PPROM

PPROM is defined as preterm rupture of membranes, in the absence of labor. PPROM is diagnosed by sterile speculum exam, during which the examiner looks for visible leakage of fluid from the cervix or pooling of fluid in the vaginal vault. During the speculum exam, swabs may be collected for additional testing: nitrazine test of vaginal pH, ferning or arborization of dried vaginal fluid on a microscope slide, or antibody detection of amniotic fluid marker proteins (such as Amnisure® or ROM Plus®).

When a diagnosis of PPROM is made, it is important to rule out placental abruption, chorioamnionitis, and abnormal fetal heart rate tracings, conditions that preclude expectant management. Then, just as with preterm labor, interventions to promote neonatal outcomes should be initiated. Appropriate interventions depend on the gestational age at which PPROM occurs and may include antibiotics to prolong latency and prevent neonatal GBS infection, magnesium sulfate for fetal neuroprotection, and corticosteroids for fetal lung maturation (ACOG, 2020).

Table 35.3   Cervical Changes and Preterm Labor Diagnosis

Digital cervical assessment	
Cervix >3 cm dilated ≥80% effaced	Preterm labor established
Cervix 2–3 cm dilated, <80% effaced	Preterm labor likely • Monitor contractions. • Repeat exam after a period of time. • If no cervical change, send previously collected fFN swab and/or conduct CL ultrasound. • Consider tocolysis if cervical change, if CL is <20 mm, or if fFN is positive.
Cervix <2 cm dilated, <80% effaced	Preterm labor uncertain • Monitor contractions. • Repeat exam in 1–2 hours. • Send previously collected fFN and/or conduct CL ultrasound. • Consider tocolysis if cervical change, if effacement reaches ≥80%, if CL is <20 mm, or if fFN is positive.

In cases of PPROM where both the pregnant person and fetus are clinically stable, the provider team should discuss with the pregnant person and family the benefits and risks of expectant management or planned PTB. Expectant management is generally advised until 34 weeks of gestation, whereas either expectant management or PTB can be considered between 34 weeks of gestation and 36 weeks 6 days (ACOG, 2020).

Diagnosis and Management of Individuals with Cervical Insufficiency

Cervical insufficiency is defined as painless cervical dilation and effacement, leading to birth of a previable or preterm fetus. As discussed above, cervical insufficiency is definitively diagnosed on the basis of reproductive history. However, it is suspected when a pregnant person presents for care with advanced dilation but no clinical signs of labor.

Management of pregnancy with a history of cervical insufficiency is discussed in the "Secondary Prevention of Spontaneous Preterm Birth" section above. For individuals with acute symptoms and exam consistent with cervical insufficiency, care is the same as for an individual who presents with preterm labor.

Interprofessional Care

Healthcare providers have a responsibility during preconception and prenatal care to evaluate each pregnant person's risk for sPTB and initiate primary prevention and secondary prevention strategies. The potential to reduce risk is greatest during the preconception and early prenatal periods, when modifiable risk factors can be addressed. Pregnant persons at high risk for sPTB and those qualifying for progesterone therapy and/or cerclage benefit from consultation with (or referral to) MFM specialists. In the case of active preterm labor, PPROM, or acute cervical insufficiency, pregnant persons should receive care from an integrated provider team. Depending on the healthcare setting, this team might include a midwife or other advanced practice provider, family medicine physician, OB/GYN physician, MFM physician, and/or neonatologist.

Summary

Preventing PTB remains one of the great challenges in perinatal care. Despite significant research and advances in treatment, PTB rates in the United States remain high. The etiologies of sPTB are complex and influenced by genetics, **epigenetics**, and environmental factors. During the course of prenatal care, risk factors should be identified and risk reduction interventions initiated. Persons with previous sPTB are at an increased risk of subsequent sPTB and may be candidates for treatment with prenatal progesterone. The greatest hopes for sPTB reduction in the United States lie in reducing chronic stress linked to socioeconomic inequality and racism and supporting the cultivation of beneficial health habits prior to pregnancy.

Resources for Clients, Families, and Healthcare Providers

Center for Disease Control and Prevention. State-specific data and many consumer and professional resources: https://www.cdc.gov/reproductivehealth/maternalin-fanthealth/pretermbirth.htm

March of Dimes. A global organization with the mission to prevent premature births: http://www.marchofdimes.com

References

Alfirevic, Z., Owen, J., Carreras Moratonas, E., Sharp, A. N., Szychowski, J. M., & Goya, M. (2013). Vaginal progesterone, cerclage or cervical pessary for preventing preterm birth in asymptomatic singleton pregnant women with a history of preterm birth and a sonographic short cervix. *Ultrasound in Obstetrics & Gynecology*, *41*(2), 146–151.

Alhusen, J. L., Bower, K. M., Epstein, E., & Sharps, P. (2016). Racial discrimination and adverse birth outcomes: An integrative review. *Journal of Midwifery & Women's Health*, *61*(6), 707–720.

American College of Obstetricians and Gynecologists (ACOG). (2014, reaffirmed 2020). Practice bulletin no.142. Cerclage for the management of cervical insufficiency. *Obstetrics & Gynecology*, *123*(2 Pt 1), 372–379.

American College of Obstetricians and Gynecologists (ACOG). (2016, reaffirmed 2020). Practice bulletin no. 171. Management of preterm labor. *Obstetrics & Gynecology*, *128*(4), e155–e164.

American College of Obstetricians and Gynecologists (ACOG). (2019). Obstetric care consensus no. 8. Interpregnancy care. *Obstetrics & Gynecology*, *133*(1), e51–e72.

American College of Obstetricians and Gynecologists (ACOG). (2020). Committee opinion no. 807. Tobacco and nicotine cessation during pregnancy. *Obstetrics & Gynecology*, *135*(5), e221–e229.

American College of Obstetricians and Gynecologists (ACOG). (2021). Practice bulletin no. 234. Prediction and prevention of spontaneous preterm birth. *Obstetrics & Gynecology*, *138*(2), e65–e90.

Angelescu, K., Nussbaumer-Streit, B., Sieben, W., Scheibler, P., & Gartlehner, G. (2016). Benefits and harms of screening for and treatment of asymptomatic bacteriuria in pregnancy: A systematic review. *BMC Pregnancy & Childbirth*, *16*(1), 336.

Appareddy, S., Pryor, J., & Bailey, B. (2016). Inter-pregnancy interval and adverse outcomes: Evidence for an additional risk in health disparate populations. *The Journal of Maternal–Fetal & Neonatal Medicine*, *30*(21), 1–5.

Baker, J. H., Rothenberger, S. D., Kline, C. E., & Okun, M. L. (2016). Exercise during early pregnancy is associated with greater sleep continuity. *Behavioral Sleep Medicine*, 1–14.

Berghella, V., Palacio, M., Ness, A., Alfirevic, Z., Nicolaides, K., & Saccone, G. (2016). Cervical length screening for prevention of preterm birth in singleton pregnancies with threatened preterm labor: A Cochrane systematic review and meta-analysis of randomized controlled trials using individual patient-level data. *Ultrasound in Obstetrics & Gynecology*, *49*(3), 322–329.

Berghella, V., & Saccone, G. (2016). Fetal fibronectin testing for prevention of preterm birth in singleton pregnancies with threatened preterm labor: A systematic review and metaanalysis of randomized controlled trials. *American Journal of Obstetrics & Gynecology*, *215*(4), 431–438.

Boggess, K. A., & Edelstein, B. L. (2006). Oral health in women during preconception and pregnancy: Implications for birth outcomes and infant oral health. *Maternal and Child Health Journal*, *10*(5 Suppl), S169–S174.

Brink, L. T., Nel, D. G., Hall, D. R., & Odendaal, H. J. (2020). Association of socioeconomic status and clinical and demographic conditions with the prevalence of preterm birth. *International Journal of Gynaecology and Obstetrics*, *149*(3), 359–369.

Buhimschi, C. S., Schatz, F., Krikun, G., Buhimschi, I. A., & Lockwood, C. J. (2010). Novel insights into molecular mechanisms of abruption-induced preterm birth. *Expert Reviews in Molecular Medicine*, *12*, e35.

Burris, H. H., & Hacker, M. R. (2017). Birth outcome racial disparities: A result of intersecting social and environmental factors. *Seminars in Perinatology*, *41*(6), 360–366.

Bushnik, T., Yang, S., Kaufman, J. S., Kramer, M. S., & Wilkins, R. (2017). Socioeconomic disparities in small-for-gestational-age birth and preterm birth. *Health Reports*, *28*(11), 3–10.

Cantor, A. G., Bougatsos, C., Dana, T., Blazina, I., & McDonagh, M. (2015). Routine iron supplementation and screening for iron deficiency anemia in pregnancy: A systematic review for the US preventive services task force: Iron supplementation and screening for iron deficiency anemia in pregnancy. *Annals of Internal Medicine*, *162*(8), 566–576.

Carter, E. B., Temming, L. A., Akin, J., Fowler, S., Macones, G. A., Colditz, G. A., & Tuuli, M. G. (2016). Group prenatal care compared with traditional prenatal care: A systematic review and metaanalysis. *Obstetrics & Gynecology*, *128*(3), 551–561.

Centers for Disease Control and Prevention (CDC). (2021). *2021 Sexually transmitted infections treatment guidelines.* https://www.cdc.gov/std/treatment-guidelines/pregnant.htm

Collins, J. W., Jr., David, R. J., Handler, A., Wall, S., & Andes, S. (2004). Very low birthweight in African American infants: The role of maternal exposure to interpersonal racial discrimination. *American Journal of Public Health*, *94*(12), 2132–2138.

Collins, J. W., Jr., David, R. J., Simon, D. M., & Prachand, N. G. (2007). Preterm birth among African American and white women with a lifelong residence in high-income Chicago neighborhoods: An exploratory study. *Ethnicity and Disease*, *17*(1), 113–117.

Collins, J. W., Jr., Rankin, K. M., & David, R. J. (2011). African American women's lifetime upward economic mobility and preterm birth: The effect of fetal programming. *American Journal of Public Health*, *101*(4), 714–719.

Conde-Agudelo, A., Romero, R., & Nicolaides, K. H. (2020). Cervical pessary to prevent preterm birth in asymptomatic high-risk women: A systematic review and meta-analysis. *American Journal of Obstetrics & Gynecology*, *223*(1), 42–65.e2.

Davey, M. A., Watson, L., Rayner, J. A., & Rowlands, S. (2015). Risk-scoring systems for predicting preterm birth with the aim of reducing associated adverse outcomes. *Cochrane Database of Systematic Reviews*, 10, CD004902.

Dunlop, A. L., Essalmi, A. G., Alvalos, L., Breton, C., Camargo, C. A., Cowell, W. J., Dabelea, D., Dager, S. R., Duarte, C., Elliott, A., Fichorova, R., Gern, J., Hedderson, M. M., Thepaksorn, E. H., Huddleston, K., Karagas, M. R., Kleinman, K., Leve, L., Li, X., . . . McGrath, M. (2021). Racial and geographic variation in effects of maternal education and neighborhood-level measures of socioeconomic status on gestational age at birth: Findings from the ECHO cohorts. *PLoS One*, *16*(1), e0245064.

Dunlop, A. L., Kramer, M. R., Hogue, C. J., Menon, R., & Ramakrishan, U. (2011). Racial disparities in preterm birth: An overview of the potential role of nutrient deficiencies. *Acta Obstetricia et Gynecologica Scandinavica*, *90*(12), 1332–1341.

East, C. E., Biro, M. A., Fredericks, S., & Lau, R. (2019). Support during pregnancy for women at increased risk of low birthweight babies. *Cochrane Database of Systematic Reviews*, 4, CD000198.

Eke, P. I., Dye, B. A., Wei, L., Slade, G. D., Thornton-Evans, G. O., Borgnakke, W. S., Taylor, G. W., Page, R. C., Beck, J. D., & Genco, R. J. (2015). Update on prevalence of periodontitis in adults in the United States: NHANES 2009 to 2012. *Journal of Periodontology*, *86*(5), 611–622.

Elimian, A., Smith, K., Williams, M., Knudtson, E., Goodman, J. R., & Escobedo, M. B. (2016). A randomized controlled trial of intramuscular versus vaginal progesterone for the prevention of recurrent preterm birth. *International Journal of Gynecology & Obstetrics*, *134*(2), 169–172.

Englund-Ogge, L., Birgisdottir, B. E., Sengpiel, V., Brantster, A. L., Haugen, M., Myhre, R., & Jacobsson, B. (2017). Meal frequency patterns and glycemic properties of maternal diet in relation to preterm delivery: Results from a large prospective cohort study. *PLoS One*, *12*(3), e0172896.

Falcao, V., Melo, C., Matias, A., & Montenegro, N. (2017). Cervical pessary for the prevention of preterm birth: Is it of any use? *Journal of Perinatal Medicine*, *45*(1), 21–27.

Felder, J. N., Baer, R. J., Rand, L., Jelliffe-Pawlowski, L. L., & Prather, A. A. (2017). Sleep disorder diagnosis during pregnancy and risk of preterm birth. *Obstetrics & Gynecology*, *130*(3), 573–581.

Field, T., Diego, M., Hernandez-Reif, M., Medina, L., Delgado, J., & Hernandez, A. (2012). Yoga and massage therapy reduce prenatal depression and prematurity. *Journal of Bodywork and Movement Therapies*, *16*(2), 204–209.

Gemmill, A., & Lindberg, L. D. (2013). Short interpregnancy intervals in the United States. *Obstetrics & Gynecology*, *122*(1), 64.

Getz, K. D., Anderka, M. T., Werler, M. M., & Case, A. P. (2012). Short interpregnancy interval and gastroschisis risk in the national birth defects prevention study. *Birth Defects Research Part A, Clinical and Molecular Teratology*, *94*, 714–720.

Girsen, A. I., Mayo, J. A., Carmichael, S. L., Phibbs, C. S., Shachar, B. Z., Stevenson, D. K., Lyell, D. J., Shaw, G. M., & Gould, J. B. (2016). Women's prepregnancy underweight as a risk factor for preterm birth: A retrospective study. *BJOG: An International Journal of Obstetrics & Gynaecology*, *123*(12), 2001–2007.

Glazier, J. D., Hayes, D., Hussain, S., D'Souza, S. W., Whitcombe, J., Heazell, A., & Ashton, N. (2018). The effect of Ramadan fasting during pregnancy on perinatal outcomes: A systematic review and meta-analysis. *BMC Pregnancy and Childbirth*, *18*(1), 421.

Goya, M., Pratcorona, L., Merced, C., Rodo, C., Valle, L., Romero, A., Juan, M., Rodriguez, A., Muñoz, B., Santacruz, B., Bello-Munoz, J. C., Llurba, E., Higueras, T., Cabero, L., & Carreras, E. (2012). Cervical pessary in pregnant women with a short cervix (PECEP): An open-label randomised controlled trial. *The Lancet*, *379*(9828), 1800–1806.

Haas, D. M., Imperiale, T. F., Kirkpatrick, P. R., Klein, R. W., Zollinger, T. W., & Golichowski, A. M. (2009). Tocolytic therapy: A metaanalysis and decision analysis. *Obstetrics & Gynecology*, *113*(3), 585–594.

Hall, E. S., & Greenberg, J. M. (2016). Estimating community-level costs of preterm birth. *Public Health*, *141*, 222–228.

Hannaford, K. E., Tuuli, M. G., Odibo, L., Macones, G. A., & Odibo, A. O. (2017). Gestational weight gain: Association with adverse pregnancy outcomes. *American Journal of Perinatology*, *34*(02), 147–154.

Hoffman, M. C., Mazzoni, S. E., Wagner, B. D., & Laudenslager, M. L. (2016). Measures of maternal stress and mood in relation to preterm birth. *Obstetrics & Gynecology*, *127*(3), 545.

Hologic. (2020). *Rapid fFN for the TLiIQ System: Information for healthcare providers.* https://www.hologic.com/package-inserts/diagnostic-products/ffn-test

Iheozor-Ejiofor, Z., Middleton, P., Esposito, M., & Glenny, A. M. (2017). Treating periodontal disease for preventing adverse birth outcomes in pregnant women. *Cochrane Database of Systematic Reviews*, 6, CD005297.

Imdad, A., & Bhutta, Z. A. (2012). Effects of calcium supplementation during pregnancy on maternal, fetal and birth outcomes. *Paediatric & Perinatal Epidemiology*, *26*, 138–152.

Jiang, S., Postovit, L., Cattaneo, A., Binder, E. B., & Aitchison, K. J. (2019). Epigenetic modifications in stress response genes associated with childhood trauma. *Frontiers in Psychiatry*, *10*, 808.

Johnson, J. D., Green, C. A., Vladutiu, C. J., & Manuck, T. A. (2020). Racial disparities in prematurity persist among women of high socioeconomic status. *American Journal of Obstetrics & Gynecology MFM*, *2*(3), 100104.

Joseph, K. S., Fahey, J., Shankardass, K., Allen, V. M., O'Campo, P., Dodds, L., Liston, R. M., & Allen, A. C. (2014). Effects of socioeconomic position and clinical risk factors on spontaneous and iatrogenic preterm birth. *BMC Pregnancy and Childbirth*, *14*, 117.

Kar, S., Wong, M., Rogozinska, E., & Thangaratinam, S. (2016). Effects of omega-3 fatty acids in prevention of early preterm delivery: A systematic review and meta-analysis of randomized studies. *European Journal of Obstetrics & Gynecology and Reproductive Biology*, *198*, 40–46.

Kazemier, B. M., Koningstein, F. N., Schneeberger, C., Ott, A., Bossuyt, P. M., de Miranda, E., Vogelvang, T. E., Verhoeven, C. J. M., Langeveld, J., Woiski, M., Oudijk, M. A., van der Ven, J. E. M., Vlegels, M. T. W., Kuiper, P. N., Feiertag, N., Pajkrt, E., de Groot, C. J. M., Mol, B.

W. J., & Geerlings, S. E. (2015). Maternal and neonatal consequences of treated and untreated asymptomatic bacteriuria in pregnancy: A prospective cohort study with an embedded randomised controlled trial. *The Lancet Infectious Diseases, 15*(11), 1324–1333.

Khalifeh, A., & Berghella, V. (2016). Universal cervical length screening in singleton gestations without a previous preterm birth: Ten reasons why it should be implemented. *American Journal of Obstetrics & Gynecology, 214*(5), 603–e1.

Kim, S., Im, E. O., Liu, J., & Ulrich, C. (2020). Maternal age patterns of preterm birth: Exploring the moderating roles of chronic stress and race/ethnicity. *Annals of Behavioral Medicine, 54*(9), 653–664.

Kirihara, N., Kamitomo, M., Tabira, T., Hashimoto, T., Taniguchi, H., & Maeda, T. (2018). Effect of probiotics on perinatal outcome in patients at high risk of preterm birth. *Journal of Obstetrics & Gynaecology Research, 44*(2), 241–247.

Koullali, B., Kamphuis, E. I., Hof, M. H., Robertson, S. A., Pajkrt, E., de Groot, C. J., Mol, B. W. J., & Ravelli, A. C. J. (2016). The effect of interpregnancy interval on the recurrence rate of spontaneous preterm birth: A retrospective cohort study. *American Journal of Perinatology, 34*(02), 174–182.

Kramer, M. S., Lydon, J., Goulet, L., Kahn, S., Dahhou, M., Platt, R. W., Sharma, S., Meaney, M. J., & Seguin, L. (2013). Maternal stress/distress, hormonal pathways and spontaneous preterm birth. *Paediatric and Perinatal Epidemiology, 27*(3), 237–246.

Leonard, S. A., Petito, L. C., Stephansson, O., Hutcheon, J. A., Bodnar, L. M., Mujahid, M. S., Cheng, Y., & Abrams, B. (2017). Weight gain during pregnancy and the black-white disparity in preterm birth. *Annals of Epidemiology, 27*(5), 323–328.

Leuthner, S. R. (2014). Borderline viability. *Clinics in Perinatology, 41*(4), 799–814.

Li, R., Zhang, J., Zhou, R., Liu, J., Dai, Z., Liu, D., Wang, Y., Zhang, J., Li, Y., & Zeng, G. (2017a). Sleep disturbances during pregnancy are associated with cesarean delivery and preterm birth. *The Journal of Maternal-Fetal & Neonatal Medicine, 30*(6), 733–738.

Li, Z., Mei, Z., Zhang, L., Li, H., Zhang, Y., Li, N., & Serdula, M. K. (2017b). Effects of prenatal micronutrients supplementation on spontaneous preterm birth: double-blind randomized controlled trial in China. *American Journal of Epidemiology, 186*(3), 318–325.

Liu, B., Xu, G., Sun, Y., Qiu, X., Ryckman, K. K., Yu, Y., Snetselaar, L. G., & Bao, W. (2020). Maternal cigarette smoking before and during pregnancy and the risk of preterm birth: A dose-response analysis of 25 million mother–infant pairs. *PLoS Medicine, 17*(8), e1003158.

Lopez, N. J., Uribe, S., & Martinez, B. (2015). Effect of periodontal treatment on preterm birth rate: A systematic review of metaanalyses. *Periodontology 2000, 67*(1), 87–130.

Lumley, J., Chamberlain, C., Dowswell, T., Oliver, S., Oakley, L., & Watson, L. (2009). Interventions for promoting smoking cessation during pregnancy. *Cochrane Database of Systematic Reviews, 3*, CD001055.

Malley, C. S., Kuylenstierna, J. C., Vallack, H. W., Henze, D. K., Blencowe, H., & Ashmore, M. R. (2017). Preterm birth associated with maternal fine particulate matter exposure: A global, regional and national assessment. *Environment International, 101*, 173–182.

Malm, H., Sourander, A., Gissler, M., Gyllenberg, D., Hinkka-Yli-Salomäki, S., McKeague, I. W., Artama, M., & Brown, A. S. (2015). Pregnancy complications following prenatal exposure to SSRIs or maternal psychiatric disorders: Results from population-based national register data. *American Journal of Psychiatry, 172*(12), 1224–1232.

March of Dimes. (2016). *Born too soon*. https://www.marchofdimes.org/mission/global-preterm.aspx

Martin, J. A., Hamilton, B. E., & Osterman, M. K. (2021). *NCHS data brief No. 418: Births in the United States, 2020*. National Center for Health Statistics. https://www.cdc.gov/nchs/data/databriefs/db418.pdf

Martin, J. A., & Osterman, M.K. (2022). *NCHC Data Brief No. 430: Exploring the decline in the singleton preterm birth rate in the United States, 2019–2020*. National Center for Health Statistics. https://www.cdc.gov/nchs/data/databriefs/db430.pdf

Medley, N., Vogel, J. P., Care, A., & Alfirevic, Z. (2018). Interventions during pregnancy to prevent preterm birth: An overview of Cochrane systematic reviews. *Cochrane Database of Systematic Reviews, 2018*(11), CD012505.

Mesches, G. A., Wisner, K. L., & Betcher, H. K. (2020). A common clinical conundrum: Antidepressant treatment of depression in pregnant women. *Seminars in Perinatology, 44*(3), 151229.

Monsanto, S. P., Daher, S., Ono, E., Pendeloski, K. P. T., Traina, E., Mattar, R., & Tayade, C. (2017). Cervical cerclage placement decreases local levels of proinflammatory cytokines in patients with cervical insufficiency. *American Journal of Obstetrics & Gynecology, 217*(4), 455–e1.

Mozurkewich, E., & Klemens, C. (2012). Omega-3 fatty acids and pregnancy: Current implications for practice. *Current Opinion in Obstetrics & Gynecology, 24*(2), 72–77.

Nelson, D. B., Rockwell, L. C., Prioleau, M. D., & Goetzl, L. (2016). The role of the bacterial microbiota on reproductive and pregnancy health. *Anaerobe, 42*, 67–73.

Nerlander, L. M., Callaghan, W. M., Smith, R. A., & Barfield, W. D. (2015). Short interpregnancy interval associated with preterm birth in US adolescents. *Maternal and Child Health Journal, 19*(4), 850–858.

Nicolaides, K. H., Syngelaki, A., Poon, L. C., Picciarelli, G., Tul, N., Zamprakou, A., & Rodriguez Calvo, J. (2016). A randomized trial of a cervical pessary to prevent preterm singleton birth. *New England Journal of Medicine, 374*(11), 1044–1052.

Okun, M. L., Luther, J. F., Wisniewski, S. R., Sit, D., Prairie, B. A., & Wisner, K. L. (2012). Disturbed sleep, a novel risk factor for preterm birth? *Journal of Women's Health, 21*(1), 54–60.

Orzechowski, K. M., Boelig, R. C., Baxter, J. K., & Berghella, V. (2014). A universal transvaginal cervical length screening program for preterm birth prevention. *Obstetrics & Gynecology, 124*(3), 520–525.

Palmer, K. T., Bonzini, M., Harris, E. C., Linaker, C., & Bonde, J. P. (2013). Work activities and risk of prematurity, low birth weight and pre-eclampsia: An updated review with meta-analysis. *Occupational and Environmental Medicine, 70*(4), 213–222.

Perunovic, N. D., Rakic, M. M., Nikolic, L. I., Jankovic, S. M., Aleksic, Z. M., Plecas, D. V., Madianos, P. N., & Cakic, S. S. (2016). The association between periodontal inflammation and labor triggers (elevated cytokine levels) in preterm birth: A cross-sectional study. *Journal of Periodontology, 87*(3), 248–256.

Rahman, M. M., Abe, S. K., Rahman, M. S., Kanda, M., Narita, S., Bilano, V., Ota, E., Gilmour, S., & Shibuya, K. (2016). Maternal anemia and risk of adverse birth and health outcomes in low-and middle-income countries: Systematic review and meta-analysis. *American Journal of Clinical Nutrition, 103*(2), 495–504.

Roberts, D., Brown, J., Medley, N., & Dalziel, S. R. (2017). Antenatal corticosteroids for accelerating fetal lung maturation for women at risk of preterm birth. *Cochrane Database of Systematic Reviews, 3*, CD004454.

Rogne, T., Tielemans, M. J., Chong, M. F. F., Yajnik, C. S., Krishnaveni, G. V., Poston, L., Jaddoe, V. W. V., Steegers, E. A. P., Joshi, S., Chong, Y., Godfrey, K. M., Yap, F., Yahyaoui, R., Thomas, T., Hay, G., Hogeveen, M., Demir, A., Saravanan, P., Skovlund, E., . . . Risnes, K. R. (2017). Associations of maternal vitamin B12 concentration in pregnancy with the risks of preterm birth and low birth weight: A systematic review and metaanalysis of individual participant data. *American Journal of Epidemiology, 185*(3), 212–223.

Romero, R., Nicolaides, K. H., Conde-Agudelo, A., O'Brien, J. M., Cetingoz, E., Da Fonseca, E., Creasy, G. W., & Hassan, S. S. (2016). Vaginal progesterone decreases preterm birth < 34 weeks of gestation in women with a singleton pregnancy and a short cervix: An updated meta-analysis including data from the OPPTIMUM study. *Ultrasound in Obstetrics & Gynecology, 48*(3), 308–317.

Runge, S. B., Pedersen, J. K., Svendsen, S. W., Juhl, M., Bonde, J. P., & Andersen, A. M. N. (2013). Occupational lifting of heavy loads and preterm birth: A study within the Danish National Birth Cohort. *Occupational and Environmental Medicine, 70*(11), 782–788. https://doi.org/10.1136/oemed-2012-101173

Sandall, J., Soltani, H., Gates, S., Shennan, A., & Devane, D. (2016). Midwife-led continuity models versus other models of care for childbearing women. *Cochrane Database of Systematic Reviews, 4*, CD004667.

Sandall, J., Soltani, H., Shennan, A., & Devane, D. (2019). *Implementing midwife-led continuity models of care and what do we still need to find out?* Evidently Cochrane. https://evidentlycochrane.net/midwife-led-continuity-of-care

Sangkomkamhang, U. S., Lumbiganon, P., Prasertcharoensuk, W., & Laopaiboon, M. (2015). Antenatal lower genital tract infection screening and treatment programs for preventing preterm delivery. *Cochrane Database of Systematic Reviews*, 2, CD006178.

Santos, S., Voerman, E., Amiano, P., Barros, H., Beilin, L. J., Bergström, A., Charles, M. A., Chatzi, L., Chevrier, C., Chrousos, G. P., Corpeleijn, E., Costa, O., Costet, N., Crozier, S., Devereux, G., Doyon, M., Eggesbø, M., Fantini, M. P., Farchi, S., . . . Jaddoe, V. (2019). Impact of maternal body mass index and gestational weight gain on pregnancy complications: An individual participant data meta-analysis of European, North American and Australian cohorts. *BJOG*, *126*(8), 984–995.

Satterfield, N., Newton, E. R., & May, L. E. (2016). Activity in pregnancy for patients with a history of preterm birth. *Clinical Medicine Insights. Women's Health*, *9*(Suppl 1), 17–21.

Smaill, F. M., & Vazquez, J. C. (2019). Antibiotics for asymptomatic bacteriuria in pregnancy. *Cochrane Database of Systematic Reviews*, 11, CD000490.

Society for Maternal-Fetal Medicine (SMFM). (2020). SMFM statement: Use of 17-alpha hydroxyprogesterone caproate for prevention of recurrent preterm birth. *American Journal of Obstetrics & Gynecology*, *223*(1), B16–B18.

Stewart, C. P., Oaks, B. M., Laugero, K. D., Ashorn, U., Harjunmaa, U., Kumwenda, C., & Dewey, K. G. (2015). Maternal cortisol and stress are associated with birth outcomes, but are not affected by lipid-based nutrient supplements during pregnancy: An analysis of data from a randomized controlled trial in rural Malawi. *BMC Pregnancy and Childbirth*, *15*(1), 346.

Talati, A. N., Hackney, D. N., & Mesiano, S. (2017). Pathophysiology of preterm labor with intact membranes. *Seminars in Perinatology*, *S41*(7), 420–426.

Traylor, C. S., Johnson, J. D., Kimmel, M. C., & Manuck, T. A. (2020). Effects of psychological stress on adverse pregnancy outcomes and nonpharmacologic approaches for reduction: An expert review. *American Journal of Obstetrics & Gynecology MFM*, *2*(4), 100229.

Tudela, F., Kelley, R., Ascher-Walsh, C., & Stone, J. L. (2016). Low cost 3d printing for the creation of cervical cerclage pessary used to prevent preterm birth: A preliminary study [26R]. *Obstetrics & Gynecology*, *127*, 154S.

US Preventive Services Task Force. (2019). Recommendation statement: Screening for asymptomatic bacteriuria in adults. *JAMA*, *322*(12), 1188–1194.

US Preventive Services Task Force. (2020). Recommendation statement: Screening for bacterial vaginosis in pregnant persons to prevent preterm delivery. *JAMA*, *323*(13), 1286–1292.

van Beukering, M. D. M., van Melick, M. J. G. J., Mol, B. W., Frings-Dresen, M. H. W., & Hulshof, C. T. J. (2014). Physically demanding work and preterm delivery: A systematic review and meta-analysis. *International Archives of Occupational and Environmental Health*, *87*(8), 809–834.

Waldorf, K. M. A., Singh, N., Mohan, A. R., Young, R. C., Ngo, L., Das, A., Tsai, J., Bansal, A., Paolella, L., Herbert, B. R., Sooranna, S. R., Gough, G. M., Astley, C., Vogel, K., Baldessari, A. E., Bammler, T. K., MacDonald, J., Gravett, M. G., Rajagopal, L., & Johnson, M. R. (2015). Uterine overdistention induces preterm labor mediated by inflammation: Observations in pregnant women and nonhuman primates. *American Journal of Obstetrics & Gynecology*, *213*(6), 830–e1.

Wallace, J. L., Aland, K. L., Blatt, K., Moore, E., & DeFranco, E. A. (2017). Modifying the risk of recurrent preterm birth: Influence of trimester-specific changes in smoking behaviors. *American Journal of Obstetrics & Gynecology*, *216*(3), 310–e1.

Wertz, R. W., & Wertz, D. C. (1989). *Lying-in: A history of childbirth in America*. Yale University Press.

Wisner, K. L., Sit, D. K., Hanusa, B. H., Moses-Kolko, E. L., Bogen, D. L., Hunker, D. F., Perel, J. M., Jones-Ivy, S., Bodnar, L. M., & Singer, L. T. (2009). Major depression and antidepressant treatment: Impact on pregnancy and neonatal outcomes. *The American Journal of Psychiatry*, *166*(5), 557–566.

World Health Organization (WHO). (2005). *Report of a WHO technical consultation on birth spacing*. https://apps.who.int/iris/handle/10665/69855

World Health Organization (WHO). (2018). *Preterm birth*. https://www.who.int/news-room/fact-sheets/detail/preterm-birth

Yang, S., Reid, G., Challis, J. R., Kim, S. O., Gloor, G. B., & Bocking, A. D. (2015). Is there a role for probiotics in the prevention of preterm birth? *Frontiers in Immunology*, *6*, 62.

Yonkers, K. A., Smith, M. V., Forray, A., Epperson, C. N., Costello, D., Lin, H., & Belanger, K. (2014). Pregnant women with posttraumatic stress disorder and risk of preterm birth. *JAMA Psychiatry*, *71*(8), 897–904.

Zhang, G., Feenstra, B., Bacelis, J., Liu, X., Muglia, L. M., Juodakis, J., & Hinds, D. A. (2017). Genetic associations with gestational duration and spontaneous preterm birth. *New England Journal of Medicine*, *2017*(377), 1156–1167.

36

Hypertensive Disorders of Pregnancy

Melissa Kitzman

The editors gratefully acknowledge Robin G. Jordan and Elizabeth Gabzdyl who authored the previous edition of this chapter.

Relevant Terms

Angiogenic factors—substances in the circulatory system that play a role in the formation and differentiation of new blood vessels

Arteriovenous nicking—a small artery is seen crossing a small vein on fundoscopic examination, causing compression of the vein with bulging on either side of the crossing; sometimes seen in hypertension and arteriosclerosis

Chronic hypertension—hypertension present prior to pregnancy, prior to 20 weeks of gestation, or hypertension that is first diagnosed during pregnancy and does not resolve in the typical postpartum period

Chronic hypertension with superimposed preeclampsia—development of preeclampsia in a person previously diagnosed with chronic hypertension

Disseminated intravascular coagulation—pathological activation of the clotting system that leads to clot formation in small vessels throughout the body; can cause multiple organ failure

Eclampsia—new-onset tonic–clonic, focal, or multifocal seizures in a pregnant or newly postpartum person with no other etiology for the seizure

Endothelium—single layer of thin flattened cells lining body cavities and organs

Gestational hypertension—hypertension in pregnancy presenting after 20 weeks of gestation without any findings associated with preeclampsia and without presence of severe features

Papilledema—optic disk swelling that is caused by increased intracranial pressure

Preeclampsia—a progressive multisystem disorder that occurs only during or after pregnancy; it is associated with new-onset hypertension that occurs after 20 weeks of gestation

Proteinuria—presence of protein in the urine and a diagnostic marker for hypertensive disorders in pregnancy

Scintillations—sparkles or flashes of light, can be experienced by people with preeclampsia due to cerebral edema

Scotomata—a blind spot or partial loss of vision, which can be experienced by people with preeclampsia due to cerebral edema

Severe features—systolic blood pressure of 160 mmHg or more, or diastolic blood pressure of 110 mmHg or more, on two occasions at least four hours apart (unless antihypertensive therapy is initiated before this time), platelet count less than 100,000, impaired liver function that is not accounted for by alternative diagnoses, renal insufficiency, pulmonary edema, new-onset headache unresponsive to medication and not accounted for by alternative diagnoses, visual disturbances

Spiral arteries—coiled branches of the uterine artery, supplying the endometrium, emptying into intervillous spaces, and thus supplying blood to the placenta

Thrombocytopenia—a decrease in platelets below 150,000/mL

Trophoblastic factors—substances and processes related to placental cells

---

Introduction

Hypertensive disorders of pregnancy (HDP) remain one of the major causes of pregnancy-related maternal and fetal morbidity and mortality worldwide. In the United States, maternal mortality is among the highest of the high-income countries with a ratio of 10 per 100,000 births. Pregnancy-related morbidity and mortality disproportionally affect birthing people who identify as Black (Ukoha et al., 2022). In 2016, the estimated maternal mortality ratio for Black American women was 41/100,000 compared to 13/100,000 for White American women (Garovic et al., 2022). Preeclampsia-related severe morbidity and mortality are also higher for Black birthing people (Garovic et al., 2022). Pregnant people who have

---

Prenatal and Postnatal Care: A Person-Centered Approach, Third Edition. Edited by Karen Trister Grace, Cindy L. Farley, Noelene K. Jeffers, and Tanya Tringali.
© 2024 John Wiley & Sons Ltd. Published 2024 by John Wiley & Sons Ltd.
Companion website: www.wiley.com/go/grace/prenatal

HDP are also at increased risk for cardiovascular disease (CVD) later in life, independent of traditional CVD risks (Garovic et al., 2022). There is a substantial and consistent body of evidence showing that a history of HDP increases the risk of future CVD (Parikh et al., 2021). CVD is very common and is the leading cause of death in women in the United States; it affects 32.7% of women of all ages (Ahmed et al., 2014).

Hypertensive disorders were responsible for 6.6% of perinatal deaths in the United States between 2014 and 2017 (Center for Disease Control and Prevention (CDC), 2017) and 18% of perinatal deaths worldwide. Hypertensive disorders in pregnancy are increasing due to increased prevalence of cardiometabolic risk factors as well as advanced age at first pregnancy (Garovic et al., 2022). HDP disproportionally affects pregnant people of color. This may be due to the overall higher prevalence of CVD risk factors, but requires a multilevel approach to identify the impact of racism and other interpersonal and societal factors (Johnson & Louis, 2022).

The greatest risks to the fetus include prematurity due to medically indicated preterm birth (PTB), fetal growth restriction (FGR), placental abruption, and stillbirth. The greatest risks to the pregnant person include stroke, myocardial infarction (MI), peripartum cardiomyopathy, pulmonary edema, and renal failure. A timely and accurate diagnosis is essential to prevent adverse perinatal outcomes. Three main goals of the care of pregnant people with hypertensive disorders include the prevention of complications, continuation of pregnancy as long as safely possible, and minimizing fetal and neonatal adverse effects. This chapter covers screening, diagnosis, and management of HDP.

Health equity key points

- Hypertensive disorders of pregnancy disproportionally affect birthing people of color; a multilevel approach to identify the impact of racism and other interpersonal and societal factors is needed.
- Standardized protocols can prevent racial health disparities by reducing bias and discrimination in care. Other strategies include telehealth, quality improvement bundles, and group prenatal care.
- Higher socioeconomic status reduces the risk of preeclampsia in White pregnant people, but not Black.

Classification of Hypertensive Disorders in Pregnancy

HDP were first classified in 1972 by the National High Blood Pressure Education Program (NHBPEP) and later modified by the American College of Obstetricians and Gynecologists (ACOG; Garovic et al., 2022). The categories of hypertensive disorders are **gestational hypertension, preeclampsia/eclampsia, chronic hypertension**, and **chronic hypertension with superimposed preeclampsia**.

Screening for Hypertensive Disorders

Blood Pressure Measurement

One of the most important steps in making an accurate diagnosis is accurately measuring the blood pressure (BP). An accurate BP reading is imperative in caring for people with HDP. The cuff size should be appropriate for the person's size and one that encircles 80% or more of the upper arm. BP is best measured after a rest period of 10 minutes or more, with the pregnant person in an upright position with cuff positioned at the level of the heart. Diagnostic criteria require that a repeat BP be done at least four hours later to verify the initial high BP measurement. This can be difficult with the realities of clinical practice. It is common for a repeat BP to be done at the conclusion of the office visit, and a working diagnosis made from both readings until confirmation can be made with a later BP reading.

BP fluctuations are normal and to be expected during pregnancy. Baseline BP measurement is obtained in the first trimester. Systemic vasodilation occurs in the second trimester, which commonly causes a decrease in BP until the third trimester, when it typically returns to the first-trimester level. Pregnant people with chronic hypertension also commonly experience a second trimester decrease, with a subsequent increase in the third trimester.

Specific guidelines are followed to obtain an accurate BP measurement.

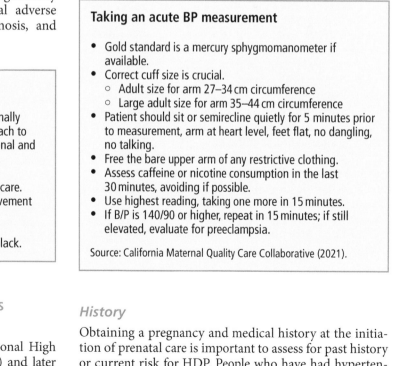

Taking an acute BP measurement

- Gold standard is a mercury sphygmomanometer if available.
- Correct cuff size is crucial.
  - Adult size for arm 27–34 cm circumference
  - Large adult size for arm 35–44 cm circumference
- Patient should sit or semirecline quietly for 5 minutes prior to measurement, arm at heart level, feet flat, no dangling, no talking.
- Free the bare upper arm of any restrictive clothing.
- Assess caffeine or nicotine consumption in the last 30 minutes, avoiding if possible.
- Use highest reading, taking one more in 15 minutes.
- If B/P is 140/90 or higher, repeat in 15 minutes; if still elevated, evaluate for preeclampsia.

Source: California Maternal Quality Care Collaborative (2021).

History

Obtaining a pregnancy and medical history at the initiation of prenatal care is important to assess for past history or current risk for HDP. People who have had hypertension or preeclampsia in a prior pregnancy are at risk for reoccurrence in subsequent pregnancies. During each prenatal visit after 20 weeks of gestation, all pregnant people are asked about signs and symptoms of preeclampsia. The presence of visual disturbances and headaches indicates potential central nervous system (CNS) involvement, and right upper quadrant pain indicates liver involvement, both indicating increasingly severe disease. Patients are asked if there is a noticeable increase in edema especially in the face; nondependent edema is more significant in preeclampsia than dependent edema, which is common in most pregnant people in later gestation.

Physical Examination

Prepregnancy weight and body mass index (BMI) determination are critical components of the physical exam as elevated BMI is a strong risk factor for the development of preeclampsia. Serial weight gain patterns can detect a sudden weight increase that may reflect fluid retention associated with preeclampsia. Observation for new-onset edema in the face, hands, and lower extremities is done with the degree of pitting noted. While not part of the clinical diagnostic criteria, significant edema can result from endothelial damage within blood vessels resulting in fluid leaking into surrounding tissues. Particular physical exam components can include ophthalmic exam to determine if there are changes such as **papilledema**, vascular spasm, or **arteriovenous nicking** related to increased edema. Abdominal palpation can assess for the presence of epigastric or right upper quadrant pain. Deep tendon reflexes can be hyperactive due to CNS irritability in the presence of preeclampsia.

Proteinuria

Presence or absence of urine protein can aid in determining the diagnosis of a hypertensive disorder in pregnancy, although dependence on protein as a diagnostic criterion has been eliminated. Preeclampsia, eclampsia, severe gestational hypertension, and/or HELLP syndrome may occur without proteinuria (California Maternal Quality Care Collaborative (CMQCC), 2021). The gold standard for evaluating **proteinuria** is a 24-hour urine collection in which excretion ≥300 mg is considered to be an abnormal value, or a protein/creatinine ratio (PCR) ≥0.3 mg/dL. A less reliable but quicker and more convenient diagnostic method is a urine dipstick. Often in clinical practice, neither a 24-hour urine collection nor a PCR is available in a timely manner, and immediate clinical management is based on dipstick assessment for proteinuria. A value of 2+ (ACOG, 2020) or greater is considered significant, and followed up with a 24-hour urine collection or PCR. Pregnant persons who present with significant proteinuria without hypertension should be evaluated for other diagnoses that may cause this finding and be monitored for the development of preeclampsia.

Gestational Hypertension

Hypertension in this disorder presents after 20 weeks of gestation and without any findings associated with preeclampsia. Antihypertensive medications are not recommended unless the BP readings are in the severe range, systolic blood pressure (SBP) ≥ 160 mmHg or diastolic blood pressure (DBP) ≥ 110 mmHg. The following surveillance is recommended by ACOG (2020):

- Fetal movement counts daily
- Awareness of warning signs of preeclampsia with prompt reporting if present
- Twice weekly BP measurement (can be combination of home and office)
- Weekly laboratory studies
  - Measure of proteinuria
  - Complete blood count (CBC) with platelet count
  - Liver enzymes
  - Serum creatinine
- 1–2 × week nonstress test (NST) with amniotic fluid measurement
- Ultrasound for fetal growth every 3–4 weeks
- Induction of labor is recommended at 37 + 0 weeks unless BPs become severe

Up to 50% of pregnant people with gestational hypertension will eventually develop proteinuria or other end-organ dysfunction consistent with a preeclampsia diagnosis (Fong et al., 2013). It is prudent to be diligent about surveillance in the event that preeclampsia develops. If evidence of preeclampsia presents, treatment guidelines for preeclampsia are followed, as discussed in the next section.

Preeclampsia/Eclampsia

Preeclampsia is a progressive, multisystem disorder characterized by hypertension and proteinuria or involvement of other organs in an exaggerated system inflammatory response that occurs only during pregnancy after 20 weeks of gestation or in the early postpartum period. Preeclampsia is variable in severity and unpredictable in progression, remaining stable or rapidly progressing to severe disease. Preeclampsia is divided into two levels: preeclampsia without **severe features** and preeclampsia with severe features (Table 36.1).

Preeclampsia can be further divided into early onset (<34 weeks of gestation) and late onset (≥34 weeks of gestation). The majority of cases are late onset, occurring after 36 weeks of gestation with slow progression and favorable outcomes. Pregnant people with severe features are at risk for liver failure, renal failure, heart failure, stroke, pulmonary edema, **disseminated intravascular coagulation** (DIC), CNS abnormalities, and significant fetal complications. People with early-onset preeclampsia typically have a more severe disease progression with higher rates of adverse perinatal outcomes.

Preeclampsia often presents during a routine prenatal visit in an asymptomatic patient. It may be difficult to clearly discern if a person is experiencing normal third-trimester pregnancy symptoms or if they are developing symptoms of preeclampsia. Symptoms can include mild nausea, headache, and edema of the face and extremities.

It is important to reiterate that while the hallmark signs of preeclampsia are proteinuria and hypertension, preeclampsia can occur with or without proteinuria; it is not mandatory for a diagnosis of preeclampsia. Preeclampsia

Table 36.1   Criteria to Diagnose Preeclampsia and Preeclampsia with Severe Features

Preeclampsia	Preeclampsia with severe features
Occurs after 20 weeks of gestation or postpartum	
• Systolic ≥140 mmHg or • Diastolic ≥90 mmHg on two BP readings at least 4 hours apart in a person with a previously normal BP **And one of the following:** • Proteinuria ≥300/mg/24-hour urine (or this amount extrapolated from a timed specimen) or ○ PCR ≥ 0.3 or ○ ≥+1 on dipstick (if no other quantitative methods available) **Or in the absence or proteinuria, new-onset hypertension with the new onset of any of the following:** • Platelet count <100,000/μL • Serum creatinine >1.1 mg/dL or a doubling of the serum creatinine in the absence of other renal disease • Liver enzymes elevated to twice normal level • Pulmonary edema • New-onset headache unresponsive to medications and not accounted for by alternative diagnoses or visual symptoms	• Systolic ≥160 mmHg or • Diastolic ≥110 mmHg on two BP readings at least 4 hours apart or sooner if antihypertensive therapy initiated • Platelet count below 100,000/μL • Evidence of impaired liver function not accounted for by alternative diagnoses ○ Liver enzymes elevated to twice normal level and/or ○ Epigastric or right upper quadrant pain that is persistent or unresponsive to medications • Evidence of worsening renal insufficiency (elevated serum creatinine >1.1 mg/dL) or a doubling of the serum creatinine in the absence of other renal disease • Pulmonary edema • New-onset headache unresponsive to medication and not accounted for by alternative diagnoses • Visual disturbances

Source: Adapted from ACOG (2020).

is most often seen prenatally; however, it can also develop postpartum. See Chapter 43, *Common Complications during the Postnatal Period*, for detailed information on postpartum preeclampsia.

Signs and symptoms of preeclampsia

- Severe headache
- Visual changes (blind spots, light flashes, and blurry)
- Right epigastric pain, indigestion, and nausea
- Increased edema
- Sudden weight gain
- Shortness of breath
- Altered mental status

Eclampsia is the onset of tonic–clonic seizures that cannot be attributed to other causes in a person with preeclampsia. Widespread availability of prenatal care has significantly reduced the incidence of eclampsia in the United States, making it a rare condition. The incidence of eclampsia is estimated to be approximately 2–8 cases per 10,000 births in higher-income countries. Eclamptic seizures can occur during the prenatal, intrapartum, and postpartum period and are typically preceded by increasingly severe preeclampsia manifestations; however, eclampsia also occurs unexpectedly in people with mild BP elevations and minimal or no proteinuria. Since this condition reflects CNS compromise, typical symptoms are headaches, **scintillations, scotomata**, and restlessness. Headache is the most common prodromal symptom (Cooray et al., 2011),

though it is a very nonspecific symptom, making it difficult to predict who will go on to develop eclampsia. Eclampsia can result in fetal distress, placental abruption, and fetal or maternal death. This is an emergency, a potentially life-threatening situation that requires immediate seizure precaution measures and urgent delivery to prevent long-term maternal or fetal sequelae. While this text does not cover detailed intrapartum management, specific steps taken when eclampsia occurs are as follows:

- Cardiorespiratory support
- Magnesium sulfate IV to prevent recurrent seizure
- Maternal hypoxemia and acidemia correction
- Severe hypertension treatment
- Planning for delivery once patient is stabilized (Bernstein et al., 2017)

Pathophysiology of Preeclampsia–Eclampsia Syndrome

Despite considerable research, the etiology of preeclampsia remains elusive. Substantial gain has been made in the understanding of preeclampsia pathophysiology; however, these advances have not yet translated into improved clinical practice.

Preeclampsia is currently considered to be primarily a disorder of placental dysfunction that leads to a syndrome of endothelial dysfunction and vasospasm. Preeclampsia develops in stages, with the last being the clinical illness. While other models to explain the development of preeclampsia exist, the two-stage model is commonly used to describe preeclampsia pathogenesis (Figure 36.1; Jim & Karumanchi, 2017).

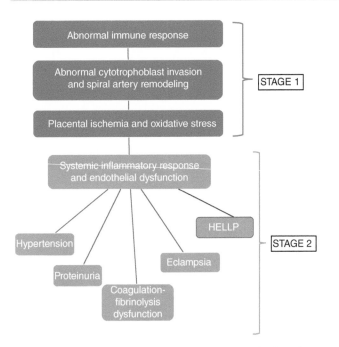

Figure 36.1 Two-stage model of preeclampsia pathophysiology.

Stage I is the development of the disease and begins early in the first trimester with placental development, well before signs and symptoms of preeclampsia develop. Abnormal placental development occurs due to altered immune responses, genetic factors, and/or early hypoxic episodes during cell differentiation. At the beginning of a normal pregnancy, the placenta should cause remodeling of the uterine **spiral arteries**, which is meant to increase the supply of oxygen and nutrients to the fetus. This remodeling is done as the cytotrophoblast cells of the developing placenta invade the **endothelium** and the maternal spiral arteries and change them into large-capacity blood vessels with low resistance for maternal–fetal exchange. In people with preeclampsia, this remodeling of the spiral arteries is incomplete. This incomplete penetration into the myometrium results in narrower blood vessels and hypoperfusion of the placenta. Placental ischemia then triggers **angiogenic factors** and **trophoblastic factors** from the placenta, which cause endothelial dysfunction and maternal inflammatory responses (Jim & Karumanchi, 2017). The coagulation–fibrinolytic system is thought to be one of the most seriously affected systems by inflammatory responses. The balance between coagulation and anticoagulation is vital to the regulation of uteroplacental circulation and organ perfusion in pregnancy. A state of hypercoagulability develops in preeclampsia, causing the blood vessels of the placenta and the pregnant person's organs to be blocked by microthrombosis (Han et al., 2014).

Stage II is the manifestation of preeclampsia that can be detected by clinical screening. Endothelial cell damage produces several factors that constrict and obstruct vascular beds, resulting in hypertension. This damage, in conjunction with an exaggerated inflammatory response in the pregnant person, causes vasospasm, increased capillary permeability, and clotting dysfunction, which

negatively affects vital organs such as the brain, liver, kidney, and placenta. The generalized hypertension, vasoconstriction, and decreased perfusion to all organ systems throughout the body result in symptoms associated with preeclampsia such as hypertension, headache, visual changes, proteinuria, and FGR (Ahmed et al., 2014).

Other immunologic factors likely play a role in the development of preeclampsia. It is theorized that the pregnant person's immune response to exposure to antigens in sperm may contribute to the alteration of placental implantation. Prior and repeated exposure to partner sperm is thought to decrease this immune response. This may explain the higher incidence of preeclampsia in very young people and in people who consistently use barrier methods of contraception (Redman & Sargent, 2010; Young et al., 2010).

Potential Problems due to Preeclampsia

The potential sequelae of preeclampsia are related to the gestational age at which it develops and the severity of the disease. Increased vascular resistance characteristic of preeclampsia leads to poor perfusion through the placenta, increasing the risk for potential problems related to uteroplacental insufficiency such as placental abruption and FGR. These potential problems include:

- Oligohydramnios
- Placental abruption
- Fetal growth restriction
- Abnormal fetal testing results
- Preterm birth

Risk factors for developing preeclampsia

Nulliparity
Multifetal gestation
Preeclampsia in a previous pregnancy
Chronic hypertension
Pregestational diabetes
Thrombophilia
Systemic lupus erythematosus (SLE)
Prepregnancy BMI > 30
Antiphospholipid syndrome (APAS)
Age 35 or older
Chronic kidney disease
Assisted reproductive technology (ART)
Obstructive sleep apnea
Family history of preeclampsia (first-degree relative)
Experience of anti-Black racism
Low socioeconomic status (SES)
History of adverse pregnancy outcome
- Stillbirth
- Placental abruption
White coat hypertension
New paternity
Pregnancy interval > 4 years
Migraine headache

Source: ACOG (2020), Garovic et al. (2022), and US Preventive Services Task Force (2021).

Risk Factors for Developing Preeclampsia

Preeclampsia is more common at the extremes of childbearing age. The increased incidence of chronic hypertension in people older than 40 years may explain the higher rates of preeclampsia in pregnant people of this age group. The incidence of preeclampsia has been rising globally, as there have been increasing medical comorbidities such as elevated BMI, pregnancy at older age, and increased use of ART; all of which have predisposed people to hypertension, preeclampsia, and renal disease (Khalil et al., 2016). Black birthing people have higher rates of preeclampsia and serious complications as a result of multigenerational racism causing health inequities (Ukoha et al., 2022). Higher socioeconomic status reduces the risk of preeclampsia in White pregnant people, but not Black, reflecting the impact of institutional, interpersonal, and internalized racism (Ross et al., 2019). Certain blood disorders such as factor V Leiden thrombophilia are implicated in some cases of severe preeclampsia, possibly due to microthrombosis in the placenta prompting a cascading inflammatory response.

Evaluation of Pregnant People with New-Onset Hypertension

Pregnant people who develop hypertension during pregnancy require additional symptom screening and laboratory evaluation for accurate diagnosis. Laboratory evaluation is a crucial component of the diagnostic workup (Table 36.2). Preeclampsia/eclampsia is a multisystem disease; thus, laboratory tests targeting multiorgan function can aid in assessing disease severity and progression. Laboratory tests used in evaluating hypertensive disorders in pregnancy vary by practice, laboratory, and the clinical picture; however, it is common practice to obtain a CBC and platelet count, lactase dehydrogenase (LDH), liver enzymes (ALT/AST), serum creatinine, and urine testing for proteinuria.

Table 36.2 Laboratory Manifestations of Preeclampsia–Eclampsia Syndrome

Laboratory indices	Diagnostic values	Trends	Comments
Renal function			
24-hour urine or PCR	Proteinuria ≥300 mg/24 hours or PCR ≥0.3	⇑	Reflects glomerular damage and renal compromise.
Blood urea nitrogen (BUN)	Increased	⇑	Elevated due to decrease in glomerular filtration rate and renal blood flow.
Serum creatinine	>1.1 mg/dL	⇑	Normal in preeclampsia without severe features; may be elevated in preeclampsia with severe features due to decreased intravascular volume and decreased glomerular filtration rate.
Hematologic function			
Hemoglobin		⇑	Increase reflects reduced plasma volume with redistribution of intravascular volume to the interstitial fluid space due to increased capillary permeability.
		⇓	Decrease reflects hemolysis in severe disease and HELLP syndrome; caused by coagulation cascade and fibrin deposits in microvessels that destroy RBCs.
Platelet count	<100,000/µL	⇑	Results from increased platelet activation, aggregation, and consumption; thrombocytopenia is the most common hematologic abnormality in people with preeclampsia.
Peripheral smear	Presence of Burr cells and schistocytes	⇑	Reflects the presence of microangiopathic hemolysis suggestive of severe disease and HELLP syndrome.
Prothrombin time (PT), partial thromboplastin time (PTT)	Elevated	⇑	Measures clotting time; can be increased in preeclampsia.
Hepatic function			
Aspartate transaminase (AST)	>70 U/L	⇑	An enzyme associated with liver parenchymal cells; reflects hepatocellular injury.
Alanine transaminase (ALT)	>70 U/L	⇑	An enzyme present in hepatocytes; increased serum levels reflect liver damage.
Lactase dehydrogenase (LDH)	>600 U/L	⇑	LDH is present in erythrocytes in high concentration. An increase may be a sign of hemolysis.

Source: Adapted from ACOG (2020), Garovic et al. (2022), and US Preventive Services Task Force (2021).

Based on the person's symptoms prior to formal diagnosis, the assessment of fetal well-being by NST and/or biophysical profile (BPP) can be done at the presenting visit. Some experts advocate for a baseline ultrasound to assess fetal growth pattern, depending on gestational age at the time of diagnosis, with follow-up at regular intervals. This is especially important in early-onset preeclampsia.

Management of Preeclampsia

The optimal management of preeclampsia depends on gestational age and disease severity. Timing of birth is based on maternal condition; in many cases, early term gestation can be reached. The only known cure for preeclampsia is giving birth since the primary source of the disorder is the placenta.

Preeclampsia without Severe Features

Some people with preeclampsia without severe features can be monitored on an outpatient basis with frequent maternal and fetal surveillance and a goal of evaluating for disease progression or evidence of impaired organ function. The current recommendations for monitoring for disease progression are (ACOG, 2020):

- daily fetal movement counting
- twice weekly BP readings
- once weekly labs
- once or twice weekly NST with amniotic fluid measurement
- growth ultrasound every three weeks

Weekly labs of CBC with platelets, liver enzymes, screening for proteinuria, and serum creatinine are often performed. The frequency of these tests can be modified based on subsequent clinical findings. If there is an initial finding of proteinuria and the diagnosis of preeclampsia, additional quantifications of proteinuria are not necessary to monitor; other lab results, BP readings, fetal status, and symptoms of severe features are used to determine when expedited birth is indicated. Since preeclampsia is progressive, hospital admission may eventually be necessary and earlier delivery discussed if the clinical picture worsens. There is increasing evidence that people with preeclampsia without severe features have improved outcomes with planned birth at 37 weeks as opposed to waiting longer (ACOG, 2020).

Discussing with pregnant people the nature of the disease and warning signs to report is a crucial component of care. Signs of worsening disease include severe headache, visual changes, shortness of breath, and epigastric pain. Pregnant people with preeclampsia are also advised to report abdominal or back pain, regular contractions, vaginal bleeding or spotting, rupture of membranes, decreased fetal movement, or any other persistent concerning or unusual symptoms.

The role of various nutrients in reducing the effects of preeclampsia has been investigated, without conclusive evidence of any benefit. Salt-restricted or protein-rich diets are not helpful and should not be advised as a treatment. Complete or partial bedrest has also been traditionally advised for people with preeclampsia. Currently, there is no evidence from randomized trials that indicate bedrest is effective in improving maternal or fetal outcomes; however, there are little quality data to support or refute its use (Bigelow & Stone, 2011; McCall et al., 2013). Prolonged bedrest increases the risk of thromboembolism and is often a significant hardship for most pregnant people and their families. Varying levels of rest may be indicated for individuals based on their clinical situation.

Preeclampsia with Severe Features

Pregnant people diagnosed with preeclampsia with severe features are immediately hospitalized. BP is stabilized with antihypertensive medications such as intravenous labetalol and hydralazine and a plan for giving birth made. Treatment with first-line medications should occur as soon as possible, ideally within 30–60 minutes of confirmed severe range BPs (BP ≥ 160/110 mmHg and persistent for at least 15 minutes) to reduce the risk of maternal stroke (ACOG, 2017). If gestation is less than 37 weeks, corticosteroids are recommended for fetal lung maturity and birth delayed, if possible, for 48 hours if the person and fetus are stable, to allow for full corticosteroid therapy effect. Birth may be expedited by induction or cesarean section, depending on fetal and maternal status and shared decision-making with the patient. Magnesium sulfate is recommended during intrapartum and early postpartum to prevent eclampsia. It is recommended to start magnesium sulfate once the diagnosis of preeclampsia or gestational hypertension with severe features is made. If either the pregnant person or fetus is showing signs of deterioration, regardless of gestational age, delivery should be planned as soon as the pregnant person is sufficiently stable, if possible, and in an environment with adequate resources to care for both the birthing person and the infant.

Prediction of Preeclampsia

Pregnant people with HDP have a 50% chance of recurrence in a subsequent pregnancy (Van Oostwaard et al., 2014). The earlier the disease manifested in a prior pregnancy, the higher the chance of recurrence is. Algorithms have been developed to predict who will go on to develop preeclampsia, though most have low predictive value. A recently developed algorithm using mean arterial pressure (MAP) and maternal factors and characteristics has shown promise (Rocha et al., 2017).

Serum biomarkers of endothelial dysfunction such as angiogenic factors are being investigated for predicting who will go on to develop symptomatic preeclampsia, allowing for earlier diagnosis and opportunities for optimizing pregnancy outcome. Serial measurement of pregnancy-associated plasma protein A (PAPP-A) and placental growth factor (PlGF) in the first trimester is emerging as predictive for early, severe preeclampsia

(Lambert-Messerlian et al., 2014). Doppler velocimetry and ultrasound are also being investigated as potential tools to predict preeclampsia. Even though there is continued research, no method has yet achieved clinical application in predicting who will develop preeclampsia (ACOG, 2020).

Prevention of Preeclampsia

Prevention of preeclampsia has been a topic that has generated much research in the last decade. Many therapies have been either disproved or have shown only minimal benefit. Nutritional interventions have been investigated with the idea that vitamin supplementation or sodium restriction may reduce the risk of preeclampsia. The majority of evidence on supplementation with vitamins C and E, omega-3 fatty acids via fish oil, garlic supplementation, vitamin D, folic acid, or sodium restriction does not support routine use for preeclampsia prevention (ACOG, 2020).

Calcium supplementation during pregnancy appears to reduce hypertension and preeclampsia in people with low baseline calcium intake; however, this is uncommon in higher-income countries (Hofmeyr et al., 2014; World Health Organization, 2014). Calcium supplements are not recommended for pregnant people as a preventive measure.

Low-dose aspirin has a modest effect on the prevention of preeclampsia in people at higher risk of developing the disease. Aspirin may prevent the cascade of physiologic events leading to preeclampsia by inhibiting the production of thromboxane, a vasoconstrictor and platelet aggregator. Daily low-dose aspirin taken at bedtime starting by 16 weeks of gestation is recommended for people at higher risk for developing preeclampsia (ACOG, 2018, 2020; Henderson et al., 2021; Rolnik et al., 2017). Pregnant people with any of the high risk factors and those with more than one moderate risk factor should receive daily low-dose (81 mg/day) aspirin for preeclampsia prophylaxis initiated between 12 and 16 weeks of gestation, and continuing until birth (ACOG, 2020; US Preventive Services Task Force, 2021). Table 36.3 displays the clinical risk assessment for preeclampsia.

Table 36.3 Clinical Risk Assessment for Preeclampsia

Risk level	Risk factors	Recommendation
High[†]	• History of preeclampsia, especially when accompanied by an adverse outcome	Recommend low-dose aspirin if the patient has one or more of these high-risk factors
	• Multifetal gestation	
	• Chronic hypertension	
	• Type 1 or 2 diabetes	
	• Renal disease	
	• Autoimmune disease (systemic lupus erythematosus, antiphospholipid syndrome)	
Moderate[‡]	• Nulliparity	Consider low-dose aspirin if the patient has more than one of these moderate-risk factors[§]
	• Obesity (body mass index greater than 30)	
	• Family history of preeclampsia (mother or sister)	
	• Sociodemographic characteristics (African American race, low socioeconomic status)	
	• Age 35 years or older	
	• Personal history factors (eg, low birthweight or small for gestational age, previous adverse pregnancy outcome, more than 10-year pregnancy interval)	
Low	• Previous uncomplicated full-term delivery	Do not recommend low-dose aspirin

[*] Includes only risk factors that can be obtained from the patient's medical history. Clinical measures, such as uterine artery Doppler ultrasonography, are not included.
[†] Single risk factors that are consistently associated with the greatest risk of preeclampsia. The preeclampsia incidence rate would be approximately 8% or more in a pregnant woman with one or more of these risk factors.
[‡] A combination of multiple moderate-risk factors may be used by clinicians to identify women at high risk of preeclampsia. These risk factors are independently associated with moderate risk of preeclampsia, some more consistently than others.
[§] Moderate-risk factors vary in their association with increased risk of preeclampsia.
Modified from LeFevre, ML. U.S. Preventive Services Task Force. Low-dose aspirin use for the prevention of morbidity and mortality from preeclampsia: U.S. Preventive Services Task Force Recommendation Statement. Ann Intern Med 2014;161:819–26.
Source: AGOC (2018) / Wolters Kluwer Health, Inc.

Prevention of racial disparities in preeclampsia and related complications can be accomplished through the standardization of protocols and procedures to prevent bias and discrimination, quality improvement bundles, use of telehealth and text messaging, and group prenatal care, which is shown to reduce implicit and explicit bias (Suresh et al., 2022).

When counseling people at risk for hypertensive disorders or with a family history of hypertensive disorders, it is appropriate to offer preconception or early pregnancy counseling. This includes general recommendations about healthful lifestyle measures, for example, working toward reaching or maintaining a healthy weight, participating in regular physical activity, and eliminating any tobacco and/or substance use.

Long-Term Sequelae of Preeclampsia

Preeclampsia has become a disease of interest as emerging evidence links preeclampsia with disease in later life. Strong associations between preeclampsia and CVD have been established. A meta-analysis including over 6 million women found that those diagnosed with preeclampsia have a fourfold risk of later hypertension and heart failure and a twofold risk of heart disease, thromboembolism, and stroke (Wu et al., 2017). These associations are even stronger in those who have experienced preeclampsia in several pregnancies. Pregnancy exerts a unique burden on the cardiovascular system and causes changes in the structure, filling capacity, and contractility of the left ventricle. With preeclampsia, this cardiac remodeling is exaggerated and persists after pregnancy: one study found that 20% of women with preeclampsia had myocardial damage (Melchiorre et al., 2011). It is unclear whether preeclampsia is an independent risk factor for future CVD or an early marker of future risk for CVD. Factors that predispose to preeclampsia are also factors associated with CVD, such as elevated BMI, insulin resistance, heightened inflammatory response, and endothelial dysfunction.

Preeclampsia may be a risk factor for permanent cerebrovascular changes. In one study, women with preeclampsia had a higher rate of white matter brain lesions and significantly reduced gray matter compared to women with normotensive pregnancies (Siepmann et al., 2017). These women also experience increased long-term structural impairment over time after pregnancy. The cerebral changes may explain increased retinal disease (Auger et al., 2017) and memory dysfunction later in life (Workman et al., 2012) found in people with a prior history of preeclampsia. It is theorized that excess production of angiogenic factors that occurs in preeclampsia may also play a role in the long-term adverse health effects (Jim & Karumanchi, 2017).

A prior history of preeclampsia is also strongly associated with chronic kidney disease (Ayansina et al., 2016) and diabetes later in life (Feig et al., 2013; Wang et al., 2012). These findings support the importance of counseling during routine health visits on disease prevention measures such as healthy diet, weight management, and exercise to reduce risk.

Risk Management Issues in the Office Setting

Because preeclampsia/eclampsia is a leading cause of death in pregnant people, appropriate recognition, treatment, and referral are vitally important issues for those providing prenatal care. Common diagnostic and treatment mistakes that can occur in the maternity triage setting include the following:

- Ignoring a BP elevation
- Not following up on proteinuria
- Misinterpreting the cause of visual changes, nausea, vomiting, malaise, or epigastric pain
- Sending a patient with preeclampsia home before verification of maternal and fetal well-being
- Failure to follow up on symptoms of disease with more frequent ambulatory visits
- Failure to reflect/implement collaborative or medical management when it is appropriate.

Chronic Hypertension

Chronic hypertension in pregnancy is defined as BP greater than or equal to 140/90 mmHg before pregnancy or detected prior to 20 weeks of gestation. Hypertension that is diagnosed for the first time during pregnancy and that does not resolve in the typical postpartum period is also classified as chronic hypertension (ACOG, 2019). Approximately 1–5% of pregnancies are complicated by chronic hypertension. The prevalence of chronic hypertension in pregnancy is rising due to (a) delayed childbearing and increased risk of hypertensive disorders with age; (b) increasing prevalence of obesity; and (c) increasing number of pregnancies with significant medical comorbidities such as pregestational diabetes, lupus, and renal disease (Ankumah & Sibai, 2017).

Chronic hypertension is classified into mild-to-moderate hypertension (140–159/90–109 Hg) and severe hypertension (systolic ≥160 mmHg, diastolic ≥110 mmHg; Podymow & August, 2017). People presenting with severe chronic hypertension in pregnancy may have a history of known hypertension and may have been on antihypertensive medications in the past.

Most people with chronic hypertension have good pregnancy outcomes; however, risk for pregnancy complications is increased and can be significant (Table 36.4). People with chronic hypertension have an eightfold increase in risk for developing superimposed preeclampsia (Bramham et al., 2014). The risk of adverse outcome is related to the severity of the hypertension.

Accurately diagnosing pregnant people with chronic hypertension can be challenging. Normotensive people entering pregnancy typically experience a decrease in BP toward the end of the first trimester. This decrease is thought to be secondary to the marked vasodilation that occurs despite the increase in plasma volume during pregnancy. BP usually falls by 5–10 mmHg and remains at this lower level throughout pregnancy until the third trimester, when it rises to return to prepregnancy values (Seely & Ecker, 2014). For most pregnant people with

Table 36.4 Potential Problems due to Chronic Hypertension

Condition	Estimated incidence or increased risk[a]
Preeclampsia	23–27% incidence with chronic hypertension
Gestational diabetes	17% incidence with chronic hypertension
Fetal growth restriction	10–20% incidence with chronic hypertension
Placental abruption	300% increased risk
Preterm birth	400–500% increased risk
Cesarean birth	300% increased risk
Postpartum hemorrhage	100% increased risk
Small for gestational age (SGA)	200% increased risk
Stillbirth	200% increased risk

Source: Adapted from ACOG (2019), Ananth et al. (2007), Hu et al. (2016), and Saunders et al. (2014).
[a] A 100% increase in risk can appear enormous, but if the risk began as 1 in 100 people, a 100% increase in risk means that 2 out of 100 will be affected.

chronic hypertension, BP changes also follow this same pattern. As a result, some hypertensive people become normotensive during early pregnancy, and others who remain hypertensive can have their antihypertensive medications tapered. These physiologic changes can confuse the diagnosis of chronic hypertension when a pregnant person begins prenatal care in the second trimester once the physiologic decrease has occurred and is now normotensive. Without first-trimester BP measurements, it is difficult to make a clear diagnosis and determine if the person has chronic hypertension. In such cases, the increase to prepregnancy values in the third trimester can mistakenly suggest gestational hypertension.

Management of Chronic Hypertension in Pregnancy

Laboratory studies as well as a comprehensive maternal and fetal evaluation should be obtained at initial evaluation, with baseline tests obtained in early pregnancy for comparison if preeclampsia is suspected later (Table 36.2; ACOG, 2019). These tests should include:

- CBC with platelets
- Serum creatinine
- LDH
- Liver enzymes (AST, ALT)
- Serum electrolytes
- BUN
- Testing for proteinuria (urine dipstick, PCR, or 24-hour urine collection)
- Electrocardiogram or echocardiogram

BP cuffs can be prescribed for a pregnant person to perform daily evaluation at home. More frequent prenatal visits are recommended for people with chronic hypertension

compared with normotensive people. Regular assessments of BPs, urine protein, fundal height, and symptoms supports early detection of complications.

Depending on BP control, prenatal visits may occur every 3 weeks until 28–30 weeks, every 2 weeks until 36 weeks, and then weekly thereafter, with more frequent visits as indicated. Early glucose screening can be considered especially for people with the additional risk factor of elevated BMI as gestational diabetes is increased in people with chronic hypertension. Pregnant people with chronic hypertension are counseled to report symptoms of preeclampsia promptly and to avoid tobacco, alcohol, and substance use, which can exacerbate risks for FGR and placental abruption.

BP control and monitoring for signs and symptoms of superimposed preeclampsia are priorities in caring for pregnant people with chronic hypertension. Medications are considered with a persistent SBP ≥ 160 mmHg and/or DBP ≥ 110 mmHg, and maintained between 120 and 160 mmHg SBP and 80–110 DBP (ACOG, 2019). The most commonly used medications include labetalol, nifedipine, and methyldopa. Caution must be maintained with antihypertensive medication use in pregnancy to avoid overcorrection of BP, which could decrease placental perfusion and increase the risk of FGR. Low-dose aspirin (81 mg) initiated between 12 and 28 weeks of gestation should be considered to prevent superimposed preeclampsia (ACOG, 2018).

Serial ultrasound evaluation of fetal growth every three weeks starting in the third trimester is recommended (ACOG, 2019). There is no consensus on routine fetal surveillance testing for people with chronic hypertension and no additional risk factors and an otherwise normal pregnancy course. With the recognition of the association between chronic hypertension and stillbirth, fetal testing is sometimes advised (ACOG, 2019). Fetal surveillance testing can include daily fetal movement counting, NST, BPP, and amniotic fluid measurement. The tests chosen, frequency of testing, and time for initiating surveillance are often based on degree and duration of hypertension, use of antihypertensive medication, evidence of underlying organ compromise related to hypertension, suspicion for FGR, and presence of pregnancy complications such as superimposed preeclampsia. Planned birth at 38 0/7 to 39 6/7 weeks of gestation is recommended for pregnant people with chronic hypertension who have no additional maternal or fetal complications and if not prescribed maintenance antihypertensive agents (ACOG, 2019; Khalil et al., 2016). For pregnant people with chronic hypertension and with no additional maternal or fetal complications supporting earlier delivery and who *are* prescribed maintenance antihypertensive medications, birth should be recommended between 37 0/7 and 38 6/7. Pregnant people with hypertension that is difficult to control are at significant risk for increased maternal and fetal morbidities. Earlier delivery may be required, along with perinatal or obstetrical interprofessional care (ACOG, 2019).

Chronic Hypertension with Superimposed Preeclampsia

Superimposed preeclampsia is the major adverse pregnancy condition associated with chronic hypertension; up to 20–50% of pregnant people with chronic hypertension go on to develop superimposed preeclampsia (ACOG, 2019). Perinatal outcomes are worsened when these conditions occur together. The clinical spectrum of chronic hypertension with superimposed preeclampsia is broad, and diagnoses can often have ambiguity; therefore, increased surveillance is warranted even if the diagnosis is only suspected (ACOG, 2019).

This complication can be challenging to diagnose, especially if a pregnant person presents late to prenatal care and demonstrates hypertension at the first visit. The acute onset of proteinuria or a sudden increase over baseline hypertension should prompt a laboratory and physical evaluation for superimposed preeclampsia. If there is evidence of preeclampsia, the individual should be treated according to established treatment guidelines.

Management of Chronic Hypertension with Superimposed Preeclampsia

Pregnant people with chronic hypertension with superimposed preeclampsia have additional perinatal risks and often require specialized perinatal care. When chronic hypertension with superimposed preeclampsia without severe features is diagnosed and the pregnant person and fetus remain stable, expectant management with birth at 37 weeks of gestation is suggested. If any severe preeclampsia features present, physician collaboration or transfer of care is indicated.

HELLP Syndrome

HELLP syndrome is a serious pregnancy complication characterized by hemolysis (H), elevated liver enzymes (EL), and low platelet count (LP). HELLP syndrome occurs in less than 1% of pregnant people but does occur in 10–20% of people with preeclampsia with severe features (Sibai & Stella, 2009). Approximately 70% of cases of HELLP develop between 27 and 37 weeks of gestation, with the remaining 30% occurring postpartum (Dusse et al., 2015). The onset and progression from early symptoms to severe disease can be rapid.

Pathophysiology and Potential Problems

HELLP syndrome is part of the disease spectrum of preeclampsia–eclampsia. It is one of the more severe forms of the disease and is associated with increased maternal morbidity and mortality (ACOG, 2020). Similar to preeclampsia, the essential phenomena in the development of HELLP syndrome is an abnormal trophoblastic invasion due to an inadequate maternal immune tolerance (Haram et al., 2009). However, the trophoblastic dysfunction is more marked and includes an acute inflammatory process targeting the liver and a greater activation of the coagulation system. The central place that the liver occupies in the disorder of HELLP syndrome is an important clue to pathogenesis. Severe epigastric/right upper quadrant pain reflects liver swelling and capsular stretch and often heralds underlying rapidly progressive disease.

Severe complications are associated with HELLP syndrome such as DIC, placental abruption, subcapsular

---

Diagnostic criteria

Chronic hypertension with superimposed preeclampsia:
- Presence of hypertension prior to 20 weeks of gestation **and** any of the following, after 20 weeks of gestation:
  - Sudden increase in BP that was previously well controlled
  - New onset or significant increase of proteinuria

Chronic hypertension with superimposed preeclampsia with severe features:
- Presence of hypertension prior to 20 weeks of gestation **and** any of the following after 20 weeks of gestation:
  - Acute persistent BP elevation of SBP $\geq$160 mmHg and/or DBP $\geq$110 mmHg
  - Platelet count <100,000/μL
  - Elevated liver transaminases (two times the upper limit of normal) or severe persistent right upper quadrant/epigastric pain unresponsive to medications
  - New-onset nausea and vomiting
  - Pulmonary edema
  - New-onset and worsening renal insufficiency—elevated serum creatinine >1.1 mg/dL or doubling of serum creatinine in absence of other renal disease
  - New-onset headache unresponsive to medication and not accounted for by alternative diagnoses
  - Visual disturbances

hematoma, and liver rupture. Maternal and fetal complications are dependent on gestational age at the onset, severity, and progression of the disease and the rapidity of intervention. DIC, also known as consumptive coagulopathy, is caused by increased fibrin deposits and other procoagulation factors that result in high production and exhaustion of platelets, leading to hemorrhage. DIC is reported to occur in approximately 20% of pregnant people with HELLP syndrome and can occur in late gestation or during the postpartum period. Placental abruption is associated with all hypertensive disorders in pregnancy, including HELLP syndrome. The reported incidence of placental abruption in people with HELLP syndrome ranges between 4% and 9% (Haram et al., 2009).

Complications associated with HELLP syndrome

In the pregnant person	In the fetus
• Disseminated intravascular coagulation (DIC) • Placental abruption • Eclampsia • Acute renal failure • Ascites • Cerebral edema • Pulmonary edema • Subcapsular liver hematoma • Liver rupture • Cerebral infarction • Cerebral hemorrhage • Postpartum hemorrhage • Death	• Preterm birth • FGR • Neonatal thrombocytopenia • Respiratory distress syndrome • Perinatal death

Diagnosis

Diagnosing HELLP syndrome can be challenging, as symptoms can be subtle and mimic those of other conditions such as gastritis, flu, acute hepatitis, gallbladder disease, and acute fatty liver of pregnancy (AFLP). Common presentation includes right upper quadrant abdominal pain or epigastric pain, nausea and vomiting, headache, or visual symptoms. The person may also report general malaise, fatigue, or flu-like symptoms (Haram et al., 2009). These nonspecific physical symptoms are experienced in 90% of people with HELLP syndrome shortly before seeking medical attention (ACOG, 2020). Nausea and vomiting, headache, and epigastric pain are prevalent. Approximately 30–60% of patients present with headache and 20% present with visual changes (Haram et al., 2009). While the majority of people with HELLP syndrome have hypertension and proteinuria, the presence and degree of both manifestations can range from absent to severe. HELLP can occur in the absence of proteinuria in approximately 10–15% of cases (Sibai et al., 2005). Epigastric tenderness on palpation can indicate hepatic involvement and reflexes can be brisk, reflecting increased CNS excitability. Because of the tendency to present with vague symptoms, delay in making the correct diagnosis of HELLP syndrome can occur. A report of malaise or feeling unwell, or of indigestion or heartburn (both symptoms common in many pregnant people), should be further investigated, especially in people with hypertension or close to term.

The diagnosis of HELLP syndrome is based on laboratory evidence of hemolytic anemia, hepatic damage, and **thrombocytopenia** in patients suspected to have preeclampsia (Table 36.5). The basic laboratory screening for people suspected of having HELLP syndrome typically includes a CBC with platelets, coagulation studies if platelet count is less than 100,000, urinalysis, serum creatinine, liver function tests, uric acid, indirect and total bilirubin levels, and peripheral smear. Thrombocytopenia may be the first indicator of disease. A platelet count less than 150,000/μL represents mild (100,000–150,000/μL), moderate (50,000–100,000/μL), or severe (<50,000/μL) thrombocytopenia in both nonpregnant and pregnant people. The trend of platelet decline is an important factor to consider because significant pathology such as hepatic hemorrhage and rupture can occur before the platelet count falls below 100,000/μL (Martin et al., 2006). It should be

Table 36.5 Laboratory Findings in HELLP Syndrome

Laboratory test	Possible result	Cause
LDH	↑	Hemolysis or liver dysfunction
AST or ALT	↑	Hemolysis or liver dysfunction/injury
Bilirubin	↑	Hemolysis
Platelets (CBC)	↓	Increased consumption
Hemoglobin/Hematocrit (CBC)	↓	Hemolysis
PT	Normal	
PTT	↑	Liver dysfunction
D-dimer	↑	Increased coagulation and secondary fibrinolysis
Fibrinogen	↓	

Source: Adapted from ACOG (2020) and Haram et al. (2017).

noted that laboratory diagnostic criteria for HELLP syndrome varies in research and in clinical practice (Haram et al., 2017).

In addition to laboratory testing, the clinical maternal status, gestational age, presence of contractions, and cervical Bishop score are determined. BP measurement, abdominal ultrasound examination, and fetal assessment testing with NST and ultrasound for growth and amniotic fluid assessment are also done. The pregnant person is stabilized with intravenous fluids, antihypertensive drugs (e.g., labetalol or nifedipine), and magnesium sulfate to prevent eclampsia. It is important to closely monitor maternal vital signs and fluid balance. Corticosteroids are administered to improve fetal lung maturity if gestational age is <37 weeks of gestation). If maternal and fetal conditions are stable and gestational age is between 27 and 34 weeks, vaginal or cesarean birth is recommended after 24–48 hours of treatment rather than immediately upon diagnosis to allow for maternal stabilization and corticosteroid efficacy; immediate delivery is indicated at 34 weeks of gestation or later (Haram et al., 2009; Martin et al., 2006). Pregnant people suspected of developing HELLP syndrome require immediate specialist evaluation and management. A diagnosis of HELLP syndrome significantly increases risk for recurrence of hypertension in some form in a subsequent pregnancy (Abildgaard & Heimdal, 2013; Leeners et al., 2011).

Interprofessional Care

Many prenatal healthcare providers, especially midwives, who provide prenatal care regularly, often manage the care of people with preeclampsia, depending on the setting. Pregnant people diagnosed with preeclampsia with severe features, with severe chronic hypertension, and with chronic hypertension who develop superimposed preeclampsia require medical consultation, interprofessional team care, or referral. Pregnant people who develop early-onset preeclampsia are best managed in a tertiary care setting with appropriate maternal–fetal medicine specialists and a neonatal intensive care unit (NICU). In practices where optimal specialty care collaboration is not possible, pregnant people are referred for management, as the risk of complications is significant in this subgroup. Providing emotional and supportive care as appropriate to the practice setting remains a responsibility of the prenatal healthcare provider.

Summary

Hypertensive disorders represent the most common medical complication of pregnancy and are a major cause of maternal and fetal morbidity and mortality in the United States and worldwide. Management depends on gestational age, symptom constellation and presentation, and maternal and fetal status. Most pregnant people with gestational hypertension or preeclampsia without severe features do not experience perinatal complications; however, the progressive and unpredictable nature of pregnancy hypertensive disorders highlights the need for regular

monitoring. Maternal and fetal complications are increased in people with gestational hypertension or preeclampsia with severe features. Hypertensive disorders in pregnancy are an important risk factor for CVD in later life. Therefore, lifestyle modifications, BP control, and control of metabolic factors are recommended after birth, to avoid complications in subsequent pregnancies and to reduce maternal cardiovascular risk in the future.

Resources for Pregnant People and Their Families

The Preeclampsia Foundation offers consumer material and information on the diagnosis and management of preeclampsia: http://www.preeclampsia.org

The March of Dimes provides an overview of preeclampsia with additional resources: https://www.marchofdimes.org/complications/preeclampsia.aspx

Resources for Healthcare Providers

The Preeclampsia Foundation offers materials on current guidelines and research for providers: https://preeclampsia.org/current-guidelines

California Maternity Quality Collaborative Maternity Care *Hypertensive Disorders of Pregnancy Toolkit* is a guide to support professionals and institutions in caring for women with preeclampsia: https://www.cmqcc.org/resources-tool-kits/toolkits/HDP

U.S. Preventive Services Task Force: Aspirin use to prevent preeclampsia and related morbidity and mortality: https://www.uspreventiveservicestaskforce.org/uspstf/recommendation/low-dose-aspirin-use-for-the-prevention-of-morbidity-and-mortality-from-preeclampsia-preventive-medication

References

Abildgaard, U., & Heimdal, K. (2013). Pathogenesis of the syndrome of hemolysis, elevated liver enzymes, and low platelet count (HELLP): A review. *European Journal of Obstetrics & Gynecology and Reproductive Biology*, *166*(2), 117–123. https://doi.org/10.1016/j.ejogrb.2012.09.026

Ahmed, R., Dunford, J., Mehran, R., Robson, S., & Kunadian, V. (2014). Pre-eclampsia and future cardiovascular risk among women. *Journal of the American College of Cardiology*, *63*(18), 1815–1822. https://doi.org/10.1016/j.jacc.2014.02.529

American College of Obstetrics and Gynecology (ACOG). (2017). Committee opinion No. 692: Emergent therapy for acute-onset, severe hypertension during pregnancy and the postpartum period. *Obstetrics & Gynecology*, *129*(4), e90–e95. https://doi.org/10.1097/AOG.0000000000002019

American College of Obstetrics and Gynecology (ACOG). (2018). Committee opinion No. 743: Low-dose aspirin use during pregnancy. *Obstetrics & Gynecology*, *132*(1), e44–e52. https://doi.org/10.1097/AOG.0000000000002708

American College of Obstetrics and Gynecology (ACOG). (2019). Practice bulletin No. 203: Chronic hypertension in pregnancy. *Obstetrics & Gynecology*, *133*(1), e237–e260.

American College of Obstetrics and Gynecology (ACOG). (2020). Practice bulletin No. 222: Gestational hypertension and preeclampsia. *American Journal of Obstetrics and Gynecology*, *135*(6), e237–e260.

Ananth, C. V., Peltier, M. R., Kinzler, W. L., Smulian, J. C., & Vintzileos, A. M. (2007). Chronic hypertension and risk of placental abruption:

Is the association modified by ischemic placental disease? *American Journal of Obstetrics and Gynecology*, 197(3), 273.e1–273.e7. https://doi.org/10.1016/j.ajog.2007.05.047

Ankumah, N.-A. E., & Sibai, B. M. (2017). Chronic hypertension in pregnancy: Diagnosis, management, and outcomes. *Clinical Obstetrics & Gynecology*, 60(1), 206–214. https://doi.org/10.1097/GRF.0000000000000255

Auger, N., Fraser, W. D., Paradis, G., Healy-Profitós, J., Hsieh, A., & Rhéaume, M.-A. (2017). Preeclampsia and long-term risk of maternal retinal disorders. *Obstetrics & Gynecology*, 129(1), 42–49. https://doi.org/10.1097/AOG.0000000000001758

Ayansina, D., Black, C., Hall, S. J., Marks, A., Millar, C., Prescott, G. J., Wilde, K., & Bhattacharya, S. (2016). Long term effects of gestational hypertension and pre-eclampsia on kidney function: Record linkage study. *Pregnancy Hypertension: An International Journal of Women's Cardiovascular Health*, 6(4), 344–349. https://doi.org/10.1016/j.preghy.2016.08.231

Bernstein, P. S., Martin, J. N., Barton, J. R., Shields, L. E., Druzin, M. L., Scavone, B. M., Frost, J., Morton, C. H., Ruhl, C., Slager, J., Tsigas, E. Z., Jaffer, S., & Menard, M. K. (2017). National Partnership for Maternal Safety: Consensus bundle on severe hypertension during pregnancy and the postpartum period. *Anesthesia & Analgesia*, 125(2), 540–547. https://doi.org/10.1213/ANE.0000000000002304

Bigelow, C., & Stone, J. (2011). Bed rest in pregnancy. *Mount Sinai Journal of Medicine: A Journal of Translational and Personalized Medicine*, 78(2), 291–302. https://doi.org/10.1002/msj.20243

Bramham, K., Parnell, B., Nelson-Piercy, C., Seed, P. T., Poston, L., & Chappell, L. C. (2014). Chronic hypertension and pregnancy outcomes: Systematic review and meta-analysis. *BMJ*, 348, g2301–g2301. https://doi.org/10.1136/bmj.g2301

California Maternal Quality Care Collaborative (CMQCC). (2021). *Hypertensive disorders of pregnancy toolkit*. https://www.cmqcc.org/resources-tool-kits/toolkits/HDP

Center for Disease Control and Prevention (CDC). (2017). *Pregnancy mortality surveillance system*. https://www.cdc.gov/reproductivehealth/maternal-mortality/pregnancy-mortality-surveillance-system.htm

Cooray, S. D., Edmonds, S. M., Tong, S., Samarasekera, S. P., & Whitehead, C. L. (2011). Characterization of symptoms immediately preceding eclampsia. *Obstetrics & Gynecology*, 118(5), 995–999. https://doi.org/10.1097/AOG.0b013e3182324570

Dusse, L. M., Alpoim, P. N., Silva, J. T., Rios, D. R. A., Brandão, A. H., & Cabral, A. C. V. (2015). Revisiting HELLP syndrome. *Clinica Chimica Acta*, 451, 117–120. https://doi.org/10.1016/j.cca.2015.10.024

Feig, D. S., Shah, B. R., Lipscombe, L. L., Wu, C. F., Ray, J. G., Lowe, J., Hwee, J., & Booth, G. L. (2013). Preeclampsia as a risk factor for diabetes: A population-based cohort study. *PLoS Medicine*, 10(4), e1001425. https://doi.org/10.1371/journal.pmed.1001425

Fong, A., Chau, C. T., Pan, D., & Ogunyemi, D. A. (2013). Clinical morbidities, trends, and demographics of eclampsia: A population-based study. *American Journal of Obstetrics and Gynecology*, 209(3), 229.e1–229.e7. https://doi.org/10.1016/j.ajog.2013.05.050

Garovic, V. D., Dechend, R., Easterling, T., Karumanchi, S. A., McMurtry Baird, S., Magee, L. A., Rana, S., Vermunt, J. V., August, P., on behalf of the American Heart Association Council on Hypertension, Council on the Kidney in Cardiovascular Disease, Kidney in Heart Disease Science Committee, Council on Arteriosclerosis, Thrombosis and Vascular Biology, Council on Lifestyle and Cardiometabolic Health, & Council on Peripheral Vascular Disease; and Stroke Council. (2022). Hypertension in pregnancy: Diagnosis, blood pressure goals, and pharmacotherapy: A scientific statement from the American Heart Association. *Hypertension*, 79(2). https://doi.org/10.1161/HYP.0000000000000208

Han, L., Liu, X., Li, H., Zou, J., Yang, Z., Han, J., Huang, W., Yu, L., Zheng, Y., & Li, L. (2014). Blood coagulation parameters and platelet indices: Changes in normal and preeclamptic pregnancies and predictive values for preeclampsia. *PLoS One*, 9(12), e114488. https://doi.org/10.1371/journal.pone.0114488

Haram, K., Mortensen, J. H., Mastrolia, S. A., & Erez, O. (2017). Disseminated intravascular coagulation in the HELLP syndrome: How much do we really know? *The Journal of Maternal-Fetal & Neonatal Medicine*, 30(7), 779–788. https://doi.org/10.1080/14767058.2016.1189897

Haram, K., Svendsen, E., & Abildgaard, U. (2009). The HELLP syndrome: Clinical issues and management. A review. *BMC Pregnancy and Childbirth*, 9(1), 8. https://doi.org/10.1186/1471-2393-9-8

Henderson, J. T., Vesco, K. K., Senger, C. A., Thomas, R. G., & Redmond, N. (2021). Aspirin use to prevent preeclampsia and related morbidity and mortality: Updated evidence report and systematic review for the US Preventive Services Task Force. *JAMA*, 326(12), 1192. https://doi.org/10.1001/jama.2021.8551

Hofmeyr, G., Belizán, J., Dadelszen, P., & the Calcium and Pre-eclampsia (CAP) Study Group. (2014). Low-dose calcium supplementation for preventing pre-eclampsia: A systematic review and commentary. *BJOG: An International Journal of Obstetrics & Gynaecology*, 121(8), 951–957. https://doi.org/10.1111/1471-0528.12613

Hu, W. S., Feng, Y., Dong, M. Y., & He, J. (2016). Comparing maternal and perinatal outcomes in pregnancies complicated by preeclampsia superimposed chronic hypertension and preeclampsia alone. *Clinical and Experimental Obstetrics & Gynecology*, 43(2), 212–215.

Jim, B., & Karumanchi, S. A. (2017). Preeclampsia: Pathogenesis, prevention, and long-term complications. *Seminars in Nephrology*, 37(4), 386–397. https://doi.org/10.1016/j.semnephrol.2017.05.011

Johnson, J. D., & Louis, J. M. (2022). Does race or ethnicity play a role in the origin, pathophysiology, and outcomes of preeclampsia? An expert review of the literature. *American Journal of Obstetrics and Gynecology*, 226(2), S876–S885. https://doi.org/10.1016/j.ajog.2020.07.038

Khalil, A., O'Brien, P., & Townsend, R. (2016). Current best practice in the management of hypertensive disorders in pregnancy. *Integrated Blood Pressure Control*, 9, 79–94. https://doi.org/10.2147/IBPC.S77344

Lambert-Messerlian, G., Eklund, E. E., Chien, E. K., Rosene-Montella, K., Neveux, L. M., Haddow, H. R. M., & Palomaki, G. E. (2014). Use of first or second trimester serum markers, or both, to predict preeclampsia. *Pregnancy Hypertension: An International Journal of Women's Cardiovascular Health*, 4(4), 271–278. https://doi.org/10.1016/j.preghy.2014.07.001

Leeners, B., Neumaier-Wagner, P. M., Kuse, S., Mütze, S., Rudnik-Schöneborn, S., Zerres, K., & Rath, W. (2011). Recurrence risks of hypertensive diseases in pregnancy after HELLP syndrome. *Journal of Perinatal Medicine*, 39(6). https://doi.org/10.1515/jpm.2011.081

Magee, L. A., Pels, A., Helewa, M., Rey, E., von Dadelszen, P., Magee, L. A., Audibert, F., Bujold, E., Côté, A.-M., Douglas, M. J., Eastabrook, G., Firoz, T., Gibson, P., Gruslin, A., Hutcheon, J., Koren, G., Lange, I., Leduc, L., Logan, A. G., . . . Sebbag, I. (2014). Diagnosis, evaluation, and management of the hypertensive disorders of pregnancy: Executive summary. *Journal of Obstetrics and Gynaecology Canada*, 36(5), 416–438. https://doi.org/10.1016/S1701-2163(15)30588-0

Martin, J. N., Rose, C. H., & Briery, C. M. (2006). Understanding and managing HELLP syndrome: The integral role of aggressive glucocorticoids for mother and child. *American Journal of Obstetrics and Gynecology*, 195(4), 914–934. https://doi.org/10.1016/j.ajog.2005.08.044

McCall, C. A., Grimes, D. A., & Lyerly, A. D. (2013). "Therapeutic" bed rest in pregnancy. *Obstetrics & Gynecology*, 121(6), 1305–1308. https://doi.org/10.1097/AOG.0b013e318293f12f

Melchiorre, K., Sutherland, G. R., Baltabaeva, A., Liberati, M., & Thilaganathan, B. (2011). Maternal cardiac dysfunction and remodeling in women with preeclampsia at term. *Hypertension*, 57(1), 85–93. https://doi.org/10.1161/HYPERTENSIONAHA.110.162321

Parikh, N. I., Gonzalez, J. M., Anderson, C. A. M., Judd, S. E., Rexrode, K. M., Hlatky, M. A., Gunderson, E. P., Stuart, J. J., Vaidya, D., On behalf of the American Heart Association Council on Epidemiology and Prevention, Council on Arteriosclerosis, Thrombosis and Vascular Biology, & Council on Cardiovascular and Stroke Nursing; and the Stroke Council. (2021). Adverse pregnancy outcomes and cardiovascular disease risk: Unique opportunities for cardiovascular disease prevention in women: A scientific statement from the American Heart Association. *Circulation*, 143(18). https://doi.org/10.1161/CIR.0000000000000961

Podymow, T., & August, P. (2017). New evidence in the management of chronic hypertension in pregnancy. *Seminars in Nephrology*, *37*(4), 398–403. https://doi.org/10.1016/j.semnephrol.2017.05.012

Redman, C. W. G., & Sargent, I. L. (2010). Immunology of pre-eclampsia. *American Journal of Reproductive Immunology*, *63*(6), 534–543. https://doi.org/10.1111/j.1600-0897.2010.00831.x

Rocha, R. S., Gurgel Alves, J. A., Bezerra Maia E Holanda Moura, S., Araujo Júnior, E., Martins, W. P., Vasconcelos, C. T. M., Da Silva Costa, F., & Oriá, M. O. B. (2017). Comparison of three algorithms for prediction preeclampsia in the first trimester of pregnancy. *Pregnancy Hypertension*, *10*, 113–117. https://doi.org/10.1016/j.preghy.2017.07.146

Rolnik, D. L., Wright, D., Poon, L. C., O'Gorman, N., Syngelaki, A., de Paco Matallana, C., Akolekar, R., Cicero, S., Janga, D., Singh, M., Molina, F. S., Persico, N., Jani, J. C., Plasencia, W., Papaioannou, G., Tenenbaum-Gavish, K., Meiri, H., Gizurarson, S., Maclagan, K., & Nicolaides, K. H. (2017). Aspirin versus placebo in pregnancies at high risk for preterm preeclampsia. *New England Journal of Medicine*, *377*(7), 613–622. https://doi.org/10.1056/NEJMoa1704559

Ross, K. M., Dunkel Schetter, C., McLemore, M. R., Chambers, B. D., Paynter, R. A., Baer, R., Feuer, S. K., Flowers, E., Karasek, D., Pantell, M., Prather, A. A., Ryckman, K., & Jelliffe-Pawlowski, L. (2019). Socioeconomic status, preeclampsia risk and gestational length in Black and White women. *Journal of Racial and Ethnic Health Disparities*, *6*(6), 1182–1191. https://doi.org/10.1007/s40615-019-00619-3

Saunders, L., Kadhel, P., Costet, N., Rouget, F., Monfort, C., Thomé, J.-P., Guldner, L., Cordier, S., & Multigner, L. (2014). Hypertensive disorders of pregnancy and gestational diabetes mellitus among French Caribbean women chronically exposed to chlordecone. *Environment International*, *68*, 171–176. https://doi.org/10.1016/j.envint.2014.03.024

Seely, E. W., & Ecker, J. (2014). Chronic hypertension in pregnancy. *Circulation*, *129*(11), 1254–1261. https://doi.org/10.1161/CIRCULATIONAHA.113.003904

Sibai, B., Dekker, G., & Kupferminc, M. (2005). Pre-eclampsia. *The Lancet*, *365*(9461), 785–799. https://doi.org/10.1016/S0140-6736(05)17987-2

Sibai, B. M., & Stella, C. L. (2009). Diagnosis and management of atypical preeclampsia-eclampsia. *American Journal of Obstetrics and Gynecology*, *200*(5), 481.e1–481.e7. https://doi.org/10.1016/j.ajog.2008.07.048

Siepmann, T., Boardman, H., Bilderbeck, A., Griffanti, L., Kenworthy, Y., Zwager, C., McKean, D., Francis, J., Neubauer, S., Yu, G. Z., Lewandowski, A. J., Sverrisdottir, Y. B., & Leeson, P. (2017). Long-term cerebral white and gray matter changes after preeclampsia. *Neurology*, *88*(13), 1256–1264. https://doi.org/10.1212/WNL.0000000000003765

Suresh, S., Amegashie, C., Patel, E., Nieman, K. M., & Rana, S. (2022). Racial disparities in diagnosis, management, and outcomes in pre-eclampsia. *Current Hypertension Reports*, *24*(4), 87–93. https://doi.org/10.1007/s11906-022-01172-x

Ukoha, E. P., Snavely, M. E., Hahn, M. U., Steinauer, J. E., & Bryant, A. S. (2022). Toward the elimination of race-based medicine: Replace race with racism as preeclampsia risk factor. *American Journal of Obstetrics and Gynecology*. https://doi.org/10.1016/j.ajog.2022.05.048

US Preventive Services Task Force. (2021). Aspirin use to prevent preeclampsia and related morbidity and mortality: US Preventive Services Task Force recommendation statement. *JAMA*, *326*(12), 1186–1191. https://doi.org/10.1001/jama.2021.14781

Van Oostwaard, M. F., Langenveld, J., Schuit, E., Wigny, K., Van Susante, H., Beune, I., Ramaekers, R., Papatsonis, D. N. M., Mol, B. W. J., & Ganzevoort, W. (2014). Prediction of recurrence of hypertensive disorders of pregnancy in the term period, a retrospective cohort study. *Pregnancy Hypertension: An International Journal of Women's Cardiovascular Health*, *4*(3), 194–202. https://doi.org/10.1016/j.preghy.2014.04.001

Wang, I.-K., Tsai, I.-J., Chen, P.-C., Liang, C.-C., Chou, C.-Y., Chang, C.-T., Kuo, H.-L., Ting, I.-W., Lin, C.-C., Chuang, F.-R., Huang, C.-C., & Sung, F.-C. (2012). Hypertensive disorders in pregnancy and subsequent diabetes mellitus: A retrospective cohort study. *The American Journal of Medicine*, *125*(3), 251–257. https://doi.org/10.1016/j.amjmed.2011.07.040

Workman, J. L., Barha, C. K., & Galea, L. A. M. (2012). Endocrine substrates of cognitive and affective changes during pregnancy and postpartum. *Behavioral Neuroscience*, *126*(1), 54–72. https://doi.org/10.1037/a0025538

World Health Organization. (2014). *WHO recommendations for prevention and treatment of pre-eclampsia and eclampsia: Implications and actions*. World Health Organization. https://apps.who.int/iris/handle/10665/119627

Wu, P., Haththotuwa, R., Kwok, C. S., Babu, A., Kotronias, R. A., Rushton, C., Zaman, A., Fryer, A. A., Kadam, U., Chew-Graham, C. A., & Mamas, M. A. (2017). Preeclampsia and future cardiovascular health: A systematic review and meta-analysis. *Circulation: Cardiovascular Quality and Outcomes*, *10*(2). https://doi.org/10.1161/CIRCOUTCOMES.116.003497

Young, B. C., Levine, R. J., & Karumanchi, S. A. (2010). Pathogenesis of preeclampsia. *Annual Review of Pathology: Mechanisms of Disease*, *5*(1), 173–192. https://doi.org/10.1146/annurev-pathol-121808-102149

37

Gestational Diabetes Mellitus

Kimberly K. Trout

Relevant Terms

Basal insulin—principal action is to reduce hepatic glucose production, thus limiting overnight (fasting) and between meal hyperglycemia

Class GDMA1—gestational diabetes in glycemic control with lifestyle interventions (medical nutrition therapy and physical activity)

Class GDMA2—gestational diabetes requiring any medication in addition to lifestyle interventions to achieve glycemic control

Dietary reference intake—provides a range for appropriate intake of nutrients

Euglycemia—normal levels of glucose in the blood

Estimated fetal weight (EFW)—clinical or sonographic estimate of fetal weight

Insulin resistance—a condition in which cells fail to respond to the normal actions of insulin, thereby increasing blood glucose levels

Large for gestational age—birth weight greater than the 90th percentile for any given gestational age in a defined population

Leptin—a hormone released from adipocytes; sends signals to the hypothalamus in the brain to help regulate food intake and energy expenditure

Macrosomia—birth weight ≥4000 g

Overt diabetes—diabetes with onset prior to pregnancy

Resistin—a cytokine secreted by adipocytes into the circulation; causes resistance of peripheral tissues to insulin

Tumor necrosis factor alpha—a multifunctional cytokine with effects on lipid metabolism, coagulation, insulin resistance, and the function of endothelial cells lining blood vessels

Introduction

Gestational diabetes mellitus (GDM) is defined as glucose intolerance that is first detected during the second or third trimester of pregnancy that was not clearly **overt diabetes** prior to gestation (ADA, 2023a). This simple definition belies the complexity of a condition that spans a spectrum of glycemia and clinical manifestations for which there is a wide diversity of opinion. GDM occurs in 7.8% of all pregnancies in the United States, representing a 30% increase since 2016 (Gregory & Ely, 2022). GDM increases with increasing maternal age, prepregnancy body mass index (BMI), and plurality (Gregory & Ely, 2022). There are wide differences noted geographically, with the lowest rate in Mississippi (4.7%) and the highest rate in Alaska (12.6%; Gregory & Ely, 2022). Data from 2020 show a larger increase in GDM with the COVID-19 pandemic onset (13%) when compared with the average annual percentage increase of the prepandemic years, 2016–2019 (5%; Gregory & Ely, 2022). The carbohydrate intolerance of GDM may be of varying degrees, with increasing perinatal problems associated with decreasing maternal blood glucose control. This, perhaps, is the only area of the study of GDM where there is agreement. There are several expert groups involved in developing guidelines for the care of pregnant people with gestational diabetes: the Endocrine Society (TES), the US Preventive Services Task Force (USPSTF), The American Diabetes Association (ADA), the American College of Obstetricians and Gynecologists (ACOG), the International Association of the Diabetes and Pregnancy Study Groups (IADPSG) and the Society for Maternal-Fetal Medicine (SMFM). Consensus on who to screen, how to screen, diagnostic methods, diagnostic criteria, fetal surveillance, and treatment of GDM remains elusive. Association between maternal glucose levels and adverse perinatal outcomes occurs on a continuum with no obvious cutoff thresholds at which risks increase (HAPO Study Cooperative Research Group et al., 2008), making the debates particularly complex.

Health equity key points

- Social determinants such as food insecurity, homelessness, language barriers, and availability of expensive blood glucose testing supplies can affect the outcomes of GDM.
- Providers should assess for barriers to following recommended treatment regimens and assist pregnant people in accessing resources for optimal success in managing GDM.
- Structural racism contributes to social conditions and environments that can make diabetes more difficult to manage.

Prenatal and Postnatal Care: A Person-Centered Approach, Third Edition. Edited by Karen Trister Grace, Cindy L. Farley, Noelene K. Jeffers, and Tanya Tringali.
© 2024 John Wiley & Sons Ltd. Published 2024 by John Wiley & Sons Ltd.
Companion website: www.wiley.com/go/grace/prenatal

Pathophysiology and Potential Problems

Pregnancy is characterized by a series of metabolic changes that promote the accumulation of adipose tissue in early pregnancy, followed by **insulin resistance** later in gestation. The hormones of pregnancy affect glucose metabolism by causing increased insulin resistance that develops around 15 weeks of gestation and continues to increase by approximately 5% per week of gestation up until 36 weeks when it tends to plateau. Thus, the effects of this increased insulin resistance manifest primarily during the late second and third trimesters (ADA, 2023b). Levels of human placental lactogen (HPL), human placental growth hormone, progesterone, cortisol, and prolactin increase and contribute to insulin resistance (Barbour et al., 2007). HPL increases up to 30-fold during pregnancy and promotes insulin release from the pancreas. **Tumor necrosis factor alpha (TNFα)** and the hormones **leptin** and **resistin** have also been implicated in the insulin resistance of pregnancy (Kirwan et al., 2002; Landon et al., 2021; Melczer et al., 2003). The increased insulin resistance during the late second and third trimesters of pregnancy poses a challenge to the maternal pancreatic β cells. For most individuals, this increase in insulin resistance has no adverse effect and actually serves a positive function to provide a steady supply of nutrients to the developing fetus. In those individuals who eventually develop GDM, there is an inability of the β cells to meet the challenge of secreting the additional amounts of insulin necessary to achieve and maintain **euglycemia** (Retnakaran et al., 2010).

Glucose passes from maternal to fetal compartments via diffusion facilitated by insulin-dependent glucose transporters. The delivery of glucose to the fetus beyond normal levels can lead to **macrosomia**, with the fetus responding to the elevated levels of glucose by becoming hyperinsulinemic. Insulin is an anabolic hormone that promotes cell growth. Most of the potential problems of GDM are related to excessive fetal growth (Table 37.1). Alterations in lipid metabolism are also thought to play a role in excessive fetal growth. In one study of women with well-controlled blood glucose levels, elevated maternal free fatty acid (FFA) concentrations correlated with increased neonatal fat mass at birth, suggesting that factors other than elevated glucose contribute to fetal macrosomia (Schafer-Graf et al., 2008). Macrosomic infants born to people with gestational diabetes typically have excessive fat on the shoulders and trunk with disproportionate chest-to-head ratios, predisposing them to shoulder dystocia or an operative birth. Evidence suggests a positive association between elevated fasting glucose levels and higher glycosylated hemoglobin (A1C) levels in early pregnancy and relative risk for shoulder dystocia (Hughes et al., 2014; Zhu et al., 2014). An increased risk for shoulder dystocia is also associated with a maternal BMI >30; however, the overall risk remains small.

The rates of stillbirth are higher in people with GDM with poor glycemic control during pregnancy (Biggio

Table 37.1 Potential Problems Related to Gestational Diabetes

Maternal
Operative birth (instrumental and cesarean)
Preeclampsia
Preterm labor
Polyhydramnios
Overt diabetes later in life
Metabolic syndrome later in life

Fetal/neonatal
Macrosomia
Large for gestational age (greater than 90th percentile)
Shoulder dystocia/birth trauma
Hypoglycemia
Polycythemia
Hyperbilirubinemia
Respiratory distress syndrome
Need for neonatal intensive care unit admission/care

Childhood/adult
Early childhood obesity
Early childhood metabolic syndrome
Type 2 diabetes during adolescence

et al., 2010). The rates of fetal anomalies are increased with pregestational diabetes but are not increased in people who develop GDM (Moore & Catalano, 2009).

Prenatal Screening and Diagnosis

All pregnant people should be screened for diabetes at the first prenatal visit by history, clinical risk factors, or lab screening of blood glucose levels. The ADA (2023a), ACOG (2018), and USPSTF (2021) recommend universal laboratory screening between 24 and 28 weeks gestation for all pregnant people. The ACOG previously supported screening based upon risk factors but acknowledged that individuals at lowest risk for GDM account for only 10% of pregnant people in the US, thus adding unnecessary complexity to the screening process (Table 37.2; ACOG, 2018).

Screening for Pregnant People at High Risk for Diabetes

For those pregnant people at high risk for developing diabetes, laboratory screening for undiagnosed diabetes should be done at the first prenatal visit before 15 weeks of gestation (Table 37.2; ADA, 2023a). The concern is that the individual may have overt diabetes (type 1 or type 2). Prior to 2017, any diabetes diagnosed during pregnancy had been defined as "gestational," but current definitions better reflect the pathophysiology of GDM, as the insulin resistance attributable to pregnancy is not a factor before 15 weeks of gestation; thus, any diabetes diagnosed prior to 15 weeks of gestation indicates overt (pregestational) diabetes rather than gestational diabetes (ADA, 2023a). A diagnosis of overt diabetes can be made in pregnant people who meet any of the standard diagnostic criteria at their initial prenatal visit (presumably occurring before 15 weeks; ADA, 2023b):

Table 37.2   Risk Factor Classification for Gestational Diabetes Screening

Low risk	Average risk	High risk

• Age < 25 years
• Prepregnancy BMI ≤25
• No known diabetes in first-degree relatives
• No history of poor obstetric outcome
• No history of prior GDM, glycosuria, or impaired carbohydrate metabolism (A_{1C} ≥ 5.7%, impaired glucose tolerance, or impaired fasting glucose)
	Any criteria not met for low-risk or high-risk status	• BMI >25, and any of the additional risk factors below:
		  ○ Prior history of GDM, glycosuria, or impaired carbohydrate metabolism (A_{1C} ≥5.7%, impaired glucose tolerance, or impaired fasting glucose)
		  ○ Physical inactivity
		  ○ Prior birth of an infant weighing >4000 g
		  ○ First-degree relative with diabetes
		  ○ HDL cholesterol <35 mg/dL
		  ○ Triglyceride level > 250 mg/dL
		  ○ History of cardiovascular disease
		  ○ History of other clinical conditions associated with insulin resistance such as polycystic ovarian syndrome, hypertension, prepregnancy BMI > 40 or acanthosis nigricans
		  ○ Prior history of stillbirth, infant with congenital anomalies, or macrosomia
		  ○ Age ≥ 40

• Laboratory screen at 24–28 weeks' gestation	• Laboratory screen at 24–28 weeks' gestation	• Laboratory screen at first visit and if normal, repeat screen 24–28 weeks' gestation

Source: Adapted from IADPSG (2010), Metzger (2007), USPSTF (2021), and ACOG (2018).

- Fasting plasma glucose ≥126 mg/dL (7.0 mmol/L) or
- A1C ≥6.5% using a standardized assay or
- Random plasma glucose ≥200 mg/dL (11.1 mmol/L) that is subsequently confirmed by elevated fasting plasma glucose or A1C or
- Two-hour plasma glucose ≥200 mg/dL following a 75 g oral glucose load[1]

Ninety percent of providers in the United States use the two-step screening process performed at 24–28 weeks (Bimson et al., 2017). If early (<15 weeks of gestation) tests are negative for overt diabetes, repeat laboratory screening with the 1-hour test is recommended at 24–28 weeks of gestation (USPSTF, 2021).

Testing for GDM has been recently reexamined by the USPSTF (2021) with affirmation of recommendations to perform GDM screening at 24–28 weeks of gestation (Grade B evidence). However, the Task Force determined that there was insufficient evidence to recommend "early GDM screening" (<24 weeks of gestation). The Task Force is quite clear that the strategy to detect undiagnosed diabetes preexisting the pregnancy (i.e., testing before 15 weeks that has been previously described in this chapter) is *not* what is being addressed as part of this recommendation. Rather, the Task Force is referring to the practice of screening a pregnant person who was not diagnosed with or screened for overt diabetes (prior to 15 weeks of gestation) for "early GDM screening" before 24 weeks (USPSTF, 2021). In other words, there is insufficient

evidence to perform "early GDM screening" between 15 and 24 weeks of pregnancy for those patients who have already had the recommended testing prior to 15 weeks to determine that they do not have overt diabetes (USPSTF, 2021). There is no clear consensus about the most appropriate test for patients who enter prenatal care between 15 and 24 weeks; people presenting for care during this time with risk factors for overt or gestational diabetes should be tested during this time with *any* of the available tests.

Screening and Diagnostic Methods

Screening and diagnostic methods lack consensus. Two methods are appropriate for use according to the ADA: the two-step method and the one-step method. The two-step method is the most common screening method used in the United States and is endorsed by ACOG and the NIH, although ACOG states that individual practices "may choose to use the IADPSG's recommendation, if appropriate, for the population they serve" (ACOG, 2018).

The two-step method begins with the 1-hour oral glucose load screening test (also commonly referred to as the 50-g glucose challenge test [GCT]), which entails administration of a 50-g oral glucose load with plasma glucose levels evaluated after 1 hour. A positive screening result is then followed up with a 3-hour oral glucose tolerance test (OGTT) for diagnosis. Screening and diagnosis occur in two separate steps. The 1-hour glucose load screening test is considered positive at levels exceeding 130, 135, or 140 mg/dL (ACOG, 2018). The screening test threshold at which a diagnostic OGTT is recommended is an arbitrary value not determined by scientific study; there are no randomized trials to support a clear benefit to one cutoff compared with others. The higher the threshold glucose level is set, the lower the sensitivity, but the better

---

1 Note that this is a diagnostic level different than that used at 24–28 weeks to diagnose GDM. The ADA also recommends that for any of the above measures, "in the absence of unequivocal hyperglycemia, diagnosis should be confirmed by two abnormal test results from the same sample or in two separate test samples" (ADA, 2023a, p. S21).

the specificity and the lower the likelihood of a false positive test result. The lower the threshold glucose level is set, the higher the sensitivity, but the higher the chance of a false positive test result, resulting in the performance of an unnecessary 3-hour diagnostic OGTT. The lower screening level of 130 mg/dL increases the sensitivity of the screening to nearly 100% but increases the false positive rate after diagnostic testing from 14% to 23%, thus increasing both costs and needless anxiety. Conversely, a higher cutoff of 140 mg/dL detects fewer people with GDM but reduces the number of false positives (Landon et al., 2021). Any of the three suggested values for defining an abnormal initial screening result can be considered correct; however, each practice should decide on a consistent measurement to be used that is based on the prevalence of GDM within their community. Individuals do not need to be fasting for this test; however, patients should be advised that a high-sugar or high-carbohydrate snack or meal just prior to the test can increase the incidence of false positive results.

The 3-hour, 100-g OGTT is the most common diagnostic test used in the United States when a 1-hour screen is positive. The test is administered in the morning after an overnight fast. There are two commonly used criteria to diagnose GDM with the 3-hour GTT.

A positive diagnosis of GDM traditionally has required that two or more threshold glucose levels on the 3-hour test be met or exceeded. However, in 2017, the ACOG recommended that one elevated value may be used to establish the diagnosis of GDM, noting that research evidence has demonstrated an increased risk for adverse perinatal outcomes with even one abnormal value. This was followed in 2018 with the caution that further research is needed on this, leaving providers with ambiguous guidance to dictate management (ACOG, 2018).

The National Diabetes Data Group (NDDG) established the diagnostic criteria for GDM in 1979. This set of values has been challenged by the Carpenter and Coustan criteria, which designate lower blood glucose values to diagnose GDM, meaning more people are diagnosed with GDM (Table 37.3). In one study comparing the NDDG criteria with the Carpenter and Coustan criteria, 3.3% of women were diagnosed with GDM under NDDG criteria as compared to 5.1% with the Carpenter and Coustan criteria (Chen et al., 2009).

Table 37.3 Criteria for Abnormal Result on 100-g, 3-Hour Oral Glucose Tolerance Test in Pregnant People

Blood sample	National Diabetes Data Group criteria	Carpenter and Coustan criteria
Fasting	105 mg/dL (5.8 mmol/L)	95 mg/dL (5.3 mmol/L)
1 h	190 mg/dL (10.5 mmol/L)	180 mg/dL (10.0 mmol/L)
2 h	165 mg/dL (9.2 mmol/L)	155 mg/dL (8.6 mmol/L)
3 h	145 mg/dL (8.0 mmol/L)	140 mg/dL (7.8 mmol/L)

Source: Adapted from ACOG (2018).

The most recent Fifth International Workshop Conference on GDM recommends using the lower Carpenter and Coustan criteria for the 3-hour glucose tolerance test (Metzger et al., 2007).

The one-step method combines screening and diagnosis in one test. A 75-g oral glucose load is administered, and plasma glucose levels are evaluated after 1 and 2 hours. *Only one abnormal value is required for a diagnosis of GDM.*

GDM diagnostic criteria—75-g 2-hour OGTT

FBS 92 mg/dL or above
1-hour: 180 mg/dL or above
2-hour: 153 mg/dL or above

Following the recommendations of the IADPSG, the ADA, in 2017, endorsed the use of the 75-g 2-hour test as a one-step test for GDM screening and diagnosis (ADA, 2017). This recommendation was based on results from the Hyperglycemia and Adverse Pregnancy Outcomes (HAPO) study, a prospective observational study of more than 23,000 pregnant women evaluated with a 75-g 2-hour OGTT (HAPO Study Cooperative Research Group et al., 2008). The investigators found a continuum of increasing risk of adverse outcomes as each of the three (fasting, 1 hour, and 2 hour) plasma glucose values increased. Because of the lower blood glucose thresholds and the fact that only one abnormal value is required for diagnosis, one-step testing would significantly increase the diagnosed prevalence of GDM, with the attendant medicalization of pregnancies and with a concomitant increase in healthcare costs both to individuals and to society. A significant criticism of the IADPSG recommendation for one-step GDM screening and diagnosis is that the decision was made based on expert opinion and consensus rather than on rigorously obtained outcome measures (Langer et al., 2013). Currently, there is no evidence that this method leads to improved maternal or fetal outcomes. One analysis found that pregnant women classified as nondiabetic by the Canadian Diabetes Association criteria but considered to have GDM according to the IADPSG criteria had similar pregnancy outcomes as women without GDM (Bodmer-Roy et al., 2012). For these reasons, the ACOG continues to recommend the two-step process, but states that either the one- or two-step processes are acceptable (ACOG, 2018). Continued support for the two-step GDM screening and diagnosis process was also reaffirmed at a National Institutes of Health Consensus Development Conference on the diagnosis of GDM in 2013. The ADA now recommends the IADPSG one-step test and diagnostic criteria, stating that the criteria for the one-step test were set "with the intent of optimizing gestational outcomes . . ." (ADA, 2023a, p. S34). Screening and testing methods for GDM continue to be the subject of ongoing investigation and debate.

Management

The majority of pregnant people diagnosed with GDM will have **class GDMA1** and do not require medication for glucose management. Basic components of lifestyle intervention management for GDMA1 are healthful eating, physical activity, and monitoring blood glucose levels.

Healthful Eating

Dietary modification is the mainstay of treatment for people with GDM and is referred to as "medical nutrition therapy" in much of the diabetes literature (ADA, 2023b). The optimal diet should provide sufficient calories and nutrients for fetal growth and maternal needs while reducing significant postprandial hyperglycemia. Patients should be advised to make an appointment with a dietician or a certified diabetes educator (CDE) for diet instruction. However, since this visit may be weeks away, it is important for healthcare providers to understand the principles of nutrition therapy for GDM since dietary modification should be initiated immediately. Surprisingly, clinical trials to date have not been conclusive in establishing the optimal diet for GDM, even though medical nutrition therapy is the cornerstone of treatment (ADA, 2023b). A dietary program of 2000–2500 kcal/day, representing approximately 30–35 kcal/kg of present pregnancy weight, is typically initiated (ADA, 2014).

Since carbohydrates are the macronutrients that appear to have the greatest effect on postprandial blood glucose levels, people with GDM are frequently advised to monitor carbohydrates more closely than other macronutrients, following a diet of approximately 33–40% complex carbohydrates, eliminating simple sugars, 20% protein, and 40% fats. Complex carbohydrate levels of 50–60% typically result in excessive weight gain and poor glucose control (ACOG, 2018). To keep blood glucose stable (less glucose variability), food is best taken in three meals with two to three snacks with carbohydrates evenly distributed throughout the day, with the exception of breakfast. Moderate use of sweeteners such as aspartame is permitted. Following these dietary guidelines, glucose levels will normalize in around 70–85% of people with GDM (ADA, 2023b).

Carbohydrates are generally less well tolerated in the morning due to hormones secreted in the early morning that contribute to wakefulness, such as cortisol and epinephrine (Trout et al., 2022). For this reason, fewer carbohydrates are recommended at breakfast than with other meals to minimize the elevation of postbreakfast blood glucose. An important part of nutrition therapy is an evening or bedtime snack, consisting of approximately 15–30 g carbohydrates, which is usually advised to prevent overnight ketosis. For the same reason, conventional wisdom has suggested that the overnight fast should not exceed 10 hours; however, this has not been rigorously tested. Henze et al. (2022) performed a rigorous crossover design study in which 68 women with GDM were randomized to three different interventions: (a) no bedtime snack; (b) a higher carbohydrate snack (yogurt and an apple); and (c) a lower carbohydrate snack (20 g of dark chocolate and 10 almonds). Blood glucose values were found to be lowest the next morning for the "no snack" group (Henze et al., 2022). However, despite statistically significant results, it remains unclear if the differences were clinically meaningful, as only a one-to-four-point difference in mean fasting blood glucose (FBG) level was detected between the groups, and fasting values were normal for all three groups (range of 87.6–90.18 mg/dL; Henze et al., 2022). Although this study does suggest that the conventional recommendation for a bedtime snack should be studied further, it would be wise to evaluate each pregnant person's response to a bedtime snack (or not) by examining the next morning's FBG level and, thus, determining recommendations based on results for that individual.

The **dietary reference intake (DRI)** for carbohydrates in pregnancy is 175 g/day, the minimal requirement to assure adequate glucose to meet fetal and maternal needs. This number is used to calculate the desired range of actual carbohydrate intake daily, depending on a person's calorie requirements. There are 4 kcal for each gram of carbohydrate, 4 kcal for each gram of protein, and 9 kcal for each gram of fat. So, for example, if a person is on a 2000-kcal diet and is attempting to consume 40% carbohydrate, the total number of kcal (2000) × 40% = 800 kcals from carbohydrates/4 = 200 g of carbohydrates daily (Tables 37.4 and 37.5).

Pregnancy weight gain within the Institute of Medicine (IOM) recommendations for BMI should be encouraged

Table 37.4   Sample Diet at 2000 calories with 35–40% Carbohydrate (CHO)

Breakfast 27 g CHO	1 scrambled egg with 1 slice (1 oz) cheese +1 tsp butter 1 piece toast (15 g CHO) 1 cup skim milk (12 g CHO) Decaf coffee or tea (no sugar)
Snack, mid am 15 g CHO	½ banana–4 oz (15 g CHO) 1 slice turkey bacon
Lunch 46 g CHO	3 oz beef or turkey burger with lettuce and tomato (30 g CHO) Carrots, cucumber, broccoli, celery (10 g CHO) 1 tbsp ranch dressing for dip ½ cup skim milk (6 g CHO)
Snack, mid pm 15 g CHO	½ cup fruit salad (15 g CHO) ¼ cup nonfat cottage cheese
Dinner 46 g CHO	3 oz baked chicken breast 1 cup green beans (10 g CHO) 1 cup mashed potatoes (30 g CHO) 2 tsp butter ½ cup skim milk (6 g CHO)
Snack, bedtime 30 g CHO	$^2/_3$ cup fat-free yogurt (12 g CHO) ¾ cup unsweetened cereal (15 g CHO) 1 tbsp sugar-free peanut butter (3 g CHO)
Total CHO 179 g	

Table 37.5 Total Daily Carbohydrates for 35–40% of Calories

Kilocalories (kcal)	35% (g)	40% (g)
2000	175	200
2200	193	220
2500	219	250

(see Chapter 9, *Nutrition during Pregnancy*). Severe caloric or carbohydrate restriction should be avoided as this can result in significant ketonuria and ketonemia. Maintaining a food log and recording daily food and fluid intake can help people with GDM monitor their food choices. The use of nutritional phone apps can make this less time-consuming and cumbersome. Interprofessional collaboration with a registered dietician or CDE on nutritional management of GDM can help the patient understand GDM and how to best manage the condition and optimize outcomes.

Physical Activity

Physical activity is an essential component of treatment for people with GDM, although it is often ignored. Regular exercise increases glucose uptake and increases insulin sensitivity, thus decreasing insulin resistance. Thirty minutes of exercise on most days can be comparable to insulin in keeping glycemic control (Brankston et al., 2004; Halse et al., 2014). The physical activity should be distributed over at least three days/week and with no more than two consecutive days without physical activity. A recent systematic review noted great heterogeneity in studies of physical activity for individuals with GDM, but essentially found that increased physical activity could possibly obviate the need for insulin treatment (Laredo-Aguilera et al., 2020).

People with GDM should be informed about the benefits of physical activity and instructed in specific exercises. Daily walking, swimming, and use of a stationary bike are excellent exercise options and can be safely recommended for individuals with no contraindications to exercise (see Chapter 20, *Physical Activity and Exercise in the Perinatal Period*). Writing out a "prescription" for the type and amount of exercise may help people recognize the importance of this therapy in managing their GDM. Keeping a daily exercise log with an app can help track their regimen, correlate activity with blood glucose levels, and emphasize the importance of regular exercise in the treatment of GDM.

Blood Glucose Monitoring

Surveillance of blood glucose levels is necessary to ascertain that glycemic control has been established. Daily self-monitoring of blood glucose consists of the FBG and 1- to 2-hour postprandial measures. Some experts advocate the 1-hour postprandial value in lieu of the 2 hours, although either one is acceptable, noting that peak glucose excursion is typically at 90 minutes after meals (ACOG, 2018). It may be reasonable to ask the pregnant person whether a 1-hour versus 2-hour option works better for them in conjunction with other aspects of their life and to tailor this recommendation individually to achieve person-centered care. Target glucose levels for control of GDM have been established largely based on expert opinion.

Target capillary blood glucose levels

Fasting: <95 mg/dL
1-hour postprandial: <140 mg/dL
2-hour postprandial: <120 mg/dL

A common schedule for self-monitoring of blood glucose is to initially test four times daily. If both fasting and postprandial measures are within normal after several weeks of testing, the testing frequency can be reduced to a schedule tailored to the person's individual situation. If postprandial blood glucose levels indicate hyperglycemia and poor glycemic control, or if FBG levels are high (diet modification most often has little effect on fasting glucose levels), then medication is required. However, there is no conclusive evidence regarding exactly how many blood glucose levels need to be elevated to initiate medication (ACOG, 2018).

While not typically used for patients with GDMA1, for patients with type 1 or type 2 diabetes, who are often advised to test more frequently than four times daily, the use of continuous glucose monitoring (CGM) systems or flash technology has been especially beneficial in facilitating blood glucose control. With CGM, a patient has a small patch with a filament placed under the skin (into subcutaneous tissue) that detects the glucose value in interstitial fluid every 5 minutes and transmits to a receiver device. Essentially, the patient is on "continuous monitoring" as opposed to the "intermittent monitoring" of capillary glucose fingersticks. The CONCEPTT randomized trial found that CGM use in women with type 1 diabetes in pregnancy resulted in improvements in HgbA1C without an increase in either maternal or neonatal hypoglycemia and with a reduction in **large for gestational age** (LGA) infants (Fieg et al., 2017). However, studies have also found that CGM is not as reliable at low blood glucose levels due to shifts in interstitial fluid that occur during pregnancy. Additionally, when blood glucose is rapidly rising or falling (for all individuals, pregnant, or nonpregnant), there is a lag time in interstitial fluid glucose values when compared with capillary blood glucose. Therefore, patients are urged to check glucose with capillary blood testing when experiencing symptoms of hypoglycemia or when it is suspected that blood glucose values are rapidly rising or falling. The use of Smartphone technology has increased the ease of recording blood glucose results (Figure 37.1). There are several phone apps available that interface well with CGM technology.

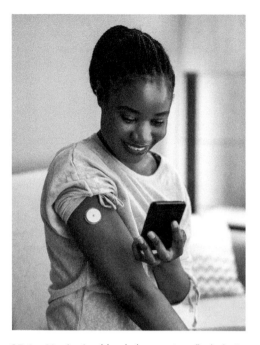

Figure 37.1 Monitoring blood glucose via a flash device. Andrey Popov/Adobe Stock.

Pharmacologic Treatments

Pregnant people with GDM requiring medication to achieve euglycemia are considered to have **class GDMA2**. Insulin is the only US Food and Drug Administration (FDA)-approved medication for the treatment of GDM, is the medication recommended by ACOG (2018), and is the first-line treatment recommended by the ADA (2023b). The Society for Maternal-Fetal Medicine (2018) considers metformin a reasonable alternative to insulin and in the United Kingdom; the National Institute for Health and Care Excellence (NICE) guidelines suggest metformin as a first-line treatment for GDM if blood glucose control is not achieved with lifestyle intervention (2015). Oral diabetic medications have several distinct advantages over insulin treatment with regard to ease of use and cost. Oral routes are preferred by many people over self-injection. Knowledge of insulin action based on the type of insulin used, peak and duration of action, and precise matching of insulin to meal timing and carbohydrate levels can be quite complex, and for some people, this complexity can be overwhelming.

The primary reason that insulin is still recommended as first-line pharmacologic treatment for GDM is the lack of long-term safety data with the use of oral agents (ACOG, 2018). Both glyburide and metformin cross the placenta, with metformin crossing in larger amounts than glyburide; insulin does not cross the placenta.

Insulin Therapy

Insulin is the only FDA-approved medication for GDM. Individuals with a BMI >40 are more likely to require insulin therapy to achieve euglycemia. The person who requires insulin treatment is also likely to have concerns about the effects of GDM on their infant's health and possible risks associated with labor and birth. While insulin initiation is typically managed by physician colleagues, midwives, nurse practitioners, and physician's assistants can play a role in the monitoring and maintenance of insulin therapy as part of an interdisciplinary team.

Insulin therapy is typically added to healthful eating and physical activity when FBG levels are consistently ≥95, if 1-hour postprandial levels are consistently ≥140, or if 2-hour postprandial levels are consistently ≥120. Insulin must be individualized with dosage determinations tailored to diet and exercise habits. The typical starting dose is 0.7–1.0 units/kg daily in divided doses, often in two to four injections (ACOG, 2018). Some clinicians will start with half of that amount in order to gauge the individual's response to the insulin dosage and not inadvertently cause hypoglycemia. Adjustments in dosages should be based on monitored blood glucose values. Establishing the correct insulin dosage is very individualized and depends on several factors, including relative degree of insulin resistance. Frequently, a combination of intermediate-acting neutral protamine Hagedorn (NPH) and fast-acting insulin such as regular or lispro is used together near breakfast and dinner to suppress gluconeogenesis in the liver, as well as to counter the rises in glucose that occur with meals (see Table 37.6). This necessitates only twice-daily injections. However, some advocate splitting the evening insulin dose, giving the short-acting insulin at dinner and then NPH at bedtime, to decrease the risk of nocturnal hypoglycemia. Some people will require only a long-acting insulin (glargine, detemir, or NPH) at night if elevated fasting levels are a problem. The advantage of glargine or detemir for **basal insulin** requirements is that there is no peak of action, thus not requiring as precisely timed meals as when NPH is used. Additionally, rapid-acting insulin analogs (aspart or lispro) can be given just prior to a meal if postprandial blood glucose values are elevated.

The ability to administer a rapid-acting insulin just prior to a meal helps avert errors in meal timing that could potentially cause inadvertent hypoglycemia. Pregnant people in general have physiologically lower FBG levels

Table 37.6 Types and Action of Insulin

Type of insulin	Onset of action	Peak of action (hours)	Duration of action (hours)
Humalog (lispro)	1–15 min	1	2–4
Novolog (aspart)	1–15 min	1	2–4
Regular insulin	30–60 min	2	4
Humulin N (NPH)	1–3 h	8	8
Lantus (glargine)	1 h	No peak	<24
Levemir (detemir)	3–4 h	No peak	12–24 (dose-dependent)

Source: Adapted from Trout and Dolin (2021).

than nonpregnant people, and if they are not on medication, they can have blood glucose levels as low as 50 mg/dL and yet be totally asymptomatic for hypoglycemia. However, once diabetes medication is initiated with the potential to produce hypoglycemia beyond the body's capacity to counter-regulate, hypoglycemia can happen quickly and can lead to coma or death if not treated promptly. Hypoglycemia is a serious risk with all insulin therapy. A rapidly absorbed glucose source should be administered immediately to any person on diabetes medication who is symptomatic with a blood glucose <80 mg/dL (symptoms include shaking, sweating, agitation, rapid heart rate, clammy skin). Treat immediately with 15 g of glucose tablets or a glass of juice. Whole milk and chocolate candy contain fat that will slow the rise in glucose and are not preferred for this purpose. However, it is appropriate to administer whatever quickly absorbed glucose source is readily available. If blood glucose is still low after 15 minutes, another dose of 15 g of glucose is administered. Glucagon should be used for those who have lost consciousness due to hypoglycemia and friends and family should be trained in its use. Glucagon is available in a kit for intramuscular injection or a newly available inhaled form (Baqsimi©) that is given in a similar manner to inhaled naloxone for an opioid overdose (Eli Lilly & Company, 2020; Rickels et al., 2016). Any person who is prescribed insulin should carry a quick source of glucose and can be prescribed a form of glucagon in case it is ever needed. It is important to know the action profiles of the various insulins, so that meals and snacks are planned accordingly, and hypoglycemia is avoided.

Oral Medications

Metformin

Metformin readily crosses the placenta with placental levels equivalent to or exceeding maternal concentrations, and the long-term effects on the fetus are unknown (Ryu et al., 2014). The primary action of metformin is to decrease glucose output from the liver. The metformin in gestational diabetes (MiG) study comparing pregnancy outcomes with metformin or insulin for the treatment of GDM demonstrated no outcome differences between the two treatments except that participants preferred oral therapy (Butalia et al., 2017). The Fifth International Workshop Conference recommended that metformin treatment for GDM is limited to clinical trials, and its use in pregnancy remains controversial (Butalia et al., 2017), although both ADA and ACOG state that its use is acceptable in pregnant persons unwilling or unable to use insulin (ACOG, 2018; ADA, 2023b). The most common side effects with metformin are gastrointestinal-related, such as abdominal pain and diarrhea. These can be minimized by increasing to optimal dosage slowly, starting with 500 mg once daily for a week, then increasing to 500 mg twice daily for a week, then further by 500 mg a week if needed up to a maximum dose of 2500 mg daily. Of note, 10–46% of pregnant women on metformin eventually require supplemental insulin to achieve adequate glycemic control (Ryu

et al., 2014). A meta-analysis by Butalia et al. (2017) found metformin to be the superior treatment when compared with both glyburide and insulin with respect to most perinatal indicators, with the exception of risk for cesarean birth (Farrar et al., 2017). The risk of LGA, macrosomia, neonatal intensive care unit (NICU) admission, neonatal hypoglycemia, and preeclampsia were all significantly reduced with metformin. Glyburide was most effective in reducing risk for cesarean birth (79.9%) as compared with insulin (10.4%) and metformin (9.7%). This meta-analysis was limited by small sample sizes in many of the studies, indicating further studies with large, well-designed trials are needed. A recent open-label trial conducted in Spain randomized 200 women with GDM to receive either insulin or metformin when not meeting blood glucose targets with lifestyle management alone (Picón-César et al., 2021). While no difference was noted for mean FBG levels, there were significantly lower postprandial blood glucose levels in the metformin group. This group also had fewer labor inductions, cesarean births, and episodes of hypoglycemia (Picón-César et al., 2021).

Metformin is appropriate for people who decline insulin therapy, those who may not be able to safely administer injections, or people who cannot afford insulin. If used, patients should be informed of placental transfer and the lack of long-term data on safety (ACOG, 2018).

Glyburide

Glyburide is a second-generation sulfonylurea oral agent that has been used more extensively than metformin, in large part because it was previously believed that glyburide did not cross the placenta in pregnancy (Moore et al., 2010; Zeng et al., 2014). The action of glyburide is to promote increased insulin secretion. Typically, glyburide is started at a dose of 2.5 mg prior to breakfast and 2.5 mg prior to the evening meal. If blood glucose values are not within goal range after one week of therapy, the evening dose is typically increased to 5 mg. Doses can be increased as needed up to 5 mg in the morning and 5 mg in the evening for a total daily dose that does not usually exceed 10 mg/day (Mazze et al., 2007). Insulin therapy is often the next step if successful blood glucose control is not achieved with doses of 10 mg/day, although the maximum daily dose is 20 mg/day. Maternal hypoglycemia is a possible side effect with glyburide, although not as commonly as with insulin. Contraindications to its use include allergy to sulfa drugs and impaired renal function. Concerns have been raised regarding slightly higher rates of NICU admission, macrosomia, and preeclampsia, but in cases of limited resources or needle phobias, glyburide offers an acceptable risk/benefit profile compared to insulin (Malek & Davis, 2016).

Social Determinants

Social determinants such as food insecurity, homelessness, language barriers, and availability of expensive blood glucose testing supplies can affect outcomes of GDM (Goldschmidt & Colletta, 2016; Trout et al., 2016). Golden

(2021) notes that historical perception of who is at risk for diabetes in the United States has changed over time and strongly relates to social constructs. Structural racism has undoubtedly been a contributing factor to social conditions that can predispose individuals to diabetes. Nonetheless, CDC data for 2020 found the lowest rate of GDM in non-Hispanic Blacks (6.5%) and the highest for non-Hispanic Asians (14.9%; Gregory and Ely, 2022). It is important for healthcare providers to understand if any barriers exist to following recommended treatment regimens, and to assist pregnant people in accessing resources for optimal success in managing GDM. Clinical social workers, CDEs, and licensed dieticians are valuable additions to the healthcare team. Enrollment in the Women, Infants, and Children (WIC) program can often provide access to these services, if not available in individual practice settings. Additionally, changes in daily diet can be difficult to make and challenging to sustain regardless of available resources. Weekends often change daily routines and glucose control may worsen. Acknowledging these challenges can improve understanding and adherence to medical nutrition therapy.

Fetal Surveillance and Timing of Birth

There is considerable variation in practice regarding third-trimester fetal surveillance for individuals with GDM who are well controlled with lifestyle interventions. When to initiate testing, what type of testing, and the benefits of testing all lack consensus. People with GDM in good glycemic control are at low risk for an intrauterine fetal death and routine nonstress testing is not advocated (Landon et al., 2021). Recommendations for pregnant people who require insulin or an oral antihyperglycemic agent to maintain euglycemia or those with additional risk factors such as hypertension, obesity, or other comorbidities are the same as for people with pregestational diabetes or other conditions placing the pregnancy at an increased risk of an adverse outcome (ACOG, 2016). Antenatal testing for people at increased risk is initiated in the mid third trimester with biophysical profile testing, nonstress testing, amniotic fluid index (AFI), and/or periodic evaluation of **estimated fetal weight** (EFW; ACOG, 2016; Yehuda et al., 2011).

Macrosomia is a recognized potential problem for the fetus and the pregnant person with GDM. Unfortunately, all the methods to estimate fetal weight are equally flawed, especially for identifying the **LGA** fetus. Fetal growth monitoring and the investigation of macrosomia is unnecessary for people with GDM controlled by lifestyle interventions, mainly because high false positive results may lead to unnecessary cesarean births (Melamed et al., 2011). Fetal weight estimated by ultrasound would have to be ≥4800 g to have at least a 50% chance of predicting an infant being born with a birth weight of 4500 kg or more (McLaren et al., 1995). If macrosomia is suspected clinically, ultrasound close to term may be done to corroborate the experienced examiners' clinical findings, which have been found to be equivalent to ultrasound findings (Melamed et al., 2011).

Labor and Birth

Both maternal and fetal factors affect the timing and type of birth for the individual with GDM. Maternal factors include degree of blood glucose control, condition of the cervix, history of any previous births, and presence or absence of any comorbidities. Fetal factors include EFW, gestational age, and evidence of fetal well-being. As is the case for individuals without GDM, spontaneous labor is the preferred option over induction of labor. There are no indications to induce labor before 40-6/7 weeks of gestation in pregnant persons with good glycemic control who are not on medication for GDM unless other maternal or fetal indications are present (ACOG, 2018). For GDM that is well controlled with medication, labor induction at 40 weeks of gestation can be appropriate (ACOG, 2018).

If maternal and fetal factors indicate that birth should be expedited and there are no contraindications to vaginal birth or cervical ripening or induction agents, induction of labor is a reasonable option to consider. The circumstances under which to offer a scheduled cesarean birth to reduce the risk of birth trauma from potential shoulder dystocia are controversial. The anthropomorphic difference in the infant of a diabetic mother increases abdominal and bisacromial diameter and increases risk for shoulder dystocia. These changes distinguish the LGA infant of a person with diabetes from other LGA infants, thus explaining why induction prior to 40 weeks of gestation or elective cesarean birth may be offered as an option at a lower EFW than in the person without diabetes. One approach is to *offer* elective cesarean birth to people with GDM and an EFW of 4500 g or more (ACOG, 2018), based on the individual's history, discussion about the risks and benefits, and shared decision-making. Estimates of fetal weight by any method can be substantially incorrect. Ultrasonic estimates of fetal abdominal circumference have been most predictive of fetal macrosomia but can vary with sonographer skill, gestational age, and time to birth interval. When counseling people with GDM about suspected fetal macrosomia, the limitations of estimating fetal weight should be included in the discussion. Ultimately, the thoughtful weighing of each individual's maternal and fetal risk profile in conjunction with the pregnant person is required to determine the best intrapartum path.

Interprofessional Care

Prenatal healthcare providers provide holistic, person-centered care to people with GDM. Midwives, nurse practitioners, and physician assistants commonly manage the care of individuals with GDM. For pregnant people with abnormal fasting glucose levels or if <80–90% of postprandial values meet glucose target levels, physician consultation regarding the need for pharmacological therapy should be considered. Collaborative management of patients on oral medications, with transfer to physician medical management if insulin therapy is initiated, can be appropriate.

Care of the Pregnant Person with Pregestational Diabetes

People with preexisting diabetes benefit from an interdisciplinary team approach to care. While there are additional risks and testing for both the pregnant person and fetus, they still have similar needs to all other pregnant people. There is a responsibility to balance the natural and normal aspects of pregnancy and maternal role development with the medical regimen dictated by the diabetic condition. Midwives, nurse practitioners, and physician assistants and other healthcare providers can and should be included in such interdisciplinary healthcare teams to help these patients achieve optimal childbearing experiences and outcomes.

Of particular importance, people with diabetes and childbearing potential should be educated about the need for good glucose control before pregnancy, utilize effective birth control methods when not planning pregnancy, and seek preconception care when planning to become pregnant (ADA, 2017; Kitzmiller et al., 2008; see Chapter 7, *Preconception and Interconception Care*). Only 30% of women with diabetes in one meta-analysis were estimated to access preconception care (Wahabi et al., 2010). Once pregnant, these patients require evaluation for diabetic nephropathy, neuropathy, and retinopathy, as well as cardiovascular disease, hypertension, dyslipidemia, depression, and thyroid disease, in addition to standard pregnancy evaluations. Frequent prenatal visits are important for adjustments in the treatment plan related to stage of pregnancy, glycemic and blood pressure control, weight gain, and the individual person's needs. See Chapter 52, *Endocrine Disorders*, for more management of pregestational diabetes in pregnancy.

Postpartum Follow-Up

Euglycemia and resolution of diabetes occurs almost immediately after the delivery of the placenta in most people with GDM. People who have been diagnosed with GDM should be advised that the diagnosis itself uncovers a greater risk for development of type 2 diabetes later in life, with many developing type 2 diabetes within five years of diagnosis (Bellamy et al., 2009). The diagnosis of GDM indicates a relative insufficiency of insulin secretion when faced with insulin resistance, which increases risk for overt diabetes. Modifiable factors that can decrease the risk of later development of type 2 diabetes should be discussed at the postpartum visit and include topics such as prolonged breastfeeding, regular physical activity, and reaching a normal BMI. The risk for GDM in a subsequent pregnancy can be greatly reduced if an individual returns to prepregnancy weight. If the person was overweight prepregnancy, a 5% weight loss has shown positive metabolic effects. Pregnancy often motivates people to adopt a healthier diet, and building on this desire in the postpartum period can help to support positive lifestyle initiatives begun in pregnancy (ADA, 2017).

A postpartum 75-g 2-hour GTT is used to determine if GDM has not resolved and if overt diabetes has developed. The ADA has changed the recommended time frame for this test to 4–12 weeks postpartum, to expand the number of people who are offered testing and may have results available for review at the postpartum visit (ADA, 2023b), but other groups still recommend testing at 6–12 weeks postpartum (ACOG, 2018; Yehuda, 2016). The diagnostic levels for the 75-g test are not the same as they are during the second and third trimesters of pregnancy, but are the diagnostic levels used for nonpregnant people. The use of glycosylated hemoglobin (A1C) for the diagnosis of persistent diabetes at the postpartum visit is not recommended, as A1C values during pregnancy are not as useful due to the shortened RBC lifespan during pregnancy (Table 37.7). People who have had GDM should be advised to undergo periodic testing for diabetes mellitus (every one to three years; ADA, 2023b).

Postpartum contraception should be discussed to avoid unintended pregnancy before the individual is ready for another baby. Allowing time to achieve a normal BMI for those people with elevated BMIs prepregnancy can help to set the stage for a healthier subsequent pregnancy and may prevent GDM in the future. The postpartum visit is also an opportunity to discuss healthy lifestyle choices to prevent development of type 2 diabetes and to discuss the importance of preconception planning before the next pregnancy (Yehuda, 2016). People who have had GDM should be encouraged to breastfeed, as several studies have shown not only beneficial effects for infants but also maternal metabolic benefits that persist beyond weaning (Ali & Dornhorst, 2011; Ley et al., 2020; Steube, 2015; Ziegler et al., 2012).

People with GDM have a higher rate of postpartum depression than the general postpartum population (Kozhimannil et al., 2009) and should be screened for depression at the postpartum visit. See Chapter 43, *Common Complications during the Postnatal Period*, for information on screening for postpartum depression.

Perspective on GDM Risk

The continuous relation between maternal glycemia and macrosomia-related perinatal risks accounts for much of the controversy in the diagnosis and management of GDM. Without a firm biological threshold for risk, it is difficult to establish a superior set of diagnostic criteria or therapeutic guidelines based on maternal glucose alone. The evidence is not clear regarding the best screening and diagnostic testing for GDM, and evidence is lacking on the utility and optimal methods of fetal surveillance in people with GDM. While GDM is a complication of pregnancy, prenatal care providers need to be mindful of the "most likely" while also being aware of the potential problems. Most people, through healthful eating, physical activity, and self-monitoring, can manage their GDM, maintain euglycemia, and are likely to have a normal pregnancy and birth course. However, the prenatal care provider's mindset on GDM may impact perspective and

Table 37.7 Recommended Time Frame for Postpartum and Beyond Follow-up of GDM

Recommendation	TES	ADA	ACOG
Postpartum testing	Screen with 2-hour, 75-g OGTT at 6–12 weeks postpartum.	Screen using nonpregnant criteria at 4–12 weeks postpartum.	Screen with FPG or 2-hour, 75-g OGTT at 4–12 weeks postpartum.
FBG, random plasma glucose, or A1C	Check periodically and before future pregnancies.	Rescreen every 1–3 years.	Rescreen every 3 years.
Other	Lifestyle counseling to prevent type 2 diabetes after GDM.	Intensive lifestyle intervention and/or metformin to prevent type 2 diabetes.	GDM history to be discussed at all healthcare encounters.

Source: Adapted from: ADA (2023b) and Yehuda (2016).

Quick GDM Summary

By Margaret Semisch McCann, MSN, WHNP-BC

Diabetes in the Context of Pregnancy: Three Entities

1. Pregestational (aka overt) diabetes: diabetes that predates the pregnancy (or diagnosed <15 weeks gestation)
2. Early gestational diabetes: pregnancy-related diabetes diagnosed at 16–24 weeks with normal first trimester or preconception diabetes testing
3. Gestational diabetes: pregnancy-related diabetes diagnosed in the second or third trimester of pregnancy (typically 24–28 weeks)

If early/initial testing is done between 16 and 24 weeks and it is positive for diabetes, it is unknown whether this represents pregestational or early gestational diabetes.

Screening Options

- First trimester/pregestational
  - A1C can be used
- 24–28 weeks
  - 2 step screening protocol:
    - 50 g glucose challenge and screening is complete if normal
    - Followed by fasting, 100-g glucose tolerance if elevated 1 hour
  - 1 step screening protocol:
    - Fasting 75-g glucose tolerance
  - Postpartum:
    - Fasting 75-g glucose tolerance is done at four weeks or greater
    - If it has been several months since birth, an A1C can be done (screen as you would in general populace)

Screening Results Criteria

- A1C
  - Normal: <5.7%
  - Prediabetes: 5.7–6.4%
  - Diabetes: 6.5% or greater
- 1-hour 50-g nonfasting glucose challenge
  - Either 130, 135, or 140 mg/dL can be used as a cutoff depending on individual practice
- 2-hour fasting 75-g gestational OGTT: 1 or more elevated values = GDM

Normal results:

- Fasting: <92
- 1 hour: <180
- 2 hour: <153
- 3-hour fasting 100-g OGTT: 2 or more elevated values = GDM

Normal results (Carpenter & Coustan):

- Fasting: <95
- 1 hour: <180
- 2 hour: <155
- 3 hour: <140

Normal results (NDDG):

- Fasting: <105
- 1 hour: <190
- 2 hour: <165
- 3 hour: <145

Glycemic Control Goals for People with GDM
Normal results:

- Fasting <95
- 1 hour postprandial <140
- 2 hour postprandial <120

People only need to check glucose levels either 1 or 2 hours after meal (not both): that is, QID (4×/day) fingersticks.

---

subsequent care. The "knowledge that a woman has GDM may modify the obstetrical practice and increase the risk of cesarean section in this pregnant patient population" (Gorgal et al., 2012, p. 158). GDM is not an indication in itself for cesarean birth; however, the cesarean rate for people diagnosed with GDM is double that of pregnant people without diabetes (Gorgal et al., 2012). To reduce this iatrogenic bias, people who remain in good glycemic control should be cared for during labor in the same way as any other individual in labor.

Summary

Reassurance is especially important for people with GDM who maintain glycemic control with the lifestyle interventions of healthful eating and increased physical activity. It is appropriate and important to reassure people diagnosed with GDM, especially those individuals with a normal BMI, that if blood glucose levels are within normal limits throughout pregnancy, the pregnancy course is likely to follow a normal path. Confidence in the body's health and strength can positively impact the birth process. An emphasis on optimizing healthful habits that are beneficial throughout the lifecycle can be empowering.

Resources for Clients and Their Families

- Phone app that maps a running route, calculates distance: http://www.mapmyrun.com
- Phone app that maps a walking route, calculates distance: http://www.mapmywalk.com
- Phone app that provides comprehensive nutrition information and tips on healthy eating and exercise: http://www.calorieking.com

Resources for Healthcare Providers

American Diabetes Association (ADA): www.diabetes.org

Centers for Disease Control and Prevention: http://www.cdc.gov/diabetes

National Institute of Diabetes and Digestive and Kidney Diseases, National Institutes of Health: http://www.niddk.nih.gov

National Institute for Health and Care Excellence: http://nice.org.uk

References

Ali, S., & Dornhorst, A. (2011). Diabetes in pregnancy: Health risks and management. *Postgraduate Medical Journal*, 87(1028), 417–427.

American College of Obstetricians and Gynecologists (ACOG). (2016). Fetal macrosomia. Practice bulletin no. 22. *Obstetrics & Gynecology*, 128(5), e195–e209.

American College of Obstetricians and Gynecologists (ACOG). (2018). Gestational diabetes mellitus. Practice bulletin no. 190. *Obstetrics & Gynecology*, 131(2), e49–e64.

American Diabetes Association (ADA). (2014). Standards of medical care in diabetes-2014. *Diabetes Care*, 37(Supplement 1), S14–S80.

American Diabetes Association (ADA). (2017). Classification and diagnosis of diabetes mellitus. *Diabetes Care*, 40(Suppl. 1), S11–S24.

American Diabetes Association (ADA). (2023a). Classification and diagnosis of diabetes: Standards of medical care in diabetes-2023. *Diabetes Care*, 46(Suppl. 1), S19–S40.

American Diabetes Association (ADA). (2023b). 15. Management of diabetes in pregnancy: Standards of medical care in diabetes-2023. *Diabetes Care*, 46(Suppl. 1), S254–S266.

Barbour, L. A., McCurdy, C. E., Hernandez, T. L., Kirwan, J. P., Catalano, P. M., & Friedman, J. E. (2007). Cellular mechanisms for insulin resistance in normal pregnancy and gestational diabetes. *Diabetes Care*, 30(Suppl. 2), S112–S119.

Bellamy, L., Casas, J.-P., Hingorani, A. D., & Williams, D. (2009). Type 2 diabetes mellitus after gestational diabetes: A systematic review and meta-analysis. *Lancet*, 373, 1773–1779.

Biggio, J. R., Chapman, V., Neely, C., Cliver, S. P., & Rouse, D. J. (2010). Fetal anomalies in obese women: The contribution of diabetes. *Obstetrics & Gynecology*, 115(2 Pt 1), 290–296.

Birnson, S. E., Rosenn, B. M., Morris, S. A., Sasso, E. B., Schwartz, R. A., & Brustman, L. E. (2017). Current trends in the diagnosis and management of gestational diabetes mellitus in the United States. *Journal of Maternal-Fetal and Neonatal Medicine*, 30(21), 2607–2612.

Bodmer-Roy, S., Morin, L., Cousinea, J., & Re, E. (2012). Pregnancy outcomes in women with and without gestational diabetes mellitus according to the international association of the diabetes and pregnancy study groups criteria. *Obstetrics & Gynecology*, 120(4), 746–752.

Brankston, G. N., Mitchell, B. F., Ryan, E. A., & Okun, N. B. (2004). Resistance exercise decreases the need for insulin in overweight women with gestational diabetes mellitus. *American Journal of Obstetrics & Gynecology*, 190, 188–193.

Butalia, S., Gutierrez, L., Lodha, A., Aitken, E., Zakariasen, A., & Donovan, L. (2017). Short-and long-term outcomes of metformin compared with insulin alone in pregnancy: A systematic review and meta-analysis. *Diabetic Medicine*, 34(1), 27–36.

Chen, Y., Block-Kurbisch, I., & Caughy, A. (2009). Carpenter-Coustan criteria compared with the National Diabetes Data Group thresholds for gestational diabetes mellitus. *Obstetrics & Gynecology*, 114(2), 326–334.

Eli Lilly and Company. (2020). *BAQSIMI: Highlights of prescribing information.* https://www.accessdata.fda.gov/drugsatfda_docs/label/2019/210134s000lbl.pdf

Farrar, D., Simmonds, M., Bryant, M., Sheldon, T. A., Tuffnell, D., Golder, S., & Lawlor, D. A. (2017). Treatments for gestational diabetes: A systematic review and meta-analysis. *BMJ Open*, 7(6), e015557.

Fieg, D. S., Donavan, L. E., Corcoy, R., Murphy, K. E., Amiel, S. A., Hunt, K. F., Asztalos, E., Barrett, J. F. R., Sanchez, J. J., de Leiva, A., Hod, M., Jovanovic, L., Keely, E., McManus, R., Hutton, E. K., Meek, C. L., Stewart, Z. A., Wysocki, T., O'Brien, R., . . . CONCEPTT Collaborative Group. (2017). Continuous glucose monitoring in pregnant women with type 1 diabetes (CONCEPTT): A multicenter international randomized controlled trial. *Lancet*, 10110(390), 2317–2359.

Golden, S. H., Joseph, J. J., & Hill-Briggs, F. (2021). Casting a health equity lens on endocrinology and diabetes. *The Journal of Clinical Endocrinology & Metabolism*, 106(4), e1908–e1916.

Goldschmidt, V. J., & Colletta, B. (2016). The challenges of providing diabetes education in resource-limited settings to women with diabetes in pregnancy: Perspectives of an educator. *Diabetes Spectrum*, 29(2), 101–104.

Gorgal, R., Gonsalves, E., Barros, M., Namora, G., Magalhaes, A., Rodrigues, T., & Montenegro, N. (2012). Gestational diabetes mellitus: A risk factor for non-elective cesarean section. *Journal of Obstetrics & Gynaecology Research*, 38, 154–159.

Gregory, C. W., & Ely, D. M. (2022). Trends and characteristics in gestational diabetes: United States, 2016–2020. *National Vital Statistics Reports*, 71(3). National Center for Health Statistics. https://doi.org/10.15620/cdc:118018

Halse, R. E., Wallman, K. E., Newnham, J. P., & Guelfi, K. J. (2014). Home-based exercise training improves capillary glucose profile in women with gestational diabetes. *Medicine and Science in Sports and Exercise*, 46(9), 1702–1709.

HAPO Study Cooperative Research Group, Metzger, B. E., Lowe, L. P., Dyer, A. R., Trimble, E. R., Chaovarindr, U., Coustan, D. R., Hadden, D. R., McCance, D. R., Hod, M., McIntyre, H. D., Oats, J. J., Persson, B., Rogers, M. S., & Sacks, D. A. (2008). Hyperglycemia and adverse pregnancy outcomes. *The New England Journal of Medicine*, 358(19), 1991–2002.

Henze, M., Burbidge, H., Nathan, E., & Graham, D. F. (2022). The effect of bedtime snacks on fasting blood glucose levels in gestational diabetes mellitus. *Diabetic Medicine*, 39, e14718.

Hughes, R. C., Moore, M. P., Gullam, J. E., Mohamed, K., & Rowan, J. (2014). An early pregnancy HbA1c ≥5.9% (41 mmol/mol) is optimal for detecting diabetes and identifies women at increased risk of adverse pregnancy outcomes. *Diabetes Care*, 37(11), 2953–2959.

International Association of Diabetes in Pregnancy Study Groups (IADPSG). (2010). International association of diabetes and pregnancy study groups recommendations on the diagnosis and classification of hyperglycemia in pregnancy. *Diabetes Care, 33*(3), 676–682.

Kirwan, J. P., Haugel-DeMouzon, S., Lepercq, J., Challier, J.-C., Huston-Presley, L., Friedman, J. E., Kalhan, S. C., & Catalano, P. M. (2002). TNF-a is a predictor of insulin resistance in human pregnancy. *Diabetes, 51*, 2207–2213.

Kitzmiller, J. L., Block, J. M., Brown, F. M., Catalano, P. M., Conway, D. L., Coustan, D. R., & Jovanovic, L. B. (2008). Managing preexisting diabetes for pregnancy. *Diabetes Care, 31*(5), 1060–1079.

Kozhimannil, K. B., Pereira, M. A., & Harlow, B. L. (2009). Association between diabetes and perinatal depression among low-income mothers. *JAMA: The Journal of the American Medical Association, 301*(8), 842.

Landon, M. B., Catalano, P. M., & Gabbe, S. G. (2021). Diabetes mellitus complicating pregnancy. In M. B. Landon, H. L. Galan, E. R. M. Jauniaux, D. A. Driscoll, V. Berghella, & W. A. Grobman (Eds.), *Gabbe's obstetrics: Normal & problem pregnancies* (8th ed., pp. 871–907). Elsevier.

Langer, O., Umans, J., & Miodovnik, M. (2013). Perspectives on the proposed gestational diabetes mellitus diagnostic criteria. *Obstetrics and Gynecology, 121*(1), 177–182.

Laredo-Aguilera, J. A., Gallardo-Bravo, M., Rabanales-Sotos, J. A., Cobo-Cuenca, A. I., & Carmona-Torres, J. M. (2020). Physical activity programs during pregnancy are effective for the control of gestational diabetes mellitus. *International Journal of Environmental Research and Public Health., 17*(17), 6151.

Ley, S. H., Chavarro, J. E., Li, M., Bao, W., Hinkle, S. N., Wander, P. L., Rich-Edwards, J., Olsen, S., Vaag, A., Damm, P., Grunnet, L. G., Mills, J. L., Hu, F. B., & Zhang, C. (2020). Lactation duration and long-term risk for incident type 2 diabetes in women with a history of gestational diabetes mellitus. *Diabetes Care, 43*, 793–798.

Malek, R., & Davis, S. N. (2016). Pharmacokinetics, efficacy and safety of glyburide for treatment of gestational diabetes mellitus. *Expert Opinion on Drug Metabolism & Toxicology, 12*(6), 691–699.

Mazze, R. S., Strock, E., Simonson, G. D., & Bergenstal, R. M. (2007). *Prevention, detection and treatment of diabetes in adults* (4th ed.). International Diabetes Center, Park Nicollet Institute.

McLaren, R. A., Puckett, J. L., & Chauhan, S. P. (1995). Estimators of birth weight in pregnant women requiring insulin: A comparison of seven sonographic models. *Obstetrics & Gynecology, 85*, 565–569.

Melamed, N., Yogev, Y., Meizner, I., Mashiach, R., Pardo, J., & Ben-Haroush, A. (2011). Prediction of fetal macrosomia: Effect of sonographic fetal weight-estimation model and threshold used. *Ultrasound in Obstetrics & Gynecology, 38*(1), 74–81.

Melczer, Z., Banhidy, F., Csomor, S., Kovacs, M., Winkler, G., & Cseh, K. (2003). Influence of leptin and the TNF system on insulin resistance in pregnancy and their effect on anthropomorphic parameters of newborns. *Acta Obstetricia et Gynecologica Scandinavica, 82*(5), 432–438.

Metzger, B. E. (2007). Long-term outcomes in mothers diagnosed with gestational diabetes mellitus and their offspring. *Clinical Obstetrics and Gynecology, 50*(4), 972–979.

Metzger, B. E., Buchanan, T. A., Coustan, D. R., De Leiva, A., Dunger, D. B., Hadden, D. R., Hod, M., Kitzmiller, J. L., Kjos, S. L., Oats, J. N., Pettitt, D. J., Sacks, D. A., & Zoupas, C. (2007). Summary and recommendations of the fifth international workshop-conference on gestational diabetes mellitus. *Diabetes Care, 30*(Supplement 2), S251–S260.

Moore, L. E., Clokey, D., Rappaport, V. J., & Curet, L. B. (2010). Metformin compared with glyburide in gestational diabetes: A randomized controlled trial. *Obstetrics & Gynecology, 115*(1), 55–59.

Moore, T. R., & Catalano, P. (2009). Diabetes in pregnancy. In R. K. Creasy, R. Resnick, J. D. Iams, C. J. Lockwood, & T. R. Moore (Eds.), *Creasy & Resnick's maternal-fetal medicine: Principles and practice* (pp. 953–994). Saunders.

Picón-Cèsar, M. J., Molina-Vega, M., Suárez-Arana, M., Gonzàlez-Mesa, E., Sola-Moyano, A. P., Roldan-López, R., Romero-Narbona, F., Olveira, G., Tinahones, F. J., & Gonzàlez-Romero, S. (2021). Metformin for gestational diabetes study: Metformin vs insulin in gestational diabetes: Glycemic control and obstetrical and perinatal outcomes: Randomized prospective trial. *American Journal of Obstetrics & Gynecology, 225*(517), e1–e17.

Retnakaran, R., Qi, Y., Sermer, M., Connelly, P. W., Hanley, A. J. G., & Zinman, B. (2010). B-Cell function declines within the first year postpartum in women with recent glucose intolerance in pregnancy. *Diabetes Care, 33*(8), 1798–1802.

Rickels, M. R., Ruedy, K. J., Foster, N. C., & T1D Exchange Intranasal Glucagon Investigators. (2016). Intranasal glucagon for treatment of insulin-induced hypoglycemia in adults with type 1 diabetes: A randomized crossover noninferiority study. *Diabetes Care, 39*, 264–270.

Ryu, R. J., Hays, K. E., & Hebert, M. F. (2014, December). Gestational diabetes mellitus management with oral hypoglycemic agents. *Seminars in Perinatology, 38*(8), 508–515.

Schafer-Graf, U. M., Graf, K., Kulbacka, I., Kjos, S. L., Dudenhausen, J., Vetter, K., & Herrara, E. (2008). Maternal lipids as strong determinants of fetal environment and growth in pregnancies with gestational diabetes mellitus. *Diabetes Care, 31*(9), 1858–1863.

Society for Maternal-Fetal Medicine Publications Committee. (2018). *SMFM Statement: Pharmacological treatment of gestational diabetes.* https://www.smfm.org/publications/252-smfm-statement-pharmacological-treatment-of-gestational-diabetes

Steube, A. M. (2015). Does breastfeeding prevent the metabolic syndrome or does the metabolic syndrome prevent breastfeeding? *Seminars in Perinatology, 39*(4), 290–295.

Trout, K. K., Compher, C. W., Dolin, C., Burns, C., Quinn, R., & Durnwald, C. (2022). Increased protein with decreased carbohydrate intake reduces postprandial blood glucose levels in women with gestational diabetes: The iPRO study. *Women's Health Report, 3*(1), 728–739. https://doi.org/10.1089/whr.2022.0012

Trout, K. K., & Dolin, C. (2021). Diabetes in pregnancy. In D. Mattison & L.-A. Halbert (Eds.), *Clinical pharmacology during pregnancy* (2nd ed., pp. 251–269). Elsevier.

Trout, K. K., Homko, C. J., Wetzel-Effinger, L., Mulla, W., Mora, R., McGrath, J., Basel-Brown, L., Arcamone, A., Sami, P., & Makambi, K. (2016). Macronutrient composition or social determinants? Impact on infant outcomes with gestational diabetes mellitus. *Diabetes Spectrum, 29*(2), 71–78.

US Preventive Services Task Force (USPSTF). (2021). Screening for gestational diabetes. US preventive services task force recommendation statement. *JAMA, 326*(6), 531–538.

Wahabi, H. A., Alzeidan, R. A., Bawazeer, G. A., Alansari, L. A., & Esmaeil, S. A. (2010). Preconception care for diabetic women for improving maternal and fetal outcomes: A systematic review and meta-analysis. *BMC Pregnancy and Childbirth, 10*(1), 63.

Yehuda, I. (2016). Implementation of preconception care for women with diabetes. *Diabetes Spectrum, 29*(2), 105–114.

Yehuda, I., Nagtalon-Ramos, J., & Trout, K. (2011). Fetal growth scans and amniotic fluid assessments in pregestational and gestational diabetes. *Journal of Obstetric, Gynecologic & Neonatal Nurses, 40*, 603–616.

Zeng, Y. C., Li, M. J., Chen, Y., Jiang, L., Wang, S. M., Mo, X. L., & Li, B. Y. (2014). The use of glyburide in the management of gestational diabetes mellitus: A meta-analysis. *Advances in Medical Sciences, 59*(1), 95–101.

Zhu, M., Cai, J., Liu, S., Huang, M., Chen, Y., Lai, X., Chen, Y., Zhao, Z., Wu, F., Wu, D., Miu, H., Lai, S., & Chen, G. (2014). Relationship between gestational fasting plasma glucose and neonatal birth weight, prenatal blood pressure and dystocia in pregnant Chinese women. *Diabetes/Metabolism Research and Reviews, 30*(6), 489–496.

Ziegler, A.-G., Wallner, M., Kaiser, I., Rossbauer, M., & Hummel, S. (2012). Long-term protective effect of lactation on the development of type 2 diabetes in women with recent gestational diabetes mellitus. *Diabetes, 61*(12), 3167–3171.

38

Multifetal Gestation

Heather M. Bradford

Relevant Terms

Amnion—the innermost membrane of the amniotic sac
Amnionicity—the number of amnions that surround the fetuses in a multifetal gestation
Chorion—the outermost membrane of the amniotic sac, contributes to the development of the placenta
Chorionicity—the number of chorions that surround the fetuses in a multifetal gestation
Dizygotic gestation—twins resulting from the fertilization of two separate eggs
Monozygotic gestation—twins resulting from the division of a single zygote produced from the fertilization of a single egg
Polyzygotic gestation—multiple gestation resulting in three or more fetuses produced by any combination of monozygotic and polyzygotic twinning
Selective reduction—the procedure of reducing the number of fetuses via selective abortion in a multifetal pregnancy, usually from three or more fetuses to two
Twin-to-twin transfusion syndrome—syndrome in which the blood of one twin is transfused to the second twin; associated with fetal anemia and discordant growth
Zygote—the cell produced by the union of two gametes before it undergoes division; a fertilized ovum
Zygosity—a description of whether two alleles have identical DNA sequence or different DNA sequences

Introduction

Multifetal gestation occurs when the uterus nurtures more than one fetus and requires additional prenatal assessment and monitoring. There are two main contributing factors to the overall higher incidence of multifetal gestations in the last four decades—the trend toward an older age at conception, when multifetal gestations are more likely to naturally occur, and the expanded use of assisted reproductive technology (ART), including ovulation-inducing drugs and *in vitro* fertilization (IVF; American College of Obstetricians and Gynecologists [ACOG], 2021a). With the increase in use of ultrasound scans in the first trimester, multifetal pregnancies are more likely to be detected early, allowing for determination of chorionicity and screening for fetal complications. Although people with twin pregnancies deliver on average at approximately 35.1 weeks of gestation, the recommendation for timing and route of delivery depends on the amnionicity and chorionicity of the pregnancy.

Health equity key points

- There is a greater risk of preterm birth among Black people carrying twin pregnancies when compared to White people, due to racism, delayed or limited access to prenatal care, and comorbidities such as diabetes, hypertension, and preeclampsia.
- Even with equal access to care, pregnant people of color carrying twin pregnancies have an increased risk of adverse perinatal outcomes, also due to racism.

Incidence

Approximately 3% of all pregnancies are multifetal, with the majority being twin pregnancies. The incidence of multifetal gestations dramatically increased over several decades beginning in the 1980s. However, the 2020 twin birth rate (births in twin deliveries per 1000 total births) was 31.1, down 8% from the 2014 high of 33.9 (Osterman et al., 2022). The 2020 twin birth rate is the lowest in almost two decades (Hamilton et al., 2015). This is most likely due to the higher rates of IVF single-embryo transfers and delay in access to sexual and reproductive healthcare due to the COVID-19 pandemic (Kavanaugh et al., 2022; US Dept of Health and Human Services, 2021). There has also been a steady decline in the triple and higher-order multiple birthrate; the rate was 79.6 per 100,000 births in 2020, down 59% compared to the 1998 peak of 193.5 per 100,000 births (Osterman et al., 2022). Even so, for the estimated 13% of reproductive-age individuals in the United States who pursue infertility treatment, the chance of a multiple pregnancy is vastly increased (US Dept of Health and Human Services, 2021).

Prenatal and Postnatal Care: A Person-Centered Approach, Third Edition. Edited by Karen Trister Grace, Cindy L. Farley, Noelene K. Jeffers, and Tanya Tringali.
© 2024 John Wiley & Sons Ltd. Published 2024 by John Wiley & Sons Ltd.
Companion website: www.wiley.com/go/grace/prenatal

Embryology

Multifetal pregnancies can be categorized by the number of ova fertilized at conception and the timing of cleavage of the embryo. **Monozygotic gestation** occurs when one egg is fertilized by one sperm and there is subsequent division of this single **zygote** into two (or more) zygotes. If it results in two zygotes, the fetuses are termed *identical twins*, with each carrying the same genetic material. The frequency of single-ovum twinning is independent of heredity, race, age, and parity.

The timing of the division of the single zygote in monozygotic twinning may result in any of three combinations, depending on whether there is one or two **amnions** (amniotic sacs) and one or two **chorions** (Figure 38.1). The **amnionicity** and **chorionicity** may be either monochorionic and monoamniotic, monochorionic and diamniotic, or dichorionic and diamniotic. Part of the chorion proliferates to form the placenta, so chorionicity determines placentation (shared or separate placentas). If the division of a zygote occurs within three days of conception, when the original zygote has not yet implanted in the uterine wall, these identical twins will have two separate placentas, two chorions, and two amnions, resulting a monozygotic, diamniotic, dichorionic (di/di) twin pregnancy. If the extra division of the zygote occurs between three and seven to eight days after conception, the identical fetuses will share a placenta but have separate amnions, resulting in a monozygotic, diamniotic, monochorionic (di/mono) twin pregnancy. If the split occurs after the eighth day following conception, the identical

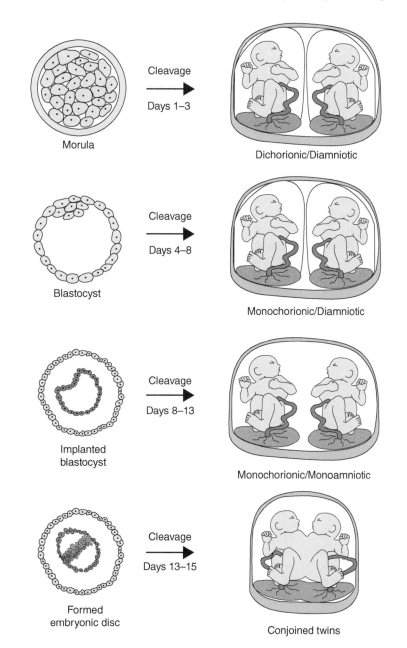

Figure 38.1 Types of amnionicity and chorionicity in multifetal gestation. Kevin Dufendach/Wikimedia Commons/CC BY 3.0.

fetuses will share the same placenta, chorion, and amnion, resulting in a monozygous, monoamniotic, monochorionic (mono/mono) twin pregnancy (Luke et al., 2017). In 99% of cases of monozygous twins, there are one chorion, one placenta, and two amniotic sacs (Posner et al., 2013). Approximately one-third of all twin pairs are monozygotic or identical (Luke et al., 2017).

Dizygotic gestation occurs when two eggs are released and fertilized by different sperm, resulting in dichorionic, diamniotic (di/di) twins. In this case, each twin has their own placenta, chorion, and amniotic sac, and the placenta may be fused or in separate locations, depending on the site of implantation. Dizygotic twins are commonly referred to as "fraternal twins" and account for two-thirds of all twins; they occur in about 1 out of every 80 pregnancies (Luke et al., 2017). These two children share similar features only to the extent that siblings of the same age would. The incidence of this occurring spontaneously is influenced by heredity, race, age, parity, and especially fertility treatment ("Multifetal Pregnancy," 2018).

Polyzygotic gestation is a result from any combination of dizygotic and monozygotic twinning and is most common with ART. While data are limited on **zygosity** among higher-order multiples, it is believed that only 6% of triplet sets are identical (Luke et al., 2017).

Conjoined twins result from the incomplete cleavage of the embryonic disc after day 13. The anatomic variations and prognosis for the pregnancy and the conjoined fetuses depend on whether there is symmetric duplication of anatomic structures and at what part of the body the structures are conjoined.

A unique condition in multifetal pregnancies is the death and resorption of one twin, known commonly as "vanishing twin syndrome." It is thought as many as 10–15% of singleton births began as a twin pregnancy. This may not be recognized, as an early first-trimester loss of one twin can present as a small amount of bleeding and cramping that resolves on its own. If one fetus dies during the second trimester, a *fetus papyraceus* can result from compression and resorption of the fetal tissue, leading to a paper-thin, mummified outline of the fetus found on the fetal surface of the placenta.

Diagnosis

One of the earliest cues that a pregnant individual is carrying more than a singleton pregnancy is a report of excessive nausea and vomiting, most likely due to the larger placental mass and higher production of human chorionic gonadotropin (HCG). Other symptoms might include extreme fatigue, an increased appetite, and rapid weight gain early in pregnancy. The uterus will measure larger than expected, and this size difference is typically evident by 14 weeks of gestation (Luke et al., 2017). However, due to trends in first-trimester ultrasound dating, ultrasound is often the initial method of diagnosing a multifetal pregnancy. Chorionicity should be determined by ultrasound at the first prenatal visit or before 14 weeks of gestation, when possible, to guide the care of the pregnant person (ACOG, 2021a).

Risks to the Pregnant Individual

Physiologic adaptations to pregnancy are heightened in a multifetal pregnancy, leading to increased risk for most pregnancy-related complications, with the exceptions of macrosomia and postterm pregnancy (Table 38.1). The risk increases proportionally with higher plurality (Newman & Unal, 2017). The mass and weight of a 25-week-gestation uterus in a multifetal pregnancy is equivalent to that of a term pregnancy. The simple mechanics of this physical increase can lead to several complications. Not only are risks for complications increased but also the conditions can present in a more severe fashion and severity can increase with higher-order multiples. Perinatal mortality is increased but remains a rare event; however, multifetal pregnancy is an independent risk factor for intensive care unit (ICU) admission of the pregnant person (Newman & Unal, 2017).

Risks to the Fetuses/Neonates and Antepartum Management

In general, all multifetal pregnancies are at increased risk for higher neonatal morbidity and mortality (Table 38.2).

Table 38.1 Risks of Multifetal Pregnancy to the Pregnant Individual

- Acute fatty liver
- Anemia
- Antepartum hemorrhage
- Cesarean birth
- Dysfunctional labor
- Early pregnancy loss of one or more fetuses
- Gestational diabetes
- Hyperemesis gravidarum
- Hypertensive disorders
- Malpresentation
- Perinatal mood disorders
- Placenta previa
- Postpartum hemorrhage
- Preeclampsia
- Pruritic urticarial papules and pustules of pregnancy (PUPPS)
- Pulmonary embolism
- Stillbirth of one or more fetuses

Table 38.2 Risks of Multifetal Pregnancy for the Fetuses/Neonates

- Anemia/polycythemia
- Aneuploidies
- Cerebral palsy
- Congenital anomalies
- Cord accidents
- Discordant fetal growth
- Fetal growth restriction
- Intrauterine demise of one or more fetuses
- Intraventricular hemorrhage
- Neonatal death
- Premature labor and birth
- Respiratory distress syndrome
- Twin-to-twin transfusion syndrome (TTTS)

The level of risk for the fetuses in a multifetal pregnancy is determined by the chorionicity. Twins that share amnions and/or chorions are at higher risk for complications (ACOG, 2021a, 2021b). Monochorionic twins are at risk for congenital anomalies, **twin-to-twin transfusion syndrome** (TTTS), and discordant growth (ACOG, 2021a). TTTS is a result of anastomoses of blood vessels on the shared placenta, compromising the blood flow to one twin, causing poor growth, while favoring the other twin. Without treatment with fetal surgery, TTTS can cause fetal death for one or both fetuses. Approximately 10–15% of monochorionic-diamniotic twins have TTTS (ACOG, 2021a).

Preterm birth (PTB) and fetal growth restriction are the major reasons for higher neonatal morbidity and mortality in multifetal gestation, with risks increasing with plurality (ACOG, 2021a). In 2020, 60% of twins were born prior to 37 weeks of gestation (Osterman et al., 2022). Because of the complications of prematurity in multifetal gestations, there is an approximate fivefold increased risk of stillbirth and a sevenfold increased risk of neonatal death as compared to singleton pregnancies. There are also disproportionate rates of PTB in twin pregnancies among varying racial/ethnic groups. Dongarwar et al. (2021) reported a five times greater risk of PTB among Black women carrying twin pregnancies when compared to white women. Multiple theories have been proposed for this disparity, including racism and comorbidities such as diabetes, hypertension, preeclampsia, and lower quality or delayed prenatal care (Dongarwar et al., 2021; Soffer et al., 2018).

The average gestational age for a twin pregnancy is 35.1 weeks (Centers for Disease Control and Prevention, 2021). Many of the decisions made in caring for individuals with multifetal pregnancy are aimed at predicting those at an increased risk for PTB and then acting to decrease that risk. However, despite extensive research, no interventions have been shown to be effective in preventing PTB in asymptomatic individuals with multifetal pregnancies. Ineffective interventions to predict or prevent PTB in asymptomatic pregnant individuals with multifetal pregnancies include: routine transvaginal ultrasonographic cervical length, digital examination, fetal fibronectin screening, home uterine monitoring, cerclage and pessary, routine hospitalization and bed rest, tocolytics, and progesterone treatment (both 17a-hydroxyprogesterone caproate and vaginal progesterone; ACOG, 2021c). Hospitalization for bed rest in asymptomatic pregnant individuals can lead to muscle atrophy and weakness, depression, decreased weight gain, and fatigue. Prolonged hospitalization has the additional stressor of separating family members and increasing anxiety in the pregnant person.

Several interventions have been found to be effective for pregnant individuals in acute preterm labor, including tocolytics, antenatal corticosteroids, and magnesium sulfate for fetal neuroprotection. A brief course of tocolysis for up to 48 hours for those in acute preterm labor may allow corticosteroids to be administered. A risk factor for the pregnant person with use of tocolytics is pulmonary edema. Although a 2020 Cochrane Review recommends further research on benefits of antenatal corticosteroids in multifetal pregnancies, current ACOG guidelines recommend the administration of antenatal corticosteroids for pregnant individuals with multifetal pregnancies between 24 and 34 weeks at risk of giving birth within 7 days (ACOG, 2021a; McGoldrick et al., 2020). Use of corticosteroids speeds fetal lung maturity and reduces the risks of neonatal death, respiratory distress syndrome, intraventricular hemorrhage, and necrotizing enterocolitis (McGoldrick et al., 2020). Depending on the embryology and gestational age (ranging from 32 to 38 6/7 weeks), as well as the presence of fetal growth restriction, the ACOG recommends a single course of betamethasone for those at risk of PTB within 7 days, assuming no prior course of antenatal corticosteroids (ACOG, 2021a). Administration of magnesium sulfate is also recommended regardless of fetal number when birth is anticipated prior to 32 weeks of gestation to reduce the risk of cerebral palsy in the infant (ACOG, 2021a).

Prenatal Care

Nutritional Counseling

Nutritional counseling is of paramount importance for pregnant individuals with multifetal gestation. Most of the complications associated with multifetal gestation have not responded to technological or pharmaceutical treatments. Optimal nutrition holds the promise of preventing or ameliorating a number of complications. A multifetal pregnancy uses nutrients at a higher metabolic rate, making a nourishing diet with vitamin and mineral supplements important for the health of the pregnant person and their fetuses. Adequate weight gain is associated with improved fetal growth, longer gestations, higher birth weight, as well as improved childhood development (Lipworth et al., 2021). Basal metabolic rate is higher in those with multifetal gestation, requiring higher caloric intake. They also experience an increase in plasma volume higher than those with singletons, causing further dilutional decreases in hemoglobin, albumin, and water-soluble vitamins (Kominarek & Rajan, 2016). There are no standard nutritional guidelines for individuals with multiple gestations; however, current recommendations are inferred from singleton data. In general, 3500 calories daily are recommended, composed of a diet with 175-g protein, 350 g of low-glycemic-index carbohydrate, and 156 g of fat per day for those with a normal prepregnancy body mass index (BMI), and apportioned accordingly for other BMI categories. It is recommended that intake be spread out over three meals and three snacks daily (Luke, 2015; Table 38.3).

The pattern of weight gain is also important (Table 38.4). It can be challenging for some to eat the amount of food needed for a healthy multifetal pregnancy, especially in the first trimester with increased nausea and vomiting and in the third trimester, when the fetuses compress the stomach. Early weight gain is especially important and should be a focus of prenatal nutrition counseling for

Table 38.3   Daily Nutrient Recommendations in Multifetal Gestation

Nutrient	Daily amount	Suggestions for source
Calories	3500 kcal	Over 3 meals and 3 snacks
Macronutrients		
Carbohydrates	350 g	Low-glycemic-index carbs
Fat	156 g	Some seafood, avocados, eggs, cheese
Protein	175 g	Animal sources recommended
Micronutrients		
Calcium	3 g	Dairy, calcium-supplemented soy milk
Folic acid	1 mg	Dark green veggies (e.g., spinach, broccoli), black-eyed peas, kidney beans, lentils
Iodine	150 ug	Some seafood, dairy, iodine-enriched breads, iodized salt
Iron	30 mg	Heme iron sources recommended (e.g., lean meats, poultry, some seafood), dark green veggies (e.g., spinach, Swiss chard), soybeans, lima beans
Magnesium	1.2 g	Nuts, legumes, fiber-rich whole grains, dairy
Omega 3 fatty acids	1000 mg	Some fish, green leafy vegetables, soybeans, wheat germ, walnuts, seeds, fish oil supplements
Vitamin D	1000 IU	Daily sunshine
Zinc	45 mg	Red meat, shellfish, legumes, some seeds

Source: Adapted from Luke (2015).

Table 38.4   Recommended Weight Gain Pattern in Twin Pregnancy by Prepregnant BMI

Gestational Period	Underweight BMI ≤ 18.5	Normal Weight BMI = 18.5–24.9	Overweight BMI = 25–29.9	Obese BMI = ≥30
<20 weeks	1.25–1.75 lb/wk	1–1.5 lb/wk	1–1.25 lb/wk	0.75–1 lb/wk
20–28 weeks	1.5–1.75 lb/wk	1.25–1.75 lb/wk	1–1.5 lb/wk	0.75–1.25 lb/wk
>29 weeks	1.25 lb/wk	1 lb/wk	1 lb/wk	0.75 lb/wk
Total (lb), assuming pregnancy duration of 37–42 weeks	*No recommendation made*	*37–54*	*31–50*	*25–42*

Source: Adapted from Institute of Medicine (2009) and Luke et al. (2017).

those with multifetal gestation. Gaining 24 pounds by 24 weeks of gestation is associated with improved fetal birth weight. Inadequate weight gain by 16–28 weeks of gestation is a strong predictor of PTB (Fox et al., 2014; Pettit et al., 2015). This offers an opportunity to promote optimal health for the pregnant person and their babies.

It is important to encourage the selection of low-glycemic-index foods whenever possible to prevent wide fluctuations in blood glucose levels and combat insulin resistance that occurs normally during pregnancy. Lower glucose levels and an exaggerated insulin response after meals are both part of normal pregnancy physiology. Pregnant individuals with multifetal gestation experience these changes to a greater degree, especially after 20 weeks of gestation (Luke, 2015). Maternal factors that influenced fetal growth in the lowest 10% of fetuses measured at 28 weeks of gestation included smoking during pregnancy, fetal reduction or fetal loss, height less than 62 inches, and low weight gain during the first half of pregnancy (Luke et al., 2017).

Additional dietary supplementation is often needed to meet increased fetal demands for micronutrient requirements, including folate (1 mg), calcium (3 g), magnesium (1.2 g), and zinc (45 mg) beyond a usual prenatal vitamin (Luke, 2015). Routine supplementation of approximately 30-mg elemental iron daily is also advised (Goodnight & Newman, 2009). Rates of iron deficiency anemia and anemia due to folate deficiency are higher in those with twins than with singleton pregnancies (Ru et al., 2016). Anemia in the first two-thirds of pregnancy is associated with a higher rate of PTB (Stanley et al., 2022).

Supplementation with omega-3 fatty acids is beneficial for fetal neurological development in twin gestation, although eating fish or other DHA-rich foods is the optimal way to obtain omega-3 fatty acids (Table 38.3). While there are no consensus recommendations, omega-3 fatty acid intake of 1000 mg daily has been suggested to accommodate increased needs in twin gestation (Luke et al., 2017).

Genetic Screening

Pregnant persons with multifetal gestations are able to screen for fetal chromosomal abnormalities. However, genetic screening tests and procedures are complex in twin and higher-order pregnancies, as the testing is less accurate. Rates of aneuploidy are increased, largely due to the association of advanced age with multifetal pregnancy. Determination of chorionicity is an important factor in determining risk of anomalies. Monochorionic twins have an increased rate of structural abnormalities, including cardiac defects, neural tube and brain defects, facial clefts, and gastrointestinal and anterior abdominal wall defects, but the risk of aneuploidy appears similar to the risk in singleton pregnancies (Audibert & Gagnon, 2017). All standard noninvasive options are reasonable to offer when calculations specific to multifetal pregnancy are able to be determined by the processing lab. Options for genetic screening include serum studies with or without ultrasound imaging and cell-free DNA testing. In a 2019 meta-analysis (n = 7 studies) of cell-free DNA testing in twin pregnancies, the detection rate for trisomy 21 was similar to singleton pregnancies (Gil et al., 2019). Nondirective counseling is important when offering invasive testing, such as chorionic villus sampling and amniocentesis, as procedures are complicated, require at least two punctures, and carry a higher risk of loss when compared to singleton pregnancies (ACOG, 2021a). Discordant results with one affected fetus and one unaffected fetus can lead to difficult decisions for the pregnant person and their family.

Anticipatory Guidance

Pregnant individuals with a multifetal pregnancy should be counseled that they will likely have an increase in the common discomforts of pregnancy due to an even greater increase in hormonal fluctuations, circulating blood volume, fetal mass, and weight gain. The increased size of the uterus may result in increased intra-abdominal pressure and difficulty in ambulation. Pregnant individuals with a multifetal gestation will also be seen more frequently for prenatal care visits and often give birth prior to term. As the pregnancy progresses and the family is preparing for the birth of the babies, special consideration should be given to identify support and resources for additional help at home. Antepartum lactation consultation can also improve the rate of postpartum breastfeeding in twin pregnancies. The demands of more than one newborn can cause increased stress and fatigue. Support for breastfeeding multiples can be sought through local agencies like Healthy Start, La Leche League, postpartum doulas, and lactation support counselors.

Fetal Growth Assessment and Surveillance

Depending on the chorionicity and amnionicity, fetal echocardiograms, anatomy surveys, and serial growth ultrasounds are recommended every two to four weeks (Behrendt & Galan, 2021). One of the most concerning findings when monitoring a multiple gestation is discordant growth. In this situation, the fetuses do not grow at comparable rates. This may occur for many reasons, including TTTS, placental problems, fetal malformation, infection, or umbilical cord differences. A difference of 20% or greater in the estimated fetal weight (as determined by ultrasound) is considered discordance (ACOG, 2021a). A multiple pregnancy complicated by this condition should be evaluated and managed by a perinatal specialist.

Birth Planning

Vaginal birth can be safely recommended for select low-risk pregnant individuals carrying twins and should be discussed prenatally (Reitter et al., 2018). Variables influencing this decision include type of twins (chorionicity), client preference, positions of twins, particularly twin A, estimated fetal weight and gestational age, provider skills, and facility resources. The most common presentation of twins at labor onset is vertex–vertex, followed by vertex–breech; these positions are favorable to vaginal birth. In fact, the opportunity to labor and give birth vaginally is appropriate for all vertex–vertex presentations, regardless of fetal weight or gestation (Barrett, 2014). When vaginal birth is attempted, it is successful in about 77% of cases (Posner et al., 2013). Factors associated with successful vaginal birth of twins are multiparity, age < 30, cephalic presentation of twin B, spontaneous labor, and BMI < 30 kg/m^2 (Mo et al., 2021).

Complications of birth are more frequent with multifetal gestation and should be included in counseling regarding birth options. At times, twin A is born vaginally without difficulty and yet changing conditions, such as a change in fetal position, cord prolapse, or abnormal fetal heart tones, necessitate an operative birth of twin B. When twin A is noncephalic, a cesarean birth is usually recommended for route of delivery. Additionally, a liberal cesarean birth policy is advocated with fetal weights estimated as <1500 grams. Cesarean birth is recommended for higher-order multiples, triplets, and beyond.

Timing of birth is another area of debate in optimal management of multifetal births. The nadir of perinatal morbidity and mortality complications occurs sooner for twins, with higher-risk profiles for monochorionic twins (ACOG, 2021a). Labor induction or cesarean birth may be planned prior to the onset of spontaneous labor. Current evidence suggests that depending on chorionicity and amnionicity, individuals carrying an uncomplicated twin pregnancy should be considered for delivery between 32 and 39 weeks of gestation (ACOG, 2021a; Behrendt & Galan, 2021).

A home birth for an individual with twins is a controversial choice. This decision is often motivated by healthcare system mistrust, concerns regarding excessive interventions, a previous negative birth experience, and limited options for current birth (Holten et al., 2018). Rather than taking a judgmental stance, healthcare providers should engage with active listening, acknowledgment of prior experiences, and respect for autonomy in finding a way forward.

Psychosocial Aspects

There are psychosocial aspects of the diagnosis, pregnancy course and birth, and parenthood of the multifetal pregnancy that are different from a singleton pregnancy.

Despite the general decline in high-order multifetal pregnancies, when these do occur naturally, parents can choose **selective reduction** via abortion of one or more fetuses in order to decrease the associated risks, such as PTB. This is a complex ethical decision, and counseling about this option and its possible medical risks and benefits should be conducted in a professional and sensitive manner. The option of selective reduction is being curtailed under recent Supreme Court rulings and state legislative restrictions on abortion.

For individuals using ART to achieve pregnancy, the adjustment to expecting multiples can be significant. There is typically a period of shock at the diagnosis of a twin or higher-order pregnancy, tempered by a desire to understand the practicalities of parenting two or more infants. Healthcare providers can assist by connecting pregnant individuals expecting multiples with other parents of multiples for tangible and emotional support during the initial adjustment and in planning for future practicalities. While individuals carrying multiples experience more physical challenges due to the physiologic changes of multifetal pregnancies, they can also be recipients of extra social support and modified expectations that enhance emotional well-being due to the special status of multifetal pregnancy.

The initial postpartum period of adjustment is challenging and a tremendous contrast to the birth of one child. Multiple births, independent of fertility treatment, can present increased stressors for families, including financial strain, emotional adjustments, relationship challenges, sleep deprivation, as well as lack of time to care for other children; all can put parents at increased risk for postpartum mood disorders (Bradshaw et al., 2022). Parents of multiples also have considerations regarding how to foster individuality and independence of each child while recognizing the unique aspects of growing up as a twin or other multiple.

Rates of breastfeeding are lower among parents of multiples due to the challenges of coordinating the needs of more than one infant; this is often further complicated by prematurity of the infants and the need for neonatal intensive care. Immediately postpartum, parents who are committed to exclusively breastfeeding multiples can benefit from education and support by healthcare personnel, practical advice from experienced parents of multiples, access to donor human milk, and referral to a lactation consultant prenatally and immediately postbirth (Whitford et al., 2017).

Summary

Approximately 3% of all pregnancies are multifetal, with the majority being twin pregnancies, although the 2020 twin birth rate is the lowest in almost two decades due to higher rates of IVF single-embryo transfers and delay in access to sexual and reproductive healthcare due to the COVID-19 pandemic. While many perinatal complications may arise with multifetal pregnancies, including fetal anomalies, anemia, preeclampsia, gestational diabetes, fetal growth restriction, and PTB, some uncomplicated twin pregnancies can result in a vaginal birth (ACOG, 2021a). Fetal risk is predominantly determined by chorionicity, and multifetal pregnancies require additional prenatal assessment and monitoring. A multidisciplinary healthcare team skilled in twin management is ideal.

Resources for Pregnant Clients and Their Families

Information about multiple gestation: http://www.acog.org/Patients/FAQs/Multiple-Pregnancy

Connecting and supporting families of multiples: http://www.multiplesofamerica.org

Clearinghouse of multiple gestation links: http://www.marvelousmultiples.com/sites.html

Tips on breastfeeding multiples: www.laleche.org.uk/twins

Nutrition recommendations in pregnancy (not specific to multiple gestations): https://www.dietaryguidelines.gov/sites/default/files/2021-12/DGA_Pregnancy_FactSheet-508c.pdf

Resources for Healthcare Providers

Society for Assisted Reproductive Technologies Practice Committee Documents: https://www.asrm.org/news-and-publications/practice-committee-documents

Twin to Twin Transfusion Foundation: http://www.ttts foundation.org/medical_professionals/index.php

UK National Institute for Health and Care Excellence (NICE). Guidelines for multiple pregnancy: www.nice.org.uk/guidance/qs46/resources/multiple-pregnancy-twin-and-triplet-pregnancies-pdf-2098670068933

References

American College of Obsetricians and Gynecologists. (2021a). Multifetal gestations: Twin, triplet, and higher-order Multifetal pregnancies: ACOG practice bulletin, number 231. *Obstetrics & Gynecology*, *137*(6), e145–e162. https://doi.org/10.1097/aog.0000000000004397

American College of Obstetricians and Gynecologists (ACOG). (2021b). Committeee opinion 831: Medically indicated late-preterm and early-term deliveries. *Obstetrics & Gynecology*, *138*(1), e35–e39. https://doi.org/10.1097/aog.0000000000004447

American College of Obstetricians and Gynecologists (ACOG). (2021c). ACOG practice bulletin number 234: Prediction and prevention of spontaneous preterm birth. *Obstetrics and Gynecology*, *138*(2), e65–e90. https://doi.org/10.1097/AOG.0000000000004479

Audibert, F., & Gagnon, A. (2017). Prenatal screening for and diagnosis of aneuploidy in twin pregnancies. *Journal of Obstetrics Gynaecology Canada*, *39*(9), e347–e361. https://doi.org/10.1016/j.jogc.2017.06.015

Barrett, J. F. (2014). Twin delivery: Method, timing and conduct. *Best Practices & Research: Clinical Obstetrics & Gynaecology*, *28*(2), 327–338. https://doi.org/10.1016/j.bpobgyn.2013.12.008

Behrendt, N., & Galan, H. L. (2021). Fetal growth in multiple gestations: Evaluation and management. *Obstetrics & Gynecology Clinics of North America*, *48*(2), 401–417. https://doi.org/10.1016/j.ogc.2021.02.009

Bradshaw, H., Riddle, J. N., Salimgaraev, R., Zhaunova, L., & Payne, J. L. (2022). Risk factors associated with postpartum depressive symptoms: A multinational study. *Journal of Affective Disorders, 301*, 345–351. https://doi.org/10.1016/j.jad.2021.12.121

Centers for Disease Control and Prevention. (2021, January 25). *About natality, 2016–2020 expanded.* CDC Wonder. https://wonder.cdc.gov/natality-expanded-current.html

Dongarwar, D., Tahseen, D., Wang, L., Aliyu, M. H., & Salihu, H. M. (2021). Temporal trends in preterm birth phenotypes by plurality: Black-white disparity over half a century. *Journal of Perinatology, 41*(2), 204–211. https://doi.org/10.1038/s41372-020-00912-8

Fox, N. S., Stern, E. M., Saltzman, D. H., Klauser, C. K., Gupta, S., & Rebarber, A. (2014). The association between maternal weight gain and spontaneous preterm birth in twin pregnancies. *Journal of Maternal & Fetal Neonatal Medicine, 27*(16), 1652–1655. https://doi.org/10.3109/14767058.2014.898058

Gil, M. M., Galeva, S., Jani, J., Konstantinidou, L., Akolekar, R., Plana, M. N., & Nicolaides, K. H. (2019). Screening for trisomies by cfDNA testing of maternal blood in twin pregnancy: Update of the Fetal Medicine Foundation results and meta-analysis. *Ultrasound in Obstetrics & Gynecology, 53*(6), 734–742. https://doi.org/10.1002/uog.20284

Goodnight, W., & Newman, R. (2009). Optimal nutrition for improved twin pregnancy outcome. *Obstetrics & Gynecology, 114*(5), 1121–1134. https://doi.org/10.1097/AOG.0b013e3181bb14c8

Hamilton, B. E., Martin, J. A., Osterman, M. J., Curtin, S. C., & Matthews, T. J. (2015). Births: Final data for 2014. *National Vital Statistics Report, 64*(12), 1–64.

Holten, L., Hollander, M., & de Miranda, E. (2018). When the hospital is no longer an option: A multiple case study of defining moments for women choosing home birth in high-risk pregnancies in The Netherlands. *Qualitative Health Research, 28*(12), 1883–1896. https://doi-org.proxy.library.vanderbilt.edu/10.1177/1049732318791535

Institute of Medicine and National Research Council. (2009). *Weight gain during pregnancy: Reexamining the guidelines.* National Academies Press. https://doi.org/10.17226/12584

Kavanaugh, M. L., Pleasure, Z. H., Pliskin, E., Zolna, M., & MacFarlane, K. (2022). Financial instability and delays in access to sexual and reproductive health care due to COVID-19. *Journal of Women's Health.* https://doi.org/10.1089/jwh.2021.0493

Kominiarek, M. A., & Rajan, P. (2016). Nutrition recommendations in pregnancy and lactation. *The Medical Clinics of North America, 100*(6), 1199–1215. https://doi-org.proxy.library.vanderbilt.edu/10.1016/j.mcna.2016.06.004

Lipworth, H., Melamed, N., Berger, H., Geary, M., McDonald, S. D., Murray-Davis, B., Murphy, K. E., Redelmeier, D. A., Yoon, E. W., Barrett, J. F. R., & Ram, M. (2021). Maternal weight gain and pregnancy outcomes in twin gestations. *American Journal of Obstetrics & Gynecology, 225*(5), 532.e531–532.e512. https://doi.org/10.1016/j.ajog.2021.04.260

Luke, B. (2015). Nutrition for multiples. *Clinical Obstetrics and Gynecology, 58*(3), 585–610. https://doi.org/10.1097/grf.0000000000000117

Luke, B., Eberlein, T., & Newman, R. (2017). *When you're expecting twins, triplets, or quads: Proven guidelines for a healthy multiple pregnancy* (4th ed.). William Morrow.

McGoldrick, E., Stewart, F., Parker, R., & Dalziel, S. R. (2020). Antenatal corticosteroids for accelerating fetal lung maturation for women at risk of preterm birth. *Cochrane Database of Systematic Reviews, 12*, Cd004454. https://doi.org/10.1002/14651858.CD004454.pub4

Mo, G. N., Cheng, Y. W., Caughey, A. B., & Yee, L. M. (2021). Disparities in trial of labor among women with twin gestations in the United States. *American Journal of Perinatology.*. https://doi.org/10.1055/s-0041-1727228

Multifetal pregnancy. (2018). In F. G. Cunningham, K. J. Leveno, S. L. Bloom, J. S. Dashe, B. L. Hoffman, B. M. Casey, C. Spong, & Y. (Eds.), *Williams obstetrics* (25th ed.). McGraw-Hill Education.

Newman, R. B., & Unal, E. R. (2017). Multiple gestations. In S. G. Gabbe, J. R. Niebyl, J. L. Simpson, M. B. Landon, H. L. Galan, E. R. Jauniaux, D. A. Driscoll, V. Berghella, & W. A. Grobman (Eds.), *Obstetrics: Normal and problem pregnancies* (7th ed.). Elsevier.

Osterman, M., Hamilton, B., Martin, J., Driscoll, A., & Valenzuela, C. (2022). *Births: Final data for 2020.* https://stacks.cdc.gov/view/cdc/112078

Pettit, K. E., Lacoursiere, D. Y., Schrimmer, D. B., Alblewi, H., Moore, T. R., & Ramos, G. A. (2015). The association of inadequate mid-pregnancy weight gain and preterm birth in twin pregnancies. *Journal of Perinatology, 35*(2), 85–89. https://doi.org/10.1038/jp.2014.160

Posner, G., Black, A., Jones, G., & Dy, J. (2013). *Oxorn-Foote human labor and birth* (6th ed.). McGraw-Hill Education.

Reitter, A., Daviss, B. A., Krimphove, M. J., Johnson, K. C., Schlößer, R., Louwen, F., & Bisits, A. (2018). Mode of birth in twins: Data and reflections. *Journal of Obstetrics & Gynaecology, 38*(4), 502–510. https://doi.org/10.1080/01443615.2017.1393402

Ru, Y., Pressman, E. K., Cooper, E. M., Guillet, R., Katzman, P. J., Kent, T. R., Bacak, S. J., & O'Brien, K. O. (2016). Iron deficiency and anemia are prevalent in women with multiple gestations. *The American Journal of Clinical Nutrition, 104*(4), 1052–1060. https://doi-org.proxy.library.vanderbilt.edu/10.3945/ajcn.115.126284

Soffer, M. D., Naqvi, M., Melka, S., Gottlieb, A., Romero, J., & Fox, N. S. (2018). The association between maternal race and adverse outcomes in twin pregnancies with similar healthcare access. *Journal of Maternal-Fetal & Neonatal Medicine, 31*(18), 2424–2428. https://doi.org/10.1080/14767058.2017.1344634

Stanley, A. Y., Wallace, J. B., Hernandez, A. M., & Spell, J. L. (2022). Anemia in pregnancy: Screening and clinical management strategies. *Maternal Child Nursing: American Journal of Maternal Child Nursing, 47*(1), 25–32. https://doi.org/10.1097/nmc.0000000000000787

US Dept of Health and Human Services. (2021). *2019 Assisted reproductive technology fertility clinic and national summary report.* https://www.cdc.gov/art/reports/2019/pdf/2019-Report-ART-Fertility-Clinic-National-Summary-h.pdf#page=40

Whitford, H. M., Wallis, S. K., Dowswell, T., West, H. M., & Renfrew, M. J. (2017). Breastfeeding education and support for women with twins or higher order multiples. *Cochrane Database Systematic Reviews, 2*, Cd012003. https://doi.org/10.1002/14651858.CD012003.pub2

39

Postterm Pregnancy

Heather M. Bradford

Relevant Terms

Amniotic fluid index (AFI)—the maximum vertical pocket (MVP) of amniotic fluid visualized by ultrasound without the presence of umbilical cord is measured in centimeters in each of the four abdominal quadrants. The AFI is the sum of those four pockets. An AFI between 5 and 24 cm is considered normal

Anovulatory cycle—menstrual cycle in which ovulation does not occur

Biophysical profile (BPP)—fetal evaluation using nonstress test and ultrasound to assess for fetal movement, fetal tone, fetal breathing movements, and quantity of amniotic fluid

Bishop score—system to evaluate cervical ripening through digital vaginal exam findings of dilation, effacement, fetal station, cervical consistency, and cervical position

Cervical ripening—a biochemical and mechanical process remodeling cervical collagen leading to its elasticity and distensibility, an antecedent to cervical dilation

Late ovulation—ovulating later than day 14 in the menstrual cycle

Late-term pregnancy—pregnancy gestation between 41 0/7 and 41 6/7 weeks

Macrosomia—defined as birth weight greater than 4000 or 4500 g. Recent literature has described it as 4000 g in a pregnant person with diabetes (of any type, due to increased

fetal abdominal circumference) or 4500 g in pregnant person without diabetes; an abdominal circumference of >35 cm identifies >90% of macrosomic infants

Meconium aspiration syndrome—condition occurring when the fetus/newborn aspirates meconium-stained amniotic fluid into the lungs; can be associated with fetal acidosis and/or pneumonia

Modified biophysical profile—fetal evaluation composed of nonstress test and amniotic fluid index

Nonstress test (NST)—assessment of fetal well-being in which the fetal heart rate (FHR) is externally monitored for the presence of accelerations

Oligohydramnios—less than normal amniotic fluid volume; variously defined as ≤200–500 mL, a maximum vertical pocket of <2 cm or an AFI of ≤5 cm

Postterm pregnancy—pregnancy lasting more than 42 weeks of gestation or 294 days from the last normal menstrual period

Stripping/Sweeping of the membranes—a mechanical technique to stimulate cervical ripening wherein the provider inserts one or two fingers into the cervix and uses a circular motion to loosen the membranes from the lower uterine segment

---

Introduction

The etiology and physiology of prolonged gestation are not completely understood. Neonatal outcomes vary with the number of completed weeks of gestation, even for those neonates born during the 5-week gestational period (37–42 weeks) considered *term*. More precise terminology and classifications have been developed to better describe outcomes and understand best care practices by gestational age. Healthcare providers, researchers, and public health officials are encouraged to use the new gestational age designations to facilitate data reporting, delivery of quality healthcare, and clinical research (Table 39.1). Most pertinent to this chapter are the classifications of **late-term** and **postterm pregnancy**. The 2020 incidences

of late-term and postterm births in the United States were 5% and 0.25%, respectively (Osterman et al., 2022). The incidence has decreased in the last decade, primarily due to an increased use of early ultrasound resulting in improved accuracy of pregnancy dating, and the increased rate of elective labor induction prior to 41 weeks of gestation (Osterman et al., 2022).

Inaccurate pregnancy dating leads to the erroneous determination of postterm pregnancy. **Late ovulation** or an **anovulatory cycle** is more common than early ovulation, thus leading to an overestimation of gestational age when using the last menstrual period as the basis for pregnancy dating. An overestimation of gestational age can lead to increased misdiagnosis of postterm pregnancy and concomitant overmanagement (Caughey, 2021).

Prenatal and Postnatal Care: A Person-Centered Approach, Third Edition. Edited by Karen Trister Grace, Cindy L. Farley, Noelene K. Jeffers, and Tanya Tringali.
© 2024 John Wiley & Sons Ltd. Published 2024 by John Wiley & Sons Ltd.
Companion website: www.wiley.com/go/grace/prenatal

Table 39.1 Classification of Term and Postterm Births by Weeks of Gestation

37 0/7 weeks through 38 6/7 weeks	Early term
39 0/7 weeks through 40 6/7 weeks	Full term
41 0/7 weeks through 41 6/7 weeks	Late term
42 0/7 weeks and beyond	Postterm

Source: Adapted from Spong (2013).

Risk factors for experiencing a postterm pregnancy include nulliparity, prior history of postterm pregnancy, elevated body mass index ($>30\,kg/m^2$), and having a family history of postterm pregnancies (Ashton et al., 2018; Caughey, 2021; Vats et al., 2021).

Genetic factors may play a role. A pregnant person with a history of one previous postterm pregnancy is two times more likely to experience a subsequent postterm pregnancy compared to those who have not had a postterm pregnancy (Kistka et al., 2007). They are almost four times as likely to have a postterm pregnancy with two previous postterm pregnancies (Norwitz, 2022).

Health equity key points

- For postterm pregnancies, lack of prenatal care is associated with higher rates of stillbirth and neonatal death, emphasizing the importance of routine prenatal care.
- Segregation of Black communities due to structural racism has led to limited access to resources such as prenatal care and birthing hospitals.

Potential Problems

There are perinatal risks associated with pregnancy after 42 weeks of gestation (Middleton et al., 2018; Murzakanova et al., 2020). Risk factors for the pregnant person include labor dystocia, infection, perineal trauma, operative vaginal birth, postpartum hemorrhage, and cesarean birth (Caughey, 2021). Some of the adverse outcomes associated with late-term and postterm pregnancies result from medical intervention when the uterus, cervix, and fetus are not ready for labor (Middleton et al., 2018). However, these complications are primarily associated with the increased risk of placental insufficiency and fetal **macrosomia** in the postterm infant. At 42 weeks of gestation, over 11% of infants will be macrosomic (Maoz et al., 2019). Fetal macrosomia increases the risk of shoulder dystocia and its associated sequelae, such as fetal birth injuries and neonatal intensive care unit (NICU) admission.

Other fetal adverse outcomes in the postterm pregnancy include meconium-stained amniotic fluid, low Apgar scores, stillbirth, the need for respiratory support and antibiotics, and oligohydramnios (Murzakanova et al., 2020). Meconium-stained fluid occurs in over 25% of postterm pregnancies, increasing the risk of **meconium aspiration syndrome** (Maoz et al., 2019). As the placenta begins to age, there are increased areas of infarction and deposition

of calcium and fiber within the placental tissue. This creates decreased placental reserve and uteroplacental insufficiency. The volume of amniotic fluid normally begins to decrease after 40 weeks of gestation, and the incidence of **oligohydramnios** is two times higher in postterm gestation (Keilman & Shanks, 2022; Maoz et al., 2019). Oligohydramnios elevates the risk of cord compression, FHR abnormalities, meconium-stained amniotic fluid, fetal distress during labor, fetal acidosis, and low Apgar scores (American College of Obstetricians and Gynecologists [ACOG], 2014). Some of these fetal risks, including meconium-stained fluid and fetal acidosis, have been found with more frequency at 41 when compared to 39 weeks of gestation, suggesting that 42 weeks does not represent a threshold for uniform risk (Caughey, 2021).

The incidence of stillbirth in the postterm infant is higher than that of the term infant (Wennerholm et al., 2019). In a meta-analysis of 15 million pregnancies, the risk of stillbirth increased with gestational age from 0.11 per 1000 at 37 weeks to 3.18 per 1000 at 42 weeks, although there was minimal risk (1 stillbirth per 1449 births) for pregnancies that advanced from 40 to 41 weeks. Neonatal mortality increased significantly (RR 1.87) for births at 42 versus 41 weeks (Muglu et al., 2019).

Prevention, Intervention, and Management Options

The most important practice for preventing postterm pregnancy and its serious risks is accurate pregnancy dating. Ultrasound dating of a pregnancy with an uncertain or unknown last menstrual period and in individuals with irregular cycles is important. First-trimester ultrasound for pregnancy dating is the most accurate and reduces the incidence of postterm pregnancy diagnosis (Caughey, 2021; see Chapter 10, *Pregnancy Diagnosis and Gestational Age Assessment*). If first-trimester ultrasound is not performed, the use of shared decision-making and mutual understanding is important early in the pregnancy when determining an estimated date of birth for the purposes of timing post-date fetal surveillance.

It is appropriate to consider and discuss management options with pregnant persons prior to the 41-week gestation mark. The management of late-term and postterm pregnancy includes the initiation of prenatal fetal surveillance and the options of (a) expectant management, (b) labor-stimulating activities, and (c) induction of labor (Figure 39.1). However, there is no interdisciplinary national guideline on fetal surveillance or management of a postterm pregnancy.

Fetal Surveillance

The goal of fetal surveillance is to minimize the risk of stillbirth (ACOG, 2021). Optimal timing to initiate postterm fetal surveillance testing is at 41 0/7 weeks of gestation, although it is unclear how often to perform fetal testing or which type of fetal surveillance is best. There is limited evidence suggesting that twice-weekly testing has superior perinatal outcomes as compared to

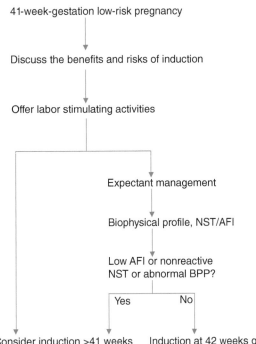

41-week-gestation low-risk pregnancy

↓

Discuss the benefits and risks of induction

↓

Offer labor stimulating activities

Expectant management

↓

Biophysical profile, NST/AFI

↓

Low AFI or nonreactive
NST or abnormal BPP?

Yes   No

Consider induction >41 weeks   Induction at 42 weeks gestation
or for indication

Figure 39.1 Algorithm for the management of late-term and postterm pregnancy.

once-weekly testing (ACOG, 2014). While no randomized prospective trials demonstrate a benefit of fetal monitoring, twice-weekly surveillance has become a generally accepted approach (Caughey, 2021).

There is no difference in testing outcomes between **biophysical profile (BPP)** and **nonstress test** (NST). However, monitoring of amniotic fluid volume via the **amniotic fluid index (AFI)** has been demonstrated as an important component of surveillance, with a recommendation for induction if the maximum vertical pocket (MVP) is 2 cm or less. It is reasonable to recommend a modified BPP (NST plus amniotic fluid assessment) twice weekly, beginning at and beyond 41 0/7 weeks of gestation (Caughey, 2021). Common fetal surveillance options used in late-term and postterm pregnancies are presented in Table 39.2.

Expectant Management

Waiting for spontaneous labor is an option for late-term and postterm low-risk pregnant persons with fetal surveillance demonstrating normal findings. Expectant management supports the physiologic processes that are preparing the body for spontaneous labor ("Supporting Healthy and Normal Physiologic Childbirth: A Consensus Statement by ACNM, MANA, and NACPM," 2013). It allows further in utero development of the fetal lungs, brain, and other organs for a smooth transition to extrauterine life for the newborn. It is also a clear preference of some to have a naturally progressing labor within the parameters of safety. Spontaneous labor offers substantial benefit to the birthing dyad, such as the option for intermittent fetal monitoring with freedom of movement. Spontaneous labor also allows for physiologic changes that support effective contractions, breastfeeding, and fetal protective processes in the transition to extrauterine life. Disruption of this process without an evidence-based medical indication represents a risk for potential harm. With fetal surveillance indicating normal findings, expectant management is an option that should be offered as late-term gestation week approaches.

Cervical Ripening and Labor-Stimulating Activities

Some pregnant persons are eager to encourage labor onset with a variety of strategies that can potentially aid **cervical ripening** and initiate contractions. **Stripping or sweeping of the membranes** is a mechanical separation of the amniotic membranes away from the wall of the uterus performed manually by the healthcare provider. The

Table 39.2 Methods of Fetal Surveillance

Method	Frequency	Comments
Fetal movement count (FMC)	Daily	If pattern of movement decreases, further testing is indicated.
Nonstress test (NST)	Twice weekly	External fetal heart rate (FHR) monitoring. If nonreactive, consultation and further testing is indicated.
Biophysical profile (BPP)	Twice weekly	Performed using external FHR monitoring and ultrasonographic exam. If AFI is low, induction of labor of term pregnancies is recommended even if all other parameters are normal. Consult for abnormal results.
Modified biophysical profile	Twice weekly	Combines NST and AFI; consult for abnormal results.
Amniotic fluid index (AFI)	Twice weekly	Performed with ultrasonographic exam; consult for oligohydramnios with maximum vertical pocket of 2 cm or less even if other fetal surveillance is normal.
Contraction stress test (CST)	Weekly	External electronic fetal monitoring of fetal response to three or more contractions in 10 minutes occurring spontaneously or induced by nipple stimulation or oxytocin administration. Because CSTs are more invasive, require prolonged periods of time to conduct, and have the risk of creating complications, they are not in common use.

cervix must be open enough to allow the insertion of the provider's finger, which is swept between the wall of the cervix and lower uterus with the intention of gently pulling the membrane slightly away from the tissue. The pregnant person needs to be informed that the intervention can be uncomfortable and may cause vaginal spotting. Overt bleeding should not occur and would need to be evaluated. In a recent Cochrane review (40 studies), women (n = 6548) who had their membranes swept versus expectant management were more likely to experience spontaneous onset of labor within 48 hours, although there was no difference in rates of cesarean or spontaneous vaginal birth and the evidence was overall weak (Finucane et al., 2020). There are no standardized recommendations on the optimal number of membrane sweeps and the timing to facilitate labor.

There are two theoretical risks to membrane sweeping. Manipulations during the process may lead to accidental rupture of the membranes, thus creating an unintended situation of prelabor rupture of the membranes. There are case reports of accidental release of amniotic fluid; however, no studies report this as a significant adverse effect. The second theoretical concern relates to Group B Streptococcus (GBS). Some healthcare providers and parents have voiced concern about bacterial seeding during the membrane stripping procedure. To date, membrane sweeping has been affirmed as a safe procedure for GBS positive persons and their babies (ACOG, 2020). Pregnant persons should be informed of the risks, benefits, and theoretical concerns associated with this intervention.

Acupuncture, theorized to stimulate the secretion of oxytocin as energy blockages are released, has been studied as a mechanism to ripen the cervix and stimulate the onset of labor. In a recent Cochrane review (n = 15 studies), the authors reported no difference in rates of cesarean birth when comparing groups who received acupuncture versus usual care. There was an increase in cervical ripening for pregnant individuals who received acupuncture, although the sample size was small (Smith et al., 2017).

Castor oil is a potent cathartic derived from the bean of the castor plant. Castor oil is one of the most popular drugs for labor induction, used by many people worldwide outside of the healthcare setting with anecdotal reports of use as a labor stimulant dating back to ancient Egypt (Montazeri et al., 2010). A metabolite of castor oil, ricinoleic acid, activates intestinal and uterine smooth muscle cell activity (Tunaru et al., 2012). In recent meta-analysis (n = 8 studies), oral administration of castor oil was effective for the promotion of cervical ripening and induction of labor, with no significant adverse outcomes (Moradi et al., 2022). A single dose of 60 cc of castor oil can be added to other liquids such as juice or ice cream milk shakes to make it more palatable. However, the expected effects can be quite uncomfortable with temporary nausea, diarrhea, and abdominal cramping. As with other labor induction methods, castor oil is not likely to be effective if the pregnant body is not yet physiologically ready for labor. A castor oil beverage is often recommended for individuals who are planning a low

intervention or community birth who reach 41+ weeks gestation. See the text box for an example of a recipe designed to minimize some of castor oil's side effects.

Castor oil beverage for labor stimulation

8 oz apricot juice
10 oz lemon verbena tea
2 tablespoons almond butter
2 tablespoons castor oil
Mix thoroughly and enjoy over ice.

Some herbal labor stimulants, such as blue and black cohosh, are associated with the potential for fetal harm and should not be used (Romm, 2018). Evening primrose oil has been used for cervical ripening and labor induction in oral or vaginal routes of administration. There is limited evidence demonstrating its effectiveness, and evening primrose oil has been associated with premature and, consequently, prolonged rupture of membranes (Kalati et al., 2018; Moradi et al., 2021).

Unprotected vaginal–penile intercourse has been suggested to trigger spontaneous onset of labor; however, the effectiveness is low (Carbone et al., 2019). Theoretically, vaginal–penile intercourse exposes the uterus to prostaglandins in semen, initiates mechanical irritation to the cervix and lower uterine segment, and releases endogenous prostaglandins in the pregnant person, similar to sweeping of the membranes, causing uterine contractions. There is also limited evidence to suggest nipple stimulation or orgasm as a labor stimulant (Carbone et al., 2019; Singh et al., 2014). Nipple stimulation is theorized to release oxytocin from the posterior pituitary gland, leading to cervical ripening and uterine contractions (Wheeler et al., 2022). Orgasm is also theorized to stimulate uterine contractility (Chayen et al., 1986).

Labor Induction

Pregnant persons at 41 weeks of gestation are candidates for labor induction. However, there is a lack of consensus on optimal management at 41 weeks of gestation and, consequently, a wide practice variation in management of postterm pregnancies (Keulen et al., 2019). A systematic review found that elective induction of labor at 41 weeks of gestation is associated with fewer cesarean births, lower rates of NICU admission and low Apgar scores, and fewer perinatal deaths, though the absolute risk of perinatal death is small (Middleton et al., 2018). Labor induction involves the use of high-alert medications and carries heightened risk of iatrogenic harm. Additionally, many cointerventions, such as tethering to the fetal monitor and IV, are used that also affect the birth process and outcomes. Induction of labor begins a cascade of interventions, each with its own inherent risks and considerations that can influence the labor and birth experience. Approach each **late-term pregnancy** within the context

Table 39.3 Bishop Cervical Scoring

	0	1	2	3
Dilation	Closed	1–2 cm	3–4 cm	>5 cm
Effacement (%)	0–30	40–50	60–70	>80
Station	–3	–2	–1	+1, +2
Cervical consistency	Firm	Medium	Soft	–
Cervical position	Posterior	Midline	Anterior	–

of the individuals' health, parity, cervical status, estimated fetal weight, and preferences for birth. A discussion of risks and benefits using shared decision-making can support each pregnant person to make an informed choice regarding their options.

As many as 80% of pregnant persons who reach 42 weeks of gestation have an unfavorable cervix for induction with a **Bishop score** of less than 7; see Table 39.3 (Caughey, 2021). When induction is planned but the cervix is not favorable, cervical ripening with a prostaglandin preparation or mechanical dilation is effective. The use of prostaglandins in the form of gel, suppository, or vaginal tablet is a common method of cervical ripening. Mechanical dilation with a Cook or Foley balloon catheter placed within the cervix is also effective (Kruit et al., 2016). The balloon catheter can be inserted in the office the afternoon before the day of the induction and the pregnant person can return home.

It is important to consider ethical concerns related to elective inductions (prior to 41 weeks of gestation; American College of Nurse-Midwives, 2016). Healthcare providers report that elective inductions of labor are primarily performed on request, for convenience or for other nonmedically indicated reasons (Jou et al., 2015). Pregnant persons have also reported that they have been encouraged or pressured to acquiesce to an induction in the absence of indications (DeClercq et al., 2013). Pregnant persons at 41 and 42 weeks of gestation and beyond who choose to proceed with awaiting spontaneous should be treated respectfully and not shamed. Biweekly testing is recommended as well as careful documentation of risks and benefits. The decision to induce labor or not requires use of informed consent and consideration of the potential for harm compared to possible benefits, including short- and long-term perinatal implications, with the pregnant person's decision respected fully.

Summary

The etiology and physiology of prolonged gestation are not completely understood. Accurate assessment of gestational age is important for appropriate management of late-term and postterm pregnancies. To prevent stillbirth, initiation of postterm fetal surveillance testing or induction of labor at 41 0/7 weeks of gestation should be considered. There are several strategies to assist with cervical ripening and initiation of uterine contractility, although

standardized recommendations are limited. Waiting for spontaneous labor is an option for late-term and postterm low-risk pregnant persons with normal fetal surveillance results. Use of informed consent and shared decision-making is important when discussing management options.

Resources for Pregnant People and Their Families

A "Share with Women" document with information about membranes sweeping: https://onlinelibrary.wiley.com/doi/10.1111/jmwh.12894

A "Share with Women" document with information about induction of labor: https://onlinelibrary.wiley.com/doi/epdf/10.1111/jmwh.12649

A consumer Web site with information about when pregnancy goes past your due date: https://www.acog.org/womens-health/faqs/when-pregnancy-goes-past-your-due-date

Resources for Healthcare Providers

A "Midwife Thinking" document with information about post-dates induction of labour and balancing risks: https://midwifethinking.com/2016/07/13/induction-of-labour-balancing-risks

References

ACNM, MANA, and NACPM. (2013, 2013). Supporting healthy and normal physiologic childbirth: A consensus statement by ACNM, MANA, and NACPM. *Journal of Perinatal Education*, *22*(1), 14–18. https://doi.org/10.1891/1058-1243.22.1.14

American College of Nurse-Midwives. (2016). *Induction of labor.* https://www.midwife.org/acnm/files/ACNMLibraryData/UPLOAD-FILENAME/000000000235/Induction-of-Labor-2016.pdf

American College of Obstetricians and Gynecologists. (2014). Practice bulletin no. 146: Management of late-term and postterm pregnancies. *Obstetrics & Gynecology*, *124*(2 Pt 1), 390–396. https://doi.org/10.1097/01.Aog.0000452744.06088.48

American College of Obstetricians and Gynecologists. (2020). Committee opinion no. 797: Prevention of group B streptococcal early-onset disease in newborns: Correction. *Obstetrics & Gynecology*, *135*(4), 978–979. https://doi.org/10.1097/aog.0000000000003824

American College of Obstetricians and Gynecologists. (2021). Antepartum fetal surveillance. Practice bulletin, no. 229. *Obstetrics & Gynecology*, *137*(6), e116–e127. https://doi.org/10.1097/aog.0000000000004410

Ashton, G., Bhattacharya, S., & Shetty, A. (2018). Repeat induction of labour for post-term pregnancy. *Journal of Obstetrics & Gynaecology*, *38*(5), 724. https://doi.org/10.1080/01443615.2018.1444393

Carbone, L., De Vivo, V., Saccone, G., D'Antonio, F., Mercorio, A., Raffone, A., Arduino, B., D'Alessandro, P., Sarno, L., Conforti, A., Maruotti, G. M., Alviggi, C., & Zullo, F. (2019). Sexual intercourse for induction of spontaneous onset of labor: A systematic review and meta-analysis of randomized controlled trials. *Journal of Sexual Medicine*, *16*(11), 1787–1795. https://doi.org/10.1016/j.jsxm.2019.08.002

Caughey, A. B. (2021). *Postterm pregnancy.* https://emedicine.medscape.com/article/261369-overview?reg=1

Chayen, B., Tejani, N., Verma, U. L., & Gordon, G. (1986). Fetal heart rate changes and uterine activity during coitus. *Acta Obstetricia et Gynecologica Scandinavica*, *65*(8), 853–855. https://doi.org/10.3109/00016348609157037

Declercq, E. R., Sakala, C., Corry, M. P., Applebaum, S., & Herrlich, A. (2013). *Listening to mothers III: Pregnancy and birth.* Childbirth Connection. https://nationalpartnership.org/wp-content/uploads/2023/02/listening-to-mothers-iii-pregnancy-and-birth-2013.pdf

Finucane, E. M., Murphy, D. J., Biesty, L. M., Gyte, G. M., Cotter, A. M., Ryan, E. M., Boulvain, M., & Devane, D. (2020). Membrane sweeping for induction of labour. *Cochrane Database of Systematic Reviews*, 2(2), Cd000451. https://doi.org/10.1002/14651858. CD000451.pub3

Jou, J., Kozhimannil, K. B., Johnson, P. J., & Sakala, C. (2015). Patient-perceived pressure from clinicians for labor induction and cesarean population-based survey of US women. *Health Services Research*, 50(4), 961–981.

Kalati, M., Kashanian, M., Jahdi, F., Naseri, M., Haghani, H., & Sheikhansari, N. (2018). Evening primrose oil and labour, is it effective? A randomised clinical trial. *Journal of Obstetrics & Gynaecology*, 38(4), 488–492. https://doi.org/10.1080/01443615.2017.1386165

Keilman, C., & Shanks, A. L. (2022). *Oligohydramnios.* StatPearls. https://www.ncbi.nlm.nih.gov/books/NBK562326

Keulen, J. K., Bruinsma, A., Kortekaas, J. C., van Dillen, J., Bossuyt, P. M., Oudijk, M. A., Duijnhoven, R. G., van Kaam, A. H., Vandenbussche, F. P., van der Post, J. A., Mol, B. W., & de Miranda, E. (2019). Induction of labour at 41 weeks versus expectant management until 42 weeks (INDEX): Multicentre, randomised non-inferiority trial. *BMJ*, 364, l344. https://doi.org/10.1136/bmj.l344

Kistka, Z. A., Palomar, L., Boslaugh, S. E., DeBaun, M. R., DeFranco, E. A., & Muglia, L. J. (2007). Risk for postterm delivery after previous postterm delivery. *American Journal of Obstetrics & Gynecology*, 196(3), 241.e241–241.e246. https://doi.org/10.1016/j.ajog.2006.10.873

Kruit, H., Heikinheimo, O., Ulander, V. M., Aitokallio-Tallberg, A., Nupponen, I., Paavonen, J., & Rahkonen, L. (2016). Foley catheter induction of labor as an outpatient procedure. *Journal of Perinatology*, 36(8), 618–622.

Maoz, O., Wainstock, T., Sheiner, E., & Walfisch, A. (2019). Immediate perinatal outcomes of postterm deliveries. *Journal of Maternal Fetal & Neonatal Medicine*, 32(11), 1847–1852. https://doi.org/10.1080/14767058.2017.1420773

Middleton, P., Shepherd, E., & Crowther, C. A. (2018). Induction of labour for improving birth outcomes for women at or beyond term. *Cochrane Database of Systematic Reviews*, 5(5), Cd004945. https://doi.org/10.1002/14651858.CD004945.pub4

Montazeri, S., Afshary, P., Souri, H., & Iravani, M. (2010). Efficacy of castor oil for induction and augmentation of labor. *Iranian Journal of Pharmaceutical Research*, 3(Suppl. 2), 38–39.

Moradi, M., Niazi, A., Heydarian Miri, H., & Lopez, V. (2021). The effect of evening primrose oil on labor induction and cervical ripening: A systematic review and meta-analysis. *Phytotherapy Research*, 35(10), 5374–5383. https://doi.org/10.1002/ptr.7147

Moradi, M., Niazi, A., Mazloumi, E., & Lopez, V. (2022). Effect of castor oil on cervical ripening and labor induction: A systematic review and meta-analysis. *Journal of Pharmacopuncture*, 25(2), 71–78. https://doi.org/10.3831/kpi.2022.25.2.71

Muglu, J., Rather, H., Arroyo-Manzano, D., Bhattacharya, S., Balchin, I., Khalil, A., Thilaganathan, B., Khan, K. S., Zamora, J., & Thangaratinam, S. (2019). Risks of stillbirth and neonatal death with advancing gestation at term: A systematic review and meta-analysis of cohort studies of 15 million pregnancies. *PLoS Medicine*, 16(7), e1002838. https://doi.org/10.1371/journal.pmed.1002838

Murzakanova, G., Räisänen, S., Jacobsen, A. F., Sole, K. B., Bjarkø, L., & Laine, K. (2020). Adverse perinatal outcomes in 665,244 term and post-term deliveries-a Norwegian population-based study. *European Journal of Obstetrics & Gynecology and Reproductive Biology*, 247, 212–218. https://doi.org/10.1016/j.ejogrb.2020.02.028

Norwitz, E. R. (2022). *Postterm pregnancy.* UpToDate. http://www.uptodate.com/contents/postterm-pregnancy.

Osterman, M., Hamilton, B., Martin, J., Driscoll, A., & Valenzuela, C. (2022). *Births: Final data for 2020.* https://stacks.cdc.gov/view/cdc/112078

Romm, A. (2018). Labor and birth. In *Botanical medicine for women's health* (2nd ed., pp. 430–435). Elsevier.

Singh, N., Tripathi, R., Mala, Y. M., & Yedla, N. (2014). Breast stimulation in low-risk primigravidas at term: Does it aid in spontaneous onset of labour and vaginal delivery? A pilot study. *Biomedical Research International*, 2014, 695037. https://doi.org/10.1155/2014/695037

Smith, C. A., Armour, M., & Dahlen, H. G. (2017). Acupuncture or acupressure for induction of labour. *Cochrane Database of Systematic Reviews*, 10(10), Cd002962. https://doi.org/10.1002/14651858.CD002962.pub4

Spong, C. (2013). Defining "term" pregnancy: Recommendations from the defining "term" pregnancy workgroup. *Journal of the American Medical Association*, 309(23), 2445–2446.

Tunaru, S., Althoff, T. F., Nusing, R. M., Diener, M., & Offermans, S. (2012). Castor oil induces laxation and uterus contractions via ricinoleic acid activation prostraglandin EP3 receptors. *Proceedings of the National Academy of Sciences*, 109(23), 9179–9184.

Vats, H., Saxena, R., Sachdeva, M. P., Walia, G. K., & Gupta, V. (2021). Impact of maternal pre-pregnancy body mass index on maternal, fetal and neonatal adverse outcomes in the worldwide populations: A systematic review and meta-analysis. *Obesity Research & Clinical Practice*, 15(6), 536–545. https://doi.org/10.1016/j.orcp.2021.10.005

Wennerholm, U. B., Saltvedt, S., Wessberg, A., Alkmark, M., Bergh, C., Wendel, S. B., Fadl, H., Jonsson, M., Ladfors, L., Sengpiel, V., Wesström, J., Wennergren, G., Wikström, A. K., Elden, H., Stephansson, O., & Hagberg, H. (2019). Induction of labour at 41 weeks versus expectant management and induction of labour at 42 weeks (SWEdish Post-term induction study, SWEPIS): Multicentre, open label, randomised, superiority trial. *BMJ*, 367, l6131. https://doi.org/10.1136/bmj.l6131

Wheeler, V., Hoffman, A., & Bybel, M. (2022). Cervical ripening and induction of labor. *American Family Physician*, 105(2), 177–186.

40

Hyperemesis Gravidarum

Ella T. Heitzler and Jennifer Wolfe

The editors gratefully acknowledge Karen Trister Grace, who authored the previous edition of this chapter.

Relevant Terms

Hyperemesis gravidarum (HG)—extreme, excessive, and persistent vomiting in pregnancy associated with weight loss (>5%), malnourishment, and dehydration

Ptyalism gravidarum—also known as sialorrhea, the excess secretion of saliva during pregnancy

Total parenteral nutrition (TPN)—intravenous nutrition including glucose, amino acids, lipids, vitamins, and minerals provided intravenously

Wernicke's encephalopathy—a disorder resulting from thiamine deficiency due to frequent vomiting

---

Introduction

Experienced by more than 70–90% of pregnant persons, nausea and vomiting are common during early pregnancy (MacGibbon et al., 2021). Although these symptoms can be distressing, they are typically benign and self-limited, with most people experiencing relief by 12–14 weeks of gestation. For a small percentage of people (about 1–2%), nausea and vomiting are severe and progress into **hyperemesis gravidarum** (HG; MacGibbon et al., 2021; Nurmi et al., 2020). HG is characterized by persistent and severe nausea and vomiting, dehydration, fluid and electrolyte imbalance, and loss of at least 5% of prepregnant weight (American College of Obstetricians and Gynecologists [ACOG], 2018). Persons with HG are deficient in intake of most nutrients and have very low caloric intake (Maslin et al., 2021). HG can negatively affect family, social, and occupational functioning as well as quality of life and is a leading cause of emergency department visits and hospitalizations during pregnancy (Castillo & Phillippi, 2015). People with HG are often unable to perform their usual daily activities and have the added psychological burden of not feeling able to manage their lives for many weeks or months.

Individuals with HG may feel helpless, incapable, and poorly supported by their families, and very concerned about fetal well-being, all of which contributes to their psychological distress (Dean et al., 2018a). Severe nausea and vomiting lead some pregnant persons to consider terminating their current pregnancy, and for three out of four, the experience of severe nausea and vomiting during pregnancy affects their willingness to consider future pregnancies (Heitmann et al., 2017).

Health equity key points

- Classism, racism, and cultural factors may impact HG risk by affecting overall health, nutrition, food access, etc.
- First-line therapy drugs for HG are quite costly. Consider lower-cost, over-the-counter alternatives that may increase access to therapies for individuals who are uninsured, underinsured, or financially challenged.

Etiology and Risk Factors

The exact cause of HG is unknown, but it likely has a multifactorial etiology (Table 40.1). Evidence suggests a strong genetic component to HG. Recurrence rates in subsequent pregnancies have been described ranging from 15% to 81% (Dean et al., 2020). Contributing factors, such as gallbladder dysfunction, *Helicobacter pylori* (*H. pylori*) infection, gastroesophageal reflux disease (GERD), and dysosmia, may worsen symptoms (Fezjo et al., 2019; MacGibbon, 2020). Risk factors include gestational trophoblastic disease, pregnancy with multifetal gestation, conception with assisted reproductive technologies, younger age, nulliparity, extremes of body mass index (BMI), and lower socioeconomic status (Castillo & Phillippi, 2015; Nurmi et al., 2020; Peled et al., 2013). Classism and bias may be a contributing factor. Compared to White individuals, Asian or Black pregnant people have

---

Prenatal and Postnatal Care: A Person-Centered Approach, Third Edition. Edited by Karen Trister Grace, Cindy L. Farley, Noelene K. Jeffers, and Tanya Tringali.
© 2024 John Wiley & Sons Ltd. Published 2024 by John Wiley & Sons Ltd.
Companion website: www.wiley.com/go/grace/prenatal

Table 40.1 Some Suggested Etiologies/Risk Factors for Hyperemesis Gravidarum

Factor	Comments
Increase in human chorionic gonadotropin (hCG)	HG is more common in multifetal gestation, gestational trophoblastic disease, and in fetuses with Down syndrome, all conditions that increase maternal levels of hCG.
Increase in estrogen	Estrogen decreases intestinal motility, leading to nausea and vomiting.
Increase in thyroid hormone production	High levels of thyroid hormone can cause gestational transient thyrotoxicosis, a condition observed in up to two-thirds of people with HG.
Genetics	HG is more common in people who have a family history of HG.
Helicobacter pylori infection	*H. pylori infection* can exacerbate NVP and is more common in people with HG (note that *H. pylori* treatment is not a recommended HG management strategy).

Source: Adapted from Castillo and Phillippi (2015), London et al. (2017), and Ng et al. (2017).

the highest risk of developing HG or having recurring HG with a subsequent pregnancy (Fiaschi et al., 2016), suggesting that racism and cultural factors may also impact HG.

Healthcare providers may make the erroneous assumption that pregnant people with severe nausea and vomiting during pregnancy are transforming psychological distress into physical symptoms. While in rare cases personality disorders and other psychogenic etiologies may be contributing factors, psychological afflictions are more likely a consequence of constant vomiting than the source (Kender et al., 2015; Magtira et al., 2015). The psychosomatic aspects of HG should be considered, but a psychopathologic etiology for HG has largely been discredited.

Potential Complications

HG can have a profound negative impact across all aspects of a pregnant person's life. Pregnant people who experience HG are at higher risk for developing new onset anxiety, depression, and post-traumatic stress disorders (Mitchell-Jones et al., 2016). Vomiting-induced esophageal rupture can result in gastrointestinal bleeding (London et al., 2017). Persistent vomiting can also cause hyponatremia. Early signs of hyponatremia, such as anorexia, headache, nausea and vomiting, and lethargy, can be missed since the clinical presentation is similar to HG itself. Some other potential complications include vitamin B6 and B12 deficiency, venous thromboembolism, retinal detachment, and splenic avulsion (Castillo & Phillippi, 2015). **Wernicke's encephalopathy**, a complication caused by a vomiting-induced thiamine deficiency, is a potentially fatal medical emergency. Thiamine acts as a

coenzyme in carbohydrate metabolism and glucose formation. Without thiamine, glucose is metabolized through less-efficient anaerobic pathways that produce lactic acid, leading to acidosis and encephalopathy. Wernicke's encephalopathy is a reversible condition that can cause persistent neurological deficits. Signs and symptoms of Wernicke's encephalopathy are weakness, loss of muscular coordination, apathy, and mental confusion.

Fetal complications may include fetal growth restriction, preterm birth, neonatal morbidity, and small-for-gestational-age (SGA) infants (Castillo & Phillippi, 2015; Peled et al., 2013). Long-term sequelae for the child of an HG pregnancy include a higher risk for emotional and behavioral disorders (Mullin et al., 2011), including autism spectrum disorders (Getahun et al., 2019).

Differential Diagnoses

Numerous differential diagnoses (Table 40.2) should be considered when an individual presents with nausea and vomiting during pregnancy (NVP). It is essential to consider when the nausea and vomiting began; nausea and vomiting experienced for the first time after nine weeks of gestation should result in careful evaluation for other conditions (ACOG, 2018). History taking is the cornerstone of diagnosing HG due to its multifactor etiology (Fezjo et al., 2019; MacGibbon, 2020).

Evaluation

Whenever a pregnant person has nausea and vomiting, evaluation should begin with a thorough history and assessment to determine the severity of the problem (see Chapter 15, *Common Discomforts of Pregnancy*). Validated measurement tools, such as the Pregnancy-Unique Quantification of Emesis and Nausea (PUQE) scale (Koren et al., 2005), the Hyperemesis Impact Questionnaire (Power et al., 2010), and the HyperEmesis Level Prediction

Table 40.2 Differential Diagnoses to Consider

System	Diagnoses to consider
Gastrointestinal	Gastroenteritis, gastroparesis, intestinal obstruction, peptic ulcer disease, *Helicobacter pylori*, pancreatitis, appendicitis, hepatitis, biliary tract disease
Genitourinary	Kidney stones, pyelonephritis, uremia, ovarian torsion, uterine leiomyoma
Endocrine/ metabolic	Diabetic ketoacidosis, thyroid disease, Addison's disease, prophyria, hyperparathyroidism
Neurological	Pseudotumor cerebri, central nervous system (CNS) tumor, migraines, vestibular lesions, lymphocytic hypophysitis
Miscellaneous	Drug toxicity, infection, molar pregnancy

Source: Adapted from ACOG (2018), Dean et al. (2018b), and MacGibbon (2020).

(HELP) Score (MacGibbon, 2020), are available to assist in the evaluation of people with HG.

Reports of extreme fatigue and exhaustion with early pregnancy onset of continuing nausea and vomiting should lead the clinician to consider HG in the differential diagnosis list. **Ptyalism gravidarum** may be present. Individuals often report an inability to go to work or to perform activities of daily living, and family relationships can suffer. Physical parameters to assess include weight changes, mucous membrane status, skin turgor, and overall appearance and energy. Physical exam findings of abdominal tenderness or fever and subjective reports of abdominal pain, diarrhea, urinary symptoms, or headache suggest etiology other than HG and warrant further evaluation.

Laboratory tests are not necessary for diagnosis but are used to determine the severity of effects of HG on the body and can include urinalysis, especially noting ketonuria, CBC, electrolytes, liver enzymes, and bilirubin levels. These tests also help rule out alternative diagnoses. If obtained, tests of thyroid function may demonstrate gestational transient thyrotoxicosis or hyperthyroxinemia; however, this is usually only present in the first half of pregnancy and the use of antithyroid drugs is not recommended (ACOG, 2018). Multifetal gestation and trophoblastic disorders should be excluded by ultrasound.

Care and Management

Patients presenting with HG have typically attempted dietary and lifestyle measures to reduce nausea and vomiting without success (see Chapter 15, *Common Discomforts of Pregnancy*). Some people with HG experience relief with acupressure and acupuncture, though evidence suggests that effectiveness is similar to placebo (Boelig et al., 2016; Matthews et al., 2015; Van den Heuvel et al., 2016). Once dietary and lifestyle measures have been attempted,

pharmacologic therapy becomes a key component of HG management (Table 40.3). Diclegis or Bonjesta (delayed release pyridoxine and doxylamine) provide a first-line therapy that may be sufficient in controlling HG symptoms. Several studies have shown this remedy to be safe and effective (Koren et al., 2015; McParlin et al., 2016b). If cost is a barrier, both doxylamine and pyridoxine (Vitamin B6) can be purchased over the counter or prescribed individually by the provider. If symptoms persist, other medications can be added.

Second-line therapies include antihistamines like dimenhydrinate and diphenhydramine. It is important to avoid antihistamines in pregnant people taking ondansetron, as it can prolong the QT interval (ACOG, 2018). Antihistamines are considered to be a safe and effective treatment for nausea and vomiting in pregnancy, with common side effects being dry mouth, sedation, and constipation (Boelig et al., 2016). If symptoms continue without improvement, a dopamine antagonist, such as metoclopramide or promethazine, can be added to the treatment plan. Although studies have shown these medications to be effective in alleviating symptoms of HG, they are not without potential risk. Both promethazine and metoclopramide have demonstrated a concern for drug-induced movement disorders, including tardive dyskinesia (Tan et al., 2010). Another option is ondansetron, a serotonin 5-HT3 inhibitor. While studies have demonstrated ondansetron to be effective in reducing symptoms of HG, it has been shown to prolong the QT interval, especially in patients with hypokalemia or other electrolyte imbalances (Freedman et al., 2014). Several recent studies have also shown a slight increase in teratogenic effects, so caution should be used with ondansetron during the first 10 weeks of gestation (Picot et al., 2020). Knowing that HG often affects electrolyte levels, ondansetron should only be used with extreme caution. Further treatment options are limited for individuals who do not respond adequately to these medications.

Table 40.3 Pharmacologic Measures to Relieve Hyperemesis Symptoms

Medication	Class/dose	Comments/side effects
Mild-to-moderate HG symptoms		
Doxylamine/pyridoxine	Antihistamine (12.5 mg q hs) + Vitamin B6 (50 mg bid)	Drowsiness; dry mouth
Dimenhydrinate	Antihistamine 25–50 mg q4–6h	Drowsiness; dry mouth
Diphenhydramine	Antihistamine 25–50 mg q4–6h	Drowsiness; dry mouth
Promethazine	Dopamine Antagonist 25 mg q8h	Drowsiness; dizziness; excitation; rash; photophobia; muscle weakness
Ondansetron	Serotonin 5-HT3 Inhibitor 4 mg q8h	Anxiety; dizziness; constipation; confusion; headache; insomnia
Metoclopramide	Dopamine Antagonist 10 mg q8h	Dystonia; drowsiness; restlessness; insomnia; dry mouth; diarrhea
Refractory HG symptoms		
Corticosteroids	PO taper/IV at various dosages	Mechanism and efficacy uncertain

Source: Adapted from ACOG (2018).

If outpatient oral medications remain ineffective, intravenous (IV) antiemetics and rehydration are important therapies in the management of people with HG. IV hydration should be used in patients who are showing signs of dehydration. IV solutions with dextrose and vitamins are recommended and can help patients feel less nauseated, though they should receive thiamine replacement prior to receiving dextrose to offset the risk of Wernicke's encephalopathy (Castillo & Phillippi, 2015; Meggs et al., 2020). Thiamine replacement is recommended with a 100-mg dose when IV fluid hydration begins, followed by 100 mg each day for two to three days (Smith et al., 2022). Other vitamins and minerals, such as potassium, magnesium, calcium, and phosphorus, should be carefully monitored and replaced if serum values are low (Smith et al., 2022). It is recommended that food is withdrawn until dehydration is corrected and vomiting is reduced. Subsequent food reintroduction is carried out gradually. When first reintroducing food, the diet should consist of bananas, rice, applesauce, and toast (BRAT diet). A more regular diet can be advanced as tolerated, ensuring that adequate protein is included to prevent nausea (Smith et al., 2022). Sleep disturbances often accompany HG, and adequate rest should be promoted with environmental management or brief pharmacological therapy if needed.

Patients with HG are often managed on an outpatient basis, even those on IV therapy. For severe and unrelenting symptoms, hospital admission can be required. **Total parenteral nutrition** (TPN) can improve symptoms in patients with refractory cases of HG. Enteric feeding for people diagnosed with HG is associated with improved maternal weight gain and fetal outcomes (Stokke et al., 2015). There is conflicting evidence on the use of corticosteroids. A tapered dose of an oral corticosteroid or short IV course may improve symptoms; however, this has typically been used as a last-resort therapy. Concern for teratogenic effects, such as oral clefts, has been demonstrated by several studies, so corticosteroids should be avoided during the first 10 weeks of the pregnancy (ACOG, 2018).

Summary

A variety of treatment options may be tried before the patient experiences relief from HG symptoms, and good communication with the clinician is key. Evidence suggests that a protocol including ongoing telehealth support can be beneficial in reducing hospital admissions (McParlin et al., 2016a).

Resources for Clients and Families

American College of Obstetrician and Gynecologists at http://www.acog.org/Patients/FAQs/Morning-Sickness-Nausea-and-Vomiting-of-Pregnancy
Hyperemesis Education & Research Foundation, Family and Friends https://www.hyperemesis.org/who-we-help/family-friends

Resource for Healthcare Providers

Hyperemesis Education & Research Foundation, Healthcare Providers at https://www.hyperemesis.org/who-we-help/healthcare-providers/

References

American College of Obstetricians and Gynecologists (ACOG). (2018). Nausea and vomiting of pregnancy. Practice bulletin no. 189. *Obstetrics & Gynecology, 131*, e15–e30.

Boelig, R. C., Barton, S. J., Saccone, G., Kelly, A. J., Edwards, S. J., & Berghella, V. (2016). Interventions for treating hyperemesis gravidarum. *The Cochrane Database of Systematic Reviews*, (5), CD010607.

Castillo, M. J., & Phillippi, J. C. (2015). Hyperemesis gravidarum. *Journal of Perinatal and Neonatal Nursing, 29*(1), 12–22.

Dean, C., Bannigan, K., & Marsden, J. (2018a). Reviewing the effect of hyperemesis gravidarum on women's lives and mental health. *British Journal of Midwifery, 26*(2), 109–119.

Dean, C. R., Bruin, C. M., O'Hara, M. E., Roseboom, T. J., Leeflang, M. M., Spijker, R., & Painter, R. C. (2020). The chance of recurrence of hyperemesis gravidarum: A systematic review. *European Journal of Obstetrics & Gynecology and Reproductive Biology: X, 5*, 100105. https://doi.org/10.1016/j.eurox.2019.100105

Dean, C. R., Shemar, M., Ostrowski, G. A. U., & Painter, R. C. (2018b). Management of severe pregnancy sickness and hyperemesis gravidarum. *BMJ, 363*. https://doi.org/10.1136/bmj.k5000

Fezjo, M. S., Trovik, J., Grooten, I. J., Sridharan, K., Rosenboom, T. J., Vikanes, A., Painter, R. C., & Mullin, P. M. (2019). Nausea and vomiting of pregnancy and hyperemesis gravidarum. *Nature Reviews, 5*, 62. https://doi.org/10.1038/s41572-019-0110-3

Fiaschi, L., Nelson-Piercy, C., & Tata, L. J. (2016). Hospital admission for hyperemesis gravidarum: A nationwide study of occurrence, reoccurrence and risk factors among 8.2 million pregnancies. *Human Reproduction, 31*(8), 1675–1684.

Freedman, S. B., Uleryk, E., Rumantir, M., & Finkelstein, Y. (2014). Ondansetron and the risk of cardiac arrhythmias: A systematic review and postmarketing analysis. *Annals of Emergency Medicine, 64*(1), 19–25.

Getahun, D., Fassett, M. J., Jacobsen, S. J., Xiang, A. H., Takhar, H. S., Wing, D. A., & Peltier, M. R. (2019). Autism spectrum disorders in children exposed in utero to hyperemesis gravidarum. *American Journal of Perinatology, 38*, 265–272.

Heitmann, K., Nordeng, H., Havnen, G. C., Solheimsnes, A., & Holst, L. (2017). The burden of nausea and vomiting during pregnancy: Severe impacts on quality of life, daily life functioning and willingness to become pregnant again—Results from a cross-sectional study. *BMC Pregnancy and Childbirth, 17*(75). https://doi.org/10.1186/s12884-017-1249-0

Kender, E. E., Yuksel, G., Ger, C., & Ozer, U. (2015). Eating attitudes, depression and anxiety levels of patients with hyperemesis gravidarum hospitalized in an obstetrics and gynecology clinic. *Dusunen Adam The Journal of Psychiatry and Neurological Sciences, 28*(2), 119–126.

Koren, G., Clark, S., Hankins, G. D., Cantis, S. N., Umans, J. G., Caritis, S. N., Umans, J. G., Miodovnik, M., Mattson, D. R., & Matok, I. (2015). Maternal safety of the delayed-release doxylamine and pyridoxine combination for nausea and vomiting of pregnancy; a randomized placebo controlled trial. *BMC Pregnancy and Childbirth, 15*(59).

Koren, G., Piwko, C., Ahn, E., Boskovic, R., Maltepe, C., Einarson, A., Navios, Y., & Ungar, W. J. (2005). Validation studies of the pregnancy unique-quantification of emesis (PUQE) scores. *Journal of Obstetrics & Gynaecology, 25*(3), 241–244.

London, V., Grube, S., Sherer, D. M., & Abulafia, O. (2017). Hyperemesis gravidarum: A review of recent literature. *Pharmacology, 100*, 161–171.

MacGibbon, K. W. (2020). Hyperemesis gravidarum: Strategies to improve outcomes. *Journal of Infusion Nursing, 43*(2), 78–96.

MacGibbon, K. W., Kim, S., Mullin, P. M., & Fezjo, M. S. (2021). Hyperemesis level prediction (HELP score) identifies patients with indicators of severe disease: A validation study. *Geburtshilfe und Frauenheilkunde, 81*(1), 90–98.

Magtira, A., Paik Schoenberg, F., MacGibbon, K., Tabsh, K., & Fejzo, M. S. (2015). Psychiatric factors do not affect recurrence risk of hyperemesis gravidarum. *Journal of Obstetrics and Gynaecology Research, 41*(4), 512–516.

Maslin, K., Shaw, V., Brown, A., Dean, C., & Shawe, J. (2021). What is known about the nutritional intake of women with hyperemesis gravidarum?: A scoping review. *European Journal of Obstetrics & Gynecology and Reproductive Biology, 257*, 76–83.

Matthews, A., Haas, D. M., O'Mathuna, D. P., & Dowswell, T. (2015). Interventions for nausea and vomiting in early pregnancy. *The Cochrane Database of Systematic Reviews, 9*, CD007575.

McParlin, C., Carrick-Sen, D., Steen, I. N., & Robson, S. C. (2016a). Hyperemesis in pregnancy study: A pilot randomised controlled trial of midwife-led outpatient care. *European Journal of Obstetrics Gynecology and Reproductive Biology, 200*, 6–10.

McParlin, C., O'Donnell, A., Robson, S. C., Beyer, F., Moloney, E., Bryant, A., Bradley, J., Muirhead, C. R., Nelson-Piercy, C., Newbury-Birch, D., Norman, J., Shaw, C., Simpson, E., Swallow, B., Yates, L., & Vale, L. (2016b). Treatments for hyperemesis gravidarum and nausea and vomiting in pregnancy: A systematic review. *Journal of the American Medical Association, 316*(13), 1392–1401.

Meggs, W. J., Lee, S. K., & Parker-Cote, J. N. (2020). Wernicke encephalopathy associated with hyperemesis gravidarum. *American Journal of Emergency Medicine, 38*(3), 690.e3–690.e5.

Mitchell-Jones, N., Gallos, I., Farren, J., Tobias, A., Bottomley, C., & Bourne, T. (2016). Psychological morbidity associated with hyperemesis gravidarum: A systematic review and meta-analysis. *BJOG: An International Journal of Obstetrics and Gynaecology, 124*, 20–30.

Mullin, P. M., Bray, A., Schoenberg, F., MacGibbon, K. W., Romero, R., Goodwin, T. M., & Fejzo, M. S. (2011). Prenatal exposure to hyperemesis gravidarum linked to increased risk of psychological and behavioral disorders in adulthood. *Journal of Developmental Origins of Health and Disease, 2*(04), 200–204.

Ng, Q. X., Venkatanarayanan, N., de Deyn, M. L. Z. Q., Ho, C. Y. X., Mo, Y., & Yeo, W. (2017). A meta-analysis of the association between *Helicobacter pylori* (*H. pylori*) infection and hyperemesis gravidarum. *Helocobacter*, e12455. https://doi.org/10.1111/hel.12455

Nurmi, M., Rautava, P., Gissler, M., Vahlberg, T., & Polo-Kantola, P. (2020). Incidence and risk factors of hyperemesis gravidarum: A national register-based study in Finland, 2005–2017. *Acta Obstetrica et Gynecologica Scandinavica, 99*, 1003–1013.

Peled, Y., Melamed, N., Hiersch, L., Hadar, E., Wiznitzer, A., & Yogev, Y. (2013). Pregnancy outcome in hyperemesis gravidarum—The role of fetal gender. *Journal of Maternal-Fetal and Neonatal Medicine, 26*(17), 1753–1757.

Picot, C., Berard, A., Grenet, G., Ripoche, E., Cucherat, M., & Cottin, J. (2020). Risk of malformation after ondansetron in pregnancy: An updated systematic review and meta-analysis. *Birth Defects Research, 112*(13), 996–1013.

Power, Z., Campbell, M., Kilcoyne, P., Kitchener, H., & Waterman, H. (2010). The hyperemesis impact of symptoms questionnaire: Development and validation of a clinical tool. *International Journal of Nursing Studies, 47*(1), 67–77.

Smith, J.A., Fox, J.A. & Clark, S.M. (2022). *Nausea and vomiting of pregnancy: Treatment and outcome.* UpToDate. Retrieved February 24, 2022. https://www.uptodate.com/contents/nausea-and-vomiting-of-pregnancy-treatment-and-outcome

Stokke, G., Gjelsvik, B. L., Flaatten, K. T., Birkeland, E., Flaatten, H., & Trovik, J. (2015). Hyperemesis gravidarum, nutritional treatment by nasogastric tube feeding: A 10-year retrospective cohort study. *Acta Obstetricia et Gynecologica Scandinavica, 94*(4), 359–367.

Tan, P. C., Khine, P. P., Vallikkannu, N., & Omar, S. Z. (2010). Promethazine compared to metoclopramide for hyperemesis gravidarum: A randomized controlled trial. *Obstetrics and Gynecology, 115*(5), 975–981.

Van den Heuvel, E., Goossens, M., Vanderhaegen, H., Sun, H. X., & Buntinx, F. (2016). Effect of acustimulation on nausea and vomiting and on hyperemesis in pregnancy: A systematic review of Western and Chinese literature. *BMC Complementary and Alternative Medicine, 16*(1), 13.

41

Abdominal Pain

Karen Trister Grace

Prenatal and Postnatal Care: A Person-Centered Approach, Third Edition. Edited by Karen Trister Grace, Cindy L. Farley, Noelene K. Jeffers, and Tanya Tringali.
© 2024 John Wiley & Sons Ltd. Published 2024 by John Wiley & Sons Ltd.
Companion website: www.wiley.com/go/grace/prenatal

Relevant Terms

Appendicitis—acute inflammation of the appendix; may be associated with complications such as gangrene, perforation, or abscess formation

Biophysical profile—fetal evaluation using ultrasound to assess for five factors: fetal movement, fetal tone, fetal breathing movements, fetal heart rate reactivity, and quantity of amniotic fluid

Kleihauer–Betke test—used to determine the presence of fetal hemoglobin, alerting the clinician to consider if RhoGAM is indicated as well as the appropriate dose

McBurney's point—the point on the lower right quadrant of the abdomen at which tenderness is maximal in cases of acute appendicitis; located 1.5–2 in from the anterior superior iliac spine on a straight line to the umbilicus

---

Introduction

Abdominal pain or discomfort is a common occurrence in pregnancy. A report of abdominal pain in pregnancy should be thoroughly investigated. Abdominal pain or discomfort in pregnancy is most often due to physiologic discomforts of pregnancy, and these conditions should be considered first in a differential diagnosis when the pain is mild to moderate. Information about comfort measures for these common conditions is found in Chapter 15, *Common Discomforts in Pregnancy*. Although normal pregnancy changes explain many cases of abdominal pain, the possibility of pathology should always be considered. A delay in diagnosis of pathological causes of abdominal pain could be life-threatening. Other sources of abdominal pain include gastroenteritis, intrahepatic cholestasis of pregnancy, and gall bladder disease, which are covered in Chapter 51, *Gastrointestinal Disorders*.

Evaluation

Evaluation of abdominal pain includes collection of thorough subjective and objective data. Obtaining an accurate history is the critical first step in determining the etiology of a patient's problem. Use the client interview to begin generating a list of differential diagnoses. Differential diagnoses to consider in the assessment of abdominal pain are listed in Table 41.1.

Health equity key points

- Implicit bias can affect evaluation and management of patients of color or from other marginalized groups who present with pain.
- The generational and lifetime experience of racism and discrimination is a direct cause of birth outcome disparities.

OLD CAARTS mnemonic

O = Onset: when and how the pain started
L = Location: Specific location of the pain. Can you put a finger on it?
D = Duration: How long does it last?
C = Characteristics: What is the pain like? (cramping, aching, stabbing, burning, tingling, itching, and so on)
A = Alleviating or aggravating factors: What makes the pain better (medication, position change, heat) and what makes it worse (specific activity, stress)?
A = Associated symptoms: Gynecologic (dyspareunia, vaginal discharge, or bleeding), gastrointestinal (constipation, diarrhea), genitourinary (dysuria, urgency, incontinence), and neurological (specific nerve involvement)
R = Radiation: Does the pain move to other body areas?
T = Temporal: What time of day is it worse and better?
S = Severity: On a scale of 1–10.

The use of "OLD CAARTS" can be helpful when collecting a history of pain symptoms. In addition to an OLD CAARTS assessment, other components of the history should include presence of fetal movement, contractions, vaginal bleeding or discharge, a recent diet history, any

Table 41.1 Differential Diagnosis of Abdominal Pain in Pregnancy

Obstetric causes	Nonobstetric causes
Chorioamnionitis (Chapter 34)	Abdominal trauma
Ectopic pregnancy (Chapter 33)	Appendicitis
Labor (Chapter 28)	Bowel obstruction
Placental abruption (Chapter 33)	Gall bladder disease (Chapter 51)
Preeclampsia/HELLP syndrome (Chapter 36)	Gastroenteritis (Chapter 51)
Preterm labor (Chapter 35)	Inflammatory bowel disease
Common discomforts of pregnancy (Chapter 15)	Nephrolithiasis (Chapter 50)
Spontaneous or threatened abortion (Chapter 33)	Pancreatitis
Uterine rupture	Peptic ulcer
	Pyelonephritis

bowel or bladder changes, change in or new onset of nausea or vomiting, exposure to any sick contacts, recent travel, fever, dysuria, and history of abdominal trauma such as fall, motor vehicle accident, or violence.

The abdominal assessment should include fetal heart tones, Leopold maneuvers, palpation for contractions, location of pain, abdominal guarding, overt or rebound tenderness, and the presence of any visible signs and symptoms of trauma. Careful documentation of any signs of trauma is vital, even if the patient denies trauma. When trauma or violence is suspected as the etiology of abdominal pain, the clinician should be aware that the medical record may ultimately be used in legal proceedings, even if the patient is not currently ready to disclose the source of their injuries. Documentation should include results of intimate partner violence (IPV) screening, lethality assessment if positive (Campbell et al., 2009), and detailed, objective description of the signs of trauma (see Chapter 26, *Violence and Trauma in the Perinatal Period*).

Objective data for diagnosis include vital signs, complete blood count (CBC), urine analysis, pancreatic enzymes, liver enzymes, a **Kleihauer–Betke test** in cases of abdominal trauma, fetal nonstress testing or **biophysical profile** depending on gestational age, ultrasound, computed tomography (CT), magnetic resonance imaging (MRI), and other exams as determined in collaboration with a consulting physician. If a pathological etiology to the report of abdominal pain is suspected, immediate consultation and possible referral of care to the hospital for physician evaluation is indicated. Normal physiologic and anatomic changes associated with pregnancy and the enlarging uterus may obscure or mimic some objective signs such as guarding, hydronephrosis, bloating, vomiting, and leukocytosis, which commonly are associated with acute abdominal emergencies (Zachariah et al., 2019).

Changes in blood volume, cardiac output, and respiratory rate can delay clinical symptoms of blood loss and hypovolemic shock (Woodhead et al., 2019).

Preterm labor and threatened abortion should be ruled out when presented with a report of abdominal pain in pregnancy, depending on gestational age. Signs and symptoms that suggest preterm labor include rhythmic abdominal pain, pressure, or low back pain after 22 weeks of gestation, leaking of amniotic fluid, or vaginal bleeding. If preterm labor is suspected, it must be ruled out before considering other etiologies of the abdominal pain.

Implicit bias among healthcare providers is as common as it is among the general population (Fitzgerald & Hurst, 2017) and may affect evaluation and management of patients of color or from other marginalized groups who present with pain. The generational and lifetime experience of racism and discrimination is a direct cause of birth outcome disparities for people of color (Alhusen et al., 2017). Recognizing these connections and taking active steps to ensure care is not impacted by bias or discrimination are essential components of management of abdominal pain in pregnancy.

Appendicitis

Appendicitis is an inflammation of the appendix, a 3.5-in-long pouch of tissue located at the junction of the large and small intestine. The incidence of appendicitis in pregnancy is low, approximately 0.5–2 per 1000 women, but is nonetheless the most common indication for nonobstetric surgeries during pregnancy, accounting for 25% of such surgeries (Weinstein et al., 2020; Zachariah et al., 2019). Risks associated with acute appendicitis in pregnancy include bowel perforation, abscess formation, and peritonitis (Snyder et al., 2018; Zachariah et al., 2019). The maternal mortality rate is as high as 4%, while fetal death is estimated at 43% in pregnancies complicated by a perforated appendix (Snyder et al., 2018; Zachariah et al., 2019). Additionally, perforated appendix with subsequent inflammatory response often leads to uterine contractions and preterm labor. Appendicitis occurs at a lower rate in the pregnant population as compared to the nonpregnant population, but the chance of rupture of the appendix is significantly higher during pregnancy (57% as compared to 4–19% of cases in nonpregnant people), indicating the need for rapid diagnosis of appendicitis during pregnancy (Weinstein et al., 2020). However, accurate diagnosis is critical, as there is a higher rate of unnecessary appendectomies in pregnancy as well (23–37% of cases in pregnancy, compared to 14–18% of cases outside of pregnancy), and also a higher rate of fetal loss when appendicitis ruptures or develops an abscess (Ali et al., 2020). These findings highlight the difficulty with diagnosing appendicitis in pregnancy. Both negative appendectomies and appendicitis itself are associated with complications such as preterm birth, fetal demise, low birth weight, and congenital anomalies (when diagnosed in the first trimester) (Aggenbach et al., 2015; Bouyou et al., 2015; Flexer et al., 2014; Weinstein et al., 2020). In some cases, conservative management of appendicitis with antibiotics may be considered, but the high rate of fetal demise associated with ruptured appendix should also guide management (Zachariah et al., 2019).

The classic presentation of abdominal pain in appendicitis is a sharp mid-abdominal pain increasing over time, becoming more localized to the right lower quadrant, and a report of nausea, vomiting, and decreased appetite. However, pregnant individuals may present with more generalized pain located in the mid- or upper-right side of the abdomen, significant heartburn, bowel irregularity, flatulence, malaise, urinary symptoms, or diarrhea.

Vital signs, including temperature and hydration status, should be evaluated by assessing mucous membranes, skin turgor, and orthostatic changes; fetal heart tones are documented. Abnormal vital signs, such as tachycardia and fever, can indicate pain and infection. Abdominal palpation may reveal rebound tenderness at **McBurney's point** and signs of an acute abdomen (such as abdominal pain with coughing and referred pain felt in one side of the abdomen when palpating the other). The appendix can move upward toward the costal margin during late pregnancy, leading to a shift in McBurney's point. Pain and tenderness are generally localized to the right side in either the upper or lower quadrant. Uterine tone and the presence of any contractions should be noted.

The diagnosis of appendicitis during pregnancy is not straightforward. Many of the symptoms of appendicitis can be easily confused with common pregnancy discomforts. General fatigue, mild or nonspecific right lower abdominal pain, nausea, vomiting, and decreased appetite are commonly reported in normal pregnancies but are also the presenting symptoms reported with appendicitis. Further complicating diagnosis is the fact that the physical location of the appendix may shift upward during pregnancy, and rebound tenderness and guarding may not be elicited in pregnant people with appendicitis, due to physiologic changes of pregnancy. Lab abnormalities, such as elevated white blood cells and C-reactive protein, may be seen with appendicitis, but may be normal despite appendicitis in pregnant people or may be elevated due to physiological changes in pregnancy (Aggenbach et al., 2015; Flexer et al., 2014). Ultrasound, CT, and MRI without contrast may be considered for diagnosis. If there is a concern of possible appendicitis, referral to a physician for definitive diagnosis and surgical management is indicated.

Abdominal Trauma

Trauma is the most common nonobstetric cause of death during the childbearing year, and occurs in about 6–8% of pregnant people (Brown & Mozurkewich, 2013), with a fetal loss rate as high as 70% (Zachariah et al., 2019) and double the risk of mortality of nonpregnant abdominal trauma victims (Greco et al., 2019). Trauma in pregnancy is most often caused by motor vehicle crashes (MVCs), falls, and violence, but trauma-related death in pregnancy is most often caused by homicide (Brown & Mozurkewich, 2013; Wallace et al., 2021). Less common causes of trauma in pregnancy include suicide, penetrating trauma, burns, animal bites, and toxic exposure (Brown & Mozurkewich, 2013; Mendez-Figueroa et al., 2013). Risk factors for trauma in pregnancy include substance abuse, younger age, and a history of IPV (Mirza et al., 2010).

MVCs cause the majority of trauma during pregnancy and are a leading cause of perinatal mortality (Greco et al., 2019). MVCs often result in blunt trauma with shearing forces on the uterus and placenta. This can lead to placental abruption, uterine rupture, and poor fetal outcomes (Greco et al., 2019). Deployment of air bags can cause trauma to the pregnant abdomen, even in an otherwise minor car accident, though there is evidence that air-bag deployment rarely results in placental abruption, especially when combined with seatbelt use (Greco et al., 2019). In many injury-causing MVCs involving pregnant people, the person was seated in the front seat, often without a safety restraint, and many involved the use of drugs and alcohol (Azar et al., 2015). This highlights the importance of discussing the proper use and positioning of seatbelts (Figure 41.1), and the effects of drug and

WHAT'S THE RIGHT WAY TO WEAR MY SEAT BELT?

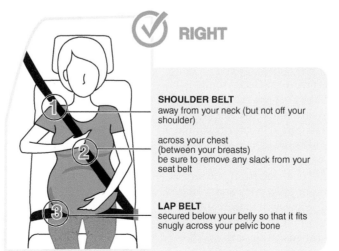

Figure 41.1   Proper positioning of seat belt in pregnancy. US Department of Transportation/Public Domain.

alcohol use with all patients during prenatal care visits. Because placental abruption can develop several hours after an accident, many clinicians will admit a pregnant person to the hospital for prolonged fetal monitoring post-MVC. While four hours of monitoring is generally sufficient after a minor accident, any more severe trauma or concerning signs such as contractions, possible rupture of membranes, bleeding, or tenderness would warrant 24 hours of monitoring or more (Greco et al., 2019).

Prevalence of IPV in pregnancy is vulnerable to underreporting and sensitivity of screening tools, but some studies report rates as high as 28% (Chisholm et al., 2017). Abusers may specifically target the abdomen, either in an attempt to harm the fetus or to conceal evidence of the abuse. IPV in pregnancy is associated with health behaviors, such as smoking or alcohol use, inadequate prenatal care, and poor maternal and fetal/neonatal outcomes (Auger et al., 2021; Chisholm et al., 2017). Clinicians should routinely screen all pregnant people for IPV at multiple points in pregnancy and provide appropriate counseling and referral (see Chapter 26, *Violence and Trauma in the Perinatal Period*).

Complications of trauma during pregnancy include cesarean birth, uterine rupture, placental abruption, preterm birth, direct fetal injury, pelvic fracture, amniotic fluid embolism, and death (Greco et al., 2019). Pregnant people with abdominal trauma should be referred for physician evaluation and management or comanagement as indicated by condition. Evaluation includes fetal assessment once the patient's status is stabilized, and possible hospital admission for prolonged monitoring. Rho(D) immune globulin can be indicated in Rh-negative people if fetomaternal hemorrhage is detected with a **Kleihauer–Betke test** (see Chapter 33, *Bleeding in Pregnancy*). Assessment should be initiated with the ability to intervene for birth if indicated and appropriate based on gestational age.

Cardiopulmonary Resuscitation in Pregnancy

Cardiopulmonary resuscitation (CPR) may be needed to save a pregnant trauma victim. Several modifications to standard CPR guidelines are recommended in the pregnant person. CPR is rarely required in pregnancy, but outcomes are similar to or better than outcomes outside of pregnancy (Bennett & Zelop, 2019). After 20 weeks of gestation, the uterus should be manually displaced to the left abdominally, to allow maximum aortocaval circulation, since left lateral position does not allow for the performance of quality chest compressions. The uterus should be pushed to the patient's left and upward, taking care not to apply downward pressure. Compression to ventilation rate and depth guidelines are not changed from outside of pregnancy. Defibrillation is safe in pregnancy and should be performed when indicated. Airway management and oxygenation are especially important in pregnancy. Fetal assessment should not be performed during active CPR as the focus should remain on maternal resuscitation and restoration of the pregnant person's pulse and blood

pressure with adequate oxygenation, and there is a theoretical electrocution risk with concurrent defibrillation (Bennett & Zelop, 2019). Evaluation of the fetal heart carries the risk of inhibiting or delaying resuscitation and monitoring, which then adversely affects the fetus. The Heimlich maneuver should be replaced with chest thrusts in the third trimester (Farinelli & Hameed, 2012).

Pancreatitis

Pancreatitis, an acute inflammatory condition, is rare in pregnancy and occurs most often in the third trimester and with multiparity (Cruciat et al., 2020). The most frequent cause of pancreatitis in pregnancy is cholelithiasis, followed by hyperlipidemia, and alcohol or medication use (Cruciat et al., 2020).

Symptoms of pancreatitis may include severe epigastric pain (often abrupt and may be relieved by leaning forward), anorexia, nausea with or without vomiting, and fever. Two of three criteria must be met for a diagnosis of pancreatitis; these include lab testing (serum amylase and/or lipase more than three times normal levels), cholelithiasis viewed on ultrasound, and severe epigastric pain (Cain et al., 2015; Mali, 2016). Though rare, risks and potential complications of pancreatitis in pregnancy are severe and include death, preterm birth, sepsis, shock, poor neonatal outcomes, and fetal demise (Cruciat et al., 2020; Gupta et al., 2022; O'Heney et al., 2021).

Cholecystectomy may be indicated in cholelithiasis-related pancreatitis, depending on gestational age. However, conservative management is usually effective, consisting of intravenous (IV) hydration, analgesics, and dietary changes such as decreased fat intake or bowel rest; hospitalization in intensive care may be indicated. See Chapter 51, *Gastrointestinal Disorders*, for the evaluation and treatment of cholelithiasis. Pregnant people with pancreatitis should be referred for physician evaluation and management or comanagement.

Resources for Healthcare Providers

CPR in pregnancy: http://www.cprcertificationonlinehq.com/cpr-pregnant-women-different-techniques-guidelines-resuscitation; www.australiawidefirstaid.com.au/resources/cpr-guide-pregnancy

Resources for Clients and Their Families

A consumer website on differentiating different types of abdominal pain during pregnancy: https://www.babycenter.com/pregnancy/your-body/cramps-during-pregnancy_204

References

Aggenbach, L., Zeeman, G. G., Cantineau, A. E. P., Gordijn, S. J., & Hofker, H. S. (2015). Impact of appendicitis during pregnancy: No delay in accurate diagnosis and treatment. *International Journal of Surgery, 15*, 84–89.

Alhusen, J. L., Bower, K. M., Epstein, E., & Sharps, P. (2017). Racial discrimination and adverse birth outcomes: An integrative review.

Journal of Midwifery & Women's Health, *61*(6), 707–720. https://doi.org/10.1111/jmwh.12490

Ali, A., Beckett, K., & Flink, C. (2020). Emergent MRI for acute abdominal pain in pregnancy—Review of common pathology and imaging appearance. *Emergency Radiology*, *27*(2), 205–214. https://doi.org/10.1007/s10140-019-01747-3

Auger, N., Low, N., Lee, G. E., Ayoub, A., & Luu, T. M. (2021). Pregnancy outcomes of women hospitalized for physical assault, sexual assault, and intimate partner violence. *Journal of Interpersonal Violence*, *37*(13-14). https://doi.org/10.1177/0886260520985496

Azar, T., Longo, C., Oddy, L., & Abenhaim, H. A. (2015). Motor vehicle collision-related accidents in pregnancy. *Journal of Obstetrics and Gynaecology Research*, *41*(9), 1370–1376.

Bennett, T. A., & Zelop, C. M. (2019). Cardiopulmonary resuscitation (CPR) in pregnancy. In J. P. Phelan, L. D. Pacheco, M. R. Foley, G. R. Saade, G. A. Dildy, & M. A. Belfort (Eds.), *Critical care obstetrics* (6th ed., pp. 183–191). Wiley. https://doi.org/10.1002/9781119129400.ch11

Bouyou, J., Gaujoux, S., Marcellin, L., Leconte, M., Goffinet, F., Chapron, C., & Dousset, B. (2015). Abdominal emergencies during pregnancy. *Journal of Visceral Surgery*, *152*(6), S105–S115.

Brown, S., & Mozurkewich, E. (2013). Trauma during pregnancy. *Obstetrics and Gynecology Clinics of North America*, *40*(1), 47–57.

Cain, M. A., Ellis, J., Vengrove, M. A., Wilcox, B., & Yankowitz, J. (2015). Gallstone and severe hypertriglyceride-induced pancreatitis in pregnancy. *Obstetrical & Gynecological Survey*, *70*(9), 577–583.

Campbell, J. C., Webster, D. W., & Glass, N. (2009). The danger assessment: validation of a lethality risk assessment instrument for intimate partner femicide. *Journal of Interpersonal Violence*, *24*, 653–674.

Chisholm, C. A., Bullock, L., Ferguson, J. E., & (Jef). (2017). Intimate partner violence and pregnancy: Epidemiology and impact. *American Journal of Obstetrics and Gynecology*, *217*(2), 141–144. https://doi.org/10.1016/j.ajog.2017.05.042

Cruciat, G., Nemeti, G., Goidescu, I., Anitan, S., & Florian, A. (2020). Hypertriglyceridemia triggered acute pancreatitis in pregnancy-diagnostic approach, management and follow-up care. *Lipids in Health and Disease*, *19*(2), 1–6. https://doi.org/10.1186/s12944-019-1180-7

Farinelli, C. K., & Hameed, A. B. (2012). Cardiopulmonary resuscitation in pregnancy. *Cardiology Clinics*, *30*(3), 453–461.

Fitzgerald, C., & Hurst, S. (2017). Implicit bias in healthcare professionals: A systematic review. *BMC Medical Ethics*, *18*(1). https://doi.org/10.1186/s12910-017-0179-8

Flexer, S. M., Tabib, N., & Peter, M. B. (2014). Suspected appendicitis in pregnancy. *The Surgeon*, *12*(2), 82–86.

Greco, P. S., Day, L. J., & Pearlman, M. D. (2019). Guidance for evaluation and management of blunt abdominal trauma in pregnancy. *Obstetrics and Gynecology*, *134*(6), 1343–1357. https://doi.org/10.1097/AOG.0000000000003585

Gupta, M., Liti, B., Barrett, C., Thompson, P. D., & Fernandez, A. B. (2022). Prevention and management of hypertriglyceridemia-induced acute pancreatitis during pregnancy: A systematic review. *The American Journal of Medicine*. https://doi.org/10.1016/j.amjmed.2021.12.006

Mali, P. (2016). Pancreatitis in pregnancy: Eetiology, diagnosis, treatment, and outcomes. *Hepatobiliary & Pancreatic Diseases International*, *15*(4), 434–438.

Mendez-Figueroa, H., Dahlke, J. D., Vrees, R. A., & Rouse, D. J. (2013). Trauma in pregnancy: An updated systematic review. *American Journal of Obstetrics & Gynecology*, *209*(1), 1–10.

Mirza, F., Devine, P., & Gaddipati, S. (2010). Trauma in pregnancy: A systematic approach. *American Journal of Perinatology*, *27*(7), 579–586.

O'Heney, J. L., Barnett, R. E., MacSwan, R. M., & Rasheed, A. (2021). Acute and chronic pancreatitis in pregnancy. *The Obstetrician & Gynaecologist*, *23*(2), 89–93. https://doi.org/10.1111/tog.12725

Snyder, M. J., Guthrie, M., & Cagle, S. (2018). Acute appendicitis: Efficient diagnosis and management. *American Family Physician*, *98*(1), 25–33.

Wallace, M., Gillispie-Bell, V., Cruz, K., Davis, K., & Vilda, D. (2021). Homicide during pregnancy and the postpartum period in the United States, 2018–2019. *Obstetrics & Gynecology*, *138*(5), 762–769. https://doi.org/10.1097/aog.0000000000004567

Weinstein, M. S., Feuerwerker, S., & Baxter, J. K. (2020). Appendicitis and cholecystitis in pregnancy. *Clinical Obstetrics and Gynecology*, *63*(2), 405–415. https://doi.org/10.1097/GRF.0000000000000529

Woodhead, N., Nkwam, O., Caddick, V., Morad, S., & Mylvaganam, S. (2019). Surgical causes of acute abdominal pain in pregnancy. *The Obstetrician & Gynaecologist*, *21*(1), 27–35. https://doi.org/10.1111/tog.12536

Zachariah, S. K., Fenn, M., Jacob, K., Arthungal, S. A., & Zachariah, S. A. (2019). Management of acute abdomen in pregnancy: Current perspectives. *International Journal of Women's Health*, *11*, 119–134. https://doi.org/10.2147/IJWH.S151501

42

Pregnancy after Infertility

Melicia Escobar and Ebony Marcelle

Relevant Terms

Assisted reproductive technologies (ARTs)—therapies in which both eggs and/or embryos and sperm are handled. These do not include treatments in which only the sperm are handled or only medications to induce ovulation are taken without the intention of retrieval

Collaborative or third-party-assisted reproduction—the use of either a sperm donor, egg donor, or gestational carrier to achieve pregnancy

Cryobanking—also known as sperm banking; a cryobank is a facility that collects and stores human sperm from a sperm donor for the purposes of future use in achieving pregnancy

Fertility—the ability to conceive and produce offspring

Gestational carrier or gestational surrogate—a person who carries a child for another couple, using their own egg and/or sperm or donor egg and/or sperm

Impaired fecundity—refers to difficulties becoming pregnant or carrying a pregnancy to term that does not meet criteria for a diagnosis of infertility

Infertility—a condition resulting in the inability to conceive and produce offspring after 12 months (or 6 months if over 35 years of age) or more of having unprotected intercourse or other assisted reproductive therapy; has known psychosocial and emotional ramifications

Fertility care—includes all care related to infertility prior to conception; this can range from counseling to testing to ART

Ovarian stimulation—a process wherein medication(s) are used to stimulate ovulation; may be used in conjunction with intrauterine insemination or *in vitro* fertilization

Primary infertility—a continuum that captures infertility having had no previous pregnancies; can be related to either sex in etiology

Recurrent pregnancy loss—having two or more failed pregnancies, distinct from infertility

Secondary infertility—a continuum that that captures infertility *after* having conceived in the past; can be related to either sex in etiology

Self-silencing—restriction of self-expression within important relationships out of concern for reprisal or in deference to the needs of others

Social infertility—the inability to conceive due to social or circumstantial factors, including being single or having a same-sex partner; grounded in the belief that reproduction is a human right

Subfertility—a term that can be used interchangeably with infertility

---

Introduction

Although the management of **infertility** is well researched and protocols for care are well defined, there is limited guidance for the provision of routine prenatal and postpartum care for those who have a history of infertility when pregnancy is finally achieved. Individuals who have experienced infertility and ultimately become pregnant will transition to prenatal care. In order to provide the most holistic care, the clinician must consider the unique context and course of the infertility, any causative pathophysiology, and resulting perinatal concerns and psychosocial implications, in addition to the common aspects of pregnancy, birth, and the postpartum experience. The care of pregnant people with a history of infertility is the focus of this chapter.

Prevalence of Infertility

Defining the scope of **impaired fecundity** and infertility is challenging given the wide range of definitions and measurements among researchers. United States data indicates that approximately 15% of women trying to become pregnant experience difficulty achieving that goal (Centers for Disease Control and Prevention (CDC), 2017; Chandra et al., 2014). The majority of these cases are **primary infertility** related to either sex in etiology. Though not all people who are infertile desire pregnancy,

Prenatal and Postnatal Care: A Person-Centered Approach, Third Edition. Edited by Karen Trister Grace, Cindy L. Farley, Noelene K. Jeffers, and Tanya Tringali.
© 2024 John Wiley & Sons Ltd. Published 2024 by John Wiley & Sons Ltd.
Companion website: www.wiley.com/go/grace/prenatal

Health equity key points

- Despite a pervasive heteronormative perspective for framing infertility, lesbian, gay, transgender, and gender-diverse individuals desire parenthood and may also experience infertility care leading up to their pregnancies.
- Being attuned to the partnering arrangements and desired terminology within the family will aid the clinician in delivering optimally inclusive care.
- Black women are twice as likely as White women to experience infertility, yet they are only half as likely to access **fertility** services.
- Disparity in infertility care is attributed to: implicit bias among clinicians including the stereotype of hyperfertility among Black women, lack of understanding of unique physiological impacts of racism (e.g., Weathering Theory), limited or restricted access to timely and appropriate infertility services and treatments, lack of representation within infertility care, lack of meaningful data collection and research to drive change in care, feelings of isolation and shame, and fear or aversion due to mistrust in the medical system stemming from a deep history of structural racism.

---

approximately 10% of women report that they or their partner has sought some form of infertility-related healthcare in hopes of achieving pregnancy (Weigel et al., 2020). Ultimately, birth rates vary depending on the level of intervention necessary to achieve pregnancy, age of the person, and etiology of infertility (CDC, American Society for Reproductive Medicine, and the Society for Assisted Reproductive Technology, 2021; Resolve, 2022; Herbert et al., 2012). Additionally, sexual and gender minorities and unpartnered individuals may face challenges achieving pregnancy defined as **social infertility** (Lo & Campo-Engelstein, 2018). This term describes a type of infertility that, rather than having a physiological etiology, is caused by social or circumstantial factors.

Context and Course of Infertility

Infertility is often conceptualized as a "couples" problem, with infertility in the person with a uterus receiving the most attention in terms of diagnosis, treatment, and care. In reality, this type of infertility accounts for up to 40% of infertility and can occur in combination with sperm-related factors. It is important to remember that nearly 50% of infertility cases are a result of an issue related to the sperm (Ramalingam et al., 2014). Infertility can also affect those opting to be single parents (Koroma & Stewart, 2012).

Despite a pervasive heteronormative perspective for framing infertility, lesbian, gay, transgender, and gender-diverse individuals desire parenthood and may also experience infertility care leading up to their pregnancies (Ellis et al., 2015; Hayman & Wilkes, 2017; Koroma & Stewart, 2012). Being attuned to the partnering arrangements and desired terminology within the family will aid the clinician in delivering optimally inclusive care

(Markus et al., 2010). Exclusionary care may promote or deepen preexisting feelings of isolation and have adverse psychosocial ramifications internally, in the partnership, and in the transition to parenthood (Babore et al., 2017; McManus et al., 2006).

People of color are also affected by infertility. Studies show that Black women are twice as likely as White women to experience infertility, yet they are only half as likely to access **fertility** services (Chandra et al., 2014). This disparity in care has been attributed to several factors: implicit bias among clinicians including the stereotype of hyperfertility, lack of understanding of unique physiological impacts of racism (e.g., Weathering Theory), limited or restricted access to timely and appropriate infertility services and treatments, lack of representation within infertility care, lack of meaningful data collection and research to drive change in care, feelings of isolation and shame, and fear or aversion due to mistrust in the medical system stemming from a deep history of structural racism (Ceballo et al., 2015; Ibrahim & Zore, 2020; Wiltshire et al., 2020). These factors are also experienced by people of color when receiving prenatal and birth care. Perpetuating these barriers can adversely affect perinatal health outcomes.

Pregnant people with a history of infertility or **subfertility** may have been engaged in **fertility care** for months to years. By the time pregnancy is diagnosed, they will likely have undergone testing and treatment, invasive physical examinations and/or procedures, and intensive follow-up with a single or small group of infertility specialists who are acutely aware of their history and journey. Once the pregnancy is established, the person transitions to routine prenatal care with a prenatal care provider, typically between 8 and 10 weeks of gestation. As a result, they can experience a "gap" in their care with less frequent, shorter visits with varied clinicians who may be unaware of their complete infertility history (French et al., 2015; Warmelink et al., 2015; Stevenson et al., 2016). The paradoxical feeling of now having a "normal" pregnancy while relinquishing the real or perceived high-risk nature of their preconception care can be a stressful transition. While some people experience relief and joy with their new pregnant state, others can feel a lack of reassurance or inability to express their fear or anxiety about the pregnancy (French et al., 2015; Warmelink et al., 2015). Further psychosocial implications of a perceived gap will be addressed later in this chapter. Table 42.1 highlights ways in which clinicians can effectively bridge the gap while providing inclusionary care.

Prior Fertility Treatments

A complete history will include the details of the infertility care and treatments the patient has undergone. Understanding what each entails will help bridge the gap from infertility care. It may also offer clues as to the degree of anxiety or other psychosocial impacts, as there is a correlation with both time spent in infertility care and also the type of treatment received (Stevenson & Sloane, 2017; Younger et al., 2015). Table 42.2 outlines a range of infertility care that patients may have experienced. Various

Table 42.1 Strategies for Bridging the Gap From Fertility Care to Routine Prenatal Care

- Examine your own attitudes and assumptions regarding family building.
- Understand that distress from infertility may likely persist.
- Review the health records with special attention to the arc of their infertility care.
- Initiate discussions about emotional response to infertility and pregnancy.
- Create space for acknowledging experience with infertility and emotions at each visit.
- Validate and normalize feelings, draw on assets they bring into the pregnancy, and reframe.
- Normalize aspects of the pregnancy where possible.
- Understand that a desire for low intervention care during pregnancy and birth may exist in response to interventive fertility treatments and interventions.
- Do not encourage sentiments of gratitude regarding the pregnancy or parenthood.
- Actively solicit information about pregnancy discomforts.
- Consider more frequent prenatal visits and increased access to care.
- Reassure the patient that clinicians will continue to check in, as feelings about being pregnant may shift as the pregnancy progresses.
- Allow extra time during prenatal visits.
- Encourage participation in prenatal and/or childbirth classes.
- Encourage continued participation in support groups.
- Include, engage, and validate the role of partners and others involved in care, including clarifying terminology to be used during the pregnancy (i.e., partner, co-parent, co-mother, etc.).
- Consider multiple and intersectional identities that each patient has, each of which may manifest differently at different times, to make care individualized and inclusive.

Source: Adapted from French et al. (2015) and Warmelink et al. (2015).

levels of intervention are associated with high out-of-pocket cost that can also impact stress. For example, one cycle of *in vitro* fertilization (IVF) can cost more than $12,000 (Macaluso et al., 2010; Weigel et al., 2020).

Preexisting Conditions and Perinatal Issues

The causes of infertility may have implications for prenatal, intrapartum, and postnatal care. Client age over 35 years and elevated body mass index (BMI) are independent contributing factors to infertility. However, one or both may further impair fertility in the presence of sex-specific etiologies (Koroma & Stewart, 2012; Luke, 2017). Unexplained infertility, wherein a cause cannot be identified, varies greatly, ranging from 8% to 28%. While there may be subclinical causes in these cases, age and individual factors account for much of this variability (Gelbaya et al., 2014). Similarly, in cases where infertility is unexplained, once pregnant, the comorbidities of advanced age and elevated BMI can also increase risk during pregnancy.

A reevaluation of all factors contributing to infertility experienced prior to pregnancy, as well as factors resulting from fertility care (e.g., multiple gestation), with the offer of continued periodic management by specialists can allow for continuity of care. This may necessitate collaborative care or comanagement with other specialists in a multidisciplinary approach. Table 42.3 lists considerations for prenatal care, intrapartum, and postnatal care related to various common etiologies that cause subfertility.

Pharmacologic Considerations

The clinician must take into consideration medications taken during the infertile period and currently. Nearly half of women treated for infertility in their lifetime report

Table 42.2 Summary of Fertility Care

Counseling	Basic counseling and reassurance are typically offered during the infertile period; as many as 74% of those identified as infertile will receive some form of counseling (Practice Committee of the American Society for Reproductive Medicine, 2015; Macaluso et al., 2010; Domar, 2015).
Fertility awareness	Couples are given education and tools to track cycles, monitor ovulation, and record basal body temperature (Koroma & Stewart, 2012); this also includes understanding individual and other risk factors, as well as societal and cultural factors involved with family planning and building (Zegers-Hochschild et al., 2017).
Diagnostic testing	Both sexes may undergo a variety of testing, including semen analysis, blood work, genetic testing, imaging studies, hysterosalpingogram, or laparoscopy (Koroma & Stewart, 2012; Practice Committee of the American Society for Reproductive Medicine, 2015).
Lifestyle modifications	The person may be engaged in several lifestyle alterations, including weight loss through diet and exercise, or weight gain, smoking cessation, etc. (Koroma & Stewart, 2012).
Complementary and alternative modalities (CAM)	The person may have used or be currently using CAM measures, including acupuncture, herbals, and supplements, or relaxation techniques (Feng et al., 2021; Koroma & Stewart, 2012; O'Reilly et al., 2014; Smith & Cochrane, 2009). They may have used these modalities alone or in conjunction with other infertility treatments.
Ovarian stimulation	Nearly half of people with infertility receive medications such as Clomid, Letrozole, and/or exogenous hormones in order to induce ovulation with the intention of timed intercourse, insemination, or ART (Koroma & Stewart, 2012; Practice Committee of the American Society for Reproductive Medicine, 2008; Macaluso et al., 2010; Zegers-Hochschild et al., 2017).

{Complex Prenatal and Postnatal Conditions

Table 42.2 (*Continued*)

Insemination	Home or self-insemination	This involves either partner or self-insertion of sperm into the vagina via needleless syringe. It is simple, no- to low-cost, and can promote comfort and autonomy. The risk of STI transmission is slightly higher if the sperm is unwashed (Markus et al., 2010).
	Intracervical insemination (ICI) and Intrauterine insemination (IUI)	Both ICI and IUI involve collection and washing of semen and then placing the concentrated sperm either in the cervix or uterine body, respectively (Koroma & Stewart, 2012; Markus et al., 2010). 13% will have utilized this method (Macaluso et al., 2010).
Assisted reproductive technology (ART)	*In vitro* fertilization (IVF)	About 3% of women receiving fertility care will have experienced some form of ART (Macaluso et al., 2010). IVF involves fertilization of an egg with sperm after extraction from the ovary and then placing the resulting embryo(s) in the uterus (CDC, ASRM, & SART, 2016).
	Gamete intrafallopian transfer (GIFT)	In this rarely used method, unfertilized egg and sperm are placed in the fallopian tubes via laparoscopy (CDC, ASRM, & SART, 2021).
	Zygote intrafallopian transfer (ZIFT)	In this method, extracted eggs are fertilized and the zygotes are placed into the fallopian tubes via laparoscopy (CDC, ASRM, and SART, 2021).
Intracytoplasmic sperm injection (ICSI)	This technique, increasingly used in conjunction with IVF, is particularly beneficial in cases of sperm-production related infertility. It involves injecting a single sperm into an extracted egg (Boulet et al., 2015).	
Collaborative or third-party-assisted reproduction	Sperm donation	Fresh donor sperm may come from a known donor, results in higher rates of conception and is a low-cost method; however, it may pose a theoretical risk for STIs due to unwashed sperm (Markus et al., 2010). Frozen donor sperm may come from either a known or unknown donor. **Cryobanking** has associated cost and carries the benefit of legal autonomy; however, it may take longer to conceive, as freezing and thawing can adversely affect essential characteristics of the sperm (Markus et al., 2010).
	Oocyte donation	Donor oocytes, or eggs, may be fertilized and/or simply implanted through ART. The person may be the recipient of a donor egg with the intent to parent the baby or may be the recipient of a donor egg with the intent to be a surrogate for another family (Greenfield, 2015).
	Gestational carrier	A process whereby a person becomes pregnant as a recipient of a donor egg and sperm through ART. Recipients are typically younger and healthier and vetted to have carried a pregnancy to term, thus have higher success rates of carrying a pregnancy; however, it can be costly and associated with multiple gestation and preterm delivery (Perkins et al., 2016).

Table 42.3 Prenatal and Postnatal Care Considerations Related to Etiologies of Subfertility

	Prenatal	Intrapartum	Postpartum
Ovulatory etiologies			
Excessive vigorous exercise Management pearl: Discuss healthy exercise in pregnancy (Chronopoulou et al., 2021)	Increased uterine contractility Decreased uterine blood flow Fetal hypoglycemia Hyperthermia	Fetal hypoglycemia	Neonatal hypoglycemia Concern for caloric intake if breast/chestfeeding
Disordered eating Management pearl: Engage a multidisciplinary team (Hecht et al., 2022)	Symptoms may improve with pregnancy Mental health issues (depression, anxiety, ambivalence about the pregnancy) Poor nutritional status Gestational diabetes Possible other comorbid behaviors (smoking, substance use, laxative and/or supplement use, self-harm behaviors) Spontaneous abortion Fetal growth restriction Neonatal microcephaly Hyperemesis Issues with weight gain or loss	Antepartum hemorrhage Miscarriage Premature birth Possible need for induction of labor or Cesarean birth Growth restriction Large for gestational age Gestational hypertension Prolonged labor	Low birth weight Low 1-minute neonatal Apgar Relapse Postpartum depression Breast/chestfeeding difficulty

Table 42.3 (*Continued*)

	Prenatal	Intrapartum	Postpartum
Pituitary tumor Management pearl: Routine prenatal care is often indicated; educate on symptoms to report (Almalki et al., 2015)	Smaller prolactinomas associated with less growth and symptoms during pregnancy Enlargement is seen with larger prolactinomas with symptoms including headache and visual changes	—	No effects on breast/chestfeeding if asymptomatic Depending on size, benefits of treatment may outweigh breast/chestfeeding as cessation is recommended prior to starting medication for treatment
Thyroid dysfunction, hypothyroid, and hyperthyroid Management pearl: Reevaluate thyroid levels serially as recommended throughout pregnancy and treat expediently and appropriately; cases of hyperthyroid will likely require interprofessional care	With hypothyroid, if effectively monitored and treated, no increased risk of complications noted If poorly controlled, spontaneous abortion, gestational hypertension, preeclampsia; additionally, with hyperthyroid, gestational diabetes, thyroid storm, and congestive heart failure are possible (Alexander et al., 2017)	If untreated, preterm birth	If effectively monitored and treated, no increased risk of complications noted If undertreated, may have difficulty lactating If untreated: Difficulties lactating Low birth weight Intellectual deficits in children
PCOS Management pearl: Metformin use may decrease the risk of spontaneous abortion and preterm birth. Increased support and vigilance may be needed for initiating breast/chestfeeding (Yu et al., 2016; Zeng et al., 2016; Vanky et al., 2008)	Spontaneous abortion Gestational diabetes Gestational hypertension Hypoglycemia Preeclampsia Perinatal death	Preterm birth Possible need for cesarean birth	May cause difficulty initiating lactation
Premature ovarian insufficiency (POI) Management pearl: Ensure the birthing person has adequate psychosocial support following oocyte donation including partnership with an oocyte donation program (Ayers & Carlson, 2020; Fraison et al., 2019)	Residual psychological distress as a result of pregnancy journey with POI	—	Pregnancy- and breast/chestfeeding-related immunosuppression may play a role in suppressing POI. Concurrent depression/anxiety, osteoporosis, and heart disease (risk factors for POI)
Tubal etiologies			
Infections (CT, GC, PID) Management pearl: Screen sexually active people with the relevant reproductive anatomy under 25 years of age and those at risk for CT/GC; encourage condom use; treat known infection (CDC, 2021)	Recurrence of infection Ectopic pregnancy Pelvic pain Vaginal bleeding	If untreated, preterm birth	
Scarring from: Endometriosis Pelvic/abdominal surgery Previous ectopic pregnancy Management pearl: Manage any pain, and be vigilant for associated risks (Farland et al., 2020)	Gestational hypertension Gestational diabetes Abdominal or pelvic pain Abnormal placentation Vaginal bleeding	Stillbirth Preterm birth Preterm PROM	Small for gestational age Risk of postpartum hemorrhage

Table 42.3   (*Continued*)

	Prenatal	Intrapartum	Postpartum
Uterine etiologies			
Fibroids Management pearl: Labor and vaginal birth may be appropriate; short-term nonsteroidal anti-inflammatory drugs (NSAIDs) (<32 weeks' gestation) and/or opioids can be used if acetaminophen fails (Ezzedine & Norwitz, 2016)	Most have no complications Depending on size and location, associated risks include: Spontaneous abortion Degeneration Torsion Vaginal bleeding Fetal growth restriction	Preterm labor Preterm birth Placental abruption Fetal malpresentation Labor dysfunction Cesarean birth	Postpartum hemorrhage Uterine inversion
Asherman's syndrome (Guo et al., 2019)	Late pregnancy loss Fetal growth restriction	Preterm birth	Retained placenta Postpartum hemorrhage
Congenital anomalies (i.e., bicornuate or septate uterus) (Hiersch et al., 2016)	Early and late pregnancy loss	PPROM Preterm birth Malpresentation Cesarean section	SGA neonate
Endometrial polyps Management pearl: Offer reassurance	Vaginal bleeding	—	—
Other etiologies involving individuals with a uterus and/or ovaries			
Advanced age: Management pearl: Assess individual risk factors; normalize where possible (ACOG & ASRM, 2014; Kenny et al., 2013; Usta & Nassar, 2008)	Aneuploidy Gestational diabetes Placenta abruption Placenta previa Spontaneous abortion Growth restriction Macrosomia	Preterm birth Malpresentation Cesarean section	Postpartum hemorrhage Postpartum depression
Other **etiologies involving sperm-producing individuals**			
Advanced paternal age: Management pearl: Offer standard screening and diagnostic testing options in pregnancy (ACOG, 2016)	Increased risk of single-gene disorders	—	—

receiving drug treatment (Macaluso et al., 2010). Ovulation-inducing agents including Clomiphene Citrate (Clomid), Letrazole (Femara), and exogenous hormones such as human chorionic gonadotropin (hCG) and follicle-stimulating hormone (FSH) are commonly used medications to treat infertility (Koroma & Stewart, 2012). Each of these medications has intensive regimens and side effects, and are typically discontinued once pregnancy is suspected or diagnosed.

People with a history of unexplained **recurrent pregnancy loss** prior to a period of **secondary infertility** may be taking a progestogen either orally, intramuscularly, or vaginally, for achieving conception and supporting early pregnancy (Saccone et al., 2017). Progestogen use may continue through the first trimester of pregnancy.

Prior to conception, metformin can be used alone or synergistically with Clomid to promote ovulation. This is particularly useful in the treatment of polycystic ovarian syndrome (PCOS) as it decreases insulin resistance and androgen concentrations and promotes ovulation (Durain & McCool, 2017). There are currently no guidelines on the use of metformin throughout pregnancy, but there is a growing body of evidence indicating it might reduce the risk of pregnancy loss and preterm birth without causing fetal or maternal harm (Zeng et al., 2016).

Other comorbidities related to chronic conditions like hypertension, diabetes, or thyroid dysfunction that may have contributed to infertility prior to pregnancy typically include medication regimens that will be continued during pregnancy. Medications to control these common chronic conditions are assessed for safety in pregnancy and are best managed within a multidisciplinary team. Refer to other chapters in this book for complete management strategies.

Patients may have used vitamin or herbal supplements in conjunction with conventional infertility treatments

(Clarke et al., 2013; Vitagliano et al., 2021) and may continue to use them in pregnancy, perceiving herbs or vitamin supplements to be relatively benign (Kennedy et al., 2016). Determining their safety in pregnancy is crucial as some are contraindicated. Black cohosh, in particular, has been studied for its use in the treatment of infertility (Clarke et al., 2013). Based on research findings regarding efficacy during labor, black cohosh is generally contraindicated in pregnancy due to stimulating effects on the uterus (Combest et al., 2017; Kennedy et al., 2016). Prenatal vitamin formulations are encouraged during pregnancy.

Lifestyle Considerations

In the course of infertility care, people often engage in lifestyle modifications to promote fertility such as weight loss or gain through dietary changes and exercise, smoking cessation, reduced alcohol and caffeine consumption, and reduced prescription and other drug use. Continued support and encouragement of positive lifestyle changes is provided.

Other complementary and alternative modalities may have been employed to support lifestyle modification, promote fertility, and address psychological and emotional issues that may arise in the course of infertility treatment (Clarke et al., 2013). Modalities most utilized include acupuncture, meditation, mindfulness, and massage. Among them, acupuncture has been most scrutinized in the literature for its efficacy when used in conjunction with IVF. Though findings are inconclusive in terms of improved fertility, an improvement in coping and reduction in anxiety have been noted (Clarke et al., 2013; Cochrane et al., 2014). Acupuncture may be beneficial to manage pregnancy nausea and vomiting, back and pelvic pain, breech presentation, and labor pain, though more high-quality studies are needed (Bergamo et al., 2018; Miranda-Garcia et al., 2019). Acupuncture has been found to be relatively safe in pregnancy with few mild side effects, if any (Park et al., 2014).

Psychological Impacts of Infertility Treatment and Transition to Pregnancy

Fertility care is highly medicalized, and in recent history, infertility has been defined as a disease state (Zeger-Hochschild et al., 2017). Infertility is unique among other disease states in that those who are ultimately diagnosed as infertile self-identify based on their desire for parenthood. It is managed as a "couples" problem rather than individual and heavily shaped by the social–cultural environment. Medicalization, high costs of treatment, and a sharp focus on achieving the desired state of pregnancy can cause stress, anxiety, and depression. Managed in the context of couples, partners and others involved likely share in this distress.

Stress, anxiety, challenges with sexual intimacy, and depression associated with infertility have been shown to carry over into pregnancy for both partners

(Stevenson & Sloane, 2017; Globevnik Velikonja et al., 2016). They may coexist with feelings of excitement, joy, peace, and gratitude for the pregnancy. These can manifest in a struggle to identify as one who is no longer infertile, fear of pregnancy loss, lack of trust in one's body, amplified pregnancy-related anxiety, ambivalence in the transition to parenthood, and increased risk of depression (Warmelink et al., 2015; French et al., 2015). **Self-silencing**, wherein a feeling of guilt develops with perceived negative feelings about the pregnancy or while pregnant, may prevent sharing and obscure distress (French et al., 2015). Self-silencing might also occur in relation to those in the patient's support network who have also struggled with infertility and other pregnant couples who cannot empathize with the experience of pregnancy after infertility. This may, in effect, reduce support structure and increase a sense of isolation (Blanchard, 2022).

Psychosocial and Emotional Care and Support

Research has shown that bridging the gap early in pregnancy between infertility care and initiation of prenatal care and intervention to mitigate psychological and emotional distress related to pregnancy after infertility promotes well-being and attachment (French et al., 2015). Table 42.1 lists best practices in fostering a healthy transition from infertility care through the rest of the pregnancy.

It is normal for people who are pregnant after experiencing infertility to exhibit a nonlinear range of emotions and feelings through the postpartum period (Globevnik Velikonja et al., 2016). Clinicians must be alert to symptoms that persist and are a barrier to wellness. These symptoms may include:

- Loss of interest in usual activities
- Continued tendency toward self-silencing
- Continued ambivalence toward pregnancy
- Strained interpersonal relationships
- High levels of anxiety
- Inability to focus
- Changes in sleep patterns
- Change in appetite or weight loss/gain
- Substance use
- Suicide ideation or attempt
- Social isolation
- Persistent feelings of pessimism or guilt

Supporting the Partner

Though not all pregnancies will involve two romantically or sexually involved partners, clinicians can support individual(s) who are supporting the pregnant patient. There is limited information about the experience of the cisgender male partner during pregnancy after infertility and even less about lesbian and gender-diverse partners. Cisgender men in heterosexual partnerships postinfertility have been found to be at increased risk of depression, particularly when they do not share their experience with others (Babore et al., 2017). Resources and support communities are generally geared to a female perspective, which may further a sense of isolation in their experience. Gender-diverse partners are also vulnerable. Feelings of isolation and invisibility may exist during fertility and prenatal care, during childbirth, and in the transition to parenthood (Dahl et al., 2013; Ellis et al., 2015; Hayman & Wilkes, 2017; McManus et al., 2006). These feelings may be perpetuated by the clinician's intentional or accidental exclusion, and the partners may lack support within their communities (McManus et al., 2006; Hayman & Wilkes, 2017). In addition to applying best practices among nonpregnant same-sex partners, a clinician may promote and support breast/chestfeeding through induced lactation to be optimally inclusive (McManus et al., 2006).

Supporting Gestational Carriers

Individuals serving as **gestational carriers** are a rare but growing component of the infertility landscape (Perkins et al., 2016). The body of research on collaborative or third-party reproduction with evidence-based recommendations on the care of a person acting as a gestational carrier is limited. A gestational carrier assumes medical risk and may perceive that their ability to exercise complete autonomy in their care is limited given that a third party is involved (Soderstrom-Anttila et al., 2016). That said, it is ethically important to ensure that autonomy is protected and that access to legal and psychosocial support services is available (Ethics Committee of the American Society for Reproductive Medicine, 2018). The clinician and receiving family may have concerns about separation difficulties after birth. These factors can warrant a shift in approach to prenatal care given this context. The limited data available suggest that most gestational carriers do not experience separation difficulties, especially when ethical legal and emotional supports were in place initially and when there was no biological connection to the fetus (Soderstrom-Anttila et al., 2016; White, 2017).

Summary

In the care of pregnant people with a history of infertility, providers must consider the physical, psychosocial, and emotional impacts of fertility care that may persist in pregnancy. Clinicians can play an important role in the transition to routine prenatal care. While provision of care may be more time intensive, offering care sensitive to the infertility history may improve perinatal outcomes.

Resources for Pregnant People and Their Families

Family Equality: https://www.familyequality.org

Fertility for Colored Girls: www.fertilityforcoloredgirls.org

RESOLVE: The National Infertility Association: http://www.resolve.org

Single Mothers by Choice: https://www.singlemothersbychoice.org/

Resources for Healthcare Providers

American Society for Reproductive Medicine: http://www.asrm.org

RESOLVE: The National Infertility Association: http://www.resolve.org

References

Alexander, E. K., Pearce, E. N., Brent, G. A., Brown, R. S., Chen, H., Dosiou, C., Grobman, W. A., Laurberg, P., Lazarus, J. H., Mandel, S. J., Peeters, R. P., & Sullivan, S. (2017). 2017 Guidelines of the American Thyroid Association for the diagnosis and management of thyroid disease during pregnancy and postpartum. *Thyroid, 27*(3), 315–389. https://doi.org/10.1089/thy.2016.0457

Almalki, M. H., Alzahrani, S., Alshahrani, F., Alsherbeni, S., Almoharib, O., Aljohani, N., & Almagamsi, A. (2015). Managing prolactinomas during pregnancy. *Frontiers in Endocrinology, 6*, 85. https://doi.org/10.3389/fendo.2015.00085

American College of Obstetricians and Gynecologists (ACOG). (2016). Practice bulletin 162: Prenatal diagnostic testing for genetic disorders. *Obstetrics & Gynecology, 127*(5), 108–122.

American College of Obstetricians and Gynecologists (ACOG) Committee on Gynecologic Practice & Practice Committee of the American Society for Reproductive Medicine (ASRM). (2014). Female age-related fertility decline, committee opinion no. 589. *Obstetrics & Gynecology, 123*, 719–721.

American Society for Reproductive Medicine (ASRM). (2008). Use of exogenous gonadotropins in anovulatory women: A technical bulletin. *Fertility and Sterility, 90*(3), s7–s12.

Ayers, C. D., & Carlson, K. S. (2020). Spontaneous pregnancy in the setting of primary ovarian insufficiency and breastfeeding: Does immunosuppression play a role? *The American Journal of Case Reports, 21*, e926980–e926981.

Babore, A., Stuppia, L., Trumello, C., Candelori, C., & Antonucci, I. (2017). Male factor infertility and lack of openness about infertility as a risk factor for depressive symptoms in males undergoing assisted reproductive technology treatment in Italy. *Fertility and Sterility, 107*(4), 1041–1047.

Bergamo, T. R., Latorraca, C. D. O. C., Pachito, D. V., Martimbianco, A. L. C., & Riera, R. (2018). Findings and methodological quality of systematic reviews focusing on acupuncture for pregnancy-related acute conditions. *Acupuncture in Medicine, 36*(3), 146–152. https://doi.org/10.1136/acupmed-2017-011436

Blanchard, A. (2022). *I'm pregnant, now what?* RESOLVE. https://resolve.org/get-help/helpful-resources-and-advice/pregnancy-after-infertility/im-pregnant-now-what

Boulet, S. L., Mehta, A. K., Kissin, D. M., Warner, L., Kawwass, J. F., & Jamieson, D. J. (2015). Trends in the use of and reproductive outcomes associated with intracytoplasmic sperm injection. *Journal of the American Medical Association, 313*(3), 255–263.

Ceballo, R., Graham, E. T., & Hart, J. (2015). Silent and infertile: An intersectional analysis of the experiences of socioeconomically diverse African American women with infertility. *Psychology of Women Quarterly, 39*(4), 497–511. https://doi.org/10.1177/0361684315581169

Centers for Disease Control and Prevention (CDC). (2017). *Key statistics from the National Survey of Family Growth [data from 2011–2015].* https://www.cdc.gov/nchs/nsfg/key_statistics/i.htm

Centers for Disease Control and Prevention (CDC). (2021). 2021 Sexual transmitted diseases treatment guidelines. *Maternal Morbidity Weekly Report, 70*(4), 94–97. https://www.cdc.gov/std/treatment-guidelines/STI-Guidelines-2021.pdf

Centers for Disease Control and Prevention, American Society for Reproductive Medicine, and the Society for Assisted Reproductive Technology. (2021). *2019 Assisted Reproductive Technology Fertility Clinic and National Summary Report.* US Dept of Health and Human Services. https://www.cdc.gov/art/reports/2019/pdf/2019-Report-ART-Fertility-Clinic-National-Summary-h.pdf

Chandra, A., Copen, C., & Stephen, E. H. (2014). Infertility and impaired fecundity in the United States, 1982–2010: Data from the National Survey of family growth. *National Health Statistics Reports, 67*, 1–18.

Chronopoulou, E., Seifalian, A., Stephenson, J., Serhal, P., Saab, W., & Seshadri, S. (2021). Preconceptual care for couples seeking fertility treatment, an evidence-based approach. *F&S Reviews, 2*(1), 57–74. https://doi.org/10.1016/j.xfnr.2020.09.001

Clarke, N. A., Will, M., Moravek, M. B., & Fisseha, S. (2013). A systematic review of the evidence for complementary and alternative medicine in infertility. *International Journal of Gynecology & Obstetrics, 122*, 202–206.

Cochrane, S., Smith, C. A., Possamai-Inesedy, A., & Bensoussan, A. (2014). Acupuncture and women's health: An overview of the role of acupuncture and its clinical management in women's reproductive health. *International Journal of Women's Health, 6*, 313–325.

Combest, Q. L., Combest, A. J., & van Olphen Fehr, J. (2017). Complementary and alternative therapies. In M. C. Brucker & T. L. King (Eds.), *Pharmacology for women's health* (2nd ed., pp. 217–236). Jones & Bartlett Learning.

Dahl, B., Fylkesnes, A. M., Sorlie, V., & Malterud, K. (2013). Lesbian women's experiences with healthcare providers in the birthing context: A meta-ethnography. *Midwifery, 29*(6), 674–681.

Domar, A. D. (2015). Creating a collaborative model of mental health counseling for the future. *Fertility and Sterility, 104*(2), 277–289.

Durain, D., & McCool, B. (2017). Pelvic and menstrual disorders. In M. C. Brucker & T. L. King (Eds.), *Pharmacology for women's health* (2nd ed., pp. 917–920). Jones & Bartlett Learning.

Ellis, S. A., Wojnar, D. M., & Pettinato, M. (2015). Conception, pregnancy, and birth experiences of male and gender variant gestational parents: It's how we could have a family. *Journal of Midwifery & Women's Health, 60*(2), 62–69.

Ethics Committee of the American Society for Reproductive Medicine. (2018). Consideration of the gestational carrier: An ethics committee opinion. *Fertility and Sterility, 110*(6), 1017–1021.

Ezzedine, D., & Norwitz, E. (2016). Are women with uterine fibroids at increased risk for adverse pregnancy outcome? *Clinical Obstetrics and Gynecology, 59*(1), 119–127.

Farland, L. V., Davidson, S., Sasamoto, N., Horne, A. W., & Missmer, S. A. (2020). Adverse pregnancy outcomes in endometriosis—myths and realities. *Current Obstetrics and Gynecology Reports, 9*, 27–35.

Feng, J., Wang, J., Zhang, Y., Zhang, Y., Jia, L., Zhang, D., Zhang, J., Han, Y., & Luo, S. (2021). The efficacy of complementary and alternative medicine in the treatment of female infertility. *Evidence-based Complementary and Alternative Medicine, 2021*, 6634309. https://doi.org/10.1155/2021/6634309

Fraison, E., Crawford, G., Casper, G., Harris, V., & Ledger, W. (2019). Pregnancy following diagnosis of premature ovarian insufficiency: a systematic review. *Reproductive BioMedicine Online, 39*(3), 467–476.

French, L. R. M., Sharp, D., & Turner, K. M. (2015). Antenatal needs of couples following fertility treatment: A qualitative study in primary care. *British Journal of General Practice, 65*(638), e570–e577.

Gelbaya, T. A., Potdar, N., Jeve, Y. B., & Nardo, L. (2014). Definition and epidemiology of unexplained infertility. *Obstetrical & Gynecological Survey, 69*(2), 109–115.

Globevnik Velikonja, V., Lozej, T., Leban, G., Verdenik, I., & Vrtacnik, B. (2016). The quality of life in pregnant women conceiving through in vitro fertilization. *Slovenian Journal of Public Health, 55*(1), 1–10.

Greenfield, D. A. (2015). Effects and outcomes of third-party reproduction: Parents. *Fertility and Sterility, 104*(3), 520–524.

Guo, E. J., Chung, J. P. W., Poon, L. C. Y., & Li, T. C. (2019). Reproductive outcomes after surgical treatment of Asherman syndrome: A systematic review. *Best Practice & Research Clinical Obstetrics & Gynaecology, 59*, 98–114. https://doi.org/10.1016/j.bpobgyn.2018.12.009

Hayman, B., & Wilkes, L. (2017). De novo families: Lesbian motherhood. *Journal of Homosexuality, 64*(5), 577–591. https://doi.org/10.1080/00918369.2016.1194119

Hecht, L. M., Hadwiger, A., Patel, S., Hecht, B. R., Loree, A., Ahmedani, B. K., & Miller-Matero, L. R. (2022). Disordered eating and eating disorders among women seeking fertility treatment: A systematic

review. *Archives of Women's Mental Health, 25*, 21–32. https://doi.org/10.1007/s00737-021-01156-x

Herbert, D. L., Lucke, J. C., & Dobson, A. J. (2012). Birth outcomes after spontaneous or assisted conception among infertile Australian women aged 28 to 36 years: A prospective, population-based study. *Fertility and Sterility, 97*(3), 630–638.

Hiersch, L., Yeoshoua, E., Miremberg, H., Krissi, H., Aviram, A., Yogev, Y., & Ashwal, E. (2016). The association between Mullerian anomalies and short-term pregnancy outcome. *The Journal of Maternal-Fetal & Neonatal Medicine, 29*(16), 2573–2578. https://doi.org/10.3109/14767058.2015.1098613

Ibrahim, Y., & Zore, T. (2020). The pervasive issue of racism and its impact on infertility patients: What can we do as reproductive endocrinologists? *Journal of Assisted Reproduction and Genetics, 37*(7), 1563–1565. https://doi.org/10.1007/s10815-020-01863-x

Kennedy, D. A., Lupattelli, A., Koren, G., & Nordeng, H. (2016). Safety classification of herbal medicines used in pregnancy in a multinational study. *BMC Complementary and Alternative Medicine, 16*(102).

Kenny, L. C., Lavender, T., McNamee, R., O'Neill, S. M., Mills, T., & Khashan, A. S. (2013). Advanced maternal age and adverse pregnancy outcome: Evidence from a large contemporary cohort. *PLoS One, 8*(2), e56583.

Koroma, L., & Stewart, L. (2012). Infertility: Evaluation and initial management. *Journal of Midwifery & Women's Health, 57*(6), 614–621.

Lo, W., & Campo-Engelstein, L. (2018). Expanding the clinical definition of infertility to include socially infertile individuals and couples. In L. Campo-Engelstein & P. Burcher (Eds.), *Reproductive ethics II*. Springer.

Luke, B. (2017). Pregnancy and birth outcomes in couples with infertility with and without assisted reproductive technology: With an emphasis on the US population-based studies. *American Journal of Obstetrics & Gynecology, 217*(3), 270–281.

Macaluso, M. M., Wright-Schnapp, T. J., Chandra, A., Johnson, R., Satterwhite, C. L., Pulver, A., Berman, S. M., Wang, R. Y., Farr, S. L., & Pollack, L. A. (2010). A public health focus on infertility prevention, detection, and management. *Fertility and Sterility, 93*(16), e11–e10.

Markus, E. B., Weingarten, A., Duplessi, Y., & Jones, J. (2010). Lesbian couples seeking pregnancy with donor insemination. *Journal of Midwifery & Women's Health, 55*(2), 124–132.

McManus, A. J., Hunter, L. P., & Renn, H. (2006). Lesbian experiences and needs during childbirth: Guidance for health care providers. *Journal of Obstetric, Gynecologic, & Neonatal Nursing, 35*(1), 13–23.

Miranda-Garcia, M., Domingo Gómez, C., Molinet-Coll, C., Nishishinya, B., Allaoui, I., Gómez Roig, M. D., & Goberna-Tricas, J. (2019). Effectiveness and safety of acupuncture and moxibustion in pregnant women with noncephalic presentation: An overview of systematic reviews. *Evidence-based Complementary and Alternative Medicine, 2019*, 7036914. https://doi.org/10.1155/2019/7036914

O'Reilly, E., Sevigny, M., Sabarre, K., & Phillips, K. P. (2014). Perspectives of complementary and alternative (CAM) practitioners in support of treatment of infertility. *BioMed Central Complementary and Alternative Medicine, 14*, 394.

Park, J., Sohn, Y., White, A. R., et al. (2014). The safety of acupuncture during pregnancy: A systematic review. *Acupuncture in Medicine, 32*, 257–266.

Perkins, K. M., Boulet, S. L., Jamieson, D. J., & Kissin, D. M. (2016). Trends and outcomes of gestational surrogacy in the United States. *Fertility and Sterility, 106*(2), 435–442.e2.

Practice Committee of the American Society for Reproductive Medicine. (2015). Diagnostic evaluation of the infertile female: A committee opinion. *Fertility and Sterility, 103*(6), e44–e50.

Ramalingam, M., Kini, S., & Mahmood, T. (2014). Male fertility and infertility. *Obstetrics, Gynaecology and Reproductive Medicine, 24*, 326–332.

RESOLVE: The National Infertility Association. (2022). *Facts, diagnosis, and risk factors*. https://resolve.org/learn/infertility-101/facts-diagnosis-and-risk-factors

Saccone, G., Schoen, C., Franasiak, J. M., Scott, R. T., & Berghella, V. (2017). Supplementation with progestogens in the first trimester of pregnancy to prevent miscarriage in women with unexplained recurrent miscarriage: A systematic review and meta-analysis of randomized, controlled trials. *Fertility and Sterility*, *107*(2), 430–438.e3.

Smith, C. A., & Cochrane, S. (2009). Does acupuncture have a place as an adjunct treatment during pregnancy? A review of randomized control trials and systemic reviews. *Birth*, *36*(3), 246–253.

Soderstrom-Anttila, V., Wennerholm, U.-B., Loft, A., Pinborg, A., Aittomaki, K., Romundstad, L. B., & Bergh, C. (2016). Surrogacy: Outcomes for surrogate mothers, children, and resulting families—A systematic review. *Human Reproduction Update*, *22*(2), 260–276.

Stevenson, E. L., & Sloane, R. (2017). Certain less invasive infertility treatments associated with different levels of pregnancy-related anxiety in pregnancies conceived via *in vitro* fertilization. *Journal of Reproduction & Infertility*, *18*(1), 190–196.

Stevenson, E. L., Trotter, K. J., Bergh, C., & Sloane, R. (2016). Pregnancy-related anxiety in women who conceive via in vitro fertilization: A mixed methods approach. *The Journal of Perinatal Education*, *25*(3), 193–200. https://doi.org/10.1891/1058-1243.25.3.193

Usta, I. M., & Nassar, A. H. (2008). Advanced maternal age. Part 1: Obstetric complications. *American Journal of Perinatology*, *25*(8), 521–534.

Vanky, E., Isaksen, H., Moen, M. H., & Carlsen, S. M. (2008). Breast-feeding in polycystic ovarian syndrome. *Acta Obstetricia et Gynecologica Scandinavica*, *87*(5), 531–535.

Vitagliano, A., Petre, G. C., Francini-Pesenti, F., De Toni, L., Di Nisio, A., Grande, G., Foresta, C., & Garolla, A. (2021). Dietary supplements for female infertility: A critical review of their composition. *Nutrients*, *13*(10), 3552.

Warmelink, J. C., Adema, W., Pranger, A., & de Cock, P. T. (2015). Client perspectives of midwifery care in the transition from subfertility to parenthood: A qualitative study in the Netherlands. *Journal of Psychosomatic Obstetrics and Gynecology*, *37*(1), 12–20.

Weigel, G., Ranji, U., Long, M., & Salganicoff, A. (2020, September) *Coverage and use of fertility services in the U.S.* Kaiser Family Foundation. https://www.kff.org/womens-health-policy/issue-brief/coverage-and-use-of-fertility-services-in-the-u-s

White, P. M. (2017). "One for sorrow, two for joy?": American embryo transfer guideline recommendations, practices, and outcomes for gestational surrogate patients. *Journal of Assisted Reproduction and Genetics*, *34*(4), 431–443.

Wiltshire, A., Ghidei, L., & Brayboy, L. M. (2020, July). Infertility and assisted reproductive technology outcomes in afro-Caribbean women. *Journal of Assisted Reproduction and Genetics*, *37*(7), 1553–1561. https://doi.org/10.1007/s10815-020-01826-2

Younger, M., Hollins-Martin, C., & Choucri, L. (2015). Individualised care for women with assisted conception pregnancies and midwifery practice implications: An analysis of the existing research and current practice. *Midwifery*, *31*(2), 265–270.

Yu, H., Chen, H., Rao, D., & Gong, J. (2016). Association between polycystic ovary syndrome and the risk of pregnancy complications: A PRISMA-compliant systematic review and meta-analysis. *Medicine*, *95*(51), e4863.

Zegers-Hochschild, F., Adamson, G. D., Dyer, S., Racowsky, C., de Mouzon, J., Sokol, R., Rienzi, L., Sunde, A., Schmidt, L., Cooke, I. D., Simpson, J. L., & van der Poel, S. (2017). The international glossary on infertility and fertility care, 2017. *Fertility and Sterility*, *108*(3), 393–406.

Zeng, X.-L., Zhang, Y.-F., Tian, Q., Xue, T., & An, R.-F. (2016). Effects of metformin on pregnancy outcomes in women with polycystic ovary syndrome: A meta-analysis. *Medicine*, *95*(36), e4526.

43

Common Complications during the Postnatal Period

Deborah Brandt Karsnitz and Linda McDaniel

Relevant Terms

Anxiety disorders—include generalized anxiety disorder, obsessive–compulsive disorder, panic disorder, and post-traumatic stress disorder

Deep vein thrombosis—inflammation of a vein located deep within a muscle secondary to a blood clot

Endometritis—postpartum uterine infection of the functional uterine lining—wall of the uterus

Maternal mortality—death while pregnant or within 42 days of termination of pregnancy, from any cause related to or aggravated by the pregnancy or its management

Puerperal fever—fever of 100.4 °F (38 °C) or greater during postpartum period caused by bacterial infection in the reproductive tract or breasts

Postpartum anxiety disorders—any of the anxiety disorders occurring in the first year postpartum

Postpartum blues—sadness, weepiness, mood swings, irritability that occurs in the first few days to 10 days postpartum; lasts less than two weeks

Postpartum depression—depression occurring within the first year postpartum that meets standard diagnostic criteria; lasts longer than two weeks

Postpartum hematoma—collection of blood in the vaginal, perineal, pelvic, or abdominal tissue, post childbirth

Postpartum (puerperal) infection—infection of the reproductive structures or abdominal incision post-cesarean section

Postpartum preeclampsia/eclampsia—postpartum-specific preeclampsia/eclampsia according to standard diagnostic criteria for increasing hypertension or proteinuria, with or without progression to seizure

Postpartum preeclampsia/eclampsia, late (LPP)—postpartum-specific preeclampsia/eclampsia that develops between 48 hours after birth and six weeks postpartum

Postpartum psychosis—psychotic episode (delusions or break with reality) occurring within the first year after birth

Psychotropics—mental health medications that affect mood, behavior, mental activity

Secondary postpartum hemorrhage—excessive bleeding occurring between 24 hours after birth until six weeks postpartum

Subinvolution—failure of the uterus to return to normal size and state after birth

Superficial venous thrombosis—inflammation of a vein located just below the skin's surface secondary to a blood clot

Thyroiditis—inflammation of the thyroid gland

Thyrotoxicosis—overproduction of thyroid hormones to toxic levels

von Willebrand's disease—an inherited bleeding disorder affecting up to 1% of the US population

---

Introduction

Postpartum, or puerperium, represents a time period of restoration and recovery after birth. Restoration and recovery follow a typical pattern of involution. Ideally, this is a time for family attachment and parental role development. Despite expected normalcy during this time frame, complications do occur and recovery can become complex. Postpartum complications include late postpartum hemorrhage, infection, postpartum preeclampsia, postpartum mood and anxiety disorders, and various medical complications directly or indirectly influenced by childbearing.

Some postpartum complications can be managed by nurse practitioners, midwives, or physician assistants, while others require physician consultation, collaboration, or referral. A significant decrease in postpartum morbidity and mortality occurred with the implementation of careful routine hand washing that prevents spread of postpartum infections, formerly called

Prenatal and Postnatal Care: A Person-Centered Approach, Third Edition. Edited by Karen Trister Grace, Cindy L. Farley, Noelene K. Jeffers, and Tanya Tringali.
© 2024 John Wiley & Sons Ltd. Published 2024 by John Wiley & Sons Ltd.
Companion website: www.wiley.com/go/grace/prenatal

childbed fever. Appropriate and timely management of complications is essential in saving lives. Unfortunately, the United States still ranks behind many other countries for **maternal mortality** (World Health Organization [WHO], 2019). This chapter will describe common postpartum complications, risk factors, assessment, and management.

Health equity key points

- Inequalities in healthcare, social determinants, and systemic racism significantly increase risk for postpartum morbidity and mortality.
- Utilization of social determinants of health screening tools is essential to provide effective healthcare and integral to prompt treatment and recovery when potential postpartum morbidity and mortality risk factors are present.
- Mental health stigma and bias can inhibit symptom disclosure and discussion between healthcare providers and individuals experiencing postpartum mood and anxiety disorders.

Postpartum Morbidity and Mortality

Postpartum recovery often includes common concerns, such as anemia, fatigue, constipation, and hemorrhoids, which are usually mild and easily managed (see Chapter 30, *Components of Postpartum Care*). Major postpartum complications, except for depression and anxiety disorders, are uncommon. Until the latter half of the twentieth century, the top three causes of maternal mortality were hemorrhage, postpartum infection, and preeclampsia. For the past several decades, the Pregnancy Mortality Surveillance System (PMSS) has collected data on pregnancy-related deaths. The most recent report (2016–2018) contains analysis of data on maternal deaths that occurred from the time of birth to one year from the end of pregnancy (Centers for Disease Control and Prevention [CDC], 2022). The PMSS analysis found an increase in maternal mortality from a low of 7.2 maternal deaths per 100,000 live births in 1987 to 17.3 in 2018 (CDC, 2022). Notably, there has been an increase in maternal mortality from indirect pregnancy-related causes, such as cardiovascular conditions and noncardiovascular medical conditions (CDC, 2022). Figure 43.1 illustrates these data.

Factors such as age, chronic health conditions, incidence of obesity, and cesarean sections impact pregnancy outcomes (Collier & Molina, 2019). In the United States, cardiovascular conditions, infection, cardiomyopathy, and hemorrhage are the leading causes of pregnancy-related mortality (CDC, 2022). Inequality, some social determinants, and systemic racism are key factors in increased risk for mortality and morbidity (CDC, 2022). The mortality ratio (maternal deaths/live births × 100,000) for non-Hispanic Black women was 41.4, more than three times the rate for White women, 13.7. The mortality ratio for American Indian/Alaskan Natives was 26.5, Asian/Pacific Islanders, 13.7, and Hispanic/Latinx women, 11.2 (CDC, 2022).

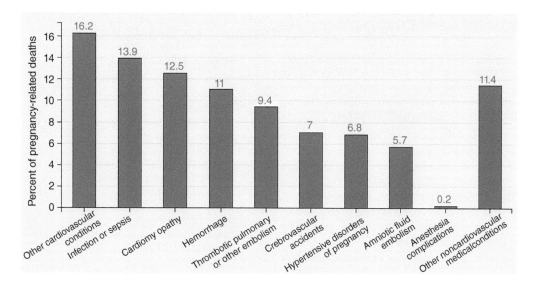

Figure 43.1   Pregnancy-related deaths in the United States, 2016–2018. Note: The cause of death is unknown for 6.0% of all 2016–2018 pregnancy-related deaths. CDC (2022)/US Department of Health and Human Services/Public Domain.

Postpartum Cultural Considerations

Most cultures have rich traditions and beliefs surrounding the postpartum period. While some cultures encourage rest and nurturing for as little as three weeks, most extend care and support for five weeks and beyond. Expectations for resumption of usual activities vary and can depend on factors such as identified needs, support, and cultural influences (Walker et al., 2019). Without adequate time for recovery, complications can occur and extend the recovery period. Healthcare providers should inquire about how healthcare decisions are made in their family. They may be shared by family members, or an individual may be chosen based on age or status within the family. Management may need to incorporate factors such as religious beliefs or traditional or herbal medicines. Discussions about mental health are important to determine if stigma is a deterrent to treatment. Feelings of sadness or despair in the postpartum period can be socially unacceptable in some cultures. An understanding of cultural influences and traditions and their impact on postpartum care is essential in order to be sensitive and effective in preventing and treating postpartum disorders. See Chapter 19, *Culture and Community*, and Chapter 30, *Components of Postpartum Care*, for further discussion of this topic.

Postpartum Disorders

Puerperal Fever (Pyrexia)

Puerperal fever is defined as a temperature of 100.4 °F (38 °C) or greater during the postpartum period and can be caused by infections. Common causes include genital tract or wound infections, and less common causes include pyelonephritis and respiratory illnesses. However, it is important to recognize that there are noninfectious causes of fever, which include breast engorgement and dehydration. In these cases, the increased temperature seldom exceeds 24 hours and will usually not increase greater than 102.2 °F (39 °C). Occasionally, a slight increase in temperature postpartum can accompany superficial or **deep vein thrombosis** (DVT). Of note, spiking a fever higher than 102 °F within 24 hours post-cesarean birth can indicate infection with group A *Streptococcus*. Any fever originating during postpartum warrants investigation for infection.

Puerperal Infection (Postpartum Infection)

Puerperal infection, usually indicated by fever, generally describes any infection in the genital tract following birth, miscarriage, or induced abortion. Since the introduction of hand washing, asepsis, and particularly antimicrobial drugs, death from puerperal infection has significantly decreased. The PMSS (2016–2018) reported that infection is one of the leading causes of maternal morbidity and mortality (13.9% of maternal deaths; CDC, 2022).

Historically dreaded for its high rate of mortality, maternal death from puerperal infection has decreased significantly because of antibiotics. However, puerperal morbidity from infection is still a significant problem. Postpartum individuals are at increased risk for infection due to wound or tissue trauma during birth, vulnerability from the placental separation site, and surgical incision from cesarean birth. Other potential sites of infection include the urinary tract, breasts, lungs, and epithelial lining in veins. Most puerperal infections occur within the first few days or weeks postpartum, a time notoriously devoid of healthcare follow-up in both lower- and higher-income countries. Infection is one of the most common reasons why individuals are readmitted to the hospital in the postpartum period, regardless of route of birth (Black et al., 2021). Postpartum infections, such as uterine and wound infections (abdominal and perineal), will be examined in this section.

Uterine Infection (Endometritis)

Uterine infection or **endometritis** is one of the most common infections to occur during the postpartum period and refers to a uterine infection that may occur in the myometrium (endomyometritis), the parametrium (endoparametritis), or both. Cesarean birth without antibiotic prophylaxis carries a high risk of postpartum uterine infection, up to 27%. Vaginal birth carries a much lower risk, approximately 1–2% (American College of Obstetricians and Gynecologists [ACOG], 2018a; Taylor & Pillarisetty, 2022). Antimicrobial prophylaxis is recommended for all individuals undergoing cesarean birth beginning within 60 minutes of initiation of surgery (Haas et al., 2020). Antimicrobial prophylaxis has dramatically decreased infection rates, though infection can still occur after cesarean birth (Haas et al., 2020).

There are a number of risk factors for infection. When several factors occur together, they can exponentially increase the risk for infection. Prolonged labor, the number of vaginal exams, and internal monitoring are individual risk factors for uterine infection. Amniotomy breaks the protective membrane barrier, which increases the risk of ascending infection and, when used in conjunction with prolonged labor and frequent vaginal exams, increases infection rates.

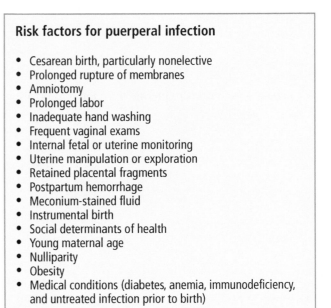

Risk factors for puerperal infection

- Cesarean birth, particularly nonelective
- Prolonged rupture of membranes
- Amniotomy
- Prolonged labor
- Inadequate hand washing
- Frequent vaginal exams
- Internal fetal or uterine monitoring
- Uterine manipulation or exploration
- Retained placental fragments
- Postpartum hemorrhage
- Meconium-stained fluid
- Instrumental birth
- Social determinants of health
- Young maternal age
- Nulliparity
- Obesity
- Medical conditions (diabetes, anemia, immunodeficiency, and untreated infection prior to birth)

Table 43.1 Common Pathogens in Uterine Infection

Aerobes		
Gram-positive	Gram-negative	Gram-variable
A, B, D streptococci	Escherichia coli	Gardnerella vaginalis
Enterococcus	Klebsiella	
Staphylococcus aureus	Enterobacter	
Staphylococcus epidermidis	Proteus species	
Anerobes		Others
Peptostreptococcus		Mycoplasma
Peptococcus		Chlamydia
Bacteroids		Neisseria gonorrhoeae
Clostridium		
Fusobacterium		

Source: Adapted from: Cunningham et al. (2022).

Once rupture of the amniotic membranes occurs during labor, the uterus becomes more susceptible to colonization and infection. Infection can occur with uterine manipulation or exploration during manual removal of the placenta or instrumental birth. Any area traumatized during birth is susceptible to infection. Infections that spread are the result of localized infections that proliferate to additional sites including other pelvic organs such as an infected incision, which can progress to endometritis if diagnosis is delayed. Uterine infections are polymicrobial. Common pathogens implicated in these infections are listed in Table 43.1.

Clinical Presentation and Management

Signs and symptoms of endometritis include elevated temperature (the degree of elevation can be indicative of severity and possible sepsis), general malaise, abdominal pain with uterine tenderness on bimanual exam, lochia with or without a foul smell, and **subinvolution**. Chills often accompany severe cases of uterine infection. On occasion, and with certain bacteria such as group A or B *Streptococcus*, early signs and symptoms may be more generalized, with fever being the only presenting symptom. Differential diagnosis includes pyelonephritis, pneumonia, and appendicitis.

Diagnosis includes physical examination, complete blood count (CBC), blood cultures, aerobic uterine culture, urinalysis, urine culture, and, if indicated, chest X-ray. Mild cases of endometritis can be treated with oral antibiotics. Culture of the wound or cervix is rarely necessary to initiate treatment. Moderate to severe cases require hospitalization and treatment with broad-spectrum antimicrobial intravenous (IV) therapy.

Physician consultation is recommended for mild cases managed with outpatient oral antimicrobials if secondary to cesarean birth. Physician collaboration or referral is indicated for moderate to severe infections requiring hospitalization (Table 43.2). Most individuals will improve markedly within 48–72 hours. Discharge from the hospital can occur after IV therapy is discontinued and the individual is afebrile and asymptomatic for 24 hours.

Wound Infection

Postpartum wound infections develop most often in the abdominal incision following cesarean birth or in a perineal laceration or episiotomy following vaginal birth. Since the advent of prophylactic antimicrobial management during cesarean birth, postsurgical infections have been dramatically reduced. Risk factors for abdominal and perineal wound infection are similar to risk factors for uterine infection.

Abdominal Wound Infection

Signs and symptoms of abdominal wound infection include localized edema, induration, and erythema, often with exudates and occasionally fever. Management includes wound care, antibiotic treatment, and drainage, if necessary. Reclosure of the wound can be indicated if dehiscence is present, although healing by secondary intention is another option, depending on the size, drainage, and other characteristics of the wound. Culture of the wound is rarely necessary for treatment. Common pathogens include *Staphylococcus aureus*, streptococci, and both aerobic and anaerobic bacilli.

Perineal Wound Infection

Infection of an episiotomy or perineal laceration most often presents with localized edema, erythema, and exudates. Management is similar to other wound infections

Table 43.2 Uterine Infection Signs, Symptoms, Diagnosis, and Treatment

Signs and symptoms (onset, duration, severity)	Diagnostics	Treatment—MD collaboration or referral for IV therapy
• Fever (chills) • General malaise • Pain/tenderness • Lochia (odor)	• CBC with differential • Urinalysis • Cultures • Radiology (if indicated) • Ultrasound (if indicated)	Antimicrobial therapy • Clindamycin 900 mg + gentamicin 1.5 mg/kg, q8 hours IV • Clindamycin 900 mg q8 hours and aztreonam—1–2 g q8 hours • Metronidazole 500 mg q12 hours, PCN, 5 million units q6 hours • Ampicillin 2 g q6 hours + gentamicin 1.5 mg/kg q8 hours

Source: Adapted from Cunningham et al. (2022).

and includes drainage, removal of sutures, and debridement of the infected area. If cellulitis is apparent, broad-spectrum antimicrobial therapy is indicated. Most infections heal without needing additional sutures. If breakdown of sutures occurs for a third- or fourth-degree laceration or episiotomy extension, repair is necessary once infection is eradicated. Some studies suggest that perineal infections after third- and fourth-degree laceration repair can be reduced with the use of prophylactic antimicrobials (Liabsuetrakul et al., 2020). However, before becoming best practice, comparative effectiveness studies are needed (Stern-Ascher, et al., 2020). Individuals with persistent fever, tachycardia, pain, and tenderness, and continuation of symptoms despite several days of treatment should be assessed for complications such as pelvic abscess, septic pelvic thrombophlebitis, and, in severe cases, septic shock.

Secondary (Late) Postpartum Hemorrhage

Hemorrhage has historically been one of the major causes of maternal mortality. Although dramatically decreased, hemorrhage continues to be a leading cause of maternal death (CDC, 2022). When it occurs between 24 hours and 12 weeks postpartum, it is considered **secondary (late) postpartum hemorrhage** (ACOG, 2017). Spiral arteries course through the layers of uterine muscle and form "living ligatures" when contracted, leading to hemostasis after childbirth. When this natural process is delayed or inhibited, hemorrhage can occur. Approximately 1% of postpartum individuals have a **secondary postpartum hemorrhage**; most occurring within the first two weeks after birth as a result of uterine atony or subinvolution (ACOG, 2017). Most cases of uterine atony occur without antecedents or risk factors; however, retained placental fragments should be considered during the diagnostic workup.

Individuals presenting with secondary postpartum hemorrhage that occurs after 48 hours should be screened for **von Willebrand's disease** (VWD), the most common inherited bleeding disorder in childbearing individuals (Byrne et al., 2021). Many factors, including von Willebrand's factor (factor VIII), a protein that causes platelets to adhere, increase in pregnant people. This effect is blunted or absent in people with VWD (Byrne et al., 2021). Factor VIII decreases in the early postpartum period, but the decrease is more dramatic in people with VWD. Bleeding is not usually a problem for the initial 48 hours. However, an increased risk for bleeding persists until approximately four months postpartum (ACOG, 2017).

Clinical Presentation and Management

Treatment for secondary postpartum hemorrhage may include uterotonic agents or curettage. Ultrasound can determine if there are significant retained placental fragments but has low sensitivity. However, echogenic masses are suspicious for retained placental fragments or clots and referral to a physician for suction evacuation may be needed to stop bleeding. Postpartum curettage is not typically performed because the uterine wall is vulnerable to perforation in the postpartum period. Most secondary postpartum hemorrhages will respond to agents such as ergonovine, methylergonovine, oxytocin, a prostaglandin analog, or tranexamic acid (ACOG, 2017).

Postpartum Hematoma

Occurrence of **postpartum hematoma** varies between 1/300 and 1/15,000 births (Rani et al., 2017). Hematoma formation most commonly is a complication of episiotomy and instrumental birth and occurs most often in nulliparous people. Hematoma formation can occur spontaneously, without laceration, and may be delayed in presentation. However, vulvar hematomas are usually related to lacerated vessels. Typically, multiple vessels are involved, and surgical repair requires drainage and suturing. If a hematoma is small, expectant management is indicated. Vaginal hematomas appear most often after instrumental assistance during birth and require surgical management (ACOG, 2017). Atypical reasons for postpartum hematoma formation include coagulopathies such as VWD. Many hematomas can be prevented with controlled, physiologic birth, and appropriate inspection and repair of lacerations or episiotomy.

Clinical Presentation and Management

Postpartum hematoma should be considered when there is evidence of blood loss such as declining hematocrit, despite normal amounts of bleeding and abdominal assessment of a firm uterus. Individuals characteristically report severe perineal or rectal pain far beyond typical postpartum pain. A hematoma can occur in the vulva, vagina, paravaginal tissues, or retroperitoneal areas.

Management varies according to presentation and site. Small hematomas can reabsorb, while moderate to larger hematomas may need incision and drainage. Subperitoneal hematomas can be more difficult to assess; bleeding, subsequent hypovolemia, and shock are of concern. Physician referral is necessary when hematoma is suspected.

Postpartum Urinary Retention

Postpartum urinary retention (PUR) is defined as the inability to void within 6 hours after giving birth. This is further categorized as *overt*—inability to void and requiring catheterization—or *covert*—inability to void more than 50% of the bladder capacity, with greater than 150 mL of residual urine postvoid. PUR can be asymptomatic, especially in individuals with covert PUR. The prevalence of PUR after vaginal birth varies widely, as there is not a standard definition. It is estimated that between 1.7% and 17.9% of individuals experience true PUR, although it is likely to be higher, as covert PUR can remain undetected (Ain et al., 2021). Epidural anesthesia, instrument-assisted birth, oxytocin infusion during labor, and third- and fourth-degree perineal tearing are associated with an increased risk of PUR (Ain et al., 2021; Biurrun et al., 2020). Prolonged bladder overdistention can lead to longer-term bladder dysfunction.

Clinical Presentation and Management

When present, symptoms can vary and include bladder pressure and discomfort, urgency, voiding small amounts, and a urine stream that is weak or intermittent. Elevated fundal height or displacement to one side, discomfort upon palpation, and inability to urinate are clinical signs of PUR. The diagnosis is made by ultrasound of the bladder to evaluate the amount of urine present. In settings where ultrasound is unavailable, clinical signs are used for diagnosis.

Clinical guidelines for managing PUR are lacking; however, straight intermittent catheterization is often the only intervention needed. Most individuals will void spontaneously within several hours of catheterization. Consider placing an indwelling catheter when there is an inability to void a second time. This is more likely to be needed by someone with significant perineal trauma or potent epidural anesthesia. The indwelling catheter is commonly taken out after 24 hours. Bladder emptying after catheter removal should be evaluated for several subsequent spontaneous voids to ensure that it is complete.

Subinvolution

Uterine involution is the physiologic process of cellular reduction and remodeling of the uterus to a nonpregnant state. Subinvolution occurs when this physiologic process is impaired. Uterine subinvolution may be secondary to retained placental fragments, uterine infection, or excessive maternal activity prohibiting proper recovery.

Clinical Presentation and Management

The diagnosis of subinvolution is made clinically. Symptoms include irregular bleeding, which can be profuse on occasion. Physical examination reveals an enlarged uterus that is often boggy upon abdominal or bimanual exam (ACOG, 2017).

If retained placental fragments and infection are ruled out, management focuses on lifestyle measures needed to support healing. Along with a short course of methylergonovine (0.2 mg po every 3–4 hours for 24–48 hours), individuals are encouraged to incorporate help at home, get proper rest, nutrition, and hydration, with follow-up in one to two weeks.

Postpartum Hypertensive Disorders

The incidence of postpartum hypertensive disorders is estimated between 0.3% and 27.5% (Redman et al., 2019). This wide range is not well understood and varies among populations, but studies show that overlapping risk factors including antepartum preeclampsia, obesity, older age, race (likely reflecting racism) and cesarean delivery are implicated (Redman et al., 2019). Postpartum hypertensive disorders are similar to antepartum hypertensive disorders, in that they can lead to devastating consequences, including maternal death. Preeclampsia is typically a prenatal condition that presents clinically during the latter half of pregnancy and generally resolves within one to two days postpartum. **Postpartum preeclampsia** or

eclampsia, also termed early postpartum preeclampsia or eclampsia, occurs within 48 hours postpartum. **Late postpartum preeclampsia–eclampsia (LPP)** develops after 48 hours and before 6 weeks postpartum and is less common (ACOG, 2020; Redman et al., 2019).

New onset and transient hypertension in the postpartum period can occur, complicating approximately 2% of pregnancies (Sharma & Kilpatrick, 2017). Individuals with postpartum hypertension share similar clinical risk factors with and have a similar antepartum plasma angiogenic profile to that of individuals with preeclampsia (Redman et al., 2019), suggesting that postpartum hypertension may represent a group of individuals with subclinical or unresolved preeclampsia. These individuals are at an increased risk for iatrogenic overload of IV fluids during labor and birth. Additionally, intravascular fluid volume increases postpartum from physiologic extravascular fluid shift. Individuals with impaired renal function from severe preeclampsia are at risk postpartum for pulmonary edema and worsening hypertension (Redman et al., 2019). Development of new-onset seizures can be prevented if prodromal symptoms of preeclampsia are recognized early.

Individuals with postpartum preeclampsia have an increased risk for pulmonary edema, eclampsia, stroke, or thromboembolism (ACOG, 2020; Redman et al., 2019). Postpartum eclampsia can develop despite treatment with magnesium sulfate during intrapartum and early postpartum. An antepartum diagnosis of preeclampsia is not a prerequisite for a postpartum diagnosis (ACOG, 2020).

Individuals who develop LPP and did not have preeclampsia during pregnancy or labor are at highest risk for eclampsia and poor outcomes especially when individuals are not provided with warning signs (Folk, 2018). Risk factors for the development of new onset LPP include age >35, body mass index (BMI) >25, gestational diabetes, pregnancy by assisted reproductive technologies (ARTs), and hypothyroidism (Folk, 2018).

Clinical Presentation and Management

Individuals diagnosed with gestational hypertension or preeclampsia need close monitoring in the early postpartum period. Evaluation includes observation for signs of worsening disease, including headache, mental confusion and visual changes, monitoring of blood pressure, oxygen saturation, respirations, fluid intake and output, and laboratory indices. Individuals most often present with headaches, visual changes, epigastric pain, or nausea and vomiting. Neurological symptoms such as headache, malaise, nausea and vomiting, shortness of breath, pedal edema and significantly abnormal laboratory markers are more often reported in individuals readmitted for postpartum preeclampsia than in individuals with intrapartum preeclampsia (Redman et al., 2019). Hypertension and proteinuria do not always present together in postpartum preeclampsia. Hypertension is defined as systolic blood pressure 140 mmHg or greater and/or diastolic blood pressure 90 mmHg or greater on two or more occasions at least 4 hours apart. Severe hypertension is defined as systolic blood pressure 160 mmHg or greater and/or diastolic blood pressure 110 mmHg or greater on 2 or more occasions repeated at a shorter interval. See Chapter 36, *Hypertensive Disorders of Pregnancy*, for detailed information on preeclampsia.

Medical management includes hospitalization and administration of magnesium sulfate, as well as antihypertensive therapy and physician referral is indicated.

All medications that can cause hypertension, such as nonsteroidal anti-inflammatory drugs (NSAIDs) and methergine, should be discontinued, and evaluation for other causes of hypertension, such as kidney disease or hypokalemia, should be conducted (ACOG, 2020; Redman et al., 2019). Severe hypertension can cause a stroke. Individuals with severe hypertension sustained over 15 minutes should be treated with fast-acting antihypertension medications. Labetalol, hydralazine, and nifedipine are all effective for acute management, although nifedipine may work the fastest. Clients should be educated on the signs and symptoms of postpartum preeclampsia prior to discharge from the birth facility.

Postpartum Venous Thromboembolism

The common practice of encouraging ambulation soon after childbirth has decreased the incidence of thromboembolic disease during the postpartum period (Figure 43.2). However, there is a 20- to 37-fold higher risk for venous thromboembolism (VTE) during the first six weeks of the postpartum period, with the first three weeks being the highest risk (Friedman, 2021). Physiologic risk factors (Table 43.3) for postpartum thrombosis include hypercoagulability, venous stasis, and inflammation known as Virchow's triad.

Thrombophlebitis is most often diagnosed in individuals with previous varicosities. However, venous stasis can occur during pregnancy secondary to the effects of progesterone. Thrombosis results from inflammation due

Table 43.3 Risk Factors for Venous Thrombosis

- Age > 35
- Cesarean birth
- Coagulopathies
- History of thrombosis or hemorrhage
- Hypercoagulability
- Immobilization
- Medical conditions (sickle cell, heart disease, and diabetes)
- Multiple pregnancy
- Obesity
- Operative vaginal birth
- Postpartum infection
- Preeclampsia
- Preterm birth
- Smoking
- Stillbirth
- Vascular trauma
- Venous stasis

to venous distension. Prevention of venous stasis during the intrapartum and postpartum periods can be accomplished by frequent positional changes and ambulation.

Clinical Presentation and Management

Superficial thrombophlebitis (SVT) presents with increased leg pain, localized edema, erythema, and warmth over the thrombotic site. Physical exam reveals an enlarged and hard, cord-like structure. SVT is managed with support stockings, analgesia (NSAIDs), leg rest, and elevation.

DVT may mimic SVT, both characterized by leg pain and inflammation. DVT, however, is usually evidenced by an abrupt onset of symptoms with increased pain elicited with movement or standing. Positive Homan's sign, increased calf pain elicited with dorsiflexion of the foot, is not a reliable diagnostic finding for DVT even when present; it can also be indicative of muscle strain from

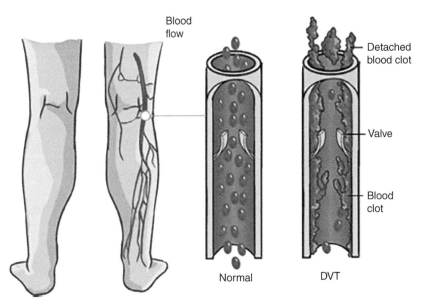

Figure 43.2 Deep vein thrombosis. National Institute of Health (NIH) Medline Plus.

childbirth. Furthermore, absence of Homan's sign does not rule out DVT. Edema may be more generalized over the leg and thigh; the affected leg may be larger than the other; and at times, a palpable cord may be present over the affected area. Differential diagnosis includes SVT, trauma, ruptured Baker's cyst (i.e., a fluid-filled cyst in the popliteal area), muscle strain, vasculitis, or lymphedema.

Compression ultrasound is the standard diagnostic test, with or without color Doppler (Stevens et al., 2021). Laboratory evaluation can include adjunct studies using D-dimer serum concentrations. Management of DVT includes anticoagulant therapy, bed rest with leg elevation, and analgesia. Support stockings should be worn until ambulation resumes. Physician management is indicated for DVT.

Postpartum Thyroiditis

Transient postpartum **thyroiditis** (inflammation of the thyroid gland) presents as either hyper- or hypothyroidism and sometimes has alternating phases of both disorders. The prevalence ranges from 1.1% to 16.7% (Rad & Deluxe, 2022). Postpartum thyroiditis can occur anytime during the first year, most commonly between one and six months postpartum. Because signs and symptoms can be vague and nonspecific, postpartum thyroiditis is sometimes mistaken for other disorders. Postpartum thyroiditis risk increases in individuals with gestational diabetes, personal or family history of thyroid disorder, and chronic hepatitis (Epp et al., 2021).

Clinical Presentation and Management

Postpartum thyroiditis can present with subtle symptoms several months postpartum, which can impede prompt diagnosis. Symptoms of postpartum thyroiditis may resemble some of the common symptoms experienced during the postpartum period, such as fatigue, insomnia, anxiety, and weight loss, leading to difficulty in diagnosis. Postpartum individuals presenting with mild dysphoria can be misdiagnosed with **postpartum depression** (PPD) or **postpartum psychosis**. Thyroid function studies should be performed when suspecting PPD or postpartum psychosis.

Treatment includes beta blockers for hyperthyroid symptoms and thyroid hormone supplementation for hypothyroid symptoms. However, most individuals have mild symptoms and do not require treatment. If indicated, treatment will not interfere with breastfeeding. Future development of hypothyroidism occurs in 20–40% of individuals diagnosed with postpartum thyroiditis (Epp et al., 2021).

Thyroid storm (**thyrotoxicosis**), although rare, is most likely to occur two to six months postpartum but may occur up to one year postpartum (Epp et al., 2021; Pearce, 2018). Thyrotoxicosis is characterized by abrupt onset, is usually short-lived, but can be life-threatening if unrecognized and untreated. Symptoms include fever, nausea, vomiting, diarrhea, tachycardia, and tremor. Cardiomyopathy and heart failure can develop secondary

to increased T_4 levels (Epp et al., 2021; Pearce, 2018; Rad & Deluxe, 2022).

Treatment includes decreasing thyroid hormone production and circulating thyroid hormones, identifying the underlying cause and providing supportive measures. Physician referral is indicated.

Postpartum Mood and Anxiety Disorders

The childbearing years are a time of increased vulnerability for mood and anxiety disorders. Mood and anxiety disorders are significant complications during the postpartum period and can result in lifelong effects for the individual and family, at times with dire outcomes.

Symptoms of depression are reported by 13% of postpartum individuals. While variation occurs among different communities (9.7–23.5%), various factors influence reporting (Bauman et al., 2020). A systematic review of individuals without a prior history of depression revealed a similar incidence of PPD of 12% with variations from 3.4% to 34% (Shorey et al., 2019).

The spectrum of **anxiety disorders** includes generalized anxiety disorder (GAD), obsessive–compulsive disorder (OCD), panic disorder (PD), and post-traumatic stress disorder (PTSD). Approximately 13–40% of individuals will experience one or more anxiety disorders during the first year postpartum (Field, 2018; Lieb et al., 2020). Anxiety disorders have been associated with depression but are more difficult to diagnose due to symptom similarities. Studies have estimated that women with depression also frequently suffer from a comorbid anxiety disorder (Pawluski et al., 2017). Most studies utilize validated screening tools to assess depression but omit assessment for comorbid postpartum mood or anxiety disorders (Lieb et al., 2020).

Mood and anxiety disorders can increase with stress, lack of social support, as well as unhealthy lifestyle choices or conditions. Coupled with hormonal influences, physiological and social stressors have been indicated as triggers for mood and anxiety disorders (Fawcett et al., 2019; Goldfinger et al., 2019). In addition to social and economic risk factors, a family or personal history of mood or anxiety disorders increases risk. When accompanied by lack of sleep, demands of a new infant, and routine family activities, risk for mood and anxiety disorders multiplies (Fawcett et al., 2019).

The pathophysiology of mood and anxiety disorders is influenced by genetics as well as environment (Pawluski et al., 2017; Stahl, 2021). Dysfunction between the hypothalamic–pituitary–adrenal (HPA) axis and the noradrenergic and serotonergic systems can result in mood and anxiety disorders. The noradrenergic system has an increased reaction to stress, while the system reacting to serotonin has a decreased response, failing to inhibit serotonin. It is theorized that norepinephrine, dopamine, and serotonin system dysfunctions may individually or in combination initiate or exacerbate underlying mood or anxiety disorders (Stahl, 2021).

A team approach provides the best opportunity for appropriate diagnosis and treatment. Mental healthcare providers have expertise in diagnosis and management options. It is important for postpartum healthcare providers to have a list of local psychologists, psychiatrists, and support groups available for postpartum individuals. Mental health stigma can inhibit symptom disclosure and discussion between healthcare providers and those experiencing postpartum mood and anxiety disorders, contributing to their underdiagnosis.

Postpartum mood and anxiety disorders affect the entire family. Appropriate interaction with an infant, such as timely and sensitive response to infant cues, is often decreased or absent in the depressed individual. Decreased maternal–infant interaction may lead to delayed cognitive skills and long-term emotional effects for the child (Rad & Deluxe, 2022). Other children can suffer emotional neglect, which may lead to behavioral problems (Furtado et al., 2018).

Treatments for most of the mood and anxiety disorders include combining **psychotropics** and psychotherapy. On occasion, benzodiazepines are effective during an acute phase but should not be used long term, as they carry a high risk of dependence (Early, 2017).

Postpartum Blues

Postpartum mood disorders occur on a spectrum. At one end, some degree of transient, short-lived mood change, called **postpartum blues,** or "baby blues," occurs in approximately 70% or more of postpartum individuals. Postpartum blues appears within the first week after birth and typically resolves within two weeks (American Psychiatric Association [APA], 2020). Symptoms include mood swings, crying, anxiety, insomnia, irritability, and loss of appetite. Mood changes can be expected in the postpartum period due to hormones, stress of new or changing roles, and neurotransmitter alterations. Additionally, a surge in levels of monoamine oxidase (MAO-A), a brain protein, is thought to contribute to postpartum blues. MAO-A breaks down serotonin, norepinephrine, and dopamine, which can lead to feelings of sadness (Dowlati et al., 2017).

During the early postpartum period, individuals can benefit from family support, periods of uninterrupted rest, exercise, adequate fluids, and nutritious meals. One small study found that a dietary supplement comprised of tryptophan, tyrosine, blueberry juice, and blueberry extract moderated the surge in MAO-A and reduced the incidence of the blues in postpartum women compared to controls (Dowlati et al., 2017). Herbal remedies and supplements may be helpful but should be discussed with a healthcare provider, as some herbal remedies can have adverse drug interactions or potential side effects. For example, St. John's wort is an herb used to alleviate symptoms of depression. However, it is a potent inducer of cytochrome P450 3A4, a major drug-metabolizing enzyme in the liver, and thus interacts with many drugs, including selective serotonin reuptake inhibitors (SSRIs). The healthcare provider's role includes active listening, risk assessment, identification, management recommendations, and follow-up. Signs and symptoms are presented in Table 43.4.

Postpartum Depression

In the middle of the spectrum is PPD, which is the most prevalent and overlooked postpartum complication. It is estimated that PPD occurs in 9.7–23.5% of postpartum women with a prevalence of 13.2% (Bauman et al., 2020). Approximately 60% of women with PPD are undiagnosed, and of those who receive a diagnosis, 50% are untreated (Ko et al., 2017). PPD presents in varying degrees, with the potential for increased severity without treatment. PPD can first appear as postpartum blues, subsequently diagnosed as depression when symptoms persist longer than two weeks.

Depression can begin during the antepartum period with subtle signs such as fatigue, anxiety, or change in sleep or appetite patterns (all common occurrences during pregnancy) and remain unrecognized until exacerbated during the postpartum period. Signs and symptoms mimic many symptoms of postpartum blues but include extremes of appetite and sleep disturbances, as well as more severe symptoms including suicidal ideations. Individuals with PPD describe feelings of overwhelming sadness and despair. Isolation may be conditional or self-induced by refusal or inability to admit suffering (Beck, 1993). In addition, recognition may be confounded by symptom similarity to normal discomforts and adjustments of postpartum. Although commonly occurring around four weeks, PPD may develop anytime within the first year. PPD typically persists for a minimum of six months if untreated.

Risk factors include a personal or family history of a mental health disorder. Individuals with a previous or present diagnosis of depression or anxiety disorders before or during pregnancy are at highest risk for PPD. Other important risk factors include an array of social and physiological factors (Bradshaw et al., 2022).

Risk factors for postpartum depression

- Previous or current mental health disorder diagnosis
  - Depression
  - Anxiety disorders
  - Bipolar
  - Eating disorder
- Prenatal depression
- Stressful life events
  - History of sexual abuse
  - Intimate partner violence
  - Death in family
  - Socioeconomic hardship, poverty
  - Relationship issues
  - Immigration
- Substance use
- Multiparity
- Twins and higher order multiples

PPD may be associated with thyroid dysfunction or exacerbated by medical conditions. Some individuals will self-medicate with alcohol or other drugs, making

Table 43.4   Postpartum Mood and Anxiety Disorders: Clinical Signs and Symptoms

Postpartum mood disorders		
Blues (symptoms early onset and <14 days)	**Depression**	**Psychosis**
Tearful	Tearful	Hallucinations (visual and auditory)
Irritability	Irritability or anger	Delusions
Mood swings	Mood swings	Inability to communicate
Fatigue	Fatigue	Rapid mood change
Appetite changes	Appetite disturbances	Paranoia
	Lack of interest in the baby	Inability to sleep
	Sleep disturbances	Hyperactivity
	Feelings of harming the baby or self	Disorganized thoughts
	Guilt or shame	Confusion
	Feelings of isolation	Bizarre behavior
	Hopelessness	Onset is rapid
	Loss of pleasure	
	Cognition impairment	

Postpartum anxiety disorders			
Generalized anxiety	**Obsessive–compulsive**	**Panic**	**Post-traumatic stress**
Excessive worry for at least 6 months	Intrusive thoughts	Fear of dying	Flashbacks or nightmares
Sleep disturbances/fatigue	Checking	Dizziness, shortness of breath anxiety	Panic attack
Appetite changes	Cleaning	Heart palpitations	Powerlessness
Feelings of dread	Hypervigilance of infant	Feeling impending doom	Increased arousal
Physical symptoms		Extreme anxiety	Avoidance of situations
Restlessness		Irritable bowel	Detachment
Lack of concentration			
Irritability			
Muscle tension			

diagnosis more challenging. Others will turn to food for comfort, and weight gain can be a feature of depression. Screening for manic episodes is an important part of assessment as bipolar disorder may present with depressive symptoms.

PPD differential diagnosis

- Mild to major depression
- Bipolar disorder
- Psychosis
- Anxiety disorders
- Thyroid dysfunction
- Substance use
- Sleep deprivation

Psychotherapy, such as cognitive behavioral therapy (CBT), is a first-line treatment recommendation for individuals with mild to moderate PPD (Vigod & Stewart, 2017). SSRIs are the first-line treatment when choosing psychotropic management. Evidence has not demonstrated one particular mode of treatment as more successful; however, psychotherapy has been shown to decrease relapse particularly in combination with psychotropics. Treatment modality depends on client preference and severity and can be adjusted according to need. Careful consideration is warranted when prescribing antidepressant treatment, as they have potential to exacerbate a manic episode in the setting of bipolar disorder and potentially trigger a psychosis (Early, 2017). It is essential to assess for suicidal or homicidal ideation. If an individual has a suicide or homicide plan, immediate action is indicated.

Screening for suicidal or homicidal ideation

Ask: Precede the initial question about suicidal and homicidal ideation with a statement normalizing such thoughts in the setting of depression:

- "It is common for people who are feeling sad and depressed to have thoughts of ending their life or of harming others. Have you. . ."
  - Thought of hurting yourself, your baby, or others?
  - Made a plan to hurt yourself, your baby, or others?
  - Made prior attempts to hurt yourself, your baby, or others?

Assess: Positive responses need immediate attention. Those at high risk for suicide or homicide express intention, plans, means, and time frame.

Act:

- Call a crisis center hotline for advice and assistance.
- Take the individual to a psychiatrist or hospital.
- Call 911 and remain with the individual until help arrives.

Source: Tharpe et al. (2022).

Postpartum Psychosis

Postpartum psychosis occurs within the first few days to one week postpartum, with a prevalence of 1–2 per 1000 (VanderKruik et al., 2017). Onset can be abrupt and unexpected, although a previous history of mental illness is a common risk factor. Women with bipolar disorder have an increased risk for psychosis, and some instances of postpartum psychosis may represent previously undiagnosed and untreated bipolar disorder or other mood or psychotic disorders (Rommel et al., 2021). Other risk factors include family history, sleep deprivation, complications of childbirth, primiparity, age >35, immune dysregulation, and other life stressors, such as limited support from family or partner (Osborne, 2018). Although diagnosis of psychosis is challenging, the clinical impression is supported by the individual's skewed sense of reality. Family members are the primary source of information and frequently describe unusual behavior and little to no sleep for an extended period of time. Postpartum psychosis is a devastating experience for a family and can have tragic outcomes if not treated. Signs and symptoms are presented in Table 43.3.

Immediate referral to a psychiatric mental health specialist for medication and inpatient treatment at a mental health facility is warranted. The role of the referring healthcare provider includes patient and family education and support, assessment, identification, and timely referral.

Generalized Anxiety Disorder

GAD is defined as an extreme amount of worry that occurs on most days and lasts for at least six months (APA, 2022). The diagnosis of postpartum GAD may be missed if not recognized in the first six months postpartum. For this reason, it is important to consider while assessing mental health history during the initial prenatal visit, as well as continued assessment during pregnancy. Signs and symptoms are presented in Table 43.3. Prevalence of GAD during postpartum is 5.7% (Dennis et al., 2017). Risk factors include past or current medical, perinatal, or family history of anxiety, depression, thyroid imbalance, hormonal fluctuations, and life stressors (Goldfinger et al., 2019).

Treatment of choice for GAD includes SSRIs and/or psychotherapy. CBT is often a first-line treatment for GAD. Once patients are able to determine specific triggers that initiate anxious episodes, coping measures, such as relaxation, can be implemented (Green et al., 2021).

Obsessive–Compulsive Disorder

OCD is characterized by an onslaught of intrusive thoughts or rituals. Individuals are debilitated by the need to perform repetitive physical or mental actions. Cleaning, checking, or counting are the activities most often performed to relieve extreme stress (APA, 2022). In a recent study, OCD had a weighted postpartum period prevalence of 16.9% with an average point prevalence of 7.0 (Fairbrother et al., 2021). When compared to prenatal OCD, both period (an interval of time) and point (at a particular time) prevalence is higher during postpartum, usually peaking by eight weeks and gradually declining during the first year (Fairbrother et al., 2021). Individuals with postpartum OCD sometimes describe intrusive thoughts of harming their baby. It is important for a healthcare provider to note that these thoughts are considered ego-dystonic (not oneself) and should be differentiated from psychosis or homicidal ideation. Ego-dystonic thoughts are self-identified, and horror and guilt are expressed for having the disturbing thoughts (Lawrence et al., 2017). Many individuals will not report symptoms of OCD unless asked by a provider.

Treatment options include SSRIs and CBT. Long-term treatment is often necessary and can require higher psychotropic dosages. Referral to a mental health specialist is indicated.

Panic Disorder

PD is exemplified by recurrences of panic attacks, often without provocation. Perinatal prevalence ranges from 0.5% to 2.9% (Beck, 2021). Individuals describe intense fear that can peak abruptly and include at least four of the following: heart palpitations, shortness of breath, dizziness, numbness, shaking, sweating, nausea, chills, hot flashes, choking, feelings of unreality, or fear of dying. Individuals with PD may live in constant fear of experiencing an attack and may avoid environments if they suspect an attack could occur. Quality of life may be influenced by an inability to hold a job or adequately care for family (APA, 2022; Beck, 2021). Hormonal fluctuations increase the risk for exacerbation in the postpartum period. PD has been indicated as a risk factor for PPD (APA, 2022). Triggers for a panic attack include caffeine, certain substances such as alcohol, and stressful events.

Post-Traumatic Stress Disorder

PTSD is derived from the experience of a real or perceived threat of death to a person (APA, 2022). Prevalence of postpartum PTSD is estimated to be 4–6% (Dekel et al., 2017; Yildiz et al., 2017). PTSD is characterized by extreme fear and helplessness when exposed to the same or similar environment where the trauma occurred. In addition, individuals report being plagued by recurring thoughts and dreams (APA, 2022). Consequences of postpartum PTSD include relationship discord, hinderance of breastfeeding, and maternal–child attachment concerns (Beck, 2017; Kjerulff et al., 2021). For many individuals, the anniversary date of the birth trauma becomes a triggering event (Beck, 2017).

While trauma can arise from a variety of past and current life situations, it is important to recognize that some births can be physically and psychologically traumatic, regardless of the outcome. Healthcare providers should take the time to ask about the birth experience and how the individual feels about what transpired. Debriefing sessions by postpartum care providers offer opportunities for the individual to describe the experience, discuss feelings, define occurrences, and obtain validation. This provides an opportunity to correct misinformation or misunderstandings about the birth and to help reframe the narrative to assist in the integration of what the individual had hoped would happen with what really happened. PTSD has also been linked to postpartum mood and anxiety disorders.

Treatment for PTSD after birth trauma can vary depending on numerous factors such as barriers to care or individual preference. There is evidence to suggest some effectiveness using psychotropic medications such as SSRIs or short-term use of benzodiazepines (Nillni et al., 2018). However, psychotherapies such as CBT, interpersonal therapy (IPT) or other debriefing and counseling sessions have been shown to be an effective treatment and can help individuals cope with their fears. Modality of treatment (web, in-person, or telephone) does not change effectiveness. Alternative or complementary therapies, such as exercise or massage, are useful tools, as well. Several studies report a significant decrease in PTSD symptoms in mothers receiving debriefing, counseling, or CBT after traumatic birth (Nillni et al., 2018; Taylor et al., 2021).

Mood and Anxiety Disorder Assessment and Screening

Assessment for mental health disorders begins at the initial preconception or prenatal visit and should continue throughout postpartum care and beyond. (see Chapter 47, *Mood and Anxiety Disorders*). Screening for perinatal mood and anxiety disorders is not standard practice, but many organizations are now recommending screening. The American College of Nurse-Midwives (ACNM) supports universal screening, treatment, and referral as part of primary care (2020). The American College of Obstetricians and Gynecologists (ACOG) recommends screening with a validated screening tool at least once during the perinatal period (2018b). The US Preventative Services Task Force (USPSTF) released guidelines recommending routine screening throughout the perinatal period (2019).

Despite a growing emphasis on screening for perinatal mood and anxiety disorders, no specific tool has been endorsed. The screening tool used most often worldwide is the Edinburgh Postnatal Depression Scale (EPDS). The EPDS has sufficient evidence to support validity and reliability (ACOG, 2018b) and has been translated into numerous languages. The EPDS is a brief, 10-item questionnaire that is easily completed in the office setting and provides a means for continued assessment. The EPDS does not specifically screen for anxiety but does include two questions that may help identify anxiety disorders. Other common screening tools include the Postpartum Depression Screening Scale (PDSS), the Center for Epidemiological Studies-Depression Scale (CED-D), the Patient Health Questionnaire (PHQ-9), and the Beck Depression Inventory (BDI).

There are few available screening tools validated to detect anxiety disorders in postpartum individuals. The generalized anxiety disorder seven-item scale (GAD-7) is commonly used to screen for anxiety in nonpregnant individuals and has been validated for use postpartum, but not widely recommended. The State–Trait Anxiety Inventory (STAI) has been used to screen for GAD in pregnancy and postpartum. This particular instrument is used to simplify the separation between feelings of anxiety and depression (Furtado et al., 2018).

Assessment for mood and anxiety disorders also includes a comprehensive history of pregnancy, labor, birth, and postpartum, including personal perceptions of events and outcomes, and coping measures. Current or history of mental health issues for the individual and their family can indicate increased risk. Social assessment should include economic and family stressors, as well as substance use and physical or emotional intimate partner violence and past or present sexual abuse.

Management of Mood and Anxiety Disorders

Management for postpartum mood and anxiety disorders should incorporate a multifaceted approach of an interdisciplinary healthcare team. Severity of condition and congruence with the individual's needs and desires guides the healthcare provider's plan. Treatment plans may include psychotropics, IPT, CBT, as well as various alternative or adjunctive therapies.

Consideration of appropriate psychotropic treatment includes past history of psychotropic medication, side effects, and tolerance. Cost of medication may be factored into the decision, as well as the individual's personal concerns regarding side effects. Postpartum individuals may have increased weight from pregnancy, feel fatigued, and have decreased sexual desire, all possible side effects of psychotropic medication. Choosing a cost-effective medication with the least side effects can increase adherence to and efficacy of the treatment plan (Green et al., 2021; Luca et al., 2020).

The US Food and Drug Administration (FDA) has replaced the formerly used pregnancy letter categories A, B, C, D, and X with a narrative risk, summarizing known data, and lactation labeling now provides three subheadings of risk, clinical considerations, and data. Prescribing of any medication should include a discussion that provides information for known risks and benefits. Some common psychotropic medications for depression and anxiety are described in Table 43.5. It is important for the provider to have access to a psychopharmacology resource to access the most current information and research. SSRIs are the most widely prescribed antidepressants as well as treatment of choice for anxiety disorders for postpartum and lactating individuals (ACOG, 2008; Early, 2017).

By inhibiting the reuptake of serotonin in the presynaptic cell, the level of serotonin increases in the synapses. There are multiple serotonin receptor cells ($5\text{-}HT_1$–$5\text{-}HT_{15}$). Each SSRI reacts differently on receptor cells, causing variable side effects (Early, 2017). Side effects typically last a few weeks and resolve once the body adapts to the medication. Most practitioners begin treatment with a lower dose, increasing after one to two weeks or as tolerated (Early, 2017; Stahl, 2021). Side effects characteristically include gastrointestinal disturbances, headaches, anorgasmia and decreased libido, weight gain or loss, sweating, vivid dreams, and agitation. Side effects play an important role in continuation of treatment and should be considered when choosing the appropriate drug therapy. Suicidal ideation has been reported in adolescents and young adults; SSRIs have an FDA black box warning for risk of suicidal thoughts for individuals 25 years and younger (Early, 2017; Stahl, 2021).

Teaching points with SSRIs include dosage, side effects, and importance of provider-guided weaning when discontinuing medication. Serotonin discontinuation syndrome can occur if the drugs are withdrawn abruptly. Symptoms of discontinuation syndrome include dizziness, confusion and tremor, and electric shock-like sensations (Early, 2017; Stahl, 2021).

Serotonin norepinephrine reuptake inhibitors (SNRIs) have a similar mechanism of action as SSRIs. In addition to inhibiting serotonin, SNRIs also inhibit norepinephrine in the neuronal synapses. Some report SRNIs begin to work more quickly. Side effects are similar to SSRIs, but some SRNIs (venlafaxine and duloxetine) can increase blood pressure (Stahl, 2021).

Norepinephrine and dopamine reuptake inhibitors (e.g., bupropion) are sometimes a good choice for PPD, as there are fewer sedative effects, and they do not cause weight gain or decrease libido. Bupropion can trigger seizures and should not be used in individuals with a seizure disorder. Although bupropion can be used for depression, it is not helpful for GAD but may be helpful in the treatment of PD (Stahl, 2021).

Tricyclic antidepressants (TCAs), once the primary medication for treatment of anxiety disorders and depression, are used less frequently today, as they have many side effects and drug interactions. Although TCAs are helpful for insomnia, individuals of childbearing age usually respond better to SSRIs. It is important to note that overdose with TCAs can be fatal (Early, 2017). Prescriptions should only be written for seven-day increments and are best managed by a mental health provider.

In 2019, the FDA approved the first medication for the treatment of PPD, Zulresso (Brexanolone). This treatment is delivered over 60 hours by IV and can cause significant sedation, therefore requiring inpatient management. Placebo-controlled studies have shown improvement in depressive symptoms at 60 hours and 30 days after initial treatment (FDA, 2019).

Psychotherapies are an important treatment modality used alone or in conjunction with pharmacotherapies. CBT utilizes specific behaviors to change a pattern of thinking or redirect negative thoughts. Postpartum individuals identify particular coping mechanisms that effectively interrupt negative or destructive thought processes (Buhagiar, 2019). IPT focuses on particular conflicts and stress-inducing situations. Postpartum individuals typically focus on infant attachment, role transition, or partner conflict and intimacy issues. A provider can facilitate IPT through phone contact, or other means, decreasing barriers to care (Nillni et al., 2018).

Peer support is gaining recognition as evidence shows a potential to prevent or decrease effects of depression (Huang et al., 2020). Peer support can be offered by various means: face-to-face groups, telephone, internet, and other media (Shorey et al., 2019). Peer support encourages sharing personal stories, postpartum or daily life stresses, and coping mechanisms. Healthcare providers can facilitate peer groups. CenteringPregnancy™ groups can extend their scheduled sessions into early postpartum and can be an important social support group for new parents. Some have continued the concept into CenteringParenting™ groups that provide emotional and tangible support for the challenges and joys of raising children.

Complementary therapies are sometimes used by individuals who are reluctant to undergo drug therapy. Omega-3 fatty acid supplements, kava root, and St. John's wort have been found to have mixed results of effectiveness, although they can ameliorate some symptoms of mental health disorders (Early, 2017; Tharpe et al., 2022). Bright light therapy, exercise, Omega-3 fatty acids, or folate are safe and can, therefore, be effective as a first-line or adjunct therapy (Tharpe et al., 2022). An assessment of alternative therapy use before starting psychotropic therapy should be done. Most complementary treatments lack an evidence base supporting their effectiveness, benefits, and risks. Teaching includes awareness of label inaccuracy as not all active ingredients and substances (leaves, stems, and roots) are described. Resources for common herbs and dietary supplements are available through the National Library of Medicine (see *Resources for Healthcare Providers*).

Table 43.5 FDA-Approved Common Medications for Depression and Anxiety Disorders

Generic (brand)	FDA-approved indications	Dosage	Common side effects	Clinical considerations
Selective serotonin reuptake inhibitors[a]				
Fluoxetine (Prozac)	MDD GAD OCD PD	Initial dose 5 mg/day in am, then increase by 5 mg each week up to 20 mg. Wait a month to assess drug effects before increasing dose, increasing by 20 mg/month; maximum dose generally 80 mg/day (Stahl, 2021)	Initial agitation/sleep disturbance, sedation at high doses, sexual dysfunction Some GI upset, but much less with low dosage and gradual increase (Stahl, 2021)	Weight neutral Take in a.m. to not interfere with sleep Decreased withdrawal symptoms if suddenly discontinued (Stahl, 2021)
Paroxetine (Paxil, Paxil CR)	GAD PTSD OCD PD MDD Social anxiety	Panic disorder: initial 10 mg/day (12.5 mg/day CR); usually wait a few weeks to assess drug effects before increasing dose but can increase by 10 mg/day (12.5 mg/day CR) once a week; maximum generally 60 mg/day (75 mg/day CR); single dose. MDD: initial 20 mg/day (25 mg/day CR); usually wait a few weeks to assess drug effects before increasing dose, but can increase by 10 mg/day (12.5 mg/day CR) once a week; maximum 60 mg/day (75 mg/day CR); single dose (Stahl, 2021)	Sedation, weight gain, sexual dysfunction (Stahl, 2021)	Most sedating SSRI (may choose to take in evening) and most potential for weight gain Difficult discontinuation A favorite first choice for GAD, PTSD (Stahl, 2021)
Escitalopram (Lexapro)	GAD MDD	Initial 5 mg/day; increase to 20 mg/day if necessary; single dose; 10 mg of escitalopram may be comparable in efficacy to 40 mg of citalopram with fewer side effects. Give an adequate trial of 10 mg prior to giving 20 mg (Stahl, 2021)	Sexual dysfunction, GI symptoms, dry mouth, insomnia, sedation, agitation, tremors, headache, dizziness, sweating, bruising, and rare bleeding Rare hyponatremia (mostly in elderly patients) (Stahl, 2021)	Relatively expensive Less GI symptoms than citalopram (Stahl, 2021)
Sertraline (Zoloft)	MDD OCD PD PTSD PMDD Social anxiety	Initial 25 mg/day; increase to 50 mg/day after 1 week; thereafter, usually wait a few weeks to assess drug effects before increasing dose; maximum generally 200 mg/day; single dose (Stahl, 2021)	GI distress, weight gain, sexual dysfunction (Stahl, 2021)	Good first choice SSRI in pregnancy
Fluvoxamine (Luvox)	OCD MDD (off-label)	Initial 50–300 mg/day. Initial 50–100 mg/day (Stahl, 2021)	GI symptoms, sexual dysfunction, difficulty sleeping. (Stahl, 2021)	Dosages higher than 100 mg/day should be in divided dosages due to short half-life. (Stahl, 2021)

(Continued)

Table 43.5 (Continued)

Generic (brand)	FDA-approved indications	Dosage	Common side effects	Clinical considerations
Tricyclic antidepressantsa				
Clomipramine (Anafranil)	OCD	Initial 25 mg/day; increase over 2 weeks to 100 mg/day maximum dose; OCD may require doses at the high end of the range (e.g., 200–250 mg/day) (Stahl, 2021)	GI upset, sedation.	Take with meals. More side effects than SSRIs (Stahl, 2021)
Doxepin (Sinequan)	Anxiety	Initial 25 mg/day at bedtime; increase by 25 mg every 3–7 days 75 mg/day; increase gradually until desired efficacy is achieved; Can be dosed once a day at bedtime or in divided doses; maximum dose 300 mg/day (Stahl, 2021)	Sedation	Helpful for anxiety with skin/hair/scalp/nail issues (scratchers and pickers) Recent FDA approval as a sleep agent. (Stahl, 2021)
Serotonin norepinephrine reuptake inhibitorsa				
Venlafaxine XR (Effexor XR)	GAD MDD PD PPD Social anxiety	Initial dose 37.5 mg once daily (extended release) or 25–50 mg divided into two to three doses (immediate release) for a week, if tolerated, increase daily dose generally no faster than 75 mg every 4 days until desired efficacy is reached; maximum dose generally 375 mg/day. Usually try doses at 75 mg increments for a few weeks prior to incrementing by an additional 75 mg. GAD—150–225 mg/day MDD—75–225 mg/day (Stahl, 2021)	Less sexual dysfunction than SSRIs (Stahl, 2021)	Difficult discontinuation Monitor for hypertension Helpful for pain syndromes (Stahl, 2021)
Duloxetine (Cymbalta)	GAD PD	For generalized anxiety, initial 60 mg once daily; maximum dose generally 120 mg/day (Stahl, 2021)	Nausea (Stahl, 2021)	Weight neutral Fewer sexual side effects/add to SSRI to decrease sexual dysfunction Hepatotoxicity—watch alcohol intake (Stahl, 2021)
Norepinephrine-dopamine reuptake inhibitors (NDRIs)a				
Bupropion (Wellbutrin)	MDD	200:450 mg in three divided doses, SR: 200–400 mg in two divided doses XL–150–450 mg/day (Stahl, 2021)	Dry mouth, GI symptoms, anorexia, headache, insomnia, sweating, rash, hypertension (Stahl, 2021)	Rise in supine BP (Stahl, 2021)

Other nonbenzodiazepines

Drug	Indication	Dosing	Side effects	Comments
Buspirone (BuSpar)	Anxiety	Initial 15 mg twice a day; increase in 5 mg/day; increments every 2–3 days until desired efficacy is reached; maximum dose generally 60 mg/day (Stahl, 2021)	Nausea, dizziness, restlessness, insomnia (Stahl, 2021)	Generally not as effective for monotherapy as other agents; may augment SSRIs; recommended as SSRI augment to reduce sexual dysfunction (Stahl, 2021)
Hydroxyzine (Vistaril)	GAD	50–100 mg four times a day (Stahl, 2021)	Sedation, dizziness (Stahl, 2021)	Can be agitating in some; Driving precautions; A good augment with SSRIs (Stahl, 2021)

Benzodiazepines[b]

Drug	Indication	Dosing	Side effects	Comments
Lorazepam (Ativan)	Occasional Situational anxiety	0.5 mg po (Stahl, 2021)	Sedation, dizziness (Stahl, 2021)	Short acting, rapid tolerance; Acute, short-term use agent; contraindicated for individuals with acute narrow-angle glaucoma, sleep apnea, myasthenia gravis; Avoid any use with history of chemical dependency (Early, 2017)
Clonazepam (Klonopin)	Short-term use while starting SSRI (2–4 weeks) (Stahl, 2021)	0.5 mg po daily, may split dose (Stahl, 2021)	Sedation, dizziness (Stahl, 2021)	Potential for dependence; Avoided with history of chemical dependency; Contraindicated for individuals with acute narrow-angle glaucoma or hepatic failure; A good choice for the first 2–4 weeks when starting an SSRI for panic symptoms (Stahl, 2021)
Alprazolam (Xanax)	Anxiety	0.25 mg po (Stahl, 2021)	Sedation, dizziness (Stahl, 2021)	Multiple drug/drug interactions; Risk of dependence is high; Avoid use except in limited situations, such as air travel, or needle phobia. Use in collaboration with a mental health specialist (Stahl, 2021)

FDA: Federal Drug Administration; GAD: generalized anxiety disorder; MDD: major depressive disorder; OCD: obsessive–compulsive disorder; PD: panic disorder; PTSD: post-traumatic stress disorder; PMDD: premenstrual dysphoric disorder; po: by mouth; mg: milligram; GI: gastrointestinal; NDRI: norepinephrine-dopamine reuptake inhibitor.

[a] Black box warning—suicidality in children, adolescents, and young adults up to 25 years (ages of some childbearing people).

[b] All benzodiazepines have the risk of tolerance and dependency and should be avoided for long-term use.

Summary

Postpartum is a time of restoration and new beginnings. Healthcare providers familiar with normal physiologic changes during postpartum will be most astute at recognition of complications. Cultural awareness should guide assessment and treatment. Provision of education, regular assessment, and follow-up will increase the likelihood of early identification and treatment. In addition to assessment, healthcare providers will diagnose and treat while recognizing when to consult, collaborate, or refer. Development of a local resource and referral list will provide individuals with options for treatment or assistance and should include supportive social and psychological services in addition to medical services.

Resources for Clients and Their Families

Postpartum Support International: Information including access to support groups and perinatal mental health specialists regarding Perinatal Mood and Anxiety Disorders: http://postpartum.net

Resources for Healthcare Providers

CenteringParenting. Centering Healthcare Institute: https://www.centeringhealthcare.org/what-we-do/centering-parenting

Council on Patient Safety in Women's Health Care: https://safehealthcareforeverywoman.org/

Edinburgh Postnatal Depression Scale (EDPS: https://perinatology.com/calculators/Edinburgh%20Depression%20Scale.htm

Generalized Anxiety Disorder 7 (GAD-7) Screening tool: https://www.mdcalc.com/calc/1727/gad7-general-anxiety-disorder7

Global Library of Women's Medicine (GLOWM): https://www.glowm.com

Medline Plus [Internet]. Bethesda, MD: National Library of Medicine (US). Herbs and supplements: http://www.nlm.nih.gov/medlineplus/druginformation.html

References

Ain, Q., Shetty, N., & Supriya, K. (2021). Postpartum urinary retention and its associated obstetric risk factors among women undergoing vaginal delivery in tertiary care hospital. *Journal of Gynecology Obstetrics and Human Reproduction, 50*(2), 101837. https://doi.org/10.1016/j.jogoh.2020.101837

American College of Nurse-Midwives (ACNM). (2020). *Position statement: Mental health during childbirth and across the lifespan.* https://www.midwife.org/acnm/files/acnmlibrarydata/uploadfilename/000000000324/PS-Mental%20Health%20During%20Childbirth%20and%20Across%20Lifespan.pdf

American College of Obstetricians and Gynecologists (ACOG). (2008, reaffirmed 2016)). Use of psychiatric medications during pregnancy and lactation: Clinical management guidelines for obstetrician-gynecologists. Practice bulletin No. 92. *Obstetrics & Gynecology, 111,* 1001–1020.

American College of Obstetricians and Gynecologists (ACOG). (2017). Postpartum hemorrhage. Practice bulletin No. 183. *Obstetrics & Gynecology, 130*(4), e168–e186.

American College of Obstetricians and Gynecologists (ACOG). (2018a). Use of prophylactic antibiotics in labor and delivery, Practice Bulletin No. 199. *Obstetrics & Gynecology, 132*(3), e103–e119. https://doi.org/10.1097/AOG.0000000000002833

American College of Obstetricians and Gynecologists (ACOG). (2018b). Screening for perinatal depression: Committee opinion No. 757. *Obstetrics & Gynecology, 132*(5), e208–e212.

American College of Obstetricians and Gynecologists (ACOG). (2020). Gestational hypertension and preeclampsia: Practice Bulletin, No. 222. *Obstetrics & Gynecology, 135*(6), e237–e260.

American Psychiatric Association. (2020). *What is peripartum depression (formerly postpartum)* https://www.psychiatry.org/patients-families/postpartum-depression/what-is-postpartum-depression

American Psychiatric Association (APA). (2022). *Diagnostic and statistical manual of mental* disorders (DSM-5-TR), 5 Text Revision, American Psychiatric Association.

Bauman, B. L., Ko, J. Y., Cox, S., D'Angelo, D. V., Warner, S., Folger, S., Tevendale, H. D., Coy, K. C., Harrison, L., & Barfield, W. D. (2020). Vital signs: Postpartum depressive symptoms and provider discussions about perinatal depression – Unites States, 2018. *Morbidity and Mortality Weekly Report, 69*(19), 575–581.

Beck, C. T. (1993). Teetering on the edge: A substantive theory of postpartum depression. *Nursing Research, 42*(1), 42–48.

Beck, C. T. (2017). The anniversary of birth trauma: A metaphor analysis. *The Journal of Perinatal Education, 26*(4), 219–228. https://doi.org/10.1891/1058-1243.26.4.219

Beck, C. T. (2021). Postpartum onset of panic disorder: A metaphor analysis. *Archives of Psychiatric Nursing, 35,* 369–374.

Biurrun, G. P., Gonzalez-Doza, E., Fernandez, C., & Corona, A. F. (2020). Postpartum urinary retention and related risk factors. *Urology, 143,* 97–102. https://doi.org/10.1016/j.urology.2020.03.061

Black, C. M., Vesco, K. K., Mehta, V., Ohman-Strickland, P., Demissie, K., & Schneider, D. (2021). Hospital readmission following delivery with and without severe maternal morbidity. *Journal of Women's Health, 30*(12), 1736–1743. https://doi.org/10.1089/jwh.2020.8815

Bradshaw, H., Riddle, J. M., Salimgaraev, R., Zhaunova, L., & Payne, J. L. (2022). Risk factors associated with postpartum depressive symptoms: A multinational study. *Journal of Affective Disorders, 15*(301), 345–351. https://doi.org/10.1016/j.jad.2021.12.121

Buhagiar, R. (2019). Psychological interventions in post-partum depression: A critical analysis. *Malta Medical Journal, 31*(3), 30–33.

Byrne, B., Ryan, K., & Lavin, M. (2021). Current challenges in the peripartum management of women with von Willebrand disease. *Seminars in Thrombosis and Hemostasis, 47*(2), 217–228. https://doi.org/10.1055/s-0041-1723797

Centers for Disease Control and Prevention (CDC). (2022). *Pregnancy mortality surveillance system.* https://www.cdc.gov/reproductivehealth/maternal-mortality/pregnancy-mortality-surveillance-system.htm

Collier, A. Y., & Molina, R. L. (2019). Maternal mortality in the United States: Updates on trends, causes, and solutions. *Neoreviews, 20*(10), e561–e574. https://doi.org/10.1542/neo.20-10-e561

Cunningham, F. G., Leveno, K. J., Dashe, J., Hoffman, B., Spong, C. Y., & Casey, B. (2022). *Williams obstetrics* (26th ed.). McGraw-Hill Co.

Dekel, S., Stuebe, C., & Dishy, G. (2017). Childbirth induced posttraumatic stress syndrome: A systematic review of prevalence and risk factors. *Frontiers in Psychology, 8,* 1–10. https://doi.org/10.3389/fpsyg.2017.00560

Dennis, C. L., Falah-Hassani, K., & Shiri, R. (2017). Prevalence of antenatal and postnatal anxiety: Systematic review and meta-analysis. *The British Journal of Psychiatry, 210*(5), 315–323.

Dowlati, Y., Ravindran, A. V., Segal, Z. V., Stewart, D. E., Steiner, M., & Meyer, J. H. (2017). Selective dietary supplementation in early postpartum is associated with high resilience against depressed mood. *PNAS, 144*(13), 3509–3514.

Early, N. K. (2017). Mental health. In M. C. Brucker & T. L. King (Eds.), *Pharmacology for women's health* (2nd ed., pp. 727–764). Jones and Bartlett.

Epp, R., Malcolm, J., Jolin-Dahel, K., Clermont, M., & Keely, E. (2021). Postpartum thyroiditis. *BMJ, 372,* n495. https://doi.org/10.1136/bmj.n495

Fairbrother, N., Collardeau, F., Albert, A. Y. K., Challacombe, F. L., Thordarson, D. S., Woody, S. R., & Janssen, P. A. (2021). High prevalence and incidence of obsessive–compulsive disorder among women across pregnancy and the postpartum. *The Journal of Clinical Psychiatry, 82*(2), e1–e8, 30368

Fawcett, E. J., Fairbrother, N., Cox, M. L., White, I. R., & Fawcett, J. M. (2019). The prevalence of anxiety disorders during pregnancy and the postpartum period: A multivariate Bayesian meta-analysis. *The Journal of Clinical Psychiatry, 80*(4), 18r12527.

Field. (2018). Postnatal anxiety prevalence, predictors and effects on development: A narrative review. *Infant Behavior and Development, 51*, 24–32.

Folk, D. (2018). Hypertensive disorders of pregnancy: Overview and current recommendations. *Journal of Midwifery and Women's Health, 63*(3), 289–300.

Food and Drug Administration. (2019). *FDA approves first drug for postpartum depression.* https://www.fda.gov/news-events/press-announcements/fda-approves-first-treatment-post-partum-depression

Friedman, A. M. (2021). Obstetric venous thromboembolism prophylaxis, risk factors and outcomes. *Current Opinions in Obstetrics and Gynecology, 33*(5), 384–390. https://doi.org/10.1097/GCO.000000000000733

Furtado, M., Chow, C. H. T., Owais, S., Frey, B. N., & Van Lieshout, R. J. (2018). Risk factors of new onset anxiety and anxiety exacerbation in the perinatal period: A systematic review and meta-analysis. *Journal of Affective Disorder, 238*, 626–635. https://doi.org/10.1016/j.jad.2018.05.073

Goldfinger, C., Green, S. M., Furtado, M., & McCabe, R. E. (2019). Characterizing the nature of worry in a sample of perinatal women with generalized anxiety disorder. *Clinical Psychology and Psychotherapy, 27*, 136–145. https://doi.org.frontier.idm.oclc.org/10.1002/cpp.2413

Green, S. M., Donegna, E., McCabe, R. E., Streiner, D. L., Furtado, M., Noble, L., Agako, A., & Frey, B. N. (2021). Cognitive behavior therapy for women with generalized anxiety disorder in the perinatal period: Impact on problematic behaviors. *Behavior Therapy, 52*(4), 907–916. https://doi.org/10.1016/j.beth.2020.11.004

Haas, D. M., Morgan, S., Contreras, K., & Kimball, S. (2020). Vaginal preparation with antiseptic solution before cesarean section for preventing postoperative infections. *Cochrane Database Systematic Review, 4*, CD007892. https://doi.org/10.1002/14651858.CD007892.pub7

Huang, R., Yan, C., Tian, Y., Lei, B., Yang, D., Liu, D., & Lei, J. (2020). Effectiveness of peer support intervention on perinatal depression: A systematic review and meta-analysis. *Journal of Affective Disorders, 276*, 788–796.

Kjerulff, K. H., Attanasio, L. B., Sznajder, K. K., & Brubaker, L. H. (2021). A prospective cohort study of post-traumatic stress disorder and maternal-infant bonding after first childbirth. *Journal of Psychosomatic Research, 144*, 110424. https://doi.org/10.1016/j.jpsychores.2021.110424

Ko, J. Y., Rockhill, K. M., Tong, V. T., Morrow, B., & Farr, S. L. (2017). Trends in postpartum depressive symptoms – 27 states, 2004, 2008, and 2012. *Morbidity & Mortality Weekly Report, 66*(6), 153–158.

Lawrence, P. J., Craske, M. G., Kempton, C., Stewart, A., & Stein, A. (2017). Intrusive thoughts and images of intentional harm to infants in the context of maternal postnatal depression, anxiety, and OCD. *British Journal of General Practice, 67*(661), 376–377. https://doi.org/10.3399/bjgp17X692105

Liabsuetrakul, T., Choobun, T., Peeyananjarassri, K., & Islam, O. M. (2020). Antibiotic prophylaxis for operative vaginal delivery. *Cochrane Database Systematic Review, 3*, CD004455. https://doi.org/10.1002/14651858.CD004455.pub5

Lieb, K., Reinstein, S., Xianhong, S., Bernstein, P. S., & Karkowsky, C. E. (2020). Adding perinatal anxiety screening to depression screening: is it worth it? *American Journal of Obstetrics and Gynecology, MFM, 2*(2), 1, 100099–8. https://doi.org/10.1016/j.ajogmf.2020.100099

Luca, D. L., Margiotta, C., Staatz, C., Garlow, E., Christensen, A., & Zivin, K. (2020). Financial toll of untreated perinatal mood and anxiety disorders among 2017 births in the United States. *American Journal of Public Health, 110*(6), 888–896. https://doi.org/10.2105/AJPH.2020.305619

Nillni, Y. I., Mehralizade, A., Mayer, L., & Milanovic, S. (2018). Treatment of depression, anxiety, and trauma-related disorders during the perinatal period: A systematic review. *Clinical Psychology Review, 66*, 136–148. https://doi.org/10.1016/j.cpr.2018.06.004

Osborne, L. M. (2018). Recognizing and managing postpartum psychosis: a clinical guide for obstetric providers. *Obstetrics and Gynecology Clinics of North America, 45*(3), 455–468. https://doi.org/10.1016/j.ogc.2018.04.005

Pawluski, J. L., Lonstein, J. D., & Fleming, A. S. (2017). The neurobiology of postpartum anxiety and depression. *Trends in Neurosciences, 40*(2), 106–120.

Pearce, E. N. (2018). Management of thyrotoxicosis: Preconception, pregnancy, and the postpartum period. *Endocrincology Practice, 25*, 62–68.

Rad, N. S., & Deluxe, L. (2022). *Postpartum thyroiditis.* StatPearls [Internet]. StatPearls Publishing. https://www.ncbi.nlm.nih.gov/books/NBK557646/

Rani, S., Verma, M., Pandher, D. K., Takkar, N., & Huria, A. (2017). Risk factors and incidence of puerperal genital haematomas. *Journal of Clinical and Diagnostic Research, 11*(5), QC01–QC03. https://doi.org/10.7860/JCDR/2017/24060.9777

Redman, E. K., Hauspurg, A., Hubel, C. A., Roberts, J. M., & Jeyabalan, A. (2019). Clinical course, associated factors, and blood pressure profile of delayed-onset postpartum preeclampsia. *Obstetrics & Gynecology, 134*(5), 995–1001. https://doi.org/10.1097/AOG.0000000000003508

Rommel, A. S., Molenaar, M. M., Gilden, J., Kushner, S., Westerbeek, N. J., Kamperman, A. M., & Bergink, V. (2021). Long-term outcome of postpartum, psychosis: A prospective clinical cohort study in 106 women. *International Journal of Bipolar Disorders, 9*(31), 1–10.

Sharma, K. J., & Kilpatrick, S. J. (2017). Postpartum hypertension: etiology, diagnosis, and management. *Obstetrical & Gynecological Survey, 72*(4), 248–252.

Shorey, S., Chee, C. Y. I., Ng, E. D., Lau, Y., Dennis, C. L., & Chan, Y. H. (2019). Evaluation of a technology-based peer-support intervention program for preventing postnatal depression (Part 1): Randomized controlled trial. *Journal of Medical Internet Research, 21*(8), e12410. https://doi.org/10.2196/12410. PMID: 31469084; PMCID: PMC6744221

Stahl, S. M. (2021). *Stahl's essential psychopharmacology: prescriber's guide* (7th ed.). Cambridge University Press.

Stern-Ascher, C. N., Huang, Y., Duffy, C. R., Andrikopoulou, M., Wright, J. D., Goffman, D., D'Alton, M. E., & Friedman, A. M. (2020). Antibiotics for 3rd and 4th edge vaginal lacerations, uterine tamponade, and manual placental extraction. *American Journal of Perinatology, 37*(01), 92–103. https://doi.org/10.1055/s-0039-3400306

Stevens, S. M., Woller, S. C., Baumann, K. L., Bounameaux, H., Doerschug, K., Geersing, G. J., Huisman, M. V., Kearon, C., King, C. S., Knighton, A. J., Lake, E., Murin, S., Vintch, J. R. E., Wells, P. S., & Moores, L. K. (2021). Executive summary: Antithrombotic therapy for VTE Disease: Second update of the CHEST guideline and expert panel report. *Chest, 160*(6), 2247–2259. ISSN 0012-3692, https://doi.org/10.1016/j.chest.2021.07.056

Taylor, M., & Pillarisetty, L. S. (2022). *Endometritis.* StatPearls [Internet]. StatPearls Publishing. https://www.ncbi.nlm.nih.gov/books/NBK553124/

Taylor, M. P. G., Sinclair, M., Gillen, P., McCullough, J. E. M., Miller, P. W., Farrell, D. P., Slater, P. F., Shaprio, E., & Klaus, P. (2021). Early psychological interventions for prevention and treatment of post-traumatic stress disorder (PTSD) and post-traumatic stress symptoms in post-partum women: A systematic review and meta-analysis. *PLoS ONE, 16*(11), e0258170. https://doi.org/10.1371/journal.pone.0258170

Tharpe, N., Farley, C. L., & Jordan, R. (2022). *Clinical practice guidelines for midwifery & women's health* (6th ed.). Jones and Bartlett Learning.

United States Preventative Task Force. (2019). Interventions to prevent perinatal depression- USPTF recommendation statement. *Journal of American Medical Society, 321*(6), 580–587. https://doi.org/10.1001/jama.2019.0007

VanderKruik, R., Barreix, M., Chou, D., Allen, T., Say, L., & Cohen, L. S., on behalf of Maternal Morbidity Working Group. (2017). The global prevalence of postpartum psychosis: A systematic review. *BMC Psychiatry*, *17*(1), 272. https://doi.org/10.1186/s12888-017-1427-7

Vigod, S. N., & Stewart, D. E. (2017). Postpartum depression. *New England Journal of Medicine*, *376*, 895. https://doi.org/10.1056/NEJMc1616547

Walker, S. B., Rossi, D. M., & Sander, T. M. (2019). Women's successful transition to motherhood during the early postnatal period: A qualitative systematic review of postnatal and midwifery home care literature. *Midwifery*, *79*, 102552. https://doi.org/10.1016/j.midw.2019.102552

World Health Organization. (2019). *Trends in maternal mortality 2000 to 2017: estimates by WHO, UNICEF, UNFPA, World Bank Group and the United Nations Population Division, executive summary*. World Health Organization. https://www.unfpa.org/featured-publication/trends-maternal-mortality-2000-2017

Yildiz, P. D., Ayers, S., & Phillips, L. (2017). The prevalence of post-traumatic stress disorder in pregnancy and after birth: A systematic review and meta-analysis. *Journal of Affective Disorders*, *208*, 634–645.

44

Common Lactation and Breastfeeding Problems

Marsha Walker

Relevant Terms

Ankyloglossia—restricted motion of the infant's tongue that interferes with feeding and can cause nipple trauma; also known as "tongue-tie"

Alternate massage—massage and compression of the breast while the infant is sucking to increase milk intake

Delayed lactogenesis II—delay in the onset of copious milk production beyond the normal interval of two to four days after birth

Engorgement—painful swelling of the breasts associated with the sudden increase in milk volume, lymphatic and vascular congestion, and interstitial edema that typically occurs during the first two weeks following childbirth

Flat or inverted nipple—a nipple that does not easily protrude from the areola, even with stimulation

Frenotomy—the procedure by which the lingual frenulum is cut when it appears unusually short or tight

Galactagogue—medication or agent that increases the milk supply

Latch—the mechanism by which the baby attaches to the breast; a correct latch delivers milk to the baby and can influence breastfeeding success

Mastitis—acute inflammation of the interlobular connective tissue of the breast that may involve an infection

Oral aversion—infant withdraws from oral stimuli such as feeding; often associated with a history of oral procedures such as suctioning, intubation, and gavage feedings

Healthy equity key points

- All breastfeeding individuals need support, but specific interventions might be needed among populations and facilities with lower breastfeeding prevalence.
- People with low resources or in rural areas may experience a lack of access to skilled lactation services, while in other areas, they are available but cost prohibitive.
- Clinicians must avoid microaggressions and stereotyping, listen closely, and pay attention to the feelings, information, plans, and thoughts of Black pregnant and breastfeeding women while being empathetic and allowing their voices to be heard and respected.
- Preterm infants cared for in neonatal intensive care units located within communities of color may utilize mother's own breastmilk less often and have less access to, or in some cases, no access to donor milk.

Introduction

Breastfeeding is the optimal method of feeding an infant and provides improved short- and long-term health outcomes; however, there are several common problems that pose a challenge to continued and exclusive breastfeeding. The most common breastfeeding problems encountered in the early postnatal period include infant problems such as failure to **latch**, fussiness or sleepiness at the breast, low weight gain, and prematurity, and maternal problems such as sore nipples, **engorgement**, **mastitis**, and low milk supply. This chapter reviews the management of these common but important breastfeeding problems.

Common Infant-Related Breastfeeding Problems

Difficulty or Failure to Latch

A definitive aspect of the mechanics of breastfeeding is the ability of the infant to draw the nipple and part of the areola into their mouth, referred to as latch or latch on. The infant opens the mouth wide such that the angle at the corner of the lips is approximately 160°, engages the extrusion reflex, grasps the nipple, exerts a vacuum to draw the elastic nipple/areola into the mouth, and forms a seal with the lips. Infants who cannot achieve an adequate latch are of concern due to the possibility of rapid weight loss, hypoglycemia, and hyperbilirubinemia. Latch difficulties may be as simple as needing extra learning time or may have its origin in more complicated issues such as medications used during labor, oral anomalies or restrictions, birth injuries, preterm birth,

Prenatal and Postnatal Care: A Person-Centered Approach, Third Edition. Edited by Karen Trister Grace, Cindy L. Farley, Noelene K. Jeffers, and Tanya Tringali.
© 2024 John Wiley & Sons Ltd. Published 2024 by John Wiley & Sons Ltd.
Companion website: www.wiley.com/go/grace/prenatal

Table 44.1 Contributors to Latch Difficulty

Maternal body position
- Leaning down over the infant
- In pain/uncomfortable
- Pushing or manipulating the breast or nipple/areola distorting its natural shape

Infant body position
- Misalignment of the head, trunk, and hips
- Not tucked close, arched back, too much flexion, or nose buried in breast tissue
- Head too high over breast
- Nose or chin not touching the breast

Mouth
- Angle of infant's mouth opening less than 160°

Tongue
- Humped (anterior to posterior)
- Not down, cupped, and forward
- Bunched (compressed in a lateral direction)
- Retracted (tip behind alveolar ridges)
- Elevated
- Flat
- Restricted lingual frenulum
- Hypotonic, protruding

Palate
- High or arched (smooth arc or "V" shaped)
- Bubble (distinct receded indentation)
- Cleft (hard or soft)

Cheeks
- Drawn in, dimpled, or hollowed with each suck
- Cheek line not in a smooth arc

Jaw
- Retrognathia or receding jaw. Can position the tongue posteriorly where it can lead to airway obstruction; can contribute to sore nipples unless the chin is brought very close to the breast
- Large jaw excursions (does not close over the areola or drops down so far that the tongue loses contact with the nipple)
- Small jaw excursions (cannot open mouth over the areola)
- Lack of graded jaw excursions heard as clicking or smacking sounds
- Jaw asymmetry or tilted jaw
- Plagiocephaly (asymmetrical distortion or flattened appearance in an area of the head) not related to fusion of the skull bones may occur from intrauterine positioning, multiple gestation, and assisted delivery. The chin may deviate from the midline, interfering with latch and sucking

Lips
- Cleft
- Poor occlusion of lips around areola (milk leaking from the sides of the mouth)
- Sucking blisters

Nipple
- Slides back and forth within the infant's mouth during a feeding
- Pops in and out of the mouth (may indicate ankyloglossia)
- Creased in a horizontal, vertical, or oblique plane
- Distorted shape or flattened
- Blanched or in spasm after the infant releases the nipple
- Pain, blisters, maceration, fissures, cracks, bleeding, and craters
- Flat, dimpled, or retracted
- Edematous areola that envelops the nipple
- Engorged breast that flattens the nipple

Patterns
- Lack of rhythmicity or coordination of suck, swallow, and breath
- Suck-to-swallow ratio more than one to three sucks per swallow
- High respiratory rate or stridor
- Coughing, gagging, or choking

use of artificial nipples, or neurological issues. Infants demonstrating latch difficulty should be checked on several parameters and corrections instituted when possible (Table 44.1).

Some latch issues can stem from an infant who is not behaviorally available to feed. The infant may be in a deep sleep state, overhungry, sedated from labor medication, shut down from too much stimulation, or have difficulty achieving the quiet alert state where they feed best. Placing the infant skin-to-skin between the mother's breasts may help the infant actively achieve a good latch. Latch can be complicated by previous or concurrent use of artificial nipples and pacifiers. Nutritive sucking patterns can be disrupted by exposure to baby bottles. The use of a baby bottle was associated with alterations in the nutritive sucking pattern at the breast, which included inadequate jaw movement and inadequate tongue cupping (Batista et al., 2019). Birth-related influences can be quite detrimental to achieving an optimal latch. Hypoxia, brachial plexus injuries, fractured clavicle, vacuum extraction, facial muscle trauma, deep or aggressive suctioning, and forceps delivery can disrupt the normal working of the facial nerves and make infant positioning challenging or painful.

Incentives at the breast may facilitate latch such as a periodontal syringe or a soft medication dropper can be placed in the side of the baby's mouth to deliver a few drops of colostrum, milk, or water (Figure 44.1). Flow regulates suck, so the establishment of a small flow of fluid may help the infant initiate the latch. Butterfly tubing attached to a 10-mL syringe and taped to the breast can also provide such incentives. An infant having difficulty opening their mouth wide enough may benefit from assistance (Figure 44.2). The mother can use their index finger to *gently* open the infant's mouth wide enough to achieve a proper latch.

Nipple shields may be a later intervention if other attempts do not achieve latch. They present a rigid, preformed teat to the infant that are not as pliable as the maternal nipple and do not taste, feel, or smell like the real thing. However, it may keep a preterm infant from continuously slipping off the nipple and provide a bridge to latching on for the term baby. Nipple shields come in several sizes, and it is important to obtain the right fit. If the height of the shield's teat is too long, the infant's jaw closure and tongue compression will fall on the shaft of the teat and not over the breast and could cause the infant to gag. If the shield is too short, it could result in the teat resting in the anterior portion of the mouth contributing to a shallow latch and impedance of milk transfer. The teat must be large enough to allow for the expansion of the

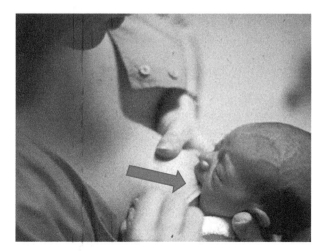

Figure 44.1   Dropper incentive for latching.

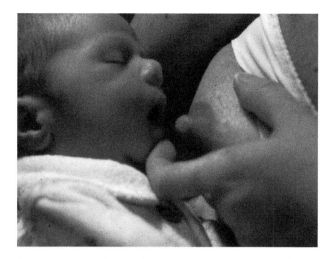

Figure 44.2   Mother gently opening infant mouth for latch on.

nipple during sucking. If the height of the teat is too short for the nipple, it may rest compressed against the inside tip of the shield. If the shield's teat is too small, the nipple may become sore. Warm the shield under hot water prior to application to help it adhere better, turn it almost inside-out to apply, hand express colostrum or milk into the teat, or use a periodontal syringe to preload the teat with milk. To encourage latch, breastmilk can be dripped onto the outside of the teat. Tubing for supplementation can be placed either inside or outside the shield.

Fussy Baby

Infants who are fussy at the breast following or in between feedings can cause a great deal of anxiety for new parents. Many interpret fussing at the breast as a sign that the infant does not "like" to breastfeed. Infants who are fretful following a feeding may be unnecessarily supplemented with formula because the mother thinks that the infant's fussiness is a sign that the infant is not getting enough milk or that her milk supply is insufficient. Failure to address the cause of a fussy infant can lead to unnecessary supplementation or weaning. Infants who are allowed to cry for prolonged periods of time may not be able to organize themselves to feed well since crying is a late sign of hunger. Factors that may contribute to fussiness include infant pain, **oral aversion**, medications, and hunger. While fussing and crying remain behaviorally appropriate for newborns and young infants, clinicians must be certain that fussing is not related to underfeeding. A chronically underfed infant may fuss directly after a feeding, when put down, shortly after a feeding and in between feedings, and be difficult to console, or never seem to settle. Complaints of a fussy, unsettled, or unsatisfied infant or an infant who "cries all the time" should be followed up with direct breastfeeding observation and verification of a measurable amount of colostrum/milk transfer, and the use of expressed colostrum/milk with alternative feeding devices if the infant cannot obtain sufficient volumes directly from the breast. This should not be minimized or ignored. Clinicians should document if swallowing has

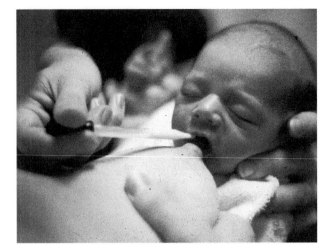

Figure 44.3 Using a dropper to stop rapid side-to-side head movement.

taken place. Some infants can mimic breastfeeding with jaw movements that do not result in milk transfer placing them at risk for weight loss, jaundice, and dehydration.

Some fussy infants exhibit a rapid side-to-side head movement as they approach the breast. This makes it difficult for the infant to establish a good latch. This behavior can be altered by placing a small dropper with colostrum or milk in it on the midline of the upper lip and move the infant onto the breast as the infant follows the dropper to the nipple (Figure 44.3). When the mouth is wide open, a couple of drops of colostrum or milk can be placed on the tongue to elicit sucking and swallowing.

Infant Pain

Infants can experience pain related to birth injuries such as a fractured clavicle or humerus, a cephalohematoma, or trauma associated with a vacuum extraction or forceps delivery. Positioning an infant with a fractured clavicle can be done with either ventral positioning or in a cradle hold on one breast, and then, the infant is kept in the same position and moved to the other breast in a cross-cradle hold, keeping the fracture site superior to the unfractured clavicle. Vacuum extraction is a significant contributor to poor feeding mechanics and is associated with lower rates of early initiation of breastfeeding (Mahfouz et al., 2022) and higher rates of breastfeeding cessation during the first 10 days after birth (Hall et al., 2002). Mothers may need to try several different positions to find one in which the baby is comfortable feeding.

Oral Aversion

Oral aversion to feeding can be caused by unpleasant oral experiences such as suctioning, gavage feeding, intubation, digital assessment of the mouth, or vigorous post tongue-tie revision exercises. Swelling or soreness in the mouth may cause the infant to fuss at the breast. Mothers can encourage infants to cuddle at the breast and taste expressed drops of colostrum or milk. Placing the infant prone on the mother's chest as they lie back in a warm bath may prove

Table 44.2 Selected Interventions for Sucking Difficulties

Type	Description
Jaw support	Dancer hand position using a "U" hold support's the infant's jaw to reduce excessive mandibular excursions.
Sublingual pressure	Thumb or forefinger placed under the infant's chin pressing up slightly under where the tongue attaches. Keeps the tongue in contact with the nipple.
Suck exercises/ suck training: To strengthen the suck	Gently place an index finger, nail side down, in the baby's mouth, allowing the infant to pull the finger into the mouth. Tug the finger with a slight downward traction against the baby's tongue as the suck develops. Let baby try to resist the pull.
Suck exercises/ suck training: To correct tongue position	Place an index finger, nail side down, into the front of the baby's mouth, allowing the infant to pull the finger into the mouth. If the baby's tongue does not curl around the finger, stroke the hard plate then gently press down on the back of the baby's tongue while stroking the tongue forward. This will pull the finger out of the baby's mouth a little. Allow them to suck it back in.

relaxing and help repattern a pleasurable experience at the breast. If the infant refuses the breast, cup feeding of expressed breastmilk can be done until the infant can be gently persuaded back to the breast.

Sucking Difficulties

Sucking difficulties may manifest as weak, erratic, ineffective, uncoordinated, or nonrhythmical. Several types of interventions may assist in improving sucking dynamics (Table 44.2).

Other suck training methods can be used for correcting differing aspects of the troubled sucking (Genna, 2017). Referral to a physical therapist or occupational therapist can be helpful to remediate sucking difficulties.

Massaging, and compressing the breast while the infant sucks or during pauses may augment milk transfer. Infants with sucking difficulties related to biomechanical issues might benefit from various forms of body work such as osteopathic treatment, craniofacial therapy, myofascial release, or chiropractic interventions (Hawk et al., 2018) as dysfunction in body structures could affect physiological functioning. These bodywork modalities have been shown to be safe and effective when performed by certified or licensed providers (Hazelbaker, 2020; Miller, 2020; Watts & Lagouros, 2020).

Medications and Breastfeeding

Most medications are compatible with breastfeeding, but a few are contraindicated or should be used with caution. For example, discontinuing breastfeeding for hours or days may be necessary with some medications such as radioactive compounds. Breastfeeding should almost always be recommended, as the risk of not breastfeeding is usually higher than the risk from most medications. Reliance on medication package inserts is an inaccurate source of information regarding the use of drugs in lactation. Often there is limited research on a given drug and its effects during lactation; shared decision-making is essential.

All medications transfer into breastmilk to some degree, and for many drugs, the amount transferred is less than 1% of the maternal dose. Medications penetrate into milk more during the colostral phase of milk production and less after the milk matures. Herbal preparations and supplements are also biologically active and should be used with caution. The purity and dosage of many herbal preparations can vary widely. Preterm or unstable infants should be evaluated carefully in terms of their ability to handle even small amounts of medication. For individuals who have been taking medications during pregnancy, the dose of medication in breastfed infants is a fraction of that received by the fetus in utero. Both over-the-counter medications and prescribed medications should be evaluated for the absolute dose received by the infant so that abandonment of breastfeeding is not suggested due to anxiety or lack of knowledge on the part of the clinician (Hale, 2021). See the resources section of this chapter for sources of drug safety during lactation.

Hunger

Hunger may be due to poor infant feeding skills or limited milk transfer. Mothers may report that the infant fusses shortly after a feeding. These infants may be hungry, as they may never have really completed a feeding. Some infants, such as late preterm infants and infants of diabetic mothers, have reduced intakes during feedings at the breast. Infants who have been exposed to artificial nipples may find it difficult to latch and transfer milk from the breast. It can take time for these infants to develop feeding skills.

Interventions should aim to increase the number of feedings per 24 hours if necessary as well as enhance the amount of colostrum/milk transferred at each feeding. Infants who cannot generate sufficient vacuum (e.g., late preterm infants, newborns affected by prenatal or labor medications, or infants with neurological challenges) can be helped to receive more milk per feeding by using breast massage and compressions. Sometimes called **alternate massage,** it is also a useful tool for sleepy infants or those who pause for long periods of time between sucking bursts. Alternate massage or breast compression is done on each breast during each feeding by massaging and compressing the breast each time the infant pauses. This type of breast compression helps elevate the positive pressure within the breast, making a more efficient pressure gradient between the breast and the low pressure within the infant's mouth.

Young infants may cluster their feedings in the late afternoon and early evening and may feed almost every hour. This is normal and these feedings should be accommodated, as some infants "fill up" with milk during this time in order to sleep longer at night.

If the infant demonstrates continued signs of hunger after feedings, consider referring the nursing couplet to an International Board Certified Lactation Consultant (IBCLC). Unresolved poor feeding can lead to infant weight loss, hypernatremia, and hyperbilirubinemia. Some of these infants may need to be supplemented with expressed breastmilk, donor human milk, or infant formula.

Sleepy Baby

Mothers may describe situations such as an infant who does not wake regularly enough to indicate hunger, or the infant falls asleep at the breast or sucks sporadically, or the infant falls asleep before taking the second breast. The sleepy infant can be a challenge to breastfeed. Sleeping is not always an indicator that an infant has received sufficient amounts of milk. Young infants often do not take both breasts at each feeding, especially during the first few days after birth. If a very young infant does not take the second breast, parents and clinicians may notice feeding readiness signs an hour or so later. Infants should be given the other breast at this time.

Some infants tend to sleep more, such as late preterm infants, jaundiced infants (including those undergoing phototherapy), infants born by cesarean section, those affected by labor medications, and heavier infants of diabetic mothers. Drowsiness at the breast may also be related to the normal release of cholecystokinin (CCK), a gastrointestinal hormone that is released in response to fat in the diet. CCK enhances gut maturation, promotes glucose-induced insulin release, enhances sedation, and is thought to play a role in regulating food intake by signaling satiety (Marchini & Linden, 1992). Breastfed infants have higher plasma concentrations of CCK during the first five days than do formula-fed infants (Marchini et al., 1993). During the breastfeeding episode, CCK has the effect of inducing sleepiness in both the mother and the infant (Uvnas-Moberg et al., 1987).

Sleepy infants should be kept skin-to-skin as much as possible during the early days. Feeding cues of sleepy infants can be quite subtle. These include rapid eye movements under the eyelids, tongue movements, hand-to-mouth movements, body movements, and small sounds. When the infant is skin-to-skin, feeding cues are more easily noted and the baby can be put quickly to the breast when the infant is most likely to feed. Some infants respond well to incentives that keep them interested in sustaining sucking throughout the feeding. A periodontal syringe or a soft medication dropper can be placed in the side of the baby's mouth to deliver a few drops of colostrum, milk, or water with each suck until the infant demonstrates sustained sucking and swallowing. Butterfly tubing attached to a 10-mL syringe and held or taped to the breast can also provide such incentives.

Slow Weight Gain

There are a number of infant and maternal factors that can contribute to slow weight gain in the breastfed infant. These factors are summarized in Tables 44.3 and 44.4 and should be assessed in an infant with slow weight gain.

Table 44.3 Infant Factors Associated with Slow Weight Gain

Factor	Effect
Gestational age and size for gestational age	Preterm, postterm, small-for-gestational-age, intrauterine growth restricted, and large-for-gestational-age infants may lack mature feeding skills, strength, and stamina to ingest an adequate amount of milk.
Oral anatomy alterations	Ankyloglossia, cleft lip, cleft palate, bubble palate, and craniofacial anomalies may interfere with suckling and result in inadequate milk intake.
Neurological alterations	Hypotonia, hypertonia, and neurological abnormalities may interfere with the infant's ability to ingest an adequate amount of milk.
Increased energy requirements	Cardiac disease, respiratory disease, and metabolic disorders may create an increased need for calories.
Infant illness or condition	Infection, cardiac abnormalities, cystic fibrosis, gastrointestinal disorders, and trisomy 21 may be associated with low endurance for feeding and/or high metabolic demands.
Maternal medications	Certain prenatal prescription medications and recreational or illicit drugs may interfere with suckling.
Intrapartum factors	Cesarean birth, fetal hypoxia during labor, medications during labor, epidural analgesia, forceps delivery, and vacuum extraction may interfere with alertness and ability to feed.
Iatrogenic factors	Separation of mothers and infants, supplementation with formula or water, inappropriate pacifier use, and inadequate breastfeeding support can result in reduced milk intake.

Table 44.4 Maternal Factors Associated with Slow Infant Weight Gain

Factor	Effect
Breast alterations	Previous breast surgery including augmentation and reduction, insufficient glandular tissue, and previous breast trauma may result in reduced milk volume.
Nipple anomalies	Flat, retracted, inverted, oddly shaped, or dimpled nipples may impair the ability to achieve correct latch and lead to reduced milk intake.
Ineffective or insufficient milk removal	Incorrect breastfeeding positions or latch, ineffective sucking, and unresolved engorgement can leave residual milk in the breast and reduce milk supply.
Delayed lactogenesis II	Individuals who are overweight, obese, diabetic, had a cesarean birth, postpartum hemorrhage, or retained placental fragments may experience delayed lactogenesis II.
Inappropriate breastfeeding management	Delayed or disrupted early feeding opportunities, separation of mother and infant, too few feedings, failure to pump milk in the absence of an infant suckling at breast, ineffective breast pump, unnecessary formula supplementation, and lack of access to skilled lactation services further contribute to the problem.
Medications	Prescription, over-the-counter, recreational and illicit drugs, labor medications, and intravenous fluids may delay lactogenesis II or may interfere with infant suckling.
Hormonal alterations	Hypothyroidism, polycystic ovarian syndrome, theca lutein cysts, pituitary disorders, diabetes insipidus, and other endocrine-related problems may interfere with milk production.
Milk ejection problems	Drugs, alcohol, smoking, stress, thyroid dysfunction, and pain can inhibit the let-down reflex and reduce the amount of milk available to the infant.
Overlapping pregnancy	Pregnancy can reduce milk production.
Other factors	Vitamin B_{12} deficiency in a vegetarian diet, inadequate weight gain during pregnancy, and anemia may contribute to an insufficient milk supply.

Slow weight gain is often a manifestation of another problem and may be the result of a combination of factors. First, a thorough history and physical exam should be conducted. Next, faulty breastfeeding management by members of the healthcare team should be considered. If pacifiers are being used, consider eliminating them as the infant may have developed a preference for it over sucking at the breast leading to excessive non-nutritive sucking.

Weak sucking is one of the most important symptoms in both breastfed and bottle-fed babies experiencing slow growth between birth and eight weeks of age (Emond et al., 2007). Exhaustion while feeding, neurological impairments, and subtle oromotor dysfunction are other markers for potentially slow weight gain.

The healthcare provider will need to determine if supplementation is necessary until the underlying problem is corrected. Indications for supplementation can be determined by the clinical condition of the infant, the amount of weight loss (greater than 10%), failure to return to birth weight by two to three weeks of age, average daily weight gain of less than 25 g, any amount of unexplained weight loss, weight and length curves that are completely flat at any age, and deceleration of head circumference that consecutively crosses percentiles (Kair & Chantry, 2021).

Supplemental feedings of the mother's own milk are ideal if their supply is sufficient. Infants can start with a minimum of 50–100 mL/kg/day divided into 6–8 feedings. If breastmilk is being expressed, recommend that the container sits in the refrigerator long enough that a fat layer forms at the top. This can be skimmed off and given to the infant as a calorie-dense supplement. If it is very thick, it can be spoon-fed to the infant. The infant can be put back to breast 30 minutes following a feeding as a supplement to the original feed to provide a bolus of higher calorie milk. Mothers can also employ breast massage while nursing or expressing to maximize milk fat content. Once supplementation has been started, the amount can be increased according to infant appetite and weight gain. When milk production has increased and the infant has attained the desired weight, supplements can gradually be reduced. A feeding tube device at the breast can be used to both deliver the supplement and increase the milk production.

Preterm Infants

Infants born before 37 weeks of pregnancy have been completed are defined as preterm. In 2019, preterm birth was seen in 1 of every 10 infants born in the United States, a 2% increase over the 2018 rate. In addition, racial and ethnic differences in preterm birth rates are of concern. In 2019, the rate of preterm birth among African American women (14.39%) was about 50% higher than the rate of preterm birth among White or Hispanic women, 9.26% and 9.97%, respectively (Martin et al., 2020). Among extremely preterm infants, 67.1% of those born to Black mothers and 60.7% of those born to American Indian/Alaska Native mothers received breastmilk, compared with approximately 75% of extremely preterm infants born to mothers of other racial/ethnic groups (Chiang et al., 2019).

All preterm infants should receive human milk, with pasteurized donor milk as a supplement rather than premature infant formula, the preferred alternative if a mother is unable to provide an adequate volume of milk (Section on Breastfeeding, 2012). These infants are vulnerable and benefit from human milk's many unique properties (Pados, 2023). Breastmilk has a microbiome of its own that provides an inoculum of microorganisms unique to the dyad and works to make sure that the succession of microbial colonization in the gut is not altered resulting in dysbiosis. Many components in preterm human milk are higher during the first four weeks following birth such as protein and bioactive factors. Parents should receive evidence-based information regarding the therapeutic effects of breastmilk and a recommendation

that human milk feeding be part of the treatment plan for the infant.

Preterm infants who are not fed breastmilk have higher levels of nosocomial infections (Schanler, 2007), are more likely to develop necrotizing enterocolitis (NEC; Meinzen-Derr et al., 2009), demonstrate lower scores on tests of visual acuity (Morales & Schanler, 2007) and cognitive performance (Belfort et al., 2016), have altered immune function (Tarcan et al., 2004), and have increased intestinal permeability and slower intestinal maturation (Reisinger et al., 2014). Lack of breastfeeding is a significant predictor of cognitive deficiencies in very preterm infants at discharge and at five years of age (Beaino et al., 2011). Vohr et al. (2006) found that every 10 mL/kg/day increase in breastmilk intake confers a 5.3 IQ point advantage for infants consuming 110 mL/kg/day. This type of effect is a long-term advantage that may optimize cognitive potential and decrease the need for costly early intervention and special education services in childhood. Provision of human milk is important because preterm infants cannot fully digest carbohydrates and proteins. Human milk provides components that aid this process. When preterm infants are fed infant formula, undigested casein can reach the gut, attract neutrophils that provoke inflammation and the opening of the tight junctions between cells, allow intact proteins to engage in systemic invasion, and further damage a fragile gut, leading to NEC (Claud & Walker, 2001).

Some infants will receive their preterm mother's milk after it is fortified. This happens when an infant's nutritional needs exceed the capacity of breastmilk to provide selected nutrients that support a particularly desired growth velocity. Protein is often the limiting factor in human milk and any shortfall in protein or other nutrients could adversely affect growth and development as well as lead to cognitive impairments.

Donor human milk is often used in a neonatal intensive care unit (NICU) to provide a predominantly human milk diet. Use of donor human milk has been shown to support in-hospital growth using predominantly human milk diets (Verd et al., 2015). Use of donor milk did not decrease the mother's own milk but it replaced formula in the first two weeks of life. The median time on oxygen and duration of mechanical ventilation was significantly higher among formula-fed infants (Verd et al., 2015). Gut microbial profiles show that donor human milk favors an intestinal microbiome more similar to the mother's own milk despite the differences between the microbial profiles of the mother's own milk compared to donor human milk (Parra-Llorca et al., 2018). Pasteurization of donor milk removes much of the microbial life, which means that the infant does not receive an inoculum of bacteria from this source. Clinicians should support as much direct feeding at the breast as possible as well as assisting the individual in expressing whatever colostrum or milk possible during those early critical weeks (Groer et al., 2015).

The use of one's own milk and donor milk in NICUs is lower in hospitals located in postal codes with more Black residents (72% vs 80%). Among hospitals with NICUs that offer donor milk in postal codes with more Black residents, the rates were 5% versus 10% in communities with fewer Black residents (Boundy et al., 2017). This suggests that disparities exist in the provision of breastmilk for high-risk infants relative to community or hospital characteristics despite breastfeeding being the optimal form of nutrition for this fragile population. Suggested hospital practices supportive of NICU breastfeeding include:

- Provide evidence-based information to families regarding the importance of breastfeeding and breastmilk as part of the therapeutic treatment plan for the infants.
- Communicate regarding how the staff values breastmilk as a form of medical therapy.
- Have a written breastfeeding policy communicated to and followed by all staff and physicians.
- Provide current and consistent breastfeeding and pumping guidelines.
- Involve the family in all feeding plans.
- Teach, assess, and monitor safe milk expression, storage, and transport.
- Encourage parents to assume responsibility for feeding tasks such as performing pre- and postfeed weights and oral colostrum care.
- Initiate skin-to-skin care as early as possible (kangaroo care).
- Introduce the breast early with frequent learning opportunities and low expectations of milk transfer.
- Work to have the first oral feeding done at the breast.
- Use a cue-based or semi-cue-based feeding strategy.
- Teach positioning; assess latch, sucking, and swallowing.
- Use assistive devices as needed.
- Measure milk transfer.
- Supplement without bottles if possible.
- Support the partner's presence and provide guidelines for help with breastfeeding.
- Refer to peer support programs or groups of other mothers with preterm infants, preferably racially concordant peers.
- Create a feeding plan for the postdischarge period.
- Refer parents to community sources for breastfeeding support that have expertise in managing complex breastfeeding situations such as IBCLCs.

In the absence of an infant at breast, mothers of preterm infants usually need to express their milk for weeks or even months until their infants are fully established at the breast or to provide as much breastmilk as possible under very trying circumstances. Mothers should consider the following:

- Secure a fully automated, multiuser (sometimes referred to as hospital grade) pump that cycles up to 60 times per minute with vacuums that do not exceed 240 mmHg, have separate controls for adjusting speed and vacuum, and that use a double collection kit to pump both breasts simultaneously (Larkin et al., 2013; Meier et al., 2016). Mothers should be instructed in the setup, cleaning, and use of the pump. Clinicians may need to help mothers secure the correct type of pump for their situation as some of the smaller personal use pumps offered by insurers may be inadequate for the needs of a pump-dependent mother of a preterm infant.
- Start milk expression within an hour of birth if possible if the infant cannot be put to breast during that time. Manual expression during the first 48 hours may yield more colostrum than using a breast pump (Ohyama et al., 2010), as the small amounts of colostrum tend to stick to sides of the flange and collection container. Mothers of preterm infants who practiced hand expression of colostrum greater than five times per day in the first three postpartum days in addition to electric pumping produced milk volumes of 860 ± 490 mL/day at six weeks and 955 ± 667 mL/day at eight weeks postpartum (Morton et al., 2009). This abundant milk supply was more than adequate to feed their preterm infants.
- Pump 8–10 times each 24 hours, especially during the first 14 days following birth. A milk production goal of 500–1,000 mL per day by the end of the first week will ensure that there is adequate milk volume to feed the infant through discharge from the NICU (Spatz, 2004).

After discharge, the infant's immature feeding skills may persist—latch difficulty, slipping off the nipple, falling asleep, undependable feeding cues, and fussing after a feeding. Tube feeding, finger feeding, and cup feeding are alternative means of providing extra milk. Use of the Dancer hand position (Figure 44.4), breast compressions, and eliciting the milk ejection reflex just prior to feeding may help increase milk transfer. A nipple shield may help the infant keep from slipping off. Some discharge instructions include a 24-hour minimum intake that the infant should consume. Pre- and postfeed weights around each breastfeeding session can be used to calculate if additional feedings or supplements are necessary.

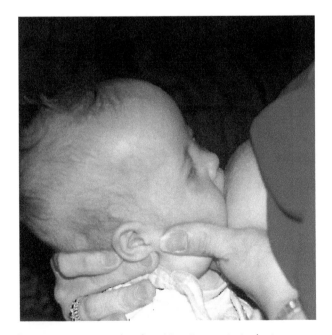

Figure 44.4 Dancer hand position. Source: La Leche League Canada/MATTOS LACTATION. Used with permission of The BreastFeeding Atlas.

Late Preterm Infants

Late preterm infants are born between 34 0/7 and 36 6/7 weeks. They can appear healthy and functional, but they remain vulnerable to many health and developmental challenges. These infants are not just a smaller version of a full-term baby. Their early birth has abruptly halted the in-utero maturation processes, leaving them physiologically, metabolically, and neurologically immature. Late preterm infants are at an increased risk for morbidities that involve most of the body's organ systems (Karnati et al., 2020) including airway instability, apnea, bradycardia, excessive sleepiness, excessive weight loss, dehydration, feeding difficulties, weak sucking, jaundice, hypoglycemia, hypothermia, immature self-regulation, respiratory distress, sepsis, prolonged infant formula supplementation, hospital readmission, and breastfeeding failure during the neonatal period.

Late preterm infants are at a disadvantage in terms of feeding skills. They are born with low energy stores and reduced subcutaneous and brown fat. They have high energy demands, poor feeding abilities, and are sleepy, with fewer and shorter awake periods. They tire easily when feeding, have a weak suck and low tone, demonstrate an inability to sustain sucking, and may have a small mouth with uncoordinated oral-motor movements. They are easily overstimulated and may shut down before consuming adequate amounts of milk or colostrum during a feeding. They may take only small volumes of milk during the early days in the hospital, which may be sufficient at that time but exhibit feeding difficulties and slow weight gain when higher volumes of milk intake become necessary for normal growth. Although some infants may demonstrate adequate muscle tone initially, this tone may be rapidly depleted during a feeding, indicating decreased endurance. Postural stability may be immature, creating a less efficient feeding pattern. Late preterm infants experience reduced tone in the muscles involved with feeding, which, coupled with neurological immaturity of the suck–swallow–breathe cycle, can result in uncoordinated and ineffective milk intake at breast. If treated like a normal newborn, they are at risk for inadequate nourishment, low weight gain, or weight loss. They may go through the motions of feeding but may transfer little if any milk for their efforts.

Infants should be positioned in a cross-cradle, clutch hold, or in a ventral position. A regular cradle hold could result in positional apnea from too much neck flexion. Mothers require specialized lactation support while in the hospital, as well as a discharge plan for feeding at home. Referral to a community-based IBCLC with expertise in managing preterm birth is advised. A sample breastfeeding plan for after hospital discharge is provided in Table 44.5.

Common Maternal Breastfeeding Problems

Breast and nipple problems, as well as insufficient milk supply, are some of the most frequently described breastfeeding challenges and are often the cause of decreasing or discontinuing breastfeeding. Even though they are common problems, they need to be addressed immediately to avoid unnecessary formula supplementation and premature weaning.

Sore Nipples

Sore nipples are one of the most common reasons for abandoning exclusive breastfeeding (Dennis et al., 2014).

Table 44.5 Sample Instructions for Breastfeeding a Late Preterm Infant

Feed your baby on cue 8–12 times each 24 hours.

Observe your baby for feeding cues. Feeding cues may not be as obvious in babies born early. Sleeping *is not* a sign that the baby is getting enough milk. Use these signs as a cue to feed if your baby is sleepy:
• sucking movements of the mouth and tongue
• rapid eye movements under the eyelids
• hand-to-mouth movements
• body movements
• small sounds

Place your baby in a clutch or cross-cradle position. If your baby has difficulty attaching to the breast, flails at the breast, or arches away from the breast, use a semireclining position with the baby prone on their tummy. Recline to a 30° angle; place your baby on their tummy with the mouth directly over the nipple. This allows gravity to bring the chin and tongue forward and helps improve latch.

As your baby latches on, make sure the mouth is wide open.

You should hear or feel your baby swallow every one to three sucks during most of the feeding.

Use alternate massage on each breast at each feeding to keep your baby sucking and increase the amount of milk they receive at each feeding. Thoroughly massage and compress each part of the breast.

If you are not sure how much milk your baby is getting at each feeding, you can weigh your baby before and after a feeding. This will help you know if you need to offer a supplement.

Record each feeding, whether a supplement is used, the number of wet diapers, and the number of bowel movements on your feeding log until your baby is feeding regularly and gaining weight. Also include the volume of milk pumped.

(Continued)

Table 44.5 *(Continued)*

If your baby does not latch, try the following:
• Gently roll your nipple between your fingers to make it easier for the baby to grasp.
• As you bring your baby to breast, have a helper place a tube feeding device or dropper in the corner of the baby's mouth and deliver a small amount of milk as the baby attempts to latch. If your baby swallows and attempts to latch again, another small amount of milk can be given. Repeat until your baby no longer attempts to latch. These practice sessions should not last longer than 10 minutes to avoid tiring both you and your baby.
• Finish the feeding by finger or cup feeding.
• If the attempts at latching do not work, you may find that a silicone nipple shield will allow the baby to latch and sustain sucking efforts. Moisten the shield with warm water, turn it almost inside-out as you apply it to the breast, apply a little milk to the outside of the shield, hand express milk into the shield tunnel, and bring the baby to breast. If the baby latches, continue using alternate massage throughout the feeding.
Babies should have at least six wet diapers and three or more bowel movements each day by the fifth day. Bowel movements should start turning yellow by day 4. Meconium diapers on day 5 or the presence of red stains in wet diapers (uric acid crystals) on day 4 may indicate that the baby is not getting enough milk.
Take your baby to see their healthcare provider two days after coming home from the hospital for a weight check and to make sure that they are not jaundiced. A weight check every three days or so ensures that your baby continues to gain about 0.5–1 oz/day.
If your baby cannot feed long enough at each feeding or is not gaining enough weight, supplements of expressed milk can be given by tube feeding at the breast, finger feeding, cup feeding, or bottle feeding. If you do not have enough milk to use as a supplement, banked donor human milk or an amino acid formula can be used until your milk production has increased.
Continue to pump your milk two to three times each day to use as a supplement and to improve your milk supply. Try "power pumping" for an hour once or twice each day. Pump for 5–10 minutes until the milk stops spraying after the first let-down. Wait for 10 minutes or so and pump again until the milk stops spraying. Almost half of the milk that is available in the breast is pumped with the first let-down. Power pumping takes advantage of these "first" letdowns to mimic frequent feedings and helps increase your milk production. Depending on how your baby is feeding, pumping should continue until they are 40–42 weeks corrected gestational age, weaning off the pump over the first month home.

Source: Adapted from Walker (2009).

The etiology of sore nipples can be multifactorial and has been attributed to the following:

- *Poor positioning and latch*. More than half of those reporting nipple pain can be helped by correcting their positioning and latch. When there is no improvement after adjustments are made, this suggests other contributing factors (Kent et al., 2015).
- *Ankyloglossia (tongue-tie)*. **Ankyloglossia** can restrict the movement of the tongue, potentially inhibiting the nipple/areolar complex from being drawn far enough into the infant's mouth to prevent pain and promote optimal milk transfer.
- *Palatal anomaly, high arched palate, or bubble palate* (Snyder, 1997).
- *Strong infant vacuum.*
- *Nipple bleb.*
- *Infection*. Common causative microbes are *Candida albicans* and *Staphylococcus aureus*, and *Herpes simplex virus*.
- *Eczema, psoriasis, contact dermatitis.*
- *Breast pump trauma.*
- *Vasospasm/Raynaud's syndrome.*
- *Anomalous shaped nipples*. These make latch difficult.
- ***Flat or inverted nipples***. These fail to protrude sufficiently when an infant latches, making it difficult to draw the nipple and areola deep enough into the mouth. They also contribute to **delayed lactogenesis II**, poor milk transfer, newborn weight loss, engorgement, and reduced milk production. (Walker, 2010). Flat nipples

can be detected when the areola is compressed, and the nipple flattens to the level of the areola or recedes back into the areola.

There is some evidence to support prenatal correction of short nipples by wearing breast cups (Chanprapaph et al., 2013) or by mechanical stretching of the nipple by suction devices such as the Supple Cup® (Bouchet-Horwitz, 2011). Supple Cups can also be used in between or immediately prior to a feeding after the baby is born to increase nipple protractility. Additional interventions that can be used prior to each feeding are described in Table 44.6.

Management of Sore Nipples

The first approach to sore nipples involves optimal positioning and latch that eliminates positional instability and a dragging force on the nipple that could exceed its ability to stretch (Douglas, 2022). Dozens of sore nipple treatments have been written about since the seventeenth century with no single agent being clearly superior to others (Morland-Schultz & Hill, 2005). Healthcare providers must identify the root cause(s). Some options treat infections, some promote healing, and others relieve pain and increase comfort. Management strategies to prevent and manage sore nipples are outlined in Table 44.7.

If a break in the nipple skin occurs and it becomes cracked or fissured, there is a high probability for colonization by bacteria and fungi. Cracked nipples also increase the risk for mastitis. *S. aureus* is a common pathogen associated with infected nipple cracks. Bacteria have a

Table 44.6   Interventions for Flat and Inverted Nipples

Apply cold compresses to the nipple area.
Shape the nipple by rolling it between the fingers.
A breast pump may help extend the nipple. However, a breast pump distributes vacuum over a wide area and may contribute to increasing edema within the nipple and areola, further contributing to latch difficulty.
Breast shells worn between feedings may help displace fluid but can damage underlying tissue if worn for long periods of time in the presence of edema.
A modified 10-mL syringe is a simple and inexpensive tool that can be fashioned by removing the plunger, cutting off the end of the syringe one-fourth of an inch above where a needle would attach, and inserting the plunger through the end that was cut. The mother then places the smooth end of the syringe directly over her nipple and pulls back gently on the plunger to her comfort for 30 seconds to a minute prior to each feeding. This procedure can be repeated several times each day between feedings to more quickly improve nipple protrusion. An FDA-approved version of this type of device is available—the Evert-It Nipple Enhancer™ (Maternal Concepts).
Flat nipples can also be caused by areolar edema. Reverse pressure softening can be used to expose the nipple in cases or areolar edema. The mother uses three or four fingertips of each hand to encircle the base of the nipple and push inward for 1–3 minutes with enough pressure to form six to eight depressions.
A nipple shield can be applied before or after reverse pressure softening if there appears to be no other way to help the infant latch to the breast.

Table 44.7   Strategies for Preventing and Managing Sore Nipples

Preventive strategies	• Instruct on optimal positioning and latch. • Assess latch, suck, swallowing and positioning. • Place infant in ventral position (prone) for gravity assistance to aid latch-on, especially if the infant is tongue-tied. • Make sure the infant's mouth is open to 160°, with lips flared outward and neck slightly extended. • If pumping, ensure that the flange is large enough to prevent nipple strangulation in the flange tunnel. • Provide relief from engorgement. • Assist mothers with flat nipples. • Avoid pacifiers until breastfeeding is well established. • Correct ankyloglossia if present (**frenotomy**). • Apply topical peppermint oil.
Sore nipples without evidence of damage	• Prevent nipple damage. • Apply warm water compresses. • Apply warm green tea bag compresses. • Apply topical coconut oil. • Apply hydrogel dressing. • Use a nipple shield if the above measures do not provide relief.
Cracked/damaged nipples	• Wash the nipples with soap and water once daily. • Apply topical mupirocin. • Avoid pacifier use or wash pacifiers thoroughly with soap and water. • Apply topical peppermint oil. • Apply topical low-strength steroids for inflammation.
Exudate, increased erythema, pus, or dry scab is present	• Initiate systemic antibiotics. • If *Candida albicans* is suspected, add 2% miconazole.
Persistent or recurrent infection	• Treat the infant with nasal mupirocin. • Culture nipple skin for small colony variants (SCVs) bacteria; send the specimen for culture and sensitivity. • If SCVs are present, switch to macrolide therapy. • Use hydrogel dressing for comfort and moist wound healing. • Be watchful for an ascending infection (mastitis).

Source: Adapted from Walker (2010).

propensity to grow and form colonies that are protected by a biofilm. Biofilms prevent antibiotics from reaching and killing the bacteria and contribute to persistent infections. To disrupt this biofilm, careful washing of the cracked nipples with soap and water daily followed by a thin application of mupirocin 2% ointment (Bactroban®) may be effective in the early stages of an infection (Livingstone et al., 1996).

The use of lanolin can be considered for sore or abraded nipples, while a hydrogel dressing may be indicated for open sores or cracks with exudate. Silver caps are small cups that are crafted with sterling silver. They help to protect and heal damaged nipples. A few drops of milk are expressed into the cup following each feeding and are placed over the nipple like a cupping glass. Silver caps have been shown to be more effective than standard education alone (Marrazzu et al., 2015). Olive oil has been shown to possess antioxidant, antifungal, and anti-inflammatory properties that help in healing. It also contains squalene, which serves as an antioxidant and emollient. Studies have shown that many women prefer extra virgin olive oil over lanolin for healing their nipple pain (Oguz et al., 2014). It is easily accessible, inexpensive, and has been reported to be extremely effective, and useful in promoting the healing of sore nipples.

Peppermint oil has been used prophylactically (Melli et al., 2007) to prevent cracked nipples and as a treatment for already damaged nipples with significantly positive effects (Akbari et al., 2014). Peppermint water has been used as a prophylactic measure and has been shown to be three times more effective than expressed breastmilk in the prevention of cracked nipples (Ismail et al., 2019). Peppermint gel is even more effective than peppermint water or lanolin in preventing cracked nipples. Coconut oil has been used for many purposes including the repair of sore, dry, and cracked nipples (Raj & Magesh, 2017). Medical-grade honey (for example, MediHoney) has been shown to be an effective wound healing agent and anti-bacterial preparation (Robson et al., 2009). An important property of medical-grade honey is its ability to penetrate bacterial biofilms, which could be helpful in treating infected wounds that are not healing (Merckoll et al., 2009). Commercial nipple creams are usually combinations of several ingredients making it difficult to separate out what might be helpful.

Breast Engorgement

Engorgement is a physiological process described as the painful swelling of the breasts associated with the sudden increase in milk volume, lymphatic and vascular congestion, and interstitial edema that occurs during the first two weeks following childbirth. Engorgement is progressive, as milk production increases rapidly and milk volume can outpace the capacity of the alveoli to store it. If the milk is not removed, engorgement progresses to alveolar overdistension, which can cause the milk-secreting cells to become flattened, drawn out, and even to rupture. The distention can partly or completely occlude the capillary blood circulation surrounding the alveolar cells. Congested blood vessels leak fluid into the surrounding tissue space, contributing to edema. Pressure and congestion obstruct lymphatic drainage of the breasts. Once the system that rids the breasts of toxins, bacteria, and castoff cell parts becomes stagnated, the breast is predisposed to mastitis (both inflammation and infection).

The areola can also become engorged or edematous and present with clinical observations of a swollen areola with tight, shiny skin, probably involving overfull lactiferous ducts as well as more interstitial edema. A puffy areola is thought to be due to tissue edema. Some degree of breast engorgement is normal.

Severe engorgement is a very painful condition that can be minimized with early frequent feedings, feeding infants on cue, no restriction on sucking times, thorough breast drainage, and correct sucking techniques. Alternate breast massage has been shown to reduce the incidence and severity of engorgement while simultaneously contributing to increased milk intake, increasing the fat content of the milk, and increasing infant weight gain (Bowles et al., 1987; Iffrig, 1968; Stutte et al., 1988). Engorgement usually occurs between three and six days after birth and declines thereafter. However, some may experience additional episodes of engorgement during the early weeks. Relief measures include the use of cold compresses, intermittent cold packs, frequent milk removal by hand expression or pumping, and anti-inflammatory medication for discomfort. The application of chilled cabbage leaves to the breasts can also be beneficial (Lim et al., 2015). Lymphatic breast drainage therapy is a gentle massage of the lymphatic drainage channels that may improve the movement of stagnated fluid and reduce edema (Wilson-Clay & Hoover, 2008). Mothers can hand express or pump milk prior to placing the baby at the breast to allow for a better latch. An edematous areola will benefit from reverse pressure softening for easier latch. Therapeutic breast massage directed toward the axilla can help reduce edema and pain and should be taught to lactating individuals (Witt et al., 2016).

Some treatments may be more promising than others for the treatment of engorgement; those include cabbage leaves, cold gel packs, herbal compresses, and massage (Zakarija-Grkovic & Stewart, 2020). Frequent breastfeeding or expressing should be encouraged, but caution should be exercised in placing a breast pump on an edematous areola as the vacuum can serve to increase tissue edema.

Plugged Ducts

Small tender lumps may present in the breasts, usually related to the blockage of a milk duct. These solid obstructions are formed by particulate matter from a mixture of casein and other materials hardened by calcium-containing salts. The lump may also have reddened skin over it, become smaller after a feeding, be warm to the touch, and lead to poor milk flow. Milk secretions that are blocked from exiting the breast can become thickened due to absorption of fluid from the milk. Plugged ducts require prompt attention because they can start a cascade of events that leads to breast inflammation and infection.

Milk expressed from the breast experiencing plugged ducts can contain material from the plug that is of a fatty composition. Strings that resemble spaghetti or lengths of fatty-looking material have been described. Observation of fatty material in milk has led clinicians to recommend the addition of lecithin to the maternal diet (Lawrence & Lawrence, 2010). Lecithin is a phospholipid used by the food industry as an emulsifier to keep fat dispersed and suspended in water rather than aggregated in a fatty mass. Lecithin has been recommended to emulsify this secretion and subsequently augment breast emptying (McGuire, 2015). One tablespoon per day of oral granular lecithin has been reported to relieve plugged ducts and prevent their recurrence (Eglash, 1998). It has become widely available in capsule form and the Academy of Breastfeeding Medicine recommends sunflower or soy lecithin at dosages of 5–10 mg/day (Mitchell et al., 2022).

Interventions for plugged ducts include warm compresses and direct massage over the lump while the baby is sucking. Massage over and/or behind the blockage can break up the material obstructing the duct and push the blockage forward. An alternate approach is to massage in front of the lump toward the nipple (Smillie, 2004). The mother begins the massage close to the nipple and repositions the massage farther back until she is massaging directly in front of the blockage (Campbell, 2006). Just as ultrasound treatment provides internal vibration of tissue, topical vibration over the blockage from an electric toothbrush, sonic face brush, or small vibrator may break apart or dislodge the material obstructing the milk duct. Anecdotally, some have tried filling a Haakaa or similar passive pumping product with warm water (some also add Epsom salts), attaching it to the breast and letting the nipple soak. It may take a few tries, but the pump's gentle continuous vacuum may help move out the clog.

Mastitis

Mastitis is an inflammatory condition of the breast that may involve an infection. *Mastitis* and *infection* are terms that are often used interchangeably; in mastitis, the inflammation is frequently treated as if it were an infection. Acute and subacute mastitis are the most prevalent forms of mastitis among breastfeeding individuals. Acute mastitis is generally obvious due to the intensity of its symptoms, namely erythema, pain, swelling, fever, and other general symptoms. *S. aureus* is usually the main causative agent in acute mastitis, producing toxins responsible for the systemic symptoms (Contreras & Rodríguez, 2011). Subacute mastitis presents with different symptomatology. *Staphylococcus epidermidis* has been identified as the predominant species responsible for subacute mastitis (Jiménez et al., 2015; Patel et al., 2017) along with other coagulase negative staphylococci and *Viridans streptococci*. Symptoms of subacute mastitis may be subtle and quite different from those of acute mastitis, leading to misdiagnosis. Bacteria responsible for subacute mastitis do not produce toxins but instead form thick biofilms in the milk ducts resulting in impedance to milk flow through the lumen of the lactiferous ducts. This pressure on the narrow, inflamed lumen causes a pain that is often described as a sharp, needlelike pain and a burning sensation. These symptoms are frequently addressed with treatments for a fungal infection, such as candidiasis, when they may represent a bacterial infection (Angelopoulou et al., 2018; Fernandez et al., 2014). Subacute mastitis results in changes to the breastmilk microenvironment, with a proinflammatory/Th1-cytokine predominant profile. During subacute mastitis, cytokine imbalances in breastmilk may have a negative impact on the mucosal immune system and gut microbiota of the infant early in life, as the infant receives milk with an altered microbiotic profile. Most clinicians rely on a cluster of signs and symptoms to presumptively diagnose mastitis due to an infection rather than culture the breastmilk. The signs and symptoms of mastitis due to an infection are listed as follows.

Signs and symptoms of mastitis due to an infection

- Fever of 101 °F (38.4 °C) or greater
- Flu-like aching, malaise
- Increased heart rate
- Nausea
- Chills
- Pain and/or swelling at the site
- Red, tender, hot area, often wedge shaped
- Red streaks on the breast extending toward the axilla
- Salty taste of the milk that might lead infant to reject the affected site

Signs and symptoms of breast problems such as engorgement, plugged ducts, and noninfectious and infectious mastitis sometimes overlap. Each process has some element related to obstructed milk flow, making the differential diagnosis difficult. When breast drainage is blocked, paracellular pathways open, allowing the leakage of cytokines, which contribute to fever, chills, muscle aches, and general malaise. This situation can give the clinical impression of an infection, whether or not that is actually the case. The reported incidence of mastitis ranges widely from 2% to 33% with the highest occurrence at two to three weeks postpartum (Jahanfar et al., 2013). However, mastitis can occur at any time during the course of lactation. Risk factors for mastitis include:

Risk factors for mastitis

- Cracked or damaged nipple
- Plugged milk ducts
- Milk stasis from unrelieved engorgement or ineffective milk removal
- Blocked nipple pore (bleb)
- Infant is a nasal carrier of *S. aureus*
- Hyperlactation or a high rate of milk synthesis
- Insulin-dependent diabetes mellitus
- Nipple piercing
- Antibiotics taken in the third trimester of pregnancy and during the postpartum period (Bergmann et al., 2014)
- Breast pump usage, often caused by Pseudomonas (Jiménez et al., 2017).

Preventive measures begin with ensuring proper positioning, latch, and milk transfer at the breast to avoid breaks in the nipple epithelium. Probiotic administration has been shown to prevent mastitis. Among women with a history of mastitis after a previous pregnancy who were taking oral *Lactobacillus salivarius* PS2, one study showed a 25% reduction in mastitis (Fernandez et al., 2016). Another study of women without a history of mastitis who took *Lactobacillus fermentum* CECT5716 saw a 50% reduction (Hurtado et al., 2017). Clinicians should note that it is the specific strains of the probiotic bacteria that produced the reported results. Consumption of fermented food products has shown to have preventive properties against mastitis. Daily consumption of kefir provided a 1.4 times greater protection against mastitis, while daily consumption of homemade or commercial yogurt provided a 1.2 times greater protection against mastitis. The greater the consumption of fermented foods, the more protective the effect. Kefir has antitumor, antifungal, antibacterial, anti-inflammatory, and antioxidant properties. Microorganisms in kefir grains produce lactic acid, antibiotics, and bactericides, inhibiting the development of degrading and pathogenic microorganisms. Microbial composition of kefir varies according to the kefir's origin (Basım & Özdenkaya, 2020).

Traditional treatment for mastitis includes recommending to continue to feed or pump on the affected side, rest, a full 10- to 14-day course of antibiotics if needed, and identifying and treating the cause or precipitating factors of the mastitis. Frequent feedings and the use of breast compressions will help relieve milk stasis. Topical application of ricinoleic acid, the main component of castor oil, has been shown to have significant analgesic and anti-inflammatory effects (Vieira et al., 2000). Mothers can preheat a heating pad. A washcloth, diaper, or breast pad is placed on a sheet of plastic wrap. A tablespoon of castor oil is poured on the cloth and spread around. This poultice is placed over the affected area of the breast with the heating pad over it while the mother lies down and rests for 20 minutes. Any oil that gets on the nipple should be washed off before the next feeding.

Conflicting recommendations regarding mastitis treatment were published by the Academy of Breastfeeding Medicine (Mitchell et al., 2022). Interventions included to avoid pumping or feeding that aimed to thoroughly drain the breast, the avoidance of deep massage, castor oil and other topical products, and the use of ice instead of heat to reduce edema.

Mastitis can recur when the bacteria are resistant or not sensitive to the prescribed antibiotic, antibiotics are not continued long enough, an incorrect antibiotic is prescribed, the individual stopped nursing on the affected side, and when the initial cause of the mastitis was not addressed. If mastitis recurs, milk culture and sensitivity testing can be done as well as cultures of the infant's nasopharynx and oropharynx. Milk cultures should be taken if the mastitis is unresponsive to antibiotics after two days because organisms can be resistant to multiple medications (Spencer, 2008). If the infection occurs more than

Table 44.8   Antibiotic treatment of mastitis

First line
Dicloxicillin or Flucloxacillin 500 mg QID for 10–14 days
Cephalexin 500 mg QID for 10–14 days
Second line
Clindamycin 300 mg QID for 10–14 days
Trimethoprim-sulfamethoxazole DS BID for 10–14 days

Source: Adapted from Mitchell et al. (2022).

two or three times in the same location, a closer follow-up and evaluation is recommended to rule out an underlying mass (Mitchell et al., 2022).

It is important to identify and address the underlying causes of inflammatory signs and symptoms in the breast, which may halt the progression to an infection. If there is a low-grade fever, aching, red splotches, and a painful area in the breast, symptom relief with the use of a nonsteroidal anti-inflammatory drug such as ibuprofen may be achieved. If the symptoms do not improve within 8–24 hours, or if the fever continues, the fever suddenly increases, flu-like symptoms or obvious signs of a bacterial infection develop, such as discharge of pus from the nipple, a 10- to 14-day course of antibiotics is recommended (Table 44.8).

Abscess

A breast abscess is a potential complication of mastitis related to untreated, delayed, inadequate, or incorrect treatment of mastitis. Further contributors to this complication are prior episodes of mastitis, avoiding feedings or not pumping on the affected breast, or acute weaning during mastitis. An abscess is a localized collection of pus that becomes walled off and lacks an outlet for the drainage of the collected material. Once this material is encapsulated, it must be drained either surgically or by needle aspiration. An abscess may appear as a well-defined area of the breast that is hard, red, and tender, or a fluctuant mass. Breast abscess occurs in about 3% of women with mastitis (Amir et al., 2004). Abscess formation is significantly increased with smoking (Gollapalli et al., 2010), and heavy smoking increases the risk of recurrent abscess formation (Bharat et al., 2009).

S. aureus is the most common organism isolated in breast abscesses with methicillin-resistant *S. aureus* (MRSA) identified in over 60% of postpartum breast abscesses (Berens, et al., 2010; Stafford et al., 2008). Other organisms are less common. Any abscess drainage should be cultured and antibiotic sensitivities determined. It is not always possible to confirm the existence of an abscess by clinical examination or mammography. A diagnostic ultrasound is typically used to confirm the presence of an abscess and to mark the site for either surgical drainage, needle, or catheter aspiration and drainage.

Surgical drainage may be necessary if the abscess is extremely large or there are multiple abscess sites. Needle aspiration or percutaneous catheter drainage offers a nonsurgical approach and better preservation of breastfeeding for selected mothers (Falco et al., 2016). Breastfeeding should continue during and after the period of treatment as it promotes drainage of the affected segment and helps resolve the infection. Weaning or not breastfeeding or pumping on the affected side can hinder the resolution of the abscess by contributing to the production of increasingly viscid fluid that may promote stasis and engorgement. Breastfeeding should continue on the affected side unless the abscess drainage site is so close to the areola that the baby's mouth would cover it during feeding. If the infant will not feed from the affected side, the breast should be pumped. Changes in protein, carbohydrate, and electrolyte concentrations from an affected breast may decrease the level of lactose and cause a rise in sodium and chloride concentrations, making the milk taste salty.

Insufficient Milk Supply

Insufficient milk supply, either real or perceived, is one of the most frequent reasons for discontinuing breastfeeding (Brown et al., 2014). The perception of insufficient milk often has its origin in the hospital or birth center during the first 48 hours following childbirth. Many healthcare providers and mothers are unaware that infants need small, frequent feedings due to their small stomach capacity (about 5–10 mL/feeding on the first day of life), and that the amount of colostrum available to the infant is small. If mothers are pumping their breasts at this time and see small amounts of colostrum, they may incorrectly assume that they have an insufficient milk supply. They may also perceive a lack of milk if the breasts do not feel full, or if the baby feeds frequently, continues to fuss after a feeding, or does not settle between feedings (Amir, 2006).

True milk insufficiency, rather than perceived low milk production, can originate from genetic, anatomical, hormonal, or environmental influences. Primary breastmilk insufficiency may result from mammary hypoplasia (insufficient glandular tissue), exposure to organochlorines in utero, polycystic ovary syndrome, thyroid dysfunction, or genetic variations or mutations. Secondary breastmilk insufficiency often includes challenges such as preterm birth, infants with latching and sucking difficulties, infrequent or inadequate breast drainage, nonmedical use of infant formula, lack of self-efficacy, and mismanagement of lactation during the early days postpartum (Table 44.9). Some medications may compromise milk sufficiency such as selective serotonin reuptake inhibitors (SSRIs; Frew, 2015; Walker et al., 2019).

People often worry about infant crying and interpret it as a sign of hunger. Those who describe insufficient milk supply most frequently do so because they perceive their infant as not satisfied after a feeding and, as a result, offer a bottle of formula after nursing, which causes the infant to sleep. While mothers most commonly report infant crying as the cue used to determine insufficient milk, milk production and infant feeding parameters are often not assessed prior to recommending supplementation. However, supplementing with formula can diminish milk production. There are many contributors to the development of perceived

Table 44.9   Contributors to Low Milk Supply

Breastfeeding mismanagement	Limiting the number of feedings, short times at the breast, scheduled feedings that do not coincide with the infant's feeding cues, failure to assess for feeding cues, unrelieved severe engorgement, inappropriate formula supplementation, and use of artificial nipples and pacifiers.
Infant problems	Poor latch, oral anomalies, ankyloglossia, neurological problems, cardiac abnormalities, preterm infants, sleepy infants, and infants who are unable to feed at the breast.
Maternal conditions	Hypoplastic breasts, obesity, diabetes, thyroid dysfunction, polycystic ovary syndrome, history of breast surgery, smoking, inverted nipples, postpartum hemorrhage, retained placental fragments, and anemia.
Breast pump issues	Use of an inadequate breast pump, poorly fitted flange on a breast pump, or not pumping frequently enough.
Genetic variations	Mutations in ZnT2 variants can alter intracellular zinc pools and the ability of milk-secreting cells to carry out their functions (Lee & Kelleher, 2016; Lee et al., 2018).
Medications	Fluoxetine (Prozac) and aripiprazole (Abilify).

insufficient milk, with the most common contributors related to misinformation and mismanagement of breastfeeding. Many of these contributing factors can be prevented and corrected with appropriate information, teaching, and support early in the postpartum period.

Insufficient milk supply should be suspected if the infant loses more than 7–10% of birth weight and fails to regain birth weight by two to three weeks. However, this may also indicate an infant with poor breastfeeding skills who is unable to transfer milk even when there is an abundant milk supply. Weight gain of less than 5 oz/week, concentrated urine in the diapers, passing of dry hard stools, lethargy, and dry mucous membranes signal a potential problem with either milk transfer or milk supply and require immediate assessment and intervention. A feeding observation is necessary for infants who sleep excessive amounts, who feed for longer than 45 minutes at a single feeding, or appear to want to nurse continuously. These dyads should be referred to a lactation specialist, ideally an IBCLC. Likewise, individuals who have been pumping regularly should also be referred to a lactation specialist. Those who are expressing milk may complain of obtaining only small amounts of milk at each expression or of an unsatisfied infant no matter how frequently they breastfeed.

Management options for insufficient milk supply depend on the cause (Table 44.10). Clinicians should first assess the infant during a breastfeeding session to see if milk transfer is occurring. Pre- and postfeed weights can

Table 44.10 Selected Interventions for Low Milk Supply

Extra feedings, extra pumpings, pumping after a feeding, improving infant positioning, and assisting milk transfer to the infant by using alternate massage.
Use of a tube feeding device at the breast to deliver supplemental milk to the baby while the baby stimulates the breast.
Mothers of preterm infants should be encouraged to engage in skin-to-skin care and pump at their infant's bedside while looking at or touching their infant.
If using a breast pump, ensure that it is an effective, electric, multiuser breast pump with a double collection kit and properly fitted breast flange. Improperly fitted flanges can impede milk flow, reduce milk yield, and cause trauma to the nipple/areola (Sakalidis et al., 2020). Check the vacuum with a vacuum gauge to ensure that the pump is operating efficiently.
People who smoke should be encouraged to quit or reduce the number of cigarettes smoked per day. Smoking should not occur directly prior to a feeding as it may inhibit the let-down reflex.
Evaluate the individual for potential endocrine abnormalities and correct if present.

verify the amount of milk transfer. Faulty sucking skills, oral anomalies, underfeeding, and poor positioning may be recognized and remedied at this time.

Medications known as **galactagogues** have been used to improve milk production. The efficacy and side effect profile of these products vary. Common pharmaceutical galactagogues include metoclopramide and domperidone.

Metoclopramide (Reglan®) is a dopamine antagonist and has been shown to stimulate basal prolactin levels, leading to increased milk production at doses of 30–45 mg/day (Drugs and Lactation Database, 2021). Metoclopramide is dose dependent, and some may not respond if their prolactin levels are normal. Abrupt discontinuation of the medication can result in a precipitous drop in milk production. Thus, tapering the dosage by decreasing it 10 mg/week is recommended. Side effects of metoclopramide include gastric cramping, diarrhea, dystonia, depression, and suicidal ideation when used for more than four weeks, ultimately limiting its usefulness as a galactagogue. Few side effects have been reported in infants (American Academy of Pediatrics [AAP], 2013). Metoclopramide should be avoided in people with a history of major depression and not used for prolonged periods during the postpartum period when the risk of postpartum depression is increased. Prescribing information questions the utility of metoclopramide as a galactagogue and contains a boxed warning that the drug can cause tardive dyskinesia (involuntary repetitive body movements) when used for longer than 12 weeks (Food and Drug Administration, 2017).

Domperidone (Motilium®) is a peripheral dopamine antagonist similar to metoclopramide, but it does not cross the blood–brain barrier. This feature reduces the likelihood of central nervous system side effects such as depression. It was developed to treat gastrointestinal disorders, but since prolactin is inhibited by dopamine, domperidone stimulates lactation and can increase milk supply. It produces increases in prolactin levels and stimulates milk production at doses of 10–20 mg three to four times daily without causing gastric side effects (Paul et al., 2015). The effects may not be seen for three to four days, with the maximum effect taking up to two to three weeks (Henderson, 2003). Not all individuals respond to the use of domperidone, but for those that do, there is a dose–response relationship with higher doses resulting in more milk production (Wan et al., 2008). Most take the medication for up to six weeks (Paul et al., 2015). Domperidone is used successfully in some hospitals for pump-dependent mothers who are not yet able to breastfeed their hospitalized preterm infants (Haase et al., 2016). A meta-analysis of domperidone used as a galactagogue reviewed five double-blinded, placebo-controlled studies of mothers with insufficient milk production and found an average increase of 94 mL in daily milk production (Taylor et al., 2019). Although not widely available in the United States, it is commonly used in other countries and compounding pharmacies might be able to formulate domperidone with a prescription. However, the Food and Drug Administration (FDA) has not approved domperidone as a galactagogue for use in the United States and has issued a safety warning to consumers and healthcare professionals recommending that the drug not be used, based primarily on information regarding the intravenous form of the medication and on its use in treating gastrointestinal disorders. People with a history of cardiac arrhythmias should not take domperidone, and all should be advised to stop taking domperidone and seek immediate medical attention if they experience signs or symptoms of an abnormal heart rate or rhythm, including dizziness, palpitations, syncope, or seizures. Domperidone should not be prescribed to those taking other medications that could alter its metabolism such as antacids, antifungal medications, macrolide antibiotics, or monoamine oxidase inhibitors. Azole antifungals and macrolide antibiotics can block the metabolism of domperidone, resulting in increased plasma concentrations of domperidone. The AAP (2013) does not promote domperidone use as its safety profile in breastfeeding couplets is not well known.

Acupuncture has been successfully used in China since ancient times for insufficient milk supply (Zhao & Guo, 2006). Clavey (1996) reports over a 90% effectiveness rate when acupuncture is initiated within 20 days of birth but less than an 85% success rate when initiated after 20 days postpartum. The earlier the postpartum treatment is begun, the quicker the results and the more likely that milk production will significantly improve. Electroacupuncture may also be very effective (Wei et al., 2008). A study using electroacupuncture demonstrated an increased serum prolactin level, infant weight gain, and increased maternal perception of milk production (Maged et al., 2020). Acupressure applied to specific pressure points has also demonstrated effectiveness in increasing milk volume (Esfahani et al., 2015). A significant increase in milk production was seen in 35 women given acupressure massage at acupoints CV17, ST18, and SI1 compared to a control group of 35 women who showed a nonsignificant increase in breastmilk production (Sulymbona et al., 2020).

Similar therapies such as auricular therapy (Chen et al., 2017), acupoint-tuina (Lu et al., 2019), reflexology (reflex zone stimulation; Aksu & Palas Karaca, 2021), as well as hypnotherapy (guided hypnosis; Anuhgera et al., 2017) have all shown improvements in milk production.

Herbal and botanical preparations have been used since antiquity to stimulate milk production. Some commonly used herbs include fenugreek, milk thistle, raspberry leaf, nettle, goat's rue, fennel seed, chaste tree seed, fireweed, anise seed, blessed thistle, stinging nettle, and cotton root. Many of these herbs are used in combination in commercial galactagogue preparations. Although there is limited science behind the use of most of these preparations or their efficacy (Anderson, 2017), many herbs and botanical preparations are widely used for improving milk output despite the lack of high-quality clinical trials and evidence supporting the safety of their use (Amer et al., 2015). Although some healthcare providers recommend the use of herbal galactagogues, herbal remedies are often used based on recommendations from family members and friends (Sim et al., 2015) and from anecdotal reports on social media sites or the Internet. In the United States, herbs are classified as nutritional supplements and do not require extensive premarketing approval from the FDA nor do manufacturers need to prove the safety and effectiveness of dietary supplements before they are marketed to the public.

Fenugreek (*Trigonella foenum-graecum*) is probably the most widely used herbal galactagogue. Fenugreek has been shown to have antianxiety effects, which may contribute to the herb's anecdotally reported effectiveness (Abascal & Yarnell, 2008). The dosage is usually 1200 mg 2–3 times daily. Fenugreek is also available as tea and has been shown to enhance milk production during the early days following birth (Turkyilmaz et al., 2011).

Goat's rue (*Galega officinalis*) is a common galactagogue (Weiss, 2001) used for insufficient milk production. Goat's rue is dosed as 1 tsp of dried herb steeped in 1 cup of water twice daily or 1–2 mL of tincture three times daily.

Other botanical preparations include fennel seed, chaste tree seed, and milk thistle. Fennel seed (*Foeniculum vulgare*) is used to increase milk production at a dose of 5–7 g of seed per day as a tea. Chaste tree seed (*Vitex adnus-castus*) is used at a dosage of 1 tsp of the berries steeped in 1 cup of water three times daily or 2.5 mL of tincture three times daily. Milk thistle (*Silybum marianum*) in a micronized 420 mg dose can significantly increase daily milk production. The micronized form improves its poor bioavailability (Di Pierro et al., 2008).

Some remedies such as beer (hops), brewer's yeast (vitamin B complex), oatmeal, and various cultural preparations and foods have also been used. Although herbal and botanical preparations are commonly employed, they require some caution. Clinicians can refer to the German Commission E Monographs for safety profiles of botanicals, the American Herbal Products Association for information on manufacturing and labeling standards, and the American Botanical Council for information on the quality of herbal products. The use of a galactagogue requires close follow-up by the clinician (Brodribb & The Academy of Breastfeeding Medicine, 2018).

Genetic variables may play a part in insufficient milk production; these factors will not respond to typical interventions, medications, or galactagogues. Mutation of the protein ZnT2, which transports zinc in specific body tissues, may result in not only decreased zinc levels in the milk but also functional problems in the development of the breast itself, leading to insufficient milk production (Lee et al., 2015). Those with decreased insulin sensitivity may experience a slower and less robust increase in milk output as a result of protein coding gene overexpression in the mammary gland (Lemay et al., 2013). These genetic alterations are not always readily apparent and can, in some cases, preclude the development of full milk production.

Delayed lactogenesis II refers to the delay in the secretory phase of lactation characterized by the perception of "milk coming in" after 72 hours postpartum. Individuals with diabetes requiring insulin treatment, obesity, primiparity, cesarean birth, and suboptimal breastfeeding in the first two days postpartum are conditions that are independently associated with a significant increase in delayed lactogenesis II (Matias et al., 2014). Even though delayed lactogenesis II may occur, breastfeeding can still be successful. Assistance with positioning and latch, frequent feeding, and lactation consultant services are important strategies to help establish a milk supply. Practices consistent with the Baby Friendly Hospital Initiative should be followed to help ensure effective breastfeeding within the first 24 hours. Some people may need to feed their infant closer to 12 times each 24 hours and clinicians need to monitor the infant for hypoglycemia, jaundice, weight loss, and hypernatremia.

The prevalence of delayed lactogenesis II has been reported to range from 33% (Dewey et al., 2003) to 44% (Nommsen-Rivers et al., 2010). There are several factors that place mothers at an increased risk for a delayed onset of lactation (Table 44.10). During delayed lactogenesis II, infants are at an increased risk for hypoglycemia, slow or no weight gain, weight loss, dehydration, and jaundice. Some of these factors are amenable to interventions such as ensuring effective infant feeding; some are correctable, such as removal of retained placental fragments, but many are conditions cannot be prevented or modified. These conditions leave the dyad in a situation of a prolonged colostral phase where more frequent feedings may be necessary as well as close follow-up after discharge. A feeding plan may include 10–12 feedings each 24 hours, use of alternate massage (massaging and compressing each breast at each feeding), hand-expressing colostrum and spoon feeding it to the infant if breastfeeding is ineffective, and the possible use of donor breastmilk, or amino-acid-based infant formula if medically necessary.

Hyperlactation

Hyperlactation (hypergalactia, galactorrhea, and oversupply) lacks a formal definition but typically refers to the production of breastmilk in excess of what a normal healthy, full-term infant would consume (450–1,200 mL/day). Those experiencing hyperlactation may complain of deep shooting pain in the breasts, breasts that never feel comfortable or fully drained, milk leakage, chronic plugged ducts, and firm or lumpy areas of the breasts. Infants may gulp or choke at the breast, especially with the first milk ejection, may arch off the breast, spit up frequently, have excessive gas, produce green, frothy, or explosive stools, exhibit reflux, or have difficulty remaining latched to the breast.

The etiology is often unknown but could originate from inducing milk production in excess of what the infant requires by excessive pumping, herbal preparations, and taking medications (including psychiatric medications that are dopamine antagonists).

Interventions include:

- Block feeding is frequently recommended as the first-line intervention for hyperlactation (Johnson et al., 2020). While there are variations of this intervention (van Veldhuizen-Staas, 2007; Eglash, 2014), block feeding typically divides the day into three-hour time blocks where the same breast is offered at each feeding during that time block. At the next three-hour time block, the other breast is offered for each feeding. Time blocks can be gradually lengthened if the condition does not improve after the first few time blocks. Time blocks are used during the day and feeding from both breasts can be done overnight (Eglash, 2014). Dyads should be closely monitored to ensure that the infant is growing appropriately, and that the mother is not experiencing additional problems or side effects from this process.
- Some herbal remedies are thought to reduce milk production such as sage and peppermint tea. Homeopathic medications are reported to decrease milk supply such as lac caninum 30C, Pulsatilla 30C, and *Ricinus communis* 30C, but evidence for effectiveness of homeopathic remedies is limited (Eglash, 2014).
- Medications such as pseudoephedrine (Sudafed) which is an over-the-counter decongestant medication that has been shown to reduce milk production (Aljazaf et al., 2003).
- A combined oral contraceptive that contains 20–35 micrograms (mcg) of estradiol could be used for a short period of time or in more extreme situations a low dose of cabergoline could be utilized (Johnson et al., 2020).
- Reclining maternal positioning with the infant prone or ventral uses gravity to reduce the fast flow of milk.
- Both breasts should be checked thoroughly for plugged milk and mastitis.

Summary

Although breastfeeding is the optimal method of infant feeding, there can be challenges for some women in establishing and maintaining breastfeeding. The most common breastfeeding problems encountered during the early postnatal period include infant problems such as failure to latch, fussiness or sleepiness at the breast, low weight gain, and prematurity, and maternal problems such as sore nipples, engorgement, mastitis, and low milk supply. All healthcare professionals who care for women and infants should be familiar with the diagnosis and management of these common breastfeeding problems so that they can provide appropriate care or referrals for the breastfeeding mother and infant.

Resources for Healthcare Providers

Books

Genna, C. W. (2017). *Supporting sucking skills in breastfeeding infants* (3rd ed.). Jones & Bartlett Learning.

Hale, T. W. (2021). *Medications and mothers' milk* (19th ed.). Springer Publishing Company.

Lauwers, J., & Swisher, A. (2021). *Counseling the nursing mother: A lactation consultant's guide* (7th ed.). Jones & Bartlett Learning.

Lawrence, R.A., & Lawrence, R.M. (2022). *Breastfeeding: A guide for the medical profession* (9th ed.). Elsevier.

Walker, M. (2023). *Breastfeeding management for the clinician: Using the evidence* (5th ed.). Jones & Bartlett Learning.

Wambach K., & Spencer, B. (2021). *Breastfeeding and human lactation* (6th ed.). Jones & Bartlett Learning.

Wilson-Clay B., & Hoover, K. (2017). *The breastfeeding atlas* (6th ed.). LactNews Press, LLC.

German Commission E Monographs for safety profiles of botanicals, the American Herbal Products Association (www.ahpa.org) for information on manufacturing and labeling standards

Web Resources for Clinicians

The melanated mammary atlas (2021). Searchable directory of various breast-related conditions on brown skin. https://www.mmatlas.com

Getting started with breastfeeding. Stanford Medicine, Newborn Nursery at Lucile Packard Children's Hospital. https://med.stanford.edu/newborns/professional-education/breastfeeding.html

American Botanical Council (www.herbalgram.org) for information on the quality of herbal products.

Pump Flange Fitting. Maymom. https://www.maymom.com/index.php/products-menu/breastshield-selection-guide

Exclusive pumping. https://exclusivepumping.com/breast-shield-sizing

Apps

Drugs and Lactation Database (LactMed). Searchable database for drug safety use during lactation. National Library of Medicine. https://www.ncbi.nlm.nih.gov/books/NBK501922

InfantRisk for healthcare professionals. Gives healthcare providers access to up-to-date and evidence-based information about prescription and nonprescription medications and their safety during pregnancy and breastfeeding. Infant Risk Center at Texas Tech University Health Sciences Center. https://www.infantrisk.com/infantrisk-center-resources

BiliTool. Designed to help clinicians assess the risks toward the development of hyperbilirubinemia or "jaundice" in newborns over 35 weeks gestational age. https://bilitool.org/?page_id=46

Newborn Weight Loss Tool (NEWT). Allows pediatric healthcare providers and parents to see how a newborn's weight during the first days and weeks following childbirth compares with a large sample of newborns, which can help with early identification of weight loss and we https://www.newbornweight.org/#:~:text=What%20is%20it%3F,gain%20issues.%22%20Ian%20M.ight gain issues

Organizations and Agencies

Academy of Breastfeeding Medicine. https://www.bfmed.org

American Academy of Pediatrics. https://www.aap.org

Baby Friendly USA. https://www.babyfriendlyusa.org

California Perinatal Quality Care Collaborative. https://www.cpqcc.org

Centers for Disease Control and Prevention. https://www.cdc.gov

Human Milk Banking Association of North America. https://www.hmbana.org

International Lactation Consultant Association. www.ilca.org

La Leche League International. https://www.llli.org

National Lactation Consultant Alliance. https://nlca.us

Office of Women's Health, US Department of Health and Human Services. https://www.womenshealth.gov

United States Breastfeeding Committee. http://www.usbreastfeeding.org

Women, Infants, and Children (WIC) Program US Department of Agriculture, Food and Nutrition Service. https://www.fns.usda.gov/wic

United States Lactation Consultant Association. www.uslca.org

Medications and Breastfeeding

Briggs, G. G., Towers, C. V., & Forinash, A. B. (2022). *Briggs drugs in pregnancy and lactation* (12th ed.). Wolters Kluwer.

Hale, T. W. (2021). *Medications and mothers' milk* (19th ed.). Springer Publishing Company.

Drugs and Lactation Database (LactMed). Searchable database for drug safety use during lactation. National Library of Medicine. https://www.ncbi.nlm.nih.gov/books/NBK501922

InfantRisk for healthcare professionals. Gives healthcare providers access to up-to-date and evidence-based information about prescription and nonprescription medications and their safety during pregnancy and breastfeeding. Infant Risk Center at Texas Tech University Health Sciences Center. https://www.infantrisk.com/infantrisk-center-resources

Nice, F. (2011). *Nonprescription drugs for the breastfeeding mother.* Praeclarus Press.

Nice, F. J., Luo, A. C., & Harrow, C.A. (2016). *Recreational drugs and drugs used to treat addicted mothers: Impact on pregnancy and breastfeeding.* Nice Breastfeeding LLC.

Resources for Clients and Families

Apps

Anya. https://anya.health/?fbclid=IwAR0z88quR4LShbE38f7rF6gatkXSUb0sdhDI6TFMHCMRuIEG81q7z_ZJOZ0

Irth. Provides prenatal, birthing, postpartum, and pediatric reviews of care for Black and brown women. https://apps.apple.com/us/app/irth-birth-without-bias/id1537466974

Pacify Health. Connects parents to a nationwide network of lactation consultants and registered nurses. https://apps.apple.com/us/app/pacify-helping-new-parents/id981698864

Books for Consumers

Marasco & West. (2019). *Making more milk* (2nd ed.). McGraw-Hill Education.

Mohrbacher & Kendall-Tackett. (2010). *Breastfeeding made simple* (2nd ed.) New Harbinger Publications.

Spangler. (2021). *Breastfeeding: A parent's guide.* Baby GooRoo. https://babygooroo.com/store/product/breastfeeding-keep-it-simple

Spangler. (2019). *Breastfeeding: Keep it simple.* Baby GooRoo. https://babygooroo.com/store/product/breastfeeding-keep-it-simple

Wiessinger et al. (2010). *The womanly art of breastfeeding* (8th ed.). Random House Publishing group.

Where to Find Help

US Lactation Consultant Association. To find a lactation consultant. https://uslca.org/resources/find-an-ibclc

ZipMilk. To find lactation care and support. https://www.zipmilk.org

WIC. Local WIC agencies.

Baby Café. Drop-in informal breastfeeding support groups. https://www.babycafeusa.org

La Leche League International. Mother-to mother support. https://www.llli.org

Mahmee. Provides care managers for personalized breastfeeding support. https://www.mahmee.com

References

Abascal, K., & Yarnell, E. (2008). Botanical galactagogues. *Alternative & Complementary Therapies, 14,* 288–294.

Akbari, S. A., Alamolhoda, S. H., Baghban, A. A., & Mirabi, P. (2014). Effects of menthol essence and breastmilk on the improvement of nipple fissures in breastfeeding women. *Journal of Research in Medical Sciences*, 19, 629–633.

Aksu, S., & Palas Karaca, P. (2021). The effect of reflexology on lactation in women who had cesarean section: A randomized controlled pilot study. *Complementary Medicine Research*, 21, 1–8.

Aljazaf, K., Hale, T. W., Ilett, K. F., Hartmann, P. E., Mitoulas, L. R., Kristensen, J. H., & Hackett, L. P. (2003). Pseudoephedrine: Effects on milk production in women and estimation of infant exposure via breastmilk. *British Journal of Clinical Pharmacology*, 56, 18–24.

Amer, M. R., Cipriano, G. C., Venci, J. V., & Gandhi, M. A. (2015). Safety of popular herbal supplements in lactating women. *Journal of Human Lactation*, 31, 348–353.

American Academy of Pediatrics. (2013). The transfer of drugs and therapeutics into human breastmilk: An update on selected topics. *Pediatrics*, 132, e796–e809.

Amir, L. H. (2006). Breastfeeding: Managing supply difficulties. *Australian Family Physician*, 35, 686–689.

Amir, L. H., Forster, D., McLachlan, H., & Lumley, J. (2004). Incidence of breast abscess in lactating women: Report from an Australian cohort. *BJOG: An International Journal of Obstetrics and Gynaecology*, 111, 1378–1381.

Anderson, P. O. (2017). Herbal use during breastfeeding. *Breastfeeding Medicine*, 12, 507–509.

Angelopoulou, A., Field, D., Ryan, C. A., Stanton, C., Hill, C., & Ross, R. P. (2018). The microbiology and treatment of human mastitis. *Medical Microbiology and Immunology*, 207, 83–94.

Anuhgera, D. E., Kuncoro, T., Sumarni, S., Mardiyono, M., & Suwondo, A. (2017). Hypnotherapy is more effective than acupressure in the production of prolactin hormone and breastmilk among women having given birth with caesarean section. *Medicine Science International Medical Journal*, 7, 25–29.

Basım, P., & Özdenkaya, Y. (2020). Can traditional fermented food products protect mothers against lactational mastitis. *Breastfeeding Medicine*, 15, 163–169.

Batista, C. L. C., Rodrigues, V. P., Ribeiro, V. S., & Nascimento, M. D. S. B. (2019). Nutritive and non-nutritive sucking patterns associated with pacifier use and bottle-feeding in full-term infants. *Early Human Development*, 132, 18–23.

Beaino, G., Khoshnood, B., Kaminski, M., Marret, S., Pierrat, V., Vieux, R., Thiriez, G., Matis, J., Picaud, J., Rozé, J., Alberge, C., Larroque, B., Bréart, G., Ancel, P., & EPIPAGE Study Group. (2011). Predictors of the risk of cognitive deficiency in very preterm infants: The EPIPAGE prospective cohort. *Acta Paediatrica*, 100, 370–378.

Belfort, M. B., Anderson, P. J., Nowak, V. A., Lee, K. J., Molesworth, C., Thompson, D. K., Doyle, L. W., & Inder, T. E. (2016). Breastmilk feeding, brain development, and neurocognitive outcomes: A 7-year longitudinal study in infants born at less than 30 weeks' gestation. *Journal of Pediatrics*, 177, 133–139.

Berens, P., Swaim, L., & Peterson, B. (2010). Incidence of methicillin-resistant *Staphylococcus aureus* in postpartum breast abscesses. *Breastfeeding Medicine*, 5, 113–115.

Bergmann, H., Rodríguez, J. M., Salminen, S., & Szajewska, H. (2014). Probiotics in human milk and probiotic supplementation in infant nutrition: A workshop report. *British Journal of Nutrition*, 112, 1119–1128.

Bharat, A., Gao, F., Aft, R. L., Gillanders, W. E., Eberlein, T. J., & Margenthaler, J. A. (2009). Predictors of primary breast abscesses and recurrence. *World Journal of Surgery*, 33, 2582–2586.

Bouchet-Horwitz, J. (2011). The use of Supple Cups for flat, retracting, and inverted nipples. *Clinical Lactation*, 2, 30–33.

Boundy, E. O., Perrine, C. G., Nelson, J. M., & Hamner, H. C. (2017). Disparities in hospital-reported breastmilk use in neonatal intensive care units—United States, 2015. *Morbidity & Mortality Weekly Report*, 66, 1313–1317.

Bowles, B. C., Stutte, P. C., & Hensley, J. (1987). Alternate breast massage: New benefits from an old technique. *Genesis*, 9, 5–9.

Brodribb, W., & The Academy of Breastfeeding Medicine. (2018). ABM clinical protocol #9: Use of galactogogues in initiating or augmenting maternal milk production, second revision 2018. *Breastfeeding Medicine*, 13, 307–314.

Brown, C. R., Dodds, L., Legge, A., Bryanton, J., & Semenic, S. (2014). Factors influencing the reasons why mothers stop breastfeeding. *Canadian Journal of Public Health*, 105(3), e179–e185.

Campbell, S. H. (2006). Recurrent plugged ducts. *Journal of Human Lactation*, 22, 340–343.

Chanprapaph, P., Luttarapakul, J., Siribariruck, S., & Boonyawanichkul, S. (2013). Outcome of non-protractile nipple correction with breast cups in pregnant women: A randomized controlled trial. *Breastfeeding Medicine*, 8, 408–412.

Chen, M. L., Tan, J. Y., & Suen, L. K. (2017). Auricular therapy for lactation: A systematic review. *Complementary Therapies in Clinical Practice*, 29, 169–184.

Chiang, K. V., Sharma, A. J., Nelson, J. M., Olson, C. K., & Perrine, C. G. (2019). Receipt of breastmilk by gestational age—United States, 2017. *Morbidity and Mortality Weekly Report*, 68, 489–493.

Claud, E. C., & Walker, W. A. (2001). Hypothesis: Inappropriate colonization of the premature intestine can cause neonatal necrotizing enterocolitis. *The FASEB Journal*, 15, 1398–1403.

Clavey, S. (1996). The use of acupuncture for the treatment of insufficient lactation (Que Ru). *American Journal of Acupuncture*, 24, 35–46.

Contreras, G. A., & Rodríguez, J. M. (2011). Mastitis: Comparative etiology and epidemiology. *Journal of Mammary Gland Biology and Neoplasia*, 16, 339–356.

Dennis, C. L., Jackson, K., & Watson, J. (2014). Interventions for treating painful nipples among breastfeeding women. *Cochrane Database of Systematic Reviews*, (12), CD007366. https://doi.org/10.1002/14651858.CD007366.pub2

Dewey, K. G., Nommsen-Rivers, L. A., Heinig, M. J., & Cohen, R. J. (2003). Risk factors for suboptimal infant breastfeeding behavior, delayed onset of lactation, and excess neonatal weight loss. *Pediatrics*, 112, 607–619.

Di Pierro, F., Callegari, A., Carotenuto, D., & Tapia, M. M. (2008). Clinical efficacy, safety and tolerability of BIO-C (micronized Silymarin) as a galactogogue. *Acta Bio-medica: Atenei Parmensis*, 79, 205–210.

Douglas, P. (2022). Re-thinking lactation-related nipple pain and damage. *Womens Health (Lond)*, 18, 17455057221087865. https://doi.org/10.1177/17455057221087865

Drugs and Lactation Database (LactMed). (2021). *Metoclopramide*. National Library of Medicine. https://www.ncbi.nlm.nih.gov/books/NBK501352

Eglash, A. (1998). Delayed milk ejection reflex and plugged ducts: Lecithin therapy. *ABM News and Views*, 4(1), 4.

Eglash, A. (2014). Treatment of maternal hypergalactia. *Breastfeeding Medicine*, 9, 423–425.

Emond, A., Drewett, R., Blair, P., & Emmett, P. (2007). Postnatal factors associated with failure to thrive in term infants in the Avon Longitudinal Study of Parents and Children. *Archives of Diseases in Children*, 92, 115–119.

Esfahani, M. S., Berenji-Sooghe, S., Valiani, M., & Ehsanpour, S. (2015). Effect of acupressure on milk volume of breastfeeding mothers referring to selected health care centers in Tehran. *Iranian Journal of Nursing & Midwifery Research*, 20(1), 7.

Falco, G., Foroni, M., Castagnetti, F., Marano, L., Bordoni, D., Rocco, N., & Ferrari, G. (2016). Ultrasound-guided percutaneous catheter drainage of large breast abscesses in lactating women: How to preserve breastfeeding safely. *Breastfeeding Medicine*, 10, 555–556.

Fernandez, L., Arroyo, R., Espinosa, I., Marin, M., Jimenez, E., & Rodriguez, J. M. (2014). Probiotics for human lactational mastitis. *Beneficial Microbes*, 5, 169–183.

Fernandez, L., Cardenas, N., Arroyo, R., Manzano, S., Jiménez, E., Martín, V., & Rodríguez, J. M. (2016). Prevention of infectious mastitis by oral administration of *Lactobacillus salivarius* PS2 during late pregnancy. *Clinical Infectious Diseases*, 62, 568–573.

Food and Drug Administration. (2017). *Highlights of prescribing information*. https://www.accessdata.fda.gov/drugsatfda_docs/label/2017/017854s062lbl.pdf

Frew, J. R. (2015). Psycopharmacology of bipolar I disorder during lactation: A case report of the used of lithium and aripiprazole in a nursing mother. *Archives of Women's Mental Health, 18*, 135–136.

Genna, C. W. (2017). *Supporting sucking skills in breastfeeding infants.* Jones & Bartlett Learning.

Gollapalli, V., Liao, J., Dudakovic, A., Sugg, S. L., Scott-Conner, C. E., & Weigel, R. J. (2010). Risk factors for development and recurrence of primary breast abscesses. *Journal of the American College of Surgeons, 211*, 41–48.

Groer, M. W., Gregory, K. E., Louis-Jacques, A., Thibeau, S., & Walker, W. A. (2015). The very low birth weight infant microbiome and childhood health. *Birth Defects Research Part C: Embryo Today, 105*, 252–264.

Haase, B., Taylor, S. N., Mauldin, J., Johnson, T. S., & Wagner, C. L. (2016). Domperidone for treatment of low milk supply in breast pump-dependent mothers of hospitalized premature infants: A clinical protocol. *Journal of Human Lactation, 32*, 373–381.

Hale, T. W. (2021). *Medications and mothers' milk* (19th ed.). Springer Publishing Company.

Hall, R. T., Mercer, A. M., Teasley, S. L., McPherson, D. M., Simon, S. D., Santos, S. R., Meyers, B. M. & Hipsh, N. E. (2002). A breastfeeding assessment score to evaluate the risk for cessation of breastfeeding by 7 to 10 days of age. *The Journal of Pediatrics, 141*(5), 659–664.

Hawk, C., Minkalis, A., Webb, C., Hogan, O., & Vallone, S. (2018). Manual interventions for musculoskeletal factors in infants with suboptimal breastfeeding: A scoping review. *Journal of Evidence-Based Integrative Medicine, 23*, 2515690X18816971. https://doi.org/10.1177/2515690X18816971

Hazelbaker, A. K. (2020). The impact of craniosacral therapy/cranial osteopathy on breastfeeding. *Clinical Lactation, 11*, 21–27.

Henderson, A. (2003). Domperidone: Discovering new choices for lactating mothers. *AWHONN Lifelines, 7*, 55–60.

Hurtado, J. A., Maldonado-Lobón, J. A., Díaz-Ropero, M. P., Flores-Rojas, K., Uberos, J., Leante, J. L., Affumicato, L., Couce, M. L., Garrido, J. M., Olivares, M., & Fonollá, J. (2017). Oral administration to nursing women of lactobacillus fermentum CECT5716 prevents lactational mastitis development: A randomized controlled trial. *Breastfeeding Medicine, 12*, 202–209.

Iffrig, M. C. (1968). Nursing care and success in breastfeeding. *The Nursing Clinics of North America, 3*, 345–354.

Ismail, N. I. A. A., Hafez, S. K., & Ghaly, A. S. (2019). Effect of breastmilk, peppermint water and breast shell on treatment of traumatic nipple in puerperal lactating mothers. *International Journal of Novel Research in Healthcare and Nursing, 6*, 692–709.

Jahanfar, S., Ng, C. J., & Teng, C. L. (2013). Antibiotics for mastitis in breastfeeding women. *Cochrane Database Systematic Reviews*, (2), CD005458. https://doi.org/10.1002/14651858.CD005458.pub3

Jiménez, E., Arroyo, R., Cardenas, N., Marín, M., Serrano, P., Fernandez, L., & Rodriguez, J. M. (2017). Mammary candidiasis: A medical condition without scientific evidence? *PLoS One, 12*, e0181071. https://doi.org/10.1371/journal.pone.0181071

Jiménez, E., de Andrés, J., Manrique, M., Pareja-Tobes, P., Tobes, R., Martínez-Blanch, J. F., Codoñer, F. M., Ramón, D., Fernandez, L., & Rodríguez, J. M. (2015). Metagenomic analysis of milk of healthy and mastitis-suffering women. *Journal of Human Lactation, 31*, 406–415.

Johnson, H. M., Eglash, A., Mitchell, K. B., Leeper, K., Smillie, C. M., Moore-Ostby, L., Manson, N., Simon, L., & Academy of Breastfeeding Medicine. (2020). ABM clinical protocol #32: Management of hyperlactation. *Breastfeeding Medicine, 15*, 129–134.

Kair, L. R., & Chantry, C. J. (2021). Low intake in the breastfed infant: Maternal and infant considerations. In K. Wambach & B. Spencer (Eds.), *Breastfeeding and human lactation* (6th ed., pp. 313–353). Jones & Bartlett Learning.

Karnati, S., Kollikonda, S., & Abu-Shaweesh, J. (2020). Late preterm infants—Changing trends and continuing challenges. *International Journal of Pediatrics & Adolescent Medicine, 7*, 36–44.

Kent, J. C., Ashton, E., Hardwick, C. M., Rowan, M. K., Chia, E. S., Fairclough, K. A., Menon, L. L., Scott, C., Mather-McCaw, G., Navarro, K., & Geddes, D. T. (2015). Nipple pain in breastfeeding mothers: Incidence, causes and treatments. *International Journal of Environmental Research and Public Health, 12*, 12247–12263.

Larkin, T., Kiehn, T., Murphy, P. K., & Uhryniak, J. (2013). Examining the use and outcomes of a new hospital-grade breast pump in exclusively pumping NICU mothers. *Advances in Neonatal Care, 13*, 75–82.

Lawrence, R. A., & Lawrence, R. M. (2010). *Breastfeeding: A guide for the medical profession* (7th ed.). Elsevier Mosby.

Lee, S., Hennigar, S. R., Alam, S., Nishida, K., & Kelleher, S. L. (2015). Essential role for zinc transporter 2 (ZnT2)-mediated zinc transport in mammary gland development and function during lactation. *Journal of Biological Chemistry, 22*, 13064–13078.

Lee, S., & Kelleher, S. L. (2016). Molecular regulation of lactation: The complex and requisite roles for zinc. *Archives of Biochemistry and Biophysics, 611*, 86–92.

Lee, S., Zhou, Y., Gill, D. L., & Kelleher, S. L. (2018). A genetic variant in SLC30A2 causes breast dysfunction during lactation by inducing ER stress, oxidative stress and epithelial barrier defects. *Scientific Reports, 8*(1), 3542. https://doi.org/10.1038/s41598-018-21505-8

Lemay, D. G., Ballard, O. A., Highes, M. A., Morrow, A. L., Horseman, N. D., & Nommsen-Rivers, L. A. (2013). RNA sequencing of the human milk fat layer transcriptome reveals distinct gene expression profiles at three stages of lactation. *PLoS One, 8*(7), e67531. https://doi.org/10.1371/journal.pone.0067531

Lim, A. R., Song, J. A., Hur, M. H., Lee, M. K., & Lee, M. S. (2015). Cabbage compression early breast care on breast engorgement in primiparous women after cesarean birth: A controlled clinical trial. *International Journal of Clinical and Experimental Medicine, 8*(11), 21335–21342.

Livingstone, V. H., Willis, C., & Berkowitz, J. (1996). *Staphylococcus aureus* and sore nipples. *Canadian Family Physician, 42*, 654–659.

Lu, P., Ye, Z. Q., Qiu, J., Wang, X. Y., & Zheng, J. J. (2019). Acupoint-Tuina therapy promotes lactation in postpartum women with insufficient milk production who underwent caesarean sections. *Medicine, 98*(35), e16456. https://doi.org/10.1097/MD.0000000000016456

Maged, A. M., Hassanin, M. E., Kamal, W. M., Abbassy, A. H., Alalfy, M., Askalani, A. N., El-Lithy, A., Nabil, M., Farouk, D., Hussein, E. A., & Hammad, B. (2020). Effect of low-level laser therapy versus electroacupuncture on postnatal scanty milk secretion: A randomized controlled trial. *American Journal of Perinatology, 37*, 1243–1249.

Mahfouz, I. A., Asali, F., Khalfieh, T., Saleem, H. A., Diab, S., Samara, B., & Jaber, H. (2022). Early initiation of breastfeeding: Antenatal, peripartum, and neonatal correlates. *Journal of Clinical Neonatology, 11*, 30–37. https://doi.org/10.4103/jcn.jcn_25_21

Marchini, G., & Linden, A. (1992). Cholecystokinin, a satiety signal in newborn infants? *Journal of Developmental Physiology, 17*, 215–219.

Marchini, G., Simoni, M. R., Bartolini, F., & Linden, A. (1993). The relationship of plasma cholecystokinin levels to different feeding routines in newborn infants. *Early Human Development, 35*, 31–35.

Marrazzu, A., Sanna, M. G., Dessole, F., Capobianco, G., Piga, M. D., & Dessole, S. (2015). Evaluation of the effectiveness of a silver-impregnated medical cap for topical treatment of nipple fissure of breastfeeding mothers. *Breastfeeding Medicine, 10*, 232–238.

Martin, J. A., Hamilton, B. E., & Osterman, M. J. K. (2020). *Births in the United States, 2019.* NCHS Data Brief, no 387. National Center for Health Statistics. https://www.cdc.gov/nchs/products/databriefs/db387.htm

Matias, S. L., Dewey, K. G., Quesenberry, C. P., & Gunderson, E. P. (2014). Maternal prepregnancy obesity and insulin treatment during pregnancy are independently associated with delayed lactogenesis in women with recent gestational diabetes mellitus. *The American Journal of Clinical Nutrition, 99*(1), 115–121.

McGuire, E. (2015). Case study: White spot and lecithin. *Breastfeeding Review, 23*, 23–25.

Meier, P. P., Patel, A. L., Hoban, R., & Engstrom, J. L. (2016). Which breast pump for which mother: An evidence-based approach to individualizing breast pump technology. *Journal of Perinatology, 36*, 493–499.

Meinzen-Derr, J., Poindexter, B., Wrage, L., Morrow, A. L., Stoll, B., & Donovan, E. F. (2009). Role of human milk in extremely low birth weight infants' risk of necrotizing enterocolitis or death. *Journal of Perinatology, 29*, 57–62.

Melli, M. S., Rashidi, M. R., Nokhoodchi, A., Tagavi, S., Farzadi, L., Sadaghat, K., Tahmasebi, Z., & Sheshvan, M. K. (2007). A randomized trial of peppermint gel, lanolin ointment, and placebo gel to prevent nipple crack in primiparous breastfeeding women. *Medical Science Monitor, 13,* CR406–CR411.

Merckoll, P., Jonassen, T. O., Vad, M. E., Jeansson, S. L., & Melby, K. K. (2009). Bacteria, biofilm and honey: A study of the effects of honey on "planktonic" and biofilm-embedded wound bacteria. *Scandinavian Journal of Infectious Diseases, 41,* 341–347.

Miller, J. (2020). Breastfeeding support teams: When to add a chiropractor. *Clinical Lactation, 11,* 7–20.

Mitchell, K., Johnson, H., Rodriguez, J., Eglash, A., Scherzinger, C., & The Academy of Breastfeeding Medicine. (2022). Academy of breastfeeding medicine clinical protocol #36: The mastitis spectrum, revised 2022. *Breastfeeding Medicine, 17*(5), 360–376. https://doi.org/10.1089/bfm.2022.29207.kbm

Morales, Y., & Schanler, R. J. (2007). Human milk and clinical outcomes in VLBW infants: How compelling is the evidence of benefit? *Seminars in Perinatology, 31,* 83–88.

Morland-Schultz, K., & Hill, P. D. (2005). Prevention of and therapies for nipple pain: A systematic review. *Journal of Obstetric Gynecologic and Neonatal Nursing, 34,* 428–437.

Morton, J., Hall, J. Y., Wong, R. J., Thairu, L., Benitz, W. E., & Rinne, W. D. (2009). Combining hand techniques with electric pumping increased milk production in mothers of preterm infants. *Journal of Perinatology, 29,* 757–764.

Nommsen-Rivers, L. A., Chantry, C. J., Peerson, J. M., Cohen, R. J., & Dewey, K. G. (2010). Delayed onset of lactogenesis among first-time mothers is related to maternal obesity and factors associated with ineffective breastfeeding. *American Journal of Clinical Nutrition, 92,* 574–584.

Oguz, S., Isık, S., Çakır Güngör, A. N., Seker, M., & Ogretmen, Z. (2014). Protective efficacy of olive oil for sore nipples during nursing. *Journal of Family Medicine and Community Health, 1,* 1021.

Ohyama, M., Watabe, H., & Hayasaka, Y. (2010). Manual expression and electric breast pumping in the first 48 h after delivery. *Pediatrics International, 52,* 39–43.

Pados, B. F. (2023). State of the science on the benefits of human milk for hospitalized, vulnerable neonates. *Nursing for Women's. Health, 27,* 121–140.

Parra-Llorca, A., Gormaz, M., Alcántara, C., Cernada, M., Nuñez-Ramiro, A., Vento, M., & Collado, M. C. (2018). Preterm gut microbiome depending on feeding type: Significance of donor human milk. *Frontiers in Microbiology, 9,* 1376. https://doi.org/10.3389/fmicb.2018.01376

Patel, S. H., Vaidya, Y. H., Patel, R. J., Pandit, R. J., Joshi, C. G., & Kunjadiya, A. P. (2017). Culture independent assessment of human milk microbial community in lactational mastitis. *Scientific Reports, 7*(1), 7804. https://doi.org/10.1038/s41598-017-08451-7

Paul, C., Zénut, M., Dorut, A., Coudoré, M. A., Vein, J., Cardot, J. M., & Balayssac, D. (2015). Use of domperidone as a galactagogue drug: A systematic review of the benefit-risk ratio. *Journal of Human Lactation, 31*(1), 57–63.

Raj, J. A., & Magesh, L. (2017). Medicinal use of coconut. *International Journal of Science and Research, 6,* 1898–1900.

Reisinger, K. W., de Vaan, L., Kramer, B. W., Wolfs, T. G., van Heurn, L. W., & Derikx, J. P. (2014). Breast-feeding improves gut maturation compared with formula feeding in preterm babies. *Journal of Pediatric Gastroenterology and Nutrition, 59,* 720–724.

Robson, V., Dodd, S., & Thomas, S. (2009). Standardized antibacterial honey (MediHoney) with standard therapy in wound care: Randomized clinical trial. *Journal of Advanced Nursing, 65,* 565–575.

Sakalidis, V. S., Ivarsson, L., Haynes, A. G., Jäger, L., Schärer-Hernández, N. G., Mitoulas, L. R., & Prime, D. K. (2020). Breast shield design impacts milk removal dynamics during pumping: A randomized controlled non-inferiority trial. *Acta Obstetricia et Gynecologica Scandinavica, 99*(11), 1561–1567.

Schanler, R. J. (2007). Mother's own milk, donor human milk, and preterm formulas in the feeding of extremely premature infants. *Journal of Pediatric Gastroenterology and Nutrition, 45*(Suppl. 3), S175–S177.

Section on Breastfeeding. (2012). Breastfeeding and the use of human milk. *Pediatrics, 129,* e827–e841.

Sim, T. F., Hattingh, H. L., Sherriff, J., & Tee, L. B. (2015). The use, perceived effectiveness and safety of herbal galactagogues during breastfeeding: A qualitative study. *International Journal of Environmental Research and Public Health, 12,* 11050–11071.

Smillie, C. M. (2004). *The prevention and treatment of plugged ducts. Clinical handout.* Breastfeeding Resources.

Snyder, J. B. (1997). Bubble palate and failure to thrive: A case report. *Journal of Human Lactation, 13,* 139–143.

Spatz, D. L. (2004). Ten steps for promoting and protecting breastfeeding for vulnerable infants. *Journal of Perinatal and Neonatal Nursing, 18,* 385–396.

Spencer, J. P. (2008). Management of mastitis in breastfeeding women. *American Family Physician, 7,* 727–731.

Stafford, I., Hernandez, J., Laibl, V., Sheffield, J., Roberts, S., & Wendel, G., Jr. (2008). Community-acquired methicillin-resistant *Staphylococcus aureus* among patients with puerperal mastitis requiring hospitalization. *Obstetrics and Gynecology, 112,* 533–537.

Stutte, P. C., Bowles, B. C., & Morman, G. Y. (1988). The effects of breast massage on volume and fat content of human milk. *Genesis (New York, N.Y.: 2000), 10,* 22–25.

Sulymbona, N., As'ad, S., Khuzaimah, A., Miskad, U. A., Ahmad, M., & Bahar, B. (2020). The effect of acupressure therapy on the improvement of breastmilk production in postpartum mothers. *Enfermeria Clinica, 30*(Suppl 2), 615–618.

Tarcan, A., Gurakan, B., Tiker, F., & Ozbek, N. (2004). Influence of feeding formula and breastmilk fortifier on lymphocyte subsets in very low birth weight premature newborns. *Biology of the Neonate, 86,* 22–28.

Taylor, A., Logan, G., Twells, L., & Newhook, L. A. (2019). Human milk expression after domperidone treatment in postpartum women: A systematic review and meta-analysis of randomized controlled trials. *Journal of Human Lactation, 35,* 501–509.

Turkyilmaz, C., Onal, E., Hirfanoglu, I. M., Turan, O., Koç, E., Ergenekon, E., & Atalay, Y. (2011). The effect of galactagogue herbal tea on breastmilk production and short-term catch-up of birth weight in the first week of life. *Journal of Alternative and Complementary Medicine, 17,* 139–142.

Uvnas-Moberg, K., Widstrom, A. M., Marchini, G., & Winberg, J. (1987). Release of GI hormones in mother and infant by sensory stimulation. *Acta Paediatrica Scandinavica, 76,* 851–860.

van Veldhuizen-Staas, C. G. (2007). Overabundant milk supply: An alternative way to intervene by full drainage and block feeding. *International Breastfeeding Journal, 2,* 11. https://doi.org/10.1186/1746-4358-2-11

Verd, S., Porta, R., Botet, F., Gutiérrez, A., Ginovart, G., Barbero, A. H., Ciurana, A., & Plata, I. I. (2015). Hospital outcomes of extremely low birth weight infants after introduction of donor milk to supplement mother's milk. *Breastfeeding Medicine, 10,* 150–155.

Vieira, C., Evangelista, S., Cirillo, R., Lippi, A., Maggi, C. A., & Manzini, S. (2000). Effect of ricinoleic acid in acute and subchronic experimental models of inflammation. *Mediators of Inflammation, 9,* 223–228.

Vohr, B. R., Poindexter, B. B., Dusick, A. M., McKinley, L. T., Wright, L. L., Langer, J. C., Poole, W. K., & NICHD Neonatal Research Network. (2006). Beneficial effects of breastmilk in the neonatal intensive care unit on the developmental outcome of extremely low birth weight infants at 18 months of age. *Pediatrics, 118,* e115–e123.

Walker, M. (2009). *Breastfeeding the late preterm infant: Improving care and outcomes.* Praeclarus Press.

Walker, M. (2010). *The nipple and areola in breastfeeding and lactation.* Praeclarus Press.

Walker, T., Coursey, C., & Duffus, A. (2019). Low dose Abilify (aripiprazole) in combination with Effexor XR (venlafaxine HCL) resulted in cessation of lactation: A case report. *Clinical Lactation, 10,* 56–58.

Wan, E. W., Davey, K., Page-Sharp, M., Hartmann, P. E., Simmer, K., & Ilett, K. F. (2008). Dose-effect study of domperidone as a galactogue in preterm mothers with insufficient milk supply, and its transfer into milk. *British Journal of Clinical Pharmacology, 66,* 283–289.

Watts, K. B., & Lagouros, M. (2020). Osteopathic manipulative treatment and breastfeeding. *Clinical Lactation, 11,* 28–33.

Wei, L., Wang, H., Han, Y., & Li, C. (2008). Clinical observation on the effects of electroacupuncture at Shaoze (SI 1) in 46 cases of postpartum insufficient lactation. *Journal of Traditional Chinese Medicine, 28,* 168–172.

Weiss, R. F. (2001). *Weiss's herbal medicine* (Classic ed.). Thieme.

Wilson-Clay, B., & Hoover, K. (2008). *The breastfeeding Atlas* (4th ed.). LactNews Press.

Witt, A. M., Bolman, M., Kredit, S., & Vanic, A. (2016). Therapeutic breast massage in lactation for the management of engorgement, plugged ducts, and mastitis. *Journal of Human Lactation, 32,* 123–131.

Zakarija-Grkovic, I., & Stewart, F. (2020). Treatments for breast engorgement during lactation. *Cochrane Database of Systematic Reviews, 9*(9), CD006946. https://doi.org/10.1002/14651858.CD006946.pub2

Zhao, Y., & Guo, H. (2006). The therapeutic effects of acupuncture in 30 cases of postpartum hypogalactia. *Journal of Traditional Chinese Medicine, 26,* 29–30.

45

Perinatal Loss and Grief

Robin G. Jordan and Holly White

Relevant Terms

Complicated grief—a form of prolonged grief with significant functional impairment, lacking psychological healing and resolution

Dilation and evacuation—dilation of the cervix and surgical evacuation of the uterus after the first trimester

Disenfranchised grief—grief that is not acknowledged by society

Early pregnancy loss—spontaneous abortion in the first trimester; more than 80% of spontaneous pregnancy losses occur during the first 12 weeks of pregnancy

Emotional cushioning—a self-protective delay in expected prenatal attachment behavior patterns seen in pregnant people who have experienced prior perinatal loss

Grief response—the anguish experience after significant loss, usually death of a beloved person, which can include physical, behavioral, spiritual, social, and cultural dimensions

Mourning—the cultural expression of grief after a loss

Miscarriage—spontaneous pregnancy loss before 20 weeks of gestation

Perinatal loss—death of a fetus through spontaneous or induced abortion, stillbirth, or early neonatal death

Stillbirth or fetal death—birth of a fetus/neonate of 20 or more completed weeks of gestation or of 400 g or more birth weight with no signs of life (no heartbeat breathing, umbilical cord pulsation, muscle movement). Early stillbirth = 20–27 completed weeks; late stillbirth = 28–36 completed weeks; term stillbirth = after 37 completed weeks of gestation

---

Introduction

> If you mention my child's name, I will cry. But if you don't, it will break my heart.
> —Author Unknown, The Compassionate Friends

Pregnancy is generally considered to be a time of happiness and anticipation, but clinicians are called on at times to be with families during heartbreaking circumstances. The loss of a desired pregnancy is a loss for the hopes and dreams of the family. Grief from **perinatal loss** can be severe and prolonged and increases risk for short- and long- term adverse health, social and psychological outcomes, including depression, anxiety, post-traumatic stress disorder, pain syndromes, and relationship and employment difficulties (Davoudian et al., 2021; Siassakos et al., 2018). Healthcare providers also experience significant emotions in the event of perinatal loss. Clinicians caring for those who have experienced stillbirth report symptoms of traumatic stress, including rage, guilt, and helplessness, which can have a profound effect on them (Gandino et al., 2019; Wahlberg et al., 2017).

Diagnosis of a pregnancy loss may come at a routine prenatal visit, when the fetal heartbeat is not auscultated or may follow a report of decreased fetal movement or trauma. The diagnosis is confirmed by the absence of a heartbeat on ultrasound. After diagnosis is confirmed, the plan is dependent in part on the gestational age at the time of the death.

Emotional support and management of physical changes and concerns are integral parts of providing quality care after the diagnosis of a perinatal loss. Although parents have built a limited relationship while the fetus was in utero and an envisioned relationship after the birth, grief after pregnancy loss does not differ significantly in intensity from other loss scenarios (Kersting & Wagner, 2012). However, unlike other categories of family loss, perinatal loss has no culturally sanctioned **mourning** rituals to assist grieving families to say goodbye and receive community support. Perinatal grief is often not deeply acknowledged by peers, community, and workplace networks (Cassidy, 2021). **Disenfranchised grief** can lead to maladaptive relationship and mental health issues for years after a loss (Grauerholz et al., 2021).

Prenatal and Postnatal Care: A Person-Centered Approach, Third Edition. Edited by Karen Trister Grace, Cindy L. Farley, Noelene K. Jeffers, and Tanya Tringali.
© 2024 John Wiley & Sons Ltd. Published 2024 by John Wiley & Sons Ltd.
Companion website: www.wiley.com/go/grace/prenatal

Table 45.3   Examples of Cultural Beliefs about Pregnancy Loss

Cultural group	Traditional beliefs[a]
Amish	Walking under a clothesline can cause a miscarriage.
Appalachian	Stillbirth can be caused by having your picture taken.
Chinese	Stillborn is buried by the parents without a ceremony. Mourning traditionally lasts 100 days for the family, after which a final prayer ceremony is held to end the mourning period.
Haitian	A miscarriage or stillbirth was caused by the sin of the mother.
Hispanic	Miscarriage is God fixing a mistake.
India	Family might view the mother as inadequate after a pregnancy loss. Loss of a female often not publicly grieved. Maternal grief is often hidden from others.
Kenya, Uganda	Loss may be attributed to God's will or witchcraft, and is viewed as a bad omen. Stillborn babies do not have the same status as those who were born live. Family and village support network often manages burial and associated tasks.
Muslim/Arabic	Pregnant person assigned blame for pregnancy loss. If either baby's parents or one of his/her Muslim relatives have passed away, then the baby will be "sent" to them so they can take care of the baby. Stillborn babies are given a name before burial; burial includes the placenta, which is considered part of the baby. Autopsy is not permitted unless required by law in the country they reside. Muslims are buried, not cremated.
Native American	Reaching over head can cause the baby to strangle on its cord. Navajo tribe elders would bury the placenta within the tribe's reservation as a binder to the ancestral land and its people. Ojibwa tribe elders would cut off the hair of the deceased infant or child and the hair would be made into a "doll of sorrow" that the mother would then carry for a year.
Orthodox Jewish	Baby showers are not given before birth for fear of jinxing the pregnancy and causing a stillbirth. Autopsies and embalming of the body may be prohibited. For a stillborn at term, full bereavement practices such as reciting Kaddish for 30 days, observing *yahrzeit*, and holding a complete *shiva*. Burial is held as soon as is possible, the baby is named at the grave.
Pakistani	A stillborn baby's body is treated differently than a newborn that dies after showing signs of life. Stillborn babies are wrapped in white sheets (kaffan) and no funeral prayers are offered.

Source: http://www.myjewishlearning.com/article/stillbirth-and-neonatal-death/4; http://stillbirthday.com/global-perspectives. Adapted from Ayebare et al. (2021), Omar et al. (2019), and Roberts et al. (2012).
[a]This table is not meant to be inclusive and represents historical possibilities for listed cultures rather than mandates or absolute beliefs and actions.

post-traumatic stress symptoms that often go unrecognized (Farren et al., 2016; Krosch & Shakespeare-Finch, 2016). Rates of psychiatric morbidity are highest in the first four months postpartum and generally decrease after the first year (Hogue et al., 2015). Individuals with a history of mental health issues have higher risk of persistent depression, anxiety, and post-traumatic stress after loss (Rich, 2018).

Rates of stillbirth are higher for Black women; Black parents experience higher levels of depression and poorer health outcomes after stillbirth (Boyden et al., 2014; Pruitt et al., 2020). Bereaved Black parents are also unlikely to receive adequate psychological service or to feel supported by the services available (Huberty et al., 2017). The high likelihood of other complicated experiences of loss, negative treatment by healthcare providers, chronic stress, economic disadvantage and experiences of racism can add heavy burdens to these families, which contribute to the experience of loss and the challenge to make meaning (Boyden et al., 2014). Healthcare providers should discuss these additional risks and stressors openly and respectfully with Black parents and seek out referrals and resources for loss support which can speak directly to this experience.

Little is known about the experiences of people in the LGBTQ+ community who have had a perinatal loss. However, given the stress process of discrimination, stigma, and consistently hostile social processes, it is likely that perinatal loss in this community has significant health consequences that are poorly addressed (Lacombe-Duncan et al., 2022; Meyer, 2003). Efforts to reduce LGBTQ+ people's experiences of erasure and discrimination should include training for staff working with pregnancy loss to reduce stigma, acknowledge LGBTQ+ reproductive experiences, use inclusive language, and respect diverse relationships (Lacombe-Duncan et al., 2022; Riggs et al., 2020).

As noted in other communities with experiences of stigma, LGBTQ+ individuals interviewed felt that their recovery was hindered by a lack of visibility and representation in healthcare institutions (Lacombe-Duncan et al., 2022; Riggs et al., 2020).

Providing effective support around pregnancy loss places high demands on clinicians who may not have adequate training or systemic support and who are often traumatized themselves. Secondary trauma is incurred through exposure to the trauma of others and may manifest the same symptoms as primary trauma. In addition, maternity care providers may experience grief, guilt, shame, isolation, fear, lost confidence, and helplessness (Aydın & Aktaş, 2021) and may even consider leaving the profession (Beck et al., 2015). Receiving institutional and peer support, establishing a work/home balance, offering support and gained insights to others in similar situations and accepting personal strengths and limitations can be steps toward regaining professional self-image after work-related trauma (Wahlberg et al., 2019).

Physical Care after Stillbirth

Provide education about the body's response after the birth, especially regarding lactation, and offer measures to decrease the discomfort of engorged breasts. Appropriate management options include the use of raw cabbage leaves inside a bra to decrease swelling or clary sage tea to help dry the milk. Acetaminophen and ibuprofen can also be used to reduce inflammation and discomfort. Pumping or milk expression for discomfort should be used sparingly or not at all, as this will encourage the body to make more milk. Some hospitals are linking individuals who have experienced a stillbirth with donor milk banks; this can be very meaningful for some in coping with their loss. Review symptoms that need to be evaluated, including fever, redness in a subscribed area on the breast, and pain in the breasts beyond engorgement.

Lochia following stillbirth will follow the expected postpartum pattern depending on gestational age of the loss. The client is informed to call with any signs and symptoms of infection or retained products such as foul-smelling lochia, lochia that is not decreasing in amount over the days after birth, fever, or abdominal pain outside of afterbirth pains.

Follow-Up Care

The initial weeks after stillbirth are especially difficult for families and often involve facing physical preparations they had made for a baby and multiple difficult conversations with family, friends, work, and acquaintances while dealing with the physical and hormonal postpartum changes. A postpartum visit or a phone call within the first week after the loss from staff known to the family can be beneficial to answer questions, evaluate their adjustment, and give referrals. Mental health screening and referrals should be a standard part of postpartum care given significant rates of depression, post-traumatic stress, and anxiety postpartum, but even higher rates occur in this population. It is also a good time to evaluate the normalcy of physical changes such as breast and uterine involution. Another visit can be scheduled at four to six weeks after birth for routine postpartum care. Within the year after a stillbirth, about 50% of women will become pregnant again, so this visit should include a discussion of plans, availability of preconception counseling, and birth control if desired (Lee et al., 2013).

If genetic testing or an autopsy was performed, a face-spiepr DHYPto-spiepr DHYPface appointment should be offered to review the results and discuss implications for future care. Although many losses have no clear reason, in cases where there is a clear cause, this discussion can help parents to feel less guilty and anxious. At this visit, it is also appropriate to assess an individual's social support system to determine if there is someone with whom the person can confide feelings, share grief, and who will be supportive. Parents grieve differently and the experience can strengthen or disrupt relationships (Avelin et al., 2013). Group interpersonal therapy led by a trained psychologist has been found to be effective in reducing symptoms of depression after pregnancy loss (Johnson et al., 2016). In-person support groups for individuals and couples experiencing early or later perinatal loss are often available locally and Internet support groups are also readily available. Web-based support groups can provide social support with a sense of privacy. It has become more common for parents to post pictures of the stillborn infant online. This can help create a social identity for the baby, reconstructing the disrupted biography of the family to include the dead infant, thereby allowing the child to be remembered, mourned, and memorialized (Godel, 2007). Some hospitals have created memorial gardens to recognize the loss. Pregnancy loss can have devastating psychological, physical, and social costs, with ongoing effects on interpersonal relationships and subsequently born children. However, with support and resolution of the loss experience, resilience and new life skills and capacities can be developed (Burden et al., 2016).

Interconception and Subsequent Pregnancy Care

Planning another pregnancy is approached from varying perspectives after a perinatal loss. Some may need to give themselves time and space to grieve before getting pregnant again. It is not uncommon for many clients to try for another pregnancy immediately, especially after an early pregnancy loss, as this may be part of the healing process for them. There is no ideal conception interval and no perinatal outcome-related or physical reason to delay pregnancy (Wong et al., 2015). Most individuals are able to move through their grief and successfully integrate the experience into their lives, and ultimately decide for themselves ideal timing for a subsequent pregnancy.

Those who have had a stillbirth often worry that this will happen again. The risk of stillbirth is twice as high following a previous stillbirth; however, the absolute risk is still low, particularly if the previous stillbirth was unexplained (Lamont et al., 2022). Preconception care and counseling can help reduce the risk of stillbirth in subsequent pregnancy. Investigation of potential physiologic reasons for perinatal loss may be part of care prior to another pregnancy. For example, testing for lupus anticoagulant as well as immunoglobulin G and immunoglobulin M for anticardiolipin and β2 glycoprotein antibodies can be recommended if it was not performed at the time of the stillbirth (Silver et al., 2013). A visit with a genetic counselor may be advisable if there is no clear cause of stillbirth or if there are indications of a genetic cause. Chronic conditions such as hypertension, diabetes, and thyroid disease should be treated and stabilized prior to achieving another pregnancy. Risk for perinatal loss can be reduced by counseling on healthy BMI, regular exercise habits, improved diet, and smoking cessation (Johnson & Gee, 2015).

Care of those who have experienced a previous perinatal loss includes acknowledging the loss and individualizing care. Clinicians should not gloss over or avoid the mention of prior losses or fail to explore the pain associated with them, nor should they imagine that a subsequent healthy pregnancy concludes the grief of a previous loss (Markin, 2016). Avoiding discussing the loss may actually increase the client's grief and cause them to feel disconnected from the provider (Moore et al., 2011). They may need to discuss the previous loss in a safe and neutral environment.

Individuals pregnant again after prior perinatal loss may fear another loss and, thus, try to protect their emotions by avoiding prenatal bonding. This phenomenon is known as **emotional cushioning** and appears to be a complex, self-protective mechanism to cope with the anxiety, uncertainty, and sense of vulnerability experienced in pregnancies after a prior loss (Côté-Arsenault, 2020). This should not be misconstrued as a lack of attachment to this baby. Clients should be reassured that this is a normal phenomenon so as not to increase their sense of anxiety. It is also appropriate to monitor and promote attachment behaviors as pregnancy progresses.

Depending on an individual's health status, increased fetal surveillance may be appropriate during a subsequent pregnancy. While there is currently no high-quality evidence for any specific protocol, twice weekly antepartum surveillance starting at 32 weeks unless other factors require closer surveillance can be offered (ACOG, 2020). Decisions about the timing of birth must be individualized with consideration also given to the risks of induction and birth prior to 39 weeks of gestation. While quality evidence exists for identifying risk factors for perinatal loss, effective models for predicting those who will experience perinatal loss remain elusive (Ishak & Khalil, 2021). It is essential to recognize that those who have experienced perinatal loss have a higher incidence of depression, anxiety disorders, and post-traumatic stress disorder in subsequent pregnancies (Gravensteen et al., 2018). This should be given weight when collaborating with the family about the birth plan (Lee et al., 2017).

Part of postpartum planning for families with prior losses should include anticipatory guidance and follow-up for mental health and attachment issues. By no means should it be assumed that the birth of a healthy infant will resolve feelings of grief from a previous loss. Prior late gestation pregnancy loss has been associated with depression for one year postpartum, self-doubt, and negative attitudes toward parenting (Côté-Arsenault et al., 2020). A mental health provider experienced in grief, attachment, and parenthood can work toward allowing and embracing the seemingly conflicting experiences of embracing a connection with a new child while honoring and embracing connection with a deceased baby (Markin, 2018).

Summary

Pregnancy as an exciting time of anticipation can turn quickly into one of profound pain and grief. The loss of an infant through **miscarriage, stillbirth,** or fetal death is recognized as one of the most stressful life events. Perinatal bereavement is a unique mourning situation. The etiology of a pregnancy loss may never be known, adding to parents' sense of guilt, confusion, and, sometimes, blame. Grief reactions can be long term with significant adverse mental health consequences. Healthcare providers must be able to therapeutically and skillfully communicate with individuals and families during the immediate crisis period as well as during the grieving and healing process when support is vital. Providing encouragement, support, and space for cultural and family grieving rituals to remember their baby can aid family healing. Individuals experiencing perinatal loss can benefit from additional follow-up and support for an extended period of time after the loss as this event can be a trigger for postpartum depression and other mood disorders. Compassionate and respectful care can help individuals and families move through their heartbreaking experience and grieve the loss in a positive manner.

Resources for Clients and Their Families

A Lost Possibility: Women on Miscarriage. Provides a resource for sharing women's common thoughts and experiences surrounding early pregnancy loss: https://thenib.com/a-lost-possibility-women-on-miscarriage-e5e4237723c3

Daily Strength. A support site for those who have experienced miscarriage: https://www.dailystrength.org/group/miscarriage

Hope After Loss. A group offering support, community, and resources for families experiencing perinatal loss with specific resources geared toward LGBTQ+ and BIPOC families: http://www.hopeafterloss.org/support/resources

Mommies Enduring Neonatal Death (MEND). A support organization providing bimonthly newsletters and support groups: (a) for those who have recently lost a baby to miscarriage, stillbirth, and infant death; (b) pregnancy group for those who are considering becoming pregnant or are currently pregnant after a loss; (c) father group: http://www.mend.org

Now I Lay Me Down to Sleep (NILMDTS). This is a non-profit organization that provides the gift of professional remembrance photography to capture images for bereaved parents in a compassionate and sensitive manner at *no charge* to the families: http://www.nowilaymedowntosleep.org

Perinatal Hospice. This group offers perinatal hospice and palliative care and support services to parents who find out during pregnancy that their baby has a life-limiting condition: http://www.perinatalhospice.org

Postpartum Support International. National center providing helpline, referrals to local resources and online support groups Helpline 1-800-944-4773. http://www.postpartum.net/get-help/loss-grief-in-pregnancy-postpartum

Shades of Blue Project. Texas based maternal mental health recourse center for birthing people of color that offers online loss support groups. https://www.shades-ofblueproject.org/online-support-groups

Share: Pregnancy and Infant Loss Support, Inc. Supportive resources for those who have experienced pregnancy or infant loss: http://nationalshare.org

Resources for Healthcare Providers

Pregnancy Loss and Infant Death Alliance. This group provides resources for healthcare providers to provide optimal support to grieving families: http://www.plida.org

Resolve Through Sharing. This nonprofit organization offers grief support materials and perinatal bereavement training to healthcare professionals https://www.gundersenhealth.org/resolve-through-sharing

References

Allanson, E. R., Copson, S., Spilsbury, K., Criddle, S., Jennings, B., Doherty, D. A., Wong, A. M., & Dickinson, J. E. (2021). Pretreatment with mifepristone compared with misoprostol alone for delivery after fetal death between 14 and 28 weeks of gestation: A randomized controlled trial. *Obstetrics & Gynecology*, 137(5), 801–809. https://doi.org/10.1097/AOG.0000000000004344

American College of Obstetricians and Gynecologists (ACOG). (2020). Management of stillbirth: Obstetric care consensus No, 10. *Obstetrics and Gynecology*, 135(3), e110–e132. https://doi.org/10.1097/AOG.0000000000003719

Avelin, P., Rådestad, I., Saflund, K., Wredling, R., & Erlandsson, K. (2013). Parental grief and relationships after the loss of a stillborn baby. *Midwifery*, 29(6), 668–673. https://doi.org/10.1016/j.midw.2012.06.007

Aydın, R., & Aktaş, S. (2021). Midwives' experiences of traumatic births: A systematic review and meta-synthesis. *European Journal of Midwifery*, 5, 31. https://doi.org/10.18332/ejm/138197

Ayebare, E., Lavender, T., Mweteise, J., Nabisere, A., Nendela, A., Mukhwana, R., Wood, R., Wakasiaka, S., Omoni, G., Birungi, S., & Mills, T. A. (2021). The impact of cultural beliefs and practices on parents' experiences of bereavement following stillbirth: A qualitative study in Uganda and Kenya. *BMC Pregnancy and Childbirth*, 21(1), 1–10. https://doi.org/10.1186/s12884-021-03912-4

Beck, C. T., LoGiudice, J., & Gable, R. K. (2015). A mixed-methods study of secondary traumatic stress in certified nurse-midwives: Shaken belief in the birth process. *Journal of Midwifery & Women's Health*, 60(1), 16–23. https://doi.org/10.1111/jmwh.12221

Bekkar, B., Pacheco, S., Basu, R., & DeNicola, N. (2020). Association of air pollution and heat exposure with preterm birth, low birth weight, and stillbirth in the US: A systematic review. *JAMA Network Open*, 3(6), e208243–e208243. https://doi.org/10.1001/jamanetworkopen.2020.8243

Boyden, J. Y., Kavanaugh, K., Issel, L. M., Eldeirawi, K., & Meert, K. L. (2014). Experiences of African American parents following perinatal or pediatric death: A literature review. *Death Studies*, 38(6–10), 374–380. https://doi.org/10.1080/07481187.2013.766656

Boyle, F. M., Horey, D., Middleton, P. F., & Flenady, V. (2020). Clinical practice guidelines for perinatal bereavement care: An overview. *Women and birth: Journal of the Australian College of Midwives*, 33(2), 107–110. https://doi.org/10.1016/j.wombi.2019.01.008

Burden, C., Bradley, S., Storey, C., Ellis, A., Heazell, A. E., Downe, S., & Siassakos, D. (2016). From grief, guilt pain and stigma to hope and pride-a systematic review and meta-analysis of mixed-method research of the psychosocial impact of stillbirth. *BMC Pregnancy and Childbirth*, 16(1), 1. https://doi.org/10.1186/s12884-016-0800-8

Cassidy, P. R. (2021). The disenfranchisement of perinatal grief: How silence, silencing and self-censorship complicate bereavement (a mixed methods study). *OMEGA-Journal of Death and Dying*, 00302228211050500. Advance online publication. https://doi.org/10.1177/00302228211050500

Centers for Disease Control and Prevention (CDC). (2020) *Facts about stillbirth*. https://www.cdc.gov/ncbddd/stillbirth/facts.html

Côté-Arsenault, D. (2020). Theoretical perspectives to guide the practice of perinatal palliative care. In E. Denney-Koelsch & D. Côté-Arsenault (Eds.), *Perinatal palliative care* (pp. 13–32). Springer Cham. https://doi.org/10.1007/978-3-030-34751-2_2

Côté-Arsenault, D., Leerkes, E. M., & Zhou, N. (2020). Individual differences in maternal, marital, parenting and child outcomes following perinatal loss: A longitudinal study. *Journal of Reproductive and Infant Psychology*, 38(1), 3–15. https://doi.org/10.1080/02646838.2019.1579897

Davoudian, T., Gibbins, K., & Cirino, N. H. (2021). Perinatal loss: The impact on maternal mental health. *Obstetrical & Gynecological Survey*, 76(4), 223–233. https://doi.org/10.1097/OGX.0000000000000874

DeSisto, C. L., Wallace, B., Simeone, R. M., Polen, K., Ko, J. Y., Meaney-Delman, D., & Ellington, S. R. (2021). Risk for stillbirth among women with and without COVID-19 at delivery hospitalization—United States, March 2020–September 2021. *Morbidity and Mortality Weekly Report*, 70(47), 1640. https://doi.org/10.15585/mmwr.mm7047e1

Ellis, A., Chebsey, C., Storey, C., Bradley, S., Jackson, S., Flenady, V., Heazell, A., & Siassakos, D. (2016). Systematic review to understand and improve care after stillbirth: A review of parents' and healthcare professionals' experiences. *BMC Pregnancy & Childbirth*, 16(1), 16. https://doi.org/10.1186/s12884-016-0806-2

Farrales, L. L., Cacciatore, J., Jonas-Simpson, C., Dharamsi, S., Ascher, J., & Klein, M. C. (2020). What bereaved parents want health care providers to know when their babies are stillborn: A community-based participatory study. *BMC Psychology*, 8(1), 1–8.

Farren, J., Jalmbrant, M., Ameye, L., Joash, K., Mitchell-Jones, N., Tapp, S., Tipperman, D., & Bourne, T. (2016). Post-traumatic stress, anxiety and depression following miscarriage or ectopic pregnancy: A prospective cohort study. *BMJ Open*, 6(11), e011864. https://doi.org/10.1136/bmjopen-2016-011864

Gandino, G., Bernaudo, A., Di Fini, G., Vanni, I., & Veglia, F. (2019). Healthcare professionals' experiences of perinatal loss: A systematic review. *Journal of Health Psychology*, 24(1), 65–78. https://doi.org/10.1177/1359105317705981

Gibbins, K. J., Pinar, H., Reddy, U. M., Saade, G. R., Goldenberg, R. L., Dudley, D. J., Drews-Botsch, C., Freedman, A., Daniels, L., Parker, C., Thoirsten, V., Bukowski, R., & Silver, R. M. (2020). Findings in stillbirths associated with placental disease. *American Journal of Perinatology*, 37(07), 708–715. https://doi.org/10.1055/s-0039-1688472

Godel, M. (2007). Images of stillbirth: Memory, mourning and memorial. *Visual Studies*, 22(3), 253–269. https://doi.org/10.1080/14725860701657159

Grauerholz, K. R., Berry, S. N., Capuano, R. M., & Early, J. M. (2021). Uncovering prolonged grief reactions subsequent to a reproductive loss: Implications for the primary care provider. *Frontiers in Psychology*, *12*. https://doi.org/10.3389/fpsyg.2021.673050

Gravensteen, I. K., Jacobsen, E. M., Sandset, P. M., Helgadottir, L. B., Rådestad, I., Sandvik, L., & Ekeberg, Ø. (2018). Anxiety, depression and relationship satisfaction in the pregnancy following stillbirth and after the birth of a live-born baby: A prospective study. *BMC Pregnancy & Childbirth*, *18*(1), 1–10. https://doi.org/10.1186/s12884-018-1666-8

Hammad, I. A., Blue, N. R., Allshouse, A. A., Silver, R. M., Gibbins, K. J., Page, J. M., Goldenberg, R. L., Reddy, U. M., Saade, G. R., Donald, J. D., Thorsten, V. R., Conway, D. L., Pinar, H., & NICHD Stillbirth Collaborative Research Group. (2020). Umbilical cord abnormalities and stillbirth. *Obstetrics & Gynecology*, *135*(3), 644. https://doi.org/10.1097/AOG.0000000000003676

Henderson, J., & Redshaw, M. (2017). Parents' experience of perinatal post-mortem following stillbirth: A mixed methods study. *PLoS One*, *12*(6), e0178475. https://doi.org/10.1371/journal.pone.0178475

Hennegan, J. M., Henderson, J., & Redshaw, M. (2018). Is partners' mental health and well-being affected by holding the baby after stillbirth? Mothers' accounts from a national survey. *Journal of Reproductive and Infant Psychology*, *36*(2), 120–131. https://doi.org/10.1080/02646838.2018.1424325

Henry, C. J., Higgins, M., Carlson, N., & Song, M. K. (2021). Racial disparities in stillbirth factors among non-Hispanic Black women and non-Hispanic White women in the United States. *MCN: The American Journal of Maternal/Child Nursing*, *46*(6), 352–359. https://doi.org/10.1186/1471-2393-12-137

Hogue, C. J., Parker, C. B., Willinger, M., Temple, J. R., Bann, C. M., Silver, R. M., Dudley, D. J., Moore, J. L., Coustan, D. R., Stoll, B. J., Reddy, U. M., Varner, M. W., Saade, G. R., Conway, D., Goldenberg, R. L., & Eunice Kennedy Shriver National Institute of Child Health and Human Development Stillbirth Collaborative Research Network Writing Group. (2015). The association of stillbirth with depressive symptoms 6-36 months post-delivery. *Paediatric and Perinatal Epidemiology*, *29*(2), 131–143. https://doi.org/10.1111/ppe.12176

Huberty, J. L., Matthews, J., Leiferman, J., Hermer, J., & Cacciatore, J. (2017). When a baby dies: A systematic review of experimental interventions for women after stillbirth. *Reproductive Sciences*, *24*(7), 967–975. https://doi.org/10.1177/1933719116670518

Ishak, M., & Khalil, A. (2021). Prediction and prevention of stillbirth: Dream or reality. *Current Opinion in Obstetrics & Gynecology*, *33*(5), 405–411. https://doi.org/10.1097/GCO.0000000000000744

Johnson, J. E., Price, A. B., Kao, J. C., Fernandes, K., Stout, R., Gobin, R. L., & Zlotnick, C. (2016). Interpersonal psychotherapy (IPT) for major depression following perinatal loss: A pilot randomized controlled trial. *Archives of Women's Mental Health*, 1–15. https://doi.org/10.1007/s00737-016-0625-5

Johnson, K. A., & Gee, R. E. (2015). Interpregnancy care. *Seminars in Perinatology*, *39*(4), 310–315. https://doi.org/10.1053/j.semperi.2015.05.011

Kang, X., Carlin, A., Cannie, M. M., Sanchez, T. C., & Jani, J. C. (2020). Fetal postmortem imaging: An overview of current techniques and future perspectives. *American Journal of Obstetrics & Gynecology*, *223*(4), 493–515. https://doi.org/10.1016/j.ajog.2020.04.034

Kapp, N., & Lohr, P. A. (2020). Modern methods to induce abortion: safety, efficacy and choice. *i Start Best Practice & Research Clinical Obstetrics & Gynaecology i End, i Start 63 i End*, 37–44.

Kavanaugh, K., & Hershberger, P. (2005). Perinatal loss in low-spiepr DHYP income African American parents. *i Start Journal of Obstetric, Gynecologic, & Neonatal Nursing i End, i Start 34 i End*, 595–605. https://doi.org/10.1177/0884217505280000

Kersting, A., & Wagner, B. (2012). Complicated grief after perinatal loss. *Dialogues in Clinical Neuroscience*, *14*(2), 187–194. https://doi.org/10.31887/DCNS.2012.14.2/akersting

Kingdon, C., Givens, J. L., O'Donnell, E., & Turner, M. (2015). Seeing and holding baby: Systematic review of clinical management and parental outcomes after stillbirth. *Birth*, *42*(3), 206–218. https://doi.org/10.1111/birt.12176

Kingdon, C., Roberts, D., Turner, M. A., Storey, C., Crossland, N., Finlayson, K. W., & Downe, S. (2019). Inequalities and stillbirth in the UK: A meta-narrative review. *BMJ Open*, *9*(9), e029672. https://doi.org/10.1136/bmjopen-2019-029672

Krosch, D. J., & Shakespeare-Finch, J. (2016). Grief, traumatic stress, and posttraumatic growth in women who have experienced pregnancy loss. *Psychological Trauma: Theory, Research, Practice, and Policy*, *9*(4), 425–433. https://doi.org/10.1037/tra0000183

Lacombe-Duncan, A., Andalibi, N., Roosevelt, L., & Weinstein-Levey, E. (2022). Minority stress theory applied to conception, pregnancy, and pregnancy loss: A qualitative study examining LGBTQ+ people's experiences. *PLoS One*, *17*(7), e0271945. https://doi.org/10.1371/journal.pone.0271945

Lamont, K., Scott, N. W., Gissler, M., Gatt, M., & Bhattacharya, S. (2022). Risk of recurrent stillbirth in subsequent pregnancies. *Obstetrics & Gynecology*, *139*(1), 31–40. https://doi.org/10.1097/AOG.0000000000004626

Lee, L., McKenzie-McHarg, K., & Horsch, A. (2013). Women's decision making and experience of subsequent pregnancy following stillbirth. *Journal of Midwifery & Women's Health*, *58*(4), 431–439. https://doi.org/10.1111/jmwh.12011

Lee, L., McKenzie-McHarg, K., & Horsch, A. (2017). The impact of miscarriage and stillbirth on maternal–fetal relationships: An integrative review. *Journal of Reproductive and Infant Psychology*, *35*(1), 32–52. https://doi.org/10.1080/02646838.2016.1239249

MacDorman, M. F., & Gregory, E. C. W. (2015). Fetal and perinatal mortality: United States, 2013. *National Vital Statistics Reports*, *64*(8), 1–24.

Markin, R. D. (2016). What clinicians miss about miscarriages: Clinical errors in the treatment of early term perinatal loss. *Psychotherapy*, *53*(3), 347. https://doi.org/10.1037/pst0000062

Markin, R. D. (2018). "Ghosts" in the womb: A mentalizing approach to understanding and treating prenatal attachment disturbances during pregnancies after loss. *Psychotherapy*, *55*(3), 275–288. https://doi.org/10.1037/pst0000186

Megli, C. J., & Coyne, C. B. (2021). Infections at the maternal–fetal interface: An overview of pathogenesis and defense. *Nature Reviews Microbiology*, 1–16. https://doi.org/10.1038/s41579-021-00610-y

Meyer, I. H. (2003). Prejudice, social stress, and mental health in lesbian, gay, and bisexual populations: Conceptual issues and research evidence. *Psychological Bulletin*, *129*(5), 674–697. https://doi.org/10.1037/0033-2909.129.5.674

Miller, E. S., Minturn, L., Linn, R., Weese-Mayer, D. E., & Ernst, L. M. (2016). Stillbirth evaluation: A stepwise assessment of placental pathology and autopsy. *American Journal of Obstetrics & Gynecology*, *214*(1), 115–e1. https://doi.org/10.1016/j.ajog.2015.08.049

Moore, T., Parrish, H., & Perry Black, B. (2011). Interconception care for couples after perinatal loss: A comprehensive review of the literature. *Journal of Perinatal & Neonatal Nursing*, *25*(1), 44–51. https://doi.org/10.1097/JPN.0b013e3182071a08

Omar, N., Major, S., Mohsen, M., Al Tamimi, H., El Taher, F., & Kilshaw, S. (2019). Culpability, blame, and stigma after pregnancy loss in Qatar. *BMC Pregnancy and Childbirth*, *19*(1), 1–8. https://doi.org/10.1186/s12884-019-2354-z

Page, J. M., Bardsley, T., Thorsten, V., Allshouse, A. A., Varner, M. W., Debbink, M. P., Dudley, D. J., Saade, G. R., Goldenberg, R. L., Stoll, B., Hogue, C. J., Bukowski, R., Conway, D., Reddy, U. M., & Silver, R. M. (2019). Stillbirth associated with infection in a diverse US cohort. *Obstetrics & Gynecology*, *134*(6), 1187–1196. https://doi.org/10.1097/AOG.0000000000003515

Page, J. M., Christiansen-Lindquist, L., Thorsten, V., Parker, C. B., Reddy, U. M., Dudley, D. J., Saade, G. R., Coustan, D., Rowland Hogue, C. J., Conway, D., Bukowski, R., Pinar, H., Heuser, C. C., Gibbins, K. J., Goldenberg, R. L., & Silver, R. M. (2017). Diagnostic tests for evaluation of stillbirth: Stillbirth collaborative research network. *Obstetrics & Gynecology*, *129*(4), 699–706. https://doi.org/10.1097/AOG.0000000000001937

Pollock, D. D., Pearson, D. E., Cooper, D. M., Ziaian, A., Foord, C., & Warland, A. (2021). Breaking the silence: Determining prevalence and understanding stillbirth stigma. *Midwifery*, *93*, 102884. https://doi.org/10.1016/j.midw.2020.102884

Pruitt, S. M., Hoyert, D. L., Anderson, K. N., Martin, J., Waddell, L., Duke, C., Honein, M. A., & Reefhuis, J. (2020). Racial and ethnic disparities in fetal deaths—United States, 2015–2017. *Morbidity and Mortality Weekly Report*, *69*(37), 1277. https://doi.org/10.15585/mmwr.mm6937a1

Ptacek, I., Sebire, N. J., Man, J. A., Brownbill, P., & Heazell, A. E. P. (2014). Systematic review of placental pathology reported in association with stillbirth. *Placenta*, *35*(8), 552–562. https://doi.org/10.1016/j.placenta.2014.05.011

Randolph, A. L., Hruby, B. T., & Sharif, S. (2015). Counseling women who have experienced pregnancy loss: A review of the literature. *Adultspan Journal*, *14*(1), 2–10. https://doi.org/10.1002/j.2161-0029.2015.00032.x

Rasmussen, T. D., Villadsen, S. F., Andersen, P. K., Jervelund, S. S., & Andersen, A. M. N. (2021). Social and ethnic disparities in stillbirth and infant death in Denmark, 2005–2016. *Scientific Reports*, *11*(1), 1–9. https://doi.org/10.1136/jech.2008.078741

Rich, D. (2018). Psychological impact of pregnancy loss: Best practice for obstetric providers. *Clinical Obstetrics and Gynecology*, *61*(3), 628–636. https://doi.org/10.1097/GRF.0000000000000369

Riggs, D. W., Pearce, R., Pfeffer, C. A., Hines, S., White, F. R., & Ruspini, E. (2020). Men, trans/masculine, and non-binary people's experiences of pregnancy loss: An international qualitative study. *BMC Pregnancy and Childbirth*, *20*(1), 482. https://doi.org/10.1186/s12884-020-03166-6

Roberts, L. R., Anderson, B. A., Lee, J. W., & Montgomery, S. B. (2012). Grief and women: Stillbirth in the social context of India. *International Journal of Childbirth*, *2*(3), 187–198. https://doi.org/10.1891/2156-5287.2.3.187

Siassakos, D., Jackson, S., Gleeson, K., Chebsey, C., Ellis, A., & Storey, C. (2018). All bereaved parents are entitled to good care after stillbirth: A mixed-methods multicentre study (INSIGHT). *BJOG: An International Journal of Obstetrics & Gynaecology*, *125*(2), 160–170. https://doi.org/10.1111/1471-0528.14765

Silver, R. M., Parker, C. B., Reddy, U. M., Goldenberg, R., Coustan, D., Dudley, D. J., Saade, G. R., Stoll, B., Koch, M. A., Conway, D., Bukowski, R., Hogue, C. J., Pinar, H., Moore, J., Willinger, M., & Branch, D. W. (2013). Antiphospholipid antibodies in stillbirth. *Obstetrics & Gynecology*, *122*(3), 641–657. https://doi.org/10.1097/AOG.0b013e3182a1060e

Wahlberg, A., Andreen Sachs, M., Johannesson, K., Hallberg, G., Jonsson, M., Skoog Svanberg, A., & Hogberg, U. (2017). Posttraumatic stress symptoms in Swedish obstetricians and midwives after severe obstetric events: A cross-sectional retrospective survey. *BJOG: An International Journal of Obstetrics & Gynaecology*, *124*(8), 1264–1271. https://doi.org/10.1111/1471-0528.14259

Wahlberg, Å., Högberg, U., & Emmelin, M. (2019). The erratic pathway to regaining a professional self-image after an obstetric work-related trauma: A grounded theory study. *International Journal of Nursing Studies*, *89*, 53–61. https://doi.org/10.1016/j.ijnurstu.2018.07.016

Williams, A. D., Wallace, M., Nobles, C., & Mendola, P. (2018). Racial residential segregation and racial disparities in stillbirth in the United States. *Health & Place*, *51*, 208–216. https://doi.org/10.1016/j.healthplace.2018.04.005

Wong, L. F., Schliep, K. C., Silver, R. M., Mumford, S. L., Perkins, N. J., Ye, A., Galai, N., Wactawski-Wende, J., Lynch, A. M., Townsend, J. M., Faraggi, D., & Schisterman, E. F. (2015). The effect of a very short interpregnancy interval and pregnancy outcomes following a previous pregnancy loss. *American Journal of Obstetrics & Gynecology*, *212*(3), 375–e11. https://doi.org/10.1016/j.ajog.2014.09.020

46

Obesity in the Perinatal Period

Cecilia M. Jevitt

Relevant Terms

Acanthosis nigricans—areas of dark, velvety skin discoloration in body folds and creases usually near axilla, groin, neck, usually associated with insulin resistance

Body mass index (BMI)—an international measurement estimating body fat content, based on a formula of height and weight (weight in pounds/[height in inches]^2 × 703) or (weight in kg/height in meters^2)

Dumping syndrome—a potential problem following bariatric surgery, particularly the Roux-en-Y procedure; a condition where undigested foods bypass the stomach quickly and enters the small intestine causing symptoms of pain, bloating, nausea, and diarrhea

Food desert—areas where grocery stores and supermarkets and the availability of fresh fruit, vegetables, and other healthful whole foods are difficult to access, generally considered to be over one mile away from an urban residence.

Food swamp—indicates the prevalence of less expensive, high-fat, high-sugar processed foods instead of fresh fruits and vegetables; beginning to replace the phrase "food desert"

Intertrigo—rash between skin folds caused by skin-on-skin friction than can harbor bacteria or fungal infections

Insulin resistance—failure of cells to respond to insulin causing an increase in blood glucose

Laparoscopic gastric banding—a reversible bariatric surgical procedure in which a device is placed around the top portion of the stomach to decrease and slow food consumption

Obesity—a condition measured by a BMI ≥ 30, divided into classes: Class I obesity BMI ≥ 30–34.9; Class II obesity BMI ≥ 35–39.9; Class III obesity BMI ≥ 40–49.9; Class IV obesity BMI ≥ 50. Class III and IV are also referred to as severe obesity.

Overweight—a weight to height classification defined as a BMI ≥ 25–29.9

Pannus—also termed panniculus; a roll of lower abdominal subcutaneous adipose tissue that can extend past the pubis or further

Roux-en-Y gastric bypass—a laparoscopic bariatric surgical procedure that creates a smaller stomach pouch; bypasses sections of the stomach and the small intestine

Introduction

Medically defined obesity is the most common condition in the perinatal period. The overall prevalence for adult obesity in the United States in 2019 was 42% with rates varying by state (Centers for Disease Control and Prevention [CDC], 2022a, 2022c; Fisher et al., 2013). Worldwide obesity rates average 13% with obesity-related complications killing more individuals than underweight complications (WHO, 2022). Pregravid obesity is a significant risk factor for adverse perinatal outcomes, and risk increases as excess weight increases; however, most individuals without prepregnancy comorbid disease, such as diabetes or hypertension, have uncomplicated perinatal courses. This chapter covers the special perinatal care issues relevant to the pregnant client with a **body mass index** (BMI) ≥30.

Obesity is a complex health issue with multifactorial origins including genetic factors, and cultural, economic, and environmental contributions. Forty years of intensive research in obesity causation and management has reframed obesity from a condition resulting from lack of willpower and overindulgence in food to a condition with multiple causes that include altered epigenomes, manufactured foods, unhealthy built environments, and changes in daily physical activity and sleep patterns. Adipose tissue is now recognized as the body's largest endocrine organ. **Obesity** was classified by the American Medical Association as a disease in 2013; however, recent research identifies individuals with obesity and normal metabolic profiles and normal vital signs (Smith et al., 2019). The classifications are tiered by risk for obesity-related chronic disease: Class 1 = high risk, Class 2 = very high risk, and Class 3 and above = extremely high risk. Clinical guidelines established by specialty medical groups focus on primary prevention of obesity and the treatment of weight-related complications such as diabetes rather than solely on weight loss (Garvey et al., 2016).

Obesity is also defined by a waist circumference greater than 35 in (88 cm) in nonpregnant clients. Abdominal

Prenatal and Postnatal Care: A Person-Centered Approach, Third Edition. Edited by Karen Trister Grace, Cindy L. Farley, Noelene K. Jeffers, and Tanya Tringali.

adipose tissue is the most metabolically active adipose tissue producing a variety of inflammatory cytokines and hormones. The greater the waist circumference, the higher the risk for obesity-related diseases. Waist circumference loses its usefulness in pregnancy; therefore, prepregnancy BMI has become the international measurement used to describe the relationship of weight to height during pregnancy. The research related to obesity in pregnancy uses prepregnancy or first-trimester BMI to analyze obesity-related risk. Most individuals in the WHO normal and **overweight** BMI ranges who gain the recommended amount of weight during pregnancy will move into the obese BMI range without changing their obesity-related risks for poor perinatal outcomes. Although many electronic medical records continue to calculate BMI as pregnancy progresses, these measurements should not be considered during advice and management planning.

Health equity key points

- Differential obesity rates reflect past population histories of oppression and inequitable access to nutritious food. Black and Hispanic clients, coming from groups with lower access to employment and income, have a higher prevalence of obesity than White clients.
- Convenience food stores stocked with highly processed, inexpensive foods with long shelf lives are often disproportionately located in low-income neighborhoods.
- Providers must consider the inequitable availability of parks, safe walking areas, and activity programs when encouraging physical activity during pregnancy.

Prevalence

Obesity during pregnancy is a common condition affecting approximately one in three pregnant clients (Deputy et al., 2018). Prior to 1970, obesity was uncommon in the United States and other industrialized nations. Between 1980 and 2000, mean pregnancy weight at the first prenatal visit increased by 20% and the incidence of clients who were obese at the first prenatal visit tripled (Lu et al., 2001). Prepregnancy obesity prevalence continues to increase in clients over aged 20 (CDC, 2022c).

Health Disparities, Nutritional Inequity, and Cultural Considerations

Significant disparities exist in obesity rates and associated health impacts across racial and ethnic groups in North America (see Table 46.1). Socioeconomic inequities and structural racism are associated with obesity, including low education attainment, low income, and environment (Jevitt, 2019). Disparities in obesity rates reflect population histories of oppression and inequitable access to nutritious food. Black and Hispanic clients, coming from groups with less access to employment and income, have a higher prevalence of obesity than White clients. Low-income levels hold people in neighborhoods with higher

Table 46.1 Prevalence of Obesity in US Adults Age ≥ 20

	Obesity all classes	Severe obesity BMI ≥ 40
Non-Hispanic Black clients	49.6%	13.8%
Non-Hispanic White clients	42.2%	9.3%
Hispanic clients	44.8%	7.9%
Non-Hispanic Asian clients	17.4%	2.0%

Source: Adapted from Hales et al. (2020).

levels of obesity-contributing stress, reduced access to nutritious foods, and endocrine disrupting chemical pollutants which alter metabolic pathways (Jevitt, 2019). Histone modification or deoxyribonucleic acid (DNA) methylation moderated by nutrition during pregnancy may lead to obesity-promoting epigenetic changes in the fetus. These epigenetic changes alter gene expression that resist later dietary or lifestyle interventions. This is a partial explanation for individual difficulty in altering weight (Fleming et al., 2018; Kaspar et al., 2020; Kwon & Kim, 2017). The elevated rate of extreme obesity in Black clients may account for a portion of the Black–White disparity in neonatal mortality (Salihu et al., 2008).

Convenience food stores stocked with highly processed, inexpensive foods with long shelf lives are often inequitably located in low-income neighborhoods. Research into food availability in these neighborhoods originally labeled them **food deserts**. This term is being replaced by the phrase **food swamp**, indicating the prevalence of less expensive, high-fat, high-sugar processed foods instead of fresh fruits and vegetables, forcing families with tight budgets to purchase less nutritious food. Transportation barriers to full-service groceries are common for low-income families. Longer distance to full-service stores and higher prices at nearby convenience stores are associated with higher rates of obesity (Ghosh-Dastidar et al., 2014).

Personal and Family Considerations

Some clients, particularly young clients and those with low incomes, have little control over their food choices. They may eat at the homes of friends or family when they have no money to buy their own food and have little choice in what is served. Clients who qualify for the Special Supplemental Food Program for Women, Infants, and Children (WIC) or the Supplemental Nutrition Assistance Program (SNAP, formerly known as food stamps) may share their food with other family members who do not qualify for assistance. The clinician can suggest that these foods be marked "for the baby" in an effort to deter this practice.

Food preferences are culturally based. Mealtimes are social opportunities. All cultures use food in celebratory ceremonies. Individuals learn to associate food with happiness and prosperity. Conversely, limiting intake or dieting can become viewed as punitive or restrictive. Food habits are among the hardest habits to change.

Obesity Physiology

Food intake greater than that used by basal metabolic needs and calories burned during daily activity are initially stored as muscle glycogen. When not used for immediate energy needs, calories are converted into stored fat. Stored fat is deposited around the body. Adipose tissue is the largest metabolically active endocrine organ, particularly retroperitoneal fat, which produces inflammatory cytokines such as tumor necrosis factor alpha (TNFa). The production of inflammatory cytokines may account for the rise in diseases, such as hypertension, with increasing BMI. Excess adipose tissue increases cardiac workload. Coupled with the increased circulatory demands of pregnancy, the increased cardiac demands of obesity increase risk for hypertensive disorders of pregnancy (Helmreich et al., 2008).

Risk factors for obesity in childbearing-aged clients

Factors Contributed by Client's Mother
- Prepregnancy BMI ≥ 30
- Any type of diabetes during pregnancy
- Excessive weight gain during pregnancy
- Excessive stress exposure

Factors Present for Client
- Birth weight > 4000 g
- Physical inactivity

Environmental Factors
- Low education
- Low income
- Food insecurity
- Food desert/swamp location
- Unsafe neighborhoods
- Partner with BMI ≥ 30
- Systemic racism
- Endocrine disrupting chemicals

Health Factors
- Hypothyroidism
- Polycystic ovary syndrome
- Psychiatric medication use

Source: Gaillard et al. (2013), Hillemeier et al. (2011), and Jevitt (2019).

Insulin is a growth hormone in pregnancy. Clients with BMIs ≥ 30 are prone to insulin resistance, and many pregnancy hormones such as estrogen and human placental lactogen promote insulin resistance. As gestation progresses, the metabolic demands of pregnancy outstrip pancreatic ability to produce insulin. **Insulin resistance** in obesity and pregnancy hormones contribute to the increased risk for gestational diabetes mellitus (GDM). Excess cytokine production, increased cardiac demand, and increasing insulin resistance contribute to a variety of conditions that often accompany obesity in pregnancy.

Psychotropic drugs are associated with weight gain especially in the first year of use (Mazereel et al., 2020). Serotonin 5-HT2C and histaminergic H1 receptor antagonism by psychotropic medications have been identified as increasing appetite and delaying satiety with resultant overeating. The association of mental health problems, low income, and food insecurity makes weight management especially challenging.

Psychiatric medications associated with weight gain

- Amisulpride
- Aripiprazole
- Clozapine
- Haloperidol
- Iloperidone
- Lamotrigine
- Lithium
- Lurasidone
- Olanzapine
- Quetiapine
- Risperidone
- Torpiramate
- Ziprasidone
- Tricyclic antidepressants
- Monoamine oxidase inhibitors
- Some selective serotonin reuptake inhibitors

Source: Adapted from Mazereel et al. (2020).

Potential Problems

The risks of adverse pregnancy outcomes increase as BMI increases beyond the normal range (Table 46.2). Conception can be more difficult for clients with obesity because they are less likely to ovulate regularly, have increased rates of polycystic ovary disease, have lower levels of gonadotropins, have decreased spontaneous pregnancy rates, and have increased risk of miscarriage (Lainez & Coss, 2019). GDM affects as many as 20% of pregnant clients with obesity, a fourfold increase compared to normal-weight clients (Kim et al., 2010). Hypertension in pregnancy is more frequent in clients with obesity. The risk of preterm birth is also elevated, likely in part because of the increased risk of preeclampsia. Obesity prior to pregnancy is one of the strongest predictors of giving birth to a macrosomic infant, even if the client did not develop GDM (Lende & Rijhsinghani, 2020; Santangeli et al., 2015). Research suggests that reducing obesity prior to pregnancy may be more effective in reducing the incidence of macrosomia than treatment for GDM (Retnakaran et al., 2012). Increasing BMI is associated with higher rates of stillbirth (ACOG, 2021). One study using the CDC's Birth Data and Fetal Death Data for 2014–2017 (n = 10,043,398 total births; including 48,799 stillbirths) found that individuals in Class II and Class III obesity were at significant increased risk for stillbirth (Obesity II ARR = 2.37 [2.07–2.72]; Obesity

Table 46.2 Potential Problems Associated with Obesity in Pregnancy

Prenatal potential problems	Intrapartum potential problems	Postpartum potential problems
• Spontaneous abortion	• Fetal macrosomia	• Delayed postpartum hemorrhage
• Fetal neural tube defects	• Dysfunctional labor	• Endometritis
• Fetal anencephaly	• Need for induction/augmentation of labor	• Deep vein thrombosis
• Anemia	• Epidural catheter placement failure	• Breastfeeding problems
• Pregestational diabetes	• Forceps- or vacuum-assisted birth	• Wound dehiscence
• Gestational diabetes	• Shoulder dystocia	• Wound infection
• Urinary tract infection	• Cesarean section	• Urinary tract infection
• Vaginitis, especially candida vaginitis	• Lower Apgar scores	• Anemia
• Essential hypertension	• Increased use of general anesthesia	• Excessive weight retention
• Hypertensive disorders of pregnancy including preeclampsia	• Immediate postpartum hemorrhage	• Dysthymia, depression and eating disorders
• Placental abruption		
• Intrauterine growth restriction		
• Prolonged pregnancy		
• Stillbirth		
• Dysthymia, depression and eating disorders		

Source: AGOC (2021) / Wolters Kluwer Health, Inc.

III ARR = 9.06 [7.61–10.78]) (Ikedionwu et al., 2020). Clients with obesity are also at an increased risk for other perinatal problems such as lower success with assisted reproductive technologies, congenital anomalies, and failure to initiate breastfeeding. Even a small weight loss prior to pregnancy can improve outcomes (ACOG, 2021). Despite the increased risk of potential perinatal problems, it should be remembered that most pregnant clients with obesity have a normal pregnancy and birth course.

Management of Pregestational Obesity

Nondiscriminatory Language

Many healthcare providers avoid discussing clients' weight, often fearing that they will cause their clients emotional harm and alienate clients from their practices (Allen-Walker et al., 2020). Weight and body image are sensitive issues; however, their effect on health can be so profound that clinicians who fail to address unhealthy weights risk ignoring their patients' most pressing healthcare needs. Studies of midwifery practice have shown that clientele expect nonjudgmental, evidence-based guidance about weight gain during pregnancy (Allen-Walker et al., 2020; Christenson et al., 2019; Daley et al., 2015; Holton et al., 2017). Nonjudgmental care includes asking the client their preferred language about weight, supporting the client's prenatal weight goals, avoiding preconceptions about the client's nutrition and physical

activity, and avoiding a focus on weight when the client has a multitude of pregnancy-related needs.

Using pejoratives such as "fatness" or "morbid obesity" is demeaning, while using euphemisms such as "big boned" or "plus sized" avoids the issue and is medically inaccurate. An international consensus group recommends using BMI descriptors or terms such as "excess weight" in place of pejorative language (Rubino, et al., 2020). The term "obesity" is used in scientific writing but may be interpreted negatively in writing for the public. Person-centered language, saying "clients with obesity" instead of "obese clients," maintains focus on the person, not the disease. The genetic, physiological, behavioral, sociocultural, economic, and environmental contributors to obesity are so complex that some professional societies promote a shift away from a focus on weight to therapies for weight-associated disease with a renaming of the medical condition termed obesity to "adiposity-based chronic disease" (Garvey et al., 2016).

Assessment of the Pregnant Client with Obesity

Problem-Focused Health History

Obesity is assessed at the first prenatal visit using height and prepregnancy weight recall, though accurate BMI calculations depend on a measured height and weight at the first prenatal visit. These measurements ideally should follow a discussion of the importance of nutrition and optimal weight gain during pregnancy, along with the risk-increasing effects of pregravid obesity and excessive gestational weight gain. This conversation can start with the question "How do you feel about your weight?" or "Would you like to discuss your weight?" to allow the healthcare provider to acknowledge and respond to any emotional issues that may be present for this client, while respecting the wishes of the client who may not be interested in addressing issues of obesity. If the first prenatal visit is within the first 12 weeks of pregnancy, the healthcare provider may decide to use the first visit weight measurement as the prepregnancy weight as some clients may not remember a prepregnancy weight. Clients should be able to measure their own weights in a private area or may wish to face away from the scale and not be told what their weight is to avoid feeling shamed or stigmatized. And clients have a right to decline to be weighed; indeed, some providers avoid weighing altogether if it is a trigger for their clients.

Waist circumference exceeding 35 in also indicates obesity. Waist measurement can be useful in diagnosing obesity during the first trimester in clients with BMIs between 28 and 35. Muscle is denser than fat, and athletic clients, such as marathon runners, may have BMIs between 25 and 30 but have little adipose tissue. A waist measurement less than 35 in paired with a BMI of 25–30 indicates increased muscle mass. Waist measurement may also be useful in the assessment of postpartum weight loss.

In addition to the elements of a routine prenatal history, a detailed diet history is taken (see Chapter 9, *Nutrition during Pregnancy*). Physical activity during the workday, frequency of fast-food meals, and eating patterns should be explored. Disordered eating patterns, such as binging, purging, lack of satiety, food-seeking behavior, night-eating, pica, and other eating habits, are evaluated (Villarejo et al., 2014). Eating disorders are associated with obesity and weight fluctuations over time (da Luz et al., 2018). Some cases of obesity and disordered eating are rooted in childhood or sexual trauma; a trauma-informed approach to care is recommended. The client's affect is assessed for signs of dysthymia or depression, such as avoidance of eye contact, flat affect, disparaging or self-deprecating comments, exhaustion, and inability to sleep. Depression screening should be done for all pregnant clients, but especially for those with obesity, as depression may be a consequence or a cause of excessive dietary intake and reduced activity (Steinig et al., 2017).

Physical Examination

Excess adipose tissue, particularly that which is deposited around the waist, may confound physical examination. In the first and early second trimesters, the healthcare provider may be unable to palpate the size of the uterus during the bimanual exam. Long speculums (6–7 in compared to 4.75 in) may be needed to visualize the cervix.

Prenatal breast growth is a common cause of shoulder and back pain in obese clients. Those with pendulous breasts should be encouraged to purchase well-fitting, supportive brassieres when breast growth is complete at about 20 weeks of gestation.

A skin exam should include assessment for **intertrigo,** which can include evidence of bacterial and/or fungal infection, **acanthosis nigricans**, hirsutism, and cellulitis and carbuncles, all of which are more common in clients with obesity (Cooper, 2016).

Ultrasound imaging is limited by obesity. Visualization during early screening, such as a 12- to 13-week nuchal translucency genetic screening, may be incomplete and may require repeat exams outside of the best screening time frame (ACOG, 2021). Fetal anatomy scans in the second trimester may need to be repeated depending on the depth of abdominal adipose tissue. Approximately 15–30% of fetal structures will be visualized poorly when maternal BMI exceeds 40 (Tsai et al., 2015). The fetal structures most likely to be seen inadequately are heart, spine, kidneys, diaphragm, and umbilical cord (Lim & Mahmood, 2015).

Doppler assessment of first-trimester fetal heart rate may be delayed depending on adipose depth. The fetal heart can be auscultated by Doppler at 10–12 weeks on clients in the 18–26 BMI range, yet may not be audible until 14–16 weeks in some clients with obesity. If the individual has a large **pannus,** the fetal heart rate might be found by having them lift the pannus and then listening for the heart tones above the pubic bone.

Fundal height measurements may be inaccurate in clients with BMIs ≥30 and often exceed 40 cm in the last trimester without indicating macrosomia. Palpation of fetal lie and position becomes more difficult as BMI exceeds 35, and the healthcare provider may be unable to reach the presenting part during vaginal exam to verify position. An ultrasound exam in late gestation may be necessary to verify position and might be useful to estimate fetal weight, although the limits of ultrasound measurements in the third trimester and in obesity must be considered.

Laboratory Testing

Clients with BMIs ≥ 35 at the first prenatal visit should have an early one-hour GDM screen (ACOG, 2021). If the first screen is normal (blood glucose ≤130–140 mg/dL, depending on practice guidelines), the screening is repeated at 24–28 weeks of gestation. Lipid screening is not done during pregnancy or lactation, as lipids are physiologically elevated during these periods. Thyroid function screening tests are not typically part of routine prenatal testing for pregnant clients; however, serum thyroid-stimulating hormone (TSH) values may be obtained early in pregnancy in clients with BMIs of 40 or greater, as they have a higher risk for overt hypothyroidism (Alexander et al., 2017).

Management Principles

International guidelines encourage people with obesity to reduce weight before starting a pregnancy through behavior modification, reducing intake, and increasing activity level (ACOG, 2021; National Institute for Care and Excellence, 2010). These guidelines do not acknowledge the difficulty of significant weight loss, especially for

Table 46.3 IOM Recommendations for Total Pregnancy Weight Gain for Individuals with BMI ≥30

Prepregnancy obesity class	Optimal weight gain
Class 1 (BMI 30.0–34.9)	11–20 lb. (5.5–9 kg)
Class 2 (BMI 35.0–39.9)	
Class 3 (BMI 40+)	

those with BMIs exceeding 35. In the absence of a successful preconception program for weight loss, helping clients achieve optimal prenatal weight gain begins at the first prenatal visit. The desired outcomes include a prenatal weight gain within the Institute of Medicine (IOM) guidelines (see Table 46.3), breastfeeding for one year, and a gradual loss of all weight gained during pregnancy by nine months postpartum. Nutritional assessments and client-centered counseling are time consuming. Some healthcare providers have clients with obesity return after the first visit for a separate nutrition counseling session. Nutrition and activity information sessions are done most efficiently in group settings whether the groups are scheduled specifically for weight gain management in addition to prenatal care or integrated into group prenatal care. Social support can be an important part of such group care experiences, as group members share successes and challenges in adopting healthier habits. Stillbirth rates are increased for those with obesity (Yao et al., 2014). New ACOG guidelines (2021) suggest offering weekly antenatal surveillance beginning by 37 0/7 weeks of gestation for those with a prepregnancy BMI between 35.0 and 39.9, and weekly surveillance for individuals whose BMIs exceed 39.9 starting at 34 0/7 weeks of gestation.

Management of obesity in pregnancy

- Ask clients how they feel about their weight and if they would like to talk about addressing it.
- Measure and document height with a stadiometer at first prenatal visit.
- Document weight. Ask the client to recall their prepregnancy weight. If the first prenatal visit is in the first trimester, consider using the weight at the first prenatal visit for the BMI calculation.
- Calculate the BMI.
- Assess psychological risk factors, depression, and potential eating disorders.
- Advise a pregnancy weight gain consistent with the current IOM recommendations (Table 46.3). Document the target weight and counseling in the medical record.
- Assess comorbidities of obesity and patterns of previous weight gain and loss.
- Perform a nutritional assessment.
- Have the client identify one to two non-nutritious foods that could be dropped or changed for more nutritious foods.
- Provide nutritional counseling. Identify weight management advantages.

- Offer nutrition and behavioral counseling referrals.
- Obtain one-hour oral glucose tolerance test at the first prenatal visit in clients without known pre-GDM. If normal, rescreen at 24–28 weeks.
- Perform a TSH screen if BMI >40.
- If the client has pre-GDM or a history of GDM, assess HgA1C at the first prenatal visit. Glycosylated hemoglobin should be less than 6%.
- Offer early screening for neural tube defects (NTDs), including early serum screening and ultrasound at 11–13 weeks to assess nuchal translucency. Obesity often limits ultrasound visualization and clients may need to return for another ultrasound one to two weeks later, past the ideal nuchal translucency evaluation time.
- Schedule frequent visits (every two weeks) for regular weight gain assessment and nutrition counseling. Visits in addition to routine prenatal visits can be coded as "other visits."
- Provide a private area for clients to weigh themselves or offer opportunity for client to face away from scale or not be told their weight.
- Consider postpartum anticoagulation for clients with Class III obesity.

Source: ACOG (2021) and Holton et al. (2017).

Nutrition

Clients with BMIs ≥ 30 have the same nutritional needs as pregnant clients with lower BMIs. Generally, pregnancy requires about an extra 340 calories per day after 16 weeks of gestation for proper fetal growth and 450 calories during the third trimester for those in the 18–26 BMI range. Those with obesity need fewer calories with 350 calories per day recommended during the third trimester. Some clients with BMIs >35 may have been eating more than 4000 calories on many days and will not need to increase food intake to gain weight. Intake should target 175 g carbohydrate per kilogram weight per day and 0.88–1.1 g protein per kilogram per day (Elliott-Sale et al., 2019).

Clients with obesity have the same elevated risk of congenital malformations as clients with type 2 diabetes, particularly neural tube and cardiac defects (Helle & Priest, 2020; Vena et al., 2021). Therefore, those with obesity ideally should start folic acid 4 mg orally daily before conceiving. If not started prenatally, extra folic acid should begin at the first prenatal visit and continue through the first trimester. Increased folic acid ingestion reduces the incidence of NTDs in obese pregnant clients; however, their risk remains elevated above clients in lower BMI ranges (McMahon et al., 2013; Ray et al., 2005).

Pregnancy Weight Gain and Management Issues

The Institute of Medicine (IOM, 2009) recommends a gain of 11- to 20-lb total for clients in the obese category, with clients in higher obesity classes gaining at the lower end of the range. This averages to approximately 0.5 (0.4–0.6) lb gain per week in the second and third trimesters.

Weight management conversations are difficult for many healthcare providers because of the cultural connections between weight and other personal attributes, including beauty, willpower, energy, and strength. Many clients have experience with prepregnancy eating and activity behaviors that can be used safely during pregnancy to manage prenatal weight gain. Research demonstrates that some behaviors are more successful in weight management (see the text box *Specific Strategies to Manage Weight*). Clinicians can discover which of these strategies clients have used in the past and encourage clients to use this experience as an advantage in preventing potential health problems associated with obesity.

Specific strategies to manage weight

- Prepare own meals (Wansink & van Kleef, 2014).
- Eat intentionally/mindfully with the TV off (Fitzpatrick et al., 2007).
- Eat low-glycemic-index foods (Juanola-Falgarona et al., 2014).
- Eat high-fiber foods (Horan et al., 2014).
- Follow the My Plate Diet.
- Eat prepackaged, portion-controlled meals.
- Weigh self regularly (Zheng et al., 2015).
- Sleep at least seven hours each night (Chaput et al., 2010).
- Engage in planned physical activity for at least 30 minutes, 5 days a week.
- Breastfeed exclusively for at least three months postpartum (Ruiz et al., 2013).

Low Weight Gain, Weight Loss, and Pregnancy Concerns

No weight gain and weight loss are not recommended during pregnancy, even for clients in the obese weight categories (ACOG, 2021). Some pregnant clients who begin eating low-fat foods and increase fruit and vegetable consumption during pregnancy reduce their daily calorie intake and lose weight. With fetal growth in the third trimester, obese clients may feel as if they do not have enough room to eat their usual prepregnancy meals. A systematic review found that obese clients with gestational weight loss instead of weight gain have a lower risk of macrosomia and large for gestational age (LGA), yet a higher risk of small for gestational age (SGA) below the third percentile (Kapadia et al., 2015). Weight gain below the IOM guidelines increases the risk of preterm birth, especially for Black clients (who have an already increased risk of preterm birth due to effects of racism) and adolescents (Berger et al., 2015). Animal studies have found chronic prenatal ketone exposure from weight loss is associated with altered anatomical and functional brain deficits in the offspring, suggesting possible adverse effects on development (Sussman et al., 2013). Given the increased risk of SGA, a key predictor of neonatal morbidity and mortality, and the unknown effects on fetal development, weight loss should not be recommended for pregnant clients with obesity.

Physical Activity

Pregnant clients with obesity are encouraged to increase physical activity. Most people can walk 30 minutes a day regardless of weight. Walking provides non-insulin-mediated glucose use by muscle, helping to stabilize blood glucose (Embaby et al., 2016; Swartz et al., 2003), and improves fitness for labor. Clients with BMIs > 40 or those with long-standing obesity should be evaluated for knee or back problems before starting a walking regimen. All clients should start additional activity gradually and increase activity as tolerated.

Walking can be done in three 10-minute periods, two 15-minute periods, or continuously for 30 minutes (CDC, 2022b). This is done in addition to any walking done during the client's regular employment. Contemporary work has become sedentary, which can significantly reduce the physical activity of pregnant clients. Providers must consider the inequitable availability of parks, safe walking areas, and activity programs when encouraging physical activity during pregnancy.

Getting more sleep instead of using some sleep time for increased physical activity may seem counterintuitive; however, sleep deprivation causes insulin resistance, lowering blood glucose levels, and increasing appetite (Wu et al., 2014; CDC, 2012). Short sleep hours and wakefulness during nighttime circadian sleep and hormone rhythms are associated with an increased risk of developing chronic conditions such as obesity, diabetes, high blood pressure, heart disease, stroke, and mental illness (Westerterp-Plantenga, 2016). Sleeping 6–8.5 hours at night facilitates weight maintenance (Westerterp-Plantenga, 2016; Liu et al., 2013). Clients should be encouraged to rearrange their daily schedules to assure a minimum of six to eight hours of sleep.

Comfort Measures

Comfort measures for clients with BMIs ≥ 30 are both psychological and physical. Clients with obesity may be reluctant to come for timely care because of the social stigma associated with excessive weight. Weight measurement should be done in a private area. Blood pressure cuffs, exam gowns, and waiting room furniture should be sized appropriately. Office settings and birthing areas should have several rooms with bariatric-sized chairs, exam tables, and beds. Healthcare providers should be aware that excess weight can amplify discomforts common in pregnancy. Pregnancy stresses joints, particularly the low back, pelvis, knees, and ankles. These joints are stressed already by excess weight. Occasional acetaminophen, hot or cold packs, or soaking in a warm tub may provide some relief.

Common pregnancy discomforts exacerbated by obesity

- Backache
- Knee pain
- Dependent edema
- Dyspnea
- Gastroesophageal reflux
- Sleep disturbances

Bariatric Surgery and Pregnancy Issues

Weight loss and maintenance of healthy weight is extremely difficult once BMI exceeds 35. Bariatric surgery is recommended when lifestyle, diet, and medication therapies have failed and BMI exceeds 35 or when BMI exceeds 30 and there are comorbid conditions such as diabetes (Garvey et al., 2016). The number of clients having weight loss surgery is increasing, especially as bariatric surgery can enhance fertility and prepregnancy health. Pregnancy in clients who have had bariatric surgery is safer than pregnancy when BMI is ≥40 (Harreiter et al., 2018). While bariatric surgery reduces maternal complications such as hypertensive disorders and GDM, it is associated with an increased risk of SGA in the neonate (Carreau et al., 2017; Johansson et al., 2015; Parker et al., 2016). It is recommended that clients wait at least 12–24 months after bariatric surgery to attempt pregnancy (Harreiter et al., 2018; Hezelgrave & Oteng-Ntim, 2011). Some researchers have found a surgery-to-pregnancy interval of less than two years is associated with a higher risk of adverse neonatal outcomes (Parent et al., 2017). A waiting time allows for the weight loss phase to be completed and nutritional deficiencies to be corrected.

There are two types of bariatric surgery procedures commonly performed in the United States: (a) restrictive (**laparoscopic gastric banding** or LAP-BAND) and (b) restrictive/malabsorptive (**Roux-en-Y gastric bypass** [RYGB]). In caring for pregnant clients who have had bariatric surgery, it is important to know the type of procedure done. LAP-BAND slippage and movement can occur during pregnancy and result in severe vomiting (Vrebosch et al., 2012). Some advocate for deflating the band prior to pregnancy to allow for adequate nutrition, though there are no guidelines or consensus.

Prenatal nutrition in clients who have had bariatric surgery is extremely important. The RYGB procedure can drastically alter the absorption of food and medications and can lead to nutritional deficiencies in iron, vitamin B_{12}, folate, vitamin D, calcium, and protein. Anemia is common and can be severe. A broad evaluation for micronutrient deficiencies should be considered at the beginning of pregnancy in clients who have had bariatric surgery, and supplements initiated if any deficits are present. If no deficits are noted, a complete blood count and measurement of B 12, iron, ferritin, calcium, and vitamin D levels every trimester should be considered (Armstrong, 2010). As with all clients, pregnancy weight gain recommendations are based on prepregnancy BMI.

Clients who have had the RYGB procedure should avoid oral glucose challenge testing due to **dumping syndrome**. Assessment for GDM can be done by either following fasting and postprandial blood glucose levels after breakfast for one week or obtaining a Hgb A1C and assuming diabetes if >6.5 for clients with prior RYGB surgery (Vrebosch et al., 2012). Fetal growth assessment by ultrasound may be appropriate in the third trimester if weight gain has been limited. Optimal care of pregnant clients after bariatric surgery includes the collaboration of multiple healthcare providers such as dieticians, midwives, and perinatal or obstetric consultants.

Prolonged Pregnancy

The incidence of pregnancies lasting longer than 294 days increases along with increasing BMI. Maternal obesity is associated with birthweight >4000 g and prolonged pregnancy >41 weeks of gestation (Stirrat et al., 2014). Inflammatory cytokines or hormones produced in adipose tissue may inhibit the onset of labor. Cortisol, involved with the onset of labor, decreases as BMI increases (Lim & Mahmood, 2015). Leptin, a hormone manufactured by adipocytes that signals satiety, is a known tocolytic (Wuntakal & Hollingworth, 2010; Tessier et al., 2013). Clients with obesity who pass their expected date of birth are candidates for fetal testing, and they are at increased risk for induction or augmentation of labor.

Intrapartum and Postpartum Issues

Obesity without comorbid conditions should not limit choice in the place of birth. Birth center and home birth planning can be offered during prenatal care for uncomplicated pregnancies (Denison et al., 2019; National Institute for Health and Care Excellence [NICE] 2019; Jevitt et al., 2021). The same physiologic mechanisms that increase the risk for prolonged pregnancy increase risk for longer induction of labor and longer stages of labor (Ellis et al., 2019). Obesity is linked with labor complications that increase the risk for operative birth or increase the difficulty of vaginal birth (Table 46.2); however, midwifery-led care during labor has been shown to improve vaginal birth outcomes for those with obesity (Carlson et al., 2017; Daemers et al., 2014; Hollowell et al., 2014; Jevitt et al., 2021; Rowe et al., 2018).

No evidence-based management recommendations have been developed to counteract the effect of obesity on labor and birth. Complications related to obesity continue in the postpartum period. The most common obesity-related complications in the postpartum period are post-cesarean wound infection and dehiscence. Incision openings must heal from the inside out, which requires daily cleaning and packing. This can be a painful, difficult process for clients, particularly those trying to establish breastfeeding. The skin incision may be below the pannus, making it impossible for the client to visually examine the wound and to pack it without assistance. If family cannot assist with wound care, assistance from a home health agency may be needed.

Postpartum deep vein thrombosis (DVT) is the most lethal obesity-related postpartum complication and is a leading cause of postpartum mortality. Prevention includes early postpartum ambulation, use of alternating pressure cuffs on lower extremities, and prenatal anticoagulation medication for those with prior thrombus formation. Clients with Class III obesity are at four times the risk for DVT as normal-weight clients

(Blondon et al., 2016). Postpartum anticoagulation is recommended, particularly those having a cesarean birth with Class III obesity and higher (ACOG, 2021).

Obesity is associated with delayed onset of milk production (lactogenesis II), maternal perception of insufficient milk supply, and early cessation of breastfeeding (Anstey & Jevitt, 2011). People with BMIs ≥ 30 need extra support in the early postpartum period. Extra stimulation with double pumping and frequent feeding can increase the supply of colostrum and later milk. Extra-large shields may be needed for breast pumps, as shields that are too small can strangulate and bruise the nipple. Chairs and beds that are large enough to comfortably position the feeding newborn with supportive pillows facilitate breastfeeding comfort (Jevitt et al., 2007).

Because lactation uses about 500 calories of energy daily, if the individual slightly limits food intake, they will have a gradual reduction in weight without affecting milk quality or infant growth (Lovelady, 2011). Breastfeeding longer than three months significantly lowers the patient's future risk for type 2 diabetes and cardiac disease (Gunderson et al., 2015). Breastfeeding is primary obesity prevention and health promotion for newborns by metabolic programming through glucose homeostasis, priming infant olfactory and gustatory senses, newborn satiety signaling, and optimizing nutrition of the infant gut microbiome (Jevitt, 2021). Providing clients with information about short- and long-term parent and newborn health benefits can encourage breastfeeding.

Interprofessional Care

Care for clients with pregestational obesity and excessive gestational weight gain without comorbidities are within the scope of practice for midwives and nurse practitioners. Collaboration, consultation, or referral to obstetric or medical services depend more on comorbid conditions such as hypertension or GDM than on pregestational obesity or excessive prenatal weight gain. Many clients with uncomplicated obesity and a weight gain within IOM ranges will have an otherwise normal pregnancy and birth. However, some obese clients are at high risk for induction, labor augmentation, and cesarean birth: conditions often requiring obstetric consultation, comanagement, or referral. Difficulty in placing intravenous and epidural catheters and intubation increase with increasing BMI; therefore, many anesthesiologists request a prenatal consult.

Legal and Liability Issues

Pregestational obesity and excessive prenatal weight gain are linked with diabetes and fetal macrosomia, which are both risk factors for shoulder dystocia. Improper management of shoulder dystocia with permanent brachial plexus injury is one of the most common claims against midwives and physicians. Tort claims have included improper management of prenatal weight gain and diabetes during pregnancy as potential contributory factors in poor birth outcomes.

Obesity should be identified at the first prenatal visit, and informed consent regarding the potential pregnancy problems related to obesity and pregnancy should be documented (ACOG, 2021). A weight gain plan also needs to be established and documented, along with associated counseling. Clients who receive appropriate weight gain counseling and who continue to gain excessive amounts of weight may be held responsible for contributory negligence in the event of a poor birth outcome that leads to legal action.

Summary

Obesity during pregnancy is a common condition that affects approximately 30% of pregnant clients in the United States. Prepregnancy obesity increases risk for birth defects, stillbirth, and prenatal complications such as hypertensive disorders and GDM. Intrapartum and postpartum risks are increased as well for clients who are obese. Risks are compounded by increasing BMI, comorbid medical disease, and increasing age; however, most individuals with prepregnancy obesity have healthy, uncomplicated pregnancies and births. Specific dietary and exercise plans are primary components of care for pregnant clients with BMIs >30. Cultural and family dietary practices as well as exercise and food availability and affordability need to be considered when counseling clients about changing eating and activity patterns. Providing respectful, nonbiased, and nonstigmatizing guidance and assistance to achieve appropriate weight gain is especially important for pregnant clients with obesity. Client-led care planning, shared decision-making between clinicians and clients, a multidisciplinary approach, and adequate time during prenatal and postnatal visits are needed to achieve optimal perinatal outcomes.

Resources for Clients and Their Families

Patient resources related to obesity are available at: http://www.cdc.gov/obesity/resources/factsheets.html

The CDC offers physical activity guidelines and tracking devices for individuals at: https://www.cdc.gov/healthy-weight/physical_activity/index.html

The US Department of Agriculture Web site contains resources for individuals, families, and healthcare providers. Included on the Choose My Plate site is a customizable program where clients can receive individualized meal plans and recipes. Data can be saved for continuous use. The program can be adjusted for pregnancy and breastfeeding. There is also a Super-Tracker that can track intake and physical activity. The healthcare provider sections contain clinical information to assist in weight management, printable nutrition handouts, and graphics. The Choose My Plate program is available at: www.myplate.gov

Resources for Healthcare Providers

The CDC offers BMI calculators as downloadable widgets that can be placed on websites or smart phones at: https://www.cdc.gov/healthyweight/assessing/bmi/

adult_bmi/english_bmi_calculator/bmi_calculator. html

The latest US obesity data are available from the Centers for Disease Control (CDC) in reports, maps, and PowerPoint slides that can be downloaded free of charge at: https://www.cdc.gov/obesity/data/prevalence-maps. html

The US Department of Agriculture provides a wealth of resources in printable, pdf format available from https://www.myplate.gov/resources/print-materials. MyPlate posters, brochures encouraging patients to make half their plate fruits and vegetables, sample meal plans for 2000 calories a day, and sample recipes are available.

References

Alexander, E. K., Pearce, E. N., Brent, G. A., Brown, R. S., Chen, H., Dosiou, C., & Peeters, R. P. (2017). 2017 Guidelines of the American Thyroid Association for the diagnosis and management of thyroid disease during pregnancy and the postpartum. *Thyroid*, *27*(3), 315–389. https://doi.org/10.1089/thy.2016.0457

Allen-Walker, V., Hunter, A. J., Holmes, V. A., & McKinley, M. C. (2020). Weighing as part of your care: A feasibility study exploring the re-introduction of weight measurements during pregnancy as part of routine antenatal care. *BMC Pregnancy and Childbirth*, *20*, 328. https://doi.org/10.1186/s12884-020-03011-w

American College of Obstetricians and Gynecologists (ACOG). (2021). Obesity in pregnancy. ACOG practice bulletin number 230. *Obstetrics & Gynecology*, *137*(6), e128–e144. https://doi.org/10.1097/AOG.0000000000004395

Anstey, E., & Jevitt, C. (2011). Maternal obesity and breastfeeding: A review of the evidence and implications for practice. *Clinical Lactation*, *2–3*, 11–16. https://doi.org/10.1891/215805311807010422

Armstrong, C. (2010). ACOG guidelines on pregnancy after bariatric surgery. *American Family Physician*, *81*(7), 905–906.

Berger, A. A., Levitan, G., Baxter, J. K., & Lerner-Geva, L. (2015). Gestational weight gain below the 2009 Institute of Medicine guidelines modifies preterm birth in obese pregnant women. *Obstetrics & Gynecology*, *125*, 102S. https://doi.org/10.1097/AOG.0000000000000818

Blondon, M., Harrington, L. B., Boehlen, F., Robert-Ebadi, H., Righini, M., & Smith, N. L. (2016). Pre-pregnancy BMI, delivery BMI, gestational weight gain and the risk of postpartum venous thrombosis. *Thrombosis Research*, *145*, 151–156. https://doi.org/10.1016/j.thromres.2016.06.026

Carlson, N. S., Corwin, E. J., & Lowe, N. K. (2017). Labor intervention and outcomes in women who are nulliparous and obese: Comparison of nurse-midwife to obstetrician intrapartum care. *Journal of Midwifery & Women's Health*, *62*(1), 29–39. https://doi.org/10.1111/jmwh.12579

Carreau, A. M., Nadeau, M., Marceau, S., Marceau, P., & Weisnagel, S. J. (2017). Pregnancy after bariatric surgery: Balancing risks and benefits. *Canadian Journal of Diabetes*, *41*(4), 432–438. https://doi.org/10.1016/j.jcjd.2016.09.005

Centers for Disease Control and Prevention (CDC). (2012). Short sleep duration among workers-United States, 2010. *MMWR. Morbidity and Mortality Weekly Report*, *61*(16), 281–285. https://pubmed.ncbi.nlm.nih.gov/22534760

Centers for Disease Control and Prevention (CDC). (2022a). *Adult obesity facts*. https://www.cdc.gov/obesity/data/adult.html

Centers for Disease Control and Prevention (CDC). (2022b). *Physical activity for healthy pregnant or postpartum clients*. http://www.cdc.gov/physicalactivity/basics/pregnancy/index.htm

Centers for Disease Control and Prevention (CDC). (2022c). *Interactive summary health statistics for adults-2019*. https://wwwn.cdc.gov/NHISDataQueryTool/SHS_adult/index.html

Chaput, J., Klingenberg, L., & Sjodin, A. (2010). Do all sedentary activities lead to weight gain: Sleep does not. *Current Opinion in Clinical Nutrition & Metabolic Care*, *13*(6), 601–607. https://doi.org/10.1016/S1499-2671(11)52110-0

Christenson, A., Johansson, E., Reynisdottir, S., Torgerson, J., & Hemmingsson, E. (2019). ". . .or else I close my ears" How women with obesity want to be approached and treated regarding gestational weight management: A qualitative interview study. *PLoS One*, *14*(9), e0222543. https://doi.org/10.1371/journal.pone.0222543

Cooper, J. (2016). Evaluation of the obese patient. In G. Steelman & E. Westman (Eds.), *Obesity: Evaluation and treatment essentials* (2nd ed., pp. 35–42). Taylor and Francis.

da Luz, F. Q., Hay, P., Touyz, S., & Sainsbury, A. (2018). Obesity with comorbid eating disorders: Associated health risks and treatment approaches. *Nutrients*, *10*(7), 829. https://doi.org/10.3390/nu10070829. PMID: 29954056; PMCID: PMC6073367

Daemers, D. O., Wijnen, H. A., van Limbeek, E. B., Budé, L. M., Nieuwenhuijze, M. J., Spaanderman, M. E., & de Vries, R. G. (2014). The impact of obesity on outcomes of midwife-led pregnancy and childbirth in a primary care population: A prospective cohort study. *BJOG: An International Journal of Obstetrics and Gynaecology*, *121*(11), 1403–1413. https://doi.org/10.1111/1471-0528.12684

Daley, A. J., Jolly, K., Jebb, S. A., Lewis, A. L., Clifford, S., Roalfe, A. K., Kenyon, S., & Aveyard, P. (2015). Feasibility and acceptability of regular weighing, setting weight gain limits and providing feedback by community midwives to prevent excess weight gain during pregnancy: Randomized controlled trial and qualitative study. *BMC Obesity*, *2*, 35. https://doi.org/10.1186/s40608-015-0061-5

Denison, F. C., Aedla, N. R., Keag, O., Hor, K., Reynolds, R. M., Milne, A., Diamond, A., & Royal College of Obstetricians and Gynaecologists. (2019). Care of women with obesity in pregnancy: Green-top guideline no. 72. *BJOG: An International Journal of Obstetrics and Gynaecology*, *126*(3), e62–e106. https://doi.org/10.1111/1471-0528.15386

Deputy, N. P., Dub, B., & Sharma, A. J. (2018). Prevalence and trends in prepregnancy normal weight—48 states, New York City, and District of Columbia, 2011–2015. *MMWR Morbidity and Mortality Weekly Report*, *66*, 1402–1407. https://doi.org/10.15585/mmwr.mm665152a3

Elliott-Sale, K. J., Graham, A., Hanley, S. J., Blumenthal, S., & Sale, C. (2019). Modern dietary guidelines for healthy pregnancy; maximising maternal and foetal outcomes and limiting excessive gestational weight gain. *European Journal of Sports Science*, *19*(1), 62–70. https://doi.org/10.1080/17461391.2018.1476591

Ellis, J. A., Brown, C. M., Barger, B., & Carlson, N. S. (2019). Influence of maternal obesity on labor induction: A systematic review and meta-analysis. *Journal of Midwifery & Women's Health*, *64*(1), 55–67. https://doi.org/10.1111/jmwh.12935

Embaby, H., Elsayed, E., & Fawzy, M. (2016). Insulin sensitivity and plasma glucose response to aerobic exercise in pregnant women at risk for gestational diabetes mellitus. *Ethiopian Journal of Health Science*, *26*(5), 409–414. https://doi.org/10.4314/ejhs.v26i5.2

Fisher, S. C., Kim, S. Y., Sharma, A. J., Rochat, R., & Morrow, B. (2013). Is obesity still increasing among pregnant clients? Prepregnancy obesity trends in 20 states, 2003–2009. *Preventive Medicine*, *56*(6), 372–378. https://doi.org/10.1016/j.ypmed.2013.02.015

Fitzpatrick, E., Edmunds, L. S., & Dennison, B. A. (2007). Positive effects of family dinner are undone by television viewing. *Journal of the American Dietetic Association*, *107*(4), 666–671. https://doi.org/10.1016/j.jada.2007.01.014

Fleming, T. P., Watkins, A. J., Velasquez, M. A., Mathers, J. C., Prentice, A. M., Stephenson, J., Barker, M., Saffery, R., Yajnik, C. S., Eckert, J. J., Hanson, M. A., Forrester, T., Gluckman, P. D., & Godfrey, K. D. (2018). Origins of lifetime health around the time of conception: Causes and consequences. *Lancet*, *391*, 1842–1852. http://10.0.3.248/S0140-6736(18)30312-X

Gaillard, R., Durmus, B., Hofman, A., Mackenbach, J. P., Steegers, E. A., & Jaddoe, V. W. (2013). Risk factors and outcomes of maternal obesity and excessive weight gain during pregnancy. *Obesity*, *21*(5), 1046–1055. https://doi.org/10.1002/oby.20088

Garvey, W. T., Mechanik, J., Brett, E., Garber, A., Hurley, D., Jastreboff, A., Nadolsky, K., Pessah-Pollack, R., & Plodkowski, R. (2016). American Association of Clinical Endocrinologists and American College of Endocrinology comprehensive clinical practice guidelines for medical care of patients with obesity. *Endocrine Practice, 22*(7), 842–884. http://10.0.16.62/EP161365.GL

Ghosh-Dastidar, B., Cohen, D., Hunter, G., Zenk, S. N., Huang, C., Beckman, R., & Dubowitz, T. (2014). Distance to store, food prices, and obesity in urban food deserts. *American Journal of Preventive Medicine, 47*(5), 587–595. https://doi.org/10.1016/j.amepre.2014.07.005

Gunderson, E., Hurston, S., Ning, X., Lo, J., Crites, Y., Walton, D., Dewey, K., Azavedo, R., Young, S., Fox, P., Elmasian, C., Salvador, N., Lum, M., Sternfeld, B., & Quesenberry, C. (2015). Lactation and progression to type 2 diabetes mellitus after gestational diabetes mellitus. *Annals of Internal Medicine, 163*(112), 889–898. https://doi.org/10.7326/M15-0807

Hales, C.M., Carroll, M.D., Fryar, C.D., & Ogden, C.L. (2020). *Prevalence of obesity and severe obesity among adults: United States, 2017–2018. NCHS Data Brief, no 360.* National Center for Health Statistics. https://www.cdc.gov/nchs/products/databriefs/db360.htm

Harreiter, J., Schindler, K., Bancher-Todesca, D., Göbl, C., Langer, F., Prager, G., Gessl, A., Leutner, M., Ludvik, B., Luger, A., Kautzky-Willer, A., & Krebs, M. (2018). Management of pregnant women after bariatric surgery. *Journal of Obesity, 2018,* 4587064. https://doi.org/10.1155/2018/4587064

Helle, E., & Priest, J. R. (2020). Maternal obesity and diabetes mellitus as risk factors for congenital heart disease in the offspring. *Journal of the American Heart Association, 9*(8), e011541. https://doi.org/10.1161/JAHA.119.011541

Helmreich, R., Hundley, V., & Varvel, P. (2008). The effect of obesity on heart rate (heart period) and physiologic parameters during pregnancy. *Biological Research for Nursing, 10,* 63–78. https://doi.org/10.1177/1099800408321077

Hezelgrave, N. I., & Oteng-Ntim, E. (2011). Pregnancy after bariatric surgery: A review. *Journal of Obesity,* 501939. https://doi.org/10.1155/2011/501939

Hillemeier, M. M., Weisman, C. S., Chuang, C., Downs, D. S., McCall-Hosenfeld, J., & Camacho, F. (2011). Transition to overweight or obesity among women of reproductive age. *Journal of Women's Health, 20*(5), 703–710. https://doi.org/10.1089/jwh.2010.2397

Hollowell, J., Pillas, D., Rowe, R., Linsell, L., Knight, M., & Brocklehurst, P. (2014). The impact of maternal obesity on intrapartum outcomes in otherwise low risk women: Secondary analysis of the Birthplace national prospective cohort study. *BJOG: An International Journal of Obstetrics and Gynaecology, 121*(3), 343–355. https://doi.org/10.1111/1471-0528.12437

Holton, S., East, C., & Fischer, J. (2017). Weight management during pregnancy: A qualitative study of women's and care providers' experiences and perspectives. *BMC Pregnancy and Childbirth, 17,* 351. https://doi.org/10.1186/s12884-017-1538-7

Horan, M. K., McGowan, C. A., Gibney, E. R., Donnelly, J. M., & McAuliffe, F. M. (2014). Maternal diet and weight at 3 months postpartum following a pregnancy intervention with a low glycaemic index diet: Results from the ROLO randomized control trial. *Nutrients, 6*(7), 2946–2955. https://doi.org/10.3390/nu6072946

Ikedionwu, C. A., Dongarwar, D., Yusuf, K. K., Ibrahimi, S., Salinas-Miranda, A. A., & Salihu, H. M. (2020). Pre-pregnancy maternal obesity, macrosomia, and risk of stillbirth: A population-based study. *European Journal of Obstetrics, Gynecology and Reproductive Biology, 252,* 1–6. https://doi.org/10.1016/j.ejogrb.2020.06.004

Institute of Medicine. (2009). *Weight gain during pregnancy: Re-examining the guidelines.* The National Academies Press.

Jevitt, C. (2021). Breastfeeding, an essential link in healthy weight promotion and obesity prevention. In S. Campbell (Ed.), *Breastfeeding as health promotion* (pp. 151–174). Jones & Bartlett Learning.

Jevitt, C., Hernandez, I., & Groer, M. (2007). Lactation complicated by overweight & obesity: Supporting the mother & newborn. *Journal of Midwifery & Women's Health, 56*(6), 606–613. https://doi.org/10.1016/j.jmwh.2007.04.006

Jevitt, C. M. (2019). Obesity and socioeconomic disparities: Rethinking causes and perinatal care. *Journal of Perinatal & Neonatal Nursing, 33*(2), 126–135. https://doi.org/10.1097/JPN.0000000000000400

Jevitt, C. M., Stapleton, S., Deng, Y., Song, X., Wang, K., & Jolles, D. R. (2021). Birth outcomes of women with obesity enrolled for care at freestanding birth centers in the United States. *Journal of Midwifery & Women's Health, 66*(1), 14–23. https://doi.org/10.1111/jmwh.13194

Johansson, K., Cnattingius, S., Naslund, I., Roos, N., Trolle Lagerros, Y., Granath, F., & Neovius, M. (2015). Outcomes of pregnancy after bariatric surgery. *New England Journal of Medicine, 372*(9), 814–824. https://doi.org/10.1056/NEJMoa1405789

Juanola-Falgarona, M., Salas-Salvado, J., Ibarrola-Jurado, N., Rabassa-Soler, A., Diaz-Lopez, A., Guasch-Ferr, M., Hernandez-Alonso, P., Balanza, R., & Bullo, M. (2014). Effect of the glycemic index of the diet on weight loss, modulation of satiety, inflammation, and other metabolic risk factors: A randomized controlled trial. *American Journal of Clinical Nutrition, 100,* 27–35. https://doi.org/10.3945/ajcn.113.081216

Kapadia, M. Z., Park, C. K., Beyene, J., Giglia, L., Maxwell, C., & McDonald, S. D. (2015). Weight loss instead of weight gain within the guidelines in obese women during pregnancy: A systematic review and meta-analyses of maternal and infant outcomes. *PLoS One, 10*(7), e0132650. https://doi.org/10.1371/journal.pone.0132650

Kaspar, D., Hastreiter, S., Irmler, M., Hrabé de Angelis, M., & Beckers, J. (2020). Nutrition and its role in epigenetic inheritance of obesity and diabetes across generations. *Mammalian Genome, 31*(5–6), 119–133. https://doi.org/10.1007/s00335-020-09839-z

Kim, S. Y., England, L., Wilson, H. G., Bish, C., Satten, G. A., & Dietz, P. (2010). Percentage of gestational diabetes mellitus attributable to overweight and obesity. *American Journal of Public Health, 100,* 1047–1052. https://ajph.aphapublications.org/doi/full/10.2105/AJPH.2009.172890

Kwon, E. J., & Kim, Y. J. (2017). What is fetal programming?: A lifetime of health is under the control of in utero health. *Obstetrics & Gynecology Science, 60*(6), 506–519. https://doi.org/10.5468/ogs.2017.60.6.506

Lainez, N. M., & Coss, D. (2019). Obesity, neuroinflammation, and reproductive function. *Endocrinology, 160*(11), 2719–2736. https://doi.org/10.1210/en.2019-00487

Lende, M., & Rijhsinghani, A. (2020). Gestational diabetes: Overview with emphasis on medical management. *International Journal of Environmental Research and Public Health, 17*(24), 9573. https://doi.org/10.3390/ijerph17249573. PMID: 33371325; PMCID: PMC7767324

Lim, C., & Mahmood, T. (2015). Obesity in pregnancy. *Best Practice & Research Clinical Obstetrics & Gynaecology, 29,* 309–319. https://doi.org/10.1016/j.bpobgyn.2014.10.008

Liu, Y., Croft, J. B., Wheaton, A. G., Perry, G. S., Chapman, D. P., Strine, T. W., McKnight-Eily, L. R., & Presley-Cantrell, L. (2013). Association between perceived insufficient sleep, frequent mental distress, obesity and chronic diseases among US adults, 2009 behavioral risk factor surveillance system. *BMC Public Health, 13*(1), 84. https://bmcpublichealth.biomedcentral.com/articles/10.1186/1471-2458-13-84

Lovelady, C. (2011). Session 1: Balancing intake and output: Food v. exercise. Balancing exercise and food intake with lactation to promote postpartum weight loss. *Proceedings of the Nutrition Society, 70*(2), 181–184. http://10.0.3.249/S002966511100005X

Lu, G. C., Rouse, D. J., DuBard, M., Cliver, S., Kimberlin, D., & Hauth, J. C. (2001). The effect of the increasing prevalence of maternal obesity on perinatal morbidity. *American Journal of Obstetrics & Gynecology, 185*(4), 845–849. https://doi.org/10.1067/mob.2001.117351

Mazereel, V., Detraux, J., Vancampfort, D., van Winkel, R., & De Hert, M. (2020). Impact of psychotropic medication effects on obesity and the metabolic syndrome in people with serious mental illness. *Frontiers in Endocrinology (Lausanne), 11,* 573479. https://doi.org/10.3389/fendo.2020.573479. PMID: 33162935; PMCID: PMC7581736

McMahon, D. M., Liu, J., Zhang, H., Torres, M. E., & Best, R. G. (2013). Maternal obesity, folate intake, and neural tube defects in offspring. *Birth Defects Research. Part A, Clinical and Molecular Teratology, 97*(2), 115–122. https://doi.org/10.1002/bdra.23113

National Institute for Health and Care Excellence (NICE). *NICE Guideline PH 27: Weight management before, during and after pregnancy. 2010, reviewed and revised 2017.* www.nice.org.uk/guidance/ph27/resources/surveillance-report-2017-weight-management-before-during-and-after-pregnancy-2010-nice-guideline-ph27-4424111104/chapter/Surveillance-decision.

National Institute for Health and Care Excellence (NICE). *Intrapartum care for women with existing medical conditions or obstetrics complications and their babies-obesity, 2019.* www.nice.org.uk/guidance/ng121/chapter/Recommendations#obesity.

Parent, B., Martopullo, I., Weiss, N. S., Khandelwal, S., Fay, E. E., & Rowhani-Rahbar, A. (2017). Bariatric surgery in clients of childbearing age, timing between an operation and birth, and associated perinatal complications. *Journal of the American Medical Association Surgery, 152*(2), 128–135.

Parker, M. H., Berghella, V., & Niijar, J. B. (2016). Bariatric surgery and associated adverse pregnancy outcomes among obese women. *Journal of Maternal, Fetal and Neonatal Medicine, 29*(11), 1747–1750. https://doi.org/10.3109/14767058.2015.1060214

Ray, J., Wyatt, P. R., Vermeulen, M. J., Meier, C., & Cole, D. E. (2005). Greater maternal weight and the ongoing risk of neural tube defects after folic acid flour fortification. *Obstetrics & Gynecology, 105*(2), 261–226. https://doi.org/10.1097/01.AOG.0000151988.84346.3e

Retnakaran, R., Ye, C., Hanley, A. J., Connelly, P. W., Sermer, M., Zinman, B., & Hamilton, J. (2012). Effect of maternal weight, adipokines, glucose intolerance and lipids on infant weight among women without gestational diabetes mellitus. *Canadian Medical Association Journal, 184*(12), 1353–1360. https://doi.org/10.1503/cmaj.111154

Rowe, R., Knight, M., Kurinczuk, J. J., & UK Midwifery Study System (UKMidSS). (2018). Outcomes for women with BMI>35 kg/m^2 admitted for labour care to alongside midwifery units in the UK: A national prospective cohort study using the UK Midwifery Study System (UKMidSS). *PLoS One, 13*(12), e0208041. https://doi.org/10.1371/journal.pone.0208041

Rubino, F., Puhl, R. M., Cummings, D. E., Eckel, R. H., Ryan, D. H., Mechanick, J. I., Nadglowski, J., Ramos Salas, X., Schauer, P. R., Twenefour, D., Apovian, C. M., Aronne, L. J., Batterham, R. L., Berthoud, H.-R., Boza, C., Busetto, L., Dicker, D., De Groot, M., Eisenberg, D., . . . Dixon, J. B. (2020). Joint international consensus statement for ending stigma of obesity. *Nature and Medicine, 26*(4), 485–497. https://doi.org/10.1038/s41591-020-0803-x

Ruiz, J. R., Perales, M., Pelaez, M., Lopez, C., Lucia, A., & Barakat, R. (2013). Supervised exercise-based intervention to prevent excessive gestational weight gain: A randomized controlled trial. *Mayo Clinic Proceedings, 88*(12), 1388–1397. https://doi.org/10.1016/j.mayocp.2013.07.020

Salihu, H., Alio, A., Wilson, R., Sharma, P., Kirby, R., & Alexander, G. (2008). Obesity and extreme obesity: New insights into the Black–White disparity in neonatal mortality. *Obstetrics & Gynecology, 111*, 1410–1416. https://doi.org/10.1097/AOG.0b013e318173ecd4

Santangeli, L., Sattar, N., & Huda, S. (2015). Impact of maternal obesity on perinatal and childhood outcomes. *Best Practice & Research Clinical Obstetrics & Gynaecology, 29*(3), 438–448. https://doi.org/10.1016/j.bpobgyn.2014.10.009

Smith, G. I., Mittendorfer, B., & Klein, S. (2019). Metabolically healthy obesity: Facts and fantasies. *The Journal of Clinical Investigation, 129*(10), 3978–3989. https://doi.org/10.1172/JCI129186

Steinig, J., Nagl, M., Linde, K., Zietlow, G., & Kersting, A. (2017). Antenatal and postnatal depression in women with obesity: A systematic review. *Archives of Women's Mental Health, 20*(4), 569–585. https://doi.org/10.1007/s00737-017-0739-4

Stirrat, L. I., O'Reilly, J. R., Riley, S. C., Howie, A. F., Beckett, G. J., Smith, R., Walker, B. R., Norman, J. E., & Reynolds, R. M. (2014). Altered maternal hypothalamic-pituitary-adrenal axis activity in obese pregnancy is associated with macrosomia and prolonged pregnancy. *Pregnancy Hypertension: An International Journal of Women's Cardiovascular Health, 4*(3), 238. https://doi.org/10.1016/j.preghy.2014.03.028

Sussman, D., Ellegood, J., & Henkelman, M. (2013). A gestational ketogenic diet alters maternal metabolic status as well as offspring physiological growth and brain structure in the neonatal mouse. *BMC Pregnancy and Childbirth, 13*(1), 198. https://doi.org/10.1186/1471-2393-13-198

Swartz, A., Strath, S., Bassett, D., Moore, J. B., Redwine, B., Groer, M., & Thompson, D. (2003). Increasing daily walking improves glucose tolerance in overweight women. *Preventive Medicine, 37*, 356–362. https://doi.org/10.1016/S0091-7435(03)00144-0

Tessier, D. R., Ferraro, Z. M., & Gruslin, A. (2013). Role of leptin in pregnancy: Consequences of maternal obesity. *Placenta, 34*(3), 205–211. https://doi.org/10.1016/j.placenta.2012.11.035

Tsai, P. J. S., Loichinger, M., & Zalud, I. (2015). Obesity and the challenges of ultrasound fetal abnormality diagnosis. *Best Practice & Research Clinical Obstetrics & Gynaecology, 29*(3), 320–327. https://doi.org/10.1016/j.bpobgyn.2014.08.011

Vena, F., D'Ambrosio, V., Paladini, V., Saluzzi, E., Di Mascio, D., Boccherini, C., Spiniello, L., Mondo, A., Pizzuti, A., & Giancotti, A. (2021). Risk of neural tube defects according to maternal body mass index: A systematic review and meta-analysis. *The Journal of Maternal-Fetal & Neonatal Medicine, 35*(25), 7296–7305. https://doi.org/10.1080/14767058.2021.1946789

Villarejo, C., Jimenez-Murcia, S., Alvarez-Moya, E., Granero, R., Penelo, E., Treasure, J., . . . Fernandez-Real, J. M. (2014). Loss of control over eating: A description of the eating disorder/obesity spectrum in women. *European Eating Disorders Review, 22*(1), 25–31. https://doi.org/10.1002/erv.2267

Vrebosch, L., Bel, S., Vansant, G., Guelinckx, I., & Devlieger, R. (2012). Maternal and neonatal outcome after laparoscopic adjustable gastric banding: A systematic review. *Obesity Surgery, 22*(10), 1568–1579. https://doi.org/10.1007/s11695-012-0740-y

Wansink, B., & van Kleef, E. (2014). Dinner rituals that correlate with child and adult BMI. *Obesity, 22*, E91–E95. https://doi.org/10.1002/oby.20629

Westerterp-Plantenga, M. S. (2016). Sleep, circadian rhythm and body weight: Parallel developments. *Proceedings of the Nutrition Society, 75*(4), 431–439. https://doi.org/10.1017/S0029665116000227

World Health Organization (WHO). (2022). *Overweight and obesity.* https://www.who.int/news-room/fact-sheets/detail/obesity-and-overweight

Wu, Y., Zhai, L., & Zhang, D. (2014). Sleep duration and obesity among adults: A meta-analysis of prospective studies. *Sleep Medicine, 15*(12), 1456–1462. https://doi.org/10.1016/j.sleep.2014.07.018

Wuntakal, R., & Hollingworth, T. (2010). Leptin-A tocolytic for the future? *Medical Hypotheses, 74*, 81–82. https://doi.org/10.1016/j.mehy.2009.07.039

Yao, R., Ananth, C. V., Park, B. Y., Pereira, L., Plante, L. A., & Perinatal Research Consortium. (2014). Obesity and the risk of stillbirth: A population-based cohort study. *American Journal of Obstetrics & Gynecology, 210*(5), 457.e1. https://doi.org/10.1016/j.ajog.2014.01.044

Zheng, Y., Klem, M. L., Sereika, S. M., Danford, C. A., Ewing, L. J., & Burke, L. E. (2015). Self-weighing in weight management: A systematic literature review. *Obesity, 23*(2), 256–265. https://doi.org/10.1002/oby.20946

47

Mood and Anxiety Disorders

Latrice Martin

The editors are grateful to Heather Shlosser, who authored the previous edition of this chapter.

Relevant Terms

Anhedonia—inability to derive pleasure from normally enjoyable activities

Cognitive behavioral therapy (CBT)—focuses on exploring relationships among a person's thoughts, feelings and behaviors; the core principles of CBT are identifying negative or false beliefs and testing or restructuring them

Hypomania—a set of distinct behaviors that are part of bipolar disorder; a milder form of mania

Interpersonal therapy—focuses on the relationships a person has with others, with a goal of improving the person's interpersonal skills by helping people evaluate their social interactions, recognize negative patterns, and ultimately learn strategies for understanding and interacting positively with others

Mania—seen in severe bipolar disorder; may include psychotic features such as hallucinations, delusions of grandeur, suspiciousness, catatonic behavior, aggression, and a preoccupation with thoughts and schemes that may lead to self-neglect

Paresthesias—the skin sensation of burning, prickling, itching, numbness, "pins and needles"

Rapid cycling—four or more episodes of depression and mania or hypomania within 12 months

Serotonin and norepinephrine reuptake inhibitors (SNRIs)—a class of medication used to treat depression and anxiety disorders, increasing the amount of serotonin and norepinephrine by blocking the reuptake process

Selective serotonin reuptake inhibitors (SSRIs)—a class of medication used to treat depression and anxiety disorders, increasing the amount of serotonin by blocking the reuptake process

---

Introduction

Mood and anxiety disorders in the antenatal and postnatal periods have become an urgent public health issue in the United States (Byatt et al., 2018). It is estimated that each year, 600,000 women suffer from perinatal depression, and this number may be higher when other mental health disorders are factored in (Postpartum Support International, 2020). The psychological distress of the global COVID-19 pandemic has weighed heavily on mental health in pregnancy (Vacaru et al., 2021). When psychiatric illness goes unrecognized or under-treated, the results can include poor adherence to prenatal care visits, exacerbation of medical issues, limited access to interpersonal and financial resources, smoking and substance use, suicide, and infanticide (Kendig et al., 2017). Subsequently, the lack of psychiatric illness identification and intervention can result in adverse maternal and neonatal outcomes, poor bonding, and other disruptions and dysfunction within the family unit. This chapter will discuss the assessment and treatment of depression, bipolar disorder, and generalized anxiety disorder (GAD) during pregnancy (Table 47.1). See Chapter 43, *Common Complications during the Postpartum Period*, for mental health disorders in the postpartum period.

Health equity key points

- People who are White are more likely to present with acute episodes of major depressive disorder; however, racial minority populations are more likely to have their daily functioning impacted by long-standing, chronic, and crippling depression.
- People of color with bipolar disorder are more likely to be misdiagnosed with schizophrenia than White individuals.
- African Americans, veterans, those with a history of trauma, substance use disorders, fear of childbirth or complications from a previous pregnancy are at higher risk for developing post-traumatic stress disorder in pregnancy.

Prenatal and Postnatal Care: A Person-Centered Approach, Third Edition. Edited by Karen Trister Grace, Cindy L. Farley, Noelene K. Jeffers, and Tanya Tringali.
© 2024 John Wiley & Sons Ltd. Published 2024 by John Wiley & Sons Ltd.
Companion website: www.wiley.com/go/grace/prenatal

Table 47.1 Definitions and classifications of select mood disorders

Major depressive disorder	Five or more of the following symptoms present during the same two-week period, represent change from previous function, cause clinically significant distress in social, occupational, or other areas of function, are not related to a medical condition or better explained by another psychiatric disorder, and have never been a manic or hypomanic episode. At least one of the symptoms is either depressed mood or loss of interest or pleasure. • Depressed mood most of the day, nearly every day • Markedly diminished interest or pleasure in all, or almost all, activities most of the day, nearly every day • Weight change (increase or decrease), not related to pregnancy or other medical conditions; loss of food enjoyment • Insomnia or hypersomnia nearly every day • Psychomotor agitation or retardation nearly every day • Fatigue or loss of energy nearly every day • Feelings of worthlessness or inappropriate guilt • Inability to think clearly or to make decisions • Recurrent thoughts of death, suicidal ideation or attempt
Persistent depressive disorder (formerly dysthymic disorder)	Depressed mood for most of the day, for more days than not for at least two years; Person has never been without the symptoms for more than two months at a time; if full criteria for MDD has been met during episode of illness, MDD diagnosis also applies. Presence of depression plus two or more of the following symptoms for at least two years: 1. Poor appetite or overeating 2. Insomnia or hypersomnia 3. Fatigue 4. Feelings of hopelessness 5. Difficulty making decisions or poor concentration 6. Low self-esteem
Manic episode	Abnormal, persistently elevated, expansive, or irritable mood lasting at least one week plus at least three symptoms. Symptoms cause marked impairment in occupational function, relationships, necessitate hospitalization, or have psychotic features. (not due to substances, medical condition): 1. Grandiosity or inflated self-esteem 2. Decreased need for sleep 3. Distractibility, attention easily drawn to irrelevant outside stimuli 4. Flight of ideas 5. Increased goal-directed activity 6. Increased talkativeness or pressure to keep talking 7. Excessive involvement in pleasurable activities with potential for painful consequences
Hypomanic episode	Abnormal, persistently elevated, expansive, or irritable mood lasting at least four days plus at least three symptoms (four if the mood is only irritable). Symptoms are not due to substances or medical condition. Episode is not severe enough to cause marked impairment in social or occupational functioning, no hospitalization, and no psychotic features: 1. Grandiosity or inflated self-esteem 2. Decreased need for sleep 3. Distractibility, attention easily drawn to irrelevant outside stimuli 4. Flight of ideas 5. Increased goal-directed activity 6. Increased talkativeness or pressure to keep talking 7. Excessive involvement in pleasurable activities with potential for painful consequences
Bipolar disorder I	One or more manic episodes; may have been preceded by or may be followed by hypomanic or MDD episodes
Bipolar disorder II	One or more MDD episodes accompanied by one or more hypomanic episodes
Cyclothymia	Chronic mood disturbance with numerous periods of relatively mild hypomanic and depressive symptoms over a two-year period

Source: Adapted from American Psychiatric Association (2022).

Care Concerns during Pregnancy

Two common factors among all mood and anxiety disorders in pregnancy are the need to balance risks of psychiatric medications in pregnancy with the risks of untreated mental health concerns, and the importance of pregnancy care providers working in close coordination with mental health providers.

Medications in Pregnancy

Informed decision-making in partnership between clients and providers regarding pharmacological interventions includes a clear discussion weighing the risks of medication use during pregnancy against the risks of untreated mood and anxiety disorders. Starting medications at a low dose and titrating slowly upward until remission is achieved is the recommended approach (National Institute for Health and Clinical Excellence [NICE], 2020). The US Food and Drug Administration (FDA) utilizes the Pregnancy Lactation Labeling Rule (PLLR), which replaced the pregnancy letter categories (A, B, C, D, and X) (Whyte, 2016), but many medications are still currently labeled under the former ABCDX category system. When determining whether to start, continue, or discontinue a medication, the provider needs to consider the patient's psychiatric history, medication history, prior nonpharmacologic treatment and effectiveness, current symptomatology, treatment preference, and risks and benefits to the client and fetus (Gorun, 2018). Shared decision-making, close follow-up, consultation, and referrals with mental health providers as needed are crucial to safely caring for pregnant people with mood and anxiety disorders. See Chapter 17, *Medication Use During Pregnancy*, for further discussion of prescribing medications for use during pregnancy.

Interprofessional Care

Initial interventions and reassessments always start with a patient safety evaluation, assessment of the most appropriate treatment environment, functional assessment, and evaluation of support systems. Frequent re-evaluation is necessary throughout pregnancy and during the postpartum period. A clear risk–benefit analysis of intervention versus nonintervention is essential and should be provided both verbally and in writing with the information being presented at the appropriate literacy level and preferred language. People with depression, bipolar disorders, or GAD in pregnancy are at a higher risk for exacerbation or new onset and could benefit from a mental health status assessment once per trimester, immediately and in the first few weeks after birth (Araji et al., 2020; NICE, 2020).

Interprofessional collaboration, referral, and/or comanagement with a mental healthcare professional is imperative for those with a high-risk score on one of the screening tools, indications of suicidal ideation, self-disclosure of concern, previous treatment in a pregnancy, or ineffective response to current regimens. Medication options and changes in pregnancy are decisions that are best made with interprofessional collaboration. For all psychological conditions occurring during pregnancy, **cognitive behavioral therapy** (CBT) or **interpersonal therapy** (IPT) should be encouraged and facilitated. A referral to a mental health specialist such as a psychiatric and mental health nurse practitioner (PMHNP), licensed clinical social worker, psychiatrist, or psychologist should be made when a person is struggling with a resistant mental health condition, is only experiencing a partial response to treatment, is a safety risk, or requires diagnostic clarification.

Depression during Pregnancy

Major depressive disorder (MDD) or clinical depression is a serious medical condition characterized by persistent feelings of sadness, apathy, and loss of interest that can lead to a range of physical and behavioral problems. Twice as many women as men are affected by depressive disorders every year (American College of Nurse-Midwives [ACNM], 2013); it is unclear if this is related to sex or gender. It is estimated that 7–20% of pregnant women globally experience MDD; however, only about one-fifth will receive adequate care (Shortis et al., 2020). People who are White are more likely to present with acute episodes of MDD; however, racial minority populations are more likely to have their daily functioning impacted by long-standing, chronic, and crippling depression (Bailey et al., 2019).

Multiple factors have been found to contribute to risk of depression in pregnancy. A prior history of depression or anxiety, extensive life or work stressors, lack of social support, unintended pregnancy, physical or sexual abuse, low socioeconomic status, limited education, smoking, lack of a partner, poor interpersonal relationships, genetics, pregestational or gestational diabetes, adolescent pregnancy, and pregnancy complications such as preterm birth and miscarriage have all been found to increase the possibility of the development or exacerbation of depression during pregnancy (American College of Obstetricians and Gynecologists [ACOG], 2018; Bailey et al., 2019; Curry, 2019).

Pregnancy itself can also be a risk factor for depression and may trigger recurrence of depressive symptoms in vulnerable people. It is unclear if elevated rates of postpartum depression are due to inadequate identification during the pregnancy versus a new disorder presenting in the postpartum period (AHRQ, 2020).

Potential Outcomes of Depression in Pregnancy

Untreated antenatal depression has been linked to adverse perinatal and neonatal outcomes in pregnant people and their children (Table 47.2). Stress related to depression may interfere with the development of the hypothalamic–pituitary–adrenal axis, the limbic system, and the prefrontal cortex in the developing fetus. Cortisol, which crosses the placenta, is a prime mediator of these effects. Increased cortisol levels that accompany depression have been implicated in higher rates of preterm birth and preeclampsia and higher rates of childhood cognitive and behavioral impairments (Jayasuriya et al., 2019; McGowan & Matthews, 2018). It is difficult to determine precise influences of prenatal depression on neonatal outcomes because of the comorbidities that often occur (e.g., substance use) and confounders (e.g., limited prenatal care and low income).

Screening for Depression in Pregnancy

Early detection of depression during pregnancy is critical since depression can cause adverse birth and neonatal health outcomes and, if left untreated, can persist after the birth.

Table 47.2 Untreated prenatal depression and potential outcomes

Outcomes in the pregnant person	Neonatal/Child outcomes
Poor nutrition	Preterm birth
Inadequate weight gain	Low birth weight
Substance use: alcohol, tobacco, drugs	Fetal growth restriction
Antepartum and postpartum hemorrhage	Low rates of breastfeeding initiation
Anxiety	Increased mental health problems: attention deficit hyperactivity disorder (ADHD), autism
Insomnia	Behavioral problems
Impaired bonding	Sleeping and eating problems
Worsening of depression	
Suicidal ideation and suicide	
Postpartum depression	
Preeclampsia	
Placental abruption	

Source: Bauman et al. (2020), Howard and Khalifeh (2020), and Miller et al. (2021).

Screening can be accomplished by routine data gathering about signs and symptoms of depression and by formalized depression inventories and should assess mental health history and current status including suicidal and homicidal thoughts, as well as social support systems and coping methods.

Screening should occur at multiple time points in pregnancy and can employ numerous screening tools, which have been validated for use during pregnancy (Table 47.3). The differential diagnosis should include bipolar disorder and other comorbid conditions such as anxiety, substance use, eating disorders, and psychosis or suicidality. Screening must be coupled with appropriate referral to a mental health professional for further evaluation and treatment as indicated.

Management of Perinatal Depression

Psychosocial Interventions

An integrative or multidisciplinary approach to treatment will offer optimal symptom relief for pregnant people with depression. A variety of effective nonpharmacological approaches exist, which can be used alone or in combination with pharmacological intervention. Discussing risks and benefits of all potential interventions, as well as risks of nontreatment, is key to optimal outcomes.

CBT and IPT are effective treatment options for mild to severe depression in pregnancy and should be part of treatment either as a sole therapy or in conjunction with medication (Howard & Khalifeh, 2020; Youssef

Table 47.3 Depression-screening tools

Screening tool description	
Personal Health Questionnaire— Depression (PHQ9)	• A nine-item depression scale based on the DSM-V (*The Diagnostic and Statistical Manual of Mental Disorders*, Fifth Edition) • MDD criteria • Used to help clinicians diagnose depression and monitor treatment • Available for free
Edinburgh Postnatal Depression Scale (EPDS)	• A 10-question self-rating scale • Efficient and effective • Available for free
Postpartum Depression Screening Scale (PDSS)	• A 35-item self-report tool • Identifies patients who are at high risk for postpartum depression • Available at cost

Source: ACOG (2018) and APA (2019).

et al., 2020). CBT and IPT may be short or long term and are typically facilitated by a clinical psychologist, psychiatrist, social worker, PMHNP, or psychotherapist. Other effective treatment modalities include facilitated self-help, mind–body modalities, exercise, and light therapy (Smith et al., 2019). Sitting in front of a specially designed light box for 30–60 minutes per day can alleviate symptoms of depression in pregnancy but is not recommended for patients with diagnosed or suspected bipolar disorder as it can induce manic or hypomanic states. Massage therapy has been found to significantly improve mood, reduce anxiety, and improve perinatal outcomes in pregnant people with depression. Yoga improves depression symptoms in nonpregnant people and can be safely used as an adjunctive therapy during pregnancy (Smith et al., 2019). Prenatal classes and group psychoeducation have also demonstrated some efficacy in the treatment of depression in pregnancy (Curry, 2019).

Effective adjunctive measures to treat depression

- Exercise
- Cognitive behavioral therapy
- Group prenatal classes, social support
- Interpersonal therapy
- Light therapy
- Massage
- Omega-3 fatty acid supplementation
- Yoga

Source: AHRQ (2020) and Curry (2019).

Starting Medications during Pregnancy

There has been a steady increase in the use of antidepressants during pregnancy, with over 14% of pregnant women filling a prescription for antidepressants in 2020 (AHRQ, 2020). For those who have been treated with antidepressants in the past and had positive symptom resolution, prescribing the same medication is a reasonable place to start. Treatment with a single medication at a higher dose is preferable to multiple medications (Table 47.4). For severe depression, pharmacotherapy with a **selective serotonin reuptake inhibitor** (SSRI), either alone or in combination with psychotherapy, is the first-line treatment (Langan & Goodbred, 2016; MacQueen et al., 2016). The SSRIs are the most widely prescribed antidepressants in pregnancy. For those with MDD and tobacco use, bupropion may be a reasonable option if anxiety is not a coexisting symptom.

Most antidepressants are FDA Pregnancy Category C, with the exception of paroxetine (Paxil), which is category D Although there is inconsistent evidence regarding association of congenital malformations with antidepressant use during pregnancy, overall, there is limited evidence of teratogenicity (Gorun, 2018; MacQueen et al., 2016; Ornoy & Koren, 2019). Exposure to SSRIs late in pregnancy has been associated with poor neonatal adaptation including symptoms of transient

neonatal complications such as jitteriness, mild respiratory distress, weak cry, poor tone, transient tachypnea, and neonatal intensive care unit admission (Gorun, 2018; MacQueen et al., 2016; Ornoy & Koren, 2019). These symptoms have been found in up to 30% of newborns exposed to SSRIs during the third trimester, and most often resolved with supportive care within a few days (MacQueen et al., 2016; Ornoy & Koren, 2019). The highest risk of poor neonatal adaptation is seen with the use of paroxetine, venlafaxine, and fluoxetine (MacQueen et al., 2016).

Mood disorders, environment, tobacco and alcohol use, social determinants, genetics, and the increasingly common treatment with SSRIs during pregnancy can all result in neurodevelopmental issues after birth, making it difficult to discern what is caused specifically by SSRI exposure. There have long been concerns around neonatal behavioral disturbances and socioemotional outcomes during the first year of life because of SSRI use during pregnancy. Recently researched areas of concern include increased risk of childhood motor development, language, mood, and autism spectrum disorders (Ornoy & Koren, 2019).

Table 47.4 Pharmacologic considerations in treating depression during pregnancy

Antidepressants
• Selective serotonin reuptake inhibitors
◦ Controlled studies have not been conducted in pregnant people
◦ Most SSRIs are pregnancy category C in the former ABCDX system
◦ Fluoxetine is the most studied SSRI in terms of general safety and efficacy; Patient registries of children exposed to fluoxetine during pregnancy do not show adverse consequences
◦ Sertraline and citalopram may be associated with an increased risk of septal heart defects; however, further studies are needed in this area
◦ Sertraline is found in very low doses in breast milk, while fluoxetine is found in high amounts (very long half-life)
◦ SSRI use in late pregnancy may cause self-limited neonatal behavioral syndrome
◦ Conflicting studies regarding the development of persistent pulmonary hypertension in the neonate exposed to SSRIs after 20 weeks of gestation
◦ Paroxetine—category D; Epidemiologic data show an increased risk of cardiovascular malformations (primarily ventricular and atrial septal defects) in infants exposed to Paroxetine during the first trimester (absolute risk is small)
• Serotonin norepinephrine reuptake inhibitor
◦ Controlled studies have not been conducted in pregnant people
◦ Venlafaxine can cause elevated blood pressure at higher doses and difficulty with withdrawal
◦ Pregnancy category C in former ABCDX System
• Norepinephrine and dopamine reuptake inhibitor—Bupropion
◦ Controlled studied have not been conducted in pregnant people
◦ Pregnancy category C in former ABCDX system
◦ Epidemiological studies do not indicate increased risk of congenital or cardiovascular malformations
◦ Not indicated for use in anxiety or panic disorder
◦ May be a good choice for people with MDD and tobacco use (aides in tobacco cessation)
◦ Higher doses can lower seizure threshold
◦ Do not use in people with anorexia, bulimia, or seizure disorder
• Tricyclic antidepressants
◦ Controlled studies have not been conducted in pregnant people
◦ Lowest known risks during pregnancy (amitriptyline, imipramine, and notriptyline)
◦ Overdose attempts with TCAs can be fatal
◦ High anticholinergic side effects
◦ Amitriptyline is pregnancy category C in former ABCDX System
◦ Clomipramine may be associated with increased risk of cardiovascular malformations

Source: NICE (2020) and Stahl (2021).

The **serotonin norepinephrine reuptake inhibitor** (SNRI) venlafaxine (Effexor) has been used in pregnancy, although on a much smaller scale compared to SSRIs. Limited data thus far suggest that this medication is not associated with congenital malformations (NICE, 2020). Tricyclic antidepressants (TCAs) have been widely studied in pregnancy and, except for clomipramine, do not appear to be associated with structural malformations in infants exposed in utero (MacQueen et al., 2016). However, due to their anticholinergic side effects and toxicity risk, they are typically reserved for treatment-resistant depression (NICE, 2020).

Continuing Antidepressant Use during Pregnancy

The decision about whether to stop or change medications is complex and should be made using shared decision-making after a discussion of potential harms and benefits. Pregnant people often feel uncertain and conflicted about making this decision. A systematic review and meta-analysis showed that up to 75% of pregnant women who use antidepressants discontinue them either on their own or after consulting with a provider, and single people and those with unplanned pregnancies are most likely to discontinue (Bayrampour et al., 2020). Interestingly, the risk of relapse was not increased during pregnancy for those who discontinued antidepressants when compared to those who continued except when depression was severe or recurrent (Bayrampour et al., 2020).

If depression is mild and the client is motivated to discontinue medication and implement lifestyle changes, this strategy can be appropriate. Withdrawal from an SSRI should be done slowly in a tapered fashion by 25% every one to two weeks to avoid SSRI discontinuation syndrome. Abrupt cessation of an SSRI can result in a wide range of physical manifestations such as flu-like symptoms, dizziness, gait instability, **paresthesias**, insomnia, and "shock-like" sensations, which typically resolve over the course of several weeks (Hengartner et al., 2020). Those who choose to discontinue medication should be advised of these transient symptoms and encouraged to use exercise, light therapy, and/or other modalities, and be monitored for signs and symptoms of recurring depression. A strategy of tapering off antidepressants in the third trimester to reduce neonatal withdrawal symptoms in people with moderate to severe depression has been reported; however, there is no evidence to support the effectiveness of this. Indeed, in some pregnant people, doses need to be increased in the second half of pregnancy because of metabolic changes during pregnancy (Bayrampour et al., 2020). It is important to review with clients that reducing their dose has not been shown to reduce fetal risk (NICE, 2020). Patients are advised to take the prescribed amount of medication to achieve remission of symptoms, and not to decrease dosage without consulting a provider (Table 47.4).

Complementary and Alternative Therapies

In an effort to reduce prenatal exposure to pharmaceuticals, pregnant people may consider herbal therapies to treat depression. St. John's wort (*Hypericum perforatum*) is a commonly used natural alterative for the treatment of depression, but studies on this herb have been short term and not well controlled (The Organization of Teratology Information Specialists [OTIS], 2020). Herbal supplements are not regulated by the FDA, and no standard for uniformity of dose or amounts and types of ingredients exists. St John's wort has a long half-life and can make other medications less effective, including some antidepressant and anticonvulsant medications (OTIS, 2020; Therapeutic Research Center [TRC], 2021). It is considered "possibly unsafe" for use in pregnancy due to some data showing teratogenicity, drowsiness, and lethargy in nursing infants and thus not recommended until more is known.

Omega-3 fatty acids have shown efficacy in improving symptoms of mild to severe prenatal depression (Grosso et al., 2016). The evidence is promising for the use of high doses, 1–2 g/day of eicosapentaenoic acid (EPA): docosahexaenoic acid (DHA) at a 2 to 1 ratio daily for those with depression and other mood disorders during pregnancy either as monotherapy or in combination with antidepressants (Bozzatello et al., 2020).

Bipolar Disorder in Pregnancy

Bipolar disorder (previously called manic depression) is a chronic condition characterized by periods of **mania**, depression, and, typically, a combination of both states. Bipolar disorder is a spectrum disorder with several different diagnostic categories. Mania and **hypomania**, a milder form of mania where the person remains able to function well in day-to-day activities, are the hallmark characteristics of bipolar disorder. Symptoms of depression become more common over the course of the illness. Bipolar disorder has an average age of onset in the mid-20s (APA, 2022; Youssef et al., 2020). The risk of relapse is not reduced during pregnancy and increases substantially in the postpartum period. Postpartum relapse of bipolar disorder ranges from 40% to 55% within the first six months postpartum and as many as 19% of people with bipolar disorder in pregnancy may experience postpartum psychosis (Perry et al., 2021).

The cause of bipolar disorder is unknown, although it is highly heritable (APA, 2022). Management of bipolar disorder in the perinatal period can be challenging due to women and caregivers' concerns about the safety of drugs during pregnancy and lactation, lack of routine screening for bipolar disorder, and misdiagnosis of bipolar disorder as MDD. People of color with bipolar disorder are more likely to be misdiagnosed with schizophrenia than White individuals (Akinhanmi et al., 2018). It is associated with an increased risk of antepartum hemorrhage, preterm birth, gestational hypertension, placenta previa, emergency cesarean birth, induction of labor and extremely small-for-gestational-age (SGA) babies (Sharma et al., 2020). People with bipolar disorder are at high risk for experiencing antepartum mood disorders and exacerbations during the postpartum period, even if they have experienced an extended period of stability prior to pregnancy. Studies showed recurrence rates ranging from 4% to 73%; however, those that remained on their mood stabilizers reported lower rates of relapse (Sharma et al., 2020). Bipolar disorder is associated with increased rates of comorbid medical and mental health conditions, and increased risk of substance abuse (alcohol, tobacco, and illicit drugs), poor nutrition and suicide, all of which increase risk for adverse effects on the fetus (Broeks et al., 2017).

Signs and Symptoms of Bipolar Disorder

Symptoms of bipolar disorder vary, depending on the phase of the illness cycle. The depressive phases tend to outnumber the manic phases, with depression lasting three or more times longer than episodes of mania or hypomania (Youssef et al., 2020). Depression symptoms with bipolar disorder are similar to those seen with MDD, such as excessive fatigue, insomnia, loss of interest, and suicidal ideation (National Institute of Mental Health [NIMH], 2020; Youssef et al., 2020). Manic episodes are characterized by periods of high activity, excitability, and impulsive behavior in varying degrees, as well as psychosis and hallucinations (Kameg, 2020). The manic phase may last from days to months. These symptoms of mania occur with bipolar disorder I. In people with bipolar disorder II, the symptoms of hypomania are similar but less intense. Psychosis does not occur in people who experience hypomania. Table 47.5 outlines the symptoms of bipolar disorder.

Mixed states or episodes in which symptoms of mania and depression occur simultaneously can be part of the disorder. High levels of energy, racing thoughts, and heightened irritability occur, along with feelings of sadness, hopelessness, and suicidal ideation. Mixed episodes are variable in length and are often followed by a phase of depression (APA, 2022).

Screening for Bipolar Disorder

Because of the variable presentation and recurrent episodes of depression, screening is often inadequate, and diagnosis delayed, sometimes for many years. The mood disorder questionnaire (MDQ) is a self-administered screening tool validated for use in the general population as well as in pregnancy, to screen for bipolar spectrum disorders (see *Resources for Healthcare Providers*). A simple screening method used in the office setting consists of asking two questions:

1. Have you ever had four continuous days in which you felt so good, high, excited, or "hyper" that other people thought you were not your usual self, or you got into trouble?
2. Have you ever had four continuous days when you were so irritable you found yourself shouting at people, or starting fights or arguments?

Those who screen positive (answer yes to either question) should be referred to a psychiatric professional for expert evaluation and treatment.

Management of Bipolar Disorder in Pregnancy

The goals of therapy for bipolar disorder are to reduce the frequency and severity of episodes, promote optimal functioning, and reduce the risk for self-harm. Both

Table 47.5   Bipolar disorder symptoms

Symptoms of a manic episode	Symptoms of a depressive episode
Mood changes	**Mood changes**
• A long period of feeling "high," or an overly happy or outgoing mood • Extremely irritable mood, agitation, feeling jumpy or wired • Increased energy • Racing thoughts • Talking a lot	• A long period of feeling worried or empty • Daily low mood or sadness • Feeling worthless, hopeless, or guilty • Loss of self-esteem
Behavioral changes	**Behavioral changes**

• Talking very fast, jumping from one idea to another, having racing thoughts
• Being easily distracted
• Increasing goal-directed activities, such as taking on new projects
• Being restless
• Sleeping little
• Poor judgment
• Poor temper control
• Having an unrealistic belief in one's abilities
• Reckless impulsive behavior
  ○ Binge eating or drinking, and/or drug use
  ○ Sex with many partners
  ○ Spending sprees
	• Feeling tired or "slowed down"
	• Having problems concentrating, remembering, and making decisions
	• Being restless or irritable
	• **Anhedonia** or loss of interest in activities once enjoyed, including sex
	• Changing eating habits
	• Trouble getting to sleep or sleeping too much
	• Pulling away from friends or activities that were once enjoyed
	• Thinking of death or suicide, or attempting suicide

Source: Adapted from NIMH (2020).

pharmacological and psychosocial interventions are used to reduce relapses and suicidal risk (Youssef et al., 2020). Pregnant people with bipolar disorder face a dilemma in determining whether to start or continue pharmacological interventions. All medication changes, including implementation, continuation, and even discontinuation, involve some risks that must be balanced against the risks associated with untreated illness.

Mood stabilizers such as lithium and antipsychotics are the mainstays of bipolar disorder treatment. Mood-stabilizing drugs are first-line medications and, in general, these medications are continued long term. Except for lithium, many of the mood-stabilizing medications are anticonvulsants, such as valproate, carbamazepine, and lamotrigine. New atypical antipsychotics like lurasidone and brexpiprazole are increasing in use, but reproductive safety data are limited (Sharma et al., 2020). Lithium is associated with an elevated risk for fetal cardiovascular anomalies, with risk increasing at higher doses (Kameg, 2020; Sharma et al., 2020). Fetal cardiac ultrasound in the second trimester should be considered in people taking lithium during pregnancy. Lithium levels need to be monitored during pregnancy with greater frequency due to the physiologic changes in blood volume (Sharma et al., 2020). Those who have been maintained on lithium and have not tolerated any alternative medications may be advised to taper off the medication with appropriate support before conception, and then restart in the second trimester if they do not plan to breastfeed (Creeley & Denton, 2019). This decision is balanced with the significant risk of bipolar symptom recurrence during pregnancy if medication is stopped.

The use of valproate in pregnancy is associated with a risk of neural tube defects, craniofacial anomalies, fetal valproate syndrome (distinctive facial appearance, anomalies and neurologic abnormalities), cognitive impairment, neonatal hepatotoxicity, coagulopathies, hypoglycemia, and withdrawal syndrome (Creeley & Denton, 2019; NICE, 2021). Table 47.6 shows the dosing schedule for lamotrigine. It is increasingly used in pregnancy for maintenance as a result of its efficacy and tolerability, as well as

Table 47.6 Dosing schedule for lamotrigine monotherapy

Weeks	Dose
Week 1 and 2	Lamotrigine 25 mg daily
Week 3 and 4	Lamotrigine 50 mg daily
Week 5	Lamotrigine 100 mg daily
Week 6	Lamotrigine 200 mg daily

- Bipolar monotherapy—200 mg is generally max daily dose
- Slow titration may reduce incidence of skin rash (Stevens-Johnson syndrome, toxic epidermal necrolysis, or drug hypersensitivity syndrome)
- If discontinuing, taper over at least two weeks to decrease risk of bipolar disorder relapse

Source: Stahl (2021)/Cambridge University Press.

increasing evidence of its safety (Creeley & Denton, 2019; Kameg, 2020).

Antidepressant medications, particularly SSRIs, are sometimes used to treat symptoms of depression in bipolar disorder. However, if they are used, they should be used cautiously because they can induce manic episodes and **rapid cycling,** four or more episodes of depression and mania or hypomania within 12 months. Antidepressant medications can also induce psychotic episodes in those with bipolar disorder. This is particularly problematic for those with undiagnosed bipolar disorder and depression symptoms.

Anxiety and Trauma-Related Disorders

As many as a quarter of pregnant people are affected by anxiety and related disorders, with negative associated outcomes including miscarriage, preeclampsia, preterm birth, low birth weight, alcohol consumption, smoking, and infants with poor self-regulation and neurodevelopmental problems (McCarthy et al., 2021; Xiong et al., 2021). During the COVID-19 pandemic, 43% of pregnant women experienced anxiety symptoms (Vacaru et al., 2021). Table 47.7 outlines characteristics of common anxiety and trauma-related disorders and their treatments.

Post-Traumatic Stress Disorder

Post-traumatic stress disorder (PTSD) prevalence in pregnancy is approximately 3% (Cook et al., 2018). In 2020, the COVID-19 pandemic contributed to an increase in rates of PTSD up to 19% (Sanjuan et al., 2021). People at particularly high risk for PTSD in pregnancy include African Americans, veterans, those with a history of trauma, substance use disorders, fear of childbirth, or complications from a previous pregnancy (Sanjuan et al., 2021). This race-based risk is proposed to be due to the impact of a long history of chronic and traumatic stress on cognitive, affective, and social resources (Gaffey et al., 2019). Early screening and intervention are key in preventing people with PTSD from being affected or triggered during the emotions and stresses common with pregnancy. The PTSD-Civilian checklist is a commonly used self-reported questionnaire validated for use in pregnancy (Gelaye et al., 2017). PTSD during pregnancy is associated with higher rates of preterm birth, postpartum depression, and impaired maternal infant bonding (Sanjuan et al., 2021).

Generalized Anxiety Disorder

GAD is a disorder characterized by excessive worries and anxieties about several different areas that are difficult to control, cause significant distress and impairment, and occur most days for at least six months. Twice as many women and adolescent girls are affected by GAD as men and adolescent boys (APA, 2022); it is unclear if this is related to sex or gender. Most individuals with GAD are found to have concomitant psychiatric disorders such as other anxiety disorders and unipolar depression and, to a lesser extent, substance use, conduct, psychotic, and neurodevelopmental disorders (APA, 2022).

Table 47.7   Common anxiety and trauma-related disorders: Characteristics and treatments

Disorder	Clinical presentation	Therapies	Pharmacological interventions
Panic disorder	• Extreme anxiety, fear, or sense of impending doom • Sudden onset of terror without warning and at times without provocation • Can occur anytime • Symptoms may mimic heart attack	• Cognitive behavioral therapy • Exposure therapy • Relaxation techniques • Pleasant mental imagery • Cognitive restructuring • Regular exercise, adequate sleep, regularly scheduled meals may help reduce attacks • Avoid caffeine or other stimulants	• SSRIs are most commonly used (Sertraline) • SNRIs are also an option • SSRIs and SNRIs can take 8–12 weeks to reach maximum therapeutic efficacy • Benzodiazepines may be considered after weighing risk versus benefit (physician consult is indicated)
OCD	• Severe anxiety, worry, or distress • Avoidant behaviors • Excessive time spent on parts of daily routine • Obsessions or compulsions • Odd or excessive behaviors • Causes significant impairment in daily life	• Exposure and response prevention therapy • Cognitive behavioral therapy • Relaxation techniques, pleasant imagery, cognitive restructuring • Regular exercise, adequate sleep, regularly scheduled meals may help reduce attacks • Avoid caffeine and other stimulants.	• SSRIs are first line (Sertraline) • Augmentation with an atypical antipsychotic may be warranted after weighing risk versus benefit in severe cases (physician consult is indicated)
PTSD	• Exposure to traumatic event • Somatic symptoms • Traumatic event is persistently re-experienced (flashbacks, dissociative states, acting or feeling as if the traumatic event is reoccurring, physiological reactivity on exposure to cues that symbolize aspects of the traumatic event) • Avoidance symptoms • Increased arousal symptoms • Causes significant distress in activities of daily living	• Cognitive behavioral therapy • Exposure therapy with response prevention • Supportive group therapy • Relaxation techniques • Eye movement desensitization and reprocessing	• SSRIs are first line • Benzodiazepines are not recommended in the treatment of PTSD • Prazosin may be used for treating nightmares (off-label) • Prazosin appears safe in pregnancy • Weigh risk versus benefit (physician consult is indicated)

Source: Stahl (2021)/Cambridge University Press.

Diagnosing GAD

Excessive anxiety, worry, and three or more of the following are needed for the diagnosis of GAD:

1. Restlessness or feeling on edge
2. Fatigue
3. Difficulty concentrating
4. Irritability
5. Muscle tension
6. Sleep disturbance

In addition, the anxiety, worry, or physical symptoms cause a significant disturbance in social, occupational, and other areas of functioning. Symptoms are not due to medications, drugs, or other physical health problems. Symptoms do not align better with another psychiatric problem such as panic disorder.

Source: Adapted from APA (2022).

Although few studies specifically focus on perinatal anxiety disorders, a growing body of literature indicates that symptoms are common. Perinatal anxiety must be differentiated from normal pregnancy-related concerns. Pathological worry usually focuses on fears about fetal well-being, uncertainties of the pregnancy, birth, and their ability to parent (Rathbone et al., 2021). Risk factors for GAD include low socioeconomic status, low self-esteem, substance abuse, adverse life events and stressors, history of physical or emotional trauma, and family history of GAD (APA, 2022; McCarthy et al., 2021). Antenatal anxiety is a strong predictor of postpartum anxiety and depression (Sinesi et al., 2019). There are few data regarding the risk to the fetus of untreated anxiety disorders during pregnancy. High levels of anxiety in pregnancy have been associated with preterm birth, SGA, spontaneous abortion, preeclampsia, excessive infant crying, postpartum depression, behavioral inhibition in infants, and less responsive and engaged interactions with the infant (Creeley & Denton, 2019; Kendig et al., 2017).

Women experience pregnancy-related anxiety (PrA) more often than they do GAD that occurs in a nonpregnant population (Araji et al., 2020). This has led to the development and use of the term PrA along with a growing body of literature. The length of time that symptoms must be present to meet the criteria for GAD complicates its diagnosis in pregnancy; thus, many pregnant people experiencing anxiety during pregnancy are not diagnosed prior to or during pregnancy. Many people who experience PrA have worries that are unique to the perinatal period and do not overlap with the typical symptoms of GAD. This separate and distinct diagnosis makes room for these specific and time-limited worries such as healthcare experiences, pregnancy-related social and financial issues, and parenting concerns. A distinguishing characteristic of PrA is that symptoms decrease in the third trimester, whereas with GAD, they increase (Araji et al., 2020).

Screening for GAD

A person's cultural background and societal norms can influence how the mind and body processes contribute to anxiety (Hofman & Hinton, 2014). There are significant cultural variations in the expression of anxiety that should be considered with all screenings and diagnostics around anxiety. Anxiety may present with physical manifestations and in other cases, cognition will be more affected (Ruscio et al., 2017). Numerous pregnancy and early-postpartum-specific self-reported scales have been found reliable and valid (Araji et al., 2020). The GAD-7 is a brief screening tool used in primary care to identify people with GAD (Sinesi et al., 2019). An excessive number of physical symptoms are often expressed by people with anxiety disorders. Therefore, people with multiple somatic symptoms in pregnancy, such as fatigue, irritability, tension, concentration issues, and insomnia, should be screened for anxiety disorders (Araji et al., 2020).

Management of GAD

Psychotherapy and medications are commonly used to treat GAD. Research has established that CBT is highly effective for anxiety disorders and should be considered first line (Araji et al., 2020). First-line medications for GAD are SSRIs and SNRIs. As with depression, sertraline, citalopram, and escitalopram should be considered as first-line agents during pregnancy.

Benzodiazepines are sometimes used to treat GAD. Benzodiazepine withdrawal syndromes may persist for several months after birth in fetuses exposed to high doses of alprazolam (Xanax), chlordiazepoxide (Librium), or diazepam (Creeley & Denton, 2019; Araji et al., 2020). Expert groups note that benzodiazepines do not pose a significant long-term risk if used in the first and second trimesters, may be safely used when needed, and tapering should be considered in the third trimester (Araji et al., 2020; Creeley & Denton, 2019). Diazepam and chlordiazepoxide are safe options to consider in the first trimester (Creeley & Denton, 2019).

Psychotropic drugs readily cross the placenta and could have effects on the developing fetus. People suffering from GAD in pregnancy may be encouraged to use additional nonpharmacological interventions such as mindfulness, meditation, exercise, and healthy diet (National Center for Complementary and Integrative Health, 2018). Treating people with GAD requires an engaged and nonjudgmental therapeutic relationship to explore worries and investigate treatment options using a patient-centered, shared decision-making approach.

Treatment of GAD	
GAD severity level	Intervention(s)
Mild	CBT, self-help reading, relaxation techniques, mindfulness/meditation
Mild to moderate	Pharmacotherapy with antidepressants (SSRI first line)
Moderate to severe	Combination pharmacotherapy with CBT
Moderate to severe, requiring more than one psychotropic, or resistant GAD	Refer to psychiatric-mental health provider

Source: Adapted from NICE (2020).

Summary

Although pregnancy can be a time of emotional well-being, as many as 20–40% of pregnant people suffer from mood or anxiety disorders. Particularly vulnerable are those with histories of psychiatric illness who discontinue psychotropic medications during pregnancy. All people should be screened for mood and anxiety disorders during pregnancy and again postpartum. Although data accumulated over the last 30 years suggest that some medications may be used safely during pregnancy, knowledge regarding the risks of prenatal exposure to psychotropic medications is incomplete. A growing body of literature suggests that the risk of adverse effects of untreated perinatal mood and anxiety disorders is high. When advising clients about treatment options, the severity of illness, history of symptoms when not taking medications, current medications, and plans for breastfeeding are important considerations. The presence of a stable support system and the availability of childcare assistance during the postpartum period are also important. Counseling is often an important component of a well-considered treatment plan. All treatment decisions should be carefully documented and discussed with the client, as well as with other collaborating or treating healthcare providers.

Resources for Pregnant People and Their Families

CDC: Depression during and after pregnancy: https://www.cdc.gov/reproductivehealth/features/maternal-depression/index.html

Health Resources and Service Administration. *Depression during and after pregnancy: A resource for women, their families, and friends*: https://mchb.hrsa.gov/sites/default/files/mchb/programs-impact/depression-during-after-pregnancy-en.pdf

National Child & Maternal Health Education Program. Action plan for depression and anxiety during pregnancy and after childbirth: https://www.nichd.nih.gov/ncmhep/initiatives/moms-mental-health-matters/moms/action-plan

National Alliance on Mental Illness: https://www.nami.org/Home

National Suicide Prevention Lifeline: http://suicidepreventionlifeline.org

Postpartum Support International. (2022). https://postpartum.net

Resources for Healthcare Providers

Center for Epidemiologic Studies Depression Scale Revised (CESD-R). : https://cesd-r.com/about-cesdr/

Edinburgh Postnatal Depression Scale (EPDS). English Version: https://perinatology.com/calculators/EdinburghDepressionScale.htm

Massachusetts General Hospital Center for Women's Mental Health: https://womensmentalhealth.org

Mood disorder Questionnaire—to screen for bipolar disorder: https://www.ohsu.edu/sites/default/files/2019-06/cms-quality-bipolar_disorder_mdq_screener.pdf

NICE *Antenatal and postnatal mental health: Clinical management and service guidance*: https://www.nice.org.uk/guidance/CG192/chapter/1-Recommendations#treating-specific-mental-health-problems-in-pregnancy-and-the-postnatal-period

Personal Health Questionnaire—Depression (PHQ-9) English Version: https://www.thenationalcouncil.org/resources/patient-health-questionnaire-phq-9/phq-9/?gclid=Cj0KCQjwuMuRBhCJARIsAHXdnqOer-AYICq6heew8K4VVmwG9wcpGPQJI0M1aOPFAsN9F5Jqv4zVk5gaAtT5EALw_wcB

References

Agency for Healthcare Research and Quality. (2020). *Maternal and fetal effects of mental health treatments in pregnant and breastfeeding women: A systematic review of pharmacological interventions*. https://effective-healthcare.ahrq.gov/products/mental-health-pregnancy/protocol

Akinhanmi, M. O., Biernacka, J. M., Strakowski, S. M., McElroy, S. L., Balls Berry, J. E., Merikangas, K. R., Assari, S., McInnis, M. G., Schulze, T. G., LeBoyer, M., Tamminga, C., Patten, C., & Frye, M. A. (2018). Racial disparities in bipolar disorder treatment and research: A call to action. *Bipolar Disorders, 20*(6), 506–514. https://doi.org/10.1111/bdi.12638

American College of Nurse-Midwives (ACNM). (2013). *Position statement: Depression in women*. https://www.midwife.org/acnm/files/ACNMLibraryData/UPLOADFILENAME/000000000061/Depression%20in%20Women%20May%202013.pdf

American College of Obstetrics and Gynecology. (2018). ACOG committee opinion no. 757: Screening for perinatal depression. *Obstetrics & Gynecology, 132*(5), e208–e212. https://doi.org/10.1097/aog.0000000000002927

American Psychiatric Association. (2022). *Diagnostic and statistical manual of mental disorders, Text revision (DSM-5-TR)* (5th ed.). American Psychiatric Association Publishing.

American Psychological Association. (2019, August). *Depression assessment instruments*. https://www.apa.org/depression-guideline/assessment

Araji, S., Griffin, A., Dixon, L., Spencer, S.-K., Peavie, C., & Wallace, K. (2020). An overview of maternal anxiety during pregnancy and the post-partum period. *Journal of Mental Health & Clinical Psychology, 4*(4), 47–56. https://doi.org/10.29245/2578-2959/2020/4.1221

Bailey, R., Mokonogho, J., & Kumar, A. (2019). Racial and ethnic differences in depression: Current perspectives. *Neuropsychiatric Disease and Treatment, 15*, 603–609. https://doi.org/10.2147/ndt.s128584

Bauman, B. L., Ko, J. Y., Cox, S., D'Angelo, D. V., Warner, L., Folger, S., Tevendale, H. D., Coy, K. C., Harrison, L., & Barfield, W. D. (2020). Vital signs: Postpartum depressive symptoms and provider discussions about perinatal depression—United States, 2018. *MMWR. Morbidity and Mortality Weekly Report, 69*(19), 575–581. https://doi.org/10.15585/mmwr.mm6919a2

Bayrampour, H., Kapoor, A., Bunka, M., & Ryan, D. (2020). The risk of relapse of depression during pregnancy after discontinuation of anti-depressants. *The Journal of Clinical Psychiatry, 81*(4), 1–9. https://doi.org/10.4088/jcp.19r13134

Bozzatello, P., De Rosa, M., Rocca, P., & Bellino, S. (2020). Effects of Omega 3 fatty acids on main dimensions of psychopathology. *International Journal of Molecular Sciences, 21*(17), 1–27. https://doi.org/10.3390/ijms21176042

Broeks, S. C., Thisted Horsdal, H., Glejsted Ingstrup, K., & Gasse, C. (2017). Psychopharmacological drug utilization patterns in pregnant patients with bipolar disorder—A nationwide register-based study. *Journal of Affective Disorders, 210*, 158–165.

Byatt, N., Carter, D., Deligiannidis, K., Epperson, C. N., Meltzer-Brody, S., Payne, J., Robinson, G., Silver, N., Stowe, Z., Sayres Van Niel, M., Wisner, K., & Yonkers, K. (2018, December). *Position statement on screening and treatment of mood and anxiety disorders during pregnancy and postpartum* [PDF]. APA Official Actions. https://www.psychnews.org/pdfs/Position Statement Screening_and_Treatment_of_Mood_and_Anxiety_Disorders_During_Pregnancy_and_Postpartum_2019.pdf

Cook, N., Ayers, S., & Horsch, A. (2018). Maternal posttraumatic stress disorder during the perinatal period and child outcomes: A systematic review. *Journal of Affective Disorders, 225*, 18–31. https://doi.org/10.1016/j.jad.2017.07.045

Creeley, C. E., & Denton, L. K. (2019). Use of prescribed psychotropics during pregnancy: A systematic review of pregnancy, neonatal, and childhood outcomes. *Brain Sciences, 9*(9), 1–42. https://doi.org/10.3390/brainsci9090235

Curry, S. J. (2019). Interventions to prevent perinatal depression. *JAMA, 321*(6), 580–587. https://doi.org/10.1001/jama.2019.0007

Gaffey, A. E., Aranda, F., Burns, J. W., Purim-Shem-Tov, Y. A., Burgess, H. J., Beckham, J. C., Bruehl, S., & Hobfoll, S. E. (2019). Race, psychosocial vulnerability and social support differences in inner-city women's symptoms of posttraumatic stress disorder. *Anxiety, Stress, & Coping, 32*(1), 18–31. https://doi.org/10.1080/10615806.2018.1532078

Gelaye, B., Zheng, Y., Medina-Mora, M. E., Rondon, M. B., Sanchez, S. E., & Williams, M. A. (2017). Validity of the posttraumatic stress disorders (PTSD) checklist in pregnant women. *BMC Psychiatry, 17*(1), 179.

Gorun, A. (2018). Choosing and discussing SSRIs for depression in pregnancy: A basic guide for residents. *The American Journal of Psychiatry Resident's Journal, 13*(6), 3–5. https://doi.org/10.1176/appi.ajp-rj.2018.130602

Grosso, G., Micek, A., Marventano, S., Castellano, S., Mistretta, A., Pajak, A., & Galvano, F. (2016). Dietary n-3 PUFA, fish consumption and depression: A systematic review and meta-analysis of observational studies. *Journal of Affective Disorders, 205*, 269–281. https://doi.org/10.1016/j.jad.2016.08.011

Hengartner, M. P., Davies, J., & Read, J. (2020). Antidepressant withdrawal – The tide is finally turning. *Epidemiology and Psychiatric Sciences, 29*, 1–3. https://doi.org/10.1017/s2045796019000465

Hofmann, S. G., & Hinton, D. E. (2014). Cross-cultural aspects of anxiety disorders. *Current Psychiatry Reports, 16*(6). https://doi.org/10.1007/s11920-014-0450-3

Howard, L. M., & Khalifeh, H. (2020). Perinatal mental health: A review of progress and challenges. *World Psychiatry, 19*(3), 313–327. https://doi.org/10.1002/wps.20769

Jayasuriya, N. A., Hughes, A. E., Sovio, U., Cook, E., Charnock-Jones, D., & Smith, G. S. (2019). A lower maternal cortisol-to-cortisone ratio precedes clinical diagnosis of preterm and term preeclampsia by many weeks. *The Journal of Clinical Endocrinology & Metabolism, 104*(6), 2355–2366. https://doi.org/10.1210/jc.2018-02312

Kameg, B. N. (2020). Bipolar disorder: Treatment strategies for women of childbearing age. *Perspectives in Psychiatric Care, 57*(3), 1244–1249. https://doi.org/10.1111/ppc.12680

Kendig, S., Keats, J. P., Hoffman, M., Kay, L. B., Miller, E. S., Moore Simas, T. A., Frieder, A., Hackley, B., Indman, P., Raines, C., Semenuk, K., Wisner, K. L., & Lemieux, L. A. (2017). Consensus bundle on maternal mental health. *Obstetrics & Gynecology, 129*(3), 422–430. https://doi.org/10.1097/aog.0000000000001902

Langan, R., & Goodbred, A. (2016). Identification and management of peripartum depression. *American Family Physician, 93*(10), 852–858.

MacQueen, G. M., Frey, B. N., Ismail, Z., Jaworska, N., Steiner, M., Van Lieshout, R. J., Kennedy, S. H., Lam, R. W., Milev, R. V., Parikh, S. V., & Ravindran, A. V. (2016). Canadian network for mood and anxiety treatments (CANMAT) 2016 clinical guidelines for the management of adults with major depressive disorder: Section 6. Special populations: Youth, women, and the elderly. *Canadian Journal of Psychiatry, 61*(9), 588–603.

McCarthy, M., Houghton, C., & Matvienko-Sikar, K. (2021). Women's experiences and perceptions of anxiety and stress during the perinatal period: A systematic review and qualitative evidence synthesis. *BMC Pregnancy and Childbirth, 21*(1), 1–12. https://doi.org/10.1186/s12884-021-04271-w

McGowan, P. O., & Matthews, S. G. (2018). Prenatal stress, glucocorticoids, and developmental programming of the stress response. *Endocrinology, 159*(1), 69–82. https://doi.org/10.1210/en.2017-00896

Miller, E. S., Grobman, W. A., Ciolino, J. D., Zumpf, K., Sakowicz, A., Gollan, J., & Wisner, K. L. (2021). Increased depression screening and treatment recommendations after implementation of a perinatal collaborative care program. *Psychiatric Services, 72*(11), 1268–1275. https://doi.org/10.1176/appi.ps.202000563

National Center for Complementary and Integrative Health. (2018, December). *Anxiety at a glance.* https://www.nccih.nih.gov/health/anxiety-at-a-glance

National Institute for Health and Care Excellence. (2021). *Pharmacological treatments for antenatal and postnatal mental health problems.* https://pathways.nice.org.uk/pathways/antenatal-and-postnatal-mental-health

National Institute for Health Care Excellence. (2020). *Antenatal and postnatal mental health: Clinical management and service guidance.* www.nice.org.uk/guidance/cg192/chapter/1-Recommendations

National Institute of Mental Health. (2020). *Bipolar disorder.* https://www.nimh.nih.gov/health/topics/bipolar-disorder

Ornoy, A., & Koren, G. (2019). SSRIs and SNRIs (SRI) in pregnancy: Effects on the course of pregnancy and the offspring: How far are we from having all the answers? *International Journal of Molecular Sciences, 20*(2370), 1–19. https://doi.org/10.3390/ijms20102370

Perry, A., Gordon-Smith, K., Di Florio, A., Craddock, N., Jones, L., & Jones, I. (2021). Mood episodes in pregnancy and risk of postpartum recurrence in bipolar disorder: The bipolar disorder research network pregnancy study. *Journal of Affective Disorders, 294*, 714–722. https://doi.org/10.1016/j.jad.2021.07.067

Postpartum Support International. (2020). *Mind the Gap: A strategic roadmap to address America's silent health crisis: untreated and unaddressed perinatal mental health disorders.* https://www.postpartum.net/wp-content/uploads/2020/06/Mind-the-Gap-National-Report-2.7.20.pdf

Rathbone, A., Prescott, J., & Cross, D. (2021). Pregnancy in a pandemic: Generalised anxiety disorder and health anxiety prevalence. *British Journal of Midwifery, 29*(8), 440–446. https://doi.org/10.12968/bjom.2021.29.8.440

Ruscio, A. M., Hallion, L. S., Lim, C., Aguilar-Gaxiola, S., Al-Hamzawi, A., Alonso, J., Andrade, L. H., Borges, G., Bromet, E. J., Bunting, B., Caldas de Almeida, J. M., Demyttenaere, K., Florescu, S., de Girolamo, G., Gureje, O., Haro, J. M., He, Y., Hinkov, H., Hu, C., . . . Scott, K. M. (2017). Cross-sectional comparison of the epidemiology of DSM-5 generalized anxiety disorder across the globe. *JAMA Psychiatry, 74*(5), 465–475. https://doi.org/10.1001/jamapsychiatry.2017.0056

Sanjuan, P. M., Fokas, K., Tonigan, J., Henry, M. C., Christian, K., Rodriguez, A., Larsen, J., Yonke, N., & Leeman, L. (2021). Prenatal maternal posttraumatic stress disorder as a risk factor for adverse birth weight and gestational age outcomes: A systematic review and meta-analysis. *Journal of Affective Disorders, 295*, 530–540. https://doi.org/10.1016/j.jad.2021.08.079

Sharma, V., Sharma, P., & Sharma, S. (2020). Managing bipolar disorder during pregnancy and the postpartum period: A critical review of current practice. *Expert Review of Neurotherapeutics, 20*(4), 373–383. https://doi.org/10.1080/14737175.2020.1743684

Shortis, E., Warrington, D., & Whittaker, P. (2020). The efficacy of cognitive behavioral therapy for the treatment of antenatal depression: A systematic review. *Journal of Affective Disorders, 272*, 485–495. https://doi.org/10.1016/j.jad.2020.03.067

Sinesi, A., Maxwell, M., O'Carroll, R., & Cheyne, H. (2019). Anxiety scales used in pregnancy: Systematic review. *BJPsych Open, 5*(1), 1–13. https://doi.org/10.1192/bjo.2018.75

Smith, C. A., Shewamene, Z., Galbally, M., Schmied, V., & Dahlen, H. (2019). The effect of complementary medicines and therapies on maternal anxiety and depression in pregnancy: A systematic review and meta-analysis. *Journal of Affective Disorders, 245*, 428–439. https://doi.org/10.1016/j.jad.2018.11.054

Stahl, S. M. (2021). *Prescriber's guide: Stahl's essential psychopharmacology* (7th ed.). Cambridge University Press.

The Organization of Teratology Information Specialists. (2020). *St. John's wort (Hypericum perforatum).* MotherToBaby. https://mothertobaby.org/fact-sheets/st-johns-wort

Therapeutic Research Center. (2021). *St. John's Wort.* Natural Medicines. https://naturalmedicines-therapeuticresearch-com.frontier.idm.oclc.org/databases/food,-herbs-supplements/professional.aspx?productid=329#pharmacokinetics

Vacaru, S., Beijers, R., Browne, P. D., Cloin, M., van Bakel, H., van den Heuvel, M. I., & de Weerth, C. (2021). The risk and protective factors of heightened prenatal anxiety and depression during the COVID-19 lockdown. *Scientific Reports, 11*(1), 1–12. https://doi.org/10.1038/s41598-021-99662-6

Whyte, J. (2016). FDA implements new labeling for medications used during pregnancy and lactation. *American Family Physician, 94*(1), 12–13.

Xiong, P., Poehlmann, J., Stowe, Z., & Antony, K. M. (2021). Anxiety, depression, and pain in the perinatal period: A review for obstetric care providers. *Obstetrical & Gynecological Survey, 76*(11), 692–713. https://doi.org/10.1097/ogx.0000000000000958

Youssef, N. A., Aquadro, E., Thomas, A., Brown, S., O'Connor, K., Hobbs, J., & Bishnoi, R. (2020). A primary care guide to bipolar depression treatment. *The Journal of Family Practice, 69*(7), 344–352. https://doi.org/10.12788/jfp.0043

48

Hematologic and Thromboembolic Disorders

Katie Daily

The editors gratefully acknowledge Jalana Lazar, Karen T. Grace, and Robin G. Jordan, who were authors of the previous edition of this chapter.

Relevant Terms

Alloimmunization/isoimmunization—the formation of antibodies in response to foreign red blood cell antigens introduced into the blood; in this chapter, this pertains to the introduction of fetal red blood cell antigens to the maternal blood

Antibody screen—an indirect Coombs test performed prenatally, screens maternal blood for IgG antibodies to a variety of erythrocyte antigens that may cause hemolytic disease of the newborn

Anti-D immunoglobulin—cold fractionated anti-D immunoglobulin used in pregnancy and postpartum to prevent alloimmunization of Rh D-negative pregnant people with Rh D-positive fetuses

Coombs test—blood test for hemolytic anemia, looks for antibodies on the surface of red blood cells (direct Coombs) or unattached to red blood cells (indirect Coombs)

Ferritin—storage form of iron; serum ferritin level is the most accurate method of assessing iron status

Fetomaternal hemorrhage—bleeding from fetal circulation into maternal circulation, most common at birth but can occur secondary to prenatal events

Folate—water-soluble B_9 vitamin, found in foods; term is often used interchangeably with folic acid

Folic acid—synthetic form of water-soluble B_9 vitamin

Hemolytic disease of the newborn (HDN)—destruction of fetal red blood cells by maternal antibodies that have crossed the placenta causing anemia, cardiac decompensation, hydrops, and fetal or neonatal death

Hydrops fetalis—an abnormal accumulation of fluid in a fetus: usually identified by ultrasound; may be associated with HDN

Kernicterus—brain damage caused by excess bilirubin (jaundice)

Kleihauer–Betke test—a blood test that measures transplacental bleeding, or how much fetal blood has crossed the placenta and mixed with maternal blood

Macrocytic anemia—a classification of anemia in which red blood cells are larger than normal (high MCV)

Mean corpuscular hemoglobin (MCH)—average amount of hemoglobin in red blood cells

Mean corpuscular volume (MCV)—average size or volume of red blood cells

Megaloblastic anemia—a type of anemia in which red blood cells are abnormally large and immature (usually seen in B_{12} or folate deficiency)

Microcytic anemia—a classification of anemia in which red blood cells are smaller than normal (low MCV)

Purpura—dark red or purple spots under the skin caused by breaking blood vessels, used interchangeably with petechia

Red cell indices—measurements of red blood cell size and hemoglobin content

Reticulocytes—immature red blood cells, reticulocyte count reflects how quickly RBCs are being produced

Rh D antigen—most immunogenic antigen belonging to the Rh blood group, historically responsible for most cases of fetal/neonatal hemolytic disease

Rh incompatibility—a condition in which a pregnant person has Rh-negative blood, and their fetus has Rh-positive blood

Rh sensitization—a response by the immune system in which Rh-negative blood is exposed to Rh-positive blood and develops antibodies to the Rh-antigen; also called alloimmunization or isoimmunization

Sickle cell disease—an autosomal recessive hemoglobinopathy in a homozygous form (hemoglobin SS or SC) in which a defect in the hemoglobin gene causes blood cells to form a sickle shape

Sickle cell trait—a heterozygous state in which a pregnant person has a combination of the normal adult form of hemoglobin (hemoglobin A) and hemoglobin S or C

Thalassemia—an inherited hemoglobinopathy that causes a reduced synthesis of hemoglobin

Thrombophilia—a group of inherited and acquired disorders that increase the likelihood of thromboembolic events

---

Prenatal and Postnatal Care: A Person-Centered Approach, Third Edition. Edited by Karen Trister Grace, Cindy L. Farley, Noelene K. Jeffers, and Tanya Tringali.
Companion website: www.wiley.com/go/grace/prenatal

Introduction

Hematologic alterations are common in pregnancy. Anemia is the most common hematologic disorder, but bleeding disorders and coagulopathies can also complicate pregnancy and postpartum care in otherwise healthy individuals. This chapter reviews the assessment, differential diagnosis, and management of the common hematologic disorders of pregnancy including anemia, alloimmunization, bleeding disorders, and coagulopathies.

Health equity key points

- Anemia affects people who are of low socioeconomic status more often, and standard education and dietary interventions are not always culturally relevant or accessible.
- Community-led interventions to address social determinants of health may be the most effective options to increase the intake of iron-rich foods, improve prenatal diet, and reduce anemia rates.
- Sickle cell disease, an inherited hematologic disorder most common among African American persons, receives far less research funding, pharmaceutical investment, and clinical center development than similar diseases common among White persons, such as cystic fibrosis.

Health Disparities in Prenatal Diet

Social determinants of health, more so than individual food choices, are primary drivers influencing pregnancy diet (McKerracher et al., 2020; Parker et al., 2019; Sabo et al., 2021). There are racial and socioeconomic disparities in the quality of prenatal dietary intake, specifically in core micronutrients such as iron, folate, and calcium (Parker et al., 2019). Providers need to be aware of the enduring legacy of racism that shapes health behaviors during pregnancy, access to healthcare, and interactions with medical professionals (Prather et al., 2018). This legacy includes the multigenerational exposure to inadequate diet that may contribute to rates of iron deficiency anemia (IDA) and associated poor birth outcomes (Prather et al., 2018).

A key federal program in the United States that attempts to address these disparities is the Special Supplemental Nutrition Program for Women, Infants, and Children (WIC). WIC provides supplemental food, nutrition education, and healthcare referrals to individuals who are low-income and pregnant or nursing, and infants (Sonchak, 2016). WIC program usage is associated with maternal weight gain in pregnancy and improved birth outcomes (Sonchak, 2016). An effective community-led intervention called Sisters Together reached out to childbearing-age African American families by offering food samples of affordable folate-rich foods in local supermarkets. The project increased awareness and intake of folate-rich foods among participants (Kannan et al., 2020). Addressing underlying issues of racism and creating community-level interventions, such as Sisters Together, hold promise to improve prenatal diets, reduce IDA, and improve childbirth outcomes.

Anemia

Physiologic Hematologic Changes in Pregnancy

Pregnancy is characterized by a dramatic increase in blood volume. The increase in blood volume includes a large increase in the plasma volume (40–50%) as well as a substantial increase in the red cell mass (15–25%; American College of Obstetricians and Gynecologists, 2021a; Blackburn, 2016; Monga & Mastrobatista, 2014). The disproportionate increase in the plasma volume in contrast to the red cell mass results in decreased hemoglobin, hematocrit, and red cell counts during pregnancy. This decrease is normal and is often described as the physiologic or dilutional anemia of pregnancy. These physiologic changes necessitate the use of different standards for evaluating common hematologic assessments such as the red blood cell (RBC) count, hemoglobin, and hematocrit during pregnancy (Table 48.1).

Table 48.1 Normal Hematologic Findings in Pregnancy

Component	Nonpregnant, female sex	First trimester	Second trimester	Third trimester
Hemoglobin (g/dL)	12–15.8	11.6–13.9	9.7–14.8	9.5–15.0
Hematocrit (%)	35.4–44.4	31.0–41.0	30.0–39.0	28.0–40.0
MCH (pg/cell)	27–32	30–32	30–33	29–32
MCV (mm)	79–93	81–96	82–97	81–99
Iron (mg/dL)	41–141	72–143	44–178	30–193
Total iron-binding capacity (mg/dL)	251–406	278–403	Not reported	359–609
Ferritin (ng/mL)	10–150	6–130	2–230	0–116
Vitamin B$_{12}$ (pg/mL)	279–966	118–438	130–656	99–526
Folate (ng/mL)	5.4–18.0	2.6–15.0	0.8–24.0	1.4–20.7

Source: Abbassi-Ghanavati et al. (2009) and Cao and O'Brien (2013).

All pregnant people should be screened for anemia at the initial prenatal care visit; screening is repeated between 24 and 28 weeks when hematologic indices are at their nadir (ACOG, 2021a). Anemia is diagnosed using a complete blood count (CBC). The laboratory diagnosis of anemia in pregnancy varies according to the trimester in pregnancy and differs from adult nonpregnant lab values due to physiologic anemia of pregnancy (ACOG, 2021a). Individual factors such as age, ethnic background, elevation from sea level, and smoking all impact hemoglobin values, yet, in practice, the same thresholds are used for the diagnosis of anemia.

Diagnosis of Anemia during Pregnancy

First trimester	Hemoglobin <11.0 g/dL	Hematocrit <33%
Second trimester	Hemoglobin <10.5 g/dL	Hematocrit <32%
Third trimester	Hemoglobin <11.0 g/dL	Hematocrit <33%

Once anemia is diagnosed, the cause of the anemia is investigated. Anemia can be categorized by whether it is inherited or acquired. Iron deficiency is the most common cause of anemia during pregnancy; however, a diagnosis of anemia should not be assumed to be caused by iron deficiency. In practice, clinicians can empirically treat for IDA with supplemental iron, while continuing the clinical evaluation of anemia. For mild to moderate anemia, RBC indices, serum iron, and ferritin levels should be evaluated. The most helpful lab value for assessing IDA is serum ferritin levels. Anemia in pregnancy may be due to deficiencies in iron, folate, or vitamin B_{12}. It may also be acquired due to chronic disease, hemolytic, aplastic, drug induced, or due to malabsorption (bariatric surgery). Anemia may also be inherited as in thalassemias, **sickle cell disease** (SCD), congenital hemolytic anemia and other hemoglobinopathies to be discussed later in this chapter.

The differential diagnosis of anemia begins with a careful examination of the **red cell indices** to evaluate the size of the RBCs and hemoglobin content of the cells, see Table 48.2. Cell size is evaluated using the **mean corpuscular volume** (MCV). If the MCV is over 100, it is considered macrocytic anemia, and in pregnancy, it is most likely related to folate deficiency. If the MCV is under 80, it is microcytic anemia and the most common cause in pregnancy is iron deficiency. Cell hemoglobin is evaluated by examining the **mean corpuscular hemoglobin** (MCH). Additional evaluation of hematologic parameters may be necessary to determine the cause of anemia. The measurements most commonly performed include serum **ferritin** to assess iron stores, hemoglobin electrophoresis to assess the types of hemoglobin present, and measurement of folate and vitamin B levels (Table 48.2).

Evaluation of the Red Blood Cell Indices

MCV	Normal 80–100 fL
	Microcytic <80 fL
	Macrocytic >100 fL
MCH	Normal 27–32 pg/cell
	Hypochromic <27 pg/cell

Iron Deficiency Anemia

IDA is the most common cause of anemia in pregnancy worldwide, accounting for 75–90% of all cases (Cantor et al., 2015). The higher incidence of IDA during pregnancy is from increased iron requirements coupled with inadequate dietary intake. Iron requirements are higher in pregnancy due to increased erythropoiesis and the growth of maternal tissues as well as fetal and placental iron requirements. Diets with a high proportion of processed food include only 15 mg of elemental daily iron and usually do not contain sufficient iron to meet the recommended daily intake of 27 mg of iron daily during pregnancy (ACOG, 2021a; Elmore & Ellis, 2022; Grieger & Clifton, 2015). Additionally, many pregnant people begin pregnancy with low iron stores due to menstruation, recent pregnancy, repeated pregnancies, as well as inadequate dietary intake and absorption. Other predisposing factors include living in poverty, malnutrition,

Table 48.2 Hematologic Conditions and Differential Laboratory Findings

Condition	MCV	MCH	Ferritin	Red blood cells
Iron deficiency	<80 but may be normal	<27 but may be normal	<12	Decreased Production
Thalassemia minor	<80	25–27	Normal range	Mild elevation
Thalassemia intermedia	<80	<25	Normal range	Moderate elevation
Thalassemia major	<80	<25	Normal range	Increased Production
Folate deficiency	>100	High end of normal range	Normal range	Decreased
Vitamin B_{12} deficiency	>100	Elevated	Normal range	Decreased

Source: Adapted from (ACOG, 2021a).

disordered eating, obesity, strict vegan or vegetarian diets, parasitic infections, or infection with *Helicobacter pylori*. Malabsorption, such as in pregnant people who have undergone gastric bypass or who have genetic malabsorption disorders, can also lead to IDA (Camaschella, 2015). This combination of a higher physiologic need for iron in pregnancy coupled with low iron stores and a diet low in iron results in most pregnant persons needing iron supplementation in pregnancy (ACOG, 2021a).

The Centers for Disease Control and Prevention (CDC) now recommends low-dose iron supplementation for all pregnant individuals due to the high rates of IDA in pregnancy (ACOG, 2021a). There are high rates of iron deficiency in people of reproductive capacity in the United States, with the highest rates in those with a parity over two, and adolescents (ACOG, 2021a). The required iron supplementation can usually be reached with adequate diet and a daily prenatal vitamin that includes an iron supplement. This approach improves maternal hemoglobin levels, decreases risks for IDA at term, and there is no known harm beyond the common gastrointestinal (GI) discomforts and side effects of iron supplements. Strategies to offset GI upset with low-dose iron supplementation are offered later in this chapter.

Pregnant people with untreated IDA are at greater risk of preterm birth, decreased milk supply, infants with low birth weight and lower mental and psychomotor performance, perinatal mortality, and cesarean birth (Abioye et al., 2016; ACOG, 2021a; Grieger & Clifton, 2015; Tran et al., 2014). Decreased iron stores have been noted in infants born to anemic people (Cao & O'Brien, 2013). IDA may also lead to higher rates of postpartum depression (ACOG, 2021a). Thus, the prevention, identification, and treatment of IDA are important during pregnancy.

IDA is a **microcytic anemia** and is the most likely cause of anemia when the MCV is less than 80 fL. Lab findings will include microcytic, hypochromic RBCs, depleted iron stores, low plasma iron levels, and low-serum ferritin levels, with a high total iron-binding capacity. Serum ferritin measurement is the most specific test that correlates with total iron stores in the body and is considered the gold standard for diagnosis of IDA. The normal range for serum ferritin levels varies during each trimester (Table 48.1). All providers should be aware of these normal changes in hematologic indices in pregnancy, so they do not overdiagnose or overtreat. When the ferritin level is lower than 12 ng/mL, the most likely diagnosis is IDA.

Symptoms reported in IDA include weakness, fatigue, dizziness, headache, shortness of breath with exertion, difficulty concentrating, restless leg syndrome, palpitations, sensitivity to cold, and irritability. Pica may also be noted. These symptoms mimic many common discomforts of pregnancy. Physical findings are usually only observed in severe iron deficiency and include angular stomatitis, glossitis, brittle, spoon-shaped fingernails, and skin pallor.

Treatment of IDA includes iron replacement and dietary changes. Iron supplementation of 30–60 mg of elemental iron daily is encouraged for all pregnant people and is easily accomplished with a daily prenatal vitamin that includes low-dose iron. For pregnant people with diagnosed IDA, daily supplementation of 60–120 mg of elemental iron is recommended, although caution should be used in areas of the world with endemic malaria as iron deficiency can be a protective factor against malarial infection (Goheen et al., 2016). Iron absorption is affected by the level of iron stores present in the body, the type of iron ingested, and whether the iron is taken with food (Camaschella, 2015). Absorption is increased if the iron is taken alone on an empty stomach, but this increases the potential for GI side effects. Thus, most providers recommend taking iron with meals. Iron will be better absorbed if taken with a food source of vitamin C, or with a vitamin C supplement. Iron will be poorly absorbed in those with an active *H. pylori* infection. Options for treatment of IDA include ferrous sulfate 65-mg elemental iron per 325-mg tablet or ferrous gluconate 34-mg elemental iron per 300-mg dose (available in a liquid form). Supplementation at 30 mg of elemental iron daily should continue for four to six months after the hemoglobin levels return to normal to rebuild iron stores. Common iron formulations are listed below.

Iron supplements

Preparation	Formulation
Ferrous gluconate	34-mg elemental iron per 300-mg tablet
	10-mg elemental iron per 10-mL liquid (Floradix®)
Ferrous sulfate	65-mg elemental iron per 325-mg tablet
Ferrous fumarate	106-mg elemental iron per 325-mg tablet
	Available in OTC preparations with vitamin C (Vitron-C®)

The most commonly reported side effects of iron supplementation are nausea, vomiting, abdominal pain, diarrhea, constipation, metallic taste, and dark stool (Camaschella, 2015). The GI side effects of iron supplements can be significant, and many people quit taking iron because of them. Intermittent dosing schedules of every other day or every three days can produce fewer side effects with similar elevations in iron stores (Pena-Rosas et al., 2015). Ferrous sulfate can be replaced by ferrous gluconate as it contains lower doses of elemental iron. Liquid iron supplements derived from plant-based sources may be better tolerated and are commercially available, such as Floradix (Tharpe et al., 2022). There are other alternative options such as black strap molasses, using cast iron cookware, and chlorophyll or alfalfa supplements to stimulate RBC production (Tharpe et al., 2022). An increase in the **reticulocyte** count is noted within several days of supplement start with stores replenished after several months of continued therapy (Pasricha et al., 2010). All iron supplements should be tightly capped and kept out of children's reach due to the potential for fatal poisoning.

There should be improvement in hematocrit and hemoglobin values after several weeks of treatment for IDA. A CBC and serum ferritin level should be repeated in 3–4 weeks to evaluate the response to therapy and possibly as soon as day 14 if the anemia is severe (Okam et al., 2016). Failure to respond to iron therapy should prompt further investigation into other disease conditions, malabsorption, and adherence to iron and diet therapy. Pregnant people may choose not to continue iron supplements if they have bothersome side effects, or they may take them with dairy products, thus reducing absorption.

Severe anemia, or IDA nonresponsive to oral iron, can be treated with intravenous (IV) iron in the second and third trimesters (Camaschella, 2015). It produces good results and leads to high maternal hemoglobin levels at term, fewer medication reactions, and greater likelihood of reaching the target hemoglobin levels that will stay at optimal levels for typically four weeks (ACOG, 2021a). IV iron should be considered in all cases when pregnant persons cannot tolerate oral iron, or those who present with moderate to severe iron deficient anemia late in pregnancy, who will not have time to build their iron stores with oral supplementation. Severe anemia is a hemoglobin level of less than 8 g/dL, as defined by the World Health Organization (WHO; McLean et al., 2009). It can also be given postpartum for quick resolution of anemia and may be used for people who hold a religious belief that prevents them from accepting blood transfusions. IV iron therapy is an effective tool to treat blood loss after postpartum hemorrhage. While parenteral iron was historically avoided because of anaphylaxis risk with older formulations, the newer formulations of parenteral iron are safer. Side effects of IV iron transfusion may include nausea or vomiting, itching, headache, or flushing. There are rare potential hypersensitive reactions with IV iron infusion; therefore, it is given as a slow infusion, with patient observation and in an environment with options for resuscitation (ACOG, 2021a; Camaschella, 2015; Wong et al., 2016).

There are rare cases of severe anemia in pregnancy that may require antepartum blood transfusions. This may be considered if maternal hemoglobin levels fall below 6 g/dL, when they are at risk for complications such as abnormal fetal oxygenation, abnormal or deteriorating fetal heart rate patterns, decreased amniotic fluid, fetal cerebral vasodilation, and fetal death. Postpartum indications for blood transfusion include severe anemia related to complications of postpartum hemorrhage in cases of instrumental delivery, uterine atony, placenta previa, retained products of conception, placental abruption, and in cases of HELLP syndrome with unstable vital signs (ACOG, 2021a).

Strategies to promote iron supplement tolerance

- Explain the need for increased iron.
- Discuss the side effects of iron and measures to avoid GI side effects.
- Increase water intake.
- Increase dietary fiber.
- Increase physical activity.
- Take supplements with food or at bedtime.
- Recommend stool softeners as needed.
- Prescribe lower dose of elemental iron or plant-derived iron.
- Change to a reduced dosing schedule if the side effects of daily dosing are intolerable.
- Take every other day.
- Replace standard pill prescription with plant-based liquid preparations.

Dietary counseling is also a mainstay of treatment for IDA (see Chapter 9, *Nutrition during Pregnancy*). Dietary iron comes in two forms: heme and nonheme. Heme iron is more readily absorbed than nonheme iron. Heme iron is found in animal products such as meat, poultry, and fish, with meat having higher iron content than fish. Nonheme iron is found in grains, cereal, eggs, vegetables, fruits, and dairy products and is consumed more than heme iron in a typical diet. Absorption of nonheme iron in the gut is reduced by other substances in nonheme iron foods. The addition of a serving of heme iron food with nonheme foods helps with the absorption of iron from the nonheme food due to the presence of meat protein factor, which facilitates iron absorption. Food sources high in heme and nonheme iron are listed in Tables 48.3 and 48.4. Those with a strict vegan or vegetarian diet are more prone to iron deficient anemia in pregnancy and postpartum.

People most at risk for IDA include individuals with a diet lacking in iron-rich foods, such as clams, oysters, liver, beef, shrimp, turkey, enriched breakfast cereals, beans, lentils, and those whose diet lacks the foods needed to absorb iron that are rich in vitamin C such as orange juice, grapefruit, strawberries, broccoli, and peppers. Some people also consume foods that prevent iron absorption, such as high amounts of dairy, soy, spinach, coffee, and tea. Other nondietary factors that contribute to IDA in pregnancy include short-interval pregnancies, GI disease, and pica. Careful diet recall with pregnant people, focusing on iron-rich foods, foods that facilitate iron absorption, and those that inhibit iron absorption should be part of counseling with all pregnant people.

Dietary counseling includes recommending a serving of meat, poultry, or fish with each meal to increase dietary iron and to aid the absorption of nonheme iron from other foods. Although organ meats such as liver are rich in iron, they are not recommended during pregnancy due to concerns for iron and vitamin A overload. Vegans and vegetarians may have more difficulty obtaining enough

Table 48.3 Food Sources of Heme Iron

Food	Milligrams per serving	Percentage of FDA daily value[a]
Oysters, canned, 3 oz	5.7	32
Beef, chuck, blade roast, lean only, braised, 3 oz	3.1	17
Turkey, dark meat, roasted, 3 oz	2.0	11
Beef, ground, 85% lean, patty, broiled, 3 oz	2.2	12
Beef, top sirloin, steak, lean only, broiled, 3 oz	1.6	9
Tuna, light, canned in water, 3 oz	1.3	7
Turkey, light meat, roasted, 3 oz	1.1	6
Chicken, dark meat, meat only, roasted, 3 oz	1.1	6
Chicken, light meat, meat only, roasted, 3 oz	0.9	5
Tuna, fresh, yellow fin, cooked, dry heat, 3 oz	0.8	4
Crab, Alaskan king, cooked, moist heat, 3 oz	0.7	4
Pork, loin chop, broiled, 3 oz	0.7	4
Shrimp, mixed species, cooked, moist heat, four large	0.3	2
Halibut, cooked, dry heat, 3 oz	0.2	1

Source: Data from Office of Dietary Supplements (2022).
[a] Based on Food and Drug Administration (FDA) recommended daily value of 18 mg.

Table 48.4 Food Sources of Nonheme Iron

Food	Milligrams per serving	Percentage of FDA daily value[a]
Ready-to-eat cereal, 100% iron fortified, ¾ cup	18.0	100
Oatmeal, instant, fortified, prepared with water, one packet	11.0	61
Soybeans, mature, boiled, 1 cup	8.8	48
Lentils, boiled, 1 cup	6.6	37
Beans, kidney, mature, boiled, 1 cup	5.2	29
Beans, lima, large, mature, boiled, 1 cup	4.5	25
Ready-to-eat cereal, 25% iron fortified, ¾ cup	4.5	25
Black-eyed peas (cowpeas), mature, boiled, 1 cup	4.3	24
Beans, navy, mature, boiled, 1 cup	4.3	24
Beans, black, mature, boiled, 1 cup	3.6	20
Beans, pinto, mature, boiled, 1 cup	3.6	21
Tofu, raw, firm, ½ cup	3.4	19
Spinach, fresh, boiled, drained, ½ cup	3.2	18
Spinach, canned, drained solids, ½ cup	2.5	14
Spinach, frozen, chopped or leaf, boiled ½ cup	1.9	11
Raisins, seedless, packed, ½ cup	1.6	9
Grits, white, enriched, quick, prepared with water, 1 cup	1.5	8
Molasses, 1 Tbsp	0.9	5
Bread, white, commercially prepared, one slice	0.9	5
Bread, whole-wheat, commercially prepared, one slice	0.7	4

Source: Adapted from Office of Dietary Supplements (2022).
[a] Percentage based on FDA recommended daily value of 18 mg.

iron from plant-based dietary iron sources, and supplements should be considered. Coffee, tea, and carbonated beverages inhibit the absorption of iron; it is recommended that these beverages not be consumed at mealtimes. Taking iron supplements with foods rich in vitamin C increases iron absorption. Daily intake of a combination of heme and nonheme foods will help improve the absorption of iron and provide a variety of foods to help balance dietary needs and improve overall nutritional status.

There are many dietary education classes, programs, and apps that exist to support pregnant people to eat a healthy diet, including iron-rich foods. Unfortunately, they are often not culturally relevant to diverse pregnant people's needs. A recent focus group study of pregnant Caribbean immigrants noted that dietary apps were not sensitive to their specific food preferences and did not offer food items that were readily accessible in their community or affordable (AlJaberi, 2018). However, there are examples of community-driven and culturally relevant nutrition programs that are meeting the needs of pregnant people. A program focused on pregnant people and school aged children living in the Navajo Nation addresses the loss of traditional foods and lifestyles that lead to less healthy diets by encouraging traditional Navajo foods, such as blue and yellow maize and cornmeals, lamb, and heirloom beans (Sundberg et al., 2020). Dietary counseling alone will not lead to healthier eating in pregnancy without considering social and cultural influences on eating habits. Care providers need to be mindful that their dietary counseling is culturally relevant to the families they serve.

It is important to build iron stores during pregnancy as the growing fetus has additional iron needs. During the second and third trimesters, the fetus is building up its own nutrient stores for extrauterine life. Iron stores accumulated in utero are the major source of iron for an infant in its first six months of life (Gernand et al., 2016). The greatest transfer of iron to the fetus occurs in the third trimester. If infants are born premature, without sufficient time to build those iron stores, or to a pregnant person with this micronutrient deficiency, it may negatively affect the infant's ability to reach normal growth and development milestones in the first six months of life (Gernand et al., 2016). Birth practices that include delayed cord clamping can help mitigate this issue by increasing infant iron stores and hemoglobin levels after birth (Elmore & Ellis, 2022).

Macrocytic Anemia

Common macrocytic anemias that affect pregnant people are related to folate and vitamin B_{12} deficiencies. These conditions should be in the differential when anemia is present with normal iron stores and with an MCV over 100. Confirmation of the type of macrocytic anemia can be done with follow-up labs for serum folic acid and vitamin B_{12} levels. Most likely, it will be folate-deficient macrocytic anemia. Treatment for this is a nutritious folate-rich diet, iron supplements, and 1-mg daily folic acid supplementation. If diagnosed with vitamin B_{12} anemia, it is often related to a history of gastric bypass surgery or underlying Crohn's disease and can be treated with vitamin B_{12} supplementation.

Folate Deficiency

The most common cause of macrocytic anemia is pregnancy is folate deficiency. **Folate** or **folic acid** is an essential micronutrient used for DNA synthesis; the need for folate is increased in pregnancy due to increased cell turnover. High rates of folate are needed in the early stages of embryogenesis between two and eight weeks of gestation when the neural tube is formed (Gernand et al., 2016). Prenatal folate deficiency is more common in pregnant people who do not consume dark leafy green vegetables, citrus fruits, and legumes. If folate deficiency is severe, **megaloblastic anemia** (formerly known as pernicious anemia of pregnancy) can develop.

Folate deficiency in early pregnancy is associated with pregnancy loss, neural tube defects, cardiac defects, preterm birth, preeclampsia, and placental abruption (Bodnar et al., 2010; Scholl & Johnson, 2000). It can have a long-lasting impact on neurologic development and is associated with smaller brain size, autism, and cognitive and behavioral problems in children of folate-deficient

pregnant people (Ars et al., 2016; Czeizel et al., 2013; Suren et al., 2013). Folate deficiency in early pregnancy has been reduced in the United States with the introduction of folic-acid-fortified foods in the early 1990s, including breakfast cereals, breads, flour, pasta, cornmeal, and white rice. However, folate deficiency can develop in pregnant people who do not consume folate-rich foods as stores are depleted starting in the second trimester. Other causes of folate deficiency include bariatric surgery, excessive alcohol consumption, and some antiseizure medications.

Symptoms of folate deficiency can be subtle. Hyperpigmentation of the digits and mucous membranes and a low-grade fever may be presenting signs and symptoms. Neurological symptoms such as numbness and tingling in the extremities, decreased metal alertness, and memory problems may be seen in folate as well as vitamin B_{12} deficiency. Vitamin B_{12} serum level should be evaluated prior to the beginning of folate supplementation as folate can mask the symptoms of a potential vitamin B_{12} deficiency.

Prevention and treatment of folate deficiency consists of supplementation and dietary changes. It can start during preconception care by recommending a folate-rich diet (Nypaver et al., 2016). A daily dose of 400-mcg (0.4-mg) folic acid is recommended for all people of childbearing age who are capable of pregnancy and throughout pregnancy. It is most important to have an adequate folate level prior to conception and in the early weeks of pregnancy to prevent neural tube defects such as anencephaly and spina bifida that can occur in the first weeks of pregnancy (Nypaver et al., 2016).

A diet rich in green leafy vegetables, lentils, beans, peanuts, and fortified breads and cereals is recommended during pregnancy to maintain adequate dietary intake of folate. Folate deficiency is treated with folic acid 5 mg daily for four months or throughout pregnancy. People able to get pregnant who are on antiseizure medications and people who have given birth to a child with a neural tube defect require doses of folic acid supplementation of 4 mg/day. Ideally, this higher dose of folate should be started in the months leading up to pregnancy to ensure adequate stores at the time of conception and into early pregnancy.

Vitamin B_{12} Deficiency

Vitamin B_{12} is needed for the production of RBCs, optimal neurological function, and DNA synthesis. During pregnancy, there is an increase in cell turnover, cell formation, and RBC production, and vitamin B_{12} stores can become depleted. Vitamin B_{12} levels decrease steadily throughout pregnancy with the lowest levels occurring near term. People at increased risk for vitamin B_{12} deficiency include those with a history of bariatric surgery or bowel conditions such as Crohn's disease, those who take metformin or proton pump-inhibitors, and those following a strict vegan diet. Dietary B_{12} is only found in animal food sources such as meat, eggs, and dairy products. While the incidence of B$_{12}$ deficiency in the United States is low, it is more common in subpopulations with limited food resources. Low maternal levels of vitamin B$_{12}$ increase the risk of adverse maternal and neonatal outcomes such as preeclampsia, recurrent pregnancy loss, fetal growth restriction, birth defects, and irreversible childhood cognitive and developmental delays (Finkelstein et al., 2015).

Symptoms of vitamin B$_{12}$ deficiency include a change in bowel habits, diarrhea, constipation, fatigue, shortness of breath, and loss of appetite. Clinical signs such as a swollen, red tongue, or bleeding gums may be present. Mental slowness, memory deficits, hallucinations, and numbness or tingling of the extremities may also be noted with vitamin B$_{12}$ deficiency. Laboratory findings include **macrocytic anemia**, MCV above 100 fL, and a low-serum vitamin B$_{12}$ level. Vitamin B$_{12}$ levels should be measured prior to the administration of folate supplements (Moll & Davis, 2017).

Dietary modifications are the best prevention for B$_{12}$ deficiency. Individuals who are diagnosed with vitamin B$_{12}$ deficiency in pregnancy are treated with supplementation, while those who follow a vegan diet or who have had bariatric surgery can benefit from vitamin B$_{12}$ supplementation as a preventive measure. Vitamin B$_{12}$ is available in multivitamin/mineral supplements, in supplements containing other B-complex vitamins, and in supplements containing only vitamin B$_{12}$. In addition to oral dietary supplements, vitamin B$_{12}$ is available in sublingual preparations as tablets or lozenges.

Alloimmunization of Pregnancy

Alloimmunization is an immune reaction against foreign antigens. It occurs in pregnancy when fetal RBC antigens are introduced to maternal RBCs, which produce antibodies against the foreign fetal antigens. In pregnancy, the most common cause of alloimmunization is related to the Rh D antigen. Mixing of maternal and fetal blood occurs most frequently during birth but can occur during other pregnancy events that cause bleeding, including early pregnancy bleeding episodes, spontaneous or induced pregnancy terminations, and incidents that lead to fetal-maternal hemorrhage at the placental site, such as trauma (see Figure 48.1).

Alloimmunization, also called **isoimmunization**, can have negative fetal and neonatal consequences. The ability to prevent alloimmunization or sensitization to Rh D-positive blood in pregnancy is perhaps one of the most important medical developments of the past century. The Rh alloimmunization program began with postpartum administration and achieved significant reductions in hemolytic disease of the fetus and newborn. Further reductions were achieved with antepartum administration of Rh D immunoglobulin. The current rate of alloimmunization in pregnancy is 0.14–0.2% and is primarily related to failure to follow established protocols (ACOG, 2021b). Universal screening of pregnant people for their Rh D status and the passive immune response elicited in Rh D-negative pregnant people via injection of Rh D immunoglobulin has resulted in a marked decrease in fetal and newborn hemolytic disease worldwide.

Rh Blood Group System

In addition to having a designated blood type (A, B, AB, or O), most human RBCs carry a Rhesus (Rh) antigen. The most significant of these Rh antigens is **Rh D antigen**. Those who carry the Rh D antigen on their blood cells are considered Rh-positive and those who lack it are Rh-negative. Approximately 15% of the US population has Rh-negative blood (ACOG, 2021b; Garratty et al., 2004).

HOW HDFN DEVELOPS

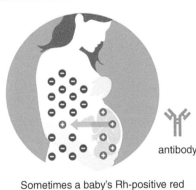

Sometimes a baby's Rh-positive red blood cells enter the Rh-negative mother's bloodstream

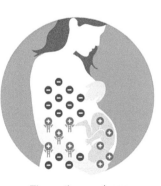

The mother produces antibodies against the baby's red blood cells. Usually, these anitbodies do not affect her first baby, but future Rh-positive babies are at risk

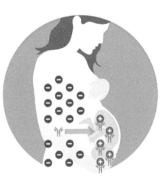

If the second baby is Rh-positive, the mother's antibodies will destroy the baby's red blood cells, putting the baby at risk for HDFN

Figure 48.1 How alloimmunization develops.

When an Rh D-negative pregnant person is carrying a fetus created from sperm by an Rh D-positive person, the fetus may have Rh D-positive blood; this is referred to as **Rh incompatibility**. Introduction of these foreign Rh D antigens into the maternal bloodstream can result in a maternal immunologic reaction of Rh D antibody formation and maternal sensitization, or alloimmunization. Maternal sensitization occurs in an unaffected pregnancy, as these newly developed antibodies are formed in maternal circulation. In future pregnancies, they are present and ready to attack the Rh D-positive fetal RBCs, resulting in **hemolytic disease of the newborn** (HDN). With each pregnancy, the severity of risk to the fetus increases. In severe cases, HDN can encompass **hydrops fetalis**, cardiac failure, and fetal death. The intrauterine fetal erythrocyte destruction can also lead to **kernicterus** of the newborn. **Rh sensitization** is not only of concern for pregnant people who have children in the future, but may also complicate cross-matching for blood transfusions. Rh-positive antibodies circulating in the bloodstream of an Rh-negative person otherwise have no adverse effects.

Not all individuals who are Rh-negative react in the same way when exposed to Rh-positive blood. In some Rh-negative individuals, only a small amount of Rh-positive blood (less than 0.1 mL) will provoke alloimmunization, and for others, sensitizing events require exposure to 30 mL or greater of fetal blood. To detect sensitization, the presence of maternal anti-Rh IgG must be identified. The indirect **Coombs test** confirms the presence of anti-D antibodies in the maternal serum and indicates if the pregnant person has been sensitized. To detect HDN, the direct Coombs test determines the presence of maternal anti-D antibodies bound to fetal RBCs.

Rh D-negative pregnant people who experience a **fetomaternal hemorrhage** are at higher risk of alloimmunization (see the text box "Causes of Fetomaternal Hemorrhage"). Other factors that increase the risk of alloimmunization include a positive **antibody screen** to another clinically significant erythrocyte, a history of a prior blood transfusion, and a history of IV drug use (Markham et al., 2016).

Causes of Fetomaternal Hemorrhage		
First trimester	Second trimester	Third trimester
Spontaneous/ induced abortion Chorionic villus sampling Ectopic or molar pregnancy	Invasive prenatal procedures such as amniocentesis, fetal surgery, or transfusion Blunt abdominal trauma	Fetal death Placental abruption Placenta previa External cephalic version Birth, vaginal or cesarean

Atypical Blood Group Incompatibilities

While Rh sensitization is responsible for the majority of HDN cases, there are more than 400 known RBC antigens, several of which can also cause HDN. Less common causes of HDN include antibodies directed at antigens of the Duffy blood group, Kidd blood group, and Kell blood group (Table 48.5). These blood antigens are screened for during routine prenatal care, but there is no immune prophylaxis available for these rare antigens.

Because of this, other blood group antigens, specifically Kell, have surpassed Rh anti-D as the leading cause of antibody-mediated HDN. Kell antigen is found on approximately 10% of the US population and has the potential to be more severe than Rh D sensitization (Goldman, et al., 2015). Anti-Kell antibodies are present in approximately 3.2 per 1000 reproductive-aged people, and prior transfusion with Kell positive blood is the primary route of sensitization (Goldman et al., 2015).

In the United States, RBCs are routinely cross-matched only for the ABO and Rh D blood groups, not Kell or other blood groups, thus making transfusion a primary source of Kell sensitization. If a pregnant person is Kell antibody positive, a titer is obtained, and if <8, serial titers are done throughout pregnancy, though it has been suggested that titers as low as 2 should be monitored in pregnant people with prior Kell sensitization (Van Wamelen et al., 2007). The American College of Obstetricians and Gynecologists (ACOG) maintains up to date guidance on

Table 48.5   Less Common Blood Group Antigens

Blood group system	Hemolytic disease–related antigen	Severity of hemolytic disease	Management
Lewis	Le(a), Le(b), Le(a-b-)	Not typically clinically significant	Routine prenatal care
Kell	K, k, Ko, Kp(a), Kp(b), Js(a), Js(b)	Mild to severe	Referral or consultation for fetal assessment
Rh (Non D)	E, C, C	Mild to severe	Referral or consultation for fetal assessment
Duffy	Fy(a), Fy(b), By(3)	Mild to severe	Referral or consultation for fetal assessment
Kidd	Jk(a), Jk(b), Jk(3)	Mild to severe	Referral or consultation for fetal assessment

Source: Adapted from (ACOG, 2018c).

management of pregnancies with Kell sensitization and practice bulletins should be reviewed for the latest management (ACOG, 2018c).

HDN can also be caused by an incompatibility of the ABO blood group. This can occur in pregnant people with type O blood carrying a fetus with a different blood type (type A, B, or AB). Type O blood contains naturally occurring anti-A and anti-B antibodies, some of which can cross the placenta. ABO incompatibility generally results in only a mild to moderate newborn jaundice, and unlike Rh D sensitization, it does not get worse with each successive pregnancy (Blackburn, 2016).

Anti-D Immunoglobulin for Prevention of Alloimmunization

Blood type (ABO and Rh) and presence of atypical antibodies is routinely determined at the first prenatal care visit. If there is presence of an anti-D antibody, then a thorough history is needed to determine if this is a passive response due to recent treatment with anti-D immunoglobulin in cases of early pregnancy bleeding, or if it is immune-mediated. If it was treatment-related, then routine prenatal care follows. If antibodies are present due to a potential sensitizing event, then protocols are followed for Rh D-alloimmunized pregnancies (see below). Pregnant people identified as a weak D blood type need prophylactic immunoglobulin and treatment as if they are Rh D negative in pregnancy.

Rh D sensitization is the only cause of HDN for which screening is routine. All Rh-negative pregnant people with a possibly Rh-positive fetus are offered Rh D antibody prophylaxis in the appropriate dosage at the appropriate time. Prenatal events that place pregnant people at risk for fetomaternal hemorrhage and sensitization include miscarriage, ectopic pregnancy, antenatal bleeding, chorionic villus sampling (CVS), amniocentesis, birth, and pregnancy-related uterine curettage. There are no adverse reactions or side effects in those Rh-positive pregnant people who mistakenly receive antibody prophylaxis or Rh-negative pregnant people who receive prophylaxis unnecessarily besides pain at the injection site, though cost and low supply may be concerns.

Anti-D immunoglobulin (RhIg; such as RhoGAM® or Rophylac®) is produced from donated human blood plasma. The plasma is donated from individuals with high-titer anti-D immunoglobulin G antibodies and goes through an extensive testing and filtration process for potential viruses (ACOG, 2021b). RhIg is given to pregnant people with Rh D-negative blood at 28 weeks of gestation and provides protection against alloimmunization for 12 weeks. The RhIg binds to Rh D antigens that may be in circulation creating, in effect, a passive immune response. All pregnant people get routine repeat antibody screening at the time of RhIg administration to evaluate for any potential missed sensitization events. Ideally, the antibody screen results are drawn and reviewed prior to giving RhIg; in practice, many administer it the same day antibody screening is done.

The antenatal RhIg dose covers the low chance of sensitization if fetal cells leak into maternal circulation in late gestation, which can occur even in the absence of a precipitating event. A repeat dose is also given within 72 hours after giving birth if the infant is determined to have Rh D-positive blood type. If the 72-hour window is missed, it is still advisable to give RhIg within 28 days of birth (Moise, 2008). There is the benefit of partial protection if given within 13 days postpartum, and some studies show partial protection for up to 28 days postpartum (ACOG, 2021b). If a pregnant person presents with risk factors requiring RhIg prior to 28 weeks of gestation, they will require a second dose 12 weeks after their initial dose to cover the possibility of a fetomaternal exchange during birth. Additionally, if pregnancy extends beyond 40 weeks, there is a theoretical need for another dose of RhIg before birth. Cases of alloimmunization with late-term pregnancies that did not receive a second dose of anti-D immune globulin have been documented, but they are very rare (Koelewijn et al., 2009). In clinical practice, it is uncommon for another dose of RhIg to be given to pregnant people with postdates pregnancies (ACOG, 2021b), but it may represent a missed opportunity. While great progress has been made in reducing Rh D alloimmunization, the cases that do occur are most often from failure to recognize a situation of possible fetomaternal hemorrhage and to recommend RhIg in a timely fashion.

When given in the second or third trimester, or after childbirth, the standard dose of RhIg is 300 mcg of anti-D immunoglobulin. This prophylactic dose covers up to 30-mL Rh D-positive fetal whole blood or 15-mL fetal RBCs (ACOG, 2021b). This dose covers routine prophylaxis for events such as a spontaneous abortion after 12 weeks. For antenatal hemorrhage events when the amount of bleeding is uncertain, or if a massive fetomaternal hemorrhage is suspected in cases such as placental abruption, manual removal of the placenta, placenta previa, intrauterine manipulation, or fetal death (ACOG, 2021b), the Kleihauer–Betke blood test can determine the amount of fetal hemorrhage and the dose necessary to cover the amount of hemorrhage (ACOG, 2021b). The **Kleihauer–Betke test** determines the percentage of fetal RBCs in maternal circulation. This test is routinely done for pregnant people who present with abdominal trauma to determine the amount of immunoglobulin required. Providers can administer multiple doses of RhIg, given IM at separate sites every 12 hours, until the full required dose is reached, or can consider IV administration.

The lower dose of 50- or 120-mcg immune globulin is given for induced medical or surgical abortions of up to 12 weeks of gestation. For terminations after 12 weeks, the standard 300 mcg should be given. Dosing is based on enough coverage for potential bleeding exposure, while limiting unnecessary use of a limited supply product.

For threatened pregnancy loss in the first 12 weeks, there is no standard evidence-based recommendation for management. It is unclear if pregnant people who experience vaginal bleeding with threatened abortion in the first trimester are at the risk of fetomaternal hemorrhage. If it does occur, the amount of exposure to fetal RBCs would be low, as the total fetal-placental blood volume at 12 weeks of gestation is approximately 3 ml (ACOG, 2021b). Since there remains a low risk of alloimmunization, and few risks of RhIg administration, many recommend the lower 50- or 120-mcg dose (ACOG, 2021b). If a smaller dose is not readily available, the larger standard dose is acceptable.

RhIg should be administered within 72 hours of a suspected fetomaternal hemorrhage event for it to be most effective. It is routinely given at the time of CVS, amniocentesis, and external cephalic version procedures, as well as with cordocentesis. Unfortunately, Rh D alloimmunization can still occur when antepartum events that could cause fetal-maternal hemorrhage are not recognized, when anti-D immune globulin is not given in the third trimester for routine prophylaxis, or when it is not properly given within 72 hours of any sensitizing event, including birth.

There are advances in fetal genetic testing that may lead to decreased need for testing and immune globulin in pregnancy and postpartum. One can determine fetal Rh status through noninvasive cell-free DNA. Care providers outside the United States are transitioning to this test-based strategy for the administration of antepartum immunoglobulin to reduce theoretical risks of exposure to plasma and reduce demand on the limited supply of this human plasma product. Other medical advances on the horizon include treatment for HDN; there are currently phase II clinical trials for monoclonal antibody treatment (ACOG, 2021b).

RhIg is a blood product and may be unacceptable to adherents of religions or cultures that refuse blood products. Rh D-negative pregnant people who are certain that their partner or sperm donor is also Rh D-negative and pregnant people who have had cell-free fetal DNA (cffDNA) tests that determine the fetal blood type to be Rh D-negative do not need RhIg. Rh D-negative pregnant people who decline RhIg should be educated about the mechanism of maternal alloimmunization and potential consequences, and their decision to decline despite this information should be carefully documented. If antenatal prophylaxis is declined, offer lab work every four weeks to monitor for sensitization.

Sensitizing events can affect a pregnant person's future health in their ability to be cross-matched for blood products. It is still of value to provide postpartum RhIg to individuals choosing to have no further children.

HDN, also referred to as erythroblastosis fetalis, is still an important cause of morbidity and mortality in countries without a program to prevent Rh D alloimmunization (ACOG, 2021b). In countries that do not have active prevention programs, 14% of affected fetuses are stillborn, and one half of affected liveborn infants suffer neonatal death or brain injury (ACOG, 2021b).

Identification and Management of Alloimmunization

If a clinically significant antibody is detected on a pregnant person's type and screen, the specific antibody and its immunoglobulin subtype (IgG or IgM) is identified.

Only IgG antibodies are of concern, as they can cross the placenta; IgM antibodies do not. If the antibody identified is known to cause HDN, the amount of antibody in maternal serum is determined and evaluated over the progression of the pregnancy. The critical titer level for each antibody differs. All pregnant people with a positive antibody screen of any clinical significance should have further evaluation, and those with critical titer levels are referred to the care of a maternal-fetal medicine specialist. Critical titers between 1:8 and 1:32 indicate significant risk for severe HDN and hydrops (ACOG, 2018c).

A sensitized Rh D-negative pregnant person who is certain about the partner or sperm donor should establish the blood type and antibody status of this person. If they are Rh-negative, no further management is necessary, because the fetus will also have Rh-negative blood, and thus be unaffected by maternal antibodies. If the partner's or donor's blood type is unknown or is Rh-positive, fetal blood group is determined by chorionic villi sampling, fetal blood sampling, or cffDNA testing, if available (Vivanti et al., 2016). If the fetus is Rh D-positive, the amount of maternal serum anti-D is monitored regularly. Additionally, serial ultrasound scans are done to evaluate the severity of HDN, including middle cerebral artery Doppler testing (ACOG, 2018c). Active hemolysis is indicated by a rising level of maternal anti-D. If a fetal blood test or antepartum surveillance confirms fetal anemia, depending on its severity, a blood transfusion can be done in utero to replace the lysed fetal RBCs.

The timing and route of birth for people who are alloimmunized are determined in partnership with the pregnant individual. Recommendations are developed from results of antenatal monitoring and determination of level of fetal hemolysis, balanced with the survival risks of premature birth. Blood transfusions may also be needed to correct anemia in the newborn period. During this period, there may also be a sharp rise in the level of bilirubin in the neonate, which can be lowered by phototherapy and exchange transfusions. These complications require the care of a specialty team that includes maternal-fetal medicine and neonatologists.

Kell antibodies (anti-K) can also cause erythroblastosis fetalis. These cases are often related to maternal exposure to a prior blood transfusion. Pregnant people with Kell antibodies need specialized fetal assessment. Alloimmunization with Kell antibodies can lead to severe fetal anemia and its course is less predictable (ACOG, 2018c).

Hemoglobinopathies

Hemoglobinopathies are inherited single-gene disorders that affect the structure, function, and production of hemoglobin. These disorders include SCD and thalassemia. Population migration has changed the geographical distribution and increased the incidence of hemoglobinopathies, while decreasing the efficacy of ethnicity as a predictor of risk. It is recommended that all pregnant people receive screening for hemoglobinopathies with red cell indices, during or before pregnancy.

Ideally, laboratory screening for hemoglobinopathies can be offered during preconception care visits to all people (ACNM, 2013; ACOG, 2017, reaffirmed 2020; Nypaver et al., 2016). The reproductive partner can be offered screening if any carrier screens present positive. If both partners are found to be carriers, they can be offered genetic counseling to review risks and options for future prenatal diagnosis and/or the use of assistive reproductive technologies (ACOG, 2020). Providers can expand opportunities for preconception health by considering every encounter with someone of reproductive age as a potential preconception visit (Nypaver et al., 2016). Screening for hemoglobinopathies starts with a complete CBC for all preconception and pregnant people to assess for anemia, and a review of their personal risk based on family history (ACOG, 2020).

Sickle Cell Hemoglobinopathies

SCD is an autosomal recessive disorder, in which a defect in the hemoglobin S gene causes blood cells to form a sickle shape. These distorted RBCs can lead to decreased tissue oxygenation, increased blood viscosity and hemolysis, and anemia. The cells can obstruct small blood vessels, blocking blood flow to vital organs and causing a vaso-occlusive crisis in the spleen, lungs, kidneys, heart, and brain. Over time, most people living with SCD lose function in the spleen leading to increased risk of infection (ACOG, 2018a).

Pregnant people who are heterozygous for the sickle cell gene carry only one copy of the abnormal hemoglobin gene. They have a combination of the normal adult form of hemoglobin (hemoglobin A) and hemoglobin S or C and are asymptomatic carriers of **sickle cell trait** (SCT). The trait is most common in people of African origin, with approximately 1 in 12 African Americans carrying SCT and 1 in 300 African American newborns diagnosed with SCD (ACOG, 2018a). Although ethnicity is a poor predictor of risk due to a changing multiethnic population, historically, SCT was common in populations of Greeks, Italians, Turks, Arabs, Southern Iranians, and Asian Indians (ACOG, 2018a). Diagnosis of SCT and SCD is made with hemoglobin electrophoresis during routine prenatal care screening.

People with SCT should be offered preconception counseling and include their partner in this visit to consider their own carrier risks (Nypaver et al., 2016). Pregnant people with SCT should receive genetic counseling regarding their infant's risk of SCD. This requires screening and genetic counseling of both biological parents. Because SCD is an autosomal recessive disorder, if both parents have SCT, there is a 50% chance that the child will have SCT and a 25% chance of SCD. If only one parent has SCT, there is a 25% chance of the fetus having SCT, but a 0% chance of SCD. In the event of both parents carrying SCT, prenatal testing of the fetus should be offered. Available options are invasive tests, such as chorionic villi sampling or amniocentesis, and noninvasive cffDNA tests (ACOG, 2018a). Pregnant people carrying a fetus diagnosed with SCD may choose pregnancy

termination or may benefit from prenatal consultation with a pediatric hematologist if they decide to continue the pregnancy. There are new advances in science in the treatment of SCD on the horizon, such as stimulating pyruvate kinase activity, a common inherited deficiency associated with SCD, and this finding holds promise to change the outlook for the disease course (Thein, 2022).

Other than offering fetal genetic testing, prenatal care of pregnant people with SCT is the same as for people with hemoglobin AA, with one exception. Though evidence is contradictory, SCT may be a risk factor for urinary tract infection in pregnancy, and people with SCT are screened at least once per trimester (Jans et al., 2010; Thurman et al., 2006). Postnatal care is similarly routine, though increased vigilance for venous thromboembolism (VTE), especially pulmonary embolism, may be warranted (Little et al., 2017).

When people have the homozygous form of this hemoglobinopathy (hemoglobin SS or SC) they have SCD. Hemoglobin SC is generally a less severe form of SCD than hemoglobin SS. Although SCD is associated with multiple acute and chronic medical problems, the majority of children born with SCD in the United States survive into adulthood. They can experience acute ischemic vaso-occlusive pain crises due to vascular occlusion caused by irregularly shaped hemoglobin molecules, which also have decreased oxygen-carrying capacity. Acute chest syndrome, spleen and liver sequestration, and overt stroke are other acute complications. Chronic health problems include hypertension, pulmonary hypertension, anemia, cholelithiasis, and renal dysfunction (Balachandren et al., 2016).

The incidence of vaso-occlusive crises with SCD may increase during pregnancy. This condition is also associated with serious pregnancy complications including infection, pulmonary complications, hypertension, preeclampsia, fetal growth restriction, low birth weight babies, spontaneous abortion, fetal demise, premature rupture of membranes, antepartum hospitalization, and preterm birth (ACOG, 2018a; Balachandren et al., 2016; Oteng-Ntim et al., 2014). Pregnant people with SCD are also at much higher risk of thromboembolic events such as acute chest syndrome (ACOG, 2018a; Balachandren et al., 2016). Their specialized prenatal care plan will include high doses of folic acid (4 mg daily) and support to avoid events that can lead to sickle crisis, including cold temperatures, heavy physical exercise, dehydration, and stress. Pregnant people living with SCD should be transferred to care by a multidisciplinary team to include a maternal-fetal medicine specialist, hematologist, and anesthesiologist and should plan to give birth in a facility with appropriate resources (ACOG, 2018a). However, it is important to remember that individuals with complex conditions still need the normal prenatal care and education provided to all pregnant people. Birth planning should include options for pain relief and route of birth based on the course of the disorder and the pregnancy.

During a preconception visit for a person with SCD, the risks of complications during pregnancy are discussed.

People with SCD should have an established relationship with a primary care doctor and maternal-fetal medicine specialist. The importance of proper hydration, avoidance of the cold, and decreasing stress in the management of sickle cell crisis are also emphasized. Medications are reviewed for possible teratogenic effects. This includes any pain medications such as nonsteroidal anti-inflammatory drugs, which should not be used before 12 weeks of gestation or after 28 weeks of gestation. People seeking pregnancy with SCD should take a folic acid supplement of 4 mg daily; prophylactic antibiotics and vitamin D supplementation may also be indicated (Balachandren et al., 2016). If the partner or sperm donor has not had genetic screening to determine the presence of hemoglobin S, this should ideally occur during the preconception period. Routine iron supplementation is not recommended for pregnant people with SCD unless there is an identified iron deficiency.

Thalassemia

Thalassemia is a genetic hemoglobinopathy caused by a decrease in the synthesis of the globulin chains of the hemoglobin molecule leading to microcytic anemia (ACOG, 2018a). The most common types of thalassemia are alpha thalassemia and beta thalassemia, which describes the specific globulin chain of the hemoglobin molecule that is affected. There are three classifications of thalassemia that describe the severity of symptoms: minor, which is the carrier or trait status, intermedia, and major, which is the most severely affected. Clinical presentation may range from mild anemia (as in alpha thalassemia minor) to severe anemia, poor growth, and childhood death (as in beta thalassemia major). The condition is most prevalent in people from the Mediterranean, Northern Africa, the Middle East, and southern Asia, but migration and interethnic relationships have made thalassemia a global issue.

Similar to other hemoglobinopathies, the recommendation is to offer genetic screening to all pregnant persons with hemoglobin electrophoresis plus a CBC. Screening is offered during preconception care and to a potential reproductive partner if trait status is identified (ACOG, 2018a). If both future parents are carriers, then preconception genetic counseling is recommended, and families offered options for reproductive assistance with embryo transfer and preimplantation genetic diagnosis.

Thalassemia should be considered as a differential diagnosis in individuals with hypochromic, microcytic anemia. An MCH is used to differentiate between thalassemia minor, major, and intermedia. In thalassemia minor, the MCH is moderately low (25–27). A person with an MCH below 25 should be screened for thalassemia major and intermedia. A ferritin level as well as a hemoglobin electrophoresis should be completed to rule out IDA and to evaluate the hemoglobin type and structure.

Pregnant people with alpha or beta thalassemia minor are at increased risk for having a child with the more severe form of thalassemia (ACOG, 2018a). Those more

at risk for alpha carrier status based on ethnicity include those of Southeast Asian, African, West Indian, or Mediterranean descent. Alpha thalassemia minor does not usually affect pregnancy beyond a diagnosis of anemia (ACOG, 2020). Beta thalassemia minor can vary in severity, though often results in similar mild asymptomatic anemia (ACOG, 2018a). Ethnic groups more at risk of beta minor thalassemia include those of Mediterranean, Middle Eastern, Hispanic, and West Indian descent (ACOG, 2018a). Overall, minor or carrier status most commonly leads to higher rates of anemia in pregnancy that can be managed routinely.

People diagnosed with thalassemia major or intermedia should be referred for specialized care, as they are at risk for cardiac failure, alloimmunization, viral infections, thrombosis, endocrine, and bone disorders (Petrakos et al., 2016). Pregnant people with alpha thalassemia major are at risk for complications such as hydrops fetalis, intrauterine fetal death, and preeclampsia (ACOG, 2018a). Improvements in medical care, specifically transfusion therapy and iron chelation, have allowed people with thalassemia (primarily beta type) to survive to reproductive age, while in the past, early mortality was common. Those living with beta thalassemia major can have severe anemia, delayed sexual development, and poor growth in childhood unless they receive early diagnosis and treatment with periodic blood transfusions (ACOG, 2018a). It is still rare to have a pregnant person with beta thalassemia major due to their disease-related complications of growth and sexual development that can often lead to infertility. They will need a multidisciplinary care team in pregnancy.

Early genetic screening of the partner or sperm donor is advised for a pregnant person with thalassemia. If both parents are confirmed carriers of the same thalassemia genetic mutation (i.e., alpha or beta), the possibility of the fetus having thalassemia major is one in four. For these cases, further genetic counseling and analysis is offered, in the same manner as couples where both are found to have SCT. Fetal diagnostic testing can be performed using CVS at 10–12 weeks of gestation or amniocentesis after 15 weeks. Many families who receive the diagnosis of an affected fetus choose to continue the pregnancy as the disease varies in severity, and it can be difficult to predict its course (ACOG, 2018a). Affected fetuses will need close surveillance and supervision by maternal-fetal medicine specialists.

Bleeding Disorders

Thrombocytopenia

Thrombocytopenia is defined as a decrease in the serum platelet count below 150,000 mm^{-3} and can have many causes when it occurs during pregnancy. An estimated 7–12% of pregnancies at term are found to be affected by thrombocytopenia (ACOG, 2019a). Normal physiologic changes in pregnancy (usually increased platelet destruction rather than decreased platelet production) can lead to a gradual decrease in platelet levels into the third trimester, and it can be normal for platelet counts to fall to ranges of 120,000–150,000 mm^{-3} without concomitant disease or pathology.

Clinically significant thrombocytopenia can be inherited or acquired through conditions such as folate deficiency, preeclampsia, HELLP syndrome, and extensive hemorrhage causing consumptive coagulopathy. It can also be drug induced. A provider can differentiate the potential causes of thrombocytopenia through detailed medical and family history, physical exam, and appropriate lab work (ACOG, 2019a).

Further investigation is required if the person has a history of thrombocytopenia prior to pregnancy, if thrombocytopenia occurs in the first or second trimester, if the platelet count is below 75,000 mm^{-3} in the third trimester, or if there are complications related to thrombocytopenia (ACOG, 2019a). This can include screening for evidence of preeclampsia, HELLP syndrome, coagulopathy, or autoimmune diseases.

Causes of thrombocytopenia in pregnancy

- Gestational thrombocytopenia (GT)
- Hypertension in pregnancy: preeclampsia-eclampsia, HELLP syndrome
- Drugs that reduce platelets (e.g., quinidine, sulfonamides, and nonsteroidal anti-inflammatory drugs [NSAIDs])
- Folate deficiency
- Immune thrombocytopenia purpura (ITP)
- Thrombotic thrombocytopenia purpura (TTP)
- Normal physiologic changes of pregnancy

GT is a benign self-limiting condition that typically occurs in the third trimester of pregnancy and resolves by one to two months postpartum. It is the most common type of thrombocytopenia in pregnancy, accounting for approximately 80% of cases, and is diagnosed by exclusion (ACOG, 2019a). If there is a new onset of thrombocytopenia in pregnancy, assess for other signs or symptoms that may indicate preeclampsia or HELLP syndrome, and be alert that it may be developing. Platelet counts often decrease before the clinical signs of preeclampsia present (ACOG, 2019a). People can start pregnancy with normal platelet counts that fall to levels generally above 75,000 mm^{-3} without symptoms. GT is managed with routine follow-up platelet counts, often at every prenatal care visit, or at least monthly, and repeated at one to three months postpartum to ensure resolution (ACOG, 2019a). No other treatment is necessary, as long as platelets range between 100,000–150,000 mm^{-3} and the person remains asymptomatic.

ITP is a rare autoimmune condition occurring more often in people assigned female at birth of reproductive capacity that can have severe consequences. It is considered as a potential diagnosis when platelet counts fall below 100,000 mm^{-3} and highly likely as the diagnosis when platelets reach the severe range of less than 50,000 mm^{-3}. ITP occurs when the body produces antibodies directed against platelet components, ultimately destroying them. It rarely causes maternal bleeding in pregnancy beyond minor mucosal or subcutaneous episodes, but can cause increased rates of postpartum hemorrhage, if platelets fall below 50,000 mm^{-3} (ACOG, 2019a). ITP can cause fetal or neonatal thrombocytopenia, the platelet equivalent of HDN, regardless of maternal severity (Neunert et al., 2011; ACOG, Bulletin 207, 2019a). ITP may not be symptomatic during pregnancy and birth, and yet within hours of birth lead to clinical signs in the neonate of generalized petechiae, ecchymosis, and intracranial hemorrhage if severe (ACOG, 2019a).

The finding of thrombocytopenia on a routine blood count may be the first indication of ITP and diagnosis often is made incidentally with routine prenatal lab tests. Clinical signs of thrombocytopenia include petechiae, ecchymosis, epistaxis, gingival bleeding, and abnormal uterine bleeding (heavy or intermenstrual). It can be difficult to distinguish ITP from GT if the thrombocytopenia is first identified during the pregnancy.

Treatment for ITP is initiated if there are symptomatic bleeding episodes or if platelets fall below 30,000 mm^{-3} (ACOG, 2019a). Prenatal management includes avoiding NSAIDs, salicylates, and trauma, and careful planning for labor and birth. There is no evidence that cesarean is safer than vaginal birth, and procedures that may increase hemorrhage risk for the fetus such as fetal scalp electrode or operative vacuum delivery should be avoided (ACOG, 2019a). In general, laboring people need a platelet count of at least 70,000 mm^{-3} to be eligible for epidural anesthesia, and at least 50,000 mm^{-3} for cesarean birth (ACOG, 2019a). Neonatologists are part of the team to develop a care plan including neonatal platelet counts, clinical assessment, and delay of intramuscular injections and circumcision (ACOG, 2019a).

Treatment of thrombocytopenia during pregnancy can consist of steroids, IV immunoglobulin, platelet transfusion, or splenectomy and is based on the urgency of treatment response, the severity of the disorder, and the presence of complications. Corticosteroids are a standard treatment option that takes weeks for clinical response, while IV immunoglobulin provides a response within one to three days. Platelet transfusions are given to prepare for urgent surgery or respond to hemorrhage (ACOG, 2019a). The purpose of treatment of thrombocytopenia in pregnancy is to minimize bleeding risks for the pregnant person associated with childbirth or regional anesthesia. People who are planning an epidural and have thrombocytopenia will benefit from evaluation and discussion with the anesthesiologist prenatally. People with severe thrombocytopenia should be closely monitored for possible complications and referred for specialized obstetric care.

TTP is a very rare disorder characterized by severe thrombocytopenia, fluctuating neurological signs such as headache and confusion, and renal impairment. During pregnancy, the clots formed by the destroyed and aggregated platelets can cause microthromboses in the placenta, leading to fetal growth restriction, and even fetal death (Scully et al., 2012).

Inherited Bleeding Disorders

Inherited bleeding disorders include von Willebrand disease (VWD), hemophilia A and B, and inherited deficiencies of coagulation factors. Inherited bleeding disorders increase the risk of significant bleeding during pregnancy, especially in the first trimester and immediately after birth (Shahbazi et al., 2012).

VWD is the most common inherited bleeding disorder in the United States, occurring in approximately 1 in 4000 pregnant people (James & Jamison, 2007). However, it can also manifest as an acquired disorder associated with onset of autoimmune disorders. Von Willebrand factor (VWF) is a glycoprotein essential for blood coagulation. Reduced levels of VWF characterize the disease, which varies greatly in severity and follows both dominant and recessive patterns of inheritance (McDonald & Austin, 2013). There are three types of VWD. Type I is a mild form of the disease involving deficiency of VWF and is the most common. Most people with Type I are asymptomatic and usually experience no additional risk during pregnancy. Type II is less common, involving abnormal VWF. Type III is very rare and involves an absence of VWF; it is associated with an increased risk of significant perinatal bleeding. Pregnant people with VWD need a multidisciplinary care team of obstetrician-gynecologists, hematologists, and midwives (ACOG, 2019b). Midwives play an essential role to maintain the standards of routine prenatal care that include patient education, support, and advocacy in complex pregnancies.

People living with VWD often have a history of abnormal uterine bleeding and heavy menses since menarche, prior to conception. They may have experienced postpartum hemorrhage with a prior childbirth. Other medical history can include episodes of epistaxis, gingival bleeding, bleeding after dental extraction, bleeding from minor cuts or abrasions, postoperative bleeding, unexplained GI bleeds, or joint bleeding (ACOG, 2019b). VWD should be included in the differential if any of these histories are present or if there is a family history of a bleeding disorder. Physical exam findings may include petechiae, ecchymoses, or other evidence of a recent bleed. If there are positive findings on history or physical exam, laboratory testing should include CBC and platelet count, prothrombin (PT) and partial prothrombin time (PTT), fibrinogen, and a hematology consult is initiated (ACOG, 2019b).

There is a physiologic increase in VWF as pregnancy progresses, which can obscure diagnosis of VWD. Those living with a mild deficiency of VWF are typically not affected in pregnancy. Those diagnosed with VWD prior to pregnancy will need evaluation of the VWF levels in the third trimester as part of birth planning (ACOG, 2019b). Treatment considerations include VFW replacement to optimize hematologic parameters for epidural placement (ACOG, 2019b). Pregnant people with VWD are at high risk for an epidural or spinal hematoma if they choose epidural anesthesia in labor (ACOG, 2019b). Vaginal birth is recommended due to lower risk for hemorrhage, with cesarean reserved for standard indications (ACOG, 2019b). The care team should strategize options for control of hemorrhage at time of birth, with VWF replacement or factor VIII as needed (ACOG, 2019b). Postpartum people with VDW are at risk for delayed hemorrhage as estrogen levels return to their normal state (ACOG, 2019b). Since there is a 50% risk of the fetus being affected by VWD, it is best to avoid the use of fetal scalp electrode or operative vaginal birth, and postpone circumcision until the newborn's status is determined (ACOG, 2019b).

Hemophilia is an X-linked recessive disorder, which means that babies with XY sex chromosomes (usually those assigned male at birth) born to hemophilia carriers have a 50% chance of inheriting the disease and babies with XX sex chromosomes (usually those assigned female at birth) have a 50% chance of being carriers. The degree of bleeding risk is related to the level of circulating clotting factors, which normally increases during pregnancy. Some people who have hemophilia or who are carriers avoid pregnancy, terminate a pregnancy with a diagnosis of hemophilia, or become parents through preimplantation diagnosis, surrogacy, or adoption.

Inherited bleeding disorders are diagnosed by the evaluation of a CBC, peripheral blood smear, PT, PTT, and platelet function activity. A family history of a bleeding disorder is especially significant. A history of easily provoked bleeding, heavy menses, epistaxis, bruising, and multiple petechiae or **purpura** also requires further evaluation. Preconception counseling and testing will help identify undiagnosed inherited bleeding disorders. This information will help the person seeking pregnancy and their partner understand the genetic implications and provides the opportunity to discuss contraception and pregnancy management.

During the antepartum period, clotting factor levels are closely monitored on a planned schedule, beginning at the first visit, and may be even more closely monitored during the third trimester. These patients are at increased risk for bleeding complications during birth and the postpartum period. A detailed plan for pain management and birth options is needed to decrease the occurrence of complications. People with bleeding disorders are best served by an interdisciplinary team with expertise in normal and complex perinatal care.

Thromboembolic Disorders

Pregnancy is a hypercoagulable state. Normal physiologic changes that lead to increased risk for formation of blood clots include increased venous stasis, decreased venous outflow, compression of the inferior vena cava and pelvic veins by the growing uterus, decreased mobility, and an increase in coagulation factors driven by rising estrogen levels. There is an increase in thrombin generation and in levels of procoagulant factors. Venous stasis increases secondary to the effects of progesterone on the blood vessels and the decrease in venous return due to increasing size of the uterus. Generalized microvascular damage can occur secondary to venous distention. All of these factors contribute to an increase in the occurrence of VTE. The risk of venous thromboembolic events is four to five times higher in pregnant people than nonpregnant people and is greatest during the last few weeks of pregnancy and the first four to six weeks postpartum (ACOG, 2018d; Heit et al., 2005; Virkus et al., 2014).

The most common types of thromboembolism in pregnancy are deep vein thromboses (DVTs) and pulmonary emboli (PE). If a DVT forms in pregnancy, it more frequently forms in the left lower extremity. If the thrombus breaks from its attachment to the blood vessel wall, it can travel toward the lungs and cause a PE, which accounted for 9.2% of US maternal deaths between 2011 and 2013 (CDC, 2017). The two types of VTE are among the leading causes of maternal mortality in the US (ACOG, 2018d).

The primary goals for thromboembolic disorders in pregnant and postpartum people are prevention for those at high risk of VTE, and prompt diagnosis and treatment of acute events (ACOG, 2018d). Prevention measures start with screening at the preconception and initial prenatal visits. All pregnant persons should be assessed for a history of a prior thrombosis, which is the greatest risk factor for developing a VTE in pregnancy, and should also be screened for a family history of thrombophilias.

Screening and Prevention of VTE

Laboratory screening for thrombophilias should be offered to people who have a personal history of a thromboembolic event, with or without recurrent risk factors, and no prior thrombophilia testing. Examples of recurrent risk factors include pregnancy and estrogen-containing contraceptives, while nonrecurrent risks include fractures, surgery, and prolonged immobilization (ACOG, 2018b). Individuals with a first degree relative with a documented high-risk thrombophilia and thrombotic event, including stroke, PE, or a blood clot unrelated to trauma should be offered screening. Laboratory tests include the more common inherited thrombophilias Factor V Leiden, prothrombin G20210A mutation, antithrombin, protein S and C deficiencies, and antiphospholipid syndrome (APS; ACOG, 2018b). Ideally, screening should take place when individuals are not pregnant, and when not taking anticoagulation or hormonal therapy, to obtain accurate results (ACOG, 2018b).

Other risks for formation of VTE include known thrombophilias, obesity, hypertension, autoimmune disease, heart disease, SCD, multiple gestation, and preeclampsia. Postpartum risk factors include cesarean birth, postpartum hemorrhage, or infection. Cesarean birth quadruples the risk of postpartum VTE (ACOG, 2018d). After a cesarean birth, care providers work together to prevent VTE using pneumatic compression devices until patient ambulates.

People who are known to have thrombophilia should be advised of the importance of non-estrogen-containing contraception and the risk of thromboembolic events during pregnancy and postpartum. Those living with inherited thrombophilias have multiple postpartum contraception options that include progestin or nonhormonal IUDs, progestin-only pills or implants, and barrier methods.

Anticoagulation Therapy

Clinicians will choose the prevention treatment regimen that fits the clinical risk profile through shared decision-making, and in partnership with a multidisciplinary team. The preferred regimen is low-molecular-weight heparin (LMWH) for both the treatment of VTE and prevention during pregnancy and postpartum due to its ease of administration and greater reliability (ACOG, 2018d). The side effects of LMWH include bleeding, thrombocytopenia, and irritation at the injection site. Treatment is typically continued for at least six weeks postpartum. Prophylactic anticoagulation may need adjustments postpartum based on risk factors and mode of birth. Providers can select an agent compatible with breastfeeding, including options for warfarin, LMWH or unfractionated heparin (ACOG, 2018d).

Management of an Acute Thromboembolic Event

Care providers should be well versed in the symptoms of a DVT and PE, in order to provide rapid and accurate diagnosis and treatment. Signs and symptoms of a thromboembolic event may mimic common discomforts of pregnancy, such as dyspnea and lower leg edema or cramping. DVT may cause a cramping pain in the calf or a feeling of heaviness in the affected leg. Dyspnea is a common symptom in pregnancy associated with normal physiologic changes, and also a leading symptom of PE.

The most common symptoms of a DVT are pain and swelling in an extremity that can encompass the entire leg with or without flank, buttock, or back pain (Rodger et al., 2015). Physical exam includes inspection, palpation, and measurement of the affected leg. If there is a difference of more than 2 cm in calf circumference, the next diagnostic step is compression ultrasound with Doppler imaging of the proximal veins. In pregnant people, it is more common to find the DVT left lower extremity and more proximal, in the iliofemoral or iliac veins (ACOG, 2018d). Anticoagulant therapy is started for positive results or if there is high clinical suspicion for DVT despite a negative ultrasound. In pregnant and postpartum people, D-dimer lab values (commonly assessed outside of pregnancy) are not helpful in the diagnosis of DVT as these levels naturally increase in the third trimester.

Blood clots that form in the lower extremities can break off and travel to the lungs and present as a PE, which is a leading cause of maternal mortality and requires prompt diagnosis and treatment. A report of chest pain, shortness of breath, a feeling of apprehension, hemoptysis, and/or unexplained tachycardia should be immediately investigated, especially in people with risk factors for thromboembolic events. The diagnosis of a PE can be made with a chest X-ray and a ventilation and perfusion (V/Q) scan. If positive, anticoagulant therapy is initiated.

All pregnant people with an acute VTE event in pregnancy require treatment with the appropriate dose-adjusted anticoagulation medications. Initial treatment typically lasts three to six months and is transitioned to intermediate or prophylactic dosing for the remainder of the pregnancy and for six weeks postpartum (ACOG, 2018d).

Inherited or Acquired Thrombophilias

The presence of inherited or acquired **thrombophilia** increases the risk of thromboembolism in pregnancy. Physiologic changes in pregnancy lead to increased clotting potential, decreased anticoagulant activity and decreased fibrinolysis, and exacerbate the risks for VTE for those living with an inherited thrombophilia. Also, both the inferior vena cava and pelvic veins are compressed by the enlarging uterus, leading to increased venous stasis of the lower extremities. Therefore, all pregnant persons should be screened through careful medical and family history taking in early pregnancy to consider the need for additional testing or specialized care.

Thrombophilias are categorized as high or low risk depending on severity of presentation, and treatment recommendations vary accordingly. Recommendations for thrombosis prophylaxis are controversial and depend on the clinical condition, the zygosity (heterozygous or homozygous for the condition), and prior or family history of thrombosis. Many pregnant people with any type of thrombophilia receive thrombosis prophylaxis (Croles et al., 2017), though some experts advocate prophylaxis be reserved for those with high-risk inherited thrombophilias (ACOG, 2018b). Those with Factor V Leiden carrier status are at increased risk for VTE in pregnancy, and the risk greatly increases if they also have a personal history of a VTE or an affected first degree relative (ACOG, 2018d). There is conflicting data regarding the efficacy of prophylaxis in preventing adverse perinatal outcomes associated with thrombophilia (Rodger et al., 2015).

Antiphospholipid Syndrome

The most common acquired thrombophilia is APS, an autoimmune disorder more common in people assigned female sex at birth of reproductive age that promotes activation of the coagulation system increasing the risk of thrombosis, and, paradoxically, thrombocytopenia. It is diagnosed through a combination of clinical features, such as recurrent fetal loss, plus laboratory confirmation of circulating antiphospholipid antibodies that can bind to the phospholipid on cell surfaces, leading to clot formation. There are three antibodies that make up the syndrome: lupus anticoagulant, anticardiolipin, and anti-B2 glycoprotein I. As lab testing can sometimes yield transient positive results, positive test results are followed with a confirmatory test at least 12 weeks later to meet diagnostic criteria.

APS is linked with complications of DVT, preeclampsia, recurrent pregnancy loss, intrauterine growth restriction (IUGR), placental insufficiency, and preterm birth (ACOG, 2012, reaffirmed 2017; Khamashta et al., 2016). The majority of pregnancy losses occur after 10 weeks of gestation, unlike in the general population of pregnant people who mainly experience fetal loss prior to 10 weeks of gestation. APS is most associated with the severe form of preeclampsia occurring at less than 34 weeks of gestation, although all pregnant people with APS are at higher risk for the spectrum of pregnancy-induced hypertensive disorders (ACOG, 2017). IUGR is found in 15–30% of pregnancies of those afflicted with this syndrome (ACOG, 2017). There is a high risk of thrombosis for pregnant and postpartum people living with APS, with some studies showing a risk of 5–12% (ACOG, 2017). Severe illness can occur postpartum as well, with such complications as heart failure, fever, renal insufficiency, and multiple thromboses (ACOG, 2017).

Criteria for APS testing include any prior arterial or VTE with unclear etiology, or a new clot formed during pregnancy, one of more fetal deaths at or beyond 10 weeks of gestation, one or more premature births prior to 34 weeks due to eclampsia or preeclampsia or features of placental insufficiency, or three or more consecutive spontaneous abortions prior to 10 weeks of gestation (in pregnancies that were morphologically normal per ultrasound or exam to ensure that there were no other chromosomal, hormonal, or maternal abnormalities that led to these pregnancy losses ACOG, 2017).

The choice to use prophylactic anticoagulants is made through shared decision-making, comprehensive discussion on risks and benefits, and the pregnant person's values and preferences (ACOG, 2018b). The use of prophylactic heparin throughout pregnancy and until six weeks postpartum is recommended for those with a history of prior thrombosis, along with low-dose aspirin (ACOG, 2017; Andreoli et al., 2017), and some also recommend prophylaxis even in the absence of prior thrombosis, especially for those with prior fetal losses. Close clinical surveillance without prophylaxis is also an option (ACOG, 2017). Antepartum surveillance often starts in the third trimester with serial growth ultrasounds and antenatal testing with nonstress tests and biophysical profiles due to increased risks for IUGR and stillbirth (ACOG, 2017; Andreoli et al., 2017).

After childbirth, people with APS should be transitioned to long-term management with an internist, hematologist, or rheumatologist. They are at a higher lifetime risk of both stroke and thrombosis and need to establish ongoing care. Postpartum care will include counseling on safe and effective contraceptive methods; estrogen-containing contraceptives should be avoided. People with APS benefit from pregnancy spacing and planned pregnancies, and shared decision-making is followed to create a reproductive life plan to meet their personal goals.

Summary

Hematologic alterations, bleeding disorders, and coagulopathies can affect pregnancy outcomes in otherwise healthy pregnant people. Anemia is the most common hematologic disorder in pregnancy. Early identification and management of bleeding disorders are key to good pregnancy outcomes. The prenatal care provider plays a key role in screening and identification of previously undiagnosed hematologic disorders, comanagement or referral of known hematologic disorders, and the prevention and identification of acute thromboembolic events.

Resources for Pregnant People and Healthcare Providers

March of Dimes: Anemia in pregnancy: https://www.marchofdimes.org/complications/anemia.aspx

March of Dimes: Rh Disease: https://www.marchofdimes.org/complications/rh-disease.aspx

National Hemophilia Foundation: https://www.hemophilia.org

WIC Nutrition: https://www.fns.usda.gov/wic

References

Abbassi-Ghanavati, M., Greer, L., & Cunningham, F. (2009). Pregnancy and laboratory studies: A reference guide for clinicians. *Obstetrics & Gynecology*, 114(6), 1326–1331. https://doi.org/10.1097/AOG.0b013e3181c2bde8

Abioye, A., Aboud, S., Premji, Z., Etheredge, A., Gunaratna, N. S., Sudfeld, C. R., Mongi, R., Meloney, L., Darling, A. M., Noor, R. A., Spiegelman, D., Duggan, C., & Fawzi, W. (2016). Iron supplementation affects hematologic biomarker concentrations and pregnancy outcomes among iron-deficient Tanzanian women. *The Journal of Nutrition*, 146, 1162–1171. https://doi.org/10.3945/jn.115.225482

AlJaberi, H. (2018). Developing culturally sensitive mHealth apps for Caribbean immigrant women to use during pregnancy: Focus group study. *JMIR Human Factors*, 5(4), e29. https://doi.org/10.2196/humanfactors.9787

American College of Nurse Midwives (ACNM). (2013). *The role of the Certified Nurse-Midwife/Certified Midwife in preconception health and health care*. https://www.midwife.org/acnm/files/ACNMLibraryData/UPLOADFILENAME/000000000081/Preconception%20Health%20and%20Health%20Care%20Feb%202013.pdf

American College of Obstetricians and Gynecologist (ACOG). (2012, reaffirmed 2017). Antiphospholipid syndrome. Practice bulletin no. 132. *Obstetrics & Gynecology*, 120, 1514–1521.

American College of Obstetricians and Gynecologists (ACOG). (2017, reaffirmed 2020). Carrier screening for genetic conditions. Committee opinion no. 691. *Obstetrics & Gynecology*, 129, e41.

American College of Obstetricians and Gynecologists (ACOG). (2007, reaffirmed 2018a). Hemoglobinopathies in pregnancy. Practice bulletin no. 78. *Obstetrics & Gynecology*, 109, 229–237.

American College of Obstetricians and Gynecologists (ACOG). (2018b). Inherited thrombophilias in pregnancy. Practice bulletin no. 197. *Obstetrics & Gynecology*, 197, e18–e34.

American College of Obstetricians and Gynecologists (ACOG). (2018c). Management of alloimmunization during pregnancy. Practice bulletin no. 192. *Obstetrics & Gynecology*, 192, e82–e90.

American College of Obstetricians and Gynecologists (ACOG). (2018d). Thromboembolism in pregnancy. Practice bulletin no. 196. *Obstetrics & Gynecology*, 132, e1–e17.

American College of Obstetricians and Gynecologists (ACOG). (2019a). Thrombocytopenia in pregnancy. Practice bulletin no. 207. *Obstetrics & Gynecology*, 133, e181–e193.

American College of Obstetricians and Gynecologists (ACOG). (2013, reaffirmed 2019b). Von Willebrand disease in women. Practice bulletin no. 580. *Obstetrics & Gynecology*, 580, 1–6.

American College of Obstetricians and Gynecologists (ACOG). (2021a). Anemia in pregnancy. ACOG practice bulletin no. 233. *Obstetrics & Gynecology*, 138, e55–e64.

American College of Obstetricians and Gynecologists (ACOG). (2017, reaffirmed 2021b). Prevention of RhD alloimmunization. Practice bulletin no. 181. *Obstetrics & Gynecology*, 130(2), e57–e70.

Andreoli, L., Bertsias, G. K., Agmon-Levin, N., Brown, S., Cervera, R., Costedoat-Chalumeau, N., Doria, A., Fischer-Betz, R., Forger, F., Moraes-Fontes, M. F., Khamashta, M., King, J., Lojacono, A., Marchiori, F., Meroni, P. L., Mosca, M., Motta, M., Ostensen, M., Pamfil, C., . . . Tincani, A. (2017). EULAR recommendations for women's health and the management of family planning, assisted reproduction, pregnancy and menopause in patients with systemic lupus erythematosus and/or antiphospholipid syndrome. *Annals of the Rheumatic Diseases*, 76(3), 476–485. https://doi.org/10.1136/annrheumdis-2016-209770

Ars, C. L., Nijs, I. M., Marroun, H. E., Muetzel, R., Schmidt, M., Steen-weg-de Graaff, J., Van Der Lugt, A., Jaddoe, V. W., Hofman, A., Steegers, E. A., Verhulst, F. C., Tiemeier, H., & White, T. (2016). Prenatal folate, homocysteine and vitamin B12 levels and child brain volumes, cognitive development and psychological functioning: The generation R study. *The British Journal of Nutrition*, 1–9. https://doi.org/10.1017/S0007114515002081

Balachandren, N., Awogbade, M., & Johns, J. (2016). Sickle cell disease in pregnancy. *Obstetrics, Gynecology and Reproductive Medicine*, 26(6), 161–166. https://doi.org/10.1016/j.ogrm.2016.03.002

Blackburn, S. (2016). *Maternal, fetal and neonatal physiology: A clinical perspective* (5th ed.). Elsevier.

Bodnar, L. M., Himes, K. P., Venkataramanan, R., Chen, J. Y., Evans, R. W., Meyer, J. L., & Simhan, H. N. (2010). Maternal serum folate species in early pregnancy and risk of preterm birth. *The American Journal of Clinical Nutrition*, 92(4), 864–871. https://doi.org/10.3945/ajcn.2010.29675

Camaschella, C. (2015). Iron-deficiency anemia. *New England Journal of Medicine*, 372, 1832–1843. https://doi.org/10.1056/NEJMra1401038

Cantor, A., Bougatsos, C., Dana, T., Blazina, I., & McDonagh, M. (2015). Routine iron supplementation and screening for iron deficiency. *Annals of Internal Medicine*, 566–576. https://doi.org/10.7326/M14-2932

Cao, C., & O'Brien, K. (2013). Pregnancy and iron homeostasis: An update. *Nutrition Reviews*, 71(1), 35–51. https://doi.org/10.1111/j.1753-4887.2012.00550.x

Centers for Disease Control and Prevention (CDC). (2017, June 29). *Reproductive health. Pregnancy mortality surveillance system*. https://www.cdc.gov/reproductivehealth/maternalin-fanthealth/pmss.html.

Croles, F. N., Nasserinejad, K., Duvekot, J. J., Kruip, M. J., Meijer, K., & Leebeek, F. W. (2017). Pregnancy, thrombophilia, and the risk of a first venous thrombosis: Systematic review and Bayesian metaanalysis. *BMJ*, 359, j4452. https://doi.org/10.1136/bmj.j4452

Czeizel, A. E., Dudas, I., Vereczkey, A., & Banhidy, F. (2013). Folate deficiency and folic acid supplementation: The prevention of neural-tube defects and congenital heart defects. *Nutrients*, 5(11), 4760–4775. https://doi.org/10.3390/nu5114760

Elmore, C., & Ellis, J. (2022). Screening, treatment, and monitoring of iron deficiency anemia in pregnancy and postpartum. *Journal of Midwifery & Women's Health*, 67, 321–331. https://doi.org/10.1111/jmwh.13370

Finkelstein, J. L., Layden, A. J., & Stover, P. J. (2015). Vitamin B-12 and perinatal health. *Advances in Nutrition: An International Review Journal*, 6(5), 552–563. https://doi.org/10.3945/an.115.008201

Garratty, G., Glynn, S. A., & McEntire, R. (2004). ABO and Rh(D) phenotype frequencies of different racial/ethnic groups in the United States. *Transfusion*, 44(5), 703–706. https://doi.org/10.1111/j.1537-2995.2004.03338.x

Gernand, A. D., Schulze, K. J., Stewart, C. P., West, K. P., & Christian, P. (2016). Micronutrient deficiencies in pregnancy worldwide: Health effects and prevention. *Nature*, 12, 279–289. https://doi.org/10.1038/nrendo.2016.37

Goheen, M. M., Wegmuller, R., Bah, A., Darboe, B., Danso, E., Affara, M., Gardner, D., Patel, J. C., Prentice, A. M., & Cerami, C. (2016). Anemia offers stronger protection than sickle cell trait against the erythrocytic stage of falciparum malaria and this protection is reversed by iron supplementation. *eBioMedicine*, 14, 123–130. https://doi.org/10.1016/j.ebiom.2016.11.011

Goldman, M., Lane, D., Webert, K., & Fallis, R. (2015). The prevalence of anti-K in Canadian prenatal patients. *Transfusion*, 55(6pt2), 1486–1491. https://doi.org/10.1111/trf.13151

Grieger, J. A., & Clifton, V. L. (2015). A review of the impact of dietary intakes in human pregnancy on infant birthweight. *Nutrients*, 7, 153–178. https://doi.org/10.3390/nu7010153

Heit, J., Kobbervig, C., James, A., et al. (2005). Trends in the incidence of venous thromboembolism during pregnancy or postpartum: A 30-year population-based study. *Annals of Internal Medicine*, 143, 697–706. https://doi.org/10.7326/0003-4819-143-10-200511150-00006

James, A., & Jamison, M. (2007). Bleeding events and other complications during pregnancy and childbirth in women with von Willebrand disease. *Journal of Thrombosis and Haemostasis*, 5(6), 1165–1169. https://doi.org/10.1111/j.1538-7836.2007.02563.x

Jans, S. M., De Jonge, P. J., & Lagro-Janssen, A. L. M. (2010). Maternal and perinatal outcomes amongst haemoglobinopathy carriers: A systematic review. *International Journal of Clinical Practice*, 64(12), 1688–1698. https://doi.org/10.1111/j.1742-1241.2010.02451.x

Kannan, S., Ranjit, N., Ganguri, H. B., Lasichak, A., Sparks, A., Scherer, H., & Schulz, A. (2020). Sisters together: Lessons learned from implementing a grocery store campaign in Michigan communities at risk for neural tube defects. *Journal of Health Care for the Poor and Underserved*, 31, 301–324. https://doi.org/10.1353/hpu.2020.0024

Khamashta, M., Taraborelli, M., Sciascia, S., & Tincani, A. (2016). Antiphospholipid syndrome. *Best Practice & Research Clinical Rheumatology*, 30(1), 133–148. https://doi.org/10.1016/j.berh.2016.04.002

Koelewijn, J. M., de Haas, M., Vrijkotte, T. G. M., van der Schoot, C. E., & Bonsel, G. J. (2009). Risk factors for Rh(D) immunisation despite antenatal and postnatal anti-D prophylaxis. *BJOG*, 116, 1307–1311. https://doi.org/10.1111/j.1471-0528.2009.02244.x

Little, I., Vinogradova, Y., Orton, E., Kai, J., & Qureshi, N. (2017). Venous thromboembolism in adults screened for sickle cell trait: A population-based cohort study with nested case-control analysis. *BMJ Open*, 7(3), e012665. https://doi.org/10.1136/bmjopen-2016-012665

Markham, K. B., Scrape, S. R., Prasad, M., Rossi, K. Q., & O'Shaughnessy, R. W. (2016). Hemolytic disease of the fetus and the newborn due to intravenous drug use. *AJP Reports*, 6(1), e129–e132.

McDonald, V., & Austin, S. K. (2013). Inherited bleeding disorders. *Medicine*, 41(4), 231–233. https://doi.org/10.1016/j.mpmed.2017.01.012

McKerracher, L., Oresnik, S., Moffat, T., Murray-Davis, B., Vickers-Manzin, J., Zalot, L., Williams, D., Sloboda, D. M., & Barker, M. E. (2020). Addressing embodied inequities in health: How do we enable improvement in women's diet in pregnancy? *Public Health Nutrition*, 23(16), 2994–3004. https://doi.org/10.1017/S1368980020001093

McLean, E., Cogswell, M., Egli, I., Wojdyla, D., & de Benoist, B. (2009). Worldwide prevalence of anaemia, WHO vitamin and mineral nutrition information system 1993–2005. *Public Health Nutrition*, 12(4), 444–454.

Moise, K. J. (2008). Fetal anemia due to non-Rhesus-D red-cell alloimmunization. *Seminars in Fetal & Neonatal Medicine*, 13, 207–214. https://doi.org/10.1016/j.siny.2008.02.007

Moll, R., & Davis, B. (2017). Iron, vitamin B12 and folate. *Medicine*, 45(4), 198–203. https://doi.org/10.1016/j.mpmed.2017.01.007

Monga, M., & Mastrobatista, J. (2014). Maternal cardiovascular, respiratory, and renal adaptation to pregnancy. In R. Creasy, R. Resnik, J. Iams, C. Lockwood, T. Moore, & M. Greene (Eds.), *Creasy and Resnik's maternal-fetal medicine: Principles and practice* (7th ed., pp. 93–99). Elsevier/Saunders.

Neunert, C., Lim, W., Crowther, M., Cohen, A., Solberg, L., & Crowther, M. A. (2011). The American Society of Hematology 2011 evidence-based practice guideline for immune thrombocytopenia. *Blood*, 117(16), 4190–4207. https://doi.org/10.1182/blood-2010-08-302984

Nypaver, C., Arbour, M., & Niederegger, E. (2016). Preconception care: Improving health of women and families. *Journal of Midwifery & Women's Health*, 61(3), 356–364. https://doi.org/10.1111/jmwh.12465

Office of Dietary Supplements. (2022). *Iron: Fact sheet for health professionals*. https://ods.od.nih.gov/factsheets/Iron-HealthProfessional

Okam, M., Koch, T., & Tran, M. (2016). Iron deficiency anemia treatment response to oral iron therapy: A pooled analysis of five randomized controlled trials. *Haematologica*, 101(1), e6–e7. https://doi.org/10.3324/haematol.2015.129114

Oteng-Ntim, E., Ayensah, B., Knight, M., & Howard, J. (2014). Pregnancy outcome in patients with sickle cell disease in the UK—A national cohort study comparing sickle cell anaemia (HbSS) with HbSC disease. *British Journal of Haematology*, 169(1), 129–137. https://doi.org/10.1111/bjh.13270

Parker, H. W., Tovar, A., McCurdy, K., & Vadiveloo, M. (2019). Socioeconomic and racial prenatal diet quality disparities in a national US sample. *Public Health Nutrition*, 23(5), 894–903. https://doi.org/10.1017/S1368980019003240

Pasricha, S. R., Flecknoe-Brown, S. C., Allen, K. J., Gibson, P. R., McMahon, L. P., Olynyk, J. K., Roger, S. D., Savoia, H. F., Tampi, R., Thomson, A. R., & Wood, E. M. (2010). Diagnosis and management of iron deficiency anaemia: A clinical update. *Medical Journal of Australia*, 193(9), 525–532. https://doi.org/10.5694/j.1326-5377.2010.tb04038.x

Pena-Rosas, J. P., De-Regil, L. M., Gomez Malave, H., Flores-Urrutia, M., & Dowswell, T. (2015). Intermittent oral iron supplementation during pregnancy. *Cochrane Database of Systematic Reviews*, (10), CD009997, 1–143. https://doi.org/10.1002/14651858.CD009997.pub2

Petrakos, G., Andriopoulos, P., & Tsironi, M. (2016). Pregnancy in women with thalassemia: Challenges and solutions. *International Journal of Women's Health*, 8, 441–451. https://doi.org/10.2147/IJWH.S89308

Prather, C., Fuller, T. R., Jeffries, W. L., Marshall, K. J., Howell, A. V., Belyue-Umole, A., & King, W. (2018). Racism, African American women, and their sexual and reproductive health: A review of historical and contemporary evidence and implications for health equity. *Health Equity*, 2(1), 249–259. https://doi.org/10.1089/heq.2017.0045

Rodger, M., Sheppard, D., Gandara, E., & Tinmouth, A. (2015). Haematological problems in obstetrics. *Best Practice & Research Clinical Obstetrics & Gynaecology*, 29(5), 671–684. https://doi.org/10.1016/j.bpobgyn.2015.02.004

Sabo, S., Wightman, P., McCue, K., Butler, M., Pilling, V., Jimenez, D. J., Celaya, M., & Rumann, S. (2021). Addressing maternal and child health equity through a community health worker home visiting intervention to reduce low birth weight: Retrospective quasi-experimental study of the Arizona Health Start Programme. *BMJ Open*, 11, e045014. https://doi.org/10.1136/bmjopen-2020-045014

Scholl, T. O., & Johnson, W. G. (2000). Folic acid: Influence on the outcome of pregnancy. *The American Journal of Clinical Nutrition*, 71(5), 1295s–1303s. https://doi.org/10.1093/ajcn/71.5.1295s

Scully, M., Hunt, B. J., Benjamin, S., Liesner, R., Rose, P., Peyvandi, F., Cheung, B., & Machin, S. J. (2012). Guidelines on the diagnosis and management of thrombotic thrombocytopenic purpura and other thrombotic microangiopathies. *British Journal of Haematology*, 158(3), 323–335. https://doi.org/10.1111/j.1365-2141.2012.09167.x

Shahbazi, S., Moghaddam-Banaem, L., Ekhtesari, F., & Ala, F. A. (2012). Impact of inherited bleeding disorders on pregnancy and postpartum hemorrhage. *Blood Coagulation & Fibrinolysis*, 23(7), 603–607. https://doi.org/10.1182/blood-2021-149673

Sonchak, L. (2016). The impact of WIC on birth outcomes: New evidence from South Carolina. *Maternal & Child Health Journal*, 20, 1518–1525. https://doi.org/10.1007/s10995-016-1951-y

Sundberg, M. A., Warren, A. C., VanWassenhove-Paetzold, J., George, C., Carroll, D. S., Becenti, L. J., Martinez, A., Jones, B., Bachman-Carter, K., Begay, M. G., Wilmot, T., Sandoval-Soland, H., MacKenzie, O., Hamilton, L., Tsosie, M., Bradburn, C. K., Ellis, E., Malone, J., Pon, J., . . . Shin, S. S. (2020). Implementation of the Navajo fruit and vegetable prescription programme to improve access to healthy foods in a rural food desert. *Public Health Nutrition*, 23(12), 2199–2210. https://doi.org/10.1017/S1368980019005068

Suren, P., Roth, C., Bresnahan, M., Haugen, M., Hornig, M., & Hirtz, D. (2013). Association between maternal use of folic acid supplements and risk of autism spectrum disorders in children. *JAMA*, 309(6), 570–577. https://doi.org/10.1001/jama.2012.155925

Tharpe, N. L., Farley, C. L., & Jordan, R. G. (Eds.) (2022). *Clinical practice guidelines for midwifery & women's health*. Jones & Bartlett Learning.

Thein, S. L., (2022). *Researchers study a new way to treat sickle cell disease.* https://www.nhlbi.nih.gov/news/2022/researchers-study-new-way-treat-sickle-cell-disease

Thurman, A. R., Steed, L. L., Hulsey, T., & Soper, D. E. (2006). Bacteriuria in pregnant women with sickle cell trait. *American Journal of Obstetrics & Gynecology*, *194*(5), 1366–1370. https://doi.org/10.1016/j.ajog.2005.11.022

Tran, T., Tran, T., Simpson, J., et al. (2014). Infant motor development in rural Vietnam and intrauterine exposures to anaemia, iron deficiency and common mental disorders: A prospective community-based study. *BMC Pregnancy and Childbirth*, *14*, 8–18. https//doi.org/10.1186/1471-2393-14-8

Van Wamelen, D. J., Klumper, F. J., De Haas, M., Meerman, R. H., van Kamp, I. L., & Oepkes, D. (2007). Obstetric history and antibody titer in estimating severity of Kell alloimmunization in pregnancy. *Obstetrics & Gynecology*, *109*(5), 1093–1098. https://doi.org/10.1097/01.AOG.0000260957.77090.4e

Virkus, R. A., Lokkegaard, E., Lidegaard, Ø., Langhoff-Roos, J., Nielsen, A. K., Rothman, K. J., & Bergholt, T. (2014). Risk factors for venous thromboembolism in 1.3 million pregnancies: A nationwide prospective cohort. *PLoS One*, *9*(5), e96495. https://doi.org/10.1371/journal.pone.0096495

Vivanti, A., Benachi, A., Huchet, F. X., Ville, Y., Cohen, H., & Costa, J. M. (2016). Diagnostic accuracy of fetal rhesus D genotyping using cell free fetal DNA during the first trimester of pregnancy. *American Journal of Obstetrics & Gynecology*, *215*(606), e1–e5. https://doi.org/10.1016/j.ajog.2016.06.054

Wong, L., Smith, S., Gilstrop, M., Derman, R., Auerbach, S., London, N., Lenowitz, S., Bahrain, H., McClintock, J., & Auerbach, M. (2016). Safety and efficacy of rapid (1,000 mg in 1 hr) intravenous iron dextran for treatment of maternal iron deficient anemia of pregnancy. *American Journal of Hematology*, *91*, 590–593. https://doi.org/10.1002/ajh.24361

49

Respiratory Disorders

Lisa Hachey and Cynthia Nypaver

The editors gratefully acknowledge Janyce C. Agruss, who was author of the previous edition of this chapter.

Relevant Terms

Forced expiratory volume in one second (FEV$_1$)—the amount of air exhaled in the first second during forced exhalation after maximal inspiration

Inspiratory capacity—the total amount of air that can be drawn into the lungs after normal expiration

Leukotriene Receptor Antagonist—medications used to treat asthma by restricting airways from narrowing caused by inflammation

Long-acting beta-agonist—medications used to provide long-term symptom relief (typically about 12 hours) of asthma symptoms; examples include salmeterol and formoterol

Peak expiratory flow rate—the maximum airflow during forced expiration beginning with the lungs fully inflated

Peak-flow meters—portable device that measures airflow or peak expiratory flow rate

Pulmonary function tests—noninvasive tests that demonstrate how well the lungs work; most basic is spirometry

Short-acting beta-agonist—medications used to provide quick relief of asthma symptoms ("rescue inhaler"); example includes albuterol sulfate inhaler

Total lung capacity—the maximum volume to which the lungs can be expanded with the greatest possible inspiratory effort

---

Introduction

When individuals are pregnant, they are not immune from experiencing some of the more common respiratory disorders such as asthma, pneumonia, and upper respiratory infections (URIs) or colds. This chapter will discuss the management of these common respiratory disorders during pregnancy.

Respiratory Physiology and Pregnancy

As the uterus enlarges, the level of the diaphragm gradually elevates to a maximum of around 4 cm, peaking at approximately 37 weeks of gestation. The anterior–posterior and transverse diameter of the thorax and chest circumference increases, and the subcostal angle widens. These changes allow lung volume and **inspiratory capacity** to increase by about 5–10% as the pregnancy progresses. This adaptation assists in preserving **total lung capacity** throughout the pregnancy as the enlarging uterus displaces the lungs.

During pregnancy, the increased level of progesterone resets the hypothalamus to accept a lower level of blood carbon dioxide (PCO_2) at closer to 32 mmHg rather than 40 mmHg. This change favors transfer of carbon dioxide from the fetus (higher PCO_2) to the pregnant person (lower PCO_2). To prevent the fetal transfer from increasing blood pH levels and causing acidosis, a mild hyperventilation to blow off excess CO_2 begins in early pregnancy. The cumulative effect of these changes is often experienced by the pregnant person as a feeling of being short of breath even without exertion. Clinicians can provide education and reassurance that this sensation is a normal and expected change in pregnancy.

Health equity key points

- The prevalence of asthma disproportionately affects people of racial and ethnic minorities and those with low income due to a higher likelihood of living in a neighborhood close to industrial facilities that emit hazardous environmental toxins.
- Structural racism in the United States housing system leads to racial and ethnic disparities in the risk for influenza, especially severe influenza, due to disproportionate numbers of people living in crowded conditions and dependent on public transportation, with little access to preventive health services, and occupations that do not support the ability to work from home, making it difficult to comply with social distancing.

Prenatal and Postnatal Care: A Person-Centered Approach, Third Edition. Edited by Karen Trister Grace, Cindy L. Farley, Noelene K. Jeffers, and Tanya Tringali.
© 2024 John Wiley & Sons Ltd. Published 2024 by John Wiley & Sons Ltd.
Companion website: www.wiley.com/go/grace/prenatal

Asthma

Asthma is a chronic inflammatory, obstructive airway disease requiring ongoing medical management. It is characterized by inflammatory hyperresponsiveness and bronchoconstriction to stimuli such as allergens, irritants, physical exertion, stress, and infections, particularly viral infections. If asthma goes untreated, then structural remodeling of the airways can occur. Symptoms are wheezing, chest tightness, dyspnea, and cough, which may worsen at night. Asthma is an episodic disease with periods of exacerbation separated by symptom-free periods. The prevalence rate of asthma in the US adult population is approximately 8.4% (CDC, 2022). Asthma is the most common lung disease in pregnancy, with prevalence of approximately 5–8% and is increasing (Bonham et al., 2018). The severity of the asthma is classified as intermittent, mild-persistent, moderate-persistent, or severe persistent and is used as the basis for treatment decisions (Table 49.1).

Disparities in asthma prevalence and outcomes persist by demographic characteristics, poverty level, and geographic location. It is more prevalent among people who identify as female ≥18 years of age, non-Hispanic Black persons, non-Hispanic multiracial persons, and Puerto Rico persons (CDC, 2021a; Pate et al., 2021). Asthma deaths are higher among adults, people who identify as female, and Black persons. Black, Brown, and Indigenous people disproportionately live in communities with poor housing and are located near industry that emits pollutants and/or environmental toxics. This form of structural racism may explain why disparities in asthma exist within minority groups and those with low incomes (Martinez et al., 2021; Ray, 2021). There is increased morbidity and mortality among persons with low family incomes and among those living in the Northeast and Midwest compared to the South and West, particularly in small and medium metropolitan areas (CDC, 2021a; Pate et al., 2021).

Potential Problems

For many years, it has been recognized that the impact of pregnancy on asthma varies, but in general, about 1/3 of people with asthma will have an improvement of their condition during pregnancy, 1/3 will worsen, and 1/3 will remain the same as it was prepregnancy (Cusack & Gauvreau, 2020; Schatz et al., 1988). A good predictor of severity of asthma during pregnancy is the severity before pregnancy. People with severe asthma during pregnancy are more likely to have exacerbations than those who have mild to moderate asthma. Asthma exacerbation during pregnancy can negatively affect the health of the parent, child, and perinatal outcomes (Robijn et al., 2021) Some individuals who have asthma find that it improves in pregnancy, and some find that it stays the same. Well-controlled asthma is not associated with significant risk to the pregnant person or fetus. For about one in three pregnant women, the changes of pregnancy will make their asthma worse (Bonham et al., 2018). Asthma exacerbations are common during pregnancy, especially in those who experience severe asthma (Roff et al., 2021).

Poorly controlled asthma can lead to maternal complications such as gestational diabetes, gestational hypertension, preeclampsia, prenatal hemorrhage, preterm birth (PTB), and intrapartum complications such as cesarean section, and, rarely, death (Wang et al., 2020). Fetal complications of severe asthma include increased risk of stillbirth, fetal growth restriction (FGR), PTB, low birthweight, and a small but significant increase in cleft lip and palate (Wang et al., 2020). The magnitude of perinatal risk is related to the asthma severity. Improving asthma control in pregnancy has the potential to improve not only the pregnant person's health but also that of the child.

Differential Diagnosis

The diagnosis of asthma during pregnancy in people without a prior history can be challenging. Other causes of cough and wheezing that may respond to asthma management therapies, such as URIs, pneumonia, or gastroesophageal reflux disease, can lead to a misdiagnosis of asthma as the etiology. Asthma is a disease that is typically diagnosed over time after multiple, chronic respiratory events. **Pulmonary function test** (PFT) to diagnose

Table 49.1　Classification of Asthma Severity

Asthma severity	Symptom frequency	Nighttime symptoms	Interference with daily activity	Peak expiratory flow (PEF) or forced expiratory volume in one second (FEV$_1$)	Pulmonary function test variability
Intermittent	2 days/week or less	<2 nights/month	None	>80% predicted	>20%
Mild-persistent	>2 but not daily	>2 nights/month	Minor limitation	>80% predicted	20–30%
Moderate-persistent	Daily, but not continual	>1 night/week, but not nightly	Moderate limitation	60–80% predicted	>30%
Severe persistent	Throughout the day	Frequent	Extreme limitation	<60% predicted	>30%

Source: National Asthma Education and Prevention Program. Expert Panel Summary Report 2007: Guidelines for the diagnosis and management of asthma (NIH publication no. 08-5846). Bethesda, MD: US Department of Health and Human Services. Public Health Service, National Institutes of Health, National Heart, Lung, and Blood Institute. Reviewed 2020; Esden and Pesta-Walsh (2018).

asthma can be performed during pregnancy; however, the provider must consider potential complications that can occur from these studies, including hyperventilation or precipitation of an asthmatic episode. The provider must weigh the benefit of information gained in determining management versus risks of the test itself.

Common Clinical Presentation and Data Gathering

The pregnant person with asthma is typically identified during the initial prenatal visit interview. Some individuals will report a history of asthma that goes back to childhood and others will report adult onset. The presentation of asthma is the same in the pregnant person as in the nonpregnant person. A thorough history includes exacerbation frequency, triggers, symptom characteristics, prior hospitalizations and interventions required (such as intubation), and type, frequency, and efficacy of medications used currently or in the past for symptom relief.

The physical examination begins with observation to evaluate breathing effort. Auscultation to assess breath sounds should be done in a quiet room with the patient seated comfortably. Abnormal lung sounds such as wheezing, a high-pitched, whistle-like sound heard mostly upon expiration, is a common finding in individuals with asthma. However, wheezing is not always present and is not required to make the diagnosis (Winland-Brown et al., 2019). Shortness of breath, a tight feeling in the chest, and coughing can be present during an exacerbation of asthma.

For people with moderate to severe asthma, evaluation of respiratory function is recommended at the time of initial prenatal visit and periodically during prenatal visits depending on the course of asthma symptoms during the prenatal period. Measurements from lung function tests, including **peak expiratory flow (PEF)** with a **peak-flow meter,** exhaled nitric oxide (FeNO) asthma control test scores, and eosinophil counts, are helpful in diagnosis and assessment of asthma (Wang et al., 2020); however, each person's asthma severity history and possible collaboration with their primary care provider should guide testing recommendations.

Management of Asthma during Pregnancy

Controlling asthma during pregnancy is a priority to ensure the well-being of both the pregnant person and the developing fetus. The main goal of treatment is to prevent asthma exacerbation and potential hypoxic episodes that can cause oxygenation deprivation in the fetus.

Pharmaceutical Asthma Management

Most pregnant people with asthma can continue using the same medications they used prior to becoming pregnant since the vast majority of asthma medications are safe to use during pregnancy and breastfeeding. Pregnant people may have concerns about fetal safety when using medications, and undertreatment of asthma exacerbations by delaying medication or reducing

medication use during pregnancy is common (Ibrahim et al., 2018). Patients should be informed that it is safer to be treated with asthma medications than to have asthma symptoms and exacerbations that may result in maternal hypoxia and inadequate fetal oxygenation (Wang et al., 2020). The choice of medication depends on asthma severity.

Inhaled, **short-acting beta-agonists** (SABAs "rescue inhalers") remain the mainstay of treating exacerbations and handling mild forms of asthma in pregnant as well as nonpregnant people. Albuterol (salbutamol) is preferred during pregnancy as it has the most well-documented safety record for use in pregnancy (National Heart, Lung, and Blood Institute [NHLBI] 2020; Wang et al., 2020). For mild-persistent and moderate-persistent asthma, a SABA combined with an inhaled corticosteroid (ICS) is recommended for treatment (ACOG & ACAAI Position Statement, 2020) (Table 49.2). ICSs, such as beclomethasone, are used to prevent acute asthma attacks and are considered the prophylactic drugs of choice during pregnancy with those who have persistent asthma (ACOG & ACAAI Position Statement, 2020). If asthma is caused by allergens, consider adding a **leukotriene receptor antagonist** (LTRA); examples are montelukast and zafirlukast. Zileuton is not recommended for use during pregnancy. Theophylline can be used during pregnancy, but the provider must monitor serum concentrations to avoid toxicity (ACOG & ACAAI Position Statement, 2020). All medication therapy is tailored to provide pregnant individuals with the lowest dose necessary to control their asthma.

The stepwise approach to medication use based on asthma severity is advocated by the NHLBI (2020). The preferred medication classifications listed in Table 49.2 have more pregnancy-use data available than other asthma medications and safety is better established. Other medications may be used safely during pregnancy, especially if the individual was well controlled by the agents prior to pregnancy. This stepwise approach to medication use allows for the dose, administration frequency, and number of medications to increase when needed and to decrease when possible. Medications are stepped up if needed and then reassessed in four to six weeks. Step-down is possible if asthma is well controlled for at least three consecutive months. Consider consultation with an asthma specialist/pulmonologist in step 2 and definitely in steps 3–6 (NHLBI, 2020).

Environmental Asthma Management

Control of environmental asthma triggers is an essential component of asthma management. The healthcare provider and the pregnant person should discuss asthma triggers and how to avoid them. Reducing proliferation of indoor allergens can be helpful for those who may not be aware of sources of allergens that trigger asthma exacerbation.

Unfair and imbalanced distribution of societal resources, such as housing, clean air, and water, and

Table 49.2   Stepwise Approach to Treatment for Asthma

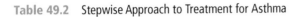

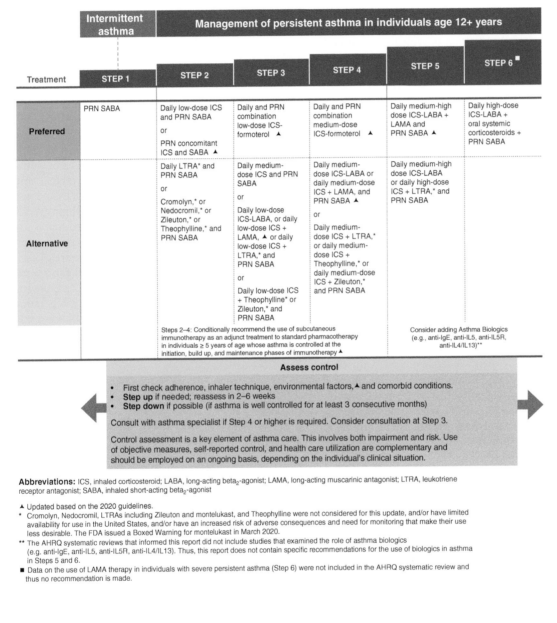

AGES 12+ YEARS: STEPWISE APPROACH FOR MANAGEMENT OF ASTHMA

Treatment	Intermittent asthma	Management of persistent asthma in individuals age 12+ years				
	STEP 1	STEP 2	STEP 3	STEP 4	STEP 5	STEP 6 ■
Preferred	PRN SABA	Daily low-dose ICS and PRN SABA or PRN concomitant ICS and SABA ▲	Daily and PRN combination low-dose ICS-formoterol ▲	Daily and PRN combination medium-dose ICS-formoterol ▲	Daily medium-high dose ICS-LABA + LAMA and PRN SABA ▲	Daily high-dose ICS-LABA + oral systemic corticosteroids + PRN SABA
Alternative		Daily LTRA* and PRN SABA or Cromolyn,* or Nedocromil,* or Zileuton,* or Theophylline,* and PRN SABA	Daily medium-dose ICS and PRN SABA or Daily low-dose ICS-LABA, or daily low-dose ICS + LAMA, ▲ or daily low-dose ICS + LTRA,* and PRN SABA or Daily low-dose ICS + Theophylline* or Zileuton,* and PRN SABA	Daily medium-dose ICS-LABA or daily medium-dose ICS + LAMA, and PRN SABA ▲ or Daily medium-dose ICS + LTRA,* or daily medium-dose ICS + Theophylline,* or daily medium-dose ICS + Zileuton,* and PRN SABA	Daily medium-high dose ICS-LABA or daily high-dose ICS + LTRA,* and PRN SABA	
		Steps 2–4: Conditionally recommend the use of subcutaneous immunotherapy as an adjunct treatment to standard pharmacotherapy in individuals ≥ 5 years of age whose asthma is controlled at the initiation, build up, and maintenance phases of immunotherapy ▲			Consider adding Asthma Biologics (e.g., anti-IgE, anti-IL5, anti-IL5R, anti-IL4/IL13)**	

Assess control

- First check adherence, inhaler technique, environmental factors, ▲ and comorbid conditions.
- **Step up** if needed; reassess in 2–6 weeks
- **Step down** if possible (if asthma is well controlled for at least 3 consecutive months)

Consult with asthma specialist if Step 4 or higher is required. Consider consultation at Step 3.

Control assessment is a key element of asthma care. This involves both impairment and risk. Use of objective measures, self-reported control, and health care utilization are complementary and should be employed on an ongoing basis, depending on the individual's clinical situation.

Abbreviations: ICS, inhaled corticosteroid; LABA, long-acting beta$_2$-agonist; LAMA, long-acting muscarinic antagonist; LTRA, leukotriene receptor antagonist; SABA, inhaled short-acting beta$_2$-agonist

▲ Updated based on the 2020 guidelines.
* Cromolyn, Nedocromil, LTRAs including Zileuton and montelukast, and Theophylline were not considered for this update, and/or have limited availability for use in the United States, and/or have an increased risk of adverse consequences and need for monitoring that make their use less desirable. The FDA issued a Boxed Warning for montelukast in March 2020.
** The AHRQ systematic reviews that informed this report did not include studies that examined the role of asthma biologics (e.g. anti-IgE, anti-IL5, anti-IL5R, anti-IL4/IL13). Thus, this report does not contain specific recommendations for the use of biologics in asthma in Steps 5 and 6.
■ Data on the use of LAMA therapy in individuals with severe persistent asthma (Step 6) were not included in the AHRQ systematic review and thus no recommendation is made.

December 2020

Source: National Heart, Lung, and Blood Institute (2020)/US Department of Health and Human Services/Public Domain.

accessible, quality healthcare (examples of some social determinants of health [SDoH]) create disparate outcome among low-income and racial/ethnic minority populations leading to poorer health in these groups (Grant et al., 2022). SDoH play a major role in disparities seen with asthma. Factors, created through US historical and ongoing structural racism in housing, that increase the risk for asthma and asthma morbidity include neighborhood violence, air pollution exposure, food insecurity, barriers to employment, social disadvantage, inequalities in wealth and education, and long-term stress (Grant et al., 2022).

Common asthma triggers

- Emotional stress
- Exercise or physical exertion
- Animal dander
- Smoking (tobacco, marijuana, and e-cigarette), including primary and secondary smoke
- Vaping
- Air pollution
- Woodburning stoves
- Pollens
- Dust mites, cockroach antigen
- Mold
- Cold air
- URI, especially viral like influenza and COVID-19
- Sulfites in foods
- Cosmetics
- Certain medications (aspirin, nonsteroidal anti-inflammatory drugs, and beta-blockers)

Reducing exposure to indoor allergens

- Keep humidity <50% to reduce dust mites.
- Use covers for mattresses, pillows, comforters, and furniture cushions.
- Reduce sources of animal dander as much as possible.
- Dust and vacuum frequently using vacuum with a high-efficiency air (HEPA) filter.
- Use cockroach traps to reduce infestation and allergen source.
- Identify and remediate household mold.
- Eliminate household smoking.
- Avoid the use of fireplaces and wood stove heaters.

Source: National Heart, Lung, and Blood Institute (2020) and Raju et al. (2020).

Smoking Cessation

Pregnant individuals with a history of asthma who also smoke should be counseled on the importance of smoking cessation. In addition to increasing maternal and fetal morbidity, smoking predisposes the pregnant person to worsening asthma and the potential for increased medication use. The perinatal morbidity of asthma is compounded by smoking, leading to an even higher risk of FGR and PTB in those with asthma who smoke during pregnancy (Bonham et al., 2018). Using the five *A's*—Ask, Advise, Assess, Assist, and Arrange—the clinician should inquire about all types of tobacco and marijuana use, including cigarette smoking, use of e-cigarettes, or vaping and advise cessation of these products, providing motivational feedback. Provide reputable resources that may be helpful with cessation and consider prescribing varenicline or bupropion (ACOG, 2020). See Chapter 18, *Substance Use during Pregnancy*, for more on the use of these medications in pregnancy.

Patient Education

Education about asthma management and how it relates to pregnancy can help individuals control their symptoms. Requesting patients to monitor their "personal best" as needed with a peak-flow meter can also assist the health-care provider in monitoring asthma status during pregnancy. Rescue therapy can be started at home if symptoms of asthma flare up, such as coughing, chest tightness, wheezing, shortness of breath, or labored breathing (ACOG, 2008, reaffirmed 2016). The information in Table 49.1 can be used during pregnancy and the postpartum period including in those who are breastfeeding. It is recommended that pregnant people receive influenza and COVID-19 vaccination because viral infections can exacerbate asthma during pregnancy.

Signs of asthma control

- Minimal or no chronic symptoms day or night
- Minimal or no exacerbations
- No limitations on activities
- Maintenance of (near) normal pulmonary function
- Minimal use of short-acting inhaled beta$_2$-agonist
- Minimal or no adverse effects from medications

Source: Winland-Brown et al. (2019)/F.A. Davis Company.

Interprofessional Care

Pregnant people with severe or poorly controlled asthma face higher perinatal risks and a referral to a physician for surveillance and medication management is recommended. A first-trimester ultrasound is often done for those with severe asthma to corroborate pregnancy dating due to the risk for PTB and FGR. Those with persistent or severe asthma, those with suboptimal asthma control, and those recovering from severe asthma exacerbation should have periodic ultrasound evaluations for fetal growth in the third trimester (ACOG, 2008, reaffirmed 2016).

Influenza

Influenza is a seasonal contagious respiratory illness that can range from mild to severe and typically occurs between late October and May in the Northern Hemisphere. Of the three viral types (A, B, and C), influenza A is the type most responsible for causing pandemics because of its high susceptibility to antigenic variation. In the United States, the incidence of influenza is approximately 8%, with a range of 3–11% depending on the season (Tokars et al., 2018). Influenza viruses are spread from person to person primarily through large-particle respiratory droplet transmission (particles ≥5 μm) and can travel up to 6 ft via coughing, sneezing, and/or speaking. The virus can also be transmitted indirectly by touching a contaminated surface (from days to weeks after contamination) followed by contact with the mucous membranes of the mouth, nose, or eyes (Otter et al., 2016).

Risk of contracting influenza is correlated with group living conditions and access to healthcare services. Increased morbidity and mortality have been associated with preexisting health conditions (Quinn et al., 2011). The typical incubation period for influenza is one to four days (Centers for Disease Control and Prevention (CDC), 2021b). The severity of any given influenza outbreak is dependent on the characteristic of the circulating viral strain, the uptake of available vaccines specific for the circulating strain, the host immune response, and individual comorbidities (Nypaver et al., 2021). Key indicators for the severity of an influenza season are classified by the CDC using the following criteria: (a) outpatient visits for influenza-like illness; (b) influenza-associated hospitalizations; and (c) influenza/pneumonia-related deaths (Biggerstaff et al., 2018).

Infection from seasonal pandemic influenza outbreaks can cause otherwise healthy pregnant and postpartum patients to have disproportionately higher rates of hospital admissions and mortality than the general population. The increased severity of influenza in pregnancy is related to physiological changes in pregnancy. Pregnancy adaptations in the cardiovascular and respiratory systems result in increased heart rate and oxygen consumption in early pregnancy and decreased lung capacity but increased efficiency near term. Immunologic alterations result in a shift away from cell-mediated immunity, predisposing pregnant people to increased susceptibility to infection and increased illness severity.

The fetal effects of prenatal influenza infection have not been well studied. Some evidence suggests that individuals with influenza during pregnancy, especially severe illness, are at increased risk of adverse outcomes such as PTB, low birthweight, small for gestational age neonates, and fetal demise (Fell et al., 2017; Giles et al., 2019). These adverse outcomes may be related to the fever and hyperthermia that usually accompanies influenza, highlighting the importance of promptly treating fever in pregnancy with acetaminophen.

Influenza is highly contagious with the same symptoms noted for pregnant and nonpregnant populations. The hallmark clinical signs of infection include an abrupt onset of fever, headache, cough, shortness of breath, congestion, sore throat, chills or sweats, myalgias, and malaise (Nypaver et al., 2021). Diagnostic tests for influenza either have low sensitivity or take time to provide results. Since it is critical to initiate appropriate treatment promptly in pregnant people, the diagnosis of influenza should be made clinically, without waiting for results from diagnostic testing. Treatment consists of symptomatic care and antiviral medications as soon as possible after symptoms are reported to reduce the severity of illness. Available data suggest no adverse fetal effects from antiviral medications (Gaitonde et al., 2019; Table 49.3).

Pregnant people with suspected influenza are advised to seek emergency care immediately if symptoms such as difficulty breathing, sudden dizziness, confusion, persistent vomiting, or fever not controlled with acetaminophen occur.

During flu season, office settings should have policy measures in place to ensure appropriate triage and care of pregnant individuals with suspected influenza.

Table 49.3   Food and Drug Administration–Approved Antiviral Influenza Medications

Influenza treatment		Use in pregnancy
Antipyretics	Acetaminophen	
Antivirals Initiate within 24 or <48 hours of symptom onset	**Neuroaminidase inhibitors** Oseltamivir (Tamiflu)—75 mg BID for 5 days (adults and children >13 y.o.) (Oral capsules or suspension) Zanamivor (Relenza)—10 mg (two inhalations) for 5 days. (2 doses should be taken on the first day of treatment, with at least 2 hours between doses) (Inhalation powder) Peramivir (Rapivab)—600 mg in a single dose (Solution for injection) **CEN inhibitors** Baloxavir (Xofluza)	First-line treatment in pregnancy. Contraindicated in people with milk allergy, underlying reactive airway disease (e.g., asthma, chronic obstructive pulmonary disease) Benefits outweigh the risk Avoid in Pregnancy
Symptomatic relief measures	Increased hydration Increased rest Acetaminophen	All are encouraged in pregnancy
Infection control	Isolation from other family members Frequent hand washing Household disinfectants used on bedside tables, doorknobs, telephones, and bathrooms while household member is sick	All are encouraged in pregnancy

Source: Gaitonde et al. (2019), Nypaver et al. (2021), and U.S. Food & Drug Administration (2022).

Advice includes reporting of signs and symptoms of influenza immediately to their healthcare provider. Empiric treatment based on telephone consultation can be considered to facilitate rapid treatment, assuming that hospitalization is not indicated. In outpatient settings, screen for respiratory symptoms at the front desk, encourage wearing of a face mask, and direct the person to a separate waiting area if they are symptomatic, to reduce exposure to others.

The Inactivated influenza vaccine (IIV) is indicated during pregnancy and should be given as soon as the vaccine is available in the fall for protection throughout the flu season. It is safe during any time in gestation, including the first trimester. Breastfeeding is not a contraindication for either the live or inactivated influenza immunization (Dehlinger et al., 2021; Gaitonde et al., 2019).

Upper Respiratory Infection

The clinical features, diagnosis, and management of URIs are generally similar in pregnant and nonpregnant populations. Changes in susceptibility to infection, physiology, and the effect of the infection and its treatment on the fetus are considerations in the evaluation and management of pregnant individuals with URI. Acute URI, also referred to as the common cold, is one of the top three acute illnesses in the outpatient setting of the United States. Patients usually present with nasal congestion, rhinorrhea, sneezing, sore throat,

cough, general malaise, and/or low-grade fever. Symptoms are self-limited with onset within 1–3 days after exposure, last for 7–10 days, and can persist for up to 3 weeks (DeGeorge et al., 2019). Upper respiratory tract infections involve the nose, sinuses, pharynx, larynx, and the large airways. Rhinovirus is the most predominant cause of acute URI and transmission occurs through contact with the nasal secretions and saliva of infected people (Thomas & Bomar, 2021). Other common URI viruses include the influenza virus, adenovirus, enterovirus, coronavirus, and respiratory syncytial virus. Approximately 5–15% of acute pharyngotonsillitis is caused by the *Streptococcus pyogenes* bacteria, Group A Streptococcus (GAS; Thomas & Bomar, 2021; Yoon et al., 2017).

Antibiotics are not indicated for treatment of the common cold or acute viral rhinosinusitis (AVRS), which should be managed with supportive care and over-the-counter medications for symptom relief, except in the small subset of patients (between 2% and 15%) with evidence of secondary acute bacterial rhinosinusitis (ABRS; Patel & Hwang, 2022; Thomas & Bomar, 2021). Analgesics, cough suppressants, decongestants, antihistamines, and expectorants are the most commonly used over-the-counter medications for relief of cold symptoms, and most are acceptable for short-term use during pregnancy (Table 49.4). An analgesic such as acetaminophen is commonly used to control fever. Nonsteroidal anti-inflammatory medication is avoided in the third trimester, as it has been associated with premature ductus arteriosus

Table 49.4   Common Treatments for the Common Cold

Dry/Inflammatory cough	**Dextromethorphan (Robitussin, Vicks 44 Cough Relief, Delsym).** 120 mg per 24 hour is maximum dose. Administer every 4–12 hours depending on formulation
Decongestants oral and nasal Short-term relief of nasal congestion and pressure	Pseudoephedrine (Sudafed) 30 mg 1–2 tables PO q 4–6 hours prn after the first trimester (risk of gastroschisis & small bowel atresia). Potential for abuse; May require RX Phenylephrine PE (10 mg) (Sudafed PE) 1 table PO every 4 hours after first trimester Phenylephrine Spray 1% 2 spray each nostril every 4 hours. Discontinue after 3 days. Short-acting phenylephrine (4 hours) Long-acting phenylephrine (Afrin spray) 2–3 sprays each nostril every 12 hours for 3 days. Risk of rebound congestion
Intranasal corticosteroid nasal and sinus congestion, rhinorrhea, and postnasal drip	Fluticasone propionate nasal (Flonase) 1–2 sprays in each nostril daily Can use for 7–14 days if needed
Antihistamines	Diphenhydramine (Benadryl) 25 mg PO every 4–6 hours prn Chlorpheniramine (Chlor-Trimeton) 4 mg PO every 4–6 hours
Expectorant: productive cough	Guaifenesin (Mucinex) 200–400 mg PO q 4–6 hours. Drink adequate water
Cough and wheezing	Albuterol (Proventil HFA) inhaler 2 puffs every 4–6 hours as needed. Only used for bronchospasms if cough is persistent and severe for short term
Fever, chills, pain, and sore throat	Acetaminophen (Tylenol). 325–1,000 mg PO every 4–6 hours Acetaminophen orally 4,000 mg per 24 hr. is maximum dose
Nasal corticosteroids	Intranasal cromolyn sodium (NasalCrom) 1 spray each nostril 3–4 times daily. Every 4–6 hours
Sore throat	Phenol oropharyngeal (chloraseptic throat spray) 1–5 sprays orally every 2 hours
Symptom relief measures	Increased humidification, rest, and fluids. Chicken or vegetable soup, warm salt water gargles, intranasal saline irrigation

Source: Levi (2019) and DeGeorge et al. (2019).

closure (Koren et al., 2006). Patients are instructed to read the labels of the over-the-counter-medication to avoid products containing alcohol and to consult with pharmacists as needed to ensure they are not taking medicine they do not require. Single-ingredient medications rather than multisymptom medications are preferred to avoid unnecessary overmedication as some have up to five medicinal ingredients. Symptoms gradually resolve over 3–10 days, although the cough may persist for longer.

Acute Bacterial Rhinosinusitis

Pregnant individuals with a common cold are at increased risk of developing ABRS, which can develop into further infection, such as acute otitis media. The increased risk for ABRS is attributed in part to congestion from hormonal effects on the nasal mucosa. Over-the-counter medications for symptom relief are recommended and the need for antibiotic therapy is evaluated. Antibiotics are generally indicated for pregnant people with any of the following characteristics: (a) persistent symptoms for 10 days without improvement, (b) severe symptoms or temperature >102.2 °F (39 °C) for several days, or (c) worsening symptoms after five to six days of improving symptoms (Table 49.5; Levi, 2019).

If an antibiotic is required, the medication is chosen based on coverage of the probable organism, community resistance, and pregnancy safety data. ABRS during pregnancy can be treated with amoxicillin 500 mg tid or 875 mg bid; or amoxicillin-clavulanate (Augmentin) 500 mg/125 mg tid or 875 mg/125 mg bid for first-line treatment (Patel & Hwang, 2022). Patients with a penicillin allergy can be treated with a third-generation oral cephalosporin (cefixime) 400 mg daily or cefpodoxime 200 mg twice daily.

Additional treatments include saline nasal spray or saline nasal irrigation. Short-term nasal corticosteroids (beclomethasone) may be initiated in those with rhinitis or ABRS in need of immediate symptom relief. Intranasal cromolyn sodium improves symptoms of a runny nose

Table 49.6 Management of Acute Bacterial Rhinosinusitis

Treatment	Dosage and duration
Supportive therapy unless symptoms persist ≥10 days	Saline nasal spray or wash 3–4 times daily, steam, fluids, and rest
First-line antibiotics	Amoxicilin 500 mg tid or 875 mg twice daily for 5–7 days or 7–10 days if risk of bacterial resistance Amoxicillin-clavulanate (Augmentin) 500 mg/125 mg tid or 875 mg/125 mg bid for 5–7 days or 7–10 days if risk of bacterial resistance
Alternative for Penicillin allergy or intolerance	Third-generation oral cephalosporins: Cefixime 400 mg daily or 200 mg bid for 10 days Cefpodoxime 200 mg bid for 10 days with food Azithromycin 500 mg PO on day 1, then 250 mg for 4 days (dictated by local resistance patterns)
Short-term nasal corticosteroids	Beclomethasone diproprionate 1–2 sprays in each nostril daily for 5–7 days. Maximum of 4 sprays in each nostril per day. Not to exceed 3 weeks of use

and sneezing and has been used safely in pregnancy (Patel & Hwang, 2022). A rapid Streptococcus screen is advised with symptoms of pharyngitis, and treatment with penicillin, erythromycin, or azithromycin is initiated with a positive diagnosis (Table 49.6).

Pneumonia

In the United States, pneumonia complicates approximately 1 per 1000 pregnancies and is the most common nonobstetric infection-related cause of maternal death (Tang et al., 2018). Pneumonia can occur independently or may follow viral URIs, such as influenza, bronchitis, or a common cold. *Streptococcus pneumoniae* and *Haemophilus influenzae* are the most common pathogens that cause pneumonia in pregnancy. While the incidence, clinical manifestations, and diagnosis of bacterial pneumonia in pregnancy are similar to the general population, physiologic changes of pregnancy increase susceptibility to viral pneumonia, including H1N1, Influenza, varicella, and COVID-19 (Annamraju & Mackillop, 2017). Severe pneumonia in pregnancy is associated with increased maternal and fetal morbidity and mortality (Tang et al., 2018). The risk of pneumonia during pregnancy is lowest during the first trimester; advanced gestational age is an independent risk factor for pneumonia (Graves, 2010). Additional risk factors and comorbidities further stress the immunocompromised person in pregnancy, including anemia, asthma, smoking, antenatal corticosteroid use, and tocolytics.

The classic symptoms of pneumonia are sudden onset of fever, shaking chills, dyspnea, and cough productive of purulent sputum, though symptom presentation varies. Chest

Table 49.5 Bacterial and Viral Sinusitis Symptoms

Bacterial sinusitis	Nonspecific symptoms of viral and bacterial sinusitis
Symptoms greater than 10 days Symptoms initially improve and then worsen May or may not have a fever Unilateral maxillary and/or tooth pain Unilateral facial pain Unilateral sinus pain with palpation or percussion No improvement with decongestants Mucopurulent anterior or posterior discharge Nasal Congestion or Obstruction	Headache Fever Malaise Generalize facial pain or tenderness Bilateral maxillary pain Postnasal drip Cough Bilateral toothache or pain

X-ray with abdominal shielding is warranted in any pregnant person suspected of having pneumonia. Pregnant individuals with pneumonia have higher rates of cardiopulmonary complications, hospitalizations, and even death, especially in the second half of pregnancy (Cantu & Tita, 2013). They also are at risk for early pregnancy loss, PTB, and other perinatal complications (Cantu & Tita, 2013). Collaborative management is indicated for pneumonia in pregnancy.

Bronchitis is a URI of the large airways (bronchi) and manifests as cough, often worse at night, that can persist for 2–3 weeks, but less than 30 days, and may be associated with bronchospasms and/or excessive mucus production (Smith et al., 2020). As with most URIs, it is caused by a virus, and antibiotic therapy is not indicated. Diagnosis is primarily clinical, and other causes for acute cough such as pneumonia, asthma, or postnasal drip should be ruled out if suspected. Bronchitis can lead to pneumonia; therefore, individuals whose symptoms worsen or persist should be reevaluated. Pregnant patients are advised to return for follow-up if there is no resolution of symptoms two to three days after the start of antibiotic therapy or if symptoms worsen.

Summary

Common respiratory disorders include asthma, influenza, URIs, and pneumonia. Symptoms of mild respiratory infections can usually be alleviated with over-the-counter or nonpharmacologic remedies. Infections and asthma that become severe likely warrant collaborative management or transfer to higher acuity care. Influenza in pregnancy increases risk of severe illness, hospitalization, and death. There is some evidence to suggest influenza during pregnancy increases adverse perinatal outcome such as early pregnancy loss and PTB. Influenza vaccination as soon as it becomes available in the fall is strongly encouraged. Pneumonia in pregnancy is potentially severe and increases risk for PTB, pulmonary edema, and death. Prenatal care providers are ideally situated for early recognition and treatment of mild to moderate respiratory disorders, thus improving the health of childbearing people and their infants.

Resources for Clients and Their Families

Flu and Pregnancy: https://www.cdc.gov/flu/pdf/freeresources/pregnant/flushot_pregnant_factsheet.pdf

Homecare for the flu: https://www.cdc.gov/flu/about/index.html

Treating Acute Bacterial Rhinosinusitis: https://www.entnet.org/wp-content/uploads/2021/04/adult-sinusitis-patient-info-treating-acute-bacterial-rhinosinusitis.pdf

Resources for Healthcare Providers

Influenza Antiviral Medications: Summary for Clinicians: https://www.cdc.gov/flu/professionals/antivirals/summary-clinicians.htm

Asthma and Allergy Foundation of America: https://www.aafa.org

Centers for Disease Control and Prevention. Influenza: Information for Health Professionals. https://www.cdc.gov/flu/professionals/index.htm

National Foundation for Infectious Diseases: Flu (Influenza). https://www.nfid.org/infectious-diseases/influenza-flu

References

American College of Obstetricians & Gynecologists (ACOG). (2020). Tobacco and nicotine cessation during pregnancy. ACOG committee opinion no. 807. *Obstetrics & Gynecology*, *135*(5), 1244–1246. https://doi.org/10.1097/AOG.0000000000003822

American College of Obstetricians & Gynecologists (ACOG), & The American College of Allergy, Asthma, and Immunology (ACAAI). (2020). The use of newer asthma and allergy medications during pregnancy: The American College of Obstetricians and Gynecologists (ACOG) and the American College of Allergy, Asthma, and Immunology (ACAAI) position statement. *Anals of Allergy, Asthma, & Immunology*, *84*(5), 475–480. https://doi.org/10.1016/S1081-1206(10)62505-7

American College of Obstetricians and Gynecologists (ACOG). (2008, reaffirmed 2016)). Asthma in pregnancy: Practice Bulletin No. 90. *Obstetrics and Gynecology*, *111*, 457–464. https://doi.org/10.1097/AOG.ob013e3181665ff4

Annamraju, H., & Mackillop, L. (2017). Respiratory disease in pregnancy. *Obstetrics, Gynaecology & Reproductive Medicine*, *27*(4), 105–111. https://doi.org/10.1016/j.ogrm.2017.01.011

Biggerstaff, M., Kniss, K., Jernigan, D. B., Brammer, L., Bresee, J., Garg, S., Burns, E., & Reed, C. (2018). Systematic assessment of multiple routine and near real-time indicators to classify the severity of influenza seasons and pandemics in the United States, 2003–2004 through 2015–2016. *American Journal of Epidemiology*, *187*(5), 1040–1050. https://doi.org/10.15585/mmwr.mm6824a3

Bonham, C. A., Patterson, K. C., & Stek, M. E. (2018). Asthma outcomes and management during pregnancy. *Chest*, *153*(2), 515–527. https://doi.org/10.1016/j.chest.2017.08.029

Cantu, J., & Tita, A. T. (2013). Management of influenza in pregnancy. *American Journal of Perinatology*, *30*(2), 99–104. https://doi.org/10.1055/s-0032-1331033

Centers for Disease Control and Prevention. (2022). *Most recent national asthma data*. https://www.cdc.gov/asthma/most_recent_national_asthma_data.htm.

Centers for Disease Control and Prevention (CDC). (2021a). *Most recent national asthma data*. https://www.cdc.gov/asthma/most_recent_national_asthma_data.htm.

Centers for Disease Control and Prevention (CDC). (2021b). *Key facts about influenza*. https://www.cdc.gov/flu/about/keyfacts.htm.

Cusack, R. P., & Gauvreau, G. M. (2020). Pharmacotherapeutic management of asthma in pregnancy and the effect of sex hormones. *Expert Opinion on Pharmacology*, *22*(3), 339–349. https://doi.org/10.1080/14656566.2020.1828863

DeGeorge, K. C., Ring, D. J., & Dalrymple, S. N. (2019). Treatment of the common cold. *American Family Physician*, *100*(5), 281–289.

Dehlinger, C., Nypaver, C., & Whiteside, J. (2021). Use of an evidence-based approach to improve influenza vaccination uptake in pregnancy. *Journal of Midwifery & Women's Health*, *66*(3), 360–365. https://doi.org/10.1111/jmwh.13227

Esden, J., & Pesta-Walsh, N. (2018). Diagnosis and treatment of asthma in nonpregnant women. *Journal of Midwifery & Women's Health*, *64*(1), 18–27. https://doi.org/10.1111/jmwh.12907

Fell, D. B., Savitz, D. A., Kramer, M. S., Gessner, B. D., Katz, M. A., Knight, M., Luteijn, J. M., Marshall, H., Bhat, N., Gravett, M. G., Skidmore, B., & Ortiz, J. R. (2017). Maternal influenza and birth outcomes: Systematic review of comparative studies. *BJOG: An International Journal of Obstetrics & Gynaecology*, *124*(1), 48–59. https://doi.org/10.1111/1471-0528.14143

Gaitonde, D. Y., Moore, F. C., & Morgan, M. K. (2019). Influenza: Diagnosis and treatment. *American Family Physician*, *100*(12), 751–758.

Giles, M. L., Krishnaswamy, S., Macartney, K., & Cheng, A. (2019). The safety of inactivated influenza vaccines in pregnancy for birth outcomes: A systematic review. *Human Vaccines & Immunotherapeutics*, *15*(3), 687–699. https://doi.org/10.1080/21645515.2018.1540807

Grant, T., Croce, E., & Matsui, E. C. (2022). Asthma and the social determinants of health. *Annals of Allergy, Asthma, & Immunology*, *128*(1), 5–11. https://doi.org/10.1016/j.anai.2021.10.002

Graves, C. R. (2010). Pneumonia in pregnancy. *Clinical Obstetrics and Gynecology*, *53*, 329–336. https://doi.org/10.1097/GRF.0b013e3181de8a6f

Ibrahim, W. H., Rasul, F., Ahmad, M., Bajwa, A. S., Alamlih, L. I., El Arabi, N. M., Dauleh, M. M., Abubekar, I. Y., Khan, M. U., Ibrahim, T. S., & Ibrahim, A. A. (2018). Asthma knowledge, care, and outcome during pregnancy: The QAKCOP study. *Chronic Respiratory Disease*, *16*. https://doi.org/10.1177/1479972318767719

Koren, G., Florescu, A., Costei, A. M., Boskovic, R., & Moretti, M. E. (2006). Nonsteroidal anti-inflammatory drugs during third trimester and the risk of premature closure of the ductus arteriosus: A meta-analysis. *The Annals of Pharmacotherapy*, *40*(5), 824–829.

Levi, M. E. (2019). Primary care management of upper respiratory infections in the wome's health care setting. *Journal of Midwifery & Wome's Health*, *64*(3), 330–336. https://doi.org/10.1111/jmwh.12938

Martinez, A., de la Rosa, R., Mujahid, M., & Thakur, N. (2021). Structural racism and its pathways to asthma and atopic dermatitis. *Journal of Allergy and Clinical Immunology*, *148*(5), 112–1120. https://doi.org/10.1016/j.jaci.2021.09.020

National Heart, Lung, and Blood Institute (NHLBI). (2020). *2020 Focused updates to the asthma management guidelines*. https://www.nhlbi.nih.gov/resources/2020-focused-updates-asthma-management-guidelines

Nypaver, C., Dehlinger, C., & Carter, C. (2021). Influenza and influenza vaccine: A review. *Journal of Midwifery & Wome's Health*, *66*(1), 45–53. https://doi.org/10.1111/jmwh.13203

Otter, J. A., Donskey, C., Yezli, S., Douthwaite, S., Goldenberg, S., & Weber, D. J. (2016). Transmission of SARS and MERS coronaviruses and influenza virus in healthcare settings: The possible role of dry surface contamination. *Journal of Hospital Infection*, *92*(3), 235–250. https://doi.org/10.1016/j.jhin.2015.08.027

Pate, C. A., Zahran, H. S., Qin, X., Johnson, C., Hummelman, E., & Malilay, J. (2021). Asthma surveillance-United States, 2006–2018: Surveillance summaries. *Morbidity and Mortality Weekly Report (MMWR)*, *70*(5), 1–32.

Patel, Z.M & Hwang, P.H. (2022). Uncomplicated acute sinusitis and rhinosinusitis in adults: Treatment. *UpToDate*. https://www.uptodate.com/contents/uncomplicated-acute-sinusitis-and-rhinosinusitis-in-adults-treatment/print

Quinn, S. C., Kumar, S., Freimuth, V. S., Musa, D., Casteneda-Angarita, N., & Kidwell, K. (2011). Racial disparities in exposure, susceptibility, and access to health care in the US H1N1 influenza pandemic. *American Journal of Public Health*, *101*(2), 285–293. https://doi.org/10.2105/AJPH.2009.188029

Raju, S., Siddharthan, T., & McCormack, M. C. (2020). Indoor air pollution and respiratory health. *Clinics in Chest Medicine*, *41*(4), 825–843. https://doi.org/10.1016/j.ccm.2020.08.014

Ray, K. (2021). In the name of racial justice: Why bioethics should care about environmental toxins. *Hastings Center Report*, *51*(3), 23–26. https://doi.org/10.1002/hast.1251

Robijn, A. L., Bokern, M. P., Jensen, D. B., Baines, K. J., & Murphy, V. E. (2021). Risk factors for asthma exacerbations during pregnancy: A systemic review and meta-analysis. *European Respiratory Review*, *31*, 220039. https://doi.org.10.1183/16000617.0039-2022

Roff, A. J., Morrison, J. L., Tai, A., Clifton, V. L., & Gatford, K. L. (2021). Maternal asthma during pregnancy and risks of allergy and asthma in progeny: A systematic review protocol. *JBI Evidence Synthesis*, *19*(8), 2007–2013. https://doi.org/10.11124/JBIES-20-00328

Schatz, M., Hayden, K., Forsythe, A., Chilingar, L., Hoffman, C., Sperling, W., & Zeiger, R. S. (1988). The course of asthma during pregnancy, post partum, and with successive pregnancies: A prospective analysis. *Journal of Allergy and Clinical Immunology*, *81*(3), 509–517.

Smith, M. P., Lown, M., Singh, S., Ireland, B., Hill, A. T., Linder, J. A., Irwin, R. S., & CHEST Expert Cough Panel. (2020). Acute cough due to acute bronchitis in immunocompetent adult outpatients: CHEST Expert Panel Report. *Chest*, *157*(5), 1256–1265.

Tang, P., Wang, J., & Song, Y. (2018). Characteristics and pregnancy outcomes of patients with severe pneumonia complicating pregnancy: A retrospective study of 12 cases and a literature review. *BMC Pregnancy & Childbirth*, *18*(1), 1–6. https://doi.org/10.1186/s12884-018-2070-0

Thomas, M., & Bomar, P. A. (2021 June 30). *Upper respiratory tract infection*. StatPearls. https://www.ncbi.nlm.nih.gov/books/NBK532961

Tokars, J. L., Olsen, S. J., & Reed, C. (2018). Seasonal incidence of symptomatic influenza in the United States. *Clinical Infectious Disease*, *66*(10), 1511–1518. https://doi.org/10.1093/cid/cix1060

U.S. Food & Drug Administration. (2022). *Influenza (flu) antiviral drugs and related information*. https://www.fda.gov/drugs/information-drug-class/influenza-flu-antiviral-drugs-and-related-information

Wang, H., Li, N., & Huang, H. (2020). Asthma in pregnancy: Pathophysiology, diagnosis, whole-course management, and medical safety. *Canadian Respiratory Journal*. https://doi.org/10.1155/2020/9046842

Winland-Brown, J. E., Beausejour, B., & Porter, B. O. (2019). Inflammatory respiratory disorders. In L. M. Dunphy, J. E. Winland-Brown, B. O. Porter, & D. J. Thomas (Eds.), *Primary care: The art and science of advanced practice nursing - An interprofessional approach* (5th ed., pp. 397–406). F.A. Davis Company.

Yoon, Y. K., Park, C. S., Kim, J. W., Hwang, K., Lee, S. Y., Kim, T. H., Park, D. Y., Kim, H. J., Kim, D. Y., Lee, H. J., Shin, H. Y., You, Y. K., Park, D. A., & Kim, S. W. (2017). Guidelines for the antibiotic use in adults with acute upper respiratory tract infections. *Infection & Chemotherapy*, *49*(4), 326–352. https://doi.org/10.3947/ic.2017.49.4.326

50

Urinary Tract Disorders

Rhonda Arthur and Nancy Pesta Walsh

Relevant Terms

Acute cystitis—infection involving the lower urinary tract

Antibiogram—a table summarizing the percent of individual bacterial pathogens susceptible to different microbial agents

Asymptomatic bacteriuria—100,000 or more colony-forming units/mL of urine in a patient without symptoms

Bacteriuria—the presence of bacteria in the urinary tract; can be symptomatic or asymptomatic

Dysuria—painful urination

Hematuria—red blood cells in the urine

Lower UTI—infection involving the bladder and urethra

Nephrolithiasis (kidney stones)—renal calculi that develop from a combination of naturally occurring chemicals in the body

Nocturia—excessive urination at night

Pyelonephritis—infection involving the renal pelves, inflammation of one or both kidneys.

Pyuria—pus or white blood cells in the urine (>7 white blood cells [WBCs]/mL)

Renal colic—pain in the lower back or abdomen usually associated with kidney stones

Upper UTI—infection involving the renal pelves

Urinary frequency—voiding at frequent intervals

Urinary tract infection (UTI)—more than 100 colony-forming units/mL of urine with accompanying pyuria in a symptomatic patient

Urinary urgency—urge to urinate immediately

Introduction

Upper and lower urinary tract disorders are common in pregnancy. Some of the most commonly encountered urinary tract disorders include **urinary tract infection** (UTI) and **pyelonephritis**. UTI during pregnancy may result in significant morbidity and mortality for both the pregnant person and the fetus, including pyelonephritis, preeclampsia, preterm birth, and low birth weight (Bookstaver et al., 2015; Habak & Griggs, 2021; Matuszkiewicz-Rowinska et al., 2015). While the occurrence of **nephrolithiasis** in pregnancy is no more common than in nonpregnant people, it poses the potential for serious complications to the person and the fetus, including hypertension, preeclampsia, preterm labor, recurrent abortions, gestational diabetes mellitus, and cesarean delivery (Lee et al., 2021). **Renal colic** is one of the most common reasons for nonobstetric hospitalization of pregnant people (Hernandez & Pais, 2016). This chapter will discuss the changes in the urinary tract, physical evaluation, diagnosis, and treatment of common pregnancy-related urinary tract complications.

Health equity key points

- Reduced access to prenatal care may result in undiagnosed UTI and may result in significant morbidity and mortality for both the pregnant person and the fetus, including pyelonephritis, preeclampsia, preterm birth, and low birth weight.
- UTIs during and outside of pregnancy are more prevalent among people with lower socioeconomic status and who are immigrants, likely due to decreased access to healthcare, antibiotic prescribing practices, nutritional status, and environmental factors.

Urinary Tract Infection

The classification of UTI depends on the presence or absence of symptoms. In the asymptomatic person, a UTI is diagnosed with the presence of 10^5 colony-forming units (cfu) per milliliter of urine (Angelescu et al., 2016; Habak & Griggs, 2021; US Preventive Services Task Force [USPSTF], 2019). This is referred to as **asymptomatic bacteriuria** (ASB) (Angelescu et al., 2016). In the symptomatic person, even growth as low as 10^2 cfu/mL could indicate infection (Chu & Lowder, 2018). These cases are sometimes called low-colony-count UTIs (Bryan, 2015).

Prenatal and Postnatal Care: A Person-Centered Approach, Third Edition. Edited by Karen Trister Grace, Cindy L. Farley, Noelene K. Jeffers, and Tanya Tringali.

Companion website: www.wiley.com/go/grace/prenatal

Prevalence and Risk Factors

The prevalence of UTI during pregnancy is approximately 1–4%, with recurrent UTI occurring more frequently during pregnancy (Ailes et al., 2016). The incidence of ASB in pregnant people ranges from 2% to 7%, and if left untreated, approximately 25–35% of these will go on to develop acute pyelonephritis (Badran et al., 2015; Habak & Griggs, 2021). UTIs during and outside of pregnancy are more prevalent among people with lower socioeconomic status and who are immigrants, likely due to decreased access to healthcare, antibiotic prescribing practices, nutritional status, and environmental factors (Casey et al., 2021; Habak & Griggs, 2021). Diabetes, obesity, sickle cell trait, and any condition that requires urinary catheterization place a person at an even greater risk of UTI (Habak & Griggs, 2021). The development of UTI is more common in the second and third trimesters. The prevalence of UTI during pregnancy increases with age.

Pathophysiology

The short urethra found in the female sex causes a higher incidence of UTI compared with the male sex, due to close proximity of the urethra to the perineum. Bacteria ascend from the colonized perineum, through the urethra, to the bladder and/or kidneys. For many people assigned female at birth, sexual activity increases risk for UTI due to minor mental trauma, which can introduce bacteria into the lower urinary tract (Quinlan & Jorgensen, 2017).

Anatomic and physiologic changes that occur with pregnancy affect the urinary tract system and further increase the risk of UTI. These normal changes include enlargement and displacement of the kidneys, dilation of the renal calyces and ureters, progesterone-related inhibition of ureteral smooth muscle contraction, bladder compression and displacement, and hyperemia, leading to increased urinary stasis and vesicoureteral reflux (Habak & Griggs, 2021). Other pregnancy-related factors contributing to UTI susceptibility include an increase in glomerular filtration rate (GFR), which decreases urine concentration, glycosuria, and the decreased ability to resist invading bacteria due to influence of progestin and estrogen that are present in the urine (Habak & Griggs, 2021). The mechanics of labor and birth, epidural anesthetics, and perineal trauma predispose the postpartum patient to UTI.

Common Pathogens

Neisseria gonorrhea and *Chlamydia trachomatis* are the most common causes of acute urethritis in the prenatal population, followed by low concentrations of coliform organisms. *Escherichia coli* is the most commonly identified pathogen in ASB and symptomatic UTI (Chotiprasitsakul et al., 2021; Habak & Griggs, 2021). This pathogen may be present in up to 82.5% of all UTIs in pregnancy (Habak & Griggs, 2021). It originates from fecal flora colonizing the periurethral area, causing an ascending infection. Other pathogens include (Chotiprasitsakul et al., 2021; Habak & Griggs, 2021):

- *Klebsiella pneumoniae*
- *Proteus mirabilis*
- *Enterobacter* species
- *Staphylococcus saprophyticus*
- Group B beta-hemolytic *Streptococcus*
- *Proteus* species

Group B streptococcus (GBS) is an important pathogen in pregnancy, as GBS colonization can result in invasive GBS disease and sepsis in the newborn. GBS **bacteriuria** occurs in approximately 2–7% of pregnant people (CDC, 2010). The presence of GBS bacteriuria in any concentration during pregnancy is associated with heavy vaginal colonization. This finding negates need for further GBS screening and is an indication for intrapartum antibiotic prophylaxis for prevention of GBS complications in infants and birthing people. The utility of treating GBS bacteriuria at colony counts $<10^5$ cfu/mL is uncertain and practice varies. The American College of Obstetricians and Gynecologists (ACOG) recommends treatment in asymptomatic patients only if the colony count is 10^5 cfu/mL or higher (ACOG, 2020).

Management of GBS bacteriuria in pregnancy

- With any colony count of GBS in the urine during the current pregnancy, the person is considered GBS positive and receives intrapartum antibiotic prophylaxis.
- GBS bacteriuria $\geq 10^5$ cfu/mL during pregnancy should be treated with a three- to seven-day course of antibiotics regardless of presence or absence of symptoms.
- All pregnant persons should undergo antepartum screening for GBS at 36 0/7–37 6/7 weeks of gestation unless intrapartum antibiotic prophylaxis is already indicated because of GBS bacteriuria during the pregnancy or previous GBS-infected newborn.
- Even if GBS bacteriuria was treated with antibiotics during pregnancy and even if subsequent cultures were negative, intrapartum antibiotic prophylaxis is still indicated.

Source: Adapted from ACOG (2020).

Asymptomatic Bacteriuria

ASB is detected with routine urine screening and occurs in approximately 2–7% of pregnant people (Habak & Griggs, 2021). If left untreated, ASB can progress to acute pyelonephritis, a complication that occurs more often during pregnancy (Nicolle et al., 2019). Screening for and treating ASB in pregnancy reduces the risk of subsequent pyelonephritis from approximately 20–35% to 1–4% (Nicolle et al., 2019).

Urine culture is the gold standard for detecting ASB in pregnancy and is recommended as a routine prenatal test by several expert groups (Habak & Griggs, 2021; Nicolle et al., 2019; United States Preventive Services Task Force [USPSTF], 2019). A diagnosis of ASB is made if the culture results indicate greater than 100,000 cfu/mL of a single organism (Habak & Griggs, 2021; Nicolle et al., 2019). The Infectious Diseases Society of America recommends a urine culture early in pregnancy (Nicolle et al., 2019). The 2019 USPSTF recommends a urine culture between 12 and 16 weeks of gestation or at the first prenatal visit if it occurs later than that time frame. There is no evidence for or against repeat screening for ASB if the initial culture is negative or after treatment of ASB (Nicolle et al., 2019). Current perinatal guidelines from the American Academy of Pediatrics and the American College of Obstetricians and Gynecologists (2017) do not recommend for or against routine screening urine culture, but state that if culture is performed and is positive, treatment is indicated and a test of cure after completion of antibiotics is recommended. In pregnancy, treatment of ASB is recommended to prevent the complications that increase perinatal morbidity and mortality (Habak & Griggs, 2021; Nicolle et al., 2019).

Urine dipstick tests are not sufficiently sensitive or specific to be used for routine prenatal bacteriuria screening in place of laboratory culture but may be more cost-effective in low-resource settings (Chotiprasitsakul et al., 2021). Urine cultures should be done every trimester in pregnant people with diabetes and sickle cell trait and can be considered in people at higher risk for preterm labor to improve the detection rate of ASB (McIsaac et al., 2005).

Acute Urethritis

Dysuria, frequency, urinary hesitancy, and purulent urethral discharge are the most common clinical manifestations of acute urethritis (Duff, 2022). Nucleic acid amplification test (NAAT) of urine or urethral discharge can identify a causative organism, which most often is chlamydia or gonorrhea (Duff, 2022). See Chapter 56, *Sexually Transmitted Infections and Vaginitis*, for treatment recommendations of these infections in pregnancy.

Acute Cystitis

Typical symptoms include dysuria, **urinary urgency**, and frequency. **Nocturia**, suprapubic pain, and **hematuria** may also be present. Some pregnant people present with vague or mild symptoms. Presenting with any combination of these symptoms indicates the need for a urine dipstick and a urine culture. **Urinary frequency** and urgency are common in normal pregnancy and are not reliable indicators of UTI (Thomas et al., 2010). Within two to four weeks of treatment, a urine culture should be repeated to ensure that the infection has cleared (Habak & Griggs, 2021). UTI is associated with increased risk for pyelonephritis, preterm birth, low birth weight, and perinatal mortality. Particularly in the third trimester, UTIs are associated with an increased risk of developing preeclampsia, possibly due to inflammatory factors (Easter et al., 2016). Pregnant people with health conditions such as immunosuppression, diabetes, sickle cell anemia, neurogenic bladder, or recurrent or persistent UTI prior to pregnancy are at an increased risk for **acute cystitis**.

Acute Pyelonephritis

Acute pyelonephritis is characterized by fever and costovertebral (CVA) tenderness in addition to significant bacteriuria. Other symptoms often include chills, myalgia, anorexia, nausea, vomiting, and low back pain. Pregnant people with acute pyelonephritis commonly appear acutely ill and require immediate care, usually including hospitalization (Habak & Griggs, 2021). Untreated pyelonephritis can lead to increased risk of maternal and fetal morbidity, including maternal sepsis, acute renal failure, acute respiratory distress, preterm birth, low birth weight, fetal growth restriction, and cesarean birth (Habak & Griggs, 2021).

Evaluation

Clinical presentation varies according to whether the person has ASB, a **lower UTI** (acute cystitis), or an **upper UTI** (pyelonephritis).

Health History

A focused health history includes determining risk factors for developing a UTI. A sexual history should be taken. Pregnant people should be queried on signs and symptoms of dysuria, urinary urgency, urinary frequency, nocturia, suprapubic pain, and hematuria. Acute UTI can also present with respiratory symptoms such as dyspnea, chest pain, and cough, and presence of these symptoms should be determined. Vaginal infections, which are common in people of reproductive age, can cause or mimic UTIs. Thus, symptoms of vaginal discharge, itching, or burning should be evaluated. If the pregnant person appears acutely ill, determining symptoms of fever, shaking chills, loss of appetite, nausea, and vomiting will increase clinical suspicion for pyelonephritis.

Risk factors for UTI in pregnancy

- Increasing parity
- Diabetes
- Sickle cell trait
- Urinary tract congenital anomaly
- History of recurring UTI
- Low socioeconomic status

Physical Examination

Physical examination findings should be considered in the context of gestational age. The differential diagnosis may change from one trimester to the next, and the increasing size of the gravid uterus may mask or mimic disease findings. Particular focus is on the abdomen and trunk, with evaluation for suprapubic tenderness and CVA tenderness. Lower UTI may present with tenderness over the bladder. Pyelonephritis signs can vary and often include fever >100.4°F (38°C), shaking chills, and CVA tenderness. Right-side flank pain is more common than left-side or bilateral flank pain due to increased ureteral dilation on the right side with resulting hydronephrosis (Talwar et al., 2021). Assessment of the fetal heart rate is included in the evaluation. If maternal fever is present, the fetal heart rate may be elevated. Depending on presentation, pelvic examination may be considered in symptomatic people to rule out vaginitis or cervicitis.

Laboratory Testing

Clinical presentation and the person's prior history will guide laboratory testing. In the office setting, urinary sediment analysis (UA) and urine dipstick testing offer speed and low cost. Urine dipstick to evaluate for UTI is based on several observations: (a) normal urine contains nitrates but not nitrites; and (b) many bacteria causing UTI can convert urinary nitrates to nitrites (Chotiprasitsakul et al., 2021). It is most useful for detecting >100,000 cfu/mL of aerobic Gram-negative rods. Additionally, the presence of white blood cells (WBCs) increases suspicion for UTI.

Urine culture is the most accurate method of diagnosing UTI; however, it requires 24–48 hours for results and is more costly. A urine specimen is obtained prior to beginning antibiotic therapy. Proper collection and handling of urine specimens includes collecting a midstream clean catch sample and prompt refrigeration. In people with disability or elevated body mass index (BMI) or who are otherwise unable to capture a clean catch urine specimen, a catheterized specimen can be collected. Routine catheterization is not recommended because of the risks of introducing bacteria into the urinary tract. Table 50.1 provides guidelines on laboratory testing during pregnancy.

A pregnant person who presents with at least two subjective symptoms of UTI and does not report vaginal discharge has a 90% probability of having acute cystitis (Grigoryan et al., 2014). People with symptoms and with positive urinalysis or dipstick can be treated empirically while awaiting culture results (Table 50.2). Antibiotics are changed as needed based on urine culture sensitivity profiles. For pregnant people without symptoms and with a positive UA or dipstick, it is appropriate to obtain a urine culture and to treat only if the culture is positive. For people presenting with signs and symptoms of pyelonephritis, workup can include a complete blood count (CBC), chemistry panel, *Chlamydia* cultures, and chest X-ray if respiratory symptoms are present (Denis et al., 2016). Other laboratory studies may be indicated, based upon patient presentation (Habak & Griggs, 2021).

Care of Urinary Tract Infections in Pregnancy

In most pregnant people with ASB or acute cystitis, the prognosis is excellent (Chen et al., 2011; Matuszkiewicz-Rowinska et al., 2015). Screening for ASB and rescreening with a repeat culture to verify cure after completion of antibiotics are key to preventing long-term sequelae.

Antibiotics are very effective at clearing UTIs in pregnancy, and complications are rare. There is little consensus on the duration of therapy or choice of antibiotic in pregnancy. Almost all antimicrobials cross the placenta, and some can be teratogenic. Commonly accepted antibiotics used in treating UTIs during pregnancy, regardless of gestational age, include

Table 50.2 Urinalysis Results

Findings	Clinical significance	Comments
Nitrites	Gram-negative bacteria like *E. coli* produce nitrites	A negative nitrite does not rule out UTI
RBCs	>5 RBCs per high-powered field indicate infection	Vaginal secretions can cause contamination
WBCs	>5 WBCs per high-powered field indicate infection	Vaginal secretions can cause contamination
WBC casts	Produced in response to cellular injury in distal convoluted tubules	Common in pyelonephritis
Leukocyte esterase	A byproduct of WBCs	A negative test means infection is unlikely

Table 50.1 Laboratory Testing for Urinary Tract Infection

Test	Timing	Comments	Significant results
Urine culture	All pregnant people at first visit or at 12–16 weeks of gestation (USPTF) Any pregnant person with UTI symptoms Every trimester in those with history of recurrent UTIs, sickle cell trait	Identifies ASB Identifies specific organisms and antibiotic sensitivities	≥100,000 cfu/mL of any single organism including GBS Any amount of GBS in clean catch midstream urine specimen (requires intrapartum prophylaxis)
Urinalysis	Pregnant people with symptoms	Faster diagnosis than culture	Positive for nitrites, WBC, RBC, and protein
Urine dipstick	Pregnant people with symptoms Often routine at prenatal care visits	Faster screening, inexpensive, unreliable	Positive for nitrites, WBC, RBC

Table 50.3   Medication Regimens for Asymptomatic Bacteriuria and Acute Cystitis in Pregnancy

Medication	Dose	Postcoital prophylaxis/ suppressive therapy Dose	Special considerations
Nitrofurantoin macrocrystals (Macrobid, Furadantin)	100 mg BID	100 mg po at bedtime	• Concentrates only in urinary tract and causes minimal resistance in Gram-negative organisms • Avoid use in the first trimester due to inconclusive studies on safety • Do not use in the last month of pregnancy
Cephalexin (Keflex)	500 mg QID	250 mg at bedtime	• High rates of bacterial resistance
Amoxicillin Ampicillin	500 mg QID or 875 mg bid	Not advised	• High rates of *E. coli* resistance • First choice for GBS in urine
Augmentin	875/125 mg BID	Not advised	• High rates of bacterial resistance
Fosfomycin	3G as a single dose	Not advised	
Trimethoprim/ Sulfamethoxazole	160/800 mg BID		• Avoid in first trimester due to risk of congenital malformations • Avoid in third trimester due to risk of kernicterus • Avoid in patients with G6PD deficiency

Source: Bookstaver et al. (2015), Duff (2022), Habak and Griggs (2021), Lassiter and Manns-James (2017), Matuszkiewicz-Rowinska et al. (2015), and Moon et al. (2010).

derivatives of penicillin and cephalosporins (Nicolle et al., 2019; Matuszkiewicz-Rowinska et al., 2015). A three- to seven-day antibiotic course is typically ordered during pregnancy to eradicate the offending bacteria; one-day courses are not recommended (Habak & Griggs, 2021). Pregnant people with asymptomatic GBS bacteriuria greater than 100,000 cfu/mL should be treated with a typical course of antibiotics to reduce the incidence of pyelonephritis, just as they would for any other organism isolated in this quantity. Several common medication regimens are noted in Table 50.3. There are no significant differences between pharmacological treatments with regard to efficacy or recurrence of infection (Smaill & Vasquez, 2019). The significant increase in microbial resistance has made appropriate antibiotic selection more challenging. For example, the resistance of *E. coli* to ampicillin and amoxicillin is 20–40%; accordingly, these agents are no longer considered optimal for treatment of UTI caused by *E. coli* (Denis et al., 2016). Providers can contact their local hospital laboratory and request an **antibiogram**. The antibiogram will indicate local antimicrobial resistance patterns and allow the provider to select antibiotics with the least likely resistance. Fluoroquinolones are not recommended as first-line treatment due to the potential teratogenic effects on the fetus (Habak & Griggs, 2021). However, if resistant or recurrent infections occur, short courses may be considered (Habak & Griggs, 2021).

For pregnant people with symptoms, phenazopyridine 200 mg TID is advised in addition to antibiotics. Phenazopyridine relieves urinary tract pain, burning, urgency, and frequent urination and is available over the counter. However, phenazopyridine is not an antibiotic and does not cure infections. Phenazopyridine is not used alone, as it will mask symptoms and allow infection to progress.

An important element of care is educating pregnant people about measures to help reduce symptoms and to prevent UTI recurrence. Patients are advised to call if symptoms worsen and given instructions on recognizing symptoms of preterm labor.

Measures to reduce risk of UTI recurrence

- Drink at least eight glasses of water per day.
- Discourage bubble baths, which can irritate the urethral opening.
- Avoid wearing thong underwear.
- Wipe front to back after defecation and urination.
- Use good hand-washing techniques.
- Void after intercourse.
- Always respond to the initial urge to void.
- Avoid bladder irritants such as coffee and carbonated beverages.
- Complete the entire course of antibiotics as prescribed.

Recurrent UTI

Approximately one-third of pregnant people diagnosed with UTI will have recurrence in that pregnancy (Foxman, 2014). Suppressive therapy can reduce the incidence of recurrence, though evidence that it is more effective than close surveillance alone is lacking (Schneeberger et al., 2015). Suppression is considered for any pregnant person with (a) a UTI that recurs after a test of cure showed successful treatment of a first infection, (b) anyone with a prepregnancy history of recurrent UTIs, or (c) pyelonephritis during the current pregnancy (Habak & Griggs, 2021). It is also reasonable to use postcoital prophylaxis (in the same dosage as daily suppression therapy) if recurrent UTIs are brought on by sexual activity, which is common. UTIs may also be persistent, meaning that infection is still present more than 48 hours after treatment initiation. This is most likely due to antibiotic resistance by the organism or noncompliance with treatment, and both should be explored.

Care of Pregnant People with Suspected Acute Pyelonephritis

Because of increased perinatal risks related to pyelonephritis, comanagement and/or referral of pregnant people with a diagnosis of pyelonephritis is warranted.

The standard treatment for pyelonephritis is hospital admission and intravenous (IV) administration of antibiotics (generally cephalosporins or gentamycin). Outpatient treatment may be an option with carefully selected patients up to 20 weeks of gestation (Duff, 2022). Pyelonephritis can cause dehydration because of nausea and vomiting and often requires IV hydration. However, due to elevated risk for pulmonary edema and acute respiratory distress syndrome (ARDS), fluids must be administered cautiously. Fever is managed with antipyretics (typically acetaminophen) and antiemetics are given for nausea and vomiting.

Nephrolithiasis

Nephrolithiasis (commonly known as kidney stones) is the presence of renal calculi that develop from a combination of naturally occurring chemicals in the body. These chemicals include calcium, oxalate, phosphate, uric acid, struvite, and cysteine (National Kidney and Urologic Diseases Information Clearinghouse, 2017). Calcium salts form the majority of the stones identified. Symptomatic nephrolithiasis is more common in the last two trimesters of pregnancy due to ureteral dilation and compression by the gravid uterus, which allows for more stones to pass through the ureter. Potential problems associated with nephrolithiasis in pregnancy include hypertension, preeclampsia, spontaneous abortion, preterm birth, and operative birth (Clennon et al., 2021; Lee et al., 2021).

Nephrolithiasis during pregnancy and postpartum commonly causes presenting symptoms of acute flank pain, abdominal pain, nausea, vomiting, and hematuria (Talwar et al., 2021). **Pyuria** may or may not be present. People with stones in the lower urinary tract may present with frequency, urgency, and **dysuria**. Approximately 50% of people with nephrolithiasis will have a concomitant UTI (Srirangam et al., 2008). Differential diagnoses include appendicitis, diverticulitis, placental abruption, pyelonephritis, and round ligament pain.

Evaluation

The problem-focused health history includes prior history of nephrolithiasis, renal disease, hypertension, and

assessment of current symptoms. Physical exam includes assessment of CVA tenderness, temperature, abdominal exam, and assessment of fetal heart rate. It should be noted that normal pregnancy-related physical changes might alter the localization of pain and obscure diagnosis (Thomas et al., 2010).

Initial laboratory testing includes UA and dipstick for red blood cells (RBCs) and WBCs to detect concomitant infection. Urine pH is also obtained, as a pH greater than 7 or less than 5 may indicate composition of the stone (Srirangam et al., 2008). Urine culture to identify the presence and sensitivity of a pathogen is also done. Renal ultrasound is the first-line imaging study to diagnose kidney stones during pregnancy.

Care of Pregnant People with Suspected Nephrolithiasis

Management of pregnant people with suspected nephrolithiasis requires consultation, collaboration, or referral for medical services, depending on the person's presentation and the clinician's expertise. A concomitant UTI is treated if the person is not in acute distress, and services to evaluate for nephrolithiasis promptly initiated. Management is determined by the size, location of stone, and gestational age. Conservative treatment of nephrolithiasis is often attempted first, which includes oral or IV hydration, pain control, and antibiotics for concomitant infection (Lee et al., 2021; Thomas et al., 2010). The majority of people will spontaneously pass kidney stones with conservative treatment (Srirangam et al., 2008), and 50% of remaining people will pass the stone in the postpartum period (Thomas et al., 2010).

Some pregnant people with stones will need active invasive intervention. Indications for enhanced intervention are the same as for nonpregnant people: intractable pain, febrile UTI, obstructive uropathy, nausea, vomiting, acute renal failure, sepsis, or obstruction of a solitary kidney (Thomas et al., 2010) as well as identification of a stone that is likely too large to pass (>1 cm) (Hernandez & Pais, 2016).

Summary

UTI, pyelonephritis, and nephrolithiasis are common in pregnancy and, if untreated, may lead to significant morbidity and mortality for both the pregnant person and the fetus. In pregnant people, UTIs are an independent risk factor for preterm birth and also are associated with preeclampsia, fetal growth restriction, and cesarean birth. Nephrolithiasis poses the potential for serious complications to the pregnant person and fetus, including hypertension, preeclampsia, preterm labor, spontaneous abortion, and cesarean birth. Interprofessional management is appropriate for significant urinary tract complications during pregnancy.

Resources for Pregnant People and Their Families

ACOG. FAQ about group B strep in pregnancy: http://www.acog.org/Patients/FAQs/Group-B-Strep-and-Pregnancy

ACOG. FAQ about urinary tract infections: https://www.acog.org/womens-health/faqs/urinary-tract-infections

CDC. Group B strep- what you need to know patient handout: https://www.cdc.gov/groupbstrep/about/

CDC. Protect your baby from group B strep handout: https://www.cdc.gov/groupbstrep/about/prevention.html

Share with Women: Group B Strep in Pregnancy. https://onlinelibrary.wiley.com/doi/epdf/10.1111/jmwh.13125

Resource for Healthcare Providers

CDC. (2010). Prevent group B strep app for obstetric and neonatal providers: https://www.cdc.gov/groupbstrep/guidelines/prevention-app.html

References

Ailes, E. C., Gilboa, S. M., Gill, S. K., Broussard, C. S., Crider, K. S., Berry, R. J., Carter, T. C., Hobbs, C. A., Interrante, J. D., & Reefhuis, J. & the National Birth Defects Prevention Study. (2016). Association between antibiotic use among pregnant women with urinary tract infections in the first trimester and birth defects, national birth defects prevention study 1997–2011. *Birth Defects Research Part A: Clinical and Molecular Teratology, 106*(11), 940–949. https://doi.org/10.1002/bdra.23570

American Academy of Pediatrics, & American College of Obstetricians and Gynecologist. (2017). *Guidelines for perinatal care* (8th ed.). Elk Grove Village.

American College of Obstetricians and Gynecologists (ACOG). (2020). Prevention of group B streptococcal early-onset disease in newborns. Committee opinion no. 797. *Obstetrics and Gynecology, 135*, e51–e72.

Angelescu, K., Nussbaumer-Streit, B., Sieben, W., Scheibler, P., & Gartlehner, G. (2016). Benefits and harms of screening for and treatment of asymptomatic bacteriuria in pregnancy: A systematic review. *BMC Pregnancy and Childbirth, 16*(336). https://doi.org/10.1186/s12884-016-1128-0

Badran, Y. A., El-Kashef, T. A., Abdelaziz, A. S., & Ali, M. M. (2015). Impact of genital hygiene and sexual activity on urinary tract infection during pregnancy. *Urology Annals, 7*(4), 478–481.

Bookstaver, P. B., Bland, C. M., Griffin, B., Stover, K. R., Eiland, L. S., & McLaughlin, M. (2015). A review of antibiotic use in pregnancy. *Pharmacotherapy, 35*(11), 1052–1062.

Bryan, C. (2015). Urinary tract infections. In R. C. Hunt (Ed.), *Microbiology and Immunology On-line.* https://microbiologybook.org/Infectious%20Disease/Urinary%20Tract%20Infections.htm

Casey, J. A., Rudolph, K. E., Robinson, S. C., Bruxvoort, K., Raphael, E., Hong, V., Pressman, A., Morello-Frosch, R., Wei, R. X., & Tartof, S. Y. (2021). Sociodemographic inequalities in urinary tract infection in 2 large California health systems. *Open Forum Infectious Diseases, 8*(6), 1–9. https://doi.org/10.1093/ofid/ofab276

Centers for Disease Control and Prevention (CDC). (2010). Prevention of perinatal group B streptococcal disease: Revised guidelines from the CDC. *MMWR. Morbidity and Mortality Weekly Report, 59*(RR10), 1–32.

Chen, Y., Chen, S., Li, H., & Lin, H. (2011). No increased risk of adverse pregnancy outcomes in women with urinary tract infections: A nationwide population-based study. *Acta Obstetricia et Gynecologica Scandinavica, 89*(7), 882–888.

Chotiprasitsakul, D., Kijnithikul, A., Uamkhayan, A., & Santanirand, P. (2021). Predictive value of urinalysis and recent antibiotic exposure to distinguish between bacteriuria, candiduria, and no-growth urine. *Infection and Drug Resistance., 14*, 5699–5709. https://doi.org/10.2147/IDR.S343021

Chu, C. M., & Lowder, J. L. (2018). Diagnosis and treatment of urinary tract infections across age groups. *American Journal of Obstetrics & Gynecology, 219*(1), 40–51. https://doi.org/10.1016/j.ajog.2017.12.231

Clennon, E. K., Garg, B., Duty, B. D., Caughey, A., & B. (2021). Obstetric outcomes of pregnancy complicated by urolithiasis: A retrospective cohort study. *Journal of Perinatal Medicine., 49*(1), 54–59. https://doi.org/10.1515/jpm-2020-0199

Denis, E., Martis, N., Guillouet-de Salvador, F., Demonchy, E., Degand, N., Carles, K., & Roger, P. M. (2016). Bacteraemic urinary tract infections may mimic respiratory infections: A nested case-control study. *European Journal of Clinical Microbiology & Infectious Diseases, 35*(10), 1601–1605.

Duff, P. (2022). UTIs in pregnancy: Managing urethritis, asymptomatic bacteriuria, cystitis, and pyelonephritis. *OBG Management. 34*(1), 42–46.

Easter, S. R., Cantonwine, D. E., Zera, C. A., Lim, K. H., Parry, S. I., & McElrath, T. F. (2016). Urinary tract infection during pregnancy, angiogenic factor profiles, and risk of preeclampsia. *American Journal of Obstetrics & Gynecology, 214*(3), 387–e1.

Foxman, B. (2014). Urinary tract infection syndromes: Occurrence, recurrence, bacteriology, risk factors, and disease burden. *Infectious Disease Clinics of North America, 28*(1), 1–13.

Grigoryan, L., Trautner, B. W., & Guptna, K. (2014). Diagnosis and management of urinary tract infections in the outpatient setting: A review. *JAMA, 312*(16), 1677–1684.

Habak, P. J. & Griggs, R. P. (2021). *Urinary tract infection in pregnancy.* StatPearls NCBI Resources. https://www.ncbi.nlm.nih.gov/books/NBK537047

Hernandez, N., & Pais, V. M. (2016). Diagnostic and management consideration for nephrolithasis in the gravid patient. *Clinical Nephrology, 85*(2), 70–76.

Lassiter, N. T., & Manns-James, L. E. (2017). Pregnancy. In M. Brucker & T. L. King (Eds.), *Pharmacology for women's health* (2nd ed., pp. 1025–1063). Jones and Bartlett.

Lee, M. S., Fenstermaker, M. A., Naoum, E. E., Chong, S., Van de Ven, C. J., Bauer, M. E., Kountanis, J. A., Ellis, J. H., Shields, J., Ambani, S., Krambeck, A. E., Roberts, W. W., & Ghani, K. R. (2021). Management of nephrolithiasis in pregnancy: Multi-disciplinary guidelines from an academic medical center. *Frontiers in Surgery, 8*, 796876. https://doi.org/10.3389/fsurg.2021.796876

Matuszkiewicz-Rowinska, J., Malyszko, J., & Wieliczko, M. (2015). Urinary tract infections in pregnancy: Old and new unresolved diagnostic and therapeutic problems. *Archives of Medical Science, 11*(1), 67–77.

McIsaac, W., Carroll, J. C., Biringer, A., Bernstein, P., Lyons, E., Low, D. E., & Permaul, J. A. (2005). Screening for asymptomatic bacteriuria in pregnancy. *Journal of Obstetrics & Gynaecology Canada, 27*, 20–24.

Moon, J., Prasad, S., & Egan, M. (2010). Treating UTIs in reproductive-age women—Proceed with caution. *Journal of Family Practice, 59*(4), 220–222.

National Kidney and Urologic Diseases Information Clearinghouse. (2017). *Definition & facts for kidney stones.* https://www.niddk.nih.gov/health-information/urologic-diseases/kidney-stones/definition-facts

Nicolle, L. E., Gupta, K., Bradley, S. F., Colgan, R., DeMuri, G. P., Drekonja, D., Ekert, L. O., Geerlings, S. E., Köves, B., Hooton, T. M., Juthani-Mehta, M., Knight, S. L., Saint, S., Schaeffer, A. J., Trautner, B., Wullt, B., & Siemieniuk, R. (2019). Clinical practice guideline for the management of asymptomatic bacteriuria: 2019 update by the Infectious Diseases Society of America. *Clinical Infectious Diseases, 68*(10), e83–e110.

Quinlan, J. D., & Jorgensen, S. D. (2017). Recurrent UTIs in women: How you can refine your care. *Journal of Family Practice*, *66*(2), 94–99.

Schneeberger, C., Geerlings, S. E., Middleton, P., & Crowther, C. A. (2015). Interventions for preventing recurrent urinary tract infection during pregnancy. *The Cochrane Library*, *7*. https://doi.org//10.1002/14651858.CD009279.pub3

Smaill, F. M., & Vasquez, J. C. (2019). Antibiotics for asymptomatic bacteriuria in pregnancy. *The Cochrane Library*, *11*. https://doi.org/10.1002/14651858.CD000490.pub4

Srirangam, S. J., Hickerton, B., & Cleynenbreugel, B. V. (2008). Management of urinary calculi in pregnancy: A review. *Journal of Endourology/Endourological Society*, *22*(5), 867–875.

Talwar, H. S., Vikas Kumar, P., Ghorai, R. P., & Ankur, M. (2021). Catastrophic complications of urolithiasis in pregnancy. *British Medical Journal Case Reports.*, *14*(5). https://doi.org/10.1136/bcr-2021-241597

Thomas, A. A., Thomas, A. Z., Campbell, S. C., & Palmer, J. S. (2010). Urologic emergencies in pregnancy. *Urology*, *76*(2), 453–460.

United States Preventive Services Task Force (USPSTF). (2019). *Guide to preventive services*. https://www.uspreventiveservicestaskforce.org/uspstf/recommendation/asymptomatic-bacteriuria-in-adults-screening

51

Gastrointestinal Disorders

Debora M. Dole

Relevant Terms

Intrahepatic cholestasis of pregnancy (ICP)—a liver condition in which bile flow is blocked from the liver resulting in excess bile acids causing severe itching on abdomen, hands, and feet

Cholecystitis—inflammatory complication of the gallbladder, commonly caused by the obstruction of the cystic duct

Cholelithiasis—formation of a stone within the gallbladder caused by accumulation of bile components, commonly known as "gallstones"

Gastroenteritis—acute or chronic inflammation of the stomach and intestine characterized by anorexia, nausea, vomiting, and/or diarrhea that may or may not be accompanied by fever

Jaundice—a yellow coloring of the skin, mucous membranes, or eyes caused by excessive unbound bilirubin in the blood

Murphy's sign—abrupt cessation of inspiration on palpation of the gallbladder (right upper quadrant of abdomen) indicates acute cholecystitis

Introduction

Approximately 50–80% of pregnant individuals will experience gastrointestinal (GI) distress during their pregnancy (Body & Christie, 2016; Gomes et al., 2018). Many of the GI symptoms reported during prenatal care are associated with normal physiologic changes of pregnancy such as nausea, vomiting, constipation, and heartburn. It is important to recognize that common GI symptoms associated with pregnancy are experienced individually and on a continuum of severity. The assessment and management of these conditions are described in Chapter 15, *Common Discomforts of Pregnancy*. Pregnancy may also be associated with a more serious form of nausea and vomiting known as hyperemesis gravidarum, which is addressed in Chapter 40, *Hyperemesis Gravidarum*. This chapter reviews the signs and symptoms, and evaluation of individuals presenting with abnormal GI conditions during pregnancy that typically have an acute onset of symptoms, including **gastroenteritis**, **intrahepatic cholestasis of pregnancy (ICP)**, and **cholecystitis**, including **cholelithiasis**. Pancreatitis and appendicitis are addressed in Chapter 41, *Abdominal Pain*.

Health equity key points

- Abdominal pain has a broad differential diagnosis including obstetric and nonobstetric etiologies, making this a common reason for pregnant people to seek emergency care.
- Disparities in health outcomes for marginalized populations have been associated with access to care barriers leading to delayed diagnosis and treatment.
- The burden of poor maternal outcomes is disproportionately carried by non-Hispanic Black pregnant people.
- Healthcare providers must examine their own biases that may impact assessment, diagnosis, and treatment.

Initial Evaluation

Initial assessment for suspected GI conditions includes the use of the "OLD CAARTS" systematic approach to gathering subjective data. General physical assessments of the GI tract are performed. These findings, in turn, guide further history, physical, and laboratory evaluation (Tables 51.1 and 51.2).

When assessing pregnant individuals for any suspected GI condition, it is important to understand how normal lab values may be altered by pregnancy (Table 51.2). For example, typical parameters for a complete blood count (CBC) can vary considerably by trimester due to hemodilution and physiologic changes of pregnancy. Indices used to assess for infection or inflammatory processes such as the white blood cell count (physiologic leukocytosis, primarily

Prenatal and Postnatal Care: A Person-Centered Approach, Third Edition. Edited by Karen Trister Grace, Cindy L. Farley, Noelene K. Jeffers, and Tanya Tringali.
© 2024 John Wiley & Sons Ltd. Published 2024 by John Wiley & Sons Ltd.
Companion website: www.wiley.com/go/grace/prenatal

an increase of neutrophils) and erythrocyte sedimentation rate (ESR) can be elevated particularly in the third trimester (Kelly & Savides, 2019; Kilpatrick & Kitahara, 2023).

Table 51.1   Data Gathering for Presentation of GI Symptoms in Pregnancy

Subjective data	Objective data
Gestational age	Maternal vital signs
Fetal movement patterns	Fetal heart rate
Uterine contractions noted	Mucous membranes, skin turgor
Current symptoms	Orthostatic changes
Recent meals	Pain rating
Recent travel	Bowel sounds
Exposure to animals	Abdominal palpation and percussion
Exposure to contaminated food/drink	Uterine palpation/tocodynamometry
Exposure to others with these symptoms	CVA tenderness
Change in diet or food tolerance	Anal sphincter tone and patency
Change in bowel habits	Urine ketones, leukocytes, and nitrites
History of GI conditions or surgeries	

Disparities in health outcomes for marginalized populations have been associated with access to care barriers leading to delayed diagnosis and treatment (Holdt Somer et al., 2017). The burden of poor maternal outcomes is disproportionately carried by non-Hispanic Black pregnant people. Healthcare providers must examine their own biases that may impact assessment, diagnosis, and treatment of other marginalized groups including immigrant populations and transgender and nonbinary individuals to ensure that equitable care is provided for everyone. Consideration must be given to each presentation and attention given to each patient's experience and description of symptoms.

Gastroenteritis

Gastroenteritis is an acute or chronic inflammation of the stomach or intestines. Acute gastroenteritis presents as a self-limiting disorder characterized by loss of appetite, nausea, vomiting, and/or diarrhea that may or may not be accompanied by fever. Gastroenteritis can be caused by infectious agents, including viruses (e.g., noroviruses), bacteria (e.g., *Escherichia coli*), and protozoa (e.g., *Giardia lamblia*). Parasitic infections and food-borne toxins may also cause gastroenteritis. Most cases of acute gastroenteritis are self-limiting and benign. However, there are more harmful bacterial causes of gastroenteritis, including *Listeria, Salmonella, E. coli, Shigella,* and *Clostridium difficile*. Chronic gastroenteritis is often a result of *Helicobacter pylori* infection and can lead to peptic ulcers and stomach cancers. Noninfective causes of

Table 51.2   Common Lab Values in Pregnancy

Lab/diagnostic testing	1st trimester	2nd trimester	3rd trimester
Total WBCs* ($\times 10^3/mm^3$)	5.7–13.6	5.6–14.8	5.9–16.9
Neutrophils = bacterial infections	3.6–10.1	3.8–12.3	3.9–13.1
Lymphocytes = viral infections	1.1–3.6	0.9–3.9	1.0–3.6
Eosinophils/Basophils = autoimmune/allergy	0–0.6	0–0.6	0–0.6
Monocytes = severe infections	0.1–1.1	0.1–1.1	0.1–1.4
Platelets ($\times 10^9/L$)	174–391	155–409	146–429
Alanine transaminase—units/L	3–30	2–33	2–25
Aspartate transaminase—units/L	3–23	3–33	4–32
Alkaline phosphatase—units/L	17–88	25–126	38–229
Amylase—units/L	24–83	16–73	15–81
Bile acids—mmol/L	0–4.9	0–9.1	0–11.3
Cryo-reactive proteins (CRP)—mg/L	0.2–3.0	0.4–20.3	0.4–8.1
Erythrocyte sedimentation rate mm/hour	4–57	7–47	13–70
INR	0.86–1.08	0.83–1.02	0.8–1.09
Lipase—units/L	21–76	26–100	41–112
Prothrombin time—seconds	9.7–13.5	9.5–13.4	9.6–12.9
Partial thromboplastin time—seconds	23–38.9	22.9–38.1	22.6–35.0

Source: Adapted from Cunningham et al. (2022).

gastroenteritis caused by stress, food sensitivities, medications, and physiologic changes of pregnancy should be given consideration and not be overlooked in the assessment and diagnosis.

Evaluation

Diagnosis of gastroenteritis is generally based on history and clinical symptoms. Gastroenteritis commonly presents as acute diarrhea, nausea, and vomiting, with or without fever (Gomes et al., 2018; Kelly & Savides, 2019). Pregnant individuals with gastroenteritis may report cramping, abdominal pain, bloating, mucus, or blood in the stool, and decreased urination. In addition to OLD CAARTS, subjective information gathered should include gestational age of the pregnancy, fetal movement patterns, presence of any uterine contractions, recent travel, exposure to animals, recent meals, anyone else in the home with same symptoms, and contact with potentially contaminated food or water. Objective data should include general status and level of distress, vital signs, mucous membranes, skin turgor, orthostatic changes, abdominal palpation for tenderness and signs of acute abdomen, fetal heart tones, and signs of uterine irritability. Patient efforts to alleviate symptoms should also be explored including homeopathic or herbal remedies.

Diagnostic Testing

Extensive diagnostic testing is not usually indicated in healthy pregnant individuals with diarrhea and GI distress but may include assessing for urinary tract infection and dehydration in the presence of urine ketones, leukocytes, and nitrites. Microbiological stool samples are considered if there are signs of more severe illness such as bloody stool, prolonged fever, or neurological involvement such as paresthesia, severe dehydration, or suspicion of exposure to food toxins (Body & Christie, 2016; Gomes et al., 2018; Zachariah et al., 2019). Differential diagnoses for gastroenteritis depend on the severity of the signs and symptoms, as well as the gestational age of the pregnancy. The differential diagnosis should be based on history and objective data and may include ectopic pregnancy, hyperemesis gravidarum, appendicitis, or urinary tract infection.

Treatment

Oral rehydration therapy is the recommended mode of administration, but this depends on the hydration status and clinical presentation. If tolerated, an over-the-counter (OTC) oral rehydration solution is recommended to replace fluids that have been lost in diarrhea. Drinking the solution slowly and consuming small amounts hourly are preferred over trying to quickly replace fluids. Intravenous fluid replacement may be indicated if the symptoms are severe, and dehydration is present. A gradual return to a normal diet, starting with bland foods, should be encouraged as symptoms subside.

Antibiotics may be required based on the results of the stool culture and sensitivity. Azithromycin is recommended to use empirically for travelers' diarrhea and is safe to use in pregnancy. It is important to note that loperamide is not recommended in pregnancy for the treatment of acute diarrhea because it may cause complications in diarrheal illnesses associated with bacterial infections such as ileus or toxic megacolon. Loperamide is also contraindicated for bloody diarrhea and immunocompromised patients. *Listeriosis* can be treated with penicillins or with sulfamethoxazole/trimethoprim if the patient has an allergy to penicillin. OTC probiotics may be recommended since they can help prevent diarrhea and restore positive flora that are often destroyed during antibiotic use (Body & Christie, 2016; Gomes et al., 2018).

Interprofessional Care

Most pregnant individuals with gastroenteritis recover without intervention or complications. Physician consultation is warranted for people presenting with severe and persistent nausea and vomiting with diarrhea, signs of preterm labor, or fetal distress.

Intrahepatic Cholestasis of Pregnancy

ICP affects approximately 0.3–5.6% of pregnant individuals (Tran et al., 2016). The incidence of ICP appears to vary by ethnicity and geographic locations, with higher rates noted in some Indigenous South American populations (Floreani & Gervasi, 2016). The disease is characterized by symptoms of severe pruritis and impaired liver function. The etiology of ICP is not known; it is thought to be a multifactorial disorder caused by hormonal, genetic, immune, and environmental factors. The condition has a strong familial component and is more common in relatives and offspring of individuals who experience ICP during pregnancy (Dixon & Williamson, 2016; Floreani & Gervasi, 2016). The normal hormonal changes of pregnancy may predispose some individuals to ICP. The elevated levels of estrogen and progesterone during pregnancy slow gallbladder emptying during pregnancy, resulting in bile stasis. The stasis may be so severe in some people that the excess bile acids can enter the circulation.

Evaluation

Typically, ICP presents in the third trimester but can begin at any time during the pregnancy. Symptoms reflect the pathophysiology of altered liver function including severe itching, especially of the hands and feet from accumulating bile salts deposited in the skin. Reports of very dark urine as the body attempts to expel excess bilirubin and light-colored bowel movements reflect altered liver function. **Jaundice** may develop but is usually seen after several weeks of ICP or in severe cases. The pruritis of ICP generally worsens at night. It can be of such intensity that it becomes intolerable and interferes with ability to function. In these cases, labor induction is considered as early as 35–37 weeks of gestation (Dixon & Williamson, 2016; Gomes et al., 2018). Questions about pruritus should be a routine component of the prenatal assessment during the last trimester of pregnancy, and when individuals report symptoms, the condition should be evaluated promptly. While maternal prognosis is good, ICP is associated with high rates of spontaneous preterm birth, fetal distress, and intrauterine fetal death (Dixon & Williamson, 2016; Gomes et al., 2018; Lee 2023). Intrauterine fetal death is described as a sudden event showing no evidence of placental insufficiency or infarct, but likely associated with fetal arrythmias caused by elevated serum bile acid levels (Lee, 2023). Fetal complications of ICP are related to elevated fetal serum bile acid levels, but the exact mechanisms are not clearly understood (Lee, 2023). Thus, prompt diagnosis and referral are imperative.

The diagnosis of ICP is based on physical examination, clinical presentation, and laboratory findings. Subjective data include degree to which the symptoms are affecting sleep and activities of daily functioning. History of other skin conditions or allergies or changes in soaps, cosmetics, or skin products should be assessed. Objective data include vital signs, fever, location, and severity of any rash, skin eruptions or excoriation, abdominal exam, and fetal assessment.

Diagnostic Testing

Elevated serum bile acid levels (above 10 µmol/L) are the primary diagnostic criterion in the evaluation of a pregnant person with suspected ICP. Laboratory testing is aimed at assessing liver function and ruling out other conditions such as HELLP (Hemolysis, Elevated Liver enzymes and Low Platelets) syndrome. Testing should include a liver panel that includes aspartate transaminase (AST), alanine transaminase (ALT), gamma-glutamyl transpeptidase (GGT), alkaline phosphatase (ALP), and total bilirubin. Coagulation studies such as prothrombin time (PT), partial thromboplastin time (PTT), and international normalized ratio (INR) should also be performed (Dixon & Williamson, 2016; Gomes et al., 2018).

Treatment

Once a diagnosis of ICP has been made, close fetal surveillance by nonstress testing and biophysical profile is indicated to monitor fetal health. In some instances when bile acid levels do not respond to treatment, induction of labor at 37 weeks of gestation is recommended to avoid increased risk of fetal death. Total serum bile acid levels are followed every two to three weeks to guide therapy and the timing of birth. Ursodeoxycholic acid (UDCA; 10–15 mg/kg body weight divided into two to three doses per day [Cunningham et al., 2022]) is the primary medication used in the treatment of ICP. It improves bile flow, thereby reducing bile stasis and resulting in improved clinical symptoms and liver parameters (Dixon & Williamson, 2016; Gomes et al., 2018). Symptomatic relief can be offered with antihistamines such as diphenhydramine (Benadryl©). Oatmeal-based lotions and baths may temporarily soothe the skin and relieve itching.

Interprofessional Care

Laboratory screening should be performed immediately for pregnant people with suspected ICP. Consultation and referral to maternal-fetal medicine services is essential if laboratory testing reveals ICP due to an increased risk of preterm birth, fetal distress, and fetal death. All individuals with ICP should have a plan for the continued assessment of fetal well-being and ongoing monitoring of maternal status and liver function. ICP has a recurrence rate of 60–70% in subsequent pregnancies (Chacko & Wolkoff, 2017; Dixon & Williamson, 2016; Floreani & Gervasi, 2016).

Cholecystitis and Cholelithiasis

Normal physiologic changes that occur during pregnancy can cause biliary stasis and elevated cholesterol levels, predisposing individuals to the formation of gallstones and the development of biliary sludge leading to a diagnosis of cholelithiasis in approximately 5–10% of pregnant people (Littlefield & Lenahan, 2019; Weinstein et al., 2020; Zachariah et al., 2019). Estrogen contributes to increased cholesterol formation and progesterone causes decreased soluble bile acid secretion, which favors the formation of gallstones. Progesterone causes decreased smooth muscle contractility of the gallbladder, which delays gallbladder emptying and exacerbates bile stasis. After birth, the more soluble forms of bile acids are secreted; however, this return to the prepregnant state may take months (Weinstein et al., 2020). The risk of gallstones increases with the number of pregnancies, weight gain, and with age.

Cholecystitis is less common than cholelithiasis (gall stones) and is acute inflammation of the gallbladder usually resulting from bile accumulation when the cystic duct becomes occluded by gallstones or biliary sludge. As the obstruction persists, the gallbladder becomes thickened and inflamed, which can lead to a secondary infection caused by organisms commonly found in the bowel, and results in necrosis or gangrene. Approximately 1 in 1000 pregnant people is affected by acute cholecystitis (Weinstein et al., 2020).

Acute cholecystitis is the second most common non-obstetrical surgical emergency in pregnant individuals after acute appendicitis (Chacko & Wolkoff, 2017; Weinstein et al., 2020). Risk factors for both conditions include obesity, high parity, high triglyceride levels, and low high-density lipoprotein (HDL) levels (Littlefield & Lenahan, 2019), and risk may be increased by high carbohydrate consumption (Wong & Ko, 2013).

Evaluation

Pregnant individuals with acute cholecystitis usually present with epigastric pain that can vary from minimal to severe. They may report colicky pain located in the upper right quadrant, nausea, vomiting, and heartburn, especially after eating a high-fat-content meal. Referred pain to the right scapular region or shoulder are also common. General appearance and level of distress should be noted and the skin and sclera observed for jaundice. A fever may be present in individuals with acute cholecystitis. The use of OLD CAARTS is particularly important in gathering subjective data when suspicious of cholecystitis or gallstones. Objective data, in addition to vital signs, include palpation of the abdomen to assess right upper quadrant tenderness and to elicit **Murphy's sign**. To elicit Murphy's sign, the examiner asks the patient to take in a deep inspiration as the examiner's fingers are placed under the liver border at the bottom of the rib cage. The inspiration causes the gallbladder to descend onto the fingers, producing pain if the gallbladder is inflamed. Abrupt cessation of inspiration, guarding, and tenderness are positive responses. The characteristic Murphy sign in nonpregnant patients with cholecystitis may not be present in pregnancy (Weinstein et al., 2020), and many people with cholelithiasis are asymptomatic.

Diagnostic Testing

Diagnoses of cholelithiasis and cholecystitis are made by ultrasound. The differential diagnosis includes appendicitis, pancreatitis, peptic ulcer disease, pyelonephritis, HELLP syndrome, hepatitis, and acute fatty liver (Weinstein et al., 2020; Zachariah et al., 2019). Laboratory testing includes CBC with differential, AST/ALT, ALP, amylase, and lipase levels. Blood work may reveal elevated white blood cells and liver function tests. Potential complications of cholelithiasis include acute gallstone pancreatitis, maternal mortality, spontaneous abortion, and complications related to diagnostic tests and surgery (Littlefield & Lenahan, 2019).

Treatment

Once a diagnosis of cholecystitis is made, clinical management is dependent on the gestational age of the pregnancy and the severity of symptoms. Warning signs of the need for intervention include fever, right upper quadrant pain, elevated white blood cell count, nausea, vomiting, and decreased appetite (Gilo et al., 2009). The addition of these symptoms in the presence of abdominal pain should prompt referral for definitive diagnosis and management. Conservative treatment includes intravenous hydration, bowel rest, broad-spectrum antibiotics, and analgesia, but is associated with a high rate of recurrence (Littlefield & Lenahan, 2019). Dietary restriction of fats is recommended. Fetal assessment and uterine monitoring are indicated, depending on the gestational age of the pregnancy. Symptomatic cholelithiasis in pregnancy is likely to require surgery, depending on gestational age. Surgical intervention may be delayed into the second trimester to avoid the risk of spontaneous pregnancy loss in the first trimester; however, surgical laparoscopic techniques have improved and are more commonly used to treat individuals with gallstones in all trimesters of pregnancy (Weinstein et al., 2020; Zachariah et al., 2019).

Interprofessional Care

A targeted evaluation by history, physical examination, and laboratory screening should be initiated immediately for pregnant individuals with suspected cholecystitis. Consultation and referral to maternal-fetal medicine services is essential since the differential diagnosis of cholecystitis includes potentially life-threatening complications such as HELLP syndrome. Additionally, the treatment plan will be determined by obstetric consultation and surgical intervention may be required.

Summary

Many of the GI symptoms reported during prenatal care are associated with normal physiologic changes of pregnancy such as nausea, vomiting, constipation, and heartburn. The healthcare provider must conduct a targeted history and physical examination in each pregnant person to rule out GI pathology. Laboratory evaluation may be required with abnormal findings. Prompt diagnosis and referral can reduce perinatal complications associated with abnormal GI conditions.

Resources for Healthcare Providers

American Gastroenterology Association website with search feature for prenatal and postnatal relevant documents: http://www.gastro.org

Resources for Pregnant Clients and Their Families

American Gastroenterology Association website with search feature for prenatal and postnatal relevant documents for patients: https://patient.gastro.org/digestive-health-topics-a-z/?category=conditions
Centers for Disease Control and Prevention. Reproductive Health https://www.cdc.gov/reproductivehealth/maternalinfanthealth/pregnancy-complications.html
Intrahepatic Cholestasis of Pregnancy Care: https://icpcare.org/intrahepatic-cholestasis-pregnancy

References

Body, C., & Christie, J. A. (2016). Gastrointestinal diseases in pregnancy. Nausea, vomiting, hyperemesis gravidarum, gastroesophageal reflux disease, constipation, and diarrhea. *Gastroenterology Clinics of North America*, 45, 267–283.

Chacko, K., & Wolkoff, A. (2017). Intrahepatic cholestasis of pregnancy: New diagnostic insights. *Annals of Hepatology*, *16*(2), 176–178.

Cunningham, F., Leveno, K. J., Dashe, J. S., Hoffman, B. L., Spong, C. Y., & Casey, B. M. (Eds.) (2022). *Williams obstetrics* (26th ed.). McGraw Hill. https://accessmedicine.mhmedical.com/content.aspx?bookid=2977&sectionid=254036061

Dixon, P. H., & Williamson, C. (2016). The pathophysiology of intrahepatic cholestasis of pregnancy. *Clinics and Research in Hepatology and Gastroenterology*, *40*(2), 141–153. https://doi.org/10.1016/j.clinre.2015.12.008

Floreani, A., & Gervasi, M. T. (2016). New insights on intrahepatic cholestasis of pregnancy. *Clinical Liver Disease*, 20, 177–189.

Gilo, N. B., Amini, D., & Landy, H. (2009). Appendicitis and cholecystitis in pregnancy. *Clinical Obstetrics and Gynecology*, *52*(4), 586–596.

Gomes, C. F., Sousa, M., Lourenço, I., Martins, D., & Torres, J. (2018). Gastrointestinal diseases during pregnancy: What does the gastroenterologist need to know? *Annals of Gastroenterology, 31*(4), 385–394. https://doi.org/10.20524/aog.2018.0264

Holdt Somer, S. J., Sinkey, R. G., & Bryant, A. S. (2017). Epidemiology of racial/ethnic disparities in severe maternal morbidity and mortality. *Seminars in Perinatology, 41*(5), 258–265.

Kelly, T., & Savides, T. (2019). Gastrointestinal disease in pregnancy. In C. J. Lockwood, T. Moore, J. Copel, R. M. Silver, & R. Resnik (Eds.), *Creasy & Resnick's maternal–fetal medicine: Principles and practice* (8th ed., pp. 1158–1171). Elsevier.

Kilpatrick, S. J., & Kitahara, S. (2023). Anemia in pregnancy. In C. J. Lockwood, J. Copel, L. Dugoff, J. Louis, T. Moore, R. M. Silver, & R. Resnick (Eds.), *Creasy & Resnick's maternal–fetal medicine: Principles and practice* (9th ed., pp. 991–1006). Elsevier.

Lee, R. H. (2023). Diseases of the liver, biliary system and pancreas. In C. J. Lockwood, J. Copel, L. Dugoff, J. Louis, T. Moore, R. M. Silver, & R. Resnick (Eds.), *Creasy & Resnick's maternal–fetal medicine: Principles and practice* (9th ed., pp. 1173–1191). Elsevier.

Littlefield, A., & Lenahan, C. (2019). Cholelithiasis: Presentation and management. *Journal of Midwifery and Women's Health, 64*(3), 289–297. https://doi.org/10.1111/jmwh.12959

Tran, T. T., Ahn, J., & Reau, N. S. (2016). ACG clinical guideline: Liver disease and pregnancy. *American Journal of Gastroenterology, 111*(2), 176–194. https://doi.org/10.1038/ajg.2015.430

Weinstein, M. S., Feuerwerker, S., & Baxter, J. K. (2020). Appendicitis and cholecystitis in pregnancy. *Clinical Obstetrics and Gynecology, 63*(2), 405–415. https://doi.org/10.1097/GRF.0000000000000529

Wong, A. C., & Ko, C. W. (2013). Carbohydrate intake as a risk factor for biliary sludge and stones during pregnancy. *Journal of Clinical Gastroenterology, 47*(8), 700–705.

Zachariah, S. K., Fenn, M., Jacob, K., Arthungal, S. A., & Zachariah, S. A. (2019). Management of acute abdomen in pregnancy: Current perspectives. *International Journal of Women's Health, 11*, 119–134. https://doi.org/10.2147/IJWH.S151501

52

Endocrine Disorders

Elizabeth Gabzdyl

Relevant Terms

Exophthalmos—eyelid lag, eyelid retraction, bulging of the eye from the orbit

Gestational diabetes—a condition in which carbohydrate intolerance develops during the latter half of pregnancy

Goiter—enlarged thyroid gland

Graves' disease—autoimmune hyperthyroid disease

Hashimoto's thyroiditis—autoimmune hypothyroid disease

Postpartum thyroiditis—a transient autoimmune thyroid dysfunction that occurs within 12 months of giving birth

Pregestational diabetes—diabetes existing prior to pregnancy

Thyroid storm—emergency thyrotoxic crisis

Type 1 diabetes—lifelong chronic disease characterized by hyperglycemia in which beta cells produce no insulin

Type 2 diabetes—chronic disease in which beta cells produce less insulin and/or the body cells are resistant to insulin

---

Introduction

The endocrine system is a network of glands that are vitally important for the regulation of many body functions including metabolism, growth, brain function, and cell and tissue activity. The most commonly encountered disorders in pregnant clients are hypothyroidism, hyperthyroidism, and diabetes, both overt (pregestational) diabetes and **gestational diabetes** mellitus (GDM). There are numerous differential diagnoses for hypothyroidism and hyperthyroidism, underscoring the necessity of complete evaluation. Referral may be necessary for additional testing such as radioactive iodine scan, thyroid ultrasound, or fine needle biopsy to rule out **Graves' disease**, **goiter**, or cancer (Hackley & Kriebs, 2017). Because management of these conditions is often complex, it is often preferable to refer the client to a healthcare provider who specializes in management of thyroid disorders in pregnancy (Kriebs & Hackley, 2019). This chapter will review the most common thyroid disorders as well as present an overview of

pregestational diabetes and pregnancy. As is the case with many chronic diseases, people with endocrine disorders can face multiple barriers to care. These may include worrying about the cost of care, not being able to get through to the office or clinic on the phone to arrange appointments, lack of transportation to an appointment, long waiting times, and inconvenient provider hours, all impacting access to care and resources (Ward, 2017).

Health equity key points

- The experience of racism increases risk for endocrine disorders such as diabetes.
- Disproportionate exposure to endocrine-disrupting chemicals may contribute to racial disparities in health outcomes.
- People with endocrine disorders face multiple barriers to care, including worrying about the cost of care, not being able to get through to the office or clinic on the phone to arrange appointments, lack of transportation to an appointment, waiting too long at the office or clinic, and inconvenient provider hours.

Thyroid Disorders in Pregnancy

Thyroid disorders are the second most common endocrinologic disorders found in pregnancy, affecting one in six pregnant clients (Dieguez et al., 2015). Since the fetal brain requires thyroid hormones for development and maturation, uncorrected maternal thyroid dysfunction in pregnancy can have adverse effects on fetal well-being potentially resulting in negative neurological sequelae if uncorrected (Coad et al., 2020). In fact, the pregnancy requires the support of the maternal thyroid for the first 20 weeks until the fetus is fully able to take over (Mayhew et al., 2022). Demand for thyroid hormones increases during pregnancy, which may cause a previously unnoticed thyroid disorder to worsen and become symptomatic for

Prenatal and Postnatal Care: A Person-Centered Approach, Third Edition. Edited by Karen Trister Grace, Cindy L. Farley, Noelene K. Jeffers, and Tanya Tringali.
© 2024 John Wiley & Sons Ltd. Published 2024 by John Wiley & Sons Ltd.
Companion website: www.wiley.com/go/grace/prenatal

Table 52.1   Causes of Thyroid Dysfunction and Expected Laboratory Findings

Diagnosis	TSH	Free T_4	Free T_3	Antibodies
Hypothyroidism				
Hashimoto's thyroiditis (autoimmune hypothyroidism)	↑	↓	Varied	Present
Subclinical hypothyroidism	↑ (slightly)	Normal	Normal	Absent
Post-thyroid ablation therapy	↑	↓	↓	Absent
Hyperthyroidism				
Graves' disease (autoimmune hyperthyroidism)	↓	↑	↑	Present
Subclinical hyperthyroidism	↓	Normal	Normal	Absent
Thyroid storm	↓↓	↑↑	↑↑	Variable
Postpartum thyroiditis	↓ fluctuates	↑ then ↓	↑ then ↓	Present

Source: Hackley and Kriebs (2017), Alexander et al. (2017), and ACOG (2020).

the first time. The common causes of thyroid dysfunction are noted in Table 52.1. A brief review of thyroid physiology during pregnancy is presented as a foundation for understanding the specific thyroid disease in pregnancy.

An emerging area of study is environmental exposure to endocrine-disrupting chemicals, or chemicals that disrupt or mimic normal hormone production, and can be associated with adverse pregnancy and neonatal outcomes such as preterm birth (PTB), low birth weight, and childhood asthma. These chemicals are found in many personal care products such as hair care products, soap, and toothpaste. Communities of color, specifically non-Hispanic Black and Hispanic communities, are disproportionately exposed to many classes of endocrine-disrupting chemicals, which may contribute to racial disparities in health outcomes (Chan et al., 2021).

Thyroid Physiology in Pregnancy

To meet the challenge of increased metabolic needs during pregnancy, the thyroid adapts through changes in thyroid hormone economy and in the regulation of the hypothalamic–pituitary–thyroid axis. Three hormones are produced by the thyroid: T_3 (triiodothyronine), T_4 (thyroxine), and calcitonin. The thyroid hormones, T_3 and T_4, are synthesized within the thyroid. Calcium metabolism is regulated by calcitonin. Thyroid-stimulating hormone (TSH) stimulates and suppresses the production of T_3 and T_4. The hypothalamic–pituitary–thyroid network produces and regulates thyroid hormones via a negative feedback control system. The hypothalamus responds to the level of circulating T_3 and T_4. If the levels are rising, it signals the pituitary to decrease production of TSH, which will decrease the production of T_3 and T_4. If decreasing levels of T_3 and T_4 are perceived, the hypothalamus will produce thyrotropin-releasing hormone (TRH), which will stimulate the pituitary to increase TSH production to produce more thyroid hormones, T_3 and T_4 (Coad et al., 2020; Hackley & Kriebs, 2017). Figure 52.1 diagrams this system.

Due to increased metabolic demands during pregnancy, the thyroid function tests of healthy pregnant people differ from those of healthy nonpregnant people.

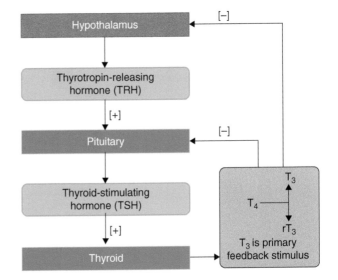

Figure 52.1   Hypothalamic–pituitary–thyroid interactions. [+], stimulation; [–], inhibition. Laposata, Aleryani, & Woodworth (2010)/McGraw Hill.

The thyroid gland is often slightly enlarged in the early weeks of pregnancy, reflecting the increased pregnancy-related metabolic demands. Pregnancy-associated goiters are much more common in iodine-deficient areas of the world and are relatively uncommon in the United States and other high-income countries. Thyroid hormones exhibit normal fluctuations during pregnancy, especially in the first trimester. This can make it especially difficult to know when it is appropriate to screen for thyroid disease and how to interpret the values. Figure 52.2 shows normal maternal thyroid hormone fluctuations.

Screening for Thyroid Disorders in Pregnancy

The universal screening of asymptomatic pregnant clients for thyroid dysfunction during the first trimester of pregnancy is not recommended by the American Thyroid Association (ATA), the American College of Obstetricians and Gynecologists (ACOG), the Endocrine Society, or the

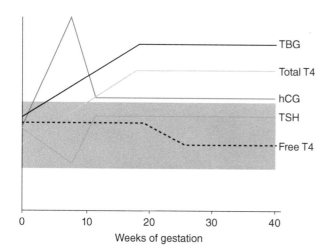

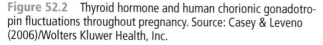

Figure 52.2   Thyroid hormone and human chorionic gonadotropin fluctuations throughout pregnancy. Source: Casey & Leveno (2006)/Wolters Kluwer Health, Inc.

American Association of Clinical Endocrinologists, as case findings do not indicate its effectiveness (Alexander et al., 2017; ACOG, 2020). In a large, randomized controlled trial of screening compared to not screening, no difference was found in neurodevelopment in the children of those with subclinical hypothyroidism (SCH; Lazarus et al., 2012). An individual's history should be reviewed at their initial prenatal visit, and if any risk factors are noted, serum TSH is recommended as the next step (ACOG, 2020; Alexander et al., 2017). This testing is indicated when a client has a history of thyroid disorder, either personal or family, a history of **type 1 diabetes** mellitus, or if a thyroid disorder is suspected based on clinical signs and/or symptoms (ACOG, 2020).

Diagnosing Thyroid Disorders

The serum TSH is a simple, accurate, and economical screening test for thyroid disorders and is used as a primary indicator when screening for thyroid disorders (ACOG, 2020; Hackley & Kriebs, 2017).

TSH screening in early pregnancy recommended in the presence of any of the following risk factors

1. A history of hypothyroidism/hyperthyroidism or current symptoms of thyroid dysfunction
2. Known thyroid antibody positivity or presence of goiter
3. History of head or neck radiation or prior thyroid surgery
4. Age >30 years
5. Type 1 diabetes or other autoimmune disorders
6. History of pregnancy loss, PTB, or infertility
7. Multiple prior pregnancies (>2)
8. Family history of autoimmune thyroid disease or thyroid dysfunction
9. Severe obesity (BMI >40 kg/m²)
10. Use of amiodarone, lithium, or recent administration of iodinated radiologic contrast
11. Residing in an area of known moderate to severe iodine insufficiency

Source: Alexander et al. (2017) and ACOG (2020).

The TSH is most reliable because it indirectly reflects thyroid hormone levels, which are sensed by the pituitary gland (ACOG, 2020). The ATA recommends that the serum TSH be used to make treatment decisions (Alexander et al., 2017). When there is an abnormal TSH result, a T_4 should be done to further clarify the diagnosis and determine if treatment is indicated (ACOG, 2020; Table 52.1). Because of the changes in thyroid physiology during pregnancy, the ATA recommends using trimester-specific reference ranges for TSH, and method and trimester-specific reference ranges for serum-free T_4 (FT_4).

The ATA's most recent (Alexander et al., 2017) guidelines for managing thyroid disease during pregnancy and postpartum recommend raising the upper limit of normal in thyroid function tests; for TSH, the upper limit was 2.5 mlU/L in the 2011 guidelines and is now 4.0 mlU/L (Alexander et al., 2017). Normal TSH ranges in pregnancy vary by country, which may be due to variations in dietary iodine availability and differences in lab assays used (Alexander et al., 2017).

The physical symptoms that many individuals experience in early pregnancy, such as fatigue and weight gain, are very similar to symptoms of thyroid disease, making diagnosis challenging (Table 52.2). It is not uncommon to have normal physical exam findings when there is thyroid disturbance. However, the results of serum thyroid function tests will assist in developing a differential diagnosis (ACOG, 2020; Alexander et al., 2017).

Overt Hypothyroidism

Overt hypothyroidism is characterized by an elevated TSH level and decreased T_4 level. **Hashimoto's thyroiditis**, also called *chronic lymphocytic thyroiditis*, is an autoimmune thyroid disorder, first described by physician Hakaru Hashimoto in 1912. Hashimoto's thyroiditis is the most common cause of overt hypothyroidism in pregnancy, occurring in approximately 2–10/1000 pregnant individuals (ACOG, 2020; Neville, 2017). In Hashimoto's thyroiditis, antithyroid peroxidase (APO) antibodies are present that destroy the thyroid gland. The ATA recommends using the upper reference range for TSH of 4.0 mlU/L (ACOG, 2020; Alexander et al., 2017). Other causes of overt hypothyroidism include insufficient iodine intake and causes related to other conditions such as pituitary adenoma or surgery such as thyroidectomy due to cancer (Hackley & Kriebs, 2017).

Maternal and Fetal Risks

Thyroid hormones are crucial for fetal brain development. With untreated overt hypothyroidism, risks may include pregnancy loss, PTB, low birth weight, and impaired cognitive ability in children resulting from these pregnancies. The most critical time is the first trimester, since a fetus does not begin to synthesize its own thyroid hormones until approximately 10–12 weeks of gestation and relies solely on the pregnant person to provide them (Coad et al., 2020; Neville, 2017). Adverse outcomes are related to the degree of thyroid hormone abnormalities,

Table 52.2 Common Signs and Symptoms of Pregnancy and Thyroid Disease

Hypothyroidism	Hyperthyroidism	Common pregnancy symptoms
Weight gain	Weight loss	Appetite increase, weight gain, muscle cramps
Cold intolerance	Heat intolerance, sweating	Increased warmth, cold intolerance
Fatigue	Nervousness/anxiety, tachycardia, palpitations	Fatigue
Depression	Insomnia	Insomnia
Constipation	Bulging of the eyes	Constipation
Dry skin, thin hair, hair loss		Skin or hair changes (thinning, thickening)
		Mild vision changes

Source: Adapted from Alexander et al. (2017).

highlighting the importance of preventing deficiency whenever possible to minimize perinatal risks. The most common maternal complications of poorly controlled hypothyroidism are hypertensive disorders, including preeclampsia and gestational hypertension. When thyroid hormone levels are well controlled, maternal and neonatal outcomes will be the same as in pregnancies without thyroid disease. Antenatal surveillance is not indicated unless hypothyroidism is poorly controlled (ACOG, 2021).

Perinatal complications of overt hypothyroidism	
Maternal	Neonatal
Preeclampsia	Low birth weight
Gestational hypertension	Prematurity
Preterm birth	Cognitive impairment
Increased rate of cesarean birth	Increased morbidity and mortality
Postpartum hemorrhage	

Clinical Presentation

When hypothyroidism is present, an enlarged thyroid (up to two to three times the normal size) may be noted. Changes in the thyroid gland may also be nonpalpable. Symptoms may include dry skin and hair, fatigue, constipation, weight gain, intolerance to cold, and hair loss (ACOG, 2020; Neville, 2017). The symptoms of hypothyroidism can sometimes be difficult to discern from symptoms of early pregnancy, making diagnosis challenging. The initial presentation can also consist of nonspecific symptoms, and subsequently, hypothyroidism may be misdiagnosed as depression, premenstrual syndrome, chronic fatigue syndrome, or fibromyalgia.

Laboratory Testing, Diagnosis, and Management

The TSH will be elevated and the T_4 will be decreased with hypothyroidism (ACOG, 2020; Alexander et al., 2017), but a TSH of 4.0 mlU/L or above is the sole finding required for a diagnosis of overt hypothyroidism.

Antithyroid antibodies will also be present in the case of Hashimoto's thyroiditis. For anyone diagnosed with pregestational hypothyroidism, early prenatal care is advised to enable early thyroid function testing and medication adjustment as necessary.

Individuals with overt hypothyroidism should be evaluated for TPO antibody status. Hypothyroidism should be treated with synthetic thyroid hormone (levothyroxine) when the TSH concentration is elevated beyond either population-based (if available) or standard reference levels. A typical starting dose is 100 mcg/day. TSH level should be assessed every four to six weeks and the levothyroxine dose should be adjusted, increasing by 25–50 mcg until the TSH value is normal (ACOG, 2020). The goal of treatment is to maintain the pregnant client's serum TSH at approximately 4.0 mlU/L, which is the upper reference limit recommended by the ATA (Alexander et al., 2017).

For someone entering prenatal care with a history of ongoing treatment for stable hypothyroidism, TSH testing should be done at the first visit. The majority of these individuals will need higher dosing of levothyroxine to maintain a normal TSH secretion during pregnancy. Total T_4 concentrations should increase by 20–50% during pregnancy in order to meet the demands of the growing fetus. In a person with hypothyroidism, the thyroid is unable to respond to the hormonal cues to increase T_4 production, resulting in a need for an increased dosage of synthetic thyroid hormone. Dose requirements may increase by as much as 50% during pregnancy, and the increase should start as soon as possible. One recommended strategy is to increase a levothyroxine by two tablets (of whatever dose is being used) *weekly* (in other words, nine doses per week instead of seven) as soon as pregnancy is confirmed (Alexander et al., 2017). The TSH should then be rechecked every four to six weeks until the TSH value is stable and within normal range (ACOG, 2020). Postpartum, the client should immediately resume taking the prepregnancy dose of levothyroxine and the TSH level should be rechecked at six weeks postpartum. Medication dose is then adjusted if indicated (Alexander et al., 2017). Figure 52.3 presents an algorithm for testing and managing TSH levels in pregnancy.

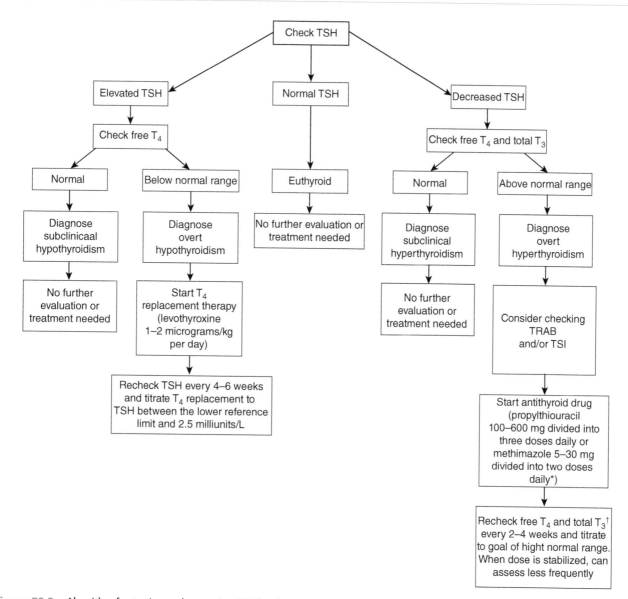

Figure 52.3   Algorithm for testing and managing TSH levels in pregnancy. ACOG (2020) / Wolters Kluwer Health, Inc.

Depending on practice protocols and the complexity of the client's hypothyroidism, the management plan will likely include consultation, collaboration, or referral.

Subclinical Hypothyroidism

Although it is well accepted that untreated overt hypothyroidism is linked to adverse perinatal outcomes, it is less clear what the potential impact of SCH is on maternal and fetal health. SCH is clinically defined as an elevated TSH with normal FT_4. SCH occurs in approximately 3.5% pregnant individuals (Dong & Stagnaro-Green, 2019). SCH has not been associated with adverse maternal or fetal outcomes; thus, both the ATA and ACOG recommend against treatment (Alexander et al., 2017; ACOG, 2020). This recommendation by the ACOG is a Level A, which is its highest recommendation based on scientific evidence rather than consensus and opinion.

Screening for Hypothyroidism in Pregnancy

At the initial prenatal appointment, the healthcare provider should determine through history taking and physical exam if the client is at risk for thyroid dysfunction and would benefit from thyroid screening. See Box 52.2 and Table 52.2 for a full list of risk factors and signs and symptoms of thyroid disease that would warrant screening.

Preconception Care of People with Hypothyroidism

It is recommended for a person with hypothyroidism planning a pregnancy to receive preconception care to ensure that their thyroid disorder is managed appropriately and is stable prior to conception. Consultation or referral to specialists in thyroid disease can be provided as needed. The target preconception serum TSH level is <2.5 mU/L (Alexander et al., 2017).

Hyperthyroidism

Overt hyperthyroidism is relatively uncommon in pregnancy, affecting less than 1% of pregnant persons (Dong & Stagnaro-Green, 2019). It is characterized by a decreased TSH and elevated T_4 level (ACOG, 2020). Up to 95% of hyperthyroidism is caused by Graves' disease, an autoimmune cause of hyperthyroidism, named for Sir Robert Graves, a surgeon who first described the condition in the early nineteenth century (Krassas et al., 2010). Ideally, Graves' hyperthyroidism is diagnosed and treated prior to conceiving. It may be advisable to postpone pregnancy during treatment and stabilization, often up to three to six months, if the person is taking medications or requires surgery to manage hyperthyroidism. If the diagnosis of Graves' disease occurs at the time of confirmation of pregnancy, accurate and prompt diagnosis, development of a management plan, and stabilization of thyroid hormones are crucial since adverse outcomes for the pregnant person and the fetus can be significant when hyperthyroidism is untreated or poorly controlled.

Maternal and Fetal Risks

Extremely high levels of thyroid-stimulating immunoglobulins (TSIs) are produced in Graves' disease, which stimulate the thyroid gland. These antibodies cross the placenta and can interact with the fetal thyroid gland, resulting in neonatal thyroid dysfunction. When excessive thyroid hormones are present during pregnancy, perinatal complications can include a significantly higher rate of spontaneous abortion, decreased birth weight, stillbirth, PTB, and neonatal mortality. Maternal adverse outcomes can include GDM, preeclampsia, maternal heart failure, and **thyroid storm** (ACOG, 2020).

Clinical Presentation

A person with hyperthyroidism may present with symptoms that may include tachycardia, palpitations, anxiety, weight loss, fine tremor, insomnia, hypertension, sweating, and heat intolerance (ACOG, 2020). In people with Graves' disease, a physical exam may reveal additional classic characteristics of an enlarged thyroid (goiter) or the presence of ophthalmopathy, such as **exophthalmos**, lid lag, or lid retraction (ACOG, 2020).

Laboratory Testing, Diagnosis, and Management

A definitive diagnosis is based on laboratory results. In hyperthyroidism, the serum TSH is suppressed and the T_3 and T_4 are elevated. Testing for thyroid receptor antibodies (TRAB) and TSI will confirm Graves' disease (ACOG, 2020). If negative, further investigation for a definitive diagnosis will be necessary to determine of further treatment is indicated. Examples of other possible causes include thyroid nodules, pituitary adenomas, and

thyroid damage from surgery, medications, or chemicals (Hackley & Kriebs, 2017).

The goal of treatment is to maintain T_4 levels as close to normal as possible. Propylthiouracil (PTU) and methimazole (MMI) are the preferred medications used to treat Graves' disease. Both block production of T_3 and T_4 (Neville, 2017). PTU is often preferred, especially in the first trimester, since use of MMI is associated with more severe fetal anomalies (ACOG, 2020). Due to the small but serious risk of liver toxicity, the US Food and Drug Administration (FDA) has recommended changing to MMI once a client is in the second trimester of pregnancy (Alexander et al., 2017; Stagnaro-Green et al., 2020). While on PTU, liver function should be monitored every three to four weeks and warning signs of serious liver problems (fever, loss of appetite, nausea, vomiting, fatigue, itchiness, abdominal pain, dark urine, light stools, yellowing of skin, or sclera) related to PTU should be reviewed with the client so that they are aware of what adverse symptoms to report (Chartwell Pharmaceuticals, 2015). Individuals with moderate to severe disease may also be treated with beta blockers to reduce symptoms (Alexander et al., 2017). After birth, depending on the stability of person's hyperthyroidism during pregnancy, the baby may have transient hypothyroidism, which usually resolves spontaneously.

Interprofessional Care

Close collaboration with or referral to maternal-fetal medicine services are recommended for people with hyperthyroidism for the development of a long-term plan of care (Alexander et al., 2017). The plan of care, especially for newly diagnosed hyperthyroidism, is often complex, and medication regimens must be determined and monitored closely. These individuals will require follow-up throughout pregnancy and postpartum.

Subclinical Hyperthyroidism

This condition is noted when the TSH is decreased and the T_4 is normal, and the individual is asymptomatic. Since there are no adverse maternal or fetal outcomes associated, no treatment is required (ACOG, 2020; Stagnaro-Green et al., 2020). In pregnant people with diagnosed subclinical hyperthyroidism, monitoring TSH and FT_4 every four to six weeks during pregnancy can assess for change to overt disease. Subclinical hyperthyroidism during pregnancy usually only requires periodic monitoring.

Thyroid Storm

Thyroid storm is a rare but life-threatening form of hyperthyroidism in which the body is in a hypermetabolic state due to an excess of thyroid hormones. This condition is very serious and must be treated quickly and aggressively. Symptoms include high fever (over 103 °F), tachycardia, nausea, and vomiting, symptoms of congestive heart failure and possible multiorgan failure. The T_4 will be very elevated and the TSH very low. Treatment is based on the constellation of presenting symptoms rather than laboratory values and should be initiated under physician care in an intensive care unit, where the individual will be given supportive therapy (ACOG, 2020).

Postpartum Thyroiditis

Postpartum thyroiditis (PPT) is a transient thyroid dysfunction that can present as hypothyroidism or hyperthyroidism and occurs in as many as 5–10% of people who are within 12 months of childbirth (ACOG, 2020; Alexander et al., 2017) with the highest incidence in the first 4 months (Neville, 2017). In most cases, symptoms will resolve spontaneously, but one third of people who experience PPT will go on to develop permanent hypothyroidism (ACOG, 2020). The most common symptoms tend to be mild and vague such as fatigue, irritability, tachycardia, dry skin, or palpitations. A mildly enlarged thyroid may be noted. Because the postpartum period can be challenging for many people, both physically and emotionally, with irregular sleep and routines, thyroid dysfunction can easily be overlooked and remain undiagnosed.

Laboratory Evaluation, Diagnosis, and Management

PPT may present with either hyperthyroidism or hypothyroidism. The thyroid becomes inflamed via an autoimmune process resulting in an overproduction of thyroid hormone. Most individuals experience a hyperthyroid phase followed by a hypothyroid phase, which may be symptomatic.

If the TSH is elevated between 4 and 10 mIU/L and a client is symptomatic, the person may require levothyroxine. Beta blockers are used for symptom management if they present with hyperthyroidism. Abnormal thyroid levels and symptoms typically resolve spontaneously within 2–12 months, and drug tapering to discontinue can be done once the client is asymptomatic and thyroid levels are stable, although there is no protocol or consensus on treatment or duration of medication. Treatment should be individualized with physician consultation or management (Karsnitz, 2019).

Iodine in Pregnancy

Iodine is an essential trace mineral. It is required for the body to synthesize the thyroid hormones, T_4 and T_3, which are essential for many physiologic functions such as reproduction, metabolism, and growth and development. Hypothyroidism can be caused by iodine deficiency, resulting in increased TSH levels, thyroid hypertrophy, and sometimes a goiter (Ferraro, 2017). When iodine deficiency occurs during pregnancy, fetal effects can be severe and may include conditions such as congenital hypothyroidism and intellectual impairment (Alexander et al., 2017). Iodine deficiency is the world's leading cause of cognitive impairment—a preventable condition.

The most common source of iodine is iodized salt. To eliminate iodine-deficiency-related hypothyroidism in the United States, salt was universally fortified with iodine in 1924. Dairy products and commercially baked breads are also good sources of dietary iodine. Small amounts of iodine are also found in other foods in varying amounts, depending on soil concentration and fertilizer used (Ferraro, 2017). Globally, iodine deficiency in pregnancy continues to be a problem. High levels of iodine deficiency have been reported in India, Pakistan, Niger, Ethiopia, Belgium, Czech Republic, Denmark, France, Latvia, Norway, Spain, and the United Kingdom (Alexander et al., 2017).

It is recommended that individuals of childbearing age and especially those planning a pregnancy make sure that their diets are sufficient in iodine and note that not all vitamins and prenatal vitamins contain iodine. The recommendation for daily iodine intake is 150 mcg during pregnancy and 220 mcg during lactation (Alexander et al., 2017; Coad et al., 2020; Ferraro, 2017).

Pregestational Diabetes Mellitus

Diabetes mellitus is a group of metabolic disorders that cause hyperglycemia and is the most common of all endocrine disorders. It is estimated that in the United States, 37.3 million people have diabetes (23.0% have not yet been diagnosed) and 96 million adults have prediabetes (approximately 38.0% of all US adults; CDC, 2022). The CDC has partnered with the Ad Council and the American Medical Association (AMA) to launch public service announcements and increase awareness of prediabetes risk in an effort to lower these concerning numbers (CDC, 2022). The two leading causes of death for people with diabetes are heart attack and stroke (CDC, 2021). Other serious complications may also be experienced, including retinopathy, chronic renal disease, and neuropathy (CDC, 2021).

Classifications

Three classifications of diabetes mellitus are considered **pregestational diabetes** (**type 1 diabetes, type 2 diabetes, and other;** Table 52.3), as defined by the ADA (2017b). Management of these conditions in pregnancy is covered in this chapter; gestational diabetes is addressed in Chapter 37, *Gestational Diabetes Mellitus*.

Type 1 diabetes (formerly known as insulin-dependent diabetes or juvenile diabetes) typically begins in childhood or adolescence. Type 1 is caused by pancreatic β cell destruction, via autoimmune process, accounting for 5–10% of all diabetes (ADA, 2017b). Insulin is always necessary for the management of type 1 diabetes and should be coordinated by a diabetes specialist (endocrinologist or general practitioner). Although the only treatment option is insulin, various injection regimens are available to reduce hypoglycemic episodes, including long-acting insulin analogs and pumps for insulin infusion.

Type 2 diabetes (formerly known as non-insulin-dependent diabetes) is the most common type of diabetes,

Table 52.3 Diabetes Mellitus Classifications, Etiology, Onset, and Usual Treatment

Classification		Etiology	Onset	Treatment options
PRE GESTATIONAL DIABETES	Type 1	• Autoimmune destruction of ß cells in pancreas. • Complete deficiency of insulin.	Childhood, adolescence, young adult	Insulin
	Type 2	• Dysfunction of insulin secretion or resistance • Dysfunction of glucose production, transport or utilization • Some continued production of insulin	Adult	Diet, medication, insulin
	Other causes: Monogenic diabetes syndromes • Neonatal diabetes • Maturity onset diabetes of the young Diseases of the exocrine pancreas • Cystic fibrosis Drug- or chemical-induced diabetes • Glucocorticoid use • HIV/AIDs treatment • After organ transplantation	• Genetic defects of ß cells, insulin action • Diseases of pancreas, endocrinopathies • Drug, infection, or chemical induced	Variable	Diet, medication, insulin
GESTATIONAL DIABETES	Gestational diabetes	The enlarging placenta secretes hormones and cytokines that result in increased insulin resistance	Second or third trimester of pregnancy	Diet, medication, insulin, exercise

Source: Adapted from ADA (2017b).

accounting for 90–95% of all cases (ADA, 2017b). Over half of people with GDM go on to develop Type 2 diabetes in subsequent years (ADA, 2017b). Although the precise etiology is not known, type 2 diabetes is characterized by insulin deficiency or resistance and a dysfunction in glucose production, transport or utilization (ACOG, 2018). Type 2 diabetes often develops gradually, and classic symptoms may be missed, increasing risk of complications such as microvascular and macrovascular disease (ADA, 2017b; Bowers & Reedy, 2017). Treatment for type 2 diabetes generally includes the oral agent metformin as a first-line drug, with insulin added if needed (ADA, 2017a).

A small number of diabetes cases are caused by other varied conditions that create a hyperglycemic state, thereby leading to diabetes mellitus and associated risks. Some examples of these include genetic defects such as neonatal diabetes or maturity onset diabetes of the young (MODY), diseases of the exocrine system such as cystic fibrosis, and drug- or chemical-induced diabetes (e.g., from glucocorticoid use, HIV/AIDS treatment or after organ transplantation; ADA, 2017b). The large-scale, longitudinal Black Women's Health Study showed a significant impact of racism on type 2 diabetes incidence (Bacon et al., 2017). These findings help explain diabetes health disparities and highlight the importance of addressing racism.

Perinatal Risks

Individuals with pregestational diabetes are at higher risk for maternal and fetal/neonatal complications, compared to people with gestational diabetes. The risk of major congenital malformations is increased in those with pregestational diabetes and is related to the degree of maternal glycemic control during the period of embryogenesis (ADA, 2017b; ACOG, 2018). Individuals with pregestational diabetes are also at risk for other comorbidities such as thyroid disease, hypertension, and cardiac disease. Collaboration or referral to perinatal care by those with expertise in diabetes during pregnancy is recommended. The optimal interprofessional team will include nurses, dieticians, and endocrinologists with referrals initiated early in pregnancy as needed. Individuals with pregestational diabetes may seek care for pregnancy-related issues unrelated to their diabetes. Midwives, nurse practitioners, and physician assistants play an important role in attending to those needs as part of a healthcare team.

Possible fetal, neonatal, and maternal complications	
Fetal, neonatal	Maternal
Spontaneous abortion	Retinopathy
Fetal malformation	Nephropathy
Fetal macrosomia	Hypertensive disorders
Fetal death	Uteroplacental insufficiency
Neonatal morbidity	Preterm birth

Source: Data from ACOG (2018).

Preconception Counseling and Care

Efforts should be made to achieve the best maternal glycemic control prior to conception to lower the risk of fetal malformation, though this can be challenging since just over 50% of pregnancies in the United States are planned. Glycated hemoglobin (A1C) values, which measure the percentage of glucose that coats hemoglobin, reflect the average blood glucose concentration over the previous 8–12 weeks, which is useful in evaluating longer-term glycemic control and important in preconception care.

Categories of preconception counseling considerations

1. **Preconception education**
   - Comprehensive nutrition assessment
   - Lifestyle recommendations
   - Self-management education
   - Diabetes in pregnancy education
   - Folic acid supplementation
2. **Medical assessment and plan**
   - General evaluation
   - Comorbidities
   - OB/Gyn history
   - Medications
3. **Screening**
   - For comorbidities (exams, labs)
   - Genetic carrier and infectious disease
4. **Immunizations**
5. **Preconception plan**
   - Nutrition and medication
   - Contraception versus timing of conception
   - General health management

Source: Adapted from ADA (2022).

Glycemic control should be achieved preconceptionally to maximize prevention of adverse outcomes. Therefore, the major goals of preconception care of clients with pregestational diabetes are to evaluate glycemic control

and to recommend adjustments in diet, medications, and lifestyle to achieve euglycemia.

Summary

Hypothyroidism, hyperthyroidism, and diabetes (both overt diabetes and GDM) are among the most commonly encountered disorders in pregnant individuals. Due to the complexity of diagnosis and management of these conditions, it is recommended that consultation or referral be obtained for all pregnant clients with an existing or new endocrine diagnosis for the development of an appropriate perinatal plan.

Resources for Pregnant People and Healthcare Providers

Agency for Healthcare Research and Quality: https://www.ahrq.gov/research/findings/factsheets/index.html

American Diabetes Association: http://www.diabetes.org

American Thyroid Association: www.thyroid.org

Centers for Disease Control and Prevention: http://www.cdc.gov/diabetes

Centers for Disease Control and Prevention: *National diabetes statistics report 2022* https://www.cdc.gov/diabetes/data/statistics-report/index.html

NIH NIDDK Clearinghouses & Health Information Center: https://www.niddk.nih.gov/health-information/community-health-outreach/information-clearinghouses

References

Alexander, E. K., Pearce, E. N., Brent, G. A., Brown, R. S., Chen, H., Dosiou, C., Grobman, W. A., Laurberg, P., Lazarus, J. H., Mandel, S. J., Peeters, R. P., & Sullivan, S. (2017). 2017 guidelines of the American Thyroid Association for the diagnosis and management of thyroid disease during pregnancy and the postpartum. *Thyroid, 27*(1), 1–162.

American College of Obstetricians and Gynecologists (ACOG). (2018). ACOG Practice bulletin No. 190: Gestational diabetes mellitus. *Obstetrics & Gynecology, 131*(2), e49–e64.

American College of Obstetricians and Gynecologists (ACOG). (2020). Thyroid disease in pregnancy. Practice bulletin, no. 223. *Obstetrics & Gynecology, 135*(6), e261–e402.

American College of Obstetricians and Gynecologists (ACOG). (2021). Indications for outpatient antenatal fetal surveillance. Committee opinion no. 828. *Obstetrics & Gynecology, 137*, e177–e197.

American Diabetes Association (ADA). (2017a). Management of diabetes in pregnancy. *Diabetes Care, 40*(Suppl. 1), S114–S119.

American Diabetes Association (ADA). (2017b). Classification and diagnosis of diabetes. *Diabetes Care, 40*(Suppl. 1), S11–S24.

American Diabetes Association (ADA) Professional Practice Committee. (2022). Management of diabetes in pregnancy: Standards of medical care in diabetes-2022. *Diabetes Care, 45*(Suppl. 1), S232–S243.

Bacon, K., Stuver, S., Cozier, Y., Palmer, J., Rosenberg, L., & Ruiz-Narvaez, E. (2017). Perceived racism and incident diabetes in the black women's health study. *Diabetologia, 60*, 2221–2225.

Bowers, E. R., & Reedy, N. J. (2017). Diabetes. In M. C. Brucker & T. L. King (Eds.), *Pharmacology for women's health* (2nd ed., pp. 491–528).

Casey, B. M., & Leveno, K. J. (2006). Thyroid diseases in pregnancy. *Obstetrics and Gynecology, 108*(5), 1284.

Centers for Disease Control and Prevention. (2021). *Put the brakes on diabetes complications.* Diabetes. Retrieved February 27, 2022 from http://www.cdc.gov/diabetes/library/features/prevent-compli cations.html

Centers for Disease Control and Prevention. (2022). *National diabetes statistics report*. Diabetes. Retrieved February 27, 2022 from https://www.cdc.gov/diabetes/data/statistics-report/index.html.

Chan, M., Mita, C., Bellavia, A., Parker, M., & James-Todd, T. (2021). Racial/ethnic disparities in pregnancy and prenatal exposure to endocrine-disrupting chemicals commonly used in personal care products. *Current Environmental Health Reports, 8*, 98–112.

Chartwell Pharmaceuticals. (2015). *Propylthiouracil tablets, USP*. https://www.accessdata.fda.gov/drugsatfda_docs/label/2016/006188s025lbl.pdf

Coad, J., Pedley, K., & Dunstall, M. (2020). *Anatomy and physiology for midwives* (4th ed.). Elsevier.

Dieguez, M., Herrero, A., Avello, N., Suarez, P., Delgado, E., & Menendez, E. (2015). Prevalence of thyroid dysfunction in women in early pregnancy: Does it increase with maternal age? *Clinical Endocrinology, 84*, 121–126.

Dong, A. C., & Stagnaro-Green, A. (2019). Differences in diagnostic criteria mask the true prevalence of thyroid disease in pregnancy: A systematic review and meta-analysis. *Thyroid, 29*(2), 278–289. https://doi.org/10.1089/thy.2018.0475

Ferraro, K. (2017). Vitamins and minerals. In M. C. Brucker & T. L. King (Eds.), *Pharmacology for women's health* (2nd ed., pp. 105–106). Jones & Bartlett Learning.

Hackley, B. K., & Kriebs, J. M. (2017). Thyroid and other endocrine disorders. In B. K. Hackley & J. M. Kriebs (Eds.), *Primary care of women* (2nd ed., pp. 435–448). Jones & Bartlett.

Karsnitz, D. B. (2019). Postpartum complications. In T. L. King, M. C. Brucker, K. Osborne, & C. M. Jevitt (Eds.), *Varney's midwifery* (6th ed., pp. 1217–1231). Jones & Bartlett Learning.

Krassas, G. E., Poppe, K., & Glinoer, D. (2010). Thyroid function and reproductive health. *Endocrine Reviews, 31*, 702–755.

Kriebs, J. M., & Hackley, B. K. (2019). Common conditions in primary care. In T. L. King, M. C. Brucker, K. Osborne, & C. M. Jevitt (Eds.), *Varney's midwifery* (6th ed., pp. 175–226). Jones & Bartlett Learning.

Laposata, M., Aleryani, S., & Woodworth, A. (2010). *Laboratory medicine: the diagnosis of disease in the clinical laboratory*, M. Weitz & R. Pancotti (Eds.). McGraw Hill.

Lazarus, J. H., Bestwick, J. P., Channon, S., Paradice, R., Maina, A., Rees, R., Chiusano, E., John, R., Guaraldo, V., George, L. M., Perona, M., Dall'Amico, D., Parkes, A. B., Joomun, M., & Wald, N. J. (2012). Antenatal thyroid screening and childhood cognitive function. *New England Journal of Medicine, 366*, 493–501.

Mayhew, C., Simonson, K., & Ellsworth Bowers, E. (2022). Antepartum care for pregnant people with overt hypothyroidism, subclinical hypothyroidism, and positive thyroid autoantibodies. *Journal of Midwifery & Women's Health, 67*(3), 295–303.

Neville, M. W. (2017). Thyroid disorders. In M. C. Brucker & T. L. King (Eds.), *Pharmacology for women's health* (2nd ed., pp. 529–547). Jones & Bartlett Learning.

Stagnaro-Green, A., Dong, A., & Stephenson, M. D. (2020). Universal screening for thyroid disease during pregnancy should be performed. *Best practice & research clinical endocrinology & metabolism, 34*(4), 1–21.

Ward, B. W. (2017). Barriers to health care for adults with multiple chronic conditions: United States, 2012–2015. *NCHS Data Brief, 275*, 1–8.

53

Neurological Disorders

Lise Hauser

Relevant Terms

Aura—sensory, motor, or visual changes that occur immediately preceding or at the onset of a migraine headache

Chronic migraine—ongoing pattern of migraine headaches occurring on 15 or more days per month for more than three months

Cluster headache—severe, unilateral headache with pattern of short duration and cluster periods of frequent headaches

Eclampsia—complication of pregnancy or early postpartum period characterized by hypertension, proteinuria, and seizures

Migraine—moderate to severe headache often with associated gastrointestinal or neurological symptoms, and may be accompanied by sensory disturbances called aura

Photophobia—sensitivity to light

Tension-type headache—usually described as achy, viselike, nonpulsatile headache of mild to moderate intensity; minimal or no associated gastrointestinal or neurological symptoms

---

Introduction

Some people have neurologic disorders that predate pregnancy, while others develop new-onset neurologic symptoms during pregnancy. The most commonly encountered neurological disorders in the pregnant client are seizure disorders, multiple sclerosis (MS), and headache. Thorough history taking and risk assessment at every visit may uncover previously unidentified incidents or symptoms that prove significant. Some preexisting neurologic conditions can be stable or have fewer relapses during pregnancy, such as migraine and MS. Preexisting hypertension can increase morbidity and mortality by increasing the risk of stroke, preeclampsia, and **eclampsia**, which can result in seizures. History of traumatic brain injury (TBI) and head and neck trauma in pregnancy is assessed during initial history, as physical trauma of any kind can increase the risk of headache. Some neurologic disorders can be managed independently, while others will require consultation, collaboration, or transfer of care to specialists. Significant

racial and ethnic inequalities exist in access to neurologic care. In the United States, Black individuals are 30% less likely and Hispanic individuals are 40% less likely to access outpatient neurologic care than their White counterparts (Saadi et al., 2017).

Health equity key points

- Significant racial and ethnic inequalities exist in access to neurologic care. Black and Hispanic individuals are less likely to access outpatient neurologic care than their White counterparts.
- Experience of migraines in pregnancy is significantly associated with exposure to violence.
- Racial and sexual minority status disparities exist in access to headache care as well as frequency of symptoms.

Seizure Disorders

It is estimated that more than 1 million people assigned female at birth have epilepsy and are of reproductive age in the United States (Mueller et al., 2022). Racial disparities exist in access to medical and surgical care for seizures as well as medication adherence and poor outcomes (Robbins et al., 2022). Epilepsy is a disease of the brain defined by at least two unprovoked seizures occurring more than 24 hours apart. Between 0.5% and 1.0% of all pregnancies occur among people with epilepsy, and epilepsy is the most commonly encountered major neurologic complication in pregnancy, as most people with epilepsy will have seizures with the same frequency in pregnancy as at baseline (Bollig & Jackson, 2018). Approximately one-third of pregnant people with epilepsy will have more frequent seizures, while up to approximately one-quarter will experience a decrease in seizures (Gerard & Samuels, 2019). The higher blood volume, nausea and vomiting, delayed gastric emptying, and increased hepatic metabolism of antiseizure medications (ASMs) during pregnancy are thought to play a significant role in increased seizure activity in some pregnant people. Some people abruptly stop taking ASMs when they discover they are pregnant, placing both themselves and the fetus at significant risk of seizure. Preconception counseling for clients with seizure disorders must include a discussion of risks associated with their current ASMs to a fetus and risks of abrupt cessation. The majority of pregnant people with a seizure disorder will have a normal pregnancy course. An interprofessional team approach including pregnancy care providers, neurologists, and pediatricians allows for optimal prenatal and postnatal care of clients with seizure disorders. The Epilepsy Foundation provides a list of older and newer terminology for seizure types and classification of epilepsies on their website (see *Resources for Clients and Their Families*).

Seizure types

Generalized onset—abnormal electrical activity originates simultaneously on both sides of the brain.
Focal onset—abnormal electrical activity originates on one side of the brain. May spread quickly to the other side of the brain.
Unknown onset—seizure onset cannot be localized.

Source: Adapted from Brodie et al. (2018).

Most seizures during pregnancy occur in clients with a preexisting seizure disorder. Other causes of seizures during pregnancy include eclampsia, acute fatty liver of pregnancy, trauma, infection, and amniotic fluid embolism. Signs and symptoms of preeclampsia are discussed in detail in Chapter 36, *Hypertensive Disorders in Pregnancy*. New onset of seizure activity in early pregnancy is suggestive of a seizure disorder, neoplasm, infection, or other acute process and mandates transfer of care to a physician. If the onset of seizure activity occurs during the third trimester of pregnancy, eclampsia is the most likely etiology, which necessitates emergent medical care. Any pregnant client with an active or uncontrolled seizure disorder should be referred to a physician for care during pregnancy.

An individual may present for prenatal care after taking ASMs for several years. They may have been declared seizure free and may have not been evaluated by a neurologist for some time. A pregnant client in this situation should be referred to a neurologist for the assessment of neurologic status and recommendations regarding appropriate ASM use. Ideally, a client with a seizure disorder will be evaluated by a neurologist before pregnancy. In addition to evaluating an individual's seizure activity and need for continued medication, the preconception period is an ideal time to change medications, to monitor the client's response to medications, and to teach the client to start taking folic acid to reduce the risk of neural tube defects. Some of the ASMs commonly used to manage seizure disorders in nonpregnant individuals are known to

Table 53.1 Risks of ASM-Induced Major Congenital Malformations

Medication	Risk
Valproate	9.3%
Phenobarbital	5.5%
Topiramate	4.2%
Carbamazepine	3%
Phenytoin	2.9%
Gabapentin	1.5%
Lamotrigine	2.1%
Levetiracetam	2%
Pregabalin	1.8%
Oxcarbazepine	1.6%

Inadequate data to accurately determine risk: Acetazolamide, Brivaracetam, Cannabidiol, Cenobamate, Clobazam, Clonazepam, Diazepam, Eslicarbazepine, Ethosuximide, Everolimus, Felbamate, Fenfluramine, Lacosamide, Lorazepam, Midazolam, Perampanel, Primidone, Rufinamide, Stiripentol, Sultiame, Tiagabine, Vigabatrin, Zonisamide.

Source: Meador & Schachter (2022)/With permission of Elsevier.

increase the risk of certain birth defects (Table 53.1). Because of the known risks of some ASMs, clients with seizure disorders should be advised to consult with their neurologist and pregnancy care provider for medication management before becoming pregnant. Additionally, it is well documented that sleep deprivation increases seizure activity; therefore, people with seizure disorders are advised to maintain a regular sleep pattern, which can be challenging in both the prenatal and postpartum periods. People with seizure disorders have an increased risk of complications during pregnancy, labor, and postpartum including preeclampsia, gestational diabetes, and preterm delivery. Their infants are more likely to be small for gestational age and require more intensive care unit (ICU) admissions (Mueller et al., 2022).

Medication Labeling in Pregnancy and Lactation

In 2015, the US Food and Drug Administration (FDA) removed the use of pregnancy categories A, B, C, D, and X from all human prescription drug labeling. Current labeling includes a general statement about medication use in pregnancy, a risk summary for the specific drug, and clinical considerations for providers to use when advising patients and prescribing in pregnancy, with subsections on lactation and use in people of reproductive potential. If there is a national pregnancy registry for the medication, FDA will include that information as well (Fantasia & Harris, 2015; Food and Drug Administration, HHS, 2014).

Antiseizure Medications during Pregnancy

Pertinent issues to address with pregnant clients who have seizure disorders include the use of ASMs and potential fetal risks, the need for genetic counseling and screening, and measures for seizure prevention (Bollig & Jackson, 2018). A pregnant person with a seizure disorder has a higher baseline risk of fetal malformations than someone without a seizure disorder, but this risk appears to be due to seizure medication exposure, rather than to the seizure disorder itself. Fetal anticonvulsant syndrome refers to the increased prevalence of major anomalies identified in children exposed to ASMs in utero. The use of some ASMs also increases the risk of neuropsychological impairments in offspring. Valproate has been shown to have the greatest detrimental effect on both physical development and cognitive ability of children exposed in utero (Meador, 2022; Tomson et al., 2019). Despite this known risk, the risk of an uncontrolled seizure disorder has the potential for even more deleterious effects on the fetus and the pregnant person.

ASMs decrease folic acid absorption, making increased folic acid supplementation imperative for prenatal clients with seizure disorders. Due to impaired folic acid absorption, evaluation for macrocytic anemia should be done preconceptionally, at the first visit, and at approximately 28 weeks of gestation. Folic acid deficiency has a well-documented association with fetal neural tube defect risk. The recommended dose for individuals at risk, including people taking ASMs, is 4 mg daily. This addition of folic acid may alter metabolism of ASMs, so it is imperative to monitor serum medication levels periodically in pregnancy. The general guideline for epilepsy therapy in people of childbearing age with the capacity for pregnancy is monotherapy at the minimum therapeutic dose to control seizures (Bollig & Jackson, 2018). Serial monitoring of ASM levels before, during, and after pregnancy may help guide appropriate dose adjustment (Gerard & Samuels, 2019). Medication levels can be monitored every trimester in clients with stable epilepsy, with more frequent evaluations in those experiencing prenatal seizure activity. Medication adjustments should be considered in prenatal clients with pregnancy-related nausea and vomiting that might adversely affect medication delivery, and it is recommended that until medication levels are stable, clients cease operation of motor vehicles due to risk of seizure. Antacids, commonly used to relieve pregnancy-related discomforts, can also interfere with absorption of ASMs. Additionally, the physiologic effects of pregnancy on serum medication concentrations vary considerably between individuals and are difficult to predict, making close ASM monitoring crucial. The North American Antiepileptic Drug Pregnancy Registry is the first hospital-based registry established to determine the safety of seizure medications during pregnancy and has enrolled over 13,500 pregnant people since 1997. The link to the Registry is provided in *Resources for Clients and Their Families*.

Clients with seizure disorders are offered early and comprehensive genetic counseling as well as screening for neural tube defects and fetal chromosomal anomalies. Ultrasound examination at 11–13 weeks for acrania and nuchal translucency can detect defects early. A comprehensive fetal ultrasound and fetal echocardiography for cardiac defects is offered at 18–22 weeks. Due to the risk of fetal growth abnormalities, fetal growth is monitored carefully.

Teaching points for pregnant people with seizure disorders

- Adequate sleep can reduce seizure risk.
- Some ASMs can increase the risk of birth defects.
- Know the benefits and risks of early genetic counseling and screening.
- Know the benefits and risks of fetal anatomy scan and fetal echocardiogram at 18–22 weeks of gestation.
- Folic acid 4.0 mg daily, ideally started preconceptionally or at pregnancy diagnosis, may prevent some birth defects.
- ASM levels will be monitored regularly.
- Antacids can decrease ASM absorption.
- A postpartum safety plan is important.
- Breastfeeding is not contraindicated with ASMs.
- Do not operate motor vehicles until medication levels are stable.

Anticipatory guidance for the pregnant client with a seizure disorder includes reassurance that vaginal birth is the safest option unless there are other complications requiring cesarean birth, and planning for safety while stable and effective medication levels are being achieved. ASMs are not a contraindication to breastfeeding (Birnbaum et al., 2020).

Postpartum clients with epilepsy need to plan for medication and seizure management in the postpartum period, in addition to the myriad challenges a new baby can bring, including sleep deprivation, hormonal shifts, and irregular hours. The ASM dose should be tapered to prepregnancy levels over the first three weeks after delivery (Bollig & Jackson, 2018). Clients are also advised that many ASMs can decrease the effectiveness of hormonal contraception; copper intrauterine devices, barrier methods, or tubal sterilization may be preferred.

Safety precautions for people with seizure disorders

- Potentially hazardous activities (e.g., ironing, cooking, or operating heavy machinery) are avoided unless another adult is present.
- Consider meal options that do not require use of the stove.
- Do not carry the baby unless another adult is present. A small folding stroller frame that carries a car seat maneuvers easily through the home.
- Bathe the baby in a tub only if another person is present and watching. Sponge baths on the floor with a separate container of water are safer.
- Perform other infant care activities (e.g., dressing and diaper changes) on the floor to decrease the risk of falls during a seizure.

A commonly asked question is whether the infant will be at an increased risk for epilepsy. Acquired seizure disorders from causes such as infection, stroke, or trauma have a lower risk of being passed on to children, as do epilepsies with later onset. But early onset seizure disorders, epilepsies associated with intellectual disabilities, and those also found in the gestational parent's first-degree relatives are more likely to be inherited. Children are more likely to inherit epilepsy from the gestational parent rather than the partner or sperm donor. The risk of passing on epilepsy is approximately 8% if the pregnant person has generalized epilepsy and 4% if they have focal epilepsy (Gerard & Samuels, 2019).

Headache

A commonly reported concern during pregnancy, especially in the first and third trimesters, is headache. Significant disparities along racial lines exist in access to headache care as well as frequency of symptoms (Robbins et al., 2022), and people with sexual minority status also experience disparities in headache symptoms, in part due to greater stress levels (Heslin, 2020). The diagnosis of headache begins with a thorough history including chronologic description of headache (frequency and duration), location and character of the pain, concurrent symptoms such as nausea, vomiting, **photophobia** and phonophobia, and any precipitating and exacerbating events. The etiology of headaches during pregnancy includes hormonal changes, an increase in blood volume, hypoglycemic episodes, tension, postural changes and related muscle strain, and preeclampsia. Headaches may also be due to trauma from accidents, assault, or intimate partner violence (IPV) during any trimester (Robbins, 2021).

Headaches are divided into two major classifications: primary and secondary. Primary headaches are disorders caused by independent mechanisms and are divided into subcategories: migraine, **tension type**, trigeminal autonomic cephalalgias, and other. Secondary headaches develop as a secondary manifestation of another problem such as trauma, infection, substance use or withdrawal, disorders of cranial, cervical or facial structures, intracranial vascular or nonvascular disorder, or psychiatric disorder (International Headache Society, 2018). Determination of headache type is the initial step in the evaluation and treatment of headaches. Self-reporting via a headache diary (Table 53.2) over the course of at least one week is useful.

Primary Headaches: Tension Type

Tension-type headaches are the most commonly reported type of headache in both pregnant and nonpregnant individuals. Tension-type headaches are generally mild to moderate in intensity, are usually perceived bilaterally, and have minimal or no associated symptoms such as nausea, visual disturbances, or photophobia. Tension-type headaches can further be categorized based on frequency (Table 53.3).

The frequency, duration, and the presence and severity of associated signs and symptoms influence the treatment plan for tension headaches. In most instances, tension-type headaches are relieved by conservative interventions such as massage, heat or ice, and oral acetaminophen. In cases where these measures do not provide adequate relief, the episodic use of opioids or acetaminophen with opioids can be considered if symptoms are severe and

Table 53.2 Items to Include in a Headache Diary

Date
Time of onset
Location of pain
Pain rating (1–10)
How long did the pain last?
Any aura or warning? Describe if present.
Describe pain (stabbing, aching, dull, sharp, pressure, etc.)
Other symptoms (nausea, sensitivity to light, etc.)
Foods and drinks before onset
Activity before and at onset
Amount of sleep last night
Stress/mood before onset
Treatments (ice, heat, medication, massage, bath, etc.)
Effectiveness of treatment(s) above
Other notes

unresponsive to more conservative treatment. Chronic tension-type headaches may be managed prophylactically in collaboration with a consulting physician specialist.

Migraines

Migraines are the third most prevalent disorder in the world and are more commonly experienced by people assigned female at birth than people assigned male, likely due to hormonal fluctuations. They account for approximately 90% of headache-related visits during pregnancy (Saldanha et al., 2021). Migraines in pregnancy have been shown to be significantly associated with a history of childhood abuse as well as current or past IPV (Gelaye et al., 2016). Migraine headaches can be divided into the subcategories of migraine with and without **aura**. Migraine with aura is preceded by transient neurologic symptoms. Some experience visual auras such as blind spots, flashes of light, zigzag lines, or temporary vision loss in one eye. Aphasia and unilateral numbness or weakness are not uncommon. Any neurologic symptom that consistently precedes a migraine headache is considered an aura. Most people find that they have a decrease in frequency and intensity of migraine headaches during pregnancy, with the most significant reduction during the second and third trimesters. Migraines may be episodic or chronic. **Chronic migraine** is characterized by ≥15 days per month with headache lasting 4 hours or longer per day. Both migraine and pregnancy are hypercoagulable conditions, increasing the risk of venous thromboembolism, stroke, and preeclampsia for prenatal clients with migraine. Those who experience worsening of migraine in pregnancy are at 13-fold higher risk of developing hypertensive disorders in pregnancy than those in whom migraine improved (Allais et al., 2019). A minority of pregnant clients will have their first migraine during pregnancy, and this is most likely to occur during the first trimester.

Table 53.3   International Headache Society Criteria for Tension Headaches

Classification	Frequency	Duration	Characteristics
Infrequent episodic tension type	• 10–12 episodes per year • <1 episode each month	30 minutes to 7 days	At least two of the following: • Bilateral location • Pressing/tightening (nonpulsating) quality • Mild/moderate intensity • Not aggravated by routine physical activity Both of the following: • No nausea or vomiting • Not attributed to another disorder Only one of the following: • Photophobia • Phonophobia
Frequent episodic tension type	• ≥10 episodes per month occurring on 1–14 days/month • Occurs for at least 3 months	30 minutes to 7 days	Same as above
Chronic tension type	• ≥15 days/month • Occurs for at least 3 months	• 30 minutes to 7 days or • Lasting hours or continuous	Same as above with the following additions: Only one of the following: • Photophobia • Phonophobia • Mild nausea

Source: Adapted from International Headache Society (2018).

Secondary Headaches: Trauma

Head trauma and TBI can occur due to IPV, accidents at home, due to sports, car or bicycle accidents, or from non-partner violence. It is estimated that 69 million people worldwide suffer TBI every year (Dewan et al., 2019). TBI is underreported to the point of being considered a "silent epidemic," due to the wide range of severity which includes very mild cases (Iaccarino et al., 2021). The client themself may not consider their injury significant until questioned by a healthcare professional. More than one in three cisgender women have experienced physical and/or sexual IPV or stalking in their lifetime (Chen et al., 2020), and the incidence is higher for transgender men (Valentine et al., 2017). Screening and ongoing risk assessment must include questions about history of trauma and violence. See Chapter 26, *Violence and Trauma in the Perinatal Period*, for detailed information on IPV. One of the strongest predictors of violence in pregnancy is a history of prepregnancy violence. It is essential to assess for other signs and symptoms of preeclampsia in any client reporting a headache in the third trimester of pregnancy (refer to Chapter 36, *Hypertensive Disorders in Pregnancy*). For clients whose headache does not have a clear etiology, completion of a headache diary (Table 53.2) can provide information on headache triggers, severity, and the impact on daily life.

Nonpharmacological Headache Management

For all headache types, nonpharmacological measures should be the first choice for pregnant clients (Table 53.4).

Ideally, nutraceutical supplementation will begin at least three months prior to conception to provide maximum effect (Parikh, 2018). Herbal supplements feverfew and butterbur have possible benefits for migraine relief but should be avoided in pregnancy. Feverfew can cause uterine contractions and butterbur can cause congenital malformations (Holdridge et al., 2022).

Lifestyle changes that support better overall health are encouraged. Maintaining regular and adequate sleep patterns will help many headache sufferers. Smoking cessation and regular exercise can also contribute to better headache control. A consistent daily routine for eating, activity, and sleeping may also be beneficial in headache prevention. Dietary modification such as not skipping meals and avoidance or minimal use of foods and beverages that can trigger headaches is often all that is needed to reduce headache frequency and intensity in pregnancy. Massage, yoga, and physical therapy can also be effective for headache relief and prevention. Prescription eyeglasses to reduce digital eye strain and taking regular breaks from working on a screen may help.

Common headache triggers

- Inadequate or excessive sleep
- Bright or flickering light
- Smoke
- Change in caffeine intake
- Stress
- Hormonal fluctuations
- Barometric pressure changes
- Digital eye strain
- Sensory overload (lights, odors, or noise)
- Very cold foods/drinks
- Foods containing histamine, monosodium glutamate (MSG), chocolate, or tyramine (examples: aged cheeses, canned or processed meats, olives, pickles)

Table 53.4 Nonpharmacological Treatment of Headaches

Treatment recommendation	Rationale	Evidence
Mind–body medicine • biofeedback • relaxation • cognitive behavioral therapy	Safe in pregnancy due to noninvasive nature	Mind–body medicine interventions have been shown to reduce headache-related disability (Seng et al., 2019)
Acupuncture	Anti-inflammatory action via neuropeptides Analgesic effects via endogenous opioid system (Zhang et al., 2020)	A systematic review of seven clinical trials compared the efficacy of acupuncture versus conventional migraine preventive treatment and found that acupuncture is just as effective and has fewer side effects than standard medications currently used (Zhang et al., 2020)
Physical therapy, massage, transcutaneous nerve stimulation (TENS), hot and cold packs, yoga	Decreasing muscle tension may decrease headache pain	Studies of yoga and physical therapy in addition to pharmacologic treatment found significant improvement in quality of life and headache frequency with minimal risk (Mehta et al., 2021)
Oxygen therapy—inhalation of normobaric oxygen through face mask	Increasing oxygen to constricted vessels will decrease pain	Weak evidence for migraine, moderately effective for cluster headache (Mo et al., 2022)
Nutraceutical supplements • Magnesium • Coenzyme Q10 • Vitamin D • Riboflavin (vitamin B2)	Oral magnesium 600 mg daily may reduce migraine frequency CoQ10 100 mg tid is anti-inflammatory Vitamin D 1,000–2,000 IU daily may modulate CGRP levels Riboflavin 400 mg has been shown to improve cellular energy metabolism, addressing one proposed mechanism of migraine exacerbation	Magnesium supplementation has a positive effect in treating migraine and enhances the effect of antimigraine medications (Domitrz & Cegielska, 2022) CoQ10 is safe in pregnancy and has been shown to reduce the risk of preeclampsia (Parikh, 2018; Teran et al., 2009) Vitamin D supplementation was shown to reduce serum levels of CGRP, known to be a significant factor in migraine pain (Ghorbani et al., 2020). Vitamin D supplementation between 1000 and 2000 IU per day is safe in pregnancy (ACOG, 2011) Riboflavin was shown to be more efficacious than placebo in preventing migraine (Parikh, 2018)

Pharmacologic Treatment of Migraine Headaches

Pharmacologic treatment of migraine includes both preventive and abortive or "rescue" medications. Consistent use of preventive treatment may reduce both the need for abortive treatment and the risk of medication overuse syndrome. Pregnant people with a history of migraine headaches should be encouraged to initiate treatment with the first onset of symptoms, when it is more likely to be effective. First-line pharmacologic treatment of migraine in pregnancy consists of analgesics such as acetaminophen and nonsteroidal anti-inflammatory drugs (NSAIDs). NSAIDs should be avoided in the first and third trimesters of pregnancy, as they have been shown to increase the risk of miscarriage in the first trimester, premature closure of the ductus arteriosus, fetal oligohydramnios in the third trimester, and increased risk for maternal bleeding and neonatal intracranial hemorrhage (Black et al., 2019; Ying et al., 2022). If the short-term use of acetaminophen is ineffective or if the headache is severe, antiemetics and opioid pain relief can be effective. Ongoing use of opioid-containing agents is avoided particularly during the third trimester due to the possibility of neonatal withdrawal syndrome. Ergot

alkaloids are contraindicated during pregnancy because of their association with fetal birth defects, uterine contractions, and hypertension.

Pregnant patients who do not respond adequately to commonly used medications and lifestyle changes are referred to a neurologist or other specialist for further evaluation and treatment. Triptans are widely used as an abortive treatment for migraine headache outside of pregnancy. Case-control and cohort studies show that the use of triptans during pregnancy does not appear to increase the rates for major congenital malformations or prematurity (Burch, 2020; Marchenko et al., 2015). Gepants are a class of migraine medication first approved by the FDA in nonpregnant people in 2018 to block calcitonin gene-related peptide (CGRP) or its receptor. The clinical efficacy of the second generation of gepants is similar to that of triptans. While animal studies and limited case reports of gepant use in pregnancy demonstrate no adverse effects on offspring, further studies are needed to assess their safety in pregnant individuals (Vig et al., 2022).

OnabotulinumtoxinA (Botox®, Allergan Inc.) was approved by the FDA in 2010 for prophylaxis of headaches in nonpregnant adult patients with **chronic migraine**. Botox has been used in the United States since 1989 for the treatment of strabismus, dystonias, and primary axillary hyperhidrosis as well as for cosmetic purposes. No adequate and well-controlled studies have been conducted using Botox in pregnancy, but retrospective reviews and case reports indicate that the incidence of fetal defects in Botox-exposed pregnancies was comparable with those expected in the general population. Data from a prospective study of 45 patients over nine years who became pregnant while receiving Botox for prevention of chronic migraine found no impact of the toxin on pregnancy outcomes (Brin et al., 2016; Wong et al., 2020). A client with migraine must weigh risks and benefits in consultation with their prenatal care provider and neurologist of continuing to receive Botox every three months through pregnancy to treat chronic migraines as compared to potential pain, depression and loss of function in daily life caused by return of debilitating migraines.

Postpartum Headaches

Postpartum headaches are very common and occur in approximately 30–40% of those in the first six weeks after delivery (Vgontzas & Robbins, 2018). Headaches in the early postpartum period must first be evaluated for the possibility of preeclampsia. If there is no indication of preeclampsia, anesthesia complications are the next diagnosis to consider, if the client had epidural pain management in the intrapartum period. If these causes are ruled out, primary headache management principles are undertaken. Nonpharmacological measures should be the primary intervention with the addition of medications as needed using acetaminophen and ibuprofen as an initial mediation choice. Safety during breastfeeding must be considered; both acetaminophen and ibuprofen are safe in breastfeeding as amounts in milk are much less than doses usually given to infants (Drugs and Lactation Database [LactMed], 2022).

Cluster Headaches

Cluster headaches are very severe and most often unilateral in nature. Patterns of cluster headaches range from short-duration headaches that occur frequently over several weeks or months followed by long headache-free periods to a more chronic pattern of daily or almost daily headaches. Cluster headaches are often associated with symptoms such as excessive tearing on the affected side and nasal stuffiness. The pregnant client with cluster headaches should be referred to a neurologist or other healthcare provider who specializes in the treatment of cluster headaches.

Multiple Sclerosis

MS is a chronic inflammatory disease of the central nervous system that occurs most frequently in people assigned female at birth due to hormonal differences linked to sex

chromosomes (Ysrraelit & Correale, 2019). It is the most common neurological disorder not caused by injury among young adults. MS causes demyelination of central nervous system myelin sheaths, which leads to neurologic symptoms such as muscle weakness, fatigue, paresthesias, and changes in vision and cognition. Diagnosis of MS is based on neurological signs and symptoms and magnetic resonance imaging (MRI) showing areas of demyelination of the central nervous system (McNicholas et al., 2018).

Preconception care should include discussions about the impact of pregnancy on the course of MS as well as the effect of MS on pregnancy, treatment options, and possible effects on the fetus. An exacerbation of MS, known as a relapse, is the occurrence of new symptoms or the worsening of old symptoms due to inflammation in the central nervous system. MS relapse rates tend to decrease during pregnancy, and recent data suggest that there may be less postpartum rebound disease activity than previously thought, due to the effect of disease-modifying treatments (Langer-Gould et al., 2020) The 1998 Pregnancy in Multiple Sclerosis (PRIMS) study found that MS does not affect the rate of miscarriage, ectopic pregnancy, stillbirth, or congenital birth defects, which has been confirmed by subsequent similar investigations (Vukusic et al., 2021). Heritability of MS is related to genetic factors responsible for immune response. The risk of passing the disease to offspring is 2–2.5% (Varytė et al., 2020). Many disease-modifying medications are contraindicated in pregnancy. If treatment is clinically necessary, interferon beta and glatiramer acetate are considered to be safe in pregnancy and lactation (Varytė et al., 2021).

The care of a pregnant client with MS can follow a normal course. A multidisciplinary team including high-risk obstetric and neurologic providers can be integrated into the care team as indicated. Prenatal care follows the usual guidelines with the added component of treatment aimed at providing symptomatic relief as needed. Pelvic floor physical therapy to optimize bladder and bowel function, and walking, water exercise, and yoga as tolerated may help with pain, balance, and spasticity (Krysko et al., 2021). Spinal and epidural anesthesia for labor and delivery are considered safe for gravidas with MS (Vukusic et al., 2021).

A unique focus of prenatal care for the pregnant person with MS is directed at teaching and preparing the client to function as a new parent while coping with treatment and management of MS symptoms. Discussions regarding the challenges that they face as a person with MS can lead to discussions about functioning as a new parent with MS. Identification of resources and support systems is encouraged.

Restless Legs Syndrome/Willis-Ekbom Disease

Restless legs syndrome (RLS), also called Willis-Ekbom disease (WED), affects up to one-third of pregnant people. Individuals report a sensation of pins and needles, an intense need to move their lower legs, and a burning or jittery feeling. The sensations occur primarily, but not exclusively, at night, and are temporarily relieved by movement. Symptoms can become very severe during pregnancy and interfere significantly with sleep. Clients are more likely to suffer from RLS in pregnancy if they experienced it prepregnancy, do not exercise regularly, have a family history of RLS, or have lower preconception folate and ferritin levels (Darvishi et al., 2020). Differential diagnosis includes leg cramps, venous stasis, and leg edema; see Chapter 15, *Common Discomforts of Pregnancy*, for additional information on diagnosis and comfort measures.

Carpal Tunnel Syndrome

Carpal tunnel syndrome (CTS) occurs in pregnancy when the median nerve at the transverse carpal ligament is compressed by increasing blood volume, weight gain, and generalized edema. Estimates of the prevalence and incidence of CTS vary widely in the general population and among pregnant people. It is the costliest upper-extremity musculoskeletal disorder in the United States in terms of loss of productivity and medical interventions. Clinical diagnosis of CTS is based on pain or paresthesia in the distribution of the median nerve (Genova et al., 2020). Treatment in pregnancy is generally limited to splinting of the affected wrist(s) at night and modification of activity such as keyboard use as possible. See Chapter 15, *Common Discomforts of Pregnancy*, for additional information on diagnosis and comfort measures.

Central Nervous System Imaging in Pregnancy and Lactation

Imaging can be an important component of diagnosis and treatment of neurological disorders. The American College of Obstetricians and Gynecologists (ACOG) guidelines for diagnostic imaging during pregnancy and lactation state that ultrasonography and MRI are not associated with known risk to the fetus or pregnant client and breastfeeding is not contraindicated after MRI or computed tomography (CT) scans with contrast (Barnes et al., 2022; Jain, 2019). If X-rays, CT scans, or other nuclear imaging studies are deemed medically necessary in pregnancy, the radiation exposure should be at a low dose to avoid fetal harm.

Summary

The most commonly encountered neurological disorders in the pregnant person are seizure disorders, headache, and MS. The pregnant person with a seizure disorder or MS can, in some instances, be managed in collaboration with a physician specialist or may require referral depending on the stability of the disorder and the time of the initial diagnosis. Headaches that occur during pregnancy are often managed independently with specialty consultation as indicated by symptoms and severity. Providers of perinatal care must maintain a current understanding of neurologic conditions and their treatments, both pharmacologic and nonpharmacologic through continuing education and professional collaboration.

Resources for Clients and Their Families

What is Epilepsy? https://www.epilepsy.com/what-is-epilepsy

Risks During Pregnancy Due to Epilepsy https://www.epilepsy.com/lifestyle/family-planning/pregnancy-risks

North American Antiepileptic Drug (NAAED) Pregnancy Registry https://www.aedpregnancyregistry.org

Common Discomforts of Pregnancy (includes headaches) http://www.marchofdimes.org/pregnancy/common-discomforts-of-pregnancy.aspx

American Migraine Foundation https://americanmigrainefoundation.org

Preconception and Prenatal Genetic Screening http://www.marchofdimes.org/professionals/pocket-facts-preconception-and-prenatal-genetic-screening.aspx

Multiple Sclerosis and Pregnancy: www.marchofdimes.org/complications/multiple-sclerosis-and-pregnancy.aspx

References

Allais, G., Chiarle, G., Sinigaglia, S., Mana, O., & Benedetto, C. (2019). Migraine during pregnancy and in the puerperium. *Neurological Sciences, 40*(S1), 81–91.

American College of Obstetricians and Gynecologists (ACOG). (2011, reaffirmed 2021). Vitamin D: Screening and supplementation during pregnancy. *Obstetrics and Gynecology, 118*(1), 197–198.

Barnes, S., Bennett, S., & Datta, S. (2022). Breastfeeding: Debunking preconceptions and removing barriers. *Obstetrics, Gynaecology & Reproductive Medicine, 32*(8), 188–192.

Birnbaum, A. K., Meador, K. J., Karanam, A., Brown, C., May, R. C., Gerard, E. E., Gedzelman, E. R., Penovich, P. E., Kalayjian, L. A., Cavitt, J., Pack, A. M., Miller, J. W., Stowe, Z. N., & Pennell, P. B. (2020). Antiepileptic drug exposure in infants of breastfeeding mothers with epilepsy. *JAMA Neurology, 77*(4), 441–450.

Black, E., Khor, K. E., Kennedy, D., Chutatape, A., Sharma, S., Vancaillie, T., & Demirkol, A. (2019). Medication use and pain management in pregnancy: A critical review. *Pain Practice, 19*(8), 875–899.

Bollig, K. J., & Jackson, D. L. (2018). Seizures in pregnancy. *Obstetrics and Gynecology Clinics of North America, 45*(2), 349–367.

Brin, M. F., Kirby, R. S., Slavotinek, A., Miller-Messana, M. A., Parker, L., Yushmanova, I., & Yang, H. (2016). Pregnancy outcomes following exposure to onabotulinumtoxin A. *Pharmacoepidemiology & Drug Safety, 25*(2), 179–187.

Brodie, M. J., Zuberi, S. M., Scheffer, I. E., & Fisher, R. S. (2018). The 2017 ILAE classification of seizure types and the epilepsies: What do people with epilepsy and their caregivers need to know? *Epileptic Disorders, 20*(2), 77–87.

Burch, R. (2020). Epidemiology and treatment of menstrual migraine and migraine during pregnancy and lactation: A narrative review. *Headache, 60*(1), 200–216.

Chen, J., Walters, M. L., Gilbert, L. K., & Patel, N. (2020). Sexual violence, stalking, and intimate partner violence by sexual orientation, United States. *Psychology of Violence, 10*(1), 110–119.

Darvishi, N., Daneshkhah, A., Khaledi-Paveh, B., Vaisi-Raygani, A., Mohammadi, M., Salari, N., Darvishi, F., Abdi, A., & Jalali, R. (2020). The prevalence of restless legs syndrome/Willis-Ekbom disease (RLS/WED) in the third trimester of pregnancy: A systematic review. *BMC Neurology*, *20*(1), 1–7.

Dewan, M. C., Rattani, A., Gupta, S., Baticulon, R. E., Hung, Y.-C., Punchak, M., Agrawal, A., Adeleye, A. O., Shrime, M. G., Rubiano, A. M., Rosenfeld, J. V., & Park, K. B. (2019). Estimating the global incidence of traumatic brain injury. *Journal of Neurosurgery*, *130*(4), 1080–1097.

Domitrz, I., & Cegielska, J. (2022). Magnesium as an important factor in the pathogenesis and treatment of migraine - from theory to practice. *Nutrients*, *14*(5), 1089. https://doi.org/10.3390/nu14051089

Drugs and Lactation Database (LactMed). (2022). National Library of Medicine. https://www.ncbi.nlm.nih.gov/books/NBK501922

Fantasia, H. C., & Harris, A. L. (2015). Changes to pregnancy and lactation risk labeling for prescription drugs. *Nursing for Women's Health*, *19*(3), 266–270.

Food and Drug Administration, HHS. (2014). Content and format of labeling for human prescription drug and biological products; requirements for pregnancy and lactation labeling. Final rule. *Federal Register*, *233*(79), 72063–72103.

Gelaye, B., Do, N., Avila, S., Carlos Velez, J., Zhong, Q.-Y., Sanchez, S. E., Lee Peterlin, B., & Williams, M. A. (2016). Childhood abuse, intimate partner violence and risk of migraine among pregnant women: An epidemiologic study. *Headache*, *56*(6), 976–986. https://doi.org/10.1111/head.12855

Genova, A., Dix, O., Saefan, A., Thakur, M., & Hassan, A. (2020). Carpal tunnel syndrome: A review of literature. *Cureus*, *12*(3), e7333.

Gerard, E. E., & Samuels, P. (2019). Neurologic disorders in pregnancy. In M. B. Landon, D. A. Driscoll, E. R. M. Jauniaux, H. L. Galan, W. A. Grobman, & V. Berghella (Eds.), *Gabbe's obstetrics essentials: Normal & problem pregnancies e-book* (7th ed., pp. 355–362). Elsevier.

Ghorbani, Z., Rafiee, P., Fotouhi, A., Haghighi, S., Magham, R. R., Ahmadi, Z. S., Djalali, M., Zareei, M., Jahromi, S. R., Shahemi, S., Mahmoudi, M., & Togha, M. (2020). The effects of vitamin D supplementation on interictal serum levels of calcitonin gene-related peptide (CGRP) in episodic migraine patients: Post hoc analysis of a randomized double-blind placebo-controlled trial. *Journal of Headache Pain*, *21*(1). https://doi.org/10.1186/s10194-020-01090-w

Heslin, K. (2020). Explaining disparities in severe headache and migraine among sexual minority adults in the United States, 2013–2018. *The Journal of Nervous and Mental Disease*, *208*(11), 876–883. https://doi.org/10.1097/NMD.0000000000001221

Holdridge, A., Donnelly, M., & Kuruvilla, D. E. (2022). Integrative, interventional, and non-invasive approaches for the treatment for migraine during pregnancy. *Current Pain and Headache Reports*, *26*, 323–330.

Iaccarino, C., Gerosa, A., & Viaroli, E. (2021). Epidemiology of traumatic brain injury. In S. Honeybul & A. G. Kolias (Eds.), *Traumatic brain injury: Science, practice, evidence and ethics* (pp. 3–11). Springer.

International Headache Society. (2018). Headache classification Committee of the International Headache Society (IHS) the international classification of headache disorders, 3rd ed. *Cephalalgia*, *38*(1), 1–211.

Jain, C. (2019). ACOG Committee opinion no. 723: Guidelines for diagnostic imaging during pregnancy and lactation. *Obstetrics & Gynecology*, *133*(1), 186.

Krysko, K. M., Bove, R., Dobson, R., Jokubaitis, V., & Hellwig, K. (2021). Treatment of women with multiple sclerosis planning pregnancy. *Current Treatment Options in Neurology*, *23*(4), 1–19.

Langer-Gould, A., Smith, J. G., Albers, K. B., Xiang, A. H., Wu, J., Kerezsi, E. H., McClearnen, K., Gonzales, E. G., Leimpeter, A. D., & Van Den Eeden, S. K. (2020). Pregnancy-related relapses and breastfeeding in a contemporary multiple sclerosis cohort. *Neurology*, *94*(18), e1939–e1949.

Marchenko, A., Etwel, F., Olutunfese, O., Nickel, C., Koren, G., & Nulman, I. (2015). Pregnancy outcome following prenatal exposure to triptan medications: A meta-analysis. *Headache*, *55*(10), 490–501.

McNicholas, N., Hutchinson, M., McGuigan, C., & Chataway, J. (2018). 2017 McDonald diagnostic criteria: A review of the evidence. *Multiple Sclerosis and Related Disorders*, *24*, 48–54.

Meador, K. J. (2022). Effects of maternal use of antiseizure medications on child development. *Neurologic Clinics*, *40*(4), 755–768.

Meador, K. J., & Schachter, S. C. (2022). *Risks during pregnancy with epilepsy*. Epilepsy Foundation. https://www.epilepsy.com/lifestyle/family-planning/pregnancy-risks

Mehta, J. N., Parikh, S., Desai, S. D., Solanki, R. C., & Pathak, A. G. (2021). Study of additive effect of yoga and physical therapies to standard pharmacologic treatment in migraine. *Journal of Neurosciences in Rural Practice*, *12*(1), 60–66.

Mo, H., Chung, S. J., Rozen, T. D., & Cho, S.-J. (2022). Oxygen therapy in cluster headache, migraine, and other headache disorders. *Journal of Clinical Neurology*, *18*(3), 271–279.

Mueller, B. A., Cheng-Hakimian, A., Crane, D. A., Doody, D. R., Schiff, M. A., & Hawes, S. E. (2022). Morbidity and rehospitalization postpartum among women with epilepsy and their infants: A population-based study. *Epilepsy & Behavior*, *136*, 108943.

Parikh, S. K. (2018). Unique populations with episodic migraine: Pregnant and lactating women. *Current Pain and Headache Reports*, *22*(20), 80. https://doi.org/10.1007/s11916-018-0737-x

Robbins, M. S. (2021). Diagnosis and Management of Headache. *JAMA*, *325*(18), 1874–1885.

Robbins, N., Charleston, L., Saadi, A., Thayer, Z., Codrington, W., Landry, A., Bernat, J., & Hamilton, R. (2022). Black patients matter in neurology. *Neurology*, *99*(3), 106–114. https://doi.org/10.1212/WNL.0000000000200830

Saadi, A., Himmelstein, D. U., Woolhandler, S., & Mejia, N. I. (2017). Racial disparities in neurologic health care access and utilization in the United States. *Neurology*, *88*(24), 2268–2275.

Saldanha, I. J., Cao, W., Bhuma, M. R., Konnyu, K. J., Adam, G. P., Mehta, S., Zullo, A. R., Chen, K. K., Roth, J. L., & Balk, E. M. (2021). Management of primary headaches during pregnancy, postpartum, and breastfeeding: A systematic review. *Headache*, *61*(1), 11–43.

Seng, E. K., Singer, A. B., Metts, C., Grinberg, A. S., Patel, Z. S., Marzouk, M., Rosenberg, L., Day, M., Minen, M. T., Lipton, R. B., & Buse, D. C. (2019). Does mindfulness-based cognitive therapy for migraine reduce migraine-related disability in people with episodic and chronic migraine? A phase 2b pilot randomized clinical trial. *Headache*, *59*(9), 1448–1467.

Teran, E., Hernandez, I., Nieto, B., Tavara, R., Ocampo, J. E., & Calle, A. (2009). Coenzyme Q10 supplementation during pregnancy reduces the risk of pre-eclampsia. *International Journal of Gynecology & Obstetrics*, *105*(1), 43–45.

Tomson, T., Battino, D., Bromley, R., Kochen, S., Meador, K., Pennell, P., & Thomas, S. V. (2019). Management of epilepsy in pregnancy: A report from the international league against epilepsy task force on women and pregnancy. *Epileptic Disorders*, *21*(6), 497–517.

Valentine, S. E., Peitzmeier, S. M., King, D. S., O'Cleirigh, C., Marquez, S. M., Presley, C., & Potter, J. (2017). Disparities in exposure to intimate partner violence among transgender/gender nonconforming and sexual minority primary care patients. *LGBT Health*, *4*(4), 260–267.

Varytė, G., Arlauskienė, A., & Ramašauskaitė, D. (2021). Pregnancy and multiple sclerosis: An update. *Current Opinion in Obstetrics & Gynecology*, *33*(5), 378–383.

Varytė, G., Zakarevičienė, J., Ramašauskaitė, D., Laužikienė, D., & Arlauskienė, A. (2020). Pregnancy and multiple sclerosis: An update on the disease modifying treatment strategy and a review of pregnancy's impact on disease activity. *Medicina*, *56*(2), 49.

Vgontzas, A., & Robbins, M. S. (2018). A hospital based retrospective study of acute postpartum headache. *Headache: The Journal of Head and Face Pain*, *58*(6), 845–851.

Vig, S. J., Garza, J., & Tao, Y. (2022). The use of erenumab for migraine prophylaxis during pregnancy: A case report and narrative review. *Headache: The Journal of Head and Face Pain*.

Vukusic, S., Michel, L., Leguy, S., & Lebrun-Frenay, C. (2021). Pregnancy with multiple sclerosis. *Revue Neurologique, 177*(3), 180–194.

Wong, H.-T., Khalil, M., & Ahmed, F. (2020). OnabotulinumtoxinA for chronic migraine during pregnancy: A real world experience on 45 patients. *The Journal of Headache and Pain, 21*(129).

Ying, X., Bao, D., Jiang, H., & Shi, Y. (2022). Maternal non-steroidal anti-inflammatory drug exposure during pregnancy and risk of miscarriage: A systematic review and meta-analysis. *European Journal of Clinical Pharmacology, 78*, 171–180.

Ysrraelit, M. C., & Correale, J. (2019). Impact of sex hormones on immune function and multiple sclerosis development. *Immunology, 156*(1), 9–22.

Zhang, N., Houle, T., Hindiyeh, N., & Aurora, S. K. (2020). Systematic review: Acupuncture vs standard pharmacological therapy for migraine prevention. *Headache, 60*(2), 309–317.

54

Dermatologic Disorders

Nell L. Tharpe

Relevant Terms

Atopic—refers to a form of allergy in which a hypersensitivity reaction such as dermatitis or asthma can occur in parts of the body not in contact with an allergen

Direct immunofluorescence—a form of laboratory testing on tissue biopsy samples used to diagnose diseases of the skin

Drug eruption—an adverse reaction of the skin to a medication; typically mild and disappears when the drug is withdrawn

Dyskeratosis—abnormal keratinization of the nails or skin

Eczema—a group of conditions resulting from genetic and environmental factors that manifest as rough, inflamed, itchy patches of skin

Extrinsic dermatitis—allergic dermatitis, characterized by allergen specific IgE, associated with asthma or food allergies

Herpetiform—resembling herpes: raised, red blisters or macules that crust to form a papule or pustule

Intrinsic dermatitis—nonallergic dermatitis, typically occurs later in life; no association with allergies or other atopic diseases

Iris or target lesions—a series of concentric rings with a dark or blistered center

Lichenification—skin that is thick or leathery

Papule or Papula—circumscribed, solid elevation of skin that does not contain pus

Plaque—broad papule or confluence of papules

Polymorphic—the ability to have more than one shape or form of a phenotype

Psoriasis—a range of inflammatory skin disorders resulting from adaptive or autoimmune responses and characterized by red, itchy, scaly areas of skin

Prurigo—the presence of intensely itchy skin lesions

Pruritic—itching quality, an unpleasant sensation of the skin that provokes the urge to scratch

Spongiosis—edema of the epidermis

Urticaria—red, raised skin rash, commonly known as hives

Vellus hair—short, slight-colored, and barely noticeable thin hair

Introduction

Characteristic skin changes often occur during pregnancy and the immediate postpartum period as a result of the significant metabolic, endocrine, and immunological changes that occur (see Chapter 5, *Physiologic Alterations during Pregnancy*, and Chapter 6, *Physiologic Alterations during the Postnatal Period*). While these physiologic skin changes are benign in nature, there are pregnancy-specific dermatoses that have the potential for adverse outcomes for the pregnant person and fetus.

The severity of preexisting dermatologic conditions can also be altered by the client's pregnant state. Conditions such as acne, **psoriasis**, and **eczema**, and cutaneous manifestations associated with allergic, autoimmune, and other health conditions such as systemic lupus erythematosus can be affected by pregnancy. Many infectious diseases commonly manifest with dermatologic lesions, necessitating that they be included in the differential diagnosis. These conditions are covered in Chapter 55, *Infectious Diseases*. All of these possibilities must be methodically considered when skin manifestations occur in pregnant people. During evaluation of skin conditions in pregnancy, a detailed history and physical examination related to skin manifestations that emerge from other serious health conditions is indicated.

Health equity key points

- Clinicians have a professional responsibility to learn how dermatologic conditions of pregnancy present in clients with skin of color.
- Health disparities can affect access to appropriate specialty care for dermatologic conditions; use shared decision-making to develop a plan to address social or economic barriers to care and access necessary resources.
- Use of telehealth can improve health equity by improving access to dermatology providers, including those of similar racial and cultural identities as the client (Rustad & Lio, 2021).

Table 54.1 Abbreviations for Pregnancy-Specific Dermatoses

Abbreviation	Current classification
AEP	Atopic eruption of pregnancy; includes: • Atopic dermatitis (AD) (new onset or flare during pregnancy) • Pruritic folliculitis of pregnancy • Prurigo of pregnancy
ICP	Intrahepatic cholestasis of pregnancy
PUPPP; PEP	Pruritic urticarial papules and plaques of pregnancy (US terminology); Polymorphic eruption of pregnancy
PG	Pemphigoid gestationis
PPP	Pustular psoriasis of pregnancy; previously known as impetigo herpetiformis

Source: Adapted from Danesh et al. (2016).

Pruritic urticarial papules and **plaques** of pregnancy (PUPPP) is known as **polymorphic** eruption of pregnancy (PEP) outside the United States (Table 54.1). PUPPP, along with **atopic** eruption of pregnancy (AEP), which includes pruritic folliculitis of pregnancy (PFP) and prurigo of pregnancy (PP), are among the most common pregnancy-related dermatoses. While there is no evidence of association of adverse effects on the health of the fetus or newborn with these conditions, they can cause significant discomfort to the pregnant person. Symptoms commonly resolve spontaneously following the birth (Chouk & Litaiem, 2021; McNulty-Brown & Vaughan-Jones, 2016; Sävervall et al., 2015).

In contrast, intrahepatic cholestasis of pregnancy (ICP), pemphigoid gestationis (PG), and pustular psoriasis of pregnancy (PPP) are all conditions that can result in adverse outcomes for the pregnant person and the fetus. Therefore, clinical recommendations include engaging with the client as an active participant in their care, and applying a methodical approach to increased antepartum surveillance when caring for clients with these conditions (Mitchell et al., 2021; Sävervall et al., 2017).

This chapter focuses on several pregnancy-specific dermatoses (Table 54.2), some of which are associated solely with significant maternal discomfort, while others hold potential for adverse fetal outcomes. Common findings of significant pregnancy-specific dermatoses are presented to aid in differentiation of these skin conditions, facilitate diagnosis, and lead to an appropriate and effective treatment plan that is acceptable to the pregnant person and can mitigate adverse outcomes.

Appropriate treatment of skin disorders during pregnancy requires a thorough history and physical

Table 54.2 Pregnancy-Specific Dermatoses: Defining Characteristics

Disorder	Defining characteristics	Diagnostic aides	Concerns
AEP (AD, PP, PFP)	• Presentation: Excoriated papules/nodules, follicular papules, pustular eruptions • Locations: Extensor surfaces of arms, legs, abdomen, chest • Timing: First and second trimesters	• Diagnosis based on history and physical examination	• No known systemic risk • Potential for scarring • Increased risk for skin infection
PUPPP/ PEP	• Presentation: Excoriated papules • Locations: Abdominal striae, thighs, buttocks, arms, legs • Timing: Third trimester or immediately postpartum	• Diagnosis based on history and physical examination	• No known systemic risk • Potential for scarring
PG	• Presentation: Severe pruritis with erythematous papules, blisters or bullae • Locations: Periumbilical area and extremities • Timing: Second or third trimester	• Diagnosis based on history, physical examination and testing • Biopsy needed for definitive diagnosis, with direct immunofluorescence (DIF)	• Increased risk of low birth weight (LBW), preterm birth (PTB), neonatal skin lesions
PPP	• Presentation: Erythematous plaques with greenish yellow pustules, no pruritis • Locations: Inner thighs, flexor surfaces, groin • Timing: Second half of pregnancy	• Diagnosis based on history, physical examination and testing • Lab measurements: ESR and WBC may be elevated • Vitamin D and calcium may be low	• Increased fetal morbidity
ICP	• Presentation: Intense pruritis without lesions • Locations: Palms of hands, soles of feet • Timing: Third trimester	• Diagnosis based on history, physical examination and testing • Laboratory measurements: Elevated serum bile acids is diagnostic; AST and ALT may be elevated; vitamin K may be low	• PTB, fetal distress, meconium-stained amniotic fluid, intrauterine fetal demise

Source: Danesh et al. (2016), McNulty-Brown and Vaughan-Jones (2016), Roth (2011), and Sävervall et al. (2015).

assessment, an accurate diagnosis, and treatment that balances the need for symptomatic relief with potential embryonic or fetal effects of any medications prescribed. Skin manifestations can appear differently in people with different skin tones. Skin of color (SOC) is the current term used during dermatologic evaluation in people of color. Specific SOC textbooks and online dermatology resources, such as *VisualDx*, can be valuable resources for the provider who is unfamiliar with the presentation of dermatologic conditions in clients of color (Lester & Taylor, 2021).

It is the clinician's responsibility to familiarize themselves with the range of presentations that can occur across skin tones. In addition, clients with SOC can have a genetic predisposition for hypertrophy of scars or formation of keloids. This becomes an important consideration for conditions associated with significant pruritis where itching and scratching can result in superficial tissue trauma and resultant scarring (Jeon et al., 2017).

Evaluation of the client with skin lesions during pregnancy

- Parity, gestational age
- Personal history
  a. Allergies and atopic disorders, including family history
  b. Usual manifestations and course
  c. Triggers; pets, household products, environmental exposures
  d. Risk factors for hepatobiliary dysfunction
  e. Travel history
  f. Concurrent illnesses or infections, STIs, HIV, hepatitis
- Client experience of symptoms
  a. Timing of onset: weeks of gestation, time of day
  b. Aggravating and alleviating factors
  c. Severity of itching or other symptoms
  d. Constitutional symptoms: appetite, sleep, malaise
  e. Relief measures used and effectiveness
- Clinical findings
  a. Location and distribution of skin lesions
  b. Characteristics of skin lesions
  c. Laboratory findings

Source: Adapted from Lee et al. (2021).

Atopic Eruption of Pregnancy

AEP includes a range of benign conditions that typically occur in the first or second trimester of pregnancy and are thought to represent either pregnancy-related atopic or immunoglobulin-E associated conditions. The significant overlap in presenting symptoms between atopic dermatitis (AD), PP, and PFP has led to the recategorization of these conditions as variations of AEP (Danesh et al., 2016); therefore, the focus of this section is on diagnosis and treatment across the spectrum of AEP.

AEP occurs in approximately 5–20% of pregnant people (McNulty-Brown & Vaughan-Jones, 2016; Sävervall et al., 2015), with up to 80% of individuals with AEP

having no prior history of eczema and the remainder having been previously diagnosed with AD (Sävervall et al., 2015). AEP typically regresses in the postpartum period and can recur in subsequent pregnancy.

While AEP includes skin conditions initially diagnosed during pregnancy, AD (also known as eczema) can predate pregnancy. AD is a chronic, relapsing, pruritic inflammatory skin condition that can be complicated by secondary infections and related scarring. AD is associated with asthma and allergic rhinitis, as well as significant food allergies, which can trigger topical or systemic manifestations. The majority of individuals with AD have a positive family history of atopic disorders resulting in characteristic inflammatory reactions, which can be exacerbated by environmental triggers (Werfel et al., 2016).

While for some people with preexisting AD, the condition improves with pregnancy, for others, symptoms worsen due to the immune, hormonal, and metabolic alterations of pregnancy (Sävervall et al., 2015). Differentiating preexisting AD from the specific dermatoses of pregnancy can present a challenge due to an absence of clear diagnostic criteria for the pruritic skin disorders that are pregnancy related.

PFP is an uncommon type of AEP that presents with papules and pustules that form within the hair follicles. Initially, the lesions appear on the shoulders, upper back, arms, chest, and abdomen (Errichetti & Stinco, 2016). PFP most commonly occurs in the second or third trimester of pregnancy with erythematous follicular papules that spontaneous regress in the early postpartum period. There are no known associated maternal or fetal complications (Errichetti & Stinco, 2016). It is considered an **intrinsic dermatitis**, rather than an **extrinsic dermatitis**, which is associated with high levels of allergy-specific immunoglobin-E, which results in the atopic conditions within the AEP classification (Roth et al., 2016). Unlike other atopic disorders of pregnancy, the histopathology of PFP demonstrates nonspecific inflammatory folliculitis.

The incidence of PFP is reported to be about 1 in every 3000 pregnancies, although the actual incidence may be higher due to co-occurrence or diagnosis of conditions with significant similarities, such as acne and bacterial folliculitis, (Roth et al., 2016). The pathophysiology of PFP is largely unknown.

Assessment and Diagnosis

With the exception of PP, the essential clinical features of AEP include pruritis, eczema, and papules of a chronic or relapsing nature, with characteristic distribution of lesions on the face, neck, flexor surfaces of the upper and lower extremities, less so on the trunk, and sparing of the groin and axilla (Eichenfield et al., 2014; McNulty-Brown & Vaughan-Jones, 2016). Onset of symptoms is usually earlier than other pregnancy-related dermatoses, occurring most commonly in the first and second trimesters. Lesions are often red, edematous, with oozing and crusting, evidence of scratching, and with skin **lichenification** typically occurring over time (Oakley, 2009). During pregnancy in clients with SOC, AEP can present with lichenified patches and plaques, which can mask the underlying erythema (Jeon et al., 2017). Lesions typically resolve within 12 weeks postpartum (Roth, 2011). Clinician inquiries regarding the impact of symptoms on the client's ability to rest, perform daily activities, and their sense of well-being are used to inform treatment decisions.

While PP is included in the AEP category, it also occurs in clients with no prior history of atopy (Agarwal et al., 2020; Ravelli et al., 2020). PP has a typical onset with itching or rash at 25–30 weeks of gestation and can persist until the client gives birth. PP affects approximately 1 in 300 to 1 in 450 pregnant people with a higher incidence demonstrated in studies performed in India (Agarwal et al., 2020). Lesions often begin on the palmar surfaces of the hands and feet and can spread to the trunk and extensor surfaces of the extremities. PP is diagnosed clinically as IgE levels can either remain within normal values or be elevated (Ravelli et al., 2020).

The lesions of PFP initially appear as small (3–5 mm) erythematous papules on the upper trunk spreading to the lower extremities. Polarized-light dermoscopic evaluation of the lesions can reveal the presence of a **vellus hair** in the center of each papule or pustule, and a central yellowish-orange hue (Errichetti & Stinco, 2016). Swabs of the lesions return with no growth, which differentiates PFP from infectious conditions with a similar appearance such as bacterial folliculitis and impetigo. Pruritus may range from absent to severe (Roth, 2011). This self-limiting disorder usually clears in the last weeks of gestation, with complete resolution in the first month postpartum. Recurrence in subsequent pregnancies is uncommon (Roth et al., 2016).

When any form of AEP presents, the clinician must remain alert for signs or symptoms of secondary bacterial, fungal, or viral infections that result from the associated inflammation and disruption of skin integrity associated with scratching (Wang et al., 2021; Werfel et al., 2016). Identification and treatment of secondary infections are an important part of the evaluation and treatment of AEP.

Differential Diagnoses

Diagnosis of AEP is based on history and clinical findings as there are no reliable biomarkers for AEP (Eichenfield et al., 2014). Onset of symptoms that occur in the first or second trimester of pregnancy is classified as an AEP (McNulty-Brown & Vaughan-Jones, 2016; Sävervall et al., 2015). Both AEP and PUPPP manifest overlapping symptoms. Differentiation of AEP from PUPPP and the other dermatoses of pregnancy is made through assessment of previous history of atopic symptoms; noting any dietary, psychosocial, or environmental triggers; examination of all skin surfaces; noting the trimester in which symptom onset occurs; and the locations and types of lesions present (Werfel et al., 2016). A useful clinical aid is SCORAD (SCORing Atopic Dermatitis; see *Resources for Healthcare Providers*), a scoring tool for AD that is used to quantify the intensity and extent of the condition and note changes over time and response to therapy (Oakley, 2009).

When making an initial diagnosis of AEP, other common dermatologic conditions should be excluded, including scabies, contact dermatitis, psoriasis, photosensitivity, and immune deficiency disorders (Eichenfield et al., 2014).

The absence of infectious matter, bullous and urticarial lesions, and the sparing of striae differentiates PFP from bacterial folliculitis, the **prurigo** lesions of atopic disorders or cholestasis, and the papular phase of PUPPP. Initial differential diagnosis is primarily clinical and relies on the follicular nature of the lesions and negative culture results (Errichetti & Stinco, 2016). Use of ample light and magnification can aid in identifying the fine vellus hairs within each lesion. An absence of comedones and lesions on the face helps differentiate this condition from acne. **Drug eruption** is also a consideration and warrants a thorough medication history. When diagnostic uncertainty exists, biopsy is recommended (Roth et al., 2016).

Treatment and Management

Treatment follows a stepwise pattern based on the type of AEP, its clinical severity, and response to treatment. With mild AEP, bathing with nonsoap cleansers and use of emollients are recommended to preserve skin integrity and reduce response to triggers (Eichenfield et al., 2014; Werfel et al., 2016).

Prenatal supplementation with probiotics can decrease development of AD in offspring of birth parents with AED, particularly for those infants who are not expected to be exclusively fed breastmilk in the first six months of life (Eichenfield et al., 2014; Panduru et al., 2015). Maternal supplementation with probiotics is helpful and can occur through diet or commercial supplements.

First-generation antihistamines (diphenhydramine and chlorpheniramine) and second-generation formulations (such as loratadine and cetirizine) are considered safe in pregnancy and can be used for symptomatic relief of the itching that accompanies AEP (Hansen et al., 2020). While use of antihistamines is accepted as a short-term measure for itch that results in sleep loss, there is insufficient evidence to recommend the use of antihistamines as a treatment modality (Eichenfield et al., 2014).

Topical steroids are used as treatment when skin care and emollients alone are insufficient to provide relief. Mild to moderate strength topical steroids can be used safely during pregnancy. They are used sparingly on affected areas during the first trimester, with judicious short-term use (two weeks) after the first trimester (Wilmer et al., 2016). Some studies have shown an association between high-potency topical steroid use and small-for-gestational-age (SGA) infants (Chi et al., 2017). Examples of topical steroids are listed in Table 54.3. Systemic steroids are reserved for treatment of severe symptoms, with avoidance during the first trimester strongly recommended, and the lowest effective dose prescribed (Wilmer et al., 2016).

Two steroid-free topical anti-inflammatory medications—classed as calcineurin inhibitors—are approved for treatment of atopic conditions and prevention of flares. Tacrolimus ointment 0.1% and pimecrolimus cream 1% can

Table 54.3 Topical Steroid Therapy for Dermatologic Conditions During Pregnancy

Potency	Medication	Examples of brand names with percent of medication and vehicle
VII (Lowest potency)	Dexamethasone	Dexamethasone topical 0.1% cream
	Hydrocortisone	LactiCare 1.0%, 2.5% AC lotion
		Hytone 2.5% cream, lotion, ointment
	Hydrocortisone acetate	Epifoam 1.0 foam spray
VI (Low potency)	Betamethasone Valerate	Betaderm 0.05%, 0.1% cream, ointment Valisone 0.1% cream
	Desonide	Desonate 0.05% gel DesOwen 0.05% cream, lotion Lokara 0.05% lotion Verdeso 0.05% foam
	Flurandrenolide	Cordran SP 0.025% cream, lotion
	Fluocinolone acetonide	Derma-smoothe/FS 0.01% body oil Synalar 0.01% solution
	Prednicarbate	Aclovate 0.05% cream, ointment
	Triamcinolone acetate	Aristocort A 0.025% cream
III (Medium potency)	Betamethasone valerate	Valisone 0.1% cream, lotion
	Fluticasone propionate	Cutivate 0.05% cream
	Hydrocortisone Valerate	Westcort 0.2% cream
	Triamcinolone Acetonide	Kenalog 0.1% lotion

Source: Chi et al. (2017), Eichenfield et al. (2014), Vandersarl Slocum (2015), and Moses (2021).

be used during pregnancy. Due to limited data on the effects of these medications during human pregnancy, they are recommended only when the benefit outweighs the potential risk, and in the smallest effective dose for the shortest duration of exposure (Eichenfield et al., 2014; Nevers et al., 2014; Werfel et al., 2016). Broad- and narrowband ultraviolet B phototherapies are another effective second-line treatment for individuals in whom response to medical treatment is insufficient (Jeon et al., 2017). Photodegradation of folic acid is associated with phototherapy; therefore, adequate supplementation of folic acid must be provided. Clients with SOC undergoing light therapy require protection of the face to prevent melasma (Jeon et al., 2017). Benzoyl peroxide wash has also been shown to be an effective treatment for PFP (Errichetti & Stinco, 2016; Roth, 2011).

In addition to instructions for treatment, client education includes information on skin care, identification and avoidance of triggers or allergens, discussion of the role of probiotics in pregnancy, and indications for additional therapy. Pregnant clients are advised that preexisting AD can improve or worsen during pregnancy and can be reassured that while uncomfortable, AD is generally considered a benign self-limiting condition. Although uncommon, client education should include warning signs of skin infections as prompt diagnosis and treatment can reduce the incidence of systemic infection (Wang et al., 2021).

Referral to or consultation with dermatology services should occur when there is diagnostic uncertainty and for

clients with significant AEP or flares of preexisting AD whose symptoms fail to improve with use of mild strength topical corticosteroid preparations. Referral or consultation is also indicated for those clients who develop significant skin or systemic infection (Wang et al., 2021).

Pruritic Urticarial Papules and Plaques of Pregnancy

PUPPP is the United States' terminology for a condition also known as PEP. PUPPP is one of the most common pregnancy-related dermatologic disorders that typically occurs near the end of the first pregnancy and resolves shortly after the birth (Chouk & Litaiem, 2021; Sävervall et al., 2015). This benign inflammatory disorder is characterized by pruritic urticarial papules and plaques that develop on the abdomen, most often originating in the striae gravidarum, which can spread to the proximal extremities. Lesions initially appear in the third trimester for more than 80% of those affected and only rarely occur postpartum (Table 54.2).

While no definitive cause for PUPPP has yet been clearly identified, it is speculated that stretching of the gravid abdomen and resultant striae lead to connective tissue damage, with mast cell mediators responding to damaged collagen contributing to an inflammatory response (Chouk & Litaiem, 2021). Multifetal pregnancy and excessive pregnancy weight gain are associated with

PUPPP, while fetal weight and sex do not appear to contribute to the development of this disorder. This theory is borne out by the rates at which PUPPP occurs: 0.5% in clients carrying singleton pregnancies, 3–16% of those with twin pregnancies, and 14–17% of those carrying triplets (Chouk & Litaiem, 2021).

Assessment

PUPPP typically develops during the late third trimester or immediately postpartum. Lesions originate most often as pruritic urticarial papules along the abdominal striae, with the periumbilical area usually spared. The eruption can spread to the thighs, buttocks, arms, and legs. The face, palms, and soles are typically spared. More than half of affected individuals later develop polymorphous features such as erythema, vesicles, urticarial abdominal plaques, and **iris or target lesions** (Chouk & Litaiem, 2021; Sävervall et al., 2015; Figure 54.1). Lesions are self-limiting and typically resolve within 4 weeks or 7–10 days after the birth without postinflammatory skin changes or scarring (Chouk & Litaiem, 2021).

Differential Diagnoses

Diagnosis of PUPPP is often a diagnosis of exclusion. There are no specific diagnostic tests for PUPPP, making timing of symptom onset and lesion location the primary clues for a clinical diagnosis. It is essential to exclude PG. The lesions of PG often occur earlier in pregnancy and typically affect the periumbilical area, while this area is spared in PUPPP. Since PUPPP can easily be mistaken for other pruritic dermatoses of pregnancy, such as AEP, PG, or ICP, laboratory testing to eliminate these conditions may be required to confirm diagnosis and direct treatment. Histopathologic findings of **dyskeratosis, spongiosis** of the epidermis, edema of the papillary dermis, and perivascular infiltrations are consistent with PUPPP (Chouk & Litaiem, 2021). **Direct immunofluorescence (DIF)** studies are negative, thus excluding PG, while

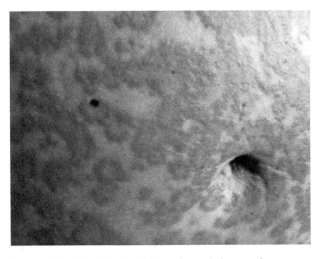

Figure 54.1 Pruritic urticarial papules and plaques of pregnancy. The papules often first localize in the abdominal striae.

normal total serum bile acid (TSBA) levels exclude ICP (Chouk & Litaiem, 2021).

Treatment and Management

Symptomatic relief is the primary goal of treatment for PUPPP. Oral antihistamines, such as loratadine, cetirizine, and fexofenadine, comprise first-line medical treatment (Sävervall et al., 2015). Topical corticosteroids, cool colloidal oatmeal baths, application of emollient creams, and topical antipruritic medications are adjunct treatments that have been shown to be safe and effective (Chouk & Litaiem, 2021). Table 54.4 lists medications and treatments for dermatologic conditions during pregnancy.

Dermatological consultation is indicated for cases of diagnostic uncertainty, or when symptoms are severe and unresponsive to usual therapy. Clients with severe pruritis with PUPPP may benefit from a short course of systemic corticosteroids.

Pemphigoid Gestationis

PG previously known as herpes gestationis is a rare autoimmune dermatosis of pregnancy associated with severe pruritis, vesiculobullous lesions, and adverse fetal outcomes (Genovese et al., 2020; Sävervall et al., 2017). Initial presentation includes urticarial papules and annular plaques, which are followed by formation of subepidermal vesicles and bullae (Sävervall et al., 2017; Figure 54.2). The condition occurs in approximately 1 in 60,000 pregnancies, most commonly in multiparous people (Genovese et al., 2020; Sävervall et al., 2017). Individuals with a history of PG have a higher incidence of autoimmune diseases, including Graves' disease, and Hashimoto thyroiditis (Sävervall et al., 2017).

The disorder typically presents during the second or third trimester of pregnancy, while a smaller percentage of pregnant people experience their initial outbreak in the first trimester or immediate postpartum period (Sävervall et al., 2017). In the majority of cases, PG worsens as birth becomes imminent and improves following the birth. Recurrences occur in approximately 50% of those with a prior history of this disorder. Recurrences are associated with an earlier onset and greater severity (Sävervall et al., 2017).

The first immunological response with PG occurs within the placenta rather than the skin. The immune response identifies a key structural protein (BP180) within the placenta as foreign. This stimulates formation of antiplacental IgG antibodies that cross-react with BP180 proteins in the skin. The antibodies bind to the basement membrane of the skin triggering the autoimmune reaction (Sävervall et al., 2017). The autoimmune response in the dermal tissues results in the accumulation of immune complexes, complement activation, and degranulation that leads to urticarial tissue response and formation of **herpetiform** lesions (Hallaji et al., 2017; Sävervall et al., 2017).

Risks to the fetus are highest when the onset of PG occurs in the first or second trimester, and when blisters

Table 54.4 Systemic Therapy for Dermatologic Conditions in Pregnancy

Medication/treatment recommendations	Indication	Period of avoidance	Adverse effects/comments
Antihistamines, first generation: diphenhydramine, chlorpheniramine; preferred choice in pregnancy	Pruritus	None; first-line agents, preferred for first trimester	Sedation, long safety history in pregnancy
Antihistamines, second generation: loratidine, cetirizine and fexofenadine; loratidine first choice for nonsedating	Pruritus	None; considered second-line agents in first trimester	Unconfirmed risk of hypospadias, lack of evidential association as teratogen
UVB phototherapy	AEP, ICP	First 28 days of pregnancy	Overheating with therapy increases risk of neural tube defects
Corticosteroids, oral; Use lowest effective dose for brief periods (~14 days) of treatment	AEP, PUPPP, PG	First trimester (organogenesis), third trimester with high doses	Possible risk of oral clefts when used before 12 weeks of gestation, association with prelabor rupture of membranes, placental insufficiency, fetal growth restriction
Cyclosporine A; Use minimum dose; monitor blood pressure and renal function	PG	None	Association with low birth weight and preterm birth in clients with additional health conditions
Ursodeoxycholic acid	ICP	None	GI side effects but no adverse effects are noted when compared with placebo

Source: Koh et al. (2019), Sävervall et al. (2015), and Wilmer et al. (2016).

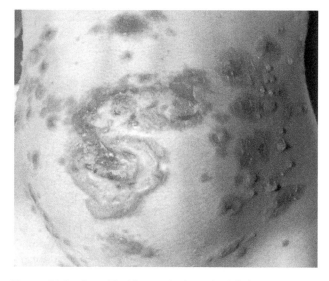

Figure 54.2 Pemphigoid gestationis: Urticarial plaques progress to generalized tense bullae on erythematous base.

or bullae are present. Fetal outcomes can include PTB, fetal growth restriction (FGR), and neonates who are SGA. In one study of 23 women with PG during pregnancy, 14 pregnancies (61%) resulted in births without complications, while 5 women experienced perinatal complications, including FGR, low birth weight (LBW), intrauterine fetal demise, and one neonate with skin involvement (Hallaji et al., 2017). Information on the remaining four pregnancies was not available. Four women experienced PTB, two women developed

preeclampsia, and five experienced flares of the disorder at the time of birth. Of the 23 women, 19 achieved clinical remission with treatment. The treatment itself can also be associated with these types of adverse perinatal outcomes, making treatment decisions and the dose and duration of medication use an important consideration when treating PG.

The passive transfer of IgG1 antibodies across the placenta to the fetus can result in approximately 10% of infants born to individuals with PG developing urticarial or vesicular skin lesions (Sävervall et al., 2017). Neonatal lesions tend to be mild and resolve spontaneously as antibodies decline during the first three months of life. Newborns can also have subclinical disease where antibody tests are positive with an absence of skin lesions. No lasting morbidity or mortality has been noted in these infants.

Assessment

The client with PG initially presents with severe pruritus and urticarial erythematous plaques or papules in the periumbilical area, which can spread to the abdomen, back, chest, and extremities (Hallaji et al., 2017; Sävervall et al., 2017). The face, palms, soles, and mucous membranes are usually unaffected. As the condition progresses, the papules evolve into plaques and tense blisters or bullae develop. Following rupture of the blisters or bullae, these areas become covered by yellowish or hemorrhagic crusts. Individuals in late pregnancy often experience a remission, which can be followed by a flare immediately after giving birth. Exacerbation can also occur postpartum with menses or hormonal contraceptive use (Genovese et al., 2020; Sävervall et al., 2017), leading to questions about the role of hormonal factors in this condition. Symptoms typically subside by six months postpartum. Clients with persistent postpartum symptoms should be evaluated for bullous pemphigoid, a skin condition that is not associated with pregnancy.

Differential Diagnosis

Other pregnancy-related diagnoses with similar presentations include PUPPP and ICP (Table 54.2). Prior to vesicle formation, it can be difficult to clinically differentiate PG from PUPPP. The timing of onset and an absence of lesions in the striae gravidarum and the presence of skin lesions in the umbilical area are suggestive of PG and can assist in ruling out PUPPP (Sävervall et al., 2017). It is also necessary to rule out other bullous conditions that are not pregnancy-specific such as varicella bullous pemphigoid, erythema multiforme, drug eruptions, and contact dermatitis.

The diagnosis of PG is reached through correlation of clinical presentation with results of DIF on bullous lesion samples. Examination of tissue from lesion margins will show characteristic changes, and DIF will show deposits along the basal membrane in 100% of samples from individuals with PG, and the presence of IgG in 25–50% of those affected. Serum enzyme-linked immunosorbent assay (ELISA) testing, with its high sensitivity (86–97%) and specificity (94–98%), can also be useful in arriving at a diagnosis (Hallaji et al., 2017; Sävervall et al., 2017). Serum levels of anti-BP180 correlate with disease activity allowing the clinician to monitor changes using ELISA testing.

Treatment and Management

The goal of treatment is to mitigate development of lesions and reduce the severity of pruritis. High-potency topical corticosteroids, along with emollients, are used in the preblistering stage to treat mild forms of PG (Table 54.3). Oral antihistamines can provide symptomatic relief of pruritus and the associated interrupted sleep. The type of antihistamine recommended will vary with the stage of pregnancy. First-generation, sedating antihistamines (e.g., chlorphenamine or diphenhydramine) are recommended in the first trimester, with newer nonsedating antihistamines (e.g., loratadine) recommended for the later trimesters.

Oral corticosteroids are the mainstay of treatment, with combination therapy (systemic corticosteroids, plus topical steroids or antihistamines) resulting in clinical remission in 83% of those treated (Genovese et al., 2020). Oral prednisone 20–60 mg/day (0.5 mg/kg/day) is the recommended therapy once blisters begin to appear (Genovese et al., 2020; Hallaji et al., 2017). This dosage should reduce pruritus and prevent the formation of new blisters. If improvement is not satisfactory, the dosage can be increased to a maximum of 1 mg/kg/day. Reevaluation should occur within two weeks of therapy initiation, or sooner if symptoms worsen, with consideration of referral if symptoms persist or worsen. Most clients on this regimen experience symptom remission in approximately two weeks. Once remission occurs, the dosage is tapered until the lowest effective dose is achieved. The client is then maintained on this lowest dose until just prior to their estimated date of birth (EDB), when the dose is again increased due to the characteristic flare-up of symptoms close to the onset of labor, birth, and the early postpartum period (Genovese et al., 2020). Flare-ups that occur with hormonal contraceptive use in individuals with a history of PG can necessitate an alternate form of contraception.

Prednisone at these doses given over a short period of time during the second or third trimester is associated with minimal adverse outcomes related to therapy. For individuals with contraindications for oral steroids or inadequate response to this therapy, referral for steroid-sparing agents is indicated. In pregnancy, intravenous (IV) immunoglobulin therapy is effective, with other immunosuppressants or immunomodulating agents being reserved for refractory cases (Genovese et al., 2020).

Interprofessional Care

An unclear diagnosis, severe symptoms, need for high-potency topical steroids, or failure to achieve remission with first-line treatments should prompt referral to a dermatologist. Due to the potential for significant adverse fetal consequences, and the potential for co-occurring conditions (Hallaji et al., 2017), collaborative care with obstetrical or perinatal specialists is preferred, with birth planned in a location with neonatal specialty care. Consultation with pediatric care providers prior to the birth can aid in planning neonatal evaluation and follow-up care.

Pustular Psoriasis of Pregnancy

Acute pustular psoriasis of pregnancy (PPP), formerly known as impetigo herpetiformis (IH), is a rare pustular form of psoriasis that is associated with life-threatening complications for the client and their fetus. The disorder typically presents in the third trimester of pregnancy with fever, neutrophilia, electrolyte imbalance, and malaise (Trivedi et al., 2018). Cutaneous symptoms include pustules that form on erythematous patches in the intertriginous areas, and rapidly coalesce into large dry plaques, followed by desquamation. The condition typically resolves within two months of the birth and can recur in subsequent pregnancies (Trivedi et al., 2018). While PPP can occur in individuals with no personal or family history of the disease, it is thought to be a variant of generalized pustular psoriasis, an immune-mediated disorder with genetic components (Trivedi et al., 2018). PPP is associated with placental insufficiency that can lead to FGR, fetal hypoxemia, and stillbirth. The actual incidence and severity of sequelae are unknown as there is a lack of data on this uncommon condition.

Assessment

The lesions of PPP appear as grouped pustules that form on the periphery of erythematous plaques (Trivedi et al., 2018). As the pustules rupture, they are replaced by crusting. Pruritus is usually absent. The lesions commonly first appear on the inner thighs, flexor areas, and groin with subsequent spread to the trunk and extremities. The face, hands, and feet may be spared. Associated signs and symptoms include fever, malaise, nausea, and lymphadenopathy (Trivedi et al., 2018). Laboratory studies include complete blood count (CBC), erythrocyte sedimentation rate (ESR), c-reactive protein, and serum chemistries. Bacterial evaluation of pustules is performed when secondary infection is suspected. When hypocalcemia is severe, severe muscle spasms can occur. Hyperpigmentation of previously inflamed areas can occur after lesions heal.

Differential Diagnosis

The diagnosis is based primarily on clinical presentation and abnormal lab findings. Laboratory findings show leukocytosis, elevated ESR, low serum calcium and albumin, and low levels of vitamin D (Yang et al., 2016). Cultures of the pustules and blood cultures are typically negative. Biopsy shows changes consistent with pustular psoriasis, and DIF skin testing is negative. PPP must be distinguished from other conditions with similar cutaneous presentations including new onset herpes, drug eruptions, eczema, lupus, and lichens simplex chronicus. Presence of fever and malaise can aid in differential diagnosis (Trivedi et al., 2018).

Treatment and Management

Early recognition and treatment of PPP is essential to mitigate the life-threatening aspects of this disorder. The first line of treatment for PPP is systemic corticosteroids. Initial treatment with prednisone at 15–30 mg/day is recommended, with the dosage titrated upward to 60–80 mg/day until relief of symptoms is achieved (Trivedi et al., 2018). When symptoms are severe or unresponsive to corticosteroids, cyclosporine is considered for treatment of PPP (Trivedi et al., 2018). The usual dose is 2–3 mg/kg body weight/day orally. Infliximab at 5 mg/kg as an IV infusion is now recognized as a first-line therapy and can be effective when steroids and cyclosporine are not (Beksac et al., 2021; Trivedi et al., 2018). Doses are repeated when necessary. Narrowband ultraviolet light B (Nb-UVB) has been used with good results in some individuals (Trivedi et al., 2018). Supportive therapy with IV fluids and electrolytes is provided, with monitoring and correction of hypocalcemia and vitamin D deficiency.

As PPP is associated with FGR and fetal and neonatal death, monitoring of fetal well-being is integral to care. Serial ultrasound is used to assess for signs of FGR and reduction in placental blood flow, with fetal kick counts and nonstress testing used to evaluate fetal well-being. Induction of labor is recommended for findings suggestive of placental insufficiency or abnormal fetal assessment.

Interprofessional Care

Because of the morbidity and mortality associated with PPP, and the potential need for preterm labor induction, collaborative care with obstetrical or perinatal specialists is recommended, with birth planned in a location with neonatal special care. Expedited labor and birth is indicated for signs of fetal compromise or worsening maternal condition. Pediatrics consultation is indicated prior to the birth when anticipating an ill newborn.

Intrahepatic Cholestasis of Pregnancy

ICP is a multifactorial liver dysfunction that occurs exclusively during pregnancy and produces dermatologic symptoms. Hormonal, environmental, and immunological factors act on genetic mutations in the biliary canal transport system, which can result in cholestasis (Jeon et al., 2017). Retention of substances normally excreted into bile, such as conjugated bilirubin and bile salts, leads to increased serum bile acids or aminotransferase levels (Jeon et al., 2017). Serum bile acids are deposited within the skin, where they cause intense pruritus. Untreated, ICP is associated with significant fetal morbidity and mortality.

ICP affects approximately 0.2–5.6% of pregnant people with rates varying based on their ethnicity, the geographic region sampled, presence of preexisting hepatobiliary disease, and the diagnostic criteria used (Lee et al., 2021; Mitchell et al., 2021). A disproportionate number of those affected are clients with SOC, particularly those of Native American or South Asian ancestry (Jeon et al., 2017), as well as Latina and Scandinavian populations (Floreani & Gervasi, 2016). Fetal complications include preterm birth, fetal asphyxia, meconium-stained amniotic fluid, associated intensive care unit admission, and stillbirth (Lee et al., 2021).

Approximately 75–80% of ICP diagnoses are made after the thirtieth week of gestation. The disorder typically manifests in the third trimester with intense pruritis of the hands and feet, accompanied by elevated liver enzymes and bilirubin (Lee et al., 2021; Li et al., 2020). While a small percentage (10–15%) of individuals affected by ICP demonstrate clinically apparent jaundice, it is more commonly a marker for other liver disorders such as hepatitis (Lee et al., 2021). Individuals with multifetal gestation are more likely to develop ICP than those with a singleton pregnancy, lending support to the theory that increased levels of estradiol and progesterone metabolites are contributing factors to the development of this condition (Ovadia & Williamson, 2016).

Elevated serum bile acids (>40 μmol/L) are associated with meconium-stained amniotic fluid, adverse fetal outcomes, and neonatal respiratory distress. Co-occurring maternal vitamin K deficiency can result in antepartal fetal hemorrhage (Ovadia & Williamson, 2016). Sudden fetal death, sometimes within hours of normal fetal heart rate tracings, is a particular concern with ICP and is thought to be related to rapid postprandial elevation of TSBA levels (Mitchell et al., 2021). The risk of intrauterine fetal demise increases as the TSBA level rises >100 μmol/L leading to recommendations for induction at 36 0/7–37 0/7 weeks for these clients (Lee et al., 2021). Maternal symptoms typically fully resolve shortly after birth. ICP has a recurrence rate of 60–70% in subsequent pregnancies (Sävervall et al., 2015).

Assessment

The classic presentation of ICP is sudden onset in the third trimester of intense, generalized pruritus of the hands and feet without associated skin lesions or rash. The pruritus tends to be more severe at night, resulting in disrupted sleep (Lee et al., 2021). The itching then becomes generalized, and secondary skin lesions can develop as a result of scratching (Li et al., 2020).

Due to the significant adverse fetal effects, ICP should be considered for all pregnant women with pruritis (Lee et al., 2021). Laboratory testing is aimed at assessing liver function while assessing for other conditions such as HELLP (Hemolysis, Elevated Liver enzymes, and Low Platelets) syndrome. The most specific and sensitive marker of ICP is TSBA; fasting TBSA levels greater than 11 μmol/L with an absence of primary skin lesions supports a diagnosis of ICP (Jeon et al., 2017). TSBA levels correlate with the severity and the duration of pruritus, and adverse fetal outcomes are associated with increasing bile acid levels. In addition to TSBA, testing can include aspartate transaminase (AST), alanine transaminase (ALT), gamma-glutamyl transpeptidase (GGT), alkaline phosphatase (ALP), and total bilirubin. Coagulation studies such a prothrombin time (PT), partial thromboplastin time (PTT), and international normalized ratio (INR) may also be performed.

Adverse fetal outcomes are associated with peak TSBA levels over 40 μmol/L. TBSA levels of 100 μmol/L or greater are associated with increased risk of stillbirth (Ovadia et al., 2021). A 2021 study evaluating postprandial TBSA levels demonstrated that peak nonfasting levels of <19 μmol/L resulted in rates of adverse fetal outcomes consistent with those of uncomplicated pregnancies (Mitchell et al., 2021). This study also demonstrated a marked spike in postprandial TSBA levels in some individuals who consistently had fasting TSBA levels below 40 μmol/L, suggesting that postprandial TSBA levels may be more effective in evaluating fetal risk than fasting levels. Monitoring the severity of the disorder requires serial levels of serum bile acids (Table 54.5). A turnaround time of three to four days for serum bile acid laboratory results is not uncommon, necessitating that immediate management decisions be based on clinical presentation.

Differential Diagnoses

Primary dermatological disorders can often be excluded from the differential diagnosis based on clinical

Table 54.5 Classification of ICP by Serum Bile Levels

Classification	Total serum bile acid level, fasting
Mild	10–19.9 μmol/L
Moderate	20–39.9 μmol/L
Severe	≥40 μmol/L

Source: Adapted from Estiu et al. (2017).

findings, while test results are pending (Table 54.2). Skin disorders unrelated to pregnancy must also be considered, including allergic dermatitis, as well as bacterial and viral rashes. Scabies infestation that occurs in pregnancy can mimic the scratch-induced excoriations of ICP. Skin biopsy is nonspecific but can be useful to rule out PG. Exclusion of these other disorders and the presence of elevated TSBA and liver enzyme levels are confirmatory for ICP (Lee et al., 2021). Individuals presenting with visible jaundice should be evaluated for other hepatobiliary conditions such as cholangitis, cytomegalovirus, hepatitis, HELLP syndrome, metabolic and hemolytic diseases, or other causes of hyperbilirubinemia (Lee et al., 2021).

Treatment and Management

When ICP is suspected, pharmacologic treatment and serial fetal evaluation should begin immediately. The goal of treatment for ICP is to reduce the severity of symptoms and improve perinatal outcomes by reducing TSBA levels to below 40 μmol/L.

Ursodeoxycholic acid (UDCA) is considered the primary medical therapy for ICP (Lee et al., 2021; Ovadia et al., 2021). This medication improves bile flow, thereby reducing bile stasis resulting in improved clinical symptoms and liver parameters. It has been demonstrated to reduce rates of preterm birth and severity of pruritis but does not affect the rate of stillbirth (Ovadia et al., 2021; Roediger & Fleckenstein, 2021). The recommended dose for UDCA is 15 mg/kg/day given in two to three divided doses and is continued until the birth (Roediger & Fleckenstein, 2021). Rifampicin can be used with UDCA to further reduce TSBA and pruritis (Roediger & Fleckenstein, 2021). Vitamin K supplements are recommended for elevated PT levels (Roediger & Fleckenstein, 2021). Mild cases of ICP may respond to supportive treatment such as soothing baths, topical antipruritics, emollients, and evening primrose oil. Antihistamine use at bedtime may help to promote sleep but is rarely effective in reducing the intense pruritis of ICP. Periodic maternal TSBA determinations and liver function tests are used to evaluate response to treatment and plan the ongoing course of care. Consideration should be given to using postprandial TSBA levels to assess ongoing client status (Mitchell et al., 2021).

Maternal-fetal surveillance is indicated with a diagnosis of ICP. Fetal movement counting, umbilical artery

Doppler studies, serial ultrasounds to evaluate fetal growth, nonstress tests, and biophysical profile testing starting at the time of diagnosis have been suggested to reduce the incidence of fetal morbidity and mortality (Estiu et al., 2017). However, fetal surveillance has limited value in predicting or preventing the sudden adverse outcomes that can occur in pregnancies where TSBA rapidly increases over 100 μmol/L. Planned birth at 36 0/7 weeks of gestation is recommended for clients with TBSA levels >100 μmol/L or earlier in the presence of prior stillbirth or worsening hepatic function (Lee et al., 2021). Birth is recommended between 36 0/7 and 39 0/7 weeks for clients with TSBA >40 μmol/L (Lee et al., 2021). Expectant management can be considered with TSBA levels consistently below 40 μmol/L and reassuring fetal surveillance findings. Timing and route of birth should be determined through shared decision-making based on the severity of the disorder and relative risks associated with preterm birth.

Interprofessional Care

Consultation and collaboration with obstetrical or perinatal specialists are recommended for moderate or severe ICP and for all pregnant people with ICP and comorbidities. Due to the need for medication management and the likelihood of planned preterm or early term birth, a team approach is recommended when ICP is suspected or diagnosed. Birth should be planned in a location with neonatal specialty care. Consultation with the pediatrics team prior to the birth is an important aspect of planning newborn care.

Summary

Changes in the skin during pregnancy can represent a temporary cosmetic condition or signify a significant underlying disorder with the potential to seriously affect maternal or fetal health. Common skin conditions during pregnancy are generally separated into three categories: hormone-related skin changes, preexisting dermatoses and health conditions with dermatologic manifestations, and pregnancy-specific dermatoses. Most of the skin changes seen in pregnancy are the result of pregnancy hormones, resolve spontaneously postpartum, and only require symptomatic treatment.

The overlapping features of the various skin conditions can present a challenge for the clinician when making a diagnosis and formulating an effective treatment plan with the client. For pregnant people demonstrating symptoms of ICP, PG, and PPP, prompt evaluation, diagnosis, and treatment are especially important as these conditions are associated with adverse effects on maternal and fetal health. In addition to pharmacotherapy and client education, shared decision-making regarding antepartum surveillance and collaboration with perinatal, medical, or dermatologic colleagues are important care components when addressing pregnancy-specific skin disorders.

Resources for Clients and Families

Atopic Eruption of Pregnancy: https://eadv.org/wp-content/uploads/2023/04/EADV-Pregnancy-TF_-Atopic-Eruption-of-pregnancy-AEP.pdf
Intrahepatic Cholestasis of Pregnancy: https://liverfoundation.org/for-patients/about-the-liver/diseases-of-the-liver/intrahepatic-cholestasis-of-pregnancy
Pruritic Urticarial Papules and Plaques of Pregnancy: https://www.babycenter.com/pregnancy/your-body/puppp-rash_40008036
Skin Diseases in Pregnancy: https://eadv.org/patient-corner/patient-leaflets/
Skin Conditions in People of Color: https://www.templehealth.org/about/blog/how-common-skin-conditions-affect-people-of-color

Resources for Healthcare Providers

Websites

Common Dermatological Conditions in Skin of Colour: https://pharmaceutical-journal.com/article/ld/common-dermatological-conditions-in-skin-of-colour
Dermatology Online Journal: an open-access, refereed publication intended to meet reference and education needs of the international dermatology community. www.odermatol.com
Dermnet Skin Disease Atlas: a searchable reference for skin diseases. www.dermnet.com
Dermnet New Zealand: the website for the New Zealand Dermatological Society, containing facts and images for numerous skin disorders. Interactive Dermatology Atlas: Offers case mode, atlas, and quizzes to improve clinical skills. https://www.dermatlas.net
Intrahepatic Cholestasis of Pregnancy: https://liverfoundation.org/liver-diseases/complications-of-liver-disease/intrahepatic-cholestasis-of-pregnancy-icp/
SCORAD (SCORing Atopic Dermatitis): https://www.dermnetnz.org/topics/scorad
Skin Conditions during Pregnancy: ACOG https://www.acog.org/womens-health/faqs/skin-conditions-during-pregnancy

Textbooks

Alexis, A. F., & Barbosa, V. H. (Eds.). (2012). *Skin of color: a practical guide to dermatologic diagnosis and treatment*. Springer Science & Business Media.
Jackson-Richards, D., & Pandya, A. G. (Eds.). (2014). *Dermatology atlas for skin of color*. Springer.
Kelly, A. P., Taylor, S. C., Lim, H. W., & Serrano, A. M. A. (Eds.). (2016). *Taylor and Kelly's dermatology for skin of color*. McGraw-Hill Medical.
Téot, L., Mustoe, T. A., Middelkoop, E., & Gauglitz, G. G. (Eds.). (2020). *Textbook on Scar Management: State of the Art Management and Emerging Technologies*. Springer International Publishing.

References

Agarwal, P., Chaudhari, S. V., Jagati, A., Rathod, S. P., & Neazee, S. T. (2020). Clinical spectrum of pregnancy related dermatoses in a tertiary care hospital in western India. *National Journal of Community Medicine*, *11*(12), 450–455. https://doi.org/10.5455/njcm.20201218045901

Beksac, B., Adisen, E., & Gurer, M. A. (2021). Treatment of generalized pustular psoriasis of pregnancy with infliximab. *Cutis*, *107*(3), E2–E5. https://doi.org/10.12788/cutis.0210

Chi, C. C., Kirtschig, G., Aberer, W., Gabbud, J. P., Lipozencic, J., Karpati, S., Haustein, U.-F., Wojnarowska, T., & Zuberbier, T. (2017). Updated evidence-based (S2e) European Dermatology Forum guideline on topical corticosteroid in pregnancy. *Journal of the European Academy of Dermatology ant Venereology*, *31*(5), 761–773.

Chouk, C., & Litaiem, N. (2021). *Pruritic urticarial papules and plaques of pregnancy*. StatPearls. https://www.ncbi.nlm.nih.gov/books/NBK539700

Danesh, M., Pomeranz, M. K., McMeniman, E., & Murase, J. E. (2016). Dermatoses of pregnancy: Nomenclature, misnomers, and myths. *Clinics in Dermatology*, *34*(3), 314–319. https://doi.org/10.1016/j.clindermatol.2016.02.002

Eichenfield, L. F., Tom, W. L., Berger, T. G., Krol, A., Paller, A. S., Schwarzenberger, K., Bergen, J. N., Chamlin, S. L., Cohen, D. E., Cooper, K. D., Cordoro, K. M., Davis, D. M., Feldmen, S. R., Hanifin, J. M., Margolis, D. J., Silverman, R. A., Simpson, E. L., Williams, H. C., Elmets, C. A., . . . Sidbury, R. (2014). Guidelines of care for the management of atopic dermatitis: Section 2. Management and treatment of atopic dermatitis with topical therapies. *Journal of the American Academy of Dermatology*, *71*(1), 116–132. https://doi.org/10.1016/j.jaad.2014.03.023

Errichetti, E., & Stinco, G. (2016). Photoletter to the editor: Dermoscopy as a diagnostic aid for pruritic folliculitis of pregnancy. *Journal of Dermatological Case Reports*, *10*(1), 19. https://doi.org/10.3315/jdcr.2016.1227

Estiu, M. C., Frailuna, M. A., Otero, C., Dericco, M., Williamson, C., Marin, J. J., & Macias, R. I. (2017). Relationship between early; onset severe intrahepatic cholestasis of pregnancy and higher risk of meconium-stained fluid. *PloS One*, *12*(4), e0176504. https://doi.org/10.1371/journal.pone.0176504

Floreani, A., & Gervasi, M. T. (2016). New insights on intrahepatic cholestasis of pregnancy. *Clinical Liver Disease*, *20*, 177–189. https://doi.org/10.1016/j.cld.2015.08.010

Genovese, G., Derlino, F., Cerri, A., Moltrasio, C., Muratori, S., Berti, E., & Marzano, A. V. (2020). A systematic review of treatment options and clinical outcomes in pemphigoid gestationis. *Frontiers in Medicine*, *7*, 604945. https://doi.org/10.3389/fmed.2020.604945

Hallaji, Z., Mortazavi, H., Ashtari, S., Nikoo, A., Abdollahi, M., & Nasimi, M. (2017). Pemphigoid gestationis: Clinical and histologic features of twenty-three patients. *International Journal of Women's Dermatology*, *3*(2), 86–90. https://doi.org/10.1016/j.ijwd.2016.11.004

Hansen, C., Desrosiers, T. A., Wisniewski, K., Strickland, M. J., Werler, M. M., & Gilboa, S. M. (2020). Use of antihistamine medications during early pregnancy and selected birth defects: The National Birth Defects Prevention Study, 1997–2011. *Birth Defects Research*, *112*(16), 1234–1252. https://doi.org/10.1002/bdr2.1749

Jeon, C., Agbai, O., Butler, D., & Murase, J. (2017). Dermatologic conditions in patients of color who are pregnant. *International Journal of Women's Dermatology*, *3*(1), 30–36. https://doi.org/10.1016/j.ijwd.2017.02.019

Koh, Y. P., Tian, E. A., & Oon, H. H. (2019). New changes in pregnancy and lactation labelling: Review of dermatologic drugs. *International Journal of Women's Dermatology*, *5*(4), 216–226. https://doi.org/10.1016/j.ijwd.2019.05.002

Lee, R. H., Greenberg, M., Metz, T. D., Pettker, C. M., & Society for Maternal-Fetal Medicine (SMFM). (2021). Society for maternal-fetal medicine consult series # 53: Intrahepatic cholestasis of pregnancy: Replaces consult# 13 April 2011. *American Journal of Obstetrics and Gynecology*, *224*(2), B2–B9. https://doi.org/10.1016/j.ajog.2020.11.002

Lester, J. C., & Taylor, S. C. (2021). Two pandemics: Opportunities for diversity, equity and inclusion in dermatology. *International Journal of Women's Dermatology*, *7*, 137–138. https://doi.org/10.1016/j.ijwd.2021.01.015

Li, R., Chen, X., Liu, Z., Chen, Y., Liu, C., Ye, L., Xiao, L., Yang, Z., He, J., Wang, W.-J., & Qi, H. (2020). Characterization of gut microbiota associated with clinical parameters in intrahepatic cholestasis of pregnancy. *BMC Gastroenterology*, *20*, 395. https://doi.org/10.1186/s12876-020-01510-w

McNulty-Brown, E., & Vaughan-Jones, S. (2016). An overview of pregnancy dermatoses. *Dermatological Nursing*, *15*(1), 24–30. https://bdng.org.uk/wp-content/uploads/2017/02/15_1_24.pdf

Mitchell, A. L., Ovadia, C., Syngelaki, A., Souretis, K., Martineau, M., Girling, J., Vasavan, T., Fan, H. M., Seed, P. T., Chambers, J., Walters, J. R. F., & Nicolaides, & Williamson, C. (2021). Re-evaluating diagnostic thresholds for intrahepatic cholestasis of pregnancy: Case–control and cohort study. *BJOG: An International Journal of Obstetrics & Gynaecology*, *128*(10), 1635–1644. https://doi.org/10.1111/1471-0528.16669

Moses, S. (2021). *Topical corticosteroid*. Family practice notebook. https://fpnotebook.com/derm/Pharm/TpclCrtcstrd.htm

Nevers, W., Pupco, A., Koren, G., & Bozzo, P. (2014). Safety of tacrolimus in pregnancy. *Canadian Family Physician*, *60*(10), 905–906. https://www.cfp.ca/content/60/10/905.full

Oakley A., (2009). *SCORAD*. DermNet NZ. http://www.dermnetnz.org/topics/scorad

Ovadia, C., Sajous, J., Seed, P. T., Patel, K., Williamson, N. J., Attilakos, G., Azzaroli, F., Bacq, Y., Batsry, L., Broom, K., Brun-Furrer, R., Bull, L., Chambers, J., Cui, Y., Ding, M., Dixon, P. H., Estiú, M. C., Gardiner, F. W., Geenes, V., Grymowicz, M., . . . Williamson, C. (2021). Ursodeoxycholic acid in intrahepatic cholestasis of pregnancy: a systematic review and individual participant data meta-analysis. *The Lancet Gastroenterology & Hepatology*, *6*(7), 547–558. https://doi.org/10.1016/S2468-1253(21)00074-1

Ovadia, C., & Williamson, C. (2016). Intrahepatic cholestasis of pregnancy: Recent advances. *Clinics in Dermatology*, *34*(3), 327–334. https://doi.org/10.1016/j.clindermatol.2016.02.004

Panduru, M., Panduru, N. M., Salavastru, C. M., & Tiplica, G. S. (2015). Probiotics and primary prevention of atopic dermatitis: A meta-analysis of randomized controlled studies. *Journal of the European Academy of Dermatology and Venereology*, *29*(2), 232–242. https://doi.org/10.1111/jdv.12496

Ravelli, F. N., Goldust, M., & Kroumpouzos, G. (2020). Assessment of prurigo of pregnancy in patients without atopic background. *International Journal of Women's Dermatology*, *6*(5), 384–389. https://doi.org/10.1016/j.ijwd.2020.06.011

Roediger, R., & Fleckenstein, J. (2021). Intrahepatic cholestasis of pregnancy: Natural history and current management. *Seminars in Liver Disease*, *41*(01), 103–108.

Roth, M. (2011). Pregnancy dermatosis: Diagnosis, management, and controversies. *American Journal of Clinical Dermatology*, *12*(1), 25–41. https://doi.org/10.2165/11532010-000000000-00000

Roth, M. M., Cristodor, P., & Kroumpouzos, G. (2016). Prurigo, pruritic folliculitis, and atopic eruption of pregnancy: Facts and controversies. *Clinics in Dermatology*, *34*(3), 392–400. https://doi.org/10.1016/j.clindermatol.2016.02.012

Rustad, A. M., & Lio, P. A. (2021). Pandemic pressure: Teledermatology and health care disparities. *Journal of Patient Experience*, *8*, 1–5. https://doi.org/10.1177/2374373521996982

Savervall, C., Sand, F. L., & Thomsen, S. F. (2015). Dermatological diseases associated with pregnancy: Pemphigoid gestationis, polymorphic eruption of pregnancy, intrahepatic cholestasis of pregnancy, and atopic eruption of pregnancy. *Dermatology Research and Practice*, *2015*, 979635. https://doi.org/10.1155/2015/979635

Sävervall, C., Sand, F. L., & Thomsen, S. F. (2017). Pemphigoid gestationis: Current perspectives. *Clinical, Cosmetic and Investigational Dermatology*, *10*, 441–449. https://doi.org/10.2147/CCID.S128144

Trivedi, M. K., Vaughn, A. R., & Murase, J. E. (2018). Pustular psoriasis of pregnancy: Current perspectives. *International Journal of Women's Health*, *10*, 109–115. https://doi.org/10.2147/IJWH.S125784

Vandersarl Slocum, B. (2015). Dermatology. In M. C. Brucker & T. L. King (Eds.), *Pharmacology for women's health* (pp. 770–772). Jones & Bartlett Publishers.

Wang, V., Boguniewicz, J., Boguniewicz, M., & Ong, P. Y. (2021). The infectious complications of atopic dermatitis. *Annals of Allergy, Asthma & Immunology*, *126*(1), 3–12. https://doi.org/10.1016/j.anai.2020.08.002

Werfel, T., Heratizadeh, A., Aberer, W., Ahrens, F., Augustin, M., Biedermann, T., Diepgen, T., Folster-Holst, R., Gieler, U., Kahle, J., Kapp, A., Nast, A., Nemat, K., Ott, H., Przybilla, B., Roecken, M., Schleager, M., Schmid-Grendelmeier, P., Schmitt, J., . . . Worm, M. (2016). S2k guideline on diagnosis and treatment of atopic dermatitis—Short version. *Allergo Journal International*, *25*(3), 82–95. https://doi.org/10.1007/s40629-016-0110-8

Wilmer, E., Chai, S., & Kroumpouzos, G. (2016). Drug safety: Pregnancy rating classifications and controversies. *Clinics in Dermatology*, *34*(3), 401–409. https://doi.org/10.1016/j.clindermatol.2016.02.013

Yang, C. S., Teeple, M., Muglia, J., & Robinson-Bostom, L. (2016). Inflammatory and glandular skin disease in pregnancy. *Clinics in Dermatology*, *34*(3), 335–343. https://doi.org/10.1016/j.clindermatol.2016.02.005

55

Infectious Diseases

Lisa Noguchi

The editors gratefully acknowledge Elizabeth A. Parr who authored the previous edition of this chapter.

Relevant Terms

Arthropathy—joint disease

Avidity testing—measures the binding strength between antibodies and pathogens, used to differentiate patients with primary and past infection

Congenital—present at birth; can be caused by a genetic mutation, the environment in the uterus, or a combination of both factors

Congenital anomaly—structural or functional health problem present at birth that varies from the standard presentation (also known as congenital abnormality, congenital malformation, or birth defect)

Enzyme-linked immunosorbent assay (ELISA)—common serological test for the presence of particular antigens (direct) or antibodies (indirect)

Epidemic—occurs when there is an increase in disease cases above normal in a limited population or area (for instance, a single country)

Herd immunity—a situation in which a sufficient proportion of a population is immune to an infectious disease (through vaccination and/or prior illness) to make its spread from person to person unlikely

Immune globulins—proteins produced by the immune system in response to antigens like bacteria and viruses; also known as antibodies

  IgM antibodies are expressed on the surface of B cells and are produced as a body's first response to a new infection or antigen, providing short-term elimination of pathogens in the early stages of humoral immunity before there is sufficient IgG.

  IgG antibodies provide the majority of antibody-based immunity against pathogens in a long-term response and

are the only antibody capable of crossing the placenta to give passive immunity to the fetus.

Pandemic—an epidemic can become a pandemic if it spreads to several different countries or continents.

Polymerase chain reaction (PCR)—diagnostic tool that facilitates the amplification and detection of DNA or RNA of pathological organisms

Protozoan—single-celled, microscopic organism that can perform all necessary functions of metabolism and reproduction

Reference laboratory—laboratory facility that provides standard and well-defined measures for testing and for interpretation of testing

Semiallograft—a partial allograft in that half of the fetal genes come from a donor of the same species as the recipient but not genetically identical; adaptation of the immune system in the gestational parent allows for successful coexistence with the semiallograft that is the fetus/placenta

Seroconversion—the new development of detectable antibodies to microorganisms in the blood serum as a result of infection or immunization, from a previously negative state

Seroprevalence—the proportion of the population that has developed antibodies in response to exposure to an infectious agent

Vertical transmission—transmission of a disease, condition, or trait either genetically or congenitally; vertical transmission of an infection, also known as perinatal transmission, occurs in utero, during the birth process, or with breastfeeding

---

Introduction

Infections acquired during pregnancy are important causes of morbidity and mortality, with incidence of many infections strongly related to gaps in health equity and social determinants of health. **Congenital** and perinatal infections can result in significant consequences, such as severe fetal anomalies, fetal loss, and/or neonatal death. Ample evidence has demonstrated the impact of such infections on early and later childhood morbidities, growth, and development. Long-term disabilities that result from **congenital**

Prenatal and Postnatal Care: A Person-Centered Approach, Third Edition. Edited by Karen Trister Grace, Cindy L. Farley, Noelene K. Jeffers, and Tanya Tringali.
© 2024 John Wiley & Sons Ltd. Published 2024 by John Wiley & Sons Ltd.
Companion website: www.wiley.com/go/grace/prenatal

anomalies have a significant impact on individuals and families, particularly in settings with inadequate systems in place to support the rights and needs of disabled persons. Importantly, the person who acquires an infection during pregnancy may be symptomatic or asymptomatic. Normal changes to the immune system during pregnancy can contribute to more serious forms of infection, including sepsis. The timing of infection and whether it is a primary or secondary infection should also be considered to determine the potential risk to the fetus. Providers must be aware of which conditions are reportable to local, state, and national agencies. As a rule, they should be prepared to assist clients who need information on local and nonlocal options for pregnancy termination, regardless of context. However, this may be especially relevant in the context of congenital infection, which in some cases may have devastating impacts on the fetus and not be apparent until later in pregnancy. Thus, to provide high-quality care, prenatal and postnatal care providers need a solid grasp of risk factors, clinical presentation, appropriate screening, diagnosis, and management strategies for a range of infections that may intersect with prenatal and postnatal care. While gender-inclusive language is used throughout this chapter, it should be noted that gender was not measured in most studies cited here. To date, inadequate attention to the ethical inclusion of pregnant and breastfeeding people in clinical research on vaccines and treatment of infections in pregnancy has contributed to evidence gaps on safety and efficacy in these populations.

This chapter discusses the infections caused by cytomegalovirus (CMV), group B *Streptococcus* (GBS), hepatitis (A, B, and C), parvovirus B19, rubella, toxoplasmosis, varicella, Ebola virus, Zika virus, and monkeypox virus. The prevention, diagnosis, and management of infections in pregnancy can be complex, with rapidly evolving evidence. Reliable online resources, such as the CDC Pink Book can provide up-to-date guidance on the epidemiology and prevention of vaccine-preventable infections, including among pregnant people (CDC, 2021a). As many infections may have adverse impacts in pregnancy outside the United States, it is critical for prenatal care providers to discuss past and planned travel with clients, so that this context can be incorporated into appropriate counseling, diagnosis, and clinical management decisions. The infection caused by SARS-CoV-2 virus, COVID-19, is given special attention because of the potential for substantial negative impact on the health of pregnant people. Prenatal and postnatal care providers must stay current on the rapidly evolving research and recommended prevention and management of these infections and be alert for new emerging infectious diseases (EIDs). When clinical decisions are not straightforward, consultation with experts in infectious disease is highly recommended, and essential when caring for those living with immune compromise.

Health equity key points

- Infections acquired during pregnancy are important causes of morbidity and mortality, with incidence of many infections strongly related to gaps in health equity and social determinants of health.
- A comprehensive approach to prevention and management of infections in pregnancy requires healthcare institutions and systems to address systemic barriers to equitable care, including racial disparities in access to primary care, vaccination, screening, diagnosis, and treatment.
- A disproportionately high number of infections and deaths due to COVID-19 in the United States occur among Black people, with substantial evidence pointing to systemic inequities in health systems and disparities in social determinants of health as key drivers.
- The damaging effects of colonialism on health systems in many countries have hampered local efforts to address prevention and management of infectious disease, including during pregnancy.

Cytomegalovirus

CMV, a member of the herpesvirus family, is the most common congenital infection (American College of Obstetricians and Gynecologists [ACOG], 2020). CMV is transmitted via bodily fluids such as blood, tears, semen, cervicovaginal secretions, saliva, urine, and breast milk (Centers for Disease Control and Prevention [CDC], 2020e). Infected children shed CMV in their urine, which is why transmission is common in daycare settings and between young children and parents or siblings (Cannon et al., 2012). Secondary infections are caused by reactivation of dormant infections or infection by different strains of CMV. Postnatal CMV infection acquired by exposure to unpasteurized breast milk is a particular concern for extremely premature newborns (Park et al., 2021).

Over 50% of adults in the United States are infected with CMV by the time they reach age 40 (CDC, 2020a). Racial and socioeconomic health disparities in **seroprevalence** of CMV and birth prevalence of congenital CMV have persisted for many years. Approximately 1–4% of pregnancies among seronegative people will be exposed to a primary CMV infection (ACOG, 2020). The overall probability of intrauterine transmission is 30–40% when there is a primary infection during the pregnancy. Most literature surrounding recurrent CMV infection resulting in a symptomatic neonate comes from case reports. Intrauterine transmission has been estimated at 0.5–2% when there is a secondary infection (Society for Maternal-Fetal Medicine [SMFM] et al., 2016; Figure 55.1). Most congenital CMV infections and related disabilities result from primary infections during pregnancy (ACOG, 2020). While the overall risk of congenital infection is much lower during the first trimester (Lazzarotto et al., 2011),

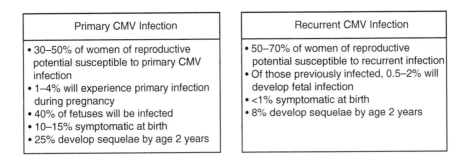

Primary CMV Infection	Recurrent CMV Infection
• 30–50% of women of reproductive potential susceptible to primary CMV infection • 1–4% will experience primary infection during pregnancy • 40% of fetuses will be infected • 10–15% symptomatic at birth • 25% develop sequelae by age 2 years	• 50–70% of women of reproductive potential susceptible to recurrent infection • Of those previously infected, 0.5–2% will develop fetal infection • <1% symptomatic at birth • 8% develop sequelae by age 2 years

Figure 55.1   Risks associated with CMV infection during pregnancy. Adapted from SMFM et al. (2016).

the most severe fetal injuries occur as a result of intrauterine transmission during this period (Pass et al., 2006).

Potential Impact

Infection with CMV is not a health concern for the general population as it usually does not result in clinical illness in adults or children. Sensorineural hearing loss is the most common CMV-related disability, and CMV is the leading nongenetic cause of childhood hearing impairment (Lazzarotto et al., 2011). About 10–15% of infants with congenital CMV are symptomatic at birth and may exhibit fetal growth restriction (FGR), low birth weight, hepatosplenomegaly, splenomegaly, jaundice, pneumonia, thrombocytopenia with resultant petechiae, microcephaly, chorioretinitis and other ophthalmologic findings, sensorineural hearing loss, encephalitis, and/or cerebral calcifications (Dreher et al., 2014; Jin et al., 2017). About 85–90% of infants with congenital CMV have no signs or symptoms at birth, but 10–15% of these will develop associated disabilities that become apparent when the child is of school age (Stagno & Whitley, 1985; Townsend et al., 2013). Infants with symptomatic congenital CMV develop neurological sequelae that may include hearing dysfunction, neuromuscular disorder, psychomotor delay, ocular abnormality, delayed language development, and intellectual disability at incidences of 65–80%, and approximately 30% of severely infected infants die (ACOG, 2020).

Clinical Presentation and Assessment

Routine screening for CMV during pregnancy is not recommended (ACOG, 2020). The person with primary or secondary CMV infection will most likely be asymptomatic. Occasionally, they will exhibit signs and symptoms that mimic mononucleosis or influenza, including malaise, **arthropathy**, persistent fever, myalgia, and cervical lymphadenopathy. A diagnosis of CMV infection should be considered in the presence of these findings. Congenital CMV should also be considered in the presence of abnormal ultrasound results that include FGR, ventriculomegaly, pleural effusion, hepatosplenomegaly, placental enlargement, oligohydramnios, or polyhydramnios, echodensities of the bowel or liver, hydrocephalus, microcephaly, ascites or hydrops, or calcified lesions in the brain (Adler, 2011, Imafuku et al., 2020).

A focused health history in this context includes household members and workplace exposures, particularly where young children or infants are present. Information regarding recent CMV infection in the home, workplace, or day care, and patient report of symptoms is elicited. A targeted physical examination consists of vital signs, including temperature, evaluation for hepatosplenomegaly, lymphadenopathy, arthralgia, and routine prenatal physical assessment, including fundal height.

In the case of suspected infection in pregnancy or abnormal ultrasound results that suggest congenital CMV, laboratory testing may be indicated (ACOG, 2020). Active infection with CMV can be diagnosed by **polymerase chain reaction (PCR)** or viral culture taken from urine, saliva, the oropharynx, or other body tissues. Serologic testing is the most common approach. Collection of serum samples three to four weeks apart with testing in parallel for anti-CMV IgG is needed for diagnosis of primary CMV infection. **Seroconversion** of **IgG antibodies** or significant (greater than fourfold) increase in anti-CMV IgG titers is diagnostic of infection, but initial seronegative data are rarely available (Adler, 2011). Serological assays for IgM and IgG antibodies are obtained when primary infection is suspected. Because IgG **avidity** has been shown to reliably detect recent primary CMV infection, this test should also be performed (Adler, 2011). Serological assays can be confusing because the IgM antibody can remain positive for four to six months following acute infection and can be detected in a subset of recurrent infections. The presence of the IgM antibody alone is not diagnostic of primary CMV infection but, together with the presence of low-avidity IgG antibodies, is considered evidence of a primary infection (ACOG, 2020). Thus, for those suspected of having primary CMV infection in pregnancy, diagnosis should be either by IgG seroconversion or with positive CMV IgM, positive IgG, and low IgG avidity.

When testing indicates primary CMV infection in the pregnant person or when a fetal anomaly is detected, congenital infection can be identified by both viral culture and PCR to detect CMV in the amniotic fluid. Amniocentesis is the best prenatal diagnostic tool to detect fetal congenital CMV infection, performed >21 weeks of gestation and >six weeks from infection in the pregnant person. However, detection of fetal CMV infection does not reliably predict newborn disease or sequelae.

Management

Treatments for CMV are either not approved for pregnant people or have not been successful in preventing or treating congenital CMV infections. A large multicenter trial found that CMV hyperimmune globulin did not decrease the incidence of congenital CMV infection or fetal or neonatal death among the offspring of people with primary CMV infection during pregnancy (Hughes et al., 2021). Some people may choose pregnancy termination in the presence of congenital CMV or fetal anomalies. Equitable access to abortion is severely limited depending on geography and the pregnant person's resources, and additional support may be needed for those who learn about the presence of anomalies at a gestational age that is near or beyond the gestational age limit for abortion in their area.

Consultation or collaboration should be considered in the presence of suspected or confirmed infection in pregnancy or fetal anomalies, for amniocentesis, serial ultrasounds, and management strategies. Counseling and support are provided, when appropriate, based on the following:

- Potential problems and resources for the parent and child can be discussed.
- With a secondary infection, congenital infection rate is very low.
- Vaginal birth and breastfeeding are appropriate options when CMV is detected.

Prevention

Most people have not heard of CMV and are unaware of how it is transmitted or the risks of congenital infection (Cannon et al., 2012). CMV vaccines are under investigation but are not yet available (CDC, 2020a). For people of reproductive age, exposure to young children under age 3 is the biggest risk factor for transmission of CMV (Adler, 2011; Cannon et al., 2012), and counseling messages have previously included a range of hygienic measures, including avoiding contact with young children's saliva and urine. However, such guidance may be difficult, impractical, and/or burdensome. At present, the value of such instruction is unclear, with recommendations differing on the potential of these strategies to reduce the risk of congenital CMV infection (ACOG, 2020; CDC 2020a, 2020e; SMFM et al., 2016).

Group B *Streptococcus*

GBS infection has for many years been a leading cause of bacteremia, sepsis, pneumonia, and meningitis in newborns (CDC, 2009). *Streptococcus agalactiae* is a Gram-positive, beta hemolytic bacterium that can cause invasive disease primarily in infants. Universal prenatal screening and antibiotic prophylaxis in GBS-positive people during labor led to a decrease in the incidence of newborn disease from 1.37 cases per 1000 live births in the 1990s to 0.22 – 0.29 cases per 1000 live births in recent years (Nanduri et al., 2019; CDC, 2020f).

Group B *Streptococci* colonize the vaginal and gastrointestinal tracts in 10–30% of healthy people (LeDoare & Heath, 2013). Colonization can be transient, intermittent, or persistent (ACOG, 2022). Neonates can acquire the organism by **vertical transmission** in utero or during the birth process. The transmission rate is 50% when the colonized person delivers vaginally, and 1–2% of infected neonates will develop GBS disease in the absence of intrapartum prophylaxis (ACOG, 2022; LeDoare & Heath, 2013). Available data do not confirm association between invasive procedures, such as membrane stripping, and GBS disease (ACOG, 2022; Kabiri et al., 2015). Pregnancy-specific GBS vaccines are in development and show promise but are not yet available (Mantel et al., 2022; Song et al., 2018).

Risk factors for early-onset GBS disease are intrapartum GBS colonization, gestational age <37 completed weeks, prolonged duration of membrane rupture, intra-amniotic infection, young age of the pregnant person, and Black race. Racial disparities persist with the incidence of GBS disease among Black infants more than twice that of white infants (CDC, 2022a). Data from 2019 also suggest that non-Hispanic Black persons with a negative antenatal screen may be more likely to convert to GBS-positive status before labor compared to non-Hispanic white pregnant persons (Spiel et al., 2019). While the precise etiologies of these differences in risk are unclear, increasing evidence points to structural and individual racism as underlying factors in all racial health disparities (Bailey et al., 2017; Williams & Mohammed, 2013).

Potential Impact

Colonization with GBS is not a clinical illness. Infection with GBS in the pregnant person is rare but can result in sepsis, amnionitis, and urinary tract infection (CDC, 2022b).

Early-onset GBS disease in infants often presents within 24 hours of the birth but may not be apparent for up to 7 days postpartum. Late-onset GBS disease becomes apparent between 7 and 89 days postpartum and can be the result of perinatal transmission or infection from another source (CDC, 2022b). Early-onset GBS disease of the newborn typically presents as sepsis or pneumonia. Meningitis can occur with early-onset disease but is more common in late-onset GBS, which is also characterized by sepsis.

Regardless of timing, GBS disease can result in hearing or visual impairment, cerebral palsy, and/or developmental disabilities (CDC, 2022b). Death due to early-onset GBS occurs primarily among preterm infants, with a case fatality rate of 19.2% among those born at less than 37 weeks of gestation; among term infants, the case fatality ratio is approximately 2.1% (Nanduri et al., 2019). Because of the continued burden of disease, the healthcare provider must be knowledgeable about current recommendations for GBS screening, prevention, and treatment. In 2018, the stewardship of and charge for updating the GBS prophylaxis guidelines were transferred from the CDC to ACOG and the American Academy of Pediatrics.

Assessment

Focused health history includes assessment of a prior history of early-onset GBS disease in another infant, history of GBS bacteriuria during any trimester of the current pregnancy, and current GBS culture results.

Antenatal screening is now recommended universally during pregnancy (regardless of planned mode of birth) at 36 0/7 to 37 6/7 weeks of gestation unless intrapartum GBS prophylaxis is already recommended due to identified risk factors (ACOG, 2022). This screening interval represents a change from previous guidelines (35–37 weeks). Cultures most accurately predict GBS colonization status at birth if GBS screening specimens are collected within five weeks before delivery. The 2020 recommendation of waiting until at least 36 0/7 weeks of gestation to collect the GBS specimen extends the predictive window for screening culture results up to 41 0/7 weeks.

Correct specimen collection is important. To collect the GBS specimen, the clinician uses a single swab to obtain a screening specimen first from the lower vagina (about 2 cm) and then from the rectum (about 1 cm) without the use of a speculum (Filkins et al., 2021). The pregnant person may prefer to obtain the culture, following appropriate instruction. Cervical, perianal, perirectal, or perineal specimens are not acceptable. Incorrect specimen collection (e.g., sampling only the vagina) is the most common GBS screening error among health care providers (Verani et al., 2014).

The American Society for Microbiology recommends that vaginal–rectal specimens are transported to the testing laboratory within 24 hours (Filkins et al., 2021). For those who are at high risk of anaphylaxis after exposure to penicillin, the laboratory requisition for prenatal GBS screening culture should indicate the presence of penicillin allergy, so that the laboratory recognizes the need to test GBS isolates for susceptibility to clindamycin (ACOG, 2022).

Management

Universal screening and the prophylactic use of antibiotics have been effective at reducing the incidence of perinatal GBS disease. When a person colonized with GBS receives antibiotics in labor, there is a 1 in 4000 risk of perinatal transmission; if the gestational parent does not receive antibiotics, the risk increases to 1 or 2 out of 100 (ACOG, 2022; Nanduri et al., 2019).

GBS screening should be done for most people at 36 0/7 to 37 6/7 weeks of gestation. People who have had a previous infant with invasive GBS disease or a positive GBS bacteriuria in the current pregnancy do not need to be screened as they qualify for intrapartum prophylaxis by history. People who plan a cesarean birth should be screened at the usual time in pregnancy to inform management in the event of prelabor rupture of membranes or unexpected vaginal birth. People who are GBS-positive during pregnancy should receive counseling and information based on the following:

Counseling pregnant people about GBS

- About one in four pregnant people carry this kind of bacteria in their body.
- Testing for GBS bacteria should occur sometime between 36 0/7 and 37 6/7 weeks of pregnancy.
- GBS is not sexually transmitted and can come and go in people's bodies without symptoms. There is no evidence to support treatment of sexual partners.
- Most cases of GBS colonization during pregnancy do not result in infant disease.
- Treatment before labor and treatment with oral antibiotics are not effective at eradicating GBS colonization.
- GBS colonization in a previous pregnancy is not predictive of colonization in the current pregnancy and screening is advised, in the absence of risk factors identified in the current pregnancy (bacteriuria).
- GBS bacteriuria in a previous pregnancy is not an indication for prophylaxis in the current pregnancy.
- Giving pregnant people antibiotics intravenously during labor can prevent most early-onset GBS disease in newborns.
- A pregnant person who tests positive for GBS bacteria and gets antibiotics during labor has only a 1 in 4000 chance of having a baby who will develop GBS disease. Without receipt of antibiotics during labor, the chance of delivering a baby who will develop GBS disease is 1 in 200.
- In the absence of known GBS status and the presence of intrapartum risk factors, for example, prolonged rupture of membranes or fever, antibiotic prophylaxis should be administered.
- Intrapartum GBS prophylaxis is not indicated when a cesarean birth is performed before the onset of labor and in the presence of intact amniotic membranes, regardless of GBS colonization status.

Prophylactic antibiotics are administered during labor when there is a positive GBS culture obtained at 36 0/7 weeks of gestation or more (unless cesarean birth is performed before labor in the presence of intact amniotic membranes), history of GBS bacteriuria in the current pregnancy during any trimester, or history of previous infant with GBS invasive disease. If screening has not been done during the pregnancy, prophylaxis is administered based on the presence of risk factors for early-onset GBS disease of the newborn (ACOG, 2022). Risk factors include substantial risk of preterm birth, preterm prelabor rupture of membranes (PPROM) or rupture of membranes for 18 or more hours at term, or intrapartum fever (temperature 100.4 °F [38 °C] or higher). Maternal antibiotic prophylaxis is most effective if initiated 4 hours or more before birth (Fairlie et al., 2013). The current ACOG recommendation for intrapartum prophylaxis is to administer penicillin, with ampicillin being an acceptable alternative. Resistance to clindamycin, the most common agent used in this population, is increasing; clindamycin is recommended only if the GBS isolate is confirmed to be susceptible to clindamycin (ACOG, 2022). Penicillin allergy testing is safe during pregnancy and can be beneficial for all pregnant people who report a penicillin allergy, particularly those that are suggestive of being IgE mediated, or of unknown severity, or both (ACOG, 2022). As most people with a reported penicillin allergy are actually penicillin tolerant, use of penicillin allergy testing is increasing as part of antibiotic stewardship initiatives, and expansion of its use has been encouraged in obstetric patients. The potential impact of immersion in water during labor and birth in individuals colonized with GBS has not been well studied. Guidelines in the UK do not advise against immersion in water during labor or birth for women colonized with GBS who have been offered appropriate intrapartum antibiotic prophylaxis if no other contraindications to water immersion are present (Hughes et al., 2017).

Alternatives to antibiotic therapy for GBS colonization do not have sufficient evidence to support their use. Current evidence supports universal screening and antibiotic therapy for GBS-positive people in labor to reduce the rate of GBS disease of the newborn (ACOG, 2022).

Hepatitis A

Hepatitis A virus (HAV) is a small RNA virus transmitted by the fecal-oral route, either by person-to-person contact or by consumption of contaminated food or water. It is typically self-limited and does not result in chronic infection. The incubation period for hepatitis A is approximately 28 days after exposure, with a range of 15–50 days (Shin & Jeong, 2018). The virus replicates in the liver and is shed in feces from two weeks before to one week after the onset of clinical symptoms. While 80% of adults infected with HAV are symptomatic, the symptoms are usually mild and nonspecific and rarely include jaundice. Infections with HAV tend to be more severe with increasing age (Auwaerter, 2020; Willner et al., 1998).

HAV was responsible for about one-third of acute hepatitis cases in the United States until vaccination programs were introduced in the 1990s. The incidence of acute HAV infection in pregnancy is very low (Rac & Sheffield, 2014). However, hepatitis A incidence increased 1325% from 2015 through 2019, due to unprecedented person-to-person outbreaks reported in 31 states primarily among people who use drugs and people experiencing homelessness (CDC, 2020b).

Risk factors for HAV include exposure to contaminated food or water, substandard hygiene or sanitation, use of drugs, and having children in day care. Those who have emigrated from or have recently traveled to certain countries are also at an increased risk for HAV. An updated list of geographic areas of concern for HAV infection is maintained by the CDC (see *Resources for Healthcare Providers*).

Potential Impact

Hepatitis A does not cause chronic liver disease, and acute liver failure is extremely rare. However, 10–15% of patients can experience prolonged or a relapse of symptoms during the six-month period after they have been acutely infected (CDC, 2020b). The course of HAV infection during pregnancy is typically similar to that in nonpregnant

individuals, although complications have been reported (Cho et al., 2013). Transmission to the fetus is uncommon (Rac & Sheffield, 2014).

Assessment

HAV is diagnosed by serological testing. IgM anti-HAV antibodies appear early in the disease process and persist for several months. IgG antibodies, which predominate during the convalescent period, persist and provide immunity for life against reinfection. IgG antibodies will also be present after vaccination.

Management

Pregnant people who have close personal (household or sexual) contact with infected individuals should receive postexposure prophylaxis by a single intramuscular dose of HAV **immune globulin** (0.02 mL/kg) and the HAV vaccine, if they have not been immunized (ACOG, 2021). Immune globulin does not pose a risk to either a pregnant person or fetus and should be administered during pregnancy if indicated. Immune globulin provides protection through passive antibody transfer. When the immune globulin is given within two weeks of exposure, it confers protection for up to three months with 80–90% efficacy. The vaccine may be as effective when given alone as when combined with immune globulin, and some experts recommend the vaccine alone for postexposure prophylaxis in people under age 40 (ACOG, 2022).

Treatment for acute HAV infection during pregnancy is typically outpatient and supportive (rest, maintaining oral intake), and the infection is usually self-limited. Care should be taken to avoid alcohol, abdominal trauma, and medications that are potentially hepatotoxic. An infant born to an infected pregnant person may be given HAV immune globulin within 48 hours of the birth to prevent infection. Infected persons can safely breastfeed their infants with appropriate infection prevention precautions, including hand hygiene.

Prevention

Vaccines against HAV are the most effective means of prevention of HAV infection and are not contraindicated in pregnancy (ACOG, 2022). Vaccines are available as a single antigen or as a combination with hepatitis B antigen. The Advisory Committee on Immunization Practices recommends that pregnant people at risk for HAV infection during pregnancy (e.g., international travelers, persons who use injection or noninjection drugs, persons who have occupational risk for infection, persons who anticipate close personal contact with an international adoptee, or persons experiencing homelessness) or for having a severe outcome from HAV infection (e.g., persons with chronic liver disease or persons with HIV infection) should be vaccinated during pregnancy if not previously vaccinated (Nelson et al., 2020). Additional preventive measures include good hygiene, ensuring clean water, and counseling travelers to countries with intermediate and high HAV endemicity regarding infection prevention precautions. Heating food to about 185 °F for one minute and disinfecting surfaces with dilute bleach can decrease the risk of food contamination (ACOG, 2022).

Hepatitis B

Hepatitis B virus (HBV) is a highly contagious small DNA virus transmitted by blood and sexual contact. The incubation period is 60–150 days from the time of initial exposure (Hoofnagle & Di Bisceglie, 1991; CDC, 2022b). HBV is transient in 95% of HBV-infected adults, and they experience complete resolution of the disease with protective antibody levels. Approximately 2–6% of infected adults will develop chronic infection (CDC, 2023b). Most individuals with chronic hepatitis are asymptomatic, although some will report fatigue, anorexia, and malaise. Individuals with chronic HBV die at younger ages and higher rates from all causes and liver-related causes compared to the general population (Bixler et al., 2019).

The incidence of HBV in the United States has declined significantly since 1991, when prevention programs for screening in pregnancy and universal vaccination at birth were implemented (CDC, 2022g). It is estimated that approximately 5% of individuals in the United States have ever been infected with HBV and less than 1% of the population has chronic HBV infection (Lim et al., 2020).

The highest concentration of HBV is found in blood, but it is also found in semen, vaginal secretions, saliva, and wound exudate. The primary risk factors for HBV are injectable drug use and sexual contact with at-risk and/or multiple partners. Sexual transmission of the virus is quite efficient, and 25% of individuals with infected sexual partners will become infected themselves. The prevalence of HBV infection is disproportionately high among immigrant populations, especially Asians and Pacific Islanders (CDC, 2020c). Others at risk include healthcare workers, hemodialysis patients, and travelers to high-risk areas.

Potential Impact

Chronic hepatitis infection carries a much higher mortality rate (15–25%) than acute hepatitis (1%; Abara et al., 2017; ACOG, 2021; CDC, 2022b). Most chronic carriers of HBV are asymptomatic and can transmit the virus unknowingly for many years. Chronic disease can persist for decades, slowly progressing to cirrhosis or hepatocellular carcinoma. More than 80% of hepatocellular carcinomas are associated with HBV (Liu, 2020).

Acute HBV is the most common cause of jaundice in pregnancy. It is usually mild and well tolerated, with only 1% of acutely infected pregnant people developing severe liver disease (Rac & Sheffield, 2014). There does not appear to be any increased risk of mortality or teratogenicity with acute HBV in pregnancy, although there are some reports of an increased incidence of low birth weight and prematurity (Rac & Sheffield, 2014; Dionne-Odom et al., 2016).

Fewer than 1% of pregnant people are infected with chronic hepatitis B (Dionne-Odom et al., 2016). Most pregnant people with chronic HBV tolerate pregnancy well, but hepatitis flares may occur. Chronic HBV in preg-nancy can be associated with an increased risk of gestational diabetes, preterm birth, and antepartum hemorrhage, but the data are not clear, and the risk of perinatal complications is low (Dionne-Odom et al., 2016; Patton & Tran, 2014).

HBV is able to cross the placenta, but transmission in utero appears to be infrequent. Most perinatal transmission occurs at the time of birth, with exposure of the infant's mucosal membranes to blood or secretions (Dionne-Odom et al., 2016). Infants who are not infected during birth are still at risk for infection during the postpartum period through close contact with the infected person, if they do not receive prophylaxis.

The risk of perinatal transmission is higher in people who are HBeAg positive (90% risk, compared to 10–20% in HBeAg negative people), have a high viral load, have threatened preterm labor, and who acquired the infection in pregnancy. The risk of neonatal transmission is highest when HBV is acquired in the third trimester (80–90%) as compared to the first trimester (10%; ACOG, 2021). Those infants who acquire HBV perinatally have a 90% chance of acquiring chronic disease. The hepatitis B vaccine series and one dose of hepatitis B immune globulin (HBIG) effectively prevent chronic HBV in 85–95% of these infants.

Assessment

Regardless of whether they have been previously tested or vaccinated, all pregnant individuals should be tested for hepatitis B surface antigen (HBsAg) at the first prenatal visit and again at delivery if at high risk for HBV infection (Workowski et al., 2021). HBV is evaluated by testing for the presence of specific antigens and antibodies, as follows:

- *Hepatitis B surface antigen*—HBsAg is present in both acute and chronic infections and indicates that the individual is infectious. It is the only serological marker that can be detected during the first three to five weeks in newly infected persons, before the onset of symptoms. HBsAg clears after acute infection in three to four months but persists in chronic carriers.
- *Antihepatitis B surface antibody (anti-HBs)*—Anti-HBs appears during convalescence from acute infection after HBsAg has cleared and continues to increase for up to 10–12 months. It can remain positive for the lifetime of those who have recovered from acute infection; it indicates immunity. It is also present in the serum of those who have been successfully vaccinated. In chronic carriers, anti-HBs is negative, but HBsAg is positive.
- *Antihepatitis B core antibody (anti-HBc)*—Anti-HBc is only present in a previous or ongoing natural infection; it is not present after vaccination. IgM anti-HBc appears with the onset of symptoms during an acute infection and persists for up to six months if the disease resolves. IgG anti-HBc appears during convalescence and usually persists for life.
- *HBe antigen (hBeAg)*—HBeAg is present in acute or chronic infection and indicates active viral replication and high infectivity.

• *Antihepatitis Be antibody (anti-HBe)*—This antibody appears during recovery of the acute phase and indicates decreased infectivity.

People at risk for HBV should be screened on admission for labor, as should those whose HBV status is unknown.

People at risk for HBV infection

- Infants born to people with HBV infection
- Sex partners of people with HBV infection
- Men who have sex with men
- People who inject drugs
- Household contacts or sexual partners of people with known chronic HBV infection
- Healthcare and public safety workers at risk for occupational exposure to blood or blood-contaminated body fluids
- Patients on hemodialysis

Pregnant people who are HBsAg negative and at risk for HBV should be vaccinated with three doses of the HBV vaccine at zero-, one-, and six-month intervals. If a pregnant person is exposed to HBV, they should have immediate screening for HBsAg and anti-HBs; if they are not immune, they should receive both HBIG and HBV vaccine (Dionne-Odom et al., 2016).

Management

Pregnant people with a positive HBsAg screen should have this result reported to state and local hepatitis prevention programs and be referred to a specialist in liver disease. Management of people who have acute HBV infection in pregnancy is primarily supportive. They are counseled to maintain good nutrition and to limit their activity to prevent upper abdominal trauma (ACOG, 2021). Periodic monitoring of liver enzymes and liver function testing is recommended. Hospitalization may be required for those who become seriously ill.

Pregnant people with chronic HBV may experience hepatitis flares, even if they were previously asymptomatic, and should be monitored for viral load and liver biochemical tests periodically. Hospitalization may be necessary with signs of liver decompensation.

Pregnant people with HBV infection should have viral load testing to help determine the risk of intrauterine infection. Antiviral therapy has been advised for pregnant individuals with HBV DNA greater than 200,000 IU/mL (7.6 log10 IU/mL; Terrault et al., 2016). Evidence indicates that antiviral therapy during pregnancy further reduces perinatal HBV transmission. The antiviral medications lamivudine, tenofovir (preferred agent), and telbivudine appear safe in pregnancy although data are limited (Brown Jr et al., 2016). Initiating antiviral medications six to eight weeks prior to birth allows time for the viral load to decline and reduces the risk of perinatal transmission (Brown Jr et al., 2016; Dionne-Odom et al., 2016). With

postexposure prophylaxis, comprised of hepatitis B vaccine and HBIG at birth, followed by completion of the hepatitis B vaccine series, 0.7–1.1% of infants develop infection (Schillie et al., 2018). These infants receive HBIG and the first dose of the hepatitis B vaccine intramuscularly in two different sites within the first 12 hours of birth. The remaining two injections in the series are administered within the first 6 months of life. If HBV status is unknown, the pregnant person should undergo screening, and the infant should receive vaccine within 12 hours of birth. Consultation and collaboration with HBV experts and pediatrics are recommended to ensure appropriate management of postvaccination serologic testing of infants born to HBsAg-positive patients and revaccination for those not responding to initial vaccination.

The risk of perinatal transmission of HBV with amniocentesis appears low, particularly in people with a low viral load; the test is offered to people when it is indicated, with appropriate counseling (Dionne-Odom et al., 2016). Vaginal birth is appropriate for people with HBV. Breastfeeding in people who are HBsAg-positive at the time of delivery is not contraindicated. Infants born to those chronically infected with HBV may breastfeed if the infant has received prophylaxis with HBIG and vaccine. People with bleeding nipples should abstain from breastfeeding until they are healed.

Prevention

All prenatal care providers should follow the national guidelines for screening and immunization (Schillie et al., 2018). The incidence of HBV infection has improved dramatically with the implementation of national prevention strategies. Routine screening of all pregnant persons is recommended because screening based on risk factors will detect only 60% of HBV carriers. When the recommended immunoprophylaxis is followed, the risk of perinatal transmission decreases from 90% to as low as 0.7–1.1% (Schillie et al., 2018). Both HBIG and the hepatitis B vaccine are safe in pregnancy. Three single antigen vaccines that contain HBsAg are licensed for use in the United States, as well as a three-antigen hepatitis B vaccine, and a combination vaccine for both hepatitis A and B. Over 95% of those vaccinated become immune (ACOG, 2021). To avoid misinterpreting a transiently positive HBsAg result during the three weeks after vaccination, HBsAg testing should be conducted before vaccine administration (Workowski et al., 2021).

HBIG contains anti-HBS and is recommended for those who experience a specific exposure to HBV, and those who have not responded to the HBV vaccine. When given within 24 hours of exposure, it provides protection for 3–6 months. Persons with chronic liver disease should be vaccinated against HBV. Unvaccinated individuals or persons known to have not responded to a complete hepatitis B vaccine series and who have been exposed to HBV through a discrete, identifiable exposure to blood or to body fluids that contain blood should receive HBIG and start the vaccine series. Immunoprophylaxis should be administered as soon as possible after exposure (preferably within 24 hours). For sexual exposures, HBIG should not be administered more than 14 days after exposure. Measures to prevent transmission of HBV to others should be discussed with people who are infected. However, it should be acknowledged that some measures (e.g., condom use) may be challenging to negotiate for some pregnant people, especially those with abusive partners.

Transmission preventive measures for HBV-positive people

- Avoid alcohol and potentially hepatotoxic medications.
- Avoid sharing household articles that could be contaminated with blood.
- Use condoms with sex partners.
- Identify household, sexual, and needle-sharing contacts so they can be tested and vaccinated.
- Inform all healthcare providers of HBV status.
- All HBsAg-positive pregnant individuals should be referred to their jurisdiction's Perinatal Hepatitis B Prevention Program for case management to ensure that their infants receive timely prophylaxis and follow-up.

Hepatitis C

Hepatitis C virus (HCV), a single-stranded RNA virus, is the most common blood-borne infection in the United States and the leading cause of chronic liver disease (Rac & Sheffield, 2014). The incidence of HCV has decreased significantly due to screening of blood donors, which has been mandated since 1992. An estimated 2.4 million people were living with chronic HCV infection in the United States during 2013–2016, and it is found in approximately 1% of pregnant people (Hofmeister et al., 2019). The majority of those infected with HCV are asymptomatic. Clinical symptoms occur in approximately 25% of exposed individuals. The onset is 2–24 weeks after exposure and can include fatigue, arthropathy, jaundice, myalgia, and generalized pruritis. The illness is generally mild and is often ignored or mistaken for transient viral illness. Chronic HCV infection develops in more than half of individuals who are positive for HCV. Most individuals with chronic HCV have no symptoms and are unaware they are infected and, thus, may unknowingly transmit HCV to others. At least 5–25% of people living with HCV infection progress to cirrhosis within 10–20 years, and of those, 20% will develop hepatocellular cancer, decades after the initial infection (CDC, 2023a).

Transmission of HCV is primarily parenteral, with risk factors being either injection drug use or having received a blood transfusion before 1992. Although it is not effectively transmitted sexually, 15–20% of those who are infected report sexual contact as their only exposure to HCV (CDC, 2023a). The risk of acquiring HCV through sexual transmission is higher in those who are living with HIV infection and have multiple sexual partners.

Risk factors for HCV infection

- History of injection drug use
- Birth to an HCV-infected gestational parent
- History of blood transfusion or transplanted organ received before 1992
- History of body tattoos or body piercings
- Healthcare workers, especially those experiencing needlestick injury
- Multiple sexual partners
- History of prior sexually transmitted infection
- HIV infection

Potential Impact

Pregnant people with HCV are at higher risk for intrahepatic cholestasis of pregnancy, prelabor rupture of membranes, preterm birth, congenital malformations, placental abruption, gestational diabetes, and overall perinatal mortality. Their infants are more likely to be of low birth weight or to be admitted to neonatal intensive care (Dunkelberg et al., 2014; Rac & Sheffield, 2014).

The risk of perinatal transmission varies; the best predictor is HCV viral load. HCV positive people who do not have detectable HCV RNA in their blood are unlikely to transmit HCV to their infants, but those who do carry a 4–8% risk of transmission. The risk of transmission is increased in people with higher viral titers (>100,000 copies/mL), people with HIV infection (two to three times higher), and those whose alanine aminotransferase (ALT) levels were elevated in the year preceding the pregnancy. Some studies suggest that perinatal transmission may be increased with invasive fetal monitoring, amniocentesis, and rupture of membranes for over six hours (Dunkelberg et al., 2014).

Assessment

As of April 2020, the CDC has recommended that prenatal care providers screen all pregnant persons for hepatitis C during each pregnancy. HCV is diagnosed by an **enzyme-linked immunosorbent assay (ELISA)** screening test for HCV-specific antibodies. HCV antibodies appear 6–10 weeks after the onset of illness and are present in more than 97% of infected persons within 6 months after exposure (CDC, 2023a). Any pregnant person testing positive for antibodies to HCV should receive a PCR test for HCV RNA, which is positive within one to three weeks after exposure. Pregnant persons with newly diagnosed HCV infection and abnormal serum aminotransferase and/or platelet levels should be promptly referred for further medical assessment to rule out liver fibrosis or injury and so antiviral treatment can be initiated at the appropriate time.

Management

There is no treatment for HCV in pregnancy other than expectant management, as the medications that are typically used, pegylated interferon and ribavirin, are contraindicated during pregnancy. At least four HCV protease inhibitors have been approved for use only in combination with other specified anti-HCV agents; however, these have not been evaluated for safety in pregnancy (US NIH, 2022). Phase 1 studies suggest that directly acting antivirals are well-tolerated and effective during pregnancy. However, large, prospective clinical trials are still needed (Curtis & Chappell, 2023). People who are infected with HCV should be referred to a specialist who treats chronic liver disease and counseled to abstain from alcohol and potentially hepatotoxic medications.

Vaginal birth and breastfeeding are encouraged and not contraindicated due to HCV. If the person has cracked or bleeding nipples, they should abstain from breastfeeding until they are healed (Rac & Sheffield, 2014).

Pregnant people infected with HCV should be counseled regarding possible transmission to sexual partners. They should not share personal items that could be contaminated with blood and should cover any open cuts. For secondary prevention of chronic liver disease, infected people should be counseled to avoid alcohol and hepatotoxic drugs, and should receive vaccinations for hepatitis A and B. Unlike hepatitis A and B, there is no effective vaccine against HCV. Providers should report HCV infection in a pregnant person to the infant's healthcare provider, as follow-up HCV testing is recommended.

Parvovirus B19

Parvovirus B19, often referred to as fifth disease, or erythema infectiosum, is a single-stranded DNA virus of the *Parvoviridae* family. Infections are more common in the winter and spring with respiratory spread as the most common route of transmission. Outbreaks often occur where there is high opportunity for exposure such as in schools and daycare centers. Transmission by hand-to-mouth contact and blood products is also possible. About 20–30% of infected individuals are asymptomatic (ACOG, 2020; Feldman et al., 2016). If symptoms are present, they are likely to be mild and nonspecific and can include fever, arthropathy, and malaise; transient aplastic crisis can occur in patients with hemoglobinopathy. In the third week after exposure, a bright facial exanthema, or rash, appears over the cheeks, giving the characteristic "slapped cheek" appearance. A lacy red rash may also appear on the trunk and extremities (Feldman et al., 2016; Society of Obstetricians & Gynaecologists of Canada [SOGC], 2014).

Potential Impact

Approximately 50–65% of women of reproductive age have developed immunity to parvovirus B19 (CDC, 2019b). Pregnant people who are not immune are at risk of contracting it. Infection with parvovirus B19 affects 1–3% of pregnant people (SOGC, 2014). The majority of pregnant people who become infected have no adverse pregnancy outcome, while less than 5% experience spontaneous abortion, severe fetal anemia, or nonimmune hydrops fetalis (CDC, 2019b). Parvovirus B19 replicates rapidly in red blood cells and is a potent inhibitor of erythropoiesis; this is the pathophysiology behind the resulting anemia and

hydrops (ACOG, 2020). Since most pregnant people who become infected with parvovirus B19 are asymptomatic, an accurate determination of the risk of fetal infection and spontaneous abortion is difficult. The highest risk of fetal infection occurs between the ninth and twentieth week of gestation and within two to four weeks of infection during pregnancy (ACOG, 2020; SOGC, 2014).

Assessment

Routine serologic screening for parvovirus B19 is not recommended for pregnant people. Laboratory testing should be performed when the pregnant person is exposed to or develops symptoms of parvovirus B19, or when abnormal ultrasound findings suggest congenital infection. Serology consists of ELISA testing for IgG and IgM antibodies. If the IgG is present but the IgM is negative, immunity is demonstrated. If both are negative, and the test was performed after the incubation period, the person is not immune and has not been infected. If both antibodies are positive, the person has been infected in the previous 7–120 days (SOGC, 2014). Pregnant people who have been exposed to parvovirus B19 during a known outbreak are understandably concerned. Counseling should address the client's concerns, with special attention to understanding potential risk and practical strategies for decreasing further risk.

Counseling pregnant people about parvovirus

- Most people of reproductive age have already been exposed and are immune.
- A lab test can determine the presence or absence of immunity.
- If no immunity is present, individuals with viral symptoms should be avoided.
- Animal strains of parvovirus do not infect humans.
- Most congenitally infected infants do not exhibit long-term sequelae.
- Handwashing can reduce risk.

Management

There is no treatment for parvovirus B19 infection. If a pregnant person is diagnosed with a recent infection, obstetrical or maternal-fetal medicine consultation is recommended (SOGC, 2014). Serial ultrasounds are done every 1–2 weeks for 8–12 weeks after exposure to evaluate for the presence of ascites, placental enlargement, cardiomegaly, hydrops, and growth restriction (ACOG, 2020). If hydrops is found, further care can include cordocentesis to determine fetal hemoglobin and reticulocyte count, possible intrauterine transfusion, and early birth.

Rubella

Rubella is typically an acute, mild disease caused by the rubella virus (RuV) that primarily affects susceptible children and young adults. Rubella, also known as German measles or three-day measles, is transmitted by direct person-to-person contact or by airborne droplets from the respiratory secretions of an infected individual. Replication of the virus occurs in the nasopharynx and regional lymph nodes (CDC, 2022c). On average, the incubation period is 17 days, with a range of 12–23 days (CDC, 2022c). Individuals are most contagious in the first days after the rash appears but can transmit the virus up to a week before and after. About 50% of rubella cases are asymptomatic and these individuals are also contagious (CDC, 2022c).

Rubella is usually a mild illness, but complications can occur and are more common in adults than in children. Complications of rubella infection include arthralgia and arthritis, which can occur in up to 70% of people (CDC, 2020d). Rarely, serious complications such as thrombocytopenic purpura and encephalitis may occur; these complications carry a high mortality rate (CDC, 2020e).

In addition to the potentially serious complications associated with rubella infection, the virus can be transmitted to the fetus during pregnancy and can cause congenital rubella syndrome (CRS; Lanzieri et al., 2023). CRS can result in spontaneous abortion, fetal death, low birth weight, and preterm birth. Hearing impairment is the most common manifestation of CRS, but other congenital anomalies including cataracts and other eye defects, cardiac anomalies, hepatosplenomegaly, and neurological abnormalities can occur. Congenital infection and sequelae are most severe early in gestation; defects are rare with infection after 20 weeks of gestation (McLean et al., 2013). Manifestations of CRS may not be apparent until early childhood when complications such as autism, progressive encephalopathy, and diabetes can be identified (WHO, 2011).

Fortunately, the rubella vaccination program has been very successful and fetal infection is relatively rare in the United States, with only 15 cases of congenital infection reported between 2005 and 2018. Despite high national coverage overall, local areas of low vaccine coverage allow outbreaks of vaccine-preventable diseases to occur, typically due to non-evidence-based concerns about vaccine safety (CDC, 2021c).

Presentation and Assessment

Rubella infection is associated with lymphadenopathy in the postauricular, deep cervical, and suboccipital lymph nodes, which persists for three weeks. Lymphadenopathy is followed by the appearance of a fine, maculopapular pink rash that begins on the face and spreads to the trunk and then the extremities. The rash resolves in the same sequence. Other presenting signs and symptoms include headache, conjunctivitis, nasal congestion, mild pyrexia, and arthralgia. An estimated 25–50% of infections are subclinical (CDC, 2022c).

CRS is not usually identified until after birth. In the case of suspected rubella, the focused health history includes the following: symptom review, rubella vaccination history, country of origin, and recent occurrence of rubella infection in the home, school, or workplace. Focused physical examination consists of vital signs,

including temperature, and evaluation for rash, lymphadenopathy, conjunctivitis, congested nose, and arthralgia.

Routine prenatal laboratory testing includes serological rubella IgG to determine whether the person has immunity to rubella. When there is suspicion of either infection in the pregnant person or CRS in the fetus in the absence of documented immunity, further laboratory testing is performed. Enzyme immunoassays are typically used for serological testing and are convenient, sensitive, and accurate. The optimum time-point for serum testing is five days after the onset of fever and rash, which is when >90% of cases will be IgM positive (CDC, 2020e). On the first day of rash appearance, approximately half of cases will be positive for IgM. Serological testing to detect IgG and **IgM antibodies** can be performed and stored in case further testing is later indicated. If the IgG is positive and the IgM is negative, the person is probably immune to rubella. If both tests are negative, they should be repeated in three to four weeks and at six weeks from the time of exposure (Roush et al., 2023).

IgM antibodies can usually be detected 4–30 days after the onset of illness, and often for longer. The presence of IgM antibodies is indicative of rubella infection. However, because the incidence of rubella is low, the presence of IgM can be a false-positive result, which can occur with illnesses with similar symptoms like parvovirus, or with a positive rheumatoid factor (CDC, 2022c). In the case of a positive IgM, the person should be retested in 5–10 days for IgM and IgG. If the IgG is positive, **avidity testing** is done. This testing can distinguish acute infection (IgM positive, low avidity, and a rise in IgG) from a false-positive or reinfection, which carries a low risk for CRS (IgG and IgM positive, high avidity).

The rubella virus can be cultured or identified by PCR analysis of specimens from the nose, throat, urine, blood, and cerebrospinal fluid, with the best results obtained from throat swabs. A positive culture or PCR analysis is considered positive evidence of rubella infection. If acute rubella infection is identified early in the pregnancy, PCR on chorionic villi sampling can identify fetal infection. Amniotic fluid or fetal blood sampling can be used later in the pregnancy (Nazme et al., 2015).

Management

There is no treatment for acute rubella except supportive care and symptomatic relief. A person with acute infection has an excellent prognosis. However, they will need counseling about the implications of CRS, and options for continuing or terminating their pregnancy, particularly if the infection is present in early pregnancy when the risk for severe birth defects is high. While some evidence has suggested that immune globulin may decrease risk of clinically evident rubella after exposure, this intervention has not been demonstrated to prevent asymptomatic infection, viremia, or CRS (Young et al., 2015).

Consultation or collaboration should be obtained when caring for a person with suspected rubella infection or fetal anomalies that may be associated with CRS. When immunity is demonstrated by serological testing, there is virtually no risk of acquiring rubella for the person or their fetus. CRS is very unlikely when infection occurs after 20 weeks of gestation.

Prevention of Rubella and CRS

Adherence to the recommended childhood immunization schedule is the first step in preventing rubella and CRS. People of reproductive age should be tested to document their rubella immunity status before becoming pregnant. The ideal times to screen people are during routine healthcare visits, family planning visits, and preconception visits. People who are not immune to rubella are offered vaccination unless they are pregnant or planning to become pregnant in the next four weeks. Vaccination is also offered to nonimmune postpartum people regardless of whether they are breastfeeding or have received Rh immune globulin. Rh immune globulin and other blood products have the theoretical potential to prevent development of antibodies after live virus vaccination; rescreening for rubella immunity three months after vaccination is recommended in those who received Rh immune globulin during or after pregnancy (CDC, 2013).

Some parents choose to decline or delay vaccinations for their children, citing concerns about adverse effects. The success of vaccines in eradicating various infectious diseases has also played a role; the current generation of parents may have no reference point for the devastating consequences of these infections. The concept of **herd immunity** may provide a false sense of security, as isolated outbreaks of these diseases do occur. If current trends in declining vaccinations continue, there is a public health concern for reemergence of these infections on a broader scale. While people have a right to decline vaccination for themselves and their children, providers should make sure that this is an informed refusal with the latest evidence available for their consideration.

Toxoplasmosis

Toxoplasmosis is a common infection caused by the **protozoan** parasite *Toxoplasma gondii,* which can be carried by many warm-blooded animals. Cats are the only animal in which *T. gondii* carries out its reproductive cycle and that shed *T. gondii* oocytes in their feces (Feldman et al., 2016). Human infection results from ingestion of raw, undercooked, or cured meats; contaminated soil or water; unpasteurized milk; contaminated seafood; transplant, transfusion, and congenital transmission, as illustrated in Figure 55.2 (CDC, 2022d).

Seroprevalence in the United States among people assigned female at birth who are of childbearing age (15–44) has been estimated at 7.5% (Jones et al., 2018). The incidence of infection during pregnancy has been estimated at 0.2 per 1000 pregnant individuals (Maldonado et al., 2017). Cases of congenital toxoplasmosis are estimated to occur at a rate of 500–5000 per year in the United States, with 400–4000 experiencing sequelae (Hampton, 2015). Congenital toxoplasmosis can occur when a previously uninfected person acquires the infection during or just prior to pregnancy. Congenital infection occurs in 20–50% of fetuses of newly infected people (ACOG, 2020; Feldman et al., 2016). The frequency of vertical transmission increases with gestational age. Approximately 750 deaths are attributable to toxoplasmosis infection yearly, and 50% of those are the result of eating contaminated meats (Furtado et al., 2011).

Potential Impact

Infection during pregnancy usually does not result in clinical illness. Symptomatic presentations are often nonspecific and mild and may include fever, chills, sweats, headaches, lymphadenopathy, myalgia, pharyngitis, hepatosplenomegaly, and/or a diffuse nonpruritic maculopapular rash.

Congenital toxoplasmosis is the primary concern. The frequency of fetal infection increases with gestational age at seroconversion; however, the overall frequency of clinical manifestations in the infant decreases with older gestational age at seroconversion. The greatest damage to the fetus results if infection occurs in the first trimester (Feldman et al., 2016). Severe sequelae can result from infection of the developing brain and include severe developmental delay, hydrocephalus, microcephaly, chorioretinitis, hepatosplenomegaly, jaundice, and seizures. Many infants are asymptomatic at birth, but most will develop learning and visual disabilities later in life if left untreated. Congenital toxoplasmosis is a significant cause of ocular infection that can result in macular retinochoroiditis later in life. Congenital infection in the first trimester can result in spontaneous abortion or stillbirth (Hampton, 2015).

Clinical Presentation and Assessment

The pregnant person with toxoplasmosis will most likely be asymptomatic but may present with self-limiting symptoms that mimic mononucleosis, including headache, fever, chills, sweats, pharyngitis, myalgia, and bilateral, symmetrical, nontender cervical lymphadenopathy. Rarely, the pregnant person may present with visual changes that result from chorioretinitis (Furtado et al., 2011) or nonspecific abnormal ultrasound findings, which could reflect other congenital infections (e.g., CMV, Zika virus infection, or genetic conditions, such as trisomy 21). In such instances, a range of possible etiologies should be investigated, in consultation with experts in reproductive infectious disease and genetics, whenever possible.

Prompt and accurate diagnosis of toxoplasmosis is important to reduce the risk to the fetus with treatment of the pregnant person. A focused health history includes recent history or habit of eating undercooked meat (especially pork, lamb, and venison), produce handling practices in the home, gardening, presence of cats in the home, and a review of pertinent symptoms. The focused physical examination consists of vital signs, including temperature; neurologic exam, including neurologic deficits, visual field deficits, gait disturbances, and

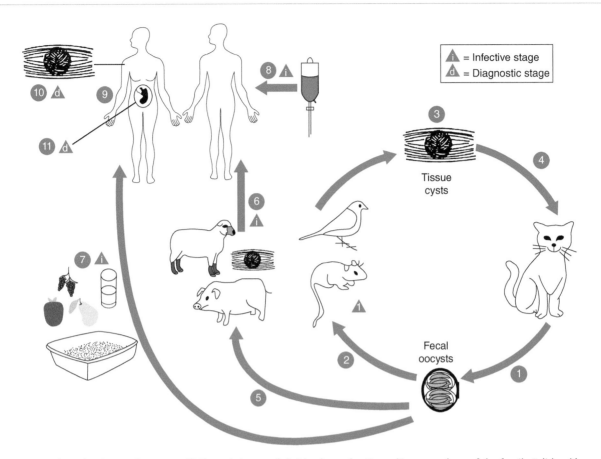

Figure 55.2 Life cycle of *Toxoplasma gondii*. The only known definitive hosts for *T. gondii* are members of the family Felidae (domestic cats and their relatives). Unsporulated oocysts are shed in the cat's feces (1). Although oocysts are usually only shed for one to two weeks, large numbers may be shed. Oocysts take one to five days to sporulate in the environment and become infective. Intermediate hosts in nature (including birds and rodents) become infected after ingesting soil, water, or plant material contaminated with oocysts (2). Oocysts transform into tachyzoites shortly after ingestion. These tachyzoites localize in neural and muscle tissue and develop into tissue cyst bradyzoites (3). Cats become infected after consuming intermediate hosts harboring tissue cysts (4). Cats may also become infected directly by ingestion of sporulated oocysts. Animals bred for human consumption and wild game may also become infected with tissue cysts after ingestion of sporulated oocysts in the environment (5). Humans can become infected by any of several routes: (a) Eating undercooked meat of animals harboring tissue cysts (6). (b) Consuming food or water contaminated with cat feces or by contaminated environmental samples (such as fecal-contaminated soil or changing the cat litter box) (7). (c) Blood transfusion or organ transplantation (8). (d) Transplacentally to the fetus (9). In the human host, the parasites form tissue cysts, most commonly in skeletal muscle, myocardium, brain, and eyes; these cysts may remain throughout the life of the host. Diagnosis is usually achieved by serology, although tissue cysts may be observed in stained biopsy specimens (10). Diagnosis of congenital infections can be achieved by detecting *T. gondii* DNA in amniotic fluid using molecular methods such as PCR (11). Image and information courtesy of DPDx of the CDC's Division of Parasitic Diseases and Malaria (2022). https://www.cdc.gov/dpdx/toxoplasmosis/index.html.

abnormalities in speech, cognitive, or affective functions; and assessment for cervical lymphadenopathy.

In the United States, where prevalence is low, prenatal testing for toxoplasmosis is not recommended routinely. Screening should be performed in people living with HIV infection and those who are immunosuppressed (ACOG, 2020). The primary diagnostic method is detection of *Toxoplasma*-specific antibodies, but, initially, IgG and IgM titers should be drawn (Table 55.1; CDC, 2022d). However, IgM antibodies appear at initial infection and may persist for years (Chaudhry et al., 2014). If the IgM result is positive, the clinician should attempt to determine whether infection occurred before or during pregnancy. Avidity testing should be pursued to help confirm the diagnosis and to clarify when the infection occurred. A high

avidity result in the first 12–16 weeks of pregnancy (time dependent upon the commercial test kit) essentially rules out an infection acquired during gestation. Estimating timing of infection is most challenging when the first serology testing is undertaken after the first trimester. If a toxoplasmosis pregnancy panel from a nonreference laboratory (e.g., commercial, clinic, or hospital laboratory) was used for initial screening, confirmatory testing should be performed by an experienced **reference laboratory**. The US Food and Drug Administration (FDA) has recommended that sera with positive IgM test results obtained at nonreference laboratories should be sent to a *Toxoplasma* reference laboratory.

When toxoplasmosis in pregnancy is suspected or diagnosed, amniocentesis and PCR after 18 weeks of gestation

Table 55.1   Interpretation of Results of Serological Tests for Toxoplasmosis

IgG result	IgM result	Interpretation
Negative	Negative	No serological evidence of infection with *Toxoplasma*.
Negative	Equivocal	Possible early acute infection or false-positive IgM reaction. Obtain a new specimen for IgG and IgM testing. If results for the second specimen remain the same, the patient is probably not infected with Toxoplasma.
Negative	Positive	Possible acute infection or false-positive IgM result. Obtain a new specimen for IgG and IgM testing. If results for the second specimen remain the same, the IgM reaction is probably a false-positive.
Equivocal	Negative	Indeterminate: obtain a new specimen for testing or retest this specimen for IgG in a different essay.
Equivocal	Equivocal	Indeterminate: obtain a new specimen for both IgG and IgM testing.
Equivocal	Positive	Possible acute infection with *Toxoplasma*. Obtain a new specimen for IgG and IgM testing. If results for the second specimen remain the same or if the IgG becomes positive, both specimens should be sent to a reference laboratory with experience in diagnosis of toxoplasmosis for further testing.
Positive	Negative	Infected with *Toxoplasma* for 6 months or more
Positive	Equivocal	Infected with Toxoplasma for probably more than 1 year or false-positive IgM reaction. Obtain a new specimen for IgM testing. If results with the second specimen remain the same, both specimens should be sent to a reference laboratory.
Positive	Positive	Possible recent infection within the last 12 months, or false-positive IgM reaction. Send the specimen to a reference laboratory with experience in the diagnosis of toxoplasmosis for further testing.

Source: Adapted from CDC (2022d).

are used for the diagnosis of congenital toxoplasmosis. Ultrasound is recommended to evaluate the presence of fetal anomalies, which are not always present, but may include central nervous system abnormalities, hydrocephaly, hepatosplenomegaly, and FGR (ACOG, 2020; Chaudhry et al., 2014). The classic triad of congenital toxoplasmosis consists of chorioretinitis, hydrocephalus, and intracranial calcifications.

Management

Prenatal treatment of people with toxoplasmosis does not prevent the fetus from becoming infected, but it can reduce the severity of sequelae in the newborn, with the most benefit from being treated promptly upon diagnosis. Antimicrobial therapy against *T. gondii* may be offered to symptomatic and asymptomatic pregnant individuals diagnosed with *T. gondii* infection acquired during pregnancy to reduce the risk of congenital infection. Consulting with experts in maternal-fetal medicine, infectious disease, and neonatology is recommended to review available data and help the pregnant person make an informed decision. The gestational age at diagnosis impacts the choice of antimicrobial regimen, with many experts favoring spiramycin when treatment begins at a gestational age less than 14 weeks, and pyrimethamine-sulfadiazine, when begun at or after 14 weeks (Maldonado et al., 2017; Peyron et al., 2019).

Prevention

Information about modes of transmission and prevention of toxoplasmosis infection should be provided during preconception visits and during routine prenatal care

(Opsteegh et al., 2015). However, it should be noted that systematic reviews have found no high-quality evidence that such information changes maternal behavior during pregnancy, and that people living with limited resources may find it challenging to avoid all risks.

Counseling pregnant people about toxoplasmosis prevention

- Avoid drinking unfiltered water.
- Wash vegetables and fruit thoroughly before consuming to reduce risk of consuming contaminated soil.
- Wash hands, utensils, and cooking surfaces after touching uncooked meat and unwashed produce.
- Avoid eating raw or undercooked meat and shellfish. Cook all meat to a safe temperature using a food thermometer. Freezing before consuming appears to be effective at reducing risk of transmission.
- Wear gloves when gardening.
- Wash hands with soap and warm water if there is contact with soil or sand.
- Keep outdoor sandboxes covered.
- Avoid changing cat litter when possible and use gloves and hand washing when it cannot be avoided.
- Indoor cats that do not hunt and are not fed raw meat pose little risk for toxoplasmosis infection. The main sources of toxoplasmosis infection in pregnancy appear to be other sources (i.e., contaminated meat, soil, seafood, water).
- There is no risk of toxoplasmosis infection through intact skin.

Varicella

Varicella zoster virus (VZV) is a highly contagious DNA herpesvirus. Primary VZV infection leads to varicella (chickenpox) and establishes latency in dorsal root ganglia. Reactivation of VZV causes herpes zoster (HZ), commonly called shingles (CDC, 2021c). VZV is transmitted by direct contact with vesicular fluid or respiratory droplets (ACOG, 2020). The incubation period is 10–21 days and the disease is infectious 48 hours before the rash appears until the vesicles have crusted over (ACOG, 2020; Lopez et al., 2015). Due to varicella vaccination programs in the United States, the mortality rate from VZV infection is as low as 0.4 per 1 million population. The incidence of varicella is uncertain, as it is not a reportable disease. Mortality rates increase with age (Hamborsky & Kroger, 2015).

It is estimated that over 90% of pregnant people are seropositive for VZV IgG antibody and are therefore immune to infection. The incidence of varicella infection in pregnancy is approximately 1–5 cases per 10,000 pregnancies (Zhang et al., 2015). Congenital varicella syndrome (CVS) is a rare complication of varicella infection. The rate of CVS is 0.4–2% of fetuses of people who become infected with VZV in the first or second trimester (ACOG, 2020; CDC, 2021c).

VZV can also manifest as shingles or HZ (CDC, 2021c). After lying dormant for years or decades, the virus can reactivate, causing a blistering, painful, unilateral rash, involving one to three adjacent dermatomes. The rash is initially erythematous and maculopapular and then forms vesicles over several days that crust over. Full resolution of zoster can take two to four weeks, but the postherpetic pain may persist and can be significant. Shingles in pregnancy is not associated with the development of congenital anomalies, although the virus can be transmitted to the newborn, leading to neonatal varicella infection, if the shingles infection is active in the last weeks of pregnancy (CDC, 2021c). Pregnant people who are not immune to varicella should avoid exposure to individuals with shingles. Such exposure can result in the pregnant person contracting chicken pox, not shingles.

Neonatal varicella is caused by varicella acquired during the last three weeks of pregnancy and occurs primarily when symptoms of infection in the pregnant person appear between five days before birth and two days after birth. This period correlates with the development of IgG antibodies in the pregnant person and is too brief to provide transplacental passive immunization to the fetus or neonate (Bapat & Koren, 2013). Neonatal varicella that occurs in the first 10–12 days of life is usually the result of transplacental transmission of the virus. When neonatal varicella occurs after this time, it is most likely due to postnatal infection (Bapat & Koren, 2013). In the absence of treatment, newborns with neonatal varicella can develop severe neonatal varicella infection.

Potential Impact

Pregnant people are at increased risk for complications from VZV infection compared to nonpregnant adults. Complications include secondary bacterial infection of the skin, central nervous system manifestations, such as meningoencephalitis or cerebellar ataxia, and pneumonia or pneumonitis, either viral or bacterial. Less common complications include hepatitis, hemorrhagic complications, thrombocytopenia, and nephritis (Lopez et al., 2015). Approximately 5–10% of pregnant people with VZV infection develop pneumonitis, particularly people who smoke or those with a profuse number of lesions (Bapat & Koren, 2013; Shrim et al., 2012). Mortality in pregnant people is higher than in nonpregnant adults, and death usually results from respiratory disease (Bapat & Koren, 2013; CDC, 2021c; Shrim et al., 2012).

If the pregnant person acquires varicella infection early in gestation (weeks 8–20), the fetus is at risk for developing CVS (Enders et al., 1994). This syndrome is characterized by limb hypoplasia, skin lesions, neurologic abnormalities, and structural eye damage. The newborn with CVS may present with low birth weight, cutaneous scars, lesions, localized absence of skin on a limb, hypoplasia of one or more limbs, malformed digits, or various ocular and central nervous system abnormalities (ACOG, 2020; Lopez et al., 2015). With current management approaches to neonatal varicella, including the postpartum administration of immune globulin, the mortality rate has decreased to about 7% (CDC, 2021c).

Clinical Presentation and Assessment

The pregnant person with primary varicella can develop a prodrome of fever, malaise, headache, and abdominal pain one to two days before a rash appears. The rash typically consists of three or more successive crops of lesions that develop over several days. Each crop progresses from macules to papules, vesicles, and pustules, then crusts over, so that any part of the body may have lesions in different stages. The rash usually starts on the face and trunk and then spreads to the extremities. It takes four to seven days for all lesions to become crusted (CDC, 2021c). Varicella infection in the pregnant person may be complicated by varicella pneumonia, which has an unpredictable clinical course with rapid progression to hypoxia and respiratory failure, leading to high rates of mortality in untreated infection.

Following maternal infection, risk for CVS may be estimated using PCR testing of fetal blood or amniotic fluid for VZV DNA, in conjunction with ultrasonography for detection of structural abnormalities in the fetus. Ultrasound findings for the fetus with CVS appear after the VZV infection has subsided and can represent virus-specific deformation or nonimmune hydrops. The deformation sequence consists of some combination of limb hypoplasia, skin lesions, microphthalmos, and abnormal positioning of limbs. Nonimmune hydrops findings include hepatosplenomegaly, ascites, pleural effusion, pericardial effusion, and liver calcification (ACOG, 2020; Shrim et al., 2012).

The incidence of varicella disease is declining as a result of vaccination programs, making clinical diagnosis uncommon and more challenging. The focused health history should include history of varicella infection in the home, school, or workplace; documentation of varicella immunity by documentation of age-appropriate vaccination, laboratory evidence of immunity, or history of varicella disease or HZ; and a review of reported symptoms or prodrome. The focused physical examination consists of vital signs, including temperature, and examination of lesions, including type and crusting.

People who report a history of chicken pox are likely immune and do not need laboratory testing (ACOG, 2020). Varicella is diagnosed based on clinical presentation, but laboratory testing can be used to determine susceptibility to varicella or confirm varicella infection. PCR testing of skin lesions is accurate and convenient. If the lesions have resolved, tissue culture can be performed, but it is less sensitive (CDC, 2021c). The use of single IgM or IgG results cannot be used to confirm infection, though in the presence of a rash and positive IgM, the clinician can interpret the findings as confirmation of varicella. A positive IgM ELISA result is suggestive of primary infection but does not exclude reinfection or reactivation of latent VZV. Serology for IgM is considerably less sensitive than PCR testing of skin lesions; commercial IgM assay may not be reliable; and false negative IgM results are common (ACOG, 2020; Lopez et al., 2015).

Management

It is recommended that pregnant people be screened for varicella at the first prenatal visit to confirm their immunity. If nonimmune, people are offered vaccination at the postpartum visit (ACOG, 2020). Varicella zoster immunoglobulin (VZIG) has been shown to lower varicella infection rates and to reduce complications in nonimmune people. VZIG is administered as soon as possible after exposure but may be effective if administered as late as 96 hours after exposure (ACOG, 2020; Bapat & Koren, 2013). The intramuscular dose for VZIG is 125 units per 10 kg, with a maximum of 625 units. Serology should, if possible, precede the use of VZIG (Lopez et al., 2015).

The pregnant person with varicella pneumonitis should be referred for treatment with antiviral agents, which may be administered orally or intravenously if the illness warrants. Acyclovir is a synthetic nucleoside analog that inhibits replication of human herpes viruses, including VZV. It crosses the placenta and can act on the virus in the fetus as well (Shrim et al., 2012). When administered within 24 hours of onset of the rash, acyclovir has been demonstrated to be effective in reducing varicella-associated morbidity and mortality in pregnant people (ACOG, 2020).

Consultation or collaboration is indicated for people who develop varicella in pregnancy for detailed ultrasound and follow-up to screen for fetal consequences of infection. If pneumonitis develops during the pregnancy,

referral to specialty care and hospital admission is warranted. The neonatal care team should be informed of peripartum varicella exposure to optimize early neonatal care with VZIG. Counseling and support are based on the following:

Key counseling points on varicella infection

- A positive IgG ELISA result indicates antibodies to VZV either from past varicella or vaccination; this test should be done at a preconception or initial prenatal care visit.
- Varicella vaccination is recommended for all nonimmune people as part of preconception or postpartum care.
- Nonpregnant people who get vaccinated should wait one month to attempt pregnancy.
- A person who acquires a varicella infection during pregnancy should be made aware of the potential adverse sequelae, the risk of transmission to the fetus, and the options for testing.
- Breastfeeding of infants infected with or exposed to VZV is encouraged.
- If siblings at home have varicella, a newborn baby should be given VZIG even if the gestational parent is seronegative.

Prevention

Varicella immunization prior to onset of pregnancy can prevent the negative effects of varicella infection on maternal, fetal, and neonatal health. Postexposure prophylaxis can be provided to pregnant people without a history of varicella and those who are seronegative in cases of significant exposure to a person with varicella or zoster. As many US adults have serologic evidence of past infection, it may be cost-effective to screen serologically prior to prophylaxis, whenever feasible.

COVID-19

Severe acute respiratory syndrome coronavirus 2 (SARS-CoV-2) is the RNA virus that causes COVID-19. As of the time of writing, the COVID-19 **pandemic** has led to over 637 million cases and over 6.6 million deaths globally (Johns Hopkins University, 2022). A disproportionately high number of infections and deaths due to COVID-19 in the United States have occurred among Black people, likely related to systemic inequities in health systems and disparities in social determinants of health (CDC, 2023c). The National Center for Health Statistics has reported an 18.4% increase in US maternal mortality between 2019 and 2020. The relative increase was 44.4% among Hispanic, 25.7% among non-Hispanic Black, and 6.1% among non-Hispanic white women, with research suggesting a possible connection to conditions directly related to COVID-19 (respiratory or viral infection) or conditions exacerbated by COVID-19 or other healthcare disruptions (diabetes or cardiovascular disease; Thoma & Declercq, 2022). Evidence regarding prevention and management of COVID-19 infection during pregnancy continues to evolve.

Potential Impact

Pregnant individuals with COVID-19 infection may be asymptomatic or symptomatic. However, those who have a symptomatic infection during pregnancy appear to have a higher risk for severe sequelae compared with nonpregnant reproductive-aged cisgender women (Berghella & Hughes, 2022). Such severe sequelae include intensive care unit (ICU) admission, need for mechanical ventilation and ventilatory support, and death (Dawood et al., 2022; Metz et al., 2021). COVID-19 infection in pregnancy has been associated with an increase in maternal death or serious morbidity related to hypertensive disorders of pregnancy, postpartum hemorrhage, or infection other than COVID-19, as well as a trend toward an increase in cesarean birth. Other impacts noted in the general population, such as increases in gender-based violence, anxiety disorders, depressive disorders, posttraumatic stress disorder, and substance use disorders, have relevance to the care of pregnant people as well.

Those who are critically ill from COVID-19 infection also may be at increased risk for preterm birth compared with uninfected or asymptomatic pregnant people (Metz et al., 2021). The true incidence of vertical transmission remains unclear, but the overall rate of congenital infection has been reported to be less than 2% of maternal infections (Allotey et al., 2022). Rates of miscarriage do not appear to be increased in pregnancies affected by COVID-19 and neonatal outcomes are typically normal. Some studies have suggested higher rates of stillbirth, possibly related to disruptions in pregnancy care.

Clinical Presentation and Assessment

The initial clinical presentation of COVID-19 during pregnancy is typically the same as in nonpregnant people. However, one systematic review has noted that fever, cough, dyspnea, and myalgia may be less frequently reported among pregnant as compared to nonpregnant people (Allotey et al., 2022). It should be noted that some signs and symptoms of COVID-19 infection overlap with those of normal pregnancy, including fatigue, shortness of breath, nasal congestion, nausea, and vomiting. A thorough assessment includes type, duration, and severity of symptoms, as well as risk factors for severe COVID-19 illness and death, which include older age (particularly ≥35 years), obesity, preexisting comorbidities (particularly hypertension, diabetes, or more than one comorbidity), and being unvaccinated (Karimi et al., 2021; Kasehagen, et al., 2021; Kleinwechter et al., 2022).

Laboratory and imaging findings are also generally the same as those in nonpregnant people, with some laboratory findings overlapping with those caused by pregnancy-related disorders; of note, thrombocytopenia and

Table 55.2   Clinical Spectrum of SARS-CoV-2 Infection

Illness Category	Criteria
Asymptomatic infection	Positive test for SARS-CoV-2 but no symptoms.
Mild illness	Any signs and symptoms (e.g., fever, cough, sore throat, malaise, headache, muscle pain) without shortness of breath, dyspnea, or abnormal chest imaging.
Moderate illness	Evidence of lower respiratory disease by clinical assessment or imaging and a saturation of oxygen (SaO$_2$) ≥94% on room air at sea level.
Severe illness	Respiratory frequency >30 breaths per minute, SaO$_2$ <94% on room air at sea level, ratio of arterial partial pressure of oxygen to fraction of inspired oxygen (PaO$_2$/FiO$_2$) <300, or lung infiltrates >50%.
Critical illness	Respiratory failure, septic shock, and/or multiple organ dysfunction.

Source: https://www.covid19treatmentguidelines.nih.gov/overview/clinical-spectrum/

elevated liver chemistries may be seen in both COVID-19 infection and HELLP (hemolysis, elevated liver enzymes, low platelets) syndrome. Acute hypertension is a common finding in patients with preeclampsia or HELLP syndrome, but not a feature of COVID-19. Observational studies of SARS-CoV-2 infection during pregnancy suggest a 62% higher odds of developing preeclampsia among patients with COVID-19 (Conde-Agudelo & Romero, 2022).

The US National Institutes of Health has categorized degrees of disease severity in nonpregnant persons (Table 55.2; National Institutes of Health [NIH], 2022). This classification may be useful for describing illness in pregnant persons as well. However, the threshold for certain interventions differs for pregnant and non-pregnant persons, e.g., oxygen supplementation for pregnant patients is typically used when SpO2 falls below 95% (on room air at sea level) to accommodate physiologic changes in oxygen demand during pregnancy and facilitate adequate oxygen delivery to the fetus.

Management

Where feasible, prenatal care practices in areas significantly impacted by COVID-19 infection should consider modifying traditional approaches to prenatal care. For further guidance on modifications to prenatal care, the ACOG and the SMFM have issued recommendations for testing and reducing risk of transmission of COVID-19, outpatient assessment, risk stratification, and modification of routine protocols for prenatal visits, including telehealth. However, it should be acknowledged that unequal access to technology may lead to inequity in telehealth services (American College of Nurse-Midwives [ACNM], 2022).

Thus, modifications to services should be undertaken with care to avoid perpetuating gaps in equity.

Over 80% of pregnant people with known or suspected COVID-19 infection have mild illness (Huntley et al., 2020). In general, those with asymptomatic, mild, or moderate illness may be managed on an outpatient basis. Home-based care is supportive and includes rest and hydration. The SMFM maintains an evidence-based summary of outpatient treatment (e.g., monoclonal antibodies, antiviral medications) for COVID-19 infection during pregnancy (SMFM, 2022), with the position that therapies otherwise recommended should not be withheld specifically due to pregnancy or lactation. Ritonavir-boosted nirmatrelvir, remdesivir, bebtelovimab, and molnupiravir fall into this category. The approach to any antenatal testing will depend on the client's gestational age, clinical, other comorbidities, and discussions with the patient and the family that consider the possibly increased risks of stillbirth and perinatal morbidities in the absence of testing.

Pregnant people with COVID-19 infection managed in outpatient settings should be monitored for progression to severe or critical disease and given instructions for infection control, symptom management, and follow-up (at least once within two weeks of COVID-19 diagnosis). Warning signs that should prompt a call to the provider or seeking emergency care include worsening dyspnea, respiratory rate $\geq$20 to 24 breaths/minute, heart rate >100 beats per minute, SpO_2 <95% (if patient has access to an over-the-counter pulse oximeter), unremitting fever >39 °C despite appropriate use of acetaminophen, inability to tolerate oral hydration and medications, persistent pleuritic chest pain, and confusion or other alterations in mentation, in addition to usual obstetric warning signs.

In the inpatient setting, pregnant individuals with COVID-19 infection should be evaluated and monitored for signs of worsening illness and comorbidities that could complicate therapy. Pregnant hospitalized patients with severe disease, an oxygen requirement, plus comorbidities or critical disease should be cared for by a multispecialty team at a level III or IV hospital with obstetric services and an adult ICU (Donders et al., 2020). Management focuses on addressing hypoxemia and managing complications. Several guidelines advise that SpO_2 be maintained at $\geq$95%, which aims to address both parental and fetal oxygen requirements. In the absence of contraindications, prophylactic-dose anticoagulation is recommended for pregnant patients hospitalized with COVID-19, with treatment generally discontinued at the time of discharge. Dexamethasone can be used safely for maternal treatment and, in pregnancies at 23–34 weeks, to induce fetal lung maturation.

Prevention

Vaccination against COVID-19 has been proven to reduce the risk of developing COVID-19 infection and reduces the severity of disease if infection occurs. All evidence to date supports the safety of administering currently available SARS-CoV-2 vaccines before, during, and after pregnancy. For pregnant people, evidence supporting efficacy of SARS-CoV-2 vaccines also includes reduced rates of perinatal death and hospitalization among infants up to six months old. Administering the vaccine earlier in gestation maximizes the duration of benefit to the pregnant person. COVID-19 vaccines may be given at the same time as other vaccines provided routinely during pregnancy, such as influenza and Tdap. Personal preventive measures such as masking, physical distancing, frequent hand washing with soap and water, and use of hand sanitizer with at least 60% alcohol are recommended similarly in pregnant and nonpregnant people.

> **Counseling pregnant people about COVID-19 infection**
>
> - Currently approved COVID-19 vaccines are safe and effective during pregnancy and have no impact on future fertility.
> - Pregnant people with COVID-19 infection have a higher risk of severe illness and death compared to nonpregnant people.
> - Avoid interacting in person with people who might have been exposed to COVID-19. If you or someone in your household is sick with COVID-19, follow recommendations for isolation.
> - You can reduce your risk of getting COVID-19 infection by wearing a mask, staying at least 6 ft away from people who do not live with you, washing your hands frequently with soap and water for at least 20 seconds or using hand sanitizer with at least 60% alcohol, and avoiding crowds and indoor spaces that do not offer fresh air from the outdoors.
> - In addition to signs of obstetric complications (e.g., preterm contractions, vaginal bleeding, leaking fluid, severe headache, visual changes, decreased fetal movement, etc.), pregnant individuals should report and/or seek care for rapid breathing, shortness of breath, feeling confused, fever that will not go away, inability to tolerate liquids, and chest pain, all of which may be signs of a worsening COVID-19 infection.

Emerging and Reemerging Infectious Diseases

An EID is an infection that has appeared and affected a population for the first time or is rapidly increasing in incidence or geographic range (WHO, 2017). Outbreaks of EID are an ongoing threat to the health and well-being of people everywhere and are monitored by national and global organizations to rapidly identify the infection, efficiently mobilize personnel and medical resources, and quickly respond to control or eradicate the infection.

Healthcare providers must remain alert to the development of EIDs and recommendations for prevention, screening, and treatment. These recommendations evolve as understanding of the EID and its impact on pregnant and breastfeeding people grows. For those who work in under-resourced settings in low- and middle-income countries, understanding of EIDs, locally circulating infectious diseases, and their effects on perinatal outcomes is essential.

The damaging effects of colonialism on health systems in many countries have hampered local efforts to address prevention and management of infectious disease. Providers who work domestically must also be aware of EIDs abroad due to global travel and immigration patterns. Three examples of EIDs and their effects on pregnancy are presented in this chapter. Depending on the travel and immigration history of clients, other infections may be relevant for clinical practice in prenatal and postnatal care (e.g., Chaga's disease, dengue virus infection, and others).

Ebola

Ebola is a *Filoviridae* RNA virus that was first identified in 1976 in the Democratic Republic of the Congo (Jamieson et al., 2014). Ebola was initially transmitted to humans through fruit bats. Due to its virulence, it can be transmitted rapidly to others through direct contact, including blood or body fluids, contaminated objects, and possibly through sexual contact with an infected partner (CDC, 2021d). Since 1976, multiple countries have experienced large outbreaks (CDC, 2021c). From September 2022 until January 2023, a confirmed outbreak of Ebola virus disease (EVD) due to *Sudan ebolavirus* occurred in Uganda.

The incubation period for Ebola ranges from 2 to 21 days. Presenting symptoms include the abrupt onset of fever, chills, malaise, myalgia, diarrhea, vomiting, abdominal pain, and unexplained hemorrhage. A symptomatic person is contagious, and the degree of infectiousness correlates with how severe the presenting symptoms are (Jamieson et al., 2014). The mortality rate is 70–90% (Bebell & Riley, 2015; Jamieson et al., 2014), with severe dehydration leading to shock and organ failure. There is no treatment for Ebola other than supportive care, which includes isolation, fluids, electrolytes, and medication to treat gastrointestinal symptoms.

It is unknown if pregnant people carry a higher risk of Ebola infection. There appears to be a higher risk for spontaneous abortion and hemorrhage during pregnancy. However, mortality for pregnant individuals with EVD does not appear to be higher compared to those in the general population with EVD (Foeller et al., 2020). A high rate of transmission to infants occurs when pregnant individuals have acute EVD, and survival has been rare for infants born to persons with EVD during pregnancy.

If EVD is suspected, it can be confirmed with laboratory testing with PCR, antigen capture ELISA, IgM ELISA, or virus isolation (Bebell & Riley, 2015; CDC, 2021d). Management of the care of pregnant people with suspected or confirmed Ebola virus infection includes sensitivity to the stigma associated with infection, awareness of the risk of hemorrhage for the person and meticulous attention to correct use of personal protective equipment of the people involved in care. Robust data on treating pregnant people with EVD by use of investigational therapeutics are lacking. Expectant management of labor is recommended, rather than cesarean birth or induction of labor, because newborns are unlikely to survive and additional health risks are present (Bebell & Riley, 2015).

Breastfeeding should be stopped if acute EVD is suspected or confirmed in a lactating person or breastfeeding child. The child should be separated from the breastfeeding parent and provided a breast milk substitute. Children without confirmed Ebola virus infection who are exposed to breast milk of someone with confirmed EVD are considered contacts and should stop breastfeeding, followed by close monitoring for 21 days (WHO, 2020). If a breastfeeding person and their child are both diagnosed with EVD, breastfeeding should be discontinued, the pair should be separated, and appropriate breast milk substitutes should be provided. However, if the child is younger than six months old and does not have access to safe and appropriate breast milk substitutes, or adequate care, then the option to continue breastfeeding can be considered. Choices related to stopping breastfeeding, or continuing after EVD recovery and testing of breast milk, should be respected and supported by healthcare workers to facilitate the choice. Detailed guidance is available from both the US Centers for Disease Control and the World Health Organization (CDC, 2021d).

Zika

The Zika virus is a flavivirus that is transmitted to humans by *Aedes aegypti* and *Aedes albopictus* mosquitos (Petersen et al., 2016). Zika was first identified in Rhesus monkeys in the Zika forest in Uganda in 1947. Zika was confined to Africa and Asia until 2015, when it was first reported in Brazil. Since then, it has quickly spread through the Americas and Caribbean (Hamel & Hughes, 2016). The CDC tracks areas with active Zika virus transmission. However, the last cases of local Zika transmission by mosquitos in the continental United States were in Florida and Texas in 2016–2017. Since 2019, no confirmed Zika virus disease cases have been reported from US territories (CDC, 2022e).

Concurrent with the spread of Zika, an increase in the incidence of fetal microcephaly was noted. In 2016, the CDC confirmed a causal relationship between Zika and brain abnormalities (Fiorentino & Montero, 2016). That same year the World Health Organization declared Zika a Public Health Emergency of International Concern and recommended a delay in childbearing in endemic areas (Hamel & Hughes, 2016). The CDC then put out the first travel advisories and has provided detailed guidelines for healthcare providers that are updated regularly.

Transmission of the Zika virus appears to occur by several means. A pregnant person who has been infected with Zika by an infected mosquito can transmit it vertically to the fetus. It can also be transmitted through sexual activity, with most but not all cases likely due to transmission via semen. The virus has been identified in semen for several months after symptom onset. There is evidence that Zika may also be transmissible through blood transfusions and needle sticks.

Potential Impact

Although understanding about the implications of Zika in pregnancy is still evolving, a direct causal relationship between Zika infection and spontaneous abortion, fetal microcephaly, and other brain abnormalities has been established (Hamel & Hughes, 2016). Reported fetal and neonatal effects of the Zika virus, in addition to microcephaly, include brain atrophy, ventricular enlargement, intracranial calcifications, and ocular defects (Meaney-Delman et al., 2016). Early studies suggest that the rate of abnormalities in infants of affected gestational parents ranges from 1 to 29%. Congenital Zika syndrome has been characterized as a pattern of abnormalities including severe microcephaly, optical damage, joint abnormalities, and rigid body tone that restrict movement (Moore et al., 2017; CDC, 2019a). In one population-based study in Brazil, the risk of death was higher among live-born children with congenital Zika syndrome compared to all live-born infants in the cohort who did not have the syndrome and persisted throughout the first three years of life (Paixao et al., 2022).

Clinical Presentation and Assessment

Only one in five individuals who are infected with Zika virus will show signs of illness. Symptoms of Zika virus are typically mild and present similarly to other viral illnesses: mild fever, rash, headache, arthropathies, myalgias, pruritis, and vomiting (Hamel & Hughes, 2016; Meaney-Delman et al., 2016). Onset of symptoms is typically 3–12 days after being bitten by an infected mosquito, with duration of 2–7 days (Hamel & Hughes, 2016). Nonpurulent conjunctivitis is more common and severe in Zika compared to other viral illness, and hospitalization and death are quite rare (Hamel & Hughes, 2016). Zika infection is confirmed by at least one of the presenting clinical symptoms along with laboratory confirmation.

Every pregnant person should be screened by history for possible Zika exposure. Possible exposure is defined as "travel to or residence in an area of active Zika virus transmission or sex without a condom with a partner who traveled to or lived in an area of active transmission." A focused health history includes screening for signs and symptoms of Zika virus, travel history, and sexual history including an assessment of partner risk.

Universal laboratory screening for Zika in pregnant people is not currently recommended (CDC, 2022f). Because Zika IgM antibodies can persist for months to years after infection, Zika virus serologic testing is not recommended for asymptomatic pregnant people. Antibodies generated by a recent dengue virus infection can also cause the Zika IgM to be falsely positive. For asymptomatic pregnant people with recent travel to an area with risk of Zika outside the United States and its territories, Zika virus testing is not routinely recommended, but nucleic acid amplification testing (NAAT) testing may still be considered up to 12 weeks after travel. In contrast, for symptomatic pregnant patients who had recent travel to areas with a risk of Zika, specimens for Zika testing should be collected as soon as possible after the onset of symptoms, up to 12 weeks after symptom onset. It is recommended that testing be performed through state health departments or the CDC to ensure that reflex testing is available if needed and that additional serum samples are stored in case later testing may be indicated.

Management

There is no treatment for Zika other than supportive measures. People with Zika infection or symptoms of Zika infection should also be tested for dengue, which is also transmitted by the *Aedes* mosquito, and presents with similar symptoms (CDC, 2022e).

Counseling regarding the current information on Zika in pregnancy, and the limitations of that knowledge, is an important part of prenatal management of Zika-infected people. Pregnancy options should be reviewed, and referrals provided to abortion services if termination is desired. People with Zika who choose to continue pregnancy should be referred to maternal-fetal medicine, and pediatric providers should be informed (Hamel & Hughes, 2016). Zika is a reportable condition; local health departments should be notified upon diagnosis (CDC, 2022e). The CDC has established a US Zika Pregnancy Registry to collect information about infections and neonatal outcomes (see *Resources for Healthcare Providers*).

Pregnant people with possible exposure but without laboratory evidence of Zika infection during pregnancy should undergo ultrasound examination as recommended for routine prenatal care. For people with confirmed or suspected Zika infection, serial ultrasounds are recommended every three to four weeks. People with Zika infection should be informed that a normal ultrasound does not guarantee that their baby will not later develop complications, as some infants who appear normal at birth may later develop microcephaly and other abnormalities (CDC, 2022e). It is important to note that microcephaly can sometimes be mistakenly diagnosed when in fact the head is constitutionally small. Amniocentesis may be suggested when fetal infection is suspected, although how to interpret such findings is unclear.

Although the Zika virus has been identified in breast milk, its transmission through breast milk has not been confirmed. The benefits of breastfeeding appear to outweigh theoretical risks, and so this practice is still recommended in people infected with Zika (Centeno-Tablante et al., 2021).

Prevention

No approved vaccine is currently available for prevention of Zika virus infection. The primary mechanism for prevention is through avoidance of mosquito bites in areas where transmission is present. The CDC (2021b) currently recommends that individuals wear long sleeved shirts and long pants, treat clothing with permethrin, and use DEET repellents. Patients should be reassured that both DEET and permethrin are considered safe in pregnancy (CDC, 2019b).

Zika virus is detectable in semen for longer periods compared to other body fluids. Sexual exposure to Zika can be avoided by either abstinence or use of internal or external condoms if a partner has traveled to or lived in endemic areas. Couples attempting pregnancy have been advised to consult with healthcare providers to consider the potential risks and consequences of travel to areas with a Zika outbreak or other areas with risk of Zika (CDC, 2021b). Recommended timeframes for delay are not the same for all couples and depend on travel history and types of sexual exposure.

Monkeypox

Monkeypox disease is caused by infection with the monkeypox virus, which is from the same family of viruses as variola, the virus that causes smallpox. While monkeypox symptoms are like smallpox symptoms, they are generally milder, and the illness is rarely fatal. As of time of publication, monkeypox outbreaks in the US have been rare. Suspected cases of monkeypox during pregnancy should be managed in consultation with local public health authorities and specialists in maternal-fetal medicine. Pregnant people can spread monkeypox virus to the fetus through the placenta. While data are limited, case reports suggest the impact on the fetus may be severe (Mbala et al., 2017). The safety and efficacy of monkeypox vaccines and treatment have not been well studied among pregnant and breastfeeding populations.

Summary

While vaccines and antibiotics have led to remarkable strides in preventing and treating the progression and serious sequelae of many infections, infectious disease remains a leading cause of death worldwide. While most deaths due to infection during pregnancy happen at the time of or shortly after birth in the form of peripartum sepsis, other infections during pregnancy can have serious consequences for the pregnant person and the fetus. Due to the normal physiologic changes in pregnancy that allow the human body to accept the **semiallograft** of the fetus, pregnant people are generally more vulnerable to infection. Incident infection during pregnancy commonly poses more risk to the fetus as well. A thorough travel history is essential when screening and evaluating clients for possible infections in pregnancy. Healthcare providers need to be aware of guidelines for routine screening and remain vigilant to signs and symptoms of infection so that they can intervene in a timely manner. A comprehensive approach to prevention and management of infections in pregnancy requires healthcare institutions to address systemic barriers to equitable care, including racial disparities in access to primary care, vaccination, screening, diagnosis, and treatment.

Resources for Clients and Their Families

Prevent to Protect: Prevent Infections for Baby's Protection: https://www.cdc.gov/ncbddd/birthdefects/infographics/prevent2protect/index.html

MedlinePlus infections and pregnancy: http://www.nlm.Nih.gov/medlineplus/infectionsandpregnancy.html

SMFM Patient Handout: CMV Infection: https://www.smfm.org/publications/227-diagnosis-and-antenatal-management-of-congenital-cytomegalovirus-infection

Resources for Healthcare Providers

CDC. About Chickenpox: https://www.cdc.gov/chickenpox/about/index.html

CDC. Clinical Evaluation and Disease: https://www.cdc.gov/zika/hc-providers/preparing-for-zika/clinicalevaluationdisease.html

CDC. Epidemiology and Prevention of Vaccine-Preventable Diseases: https://www.cdc.gov/vaccines/pubs/pinkbook/index.html

CDC. Infectious Diseases Travel Alerts: https://wwwnc.cdc.gov/travel

CDC. Interpretation of Hepatitis B Serological Results: http://www.cdc.gov/hepatitis/HBV/PDFs/SerologicChartv8.pdf

CDC. Screening and Referral Algorithm for Hepatitis B Virus (HBV) Infection Among Pregnant Women: https://www.cdc.gov/hepatitis/hbv/pdfs/PrenatalHBsAgTesting_508.pdf

CDC. Sexually Transmitted Infections Treatment Guidelines, 2021: https://www.cdc.gov/std/treatment-guidelines/STI-Guidelines-2021.pdf

CDC. Viral Hepatitis in Pregnancy: https://www.cdc.gov/hepatitis/hbv/hbvfaq.htm

CDC. World Map of Zika Outbreak Areas: https://wwwnc.cdc.gov/travel/page/world-map-areas-with-zika

National Institute of Allergy and Infectious Diseases: http://www.niaid.nih.gov/Pages/default.aspx

World Health Organization. Introductory-level online course on pandemic and **epidemic**-prone diseases: https://openwho.org/courses/pandemic-epidemic-diseases

References

Abara, W. E., Qaseem, A., Schillie, S., McMahon, B. J., Harris, A. M., High Value Care Task Force of the American College of Physicians and the Centers for Disease Control and Prevention, Abraham, G. M., Centor, R., DeLong, D. M., Gantzer, H. E., Horwitch, C. A., Humphrey, L. L., Jokela, J. A., Li, J. M. W., Lohr, R. H., López, A. M., & McLean, R. M. (2017). Hepatitis B vaccination, screening, and linkage to care: Best practice advice from the American College of Physicians and the Centers for Disease Control and Prevention. *Annals of Internal Medicine, 167*(11), 794–804.

Adler, S. P. (2011). Screening for cytomegalovirus during pregnancy. *Infectious Diseases in Obstetrics and Gynecology, 2011*, 942937.

Allotey, J., Chatterjee, S., Kew, T., Gaetano, A., Stallings, E., Fernández-García, S., Yap, M., Sheikh, J., Lawson, H., Coomar, D., Dixit, A., Zhou, D., Balaji, R., Littmoden, M., King, Y., Debenham, L., Llavall, A. C., Ansari, K., Sandhu, G., et al. PregCOV-19 Living Systematic Review Consortium(2022). SARS-CoV-2 positivity in offspring and timing of mother-to-child transmission: Living systematic review and meta-analysis. *BMJ (Clinical Research Ed.), 376*, e067696. https://doi.org/10.1136/bmj-2021-067696

American College of Nurse-Midwives (ACNM). (2022). *Position statement: The use of telehealth in midwifery*. https://www.midwife.org/acnm/files/acnmlibrarydata/uploadfilename/000000000330/(FORMATTED)%202022_The%20Use%20of%20Telehealth%20in%20Midwifery.pdf.

American College of Obstetricians and Gynecologists (ACOG). (2020). Cytomegalovirus, parvovirus B19, varicella zoster, and toxoplasmosis in pregnancy. Practice bulletin no. 151. *Obstetrics & Gynecology, 125*(6), 1510–1525.

American College of Obstetricians and Gynecologists (ACOG). (2021). Viral hepatitis in pregnancy. Practice bulletin no. 86. *Obstetrics & Gynecology, 110*(4), 941–956.

American College of Obstetricians and Gynecologists (ACOG). (2022). Prevention of group B streptococcal early-onset disease in newborns. Committee opinion no. 797. *Obstetrics & Gynecology, 135*, e51–e72.

Auwaerter, P. (2020). Hepatitis A. Johns Hopkins ABX Guide. The Johns Hopkins University. https://www.hopkinsguides.com/hopkins/view/Johns_Hopkins_ABX_Guide/540260/all/Hepatitis_A.

Bailey, Z. D., Krieger, N., Agénor, M., Graves, J., Linos, N., & Bassett, M. T. (2017). Structural racism and health inequities in the USA: Evidence and interventions. *Lancet, 389*(10077), 1453–1463.

Bapat, P., & Koren, G. (2013). The role of VariZIG in pregnancy. *Expert Review of Vaccines, 12*(11), 1243–1248.

Bebell, L. M., & Riley, L. E. (2015). Ebola virus disease and Marburg disease in pregnancy. *Obstetrics & Gynecology, 125*(6), 1293–1298.

Berghella, V., & Hughes, B. (2022). COVID-19: Overview of pregnancy issues. In C. J. Lockwood (Ed.), *UpToDate*.

Bixler, D., Zhong, Y., Ly, K. N., Moorman, A. C., Spradling, P. R., Teshale, E. H., Rupp, L. B., Gordon, S. C., Boscarino, J. A., Schmidt, M. A., Daida, Y. G., & Holmberg, S. D. CHeCS Investigators(2019). Mortality among patients with chronic hepatitis B infection: The chronic hepatitis cohort study (CHeCS). *Clinical Infectious Diseases, 68*(6), 956–963.

Brown, R. S., Jr., McMahon, B. J., Lok, A. S., Wong, J. B., Ahmed, A. T., Mouchli, M. A., Wang, Z., Prokop, L. J., Murad, M. H., & Mohammed, K. (2016). Antiviral therapy in chronic hepatitis B viral infection during pregnancy: A systematic review and meta-analysis. *Hepatology, 63*(1), 319–333.

Cannon, M. J., Westbrook, K., Levis, D., Schleiss, M. R., Thackeray, R., & Pass, R. F. (2012). Awareness of and behaviors related to child-to-mother transmission of cytomegalovirus. *Preventive Medicine, 54*(5), 351–357.

Centeno-Tablante, E., Medina-Rivera, M., Finkelstein, J. L., Herman, H. S., Rayco-Solon, P., Garcia-Casal, M. N., Rogers, L., Ghezzi-Kopel, K., Zambrano Leal, M. P., Andrade Velasquez, J. K., Chang Asinc, J. G., Peña-Rosas, J. P., & Mehta, S. (2021). Update on the transmission of Zika virus through breast milk and breastfeeding: A systematic review of the evidence. *Viruses, 13*(1), 123.

Centers for Disease Control and Prevention (CDC). (2009). Trends in perinatal group B streptococcal disease—United States, 2000–2006. *MMWR: Morbidity & Mortality Weekly Report, 58*(5), 109–112.

Centers for Disease Control and Prevention (CDC). (2013). Prevention of measles, rubella, congenital rubella syndrome, and mumps, 2013: Summary recommendations of the Advisory Committee on Immunization Practices (ACIP). *MMWR: Morbidity & Mortality Weekly Report, 62*(4), 1–34.

Centers for Disease Control and Prevention (CDC). (2019a). *Microcephaly & other birth defects*. https://www.cdc.gov/zika/healtheffects/birth_defects.html

Centers for Disease Control and Prevention (CDC). (2019b). *Parvovirus B19 and fifth disease: Pregnancy and fifth disease*. http://www.cdc.gov/parvovirusb19/pregnancy.html

Centers for Disease Control and Prevention (CDC). (2020a). *Cytomegalovirus (CMV) and congenital CMV infection: For healthcare providers*. https://www.cdc.gov/cmv/clinical/overview.html

Centers for Disease Control and Prevention (CDC). (2020b). *Hepatitis A*. http://www.cdc.gov/hepatitis/hav/index.htm.

Centers for Disease Control and Prevention (CDC). (2020c). *People born outside of the United States and viral hepatitis*. https://www.cdc.gov/hepatitis/populations/Born-Outside-United-States.htm

Centers for Disease Control and Prevention (CDC). (2020d). *Rubella (German measles, three-day measles): For healthcare professionals*. https://www.cdc.gov/rubella/hcp.html

Centers for Disease Control and Prevention (CDC). (2020e). *About Cytomegalovirus*. http://www.cdc.gov/cmv/overview.html.

Centers for Disease Control and Prevention (CDC). (2020f). *Active bacterial core surveillance report, emerging infections program network, Group B Streptococcus, 2020*. www.cdc.gov/abcs/downloads/GBS_Surveillance_Report_2020.pdf

Centers for Disease Control and Prevention (CDC). (2021a). *Epidemiology and prevention of vaccine-preventable diseases*, (14th ed.). https://www.cdc.gov/vaccines/pubs/pinkbook/index.html

Centers for Disease Control and Prevention (CDC). (2021b). *Zika virus*. https://www.cdc.gov/zika/prevention/index.html.

Centers for Disease Control and Prevention (CDC). (2021c). *2019 viral hepatitis surveillance report – United States*. https://www.cdc.gov/hepatitis/statistics/2019surveillance/index.htm.

Centers for Disease Control and Prevention (CDC). (2021d). *What is Ebola virus disease?* https://www.cdc.gov/vhf/ebola/about.html.

Centers for Disease Control and Prevention (CDC). (2022a). *ABCs bact facts interactive data dashboard*. https://www.cdc.gov/abcs/bact-facts-interactive-dashboard.html.

Centers for Disease Control and Prevention (CDC). (2022b). *Group B Strep: Clinical overview*. https://www.cdc.gov/groupbstrep/clinicians/index.html.

Centers for Disease Control and Prevention (CDC). (2022c). *Manual for the surveillance of vaccine-preventable diseases*. Centers for Disease Control and Prevention.

Centers for Disease Control and Prevention (CDC). (2022d). *Toxoplasmosis*. https://www.cdc.gov/dpdx/toxoplasmosis/index.html.

Centers for Disease Control and Prevention (CDC). (2022e). *Areas at risk for Zika*. https://www.cdc.gov/zika/geo/index.html.

Centers for Disease Control and Prevention (CDC). (2022f). *Testing guidance*. https://www.cdc.gov/zika/hc-providers/testing-guidance.html.

Centers for Disease Control and Prevention (CDC). (2022g). *Frequently asked questions for health professionals*. https://www.cdc.gov/hepatitis/hbv/hbvfaq.htm

Centers for Disease Control and Prevention (CDC). (2023a). *Hepatitis C*. http://www.cdc.gov/hepatitis/hcv.

Centers for Disease Control and Prevention (CDC). (2023b). *Hepatitis B information*. https://www.cdc.gov/hepatitis/hbv/index.htm.

Centers for Disease Control and Prevention (CDC). (2023c). *Risk for COVID-19 infection, hospitalization, and death by race/ethnicity*. https://www.cdc.gov/coronavirus/2019-ncov/covid-data/investigations-discovery/hospitalization-death-by-race-ethnicity.html.

Chaudhry, S. A., Gad, N., & Koren, G. (2014). Toxoplasmosis and pregnancy. *Canadian Family Physician, 60*, 334–336.

Cho, G. J., Kim, Y. B., Kim, S. M., Hong, H. R., Kim, J. H., Seol, H. J., Hong, S. C., Oh, M. J., & Kim, H. J. (2013). Hepatitis A virus infection during pregnancy in Korea: Hepatitis A infection in pregnant women. *Obstetrics & Gynecology Science, 56*(6), 368–374.

Conde-Agudelo, A., & Romero, R. (2022). SARS-CoV-2 infection during pregnancy and risk of preeclampsia: A systematic review and meta-analysis. *American Journal of Obstetrics & Gynecology, 226*, 68.

Curtis, M. R., & Chappell, C. (2023). Evidence for implementation: HIV/HCV coinfection and pregnancy. *Current HIV/AIDS Reports, 20*(1), 1–8.

Dawood, F. S., Varner, M., Tita, A., Newes-Adeyi, G., Gyamfi-Bannerman, C., Battarbee, A., Bruno, A., Daugherty, M., Reichle, L., Vorwaller, K., Vargas, C., Parks, M., Powers, E., Lucca-Susana, M., Gibson, M., Subramaniam, A., Cheng, Y. J., Feng, P. J., Ellington, S., . . . Stockwell, M. S. (2022). Incidence and clinical characteristics of and risk factors for severe acute respiratory syndrome Coronavirus 2 (SARS-CoV-2) infection among pregnant individuals in the United States. *Clinical Infectious Diseases, 74*(12), 2218–2226.

Dionne-Odom, J., Tita, A. T., & Silverman, N. S. (2016). #38: Hepatitis B in pregnancy screening, treatment, and prevention of vertical transmission. *American Journal of Obstetrics & Gynecology, 214*(1), 6–14.

Donders, F., Lonnée-Hoffmann, R., Tsiakalos, A., Mendling, W., Martinez de Oliveira, J., Judlin, P., Xue, F., & Donders, G. Isidog Covid-Guideline Workgroup(2020). ISIDOG recommendations concerning COVID-19 and pregnancy. *Diagnostics, 10*(4), 243.

Dreher, A. M., Arora, N., Fowler, K. B., Novak, Z., Britt, W. J., Boppana, S. B., & Ross, S. A. (2014). Spectrum of disease and outcome in children with symptomatic congenital cytomegalovirus infection. *The Journal of Pediatrics, 164*(4), 855–859.

Dunkelberg, J. C., Berkley, E. M., Thiel, K. W., & Leslie, K. K. (2014). Hepatitis B and C in pregnancy: A review and recommendations for care. *Journal of Perinatology, 34*(12), 882–891.

Enders, G., Miller, E., Cradock-Watson, J., Bolley, I., & Ridehalgh, M. (1994). Consequences of varicella and herpes zoster in pregnancy: Prospective study of 1739 cases. *The Lancet, 343*(8912), 1548–1551.

Fairlie, T., Zell, E. R., & Schrag, S. (2013). Effectiveness of intrapartum antibiotic prophylaxis for prevention of early-onset group B streptococcal disease. *Obstetrics & Gynecology*, 121(3), 570–577.

Feldman, D. M., Keller, R., & Borgida, A. F. (2016). Toxoplasmosis, parvovirus, and cytomegalovirus in pregnancy. *Clinics in Laboratory Medicine*, 36(2), 407–419.

Filkins, L., Hauser, J., Robinson-Dunn, B., Tibbetts, R., Boyanton, B., Revell, P., on behalf of the American Society for Microbiology Clinical and Public Health Microbiology Committee, Subcommittee on Laboratory Practices. (2021, July 23). *Guidelines for the detection and identification of Group B Streptococcus*. https://asm.org/Guideline/Guidelines-for-the-Detection-and-Identification-of

Fiorentino, D. G., & Montero, F. J. (2016). The zika virus and pregnancy. *Current Obstetrics and Gynecology Reports*, 5(3), 234238.

Foeller, M. E., do Valle, C. C. R., Foeller, T. M., Oladapo, O. T., Roos, E., & Thorson, A. E. (2020). Pregnancy and breastfeeding in the context of Ebola. *Lancet Infectious Disease*, 20, e149–e158.

Furtado, J. M., Smith, J. R., Belfort, R., Gattey, D., & Winthrop, K. L. (2011). Toxoplasmosis: A global threat. *Journal of Global Infectious Diseases*, 3(3), 281–284.

Hamborsky, J., & Kroger, A. (Eds.) (2015). *Epidemiology and prevention of vaccine-preventable diseases, e-book: The pink book*. Public Health Foundation.

Hamel, M. S., & Hughes, B. (2016). Zika infection in pregnancy. *Contemporary OB/GYN*, 61(8), 16–18, 20, 22, 42

Hampton, M. M. (2015). Congenital toxoplasmosis: A review. *Neonatal Network*, 34(5), 274–278.

Hofmeister, M. G., Rosenthal, E. M., Barker, L. K., Rosenberg, E. S., Barranco, M. A., Hall, E. W., Edlin, B. R., Mermin, J., Ward, J. W., & Ryerson, A. B. (2019). Estimating prevalence of hepatitis C virus infection in the United States, 2013–2016. *Hepatology*, 69(3), 1020–1031.

Hoofnagle, J. H., & Di Bisceglie, A. M. (1991). Serologic diagnosis of acute and chronic viral hepatitis. *Seminars in Liver Disease*, 11(2), 73–83.

Hughes, B. L., Clifton, R. G., Rouse, D. J., Saade, G. R., Dinsmoor, M. J., Reddy, U. M., Pass, R., Allard, D., Mallett, G., Fette, L. M., Gyamfi-Bannerman, C., Varner, M. W., Goodnight, W. H., Tita, A. T. N., Costantine, M. M., Swamy, G. K., Gibbs, R. S., Chien, E. K., Chauhan, S. P., et al. Eunice Kennedy Shriver National Institute of Child Health and Human Development Maternal–Fetal Medicine Units Network(2021). A trial of hyperimmune globulin to prevent congenital cytomegalovirus infection. *The New England Journal of Medicine*, 385(5), 436–444.

Hughes, R. G., Brocklehurst, P., Steer, P. J., Heath, P., & Stenson, B. M. on behalf of the Royal College of Obstetricians and Gynaecologists(2017). Prevention of early-onset neonatal group B streptococcal disease. Green-top guideline no. 36. *BJOG*, 124, e280–e305.

Huntley, B. J. F., Huntley, E. S., Di Mascio, D., Chen, T., Berghella, V., & Chauhan, S. P. (2020). Rates of maternal and perinatal mortality and vertical transmission in pregnancies complicated by severe acute respiratory syndrome Coronavirus 2 (SARS-Co-V-2) infection: A systematic review. *Obstetrics & Gynecology*, 136(2), 303.

Imafuku, H., Yamada, H., Uchida, A., et al. (2020). Clinical and ultrasound features associated with congenital cytomegalovirus infection as potential predictors for targeted newborn screening in high-risk pregnancies. *Scientific Reports*, 10, 19706.

Jamieson, D. J., Uyeki, T. M., Callaghan, W. M., Meaney-Delman, D., & Rasmussen, S. A. (2014). What obstetrician-gynecologists should know about Ebola. *Obstetrics & Gynecology*, 124(5), 1005–1010.

Jin, H. D., Demmler-Harrison, G. J., Coats, D. K., Paysse, E. A., Bhatt, A., Edmond, J. C., Yen, K. G., Steinkuller, P., & Miller, J. Congenital CMV Longitudinal Study Group(2017). Long-term visual and ocular sequelae in patients with congenital Cytomegalovirus infection. *The Pediatric Infectious Disease Journal*, 36(9), 877–882.

Johns Hopkins University. (2022). *COVID-19 dashboard*. https://coronavirus.jhu.edu/map.html.

Jones, J. L., Kruszon-Moran, D., Elder, S., Rivera, H. N., Press, C., Montoya, J. G., & McQuillan, G. M. (2018). Toxoplasma gondii infection in the United States, 2011–2014. *American Journal of Tropical Medicine & Hygiene*, 98(2), 551.

Kabiri, D., Hants, Y., Yarkoni, T. R., Shaulof, E., Friedman, S. E., Paltiel, O., Nir-Paz, R., Aljamal, W. E., & Ezra, Y. (2015). Antepartum membrane stripping in GBS carriers, is it safe? (The STRIP-G study). *PLoS One*, 10(12), e0145905.

Karimi, L., Makvandi, S., Vahedian-Azimi, A., Sathyapalan, T., & Sahebkar, A. (2021). Effect of COVID-19 on mortality of pregnant and postpartum women: A systematic review and meta-analysis. *Journal of Pregnancy*, 2021, 8870129.

Kasehagen, L., Byers, P., Taylor, K., Kittle, T., Roberts, C., Collier, C., Rust, B., Ricaldi, J. N., Green, J., Zapata, L. B., Beauregard, J., & Dobbs, T. (2021). COVID-19-associated deaths after SARS-CoV-2 infection during pregnancy – Mississippi, March 1, 2020-October 6, 2021. *MMWR Reports*, 70, 1646.

Kleinwechter, H. J., Weber, K. S., Mingers, N., Ramsauer, B., Schaefer-Graf, U. M., Groten, T., Kuschel, B., Backes, C., Banz-Jansen, C., Berghaeuser, M. A., Brotsack, I. A., Dressler-Steinbach, I., Engelbrecht, C., Engler-Hauschild, S., Gruber, T. M., Hepp, V., Hollatz-Galuschki, E., Iannaccone, A., Jebens, A., et al. COVID-19-Related Obstetric and Neonatal Outcome Study (CRONOS) Network(2022). Gestational diabetes mellitus and COVID-19: Results from the COVID-19-Related Obstetric and Neonatal Outcome Study (CRONOS). *American Journal of Obstetrics and Gynecology*, 227(4), 631.

Lanzieri, T., Redd, S., Abernathy, E., & Icenogle, J. (2023). Congenital rubella syndrome. In S. W. Roush, L. McIntyre, & L. M. Baldy (Eds.), *Manual for the surveillance of vaccine-preventable diseases* (pp. 1–7). Centers for Disease Control and Prevention. https://www.cdc.gov/vaccines/pubs/surv-manual/chpt15-crs.html

Lazzarotto, T. T., Guerra, B. B., Gabrielli, L. L., Lanari, M. M., & Landini, M. P. (2011). Update on the prevention, diagnosis and management of cytomegalovirus infection in pregnancy. *Clinical Microbiology and Infection*, 17(9), 1285–1293.

LeDoare, K., & Heath, P. T. (2013). An overview of global GBS epidemiology. *Vaccine Supplement*, 4, D7–D12.

Lim, J. K., Nguyen, M. H., Kim, W. R., Gish, R., Perumalswami, P., & Jacobson, I. M. (2020). Prevalence of chronic hepatitis B virus infection in the United States. *The American Journal of Gastroenterology*, 115(9), 1429–1438.

Liu, L. (2020). Clinical features of hepatocellular carcinoma with hepatitis B virus among patients on Nucleos(t)ide analog therapy. *Infectious Agents & Cancer*, 15, 8.

Lopez, A., Scmid, S., & Bialek, S. (2015). Varicella. In S. W. Roush, L. McIntyre, & L. M. Baldy (Eds.), *Manual for the surveillance of vaccine-preventable diseases* (pp. 1–7). Centers for Disease Control and Prevention. https://www.cdc.gov/vaccines/pubs/surv-manual/chpt17-varicella.html

Maldonado, Y. A., & Read, J. S. Committee on Infectious Diseases. (2017). Diagnosis, treatment, and prevention of congenital toxoplasmosis in the United States. *Pediatrics*, 139(2), e20163860.

Mantel, C., Cherian, T., Ko, M., Malvolti, S., Mason, E., Giles, M., & Lambach, P. (2022). Stakeholder perceptions about group B streptococcus disease and potential for maternal vaccination in low- and middle-income countries. *Clinical Infectious Diseases*, 74(Supplement_1), S80–S87.

Mbala, P. K., Huggins, J. W., Riu-Rovira, T., Ahuka, S. M., Mulembakani, P., Rimoin, A. W., Martin, J. W., & Muyembe, J. T. (2017). Maternal and fetal outcomes among pregnant women with human monkeypox infection in the Democratic Republic of Congo. *Journal of Infectious Disease*, 216(7), 824–828.

McLean, H. Q., Fiebelkorn, A. P., Temte, J. L., Wallace, G. S., & Centers for Disease Control and Prevention. (2013). Prevention of measles, rubella, congenital rubella syndrome, and mumps, 2013: Summary recommendations of the Advisory Committee on Immunization Practices (ACIP). *MMWR Recommendations and Reports*, 62(RR-04), 1–34. Erratum in: *MMWR Recommendations and Reports* 2015 Mar 13;64(9):259. PMID: 23760231

Meaney-Delman, D., Rasmussen, S. A., Staples, J. E., Oduyebo, T., Ellington, S. R., Petersen, E. E., Fischer, M., & Jamieson, D. J. (2016). Zika virus and pregnancy: What obstetric health care providers need to know. *Obstetrics & Gynecology*, 127(4), 642–648.

Metz, T. D., Clifton, R. G., Hughes, B. L., Sandoval, G., Saade, G. R., Grobman, W. A., Manuck, T. A., Miodovnik, M., Sowles, A., Clark, K., Gyamfi-Bannerman, C., Mendez-Figueroa, H., Sehdev, H. M., Rouse, D. J., Tita, A. T. N., Bailit, J., Costantine, M. M., Simhan, H. N., & Macones, G. A. Eunice Kennedy Shriver National Institute of Child Health and Human Development (NICHD) Maternal-Fetal Medicine Units (MFMU) Network. (2021). Disease severity and perinatal outcomes of pregnant patients with Coronavirus Disease 2019 (COVID-19). *Obstetrics & Gynecology, 137*(4), 571–580.

Moore, C. A., Staples, J. E., Dobyns, W. B., Pessoa, A., Ventura, C. V., Borges da Fonseca, E., Marques Ribeiro, E., Ventura, L. O., Neto, N. N., Arena, J. F., & Rasmussen, S. A. (2017). Characterizing the pattern of anomalies in congenital Zika syndrome for pediatric clinicians. *JAMA Pediatrics, 171*(3), 288–295. https://doi.org/10.1001/jamapediatrics.2016.3982

Nanduri, S. A., Petit, S., Smelser, C., Apostol, M., Alden, N. B., Harrison, L. H., Lynfield, R., Vagnone, P. S., Burzlaff, K., Spina, N. L., Dufort, E. M., Schaffner, W., Thomas, A. R., Farley, M. M., Jain, J. H., Pondo, T., McGee, L., Beall, B. W., & Schrag, S. J. (2019). Epidemiology of invasive early-onset and late-onset group B streptococcal disease in the United States, 2006 to 2015: Multistate laboratory and population-based surveillance. *JAMA Pediatrics, 173*(3), 224–233.

National Institutes of Health (NIH). (2022). *Clinical spectrum of SARS-CoV-2 infection.* NIH COVID-19 Treatment Guidelines. https://www.covid19treatmentguidelines.nih.gov/overview/clinical-spectrum/

Nazme, N. I., Hussain, M., & Das, A. C. (2015). Congenital rubella syndrome—A major review and update. *Delta Medical College Journal, 3*(2), 89.

Nelson, N. P., Weng, M. K., Hofmeister, M. G., Moore, K. L., Doshani, M., Kamili, S., Koneru, A., Haber, P., Hagan, L., Romero, J. R., Schillie, S., & Harris, A. M. (2020). Prevention of hepatitis A virus infection in the United States: Recommendations of the Advisory Committee on Immunization Practices, 2020. *Morbidity and Mortality Weekly Report, 69*(5), 1–38.

Opsteegh, M., Kortbeek, T. M., Havelaar, A. H., & van der Giessen, J. W. (2015). Intervention strategies to reduce human toxoplasma gondii disease burden. *Clinical Infectious Disease, 60*(1), 101.

Paixao, E. S., Cardim, L. L., Costa, M. C. N., Brickley, E. B., de Carvalho-Sauer, R. C. O., Carmo, E. H., Andrade, R. F. S., Rodrigues, M. S., Veiga, R. V., Costa, L. C., Moore, C. A., França, G. V. A., Smeeth, L., Rodrigues, L. C., Barreto, M. L., & Teixeira, M. G. (2022). Mortality from congenital Zika syndrome – Nationwide Cohort Study in Brazil. *The New England Journal of Medicine, 386*(8), 757–767.

Park, H. W., Cho, M. H., Bae, S. H., Lee, R., & Kim, K. S. (2021). Incidence of postnatal CMV infection among breastfed preterm infants: A systematic review and meta-analysis. *Journal of Korean Medical Science, 36*(12), e84.

Pass, R. F., Fowler, K. B., Boppana, S. B., Britt, W. J., & Stagno, S. (2006). Congenital cytomegalovirus infection following first trimester maternal infection: Symptoms at birth and outcome. *Journal of clinical virology : the official publication of the Pan American Society for Clinical Virology, 35*(2), 216–220.

Patton, H., & Tran, T. T. (2014). Management of hepatitis B during pregnancy. *Nature Reviews Gastroenterology & Hepatology, 11*(7), 402–409.

Petersen, L. R., Jamieson, D. J., & Honein, M. A. (2016). Zika virus. *The New England Journal of Medicine, 375*(3), 294–295.

Peyron, F., L'ollivier, C., Mandelbrot, L., Wallon, M., Piarroux, R., Kieffer, F., Hadjadj, E., Paris, L., & Garcia-Meric, P. (2019). Maternal and congenital toxoplasmosis: Diagnosis and treatment recommendations of a French multidisciplinary working group. *Pathogens, 8*(1), 24.

Rac, M. W., & Sheffield, J. S. (2014). Prevention and management of viral hepatitis in pregnancy. *Obstetrics & Gynecology Clinics of North America, 41*(4), 573–592.

Roush, S., Beall, B., McGee, L., Bowen, M., Oberste, S., Payne, D., Rota, P., Hickman, C., Tondella, M. L., Wasley, A., & Wang, X. (2023). Chapter 22: Laboratory Support for the Surveillance of Vaccine-Preventable Diseases. In S. W. Roush, L. McIntyre, & L. M. Baldy (Eds.), *Manual for the surveillance of vaccine-preventable diseases* (pp. 1–7). Centers for Disease Control and Prevention. https://www.cdc.gov/vaccines/pubs/surv-manual/chpt22-lab-support.html

Schillie, S., Vellozzi, C., Reingold, A., Harris, A., Haber, P., Ward, J. W., & Nelson, N. P. (2018). Prevention of hepatitis B virus infection in the United States: Recommendations of the Advisory Committee on Immunization Practices. *MMWR Recommendations & Reports, 67*(1), 1–31.

Shin, E. C., & Jeong, S. H. (2018). Natural history, clinical manifestations, and pathogenesis of hepatitis A. *Cold Spring Harbor Perspectives in Medicine, 8*, a031708.

Shrim, A., Koren, G., Yudin, M. H., Farine, D., Gagnon, R., Hudon, L., & Delisle, M. F. (2012). Management of varicella infection (chickenpox) in pregnancy. *Journal of Obstetrics and Gynaecology Canada, 34*(3), 287–292.

Society for Maternal-Fetal Medicine (SMFM). (2022). *COVID-19 outpatient treatment for pregnant patients.* https://s3.amazonaws.com/cdn.smfm.org/media/3526/COVID_treatment_table_6-21-22_%28final%29.pdf

Society for Maternal-Fetal Medicine (SMFM), Hughes, B. L., & Gyamfi-Bannerman, C. (2016). Diagnosis and antenatal management of congenital cytomegalovirus infection. *American Journal of Obstetrics and Gynecology, 214*(6), B5–B11.

Society of Obstetricians and Gynaecologists of Canada (SOGC). (2014). Parvovirus B19 infection in pregnancy. SOGC clinical practice guidelines, no. 316119. *Journal of Obstetrics and Gynaecology Canada, 36*(12), 1107–1116.

Song, J. Y., Lim, J. H., Lim, S., Yong, Z., & Seo, H. S. (2018). Progress toward a group B streptococcal vaccine. *Human Vaccines & Immunotherapeutics, 14*(11), 2669–2681.

Spiel, M. H., Hacker, M. R., Haviland, M. J., Mulla, B., Roberts, E., Dodge, L. E., & Young, B. C. (2019). Racial disparities in intrapartum group B Streptococcus colonization: A higher incidence of conversion in African American women. *Journal of Perinatology, 39*(3), 433–438.

Stagno, S., & Whitley, R. J. (1985). Herpesvirus infections of pregnancy: Cytomegalovirus and Epstein–Barr virus infections. *New England Journal of Medicine, 313*(20), 1270–1274.

Terrault, N. A., Bzowej, N. H., Chang, K. M., Hwang, J. P., Jonas, M. M., & Murad, M. H. (2016). AASLD guidelines for treatment of chronic hepatitis B. *Hepatology, 63*, 261–283.

Thoma, M. E., & Declercq, E. R. (2022). All-cause maternal mortality in the US before vs. during the COVID-19 pandemic. *JAMA Network Open, 5*(6), e2219133.

Townsend, C. L., Forsgren, M., Ahlfors, K., Ivarsson, S. A., Tookey, P. A., & Peckham, C. S. (2013). Long-term outcomes of congenital cytomegalovirus infection in Sweden and the United Kingdom. *Clinical Infectious Diseases, 56*(9), 1232–1239.

US National Institutes of Health. (2022). *LiverTox: Clinical and research information on drug-induced liver injury.* National Institute of Diabetes and Digestive and Kidney Diseases; https://www.ncbi.nlm.nih.gov/books/NBK548887

Verani, J. R., Spina, N. L., Lynfield, R., Schaffner, W., Harrison, L. H., Holst, A., & Schrag, S. J. (2014). Early-onset Group B streptococcal disease in the United States. *Obstetrics & Gynecology, 123*(4), 828–837.

Williams, D. R., & Mohammed, S. A. (2013). Racism and health I: Pathways and scientific evidence. *American Behavioral Scientist, 57*(8), 1152–1173.

Willner, I. R., Uhl, M. D., Howard, S. C., Williams, E. Q., Riely, C. A., & Waters, B. (1998). Serious hepatitis A: An analysis of patients hospitalized during an urban epidemic in the United States. *Annals of Internal Medicine, 128*(2), 111–114.

Workowski, K. A., Bachmann, L. H., Chan, P. A., Johnston, C. M., Muzny, C. A., Park, I., Reno, H., Zenilman, J. M., & Bolan, G. A. (2021). Sexually transmitted infections treatment guidelines, 2021. *MMWR Recommendations and Reports, 70*(4), 1–187.

World Health Organization. (2011). *WHO position paper: Rubella vaccines.* World Health Organization. http://www.who.int/wer/2011/wer8629.pdf.

World Health Organization. (2017). *Pandemic and epidemic diseases.* http://www.who.int/csr/disease/en.

World Health Organization. (2020). Guidelines for the management of pregnant and breastfeeding women in the context of Ebola virus disease. https://www.who.int/publications/i/item/9789240001381

Young, M. K., Cripps, A. W., Nimmo, G. R., & van Driel, M. L. (2015). Post-exposure passive immunisation for preventing rubella and congenital rubella syndrome. *The Cochrane Database of Systematic Reviews, 2015*(9), CD010586.

Zhang, H. J., Patenaude, V., & Abenhaim, H. A. (2015). Maternal outcomes in pregnancies affected by varicella zoster virus infections: Population-based study on 7.7 million pregnancy admissions. *Journal of Obstetrics & Gynaecology Research, 41*, 62–68.

56

Sexually Transmitted Infections and Vaginitis

Gina M. Fullbright

The editors gratefully acknowledge Eva M. Fried and Cindy L. Farley, who were authors of the previous edition of this chapter.

Relevant Terms

Acquired immunodeficiency syndrome (AIDS)—a chronic immune system disease caused by HIV

Antibodies—proteins in the blood produced in reaction to foreign substances, such as bacteria and viruses that cause infection

Bacterial vaginosis—an imbalance of the naturally occurring bacteria in the vagina, with a decrease in lactobacilli and overgrowth of the various other vaginal flora leading to symptoms of a fishy odor and thin whitish gray discharge

Chancre—a sore caused by syphilis and appearing during the primary phase of infection

Chlamydia—the most frequently reported bacterial sexually transmitted infection (STI) in the United States; caused by *Chlamydia trachomatis*

Expedited partner therapy—treatment of sex partners of individuals diagnosed with STIs

Gonorrhea—STI caused by infection with the *Neisseria gonorrhoeae* bacterium; infects the mucous membranes of the reproductive tract and the mucous membranes of the mouth, throat, eyes, and anus

Herpes simplex virus—STI caused by the herpes simplex virus type 1 or herpes simplex virus type 2

Human immunodeficiency virus (HIV)—a virus that attacks the immune system

Human papillomavirus (HPV)—genital HPV is the most common viral STI; there are more than 40 HPV types that can infect genitalia, including high-risk HPV types that can cause cervical cancer and low-risk HPV types that can cause genital warts

Pelvic inflammatory disease (PID)—an infection of the uterus, fallopian tubes, and nearby pelvic structures

Sexually transmitted infections—also known as sexually transmitted diseases; these are infections that are spread by sexual contact

Syphilis—STI caused by the spirochete bacterium *Treponema pallidum*

Trichomoniasis—STI caused by a protozoan parasite called *Trichomonas vaginalis*

Vertical transmission—transmission of a disease, condition, or trait either genetically or congenitally; vertical transmission of an infection, also known as perinatal transmission, occurs in utero, during the birth process, or with breastfeeding

Vulvovaginal candidiasis—a fungal infection that causes irritation, discharge, and intense itchiness of the vagina and the vulva

---

Introduction

The intimate nature of interpersonal relationships before, during, and after pregnancy provides opportunities for the spread of infectious pathogens. Intercourse, birth, and breastfeeding break down usual physical barriers that protect against infection. Five of the top 10 reportable diseases in the United States are **sexually transmitted infections (STIs)**. Normal changes in the immune system during pregnancy increase susceptibility to STIs. There are four major classes of infectious agents: bacterial, viral, fungal, and parasitic. Sexual and reproductive health can be adversely affected by any of these. Infectious diseases have been implicated in many pregnancy complications including spontaneous abortion, prelabor rupture of membranes, preterm birth (PTB), chorioamnionitis, cesarean birth, and postpartum infection. Infectious disease is also associated with an increased risk of complication in the fetus and neonate including congenital anomalies, fetal infection, fetal growth restriction, neonatal conjunctivitis, and perinatal mortality.

Social determinants of health play a significant role in STI transmission, prevention, and management. The increasing rates of STIs are fueled by a multitude of underlying social and structural determinants. These can include poverty, health literacy, racism, disability, geographic location, healthcare access, education, gender imbalances, and stigma. These factors may limit access to appropriate and

Prenatal and Postnatal Care: A Person-Centered Approach, Third Edition. Edited by Karen Trister Grace, Cindy L. Farley, Noelene K. Jeffers, and Tanya Tringali.
© 2024 John Wiley & Sons Ltd. Published 2024 by John Wiley & Sons Ltd.
Companion website: www.wiley.com/go/grace/prenatal

quality STI testing, treatment, and management. The nature of these disparities demands interventions on multiple levels through partnerships and collaborations to promote sexual health at the individual, community, and policy levels (Friedman, et al., 2014; Hamilton & Morris, 2015; Hogben & Leichliter, 2008; Sutton et al., 2021). Populations that are marginalized carry a disproportionate disease burden related to STIs. In particular, racial disparities can be noted in the rates of all reportable STIs (Hamilton & Morris, 2015). Sexual behaviors and risks for STIs vary by cultural and ethnic norms as well as by access to comprehensive sexual education and healthcare.

Health equity key points

- STIs have a disproportionate impact on populations that are marginalized in the United States.
- STIs transmitted perinatally can have significant consequences for pregnant people and their fetus/newborn.
- Racial disparities can be seen in the rates of all reportable STIs.
- Limited access to quality sexual healthcare contributes to these inequities.
- Clinicians must continue to work toward improved outcomes for individuals by addressing the structural racism, biases, and social conditions that contribute to STI care disparities.

Pregnancy is a frequent point of entry into the healthcare system, and screening for STIs is a routine part of prenatal care. Some screening recommendations apply to all pregnant individuals, while others are specific to those at increased risk for STIs. Additionally, a specific geographic area may be a high prevalence area for a certain STI. Providers can consult their local health departments for guidance in this regard. The Centers for Disease Control and Prevention (CDC, 2021c) recommends that all pregnant individuals and their sex partners be counseled about the risks of STIs in pregnancy. Providers should also keep in mind that some STIs increase the risk of HIV infection due to their effect on genital tissue.

This chapter will review STIs including **chlamydia, gonorrhea, syphilis, herpes simplex virus (HSV), human immunodeficiency virus (HIV)/acquired immunodeficiency syndrome (AIDS), human papillomavirus (HPV),**

Risk factors for STIs

- Sexually active individuals with a cervix, age 25 and under
- Current or recent STI
- A new sex partner
- A partner who has other partners
- Individuals having penile to anal intercourse
- Use of injection drugs or a sex partner who does
- Exchange of sex for drugs or money
- Inconsistent use of barrier methods in a relationship that is not mutually monogamous
- Sexually active with multiple partners

---

and **trichomoniasis**. **Bacterial vaginosis (BV)** and **vulvovaginal candidiasis (VVC)** are common vaginal conditions in pregnancy and are covered in this chapter.

Sexually Transmitted Bacterial Infections

Chlamydia Trachomatis

Chlamydia is frequently an asymptomatic STI. Presenting symptoms can include vaginal discharge, postcoital bleeding, dysuria, dyspareunia, intermenstrual bleeding, and vague lower abdominal pain. Mucopurulent cervical discharge and tenderness on bimanual exam may be present. Numerous white blood cells may be noted on microscopic examination of vaginal discharge, though this is not diagnostic.

The greatest disease burden of chlamydia is among adolescents and young adults. *C. trachomatis* has been associated with multiple sequelae including **pelvic inflammatory disease** (PID), ectopic pregnancy, and infertility. Past infection can destroy tubal cilia and lead to fibrosis of the fallopian tubes, resulting in increased risk of ectopic pregnancy and fertility issues. For pregnant individuals, chlamydial infection can cause spontaneous abortion, prelabor rupture of the membranes, postpartum endometritis, PTB, and stillbirth (Clennon et al., 2017). In the newborn, it can lead to neonatal conjunctivitis, pneumonia up to three months after birth and increased neonatal mortality (CDC, 2021c). Generally, neonatal infection is associated with vaginal birth but may also occur following cesarean birth, especially after prolonged rupture of membranes. Those individuals with active chlamydial infection at the time of vaginal birth have a 50–75% chance of passing the infection to the neonate (CDC, 2021c).

Pregnancy Testing and Treatment

The CDC recommends that pregnant individuals at increased risk for chlamydia due to age or sexual practice, such as those with a new sex partner, self or partner with more than one partner, or sex partner with an STI, be tested at the first prenatal visit; however, it is common to test all pregnant individuals at the first prenatal visit. Nucleic acid amplification testing (NAAT) with an endocervical or vaginal swab is sensitive and specific (CDC, 2021c). In addition, self-collection with a vaginal swab by the patient is shown to be equally reliable to clinician collection (CDC, 2021c). First-catch urine testing can also be done, but may not detect as many infections as the swab collection method (CDC, 2021c). Individuals who are at high risk for chlamydia, including those whose age is less than 25 years, individuals who test positive at any time during pregnancy, and those that meet any of the criteria for increased risk listed above, are retested in the third trimester (CDC, 2021c). Further, pregnant individuals who are treated for chlamydia should have a test of cure at four weeks after treatment. This is because a NAAT may read positive for up to three weeks following treatment. A test of reinfection approximately three months following the test of cure is suggested (CDC, 2021c).

Recommended treatment regimens in pregnancy are listed in the box below; one is chosen after reviewing history and allergies.

Recommended treatments for chlamydia in pregnancy

- Azithromycin 1 g as a one-dose treatment (preferred)
- Amoxicillin 500 mg three times daily for seven days

Source: Adapted from CDC (2021c).

Sex partners should receive testing for chlamydia, gonorrhea, and HIV, as well as treatment if positive. Patient and partners should abstain from sexual contact, unless a reliable barrier method is used, until seven days after completion of antibiotic therapy. Extragenital chlamydia screening for individuals at the rectal and oropharyngeal sites can be considered based on reported sexual practices through shared clinical decision making between the provider and the patient (CDC, 2021c).

Neisseria gonorrhoeae

Like chlamydia, gonorrhea is often asymptomatic. Individuals presenting with symptoms report vaginal discharge, dysuria, urinary frequency, and tenderness in the area of Bartholin's or Skene's glands and lower abdominal tenderness. Mucopurulent discharge and tenderness on abdominal exam may be noted.

Gonorrhea is associated with PTB in a limited number of studies. It has also been linked to fetal growth restriction in populations with high rates of infection (Heumann et al., 2017). Past infection is also associated with ectopic pregnancy. **Vertical transmission** occurs during vaginal birth at rates of 30–50% (Heumann et al., 2017). The neonatal conjunctiva is the most common site of infection. Other neonatal manifestations include polyarticular arthritis, gonococcemia, and genital infection. In the United States, routine screening for chlamydia and gonorrhea and routine newborn erythromycin eye prophylaxis have dramatically decreased neonatal ophthalmic infection.

Pregnancy Testing and Treatment

As with chlamydia, the CDC recommends that pregnant individuals at increased risk for gonorrhea due to age or sexual practice be tested at the first prenatal visit; however, screening is common for all individuals at the first prenatal visit. Concurrent chlamydia is typically tested using the same sample with the NAAT test as these infections have similar presentations and persons affected by one pathogen are often infected with the other. For pregnant individuals testing positive, a test of cure is not recommended unless the infection is pharyngeal; however, a test for reinfection is performed after three months (CDC, 2021c). Healthcare providers should consider repeat testing during the third trimester for individuals under 25 and anyone with high-risk sexual behaviors (CDC, 2021c).

Chlamydia infection often accompanies gonorrhea; therefore, treatment for both is recommended, unless chlamydia infection has been excluded (CDC, 2021c). Recommended treatments are listed in the following box. Partners should be tested for chlamydia and HIV and receive treatment as outlined previously, and patient and partners should abstain from sex until seven days after treatment, unless a reliable barrier method is used.

Recommended treatments for gonorrhea in pregnancy

- Ceftriaxone 500 mg intramuscularly, and 1 g azithromycin if chlamydia infection has not been excluded (preferred)
- If allergic to cephalosporins, consult an infectious disease specialist

Source: Adapted from CDC (2021c).

Because the burden and disease resistance of gonorrhea varies among communities, healthcare providers need to consider these factors when making decisions about the frequency of screening (CDC, 2021c). Extragenital gonorrhea screening for individuals at the rectal and oropharyngeal sites can be considered based on reported sexual practices through shared clinical decision making between the provider and the patient (CDC, 2021c).

Syphilis

Syphilis is caused by the Gram-negative spirochete bacterium *Treponema palladium*. After decades of decline, a marked resurgence of syphilis has been noted worldwide. The incidence of syphilis has more than quadrupled in the United States since 2000, with the highest increases seen in men who have sex with men (Schmidt et al., 2019). However, rates of syphilis are rising in women, and congenital syphilis rates are increasing exponentially as well. The rate of congenital syphilis increased 291% between 2015 and 2019. Syphilis rates are increasing across the United States impacting all demographic groups, but disproportionately impacting communities of color and sexual and gender minority groups (CDC, 2020a). The history of the treatment of syphilis is replete with unethical experiments on marginalized populations, such as the infamous Tuskegee experiment that withheld treatment from men of color inoculated with *Treponema palladium* for 40 years (McNamara & Yingling, 2020). This historical trauma left communities of color with an understandable mistrust of medical professionals. Medical mistrust can, in turn, accelerate disparities due to decreased healthcare utilization.

Syphilis is known as the "great imitator" because symptoms can present in varying forms and in time frames that are remote from exposure (McNamara & Yingling, 2020). Classic primary syphilis presents as a **chancre**, a painless ulcer that has a raised, indurated border found at the site of infection, usually the genitals. It resolves spontaneously in three to six weeks. Infected people may be unaware of lesions especially inside the vagina or on the cervix. Secondary syphilis presents within weeks or months of the primary phase. It is a systemic disease characterized by a maculopapular rash especially on the palms, soles, and mucous membranes. Adenopathy, fever, anorexia, weight loss, and flesh-colored genital lesions called condylomata lata that are highly infectious may also be present. Symptoms resolve spontaneously in two to six weeks. Tertiary syphilis is a rare complication characterized by gummatous lesions, aortic aneurysm, seizures, and dementia. Recognizing how syphilis presents clinically and understanding how it moves from latent to active infection can be challenging even for experienced clinicians. It does not always move through consecutive clinical stages, and a person with secondary or tertiary syphilis may present with no recollection of prior symptoms. Individuals testing positive for syphilis should be offered testing for other STIs including HIV, hepatitis B, and hepatitis C.

Syphilis easily crosses the placenta and is devastating to the developing fetus. Congenital syphilis can affect any organ system but is often associated with infections of the bone, brain, heart, lungs, and abdominal organs. Infected neonates may also be asymptomatic with signs not developing until weeks or years after birth (CDC, 2021d). Maternal syphilis is associated with multiple increased risks for the pregnant client and fetus—21% increased risk for stillbirth, 6% increased risk for PTB, and 9% increased risk for neonatal death (Adhikari, 2021). Approximately 1 million pregnancies are affected worldwide by syphilis annually with nearly half ending in miscarriage or neonatal death, one-quarter ending in PTB, and one-quarter of neonates acquiring congenital syphilis (Tsimis & Sheffield, 2017).

Pregnancy Testing and Treatment

Unlike screening guidelines for many other STIs, which are based on risk factors and prevalence, screening guidelines for syphilis are based on the knowledge that this relatively uncommon infection is easily treated and has potential for devastating consequences for the fetus. A serological test for syphilis is universally recommended at the first prenatal visit. Some states and areas where syphilis is more common require repeat testing after 28 weeks of gestation and/or upon hospital admission for labor (CDC, 2021c). Additionally, any pregnant person who has a fetal death after 20 weeks should be tested for syphilis. Pregnant individuals with inadequate prenatal care and no documented maternal serologic status should be tested during their hospital stay for labor, birth, and postpartum care (CDC, 2021c). The majority of states have enacted specific laws requiring prenatal syphilis testing. Providers should be familiar with current guidelines and adhere to regulations for the state in which they practice (CDC, 2020c). Furthermore, the CDC (2021c) recommends confirmation of serologic status of the mother prior to discharge of the neonate from the hospital.

Commercially available serological screening tests for syphilis measure IgG and IgM **antibodies**. These are called nontreponemal tests because they do not directly measure the presence of the bacteria and include rapid plasma reagin (RPR) and Venereal Disease Research Laboratory (VDRL) tests. Positive results on a nontreponemal test are followed by a diagnostic confirmatory treponemal test, such as Fluorescent Treponemal Antibody-Absorption (FTA-ABS), Serodia *Treponema Pallidum* Passive Particle Agglutination (TP-PA), or *Treponema pallidum* hemagglutination assay (TPHA). Pregnant individuals who are seropositive for syphilis should be considered infected unless adequate treatment history is documented in medical records (CDC, 2021c). Current tests are unable to distinguish between recent or remote infections or among the various stages of infection. A new reverse sequence testing algorithm is recommended by the CDC (2021c), which begins with a treponemal test, and if positive is followed by a nontreponemal test. This sequence is thought to more accurately diagnose chronic, untreated syphilis, but implementation of this algorithm is hampered by cost and resource considerations. Rapid point-of-care (POC) testing for syphilis via fingerstick blood samples has recently become more readily available. These tests may be treponemal, nontreponemal, or both (Angel-Müller et al., 2018). The rapid POC testing offers the opportunity for rapid diagnosis, prompt treatment, and prevention of vertical transmission to the fetus (Gaydos et al., 2017).

Treatment recommendation for parenteral penicillin is based on decades of clinical experience and past treatment success, as defined by clinical resolution of symptoms and prevention of sexual transmission. No alternative to penicillin treatment is considered adequate in pregnancy (CDC, 2021c). Pregnant individuals who report penicillin allergy should have skin testing to confirm allergy. If true allergy exists, the person will undergo desensitization therapy prior to treatment.

Individuals treated for syphilis should be aware of the possibility of a Jarisch-Herxheimer reaction, a reaction that includes fever, headache, and myalgia, which may occur within the first 24 hours after treatment. This reaction and associated symptoms should not be confused with an allergic reaction to the medication. During pregnancy, the Jarisch-Herxheimer reaction might cause fetal distress or induce early labor. This should not, however, delay or prevent treatment (CDC, 2021c). A team of care providers should be involved to treat the infection and safeguard maternal-fetal health.

Recommended treatments for syphilis in pregnancy

Primary and secondary syphilis	Benzathine penicillin G 2.4 million unit single dose
Early latent syphilis	Benzathine penicillin G 2.4 million unit single dose
Late latent syphilis or syphilis of unknown duration	Benzathine penicillin G 2.4 million units once weekly for three weeks

Source: Adapted from CDC (2021c).

Sexually Transmitted Viral Infections

Herpes Simplex

HSV is one of the most prevalent STIs, affecting more than one in six people aged 14–49 years, and it is common in pregnancy. Studies show 22% of pregnant women are seropositive for herpes simplex virus type 2 (HSV-2), 63% for herpes simplex virus type 1 (HSV-1), and 13% for both HSV-1 and HSV-2 (CDC, 2021c; Stephenson-Famy & Gardella, 2014). The HSV viruses are in the same class of viruses that cause varicella zoster shingles. After an initial infection, the virus moves to nerve cells where it remains dormant until a recurrence is triggered. Infected persons can transmit the infection during periods of asymptomatic viral shedding. Transmission of HSV to infants is frequently from pregnant clients with no known history of genital herpes (James & Kimberlin, 2015). Primary infection with HSV may present as genital or rectal sores accompanied by one or more of the following: pruritis, pain, burning, edema, dysuria, myalgia, headache, and fever. Subsequent outbreaks tend to be mild and have fewer systemic symptoms. Lesions or vesicles may be noted on inspection, and tender inguinal lymph nodes may be present. The occurrence of primary HSV-2 infection during pregnancy is of concern as primary lesions have a higher risk of transmitting HSV to the fetus than recurrent ones (James & Kimberlin, 2015). While historically HSV-2 has been associated with genital lesions and HSV-1 with oral lesions, HSV-1 is increasingly the cause of genital lesions (Sampath et al., 2016).

Classification of genital HSV infection can be divided into three categories: primary, nonprimary first episode, or recurrent (Table 56.1). The incidence of primary HSV infection during pregnancy is approximately 2% (Rogan & Beigi, 2019). There are multiple strains of HSV-2, and infection with one does not confer immunity to others.

Primary HSV infection may be asymptomatic, minor, or severe. Generally, symptomatic primary HSV infections have an incubation period of about 4 days and lesions may occur 2–12 days after exposure. Lesions during a primary infection tend to be larger, more numerous, pustular, ulcerating, and bilateral as compared to lesions

Table 56.1 Classification of Genital HSV Infections

Clinical designation	Description
Primary genital HSV infection	Newly acquired antibodies to HSV-1 or HSV-2 in the absence of preexisting antibodies
Nonprimary first-episode genital HSV infection	Newly acquired antibodies to HSV-2 in the presence of preexisting antibodies to HSV-1
Recurrent genital HSV infection	Reactivation of genital HSV with HSV type recovered from the lesion the same as serum HSV type

Source: Adapted from Westhoff et al. (2011) and Hammad and Konje (2021).

in individuals with HSV antibodies but no prior outbreak or in recurrent infections. Lesions generally disappear after three weeks. Most individuals with symptomatic primary infection also present with systemic symptoms including fever, headache, malaise, and myalgia.

Nonprimary, first-episode infection occurs most frequently when a person has a newly acquired HSV-2 infection in the presence of a preexisting HSV-1 infection. HSV-1 antibodies can be partially protective against HSV-2. Conversely, HSV-2 antibodies are highly protective against new HSV-1 infection (Hammad & Konje, 2021; Westhoff et al., 2011), making nonprimary, first-episode infection with HSV-1 very unlikely. Nonprimary first-episode infections tend to have fewer systemic symptoms, less pain, a shorter period of viral shedding, and a more rapid resolution of symptoms.

Recurrent genital infections are more common with HSV-2 than with HSV-1. Individuals with HSV-2 have an average of four recurrences in the first year after infection compared to one recurrence for individuals infected with HSV-1 (Hammad & Konje, 2021; Westhoff et al., 2011). Recurrent infections are typically less severe. Prodromal symptoms of tingling, shooting pain, burning, or itching at the site of infection are common. Recurrent infections also tend to be unilateral and have fewer lesions. These lesions may not have the classic vesicular appearance and instead appear as fissures or simply vulvar irritation. Approximately 75% of pregnant individuals infected with HSV2 experience at least one recurrence during pregnancy, and 14% will have prodromal symptoms or genital lesions at the onset of labor (Stephenson-Famy & Gardella, 2014).

Fetal HSV infection is more likely in the setting of recent maternal primary HSV infection, prolonged rupture of membranes, or disruption of fetal skin or mucous membranes during labor or birth. Fetal infection can occur in utero by transmission of the virus through the placenta. Fetal infection from transplacental HSV is called congenital herpes, and neonatal infection acquired during birth is called neonatal herpes. Intrauterine infection is associated with spontaneous abortion and stillbirth as well as neurological damage, congenital cataracts, and skin vesicles. About 30% of neonates with disseminated disease will die; many who survive are left with significant morbidities (Stephenson-Famy & Gardella, 2014).

Pregnancy Testing and Treatment

Pregnant individuals presenting with symptoms of HSV infection should have serological testing for HSV-1 and HSV-2 IgG and IgM in addition to viral culture, polymerase chain reaction (PCR), or direct antibody fluorescence to identify the subtype of HSV infection (ACOG, 2020; Hammad & Konje, 2021). The latter two tests have limited availability. IgG and IgM can help determine whether the episode is primary or recurrent as well as identify the infection subtype to better characterize the risk of vertical transmission. Antibodies to HSV infection develop relatively late, up to 12–16 weeks after infection, and cannot be used alone to diagnose acute infection.

Currently, universal screening for HSV is not recommended in asymptomatic pregnant individuals (CDC, 2021c). However, screening can be useful for individuals who do not have a history of genital herpes but who have a partner that does, as it can guide their decisions about having intercourse and risking a primary infection in late pregnancy. During the third trimester, individuals with a partner with known or suspected genital herpes should be counseled to abstain from vaginal intercourse, whether or not the patient has known history of genital herpes (CDC, 2021c).

The mainstays of antenatal treatment for HSV are famicyclovir, acyclovir, and valacyclovir (Table 56.2). These drugs are not associated with adverse neonatal or fetal effects and are considered safe in all trimesters. Suppressive therapy starting at 36 weeks of pregnancy, using the same medications for pregnant individuals with primary or recurrent HSV, has demonstrated effectiveness in reducing the risk of HSV recurrence at the time of labor (Stephenson-Famy & Gardella, 2014). Individuals with any history of genital HSV outbreaks are offered suppressive therapy starting at 36 weeks, as this reduces the incidence of cesarean birth due to herpes outbreak (Stephenson-Famy & Gardella, 2014).

The primary goal of prenatal and intrapartum care for pregnant people with a history of genital HSV infection is to prevent transmission to the neonate and limit the necessity of cesarean birth. As with other STIs, vertical transmission of HSV can be associated with several risk factors, such as maternal type of infection and serologic status, birth route (vaginal or cesarean), the specific type of HSV genital lesion, the duration of membrane rupture, and the use of fetal scalp electrodes (Samies & James, 2020). Vertical transmission is thought to be almost exclusively through contact with virus-containing vaginal secretions during birth, although in utero and postnatal infection may occur rarely. While much of the effort toward preventing vertical transmission is aimed at individuals with recurrent HSV-2, this is not the primary etiology of the estimated 1500 cases of neonatal HSV infection that occur annually in the United States (Hammad & Konje, 2021; Westhoff et al., 2011). It is thought that <1% of neonatal infection is due to recurrent, as opposed to primary, HSV-2, and this suggests a significant protective role for maternal antibodies.

The greatest risk of vertical transmission is for seronegative pregnant individuals who contract either HSV-1 or HSV-2 near term. In this population, the risk of transmission is estimated between 20% and 50% (Westhoff et al., 2011). Infection with HSV-1, either primary or recurrent, appears to be more easily transmitted to the neonate than HSV-2 (Hammad & Konje, 2021; Westhoff et al., 2011). Other risks for HSV transmission during labor and birth include internal fetal monitoring, birth prior to 38 weeks of gestation, and HSV isolated from the cervix.

When individuals with a history of HSV infection present in labor, a careful examination of the vulva, vagina, and cervix is performed and a detailed history of the presence of prodromal symptoms obtained. Vaginal birth is an appropriate option for pregnant individuals presenting with lesions near but not on the genital area, such as the buttocks; an occlusive dressing over the site is recommended. Asymptomatic viral shedding at the time of birth is a theoretical concern; however, studies of PCR testing in labor to screen for this have failed to demonstrate a health or cost benefit (Westhoff et al., 2011). Pregnant individuals at term or in labor with active lesions or prodromal symptoms such as vulvar pain or burning should be counseled to have a cesarean birth to reduce the risk of neonatal transmission (ACOG, 2020).

Human Immunodeficiency Virus

The HIV causes an acute viral illness that affects the immune system by destroying CD4+ T lymphocytes.

Table 56.2 Recommended Treatments for HSV in Pregnancy

Indication	Drug	Dosage	Duration	Alternative
Suppressive therapy	Acyclovir	400 mg TID	Begin at 36 weeks, continue until birth	
	Valacyclovir	500 mg BID	Begin at 36 weeks, continue until birth	
Primary infection	Acyclovir	400 mg TID	7–10 days	200 mg five times daily
	Valacyclovir	1000 mg BID	7–14 days	
	Famciclovir	400 mg TID	7–14 days or until lesions disappear	
Recurrent infection	Acyclovir	400 mg TID	5 days	200 mg five times daily or 800 mg qid × 5–10 days
	Valacyclovir	500 mg BID	3 days	800 mg BID for 5 days or
	Famciclovir	250 mg BID	5 days	1000 mg daily for 5 days
Severe infection	Acyclovir	5–10 mg/kg	2–7 days or until clinical improvement	
		IV Q8h	followed by oral acyclovir for a total of 10 treatment days	

Source: Adapted from Westhoff et al. (2011) and Hammad and Konje (2021).

Acquired immunodeficiency syndrome (AIDS) develops with sharply decreased numbers of CD4+ T lymphocytes. If left untreated, HIV leads to AIDS at a variable progression, depending on viral, host, and environmental factors. However, early diagnosis and treatment of HIV with antiretroviral therapy prolongs life expectancy, resulting in a near normal lifespan, and reduces the rate of transmission to others (CDC, 2021c). With advances in treatment, HIV has become a chronic illness, rather than a lethal disease. In addition to occupational transmission, such as needlestick injuries, HIV can be transmitted sexually during penetrative intercourse, via oral-genital or digital-genital contact with an infected partner, and through HIV-contaminated needles during injection drug use.

Pregnancy Screening and Treatment

Screening for HIV is recommended for all pregnant individuals upon entry to prenatal care regardless of previous screening. Pregnant individuals are notified that HIV screening is included in the standard prenatal testing profile, and the individual's decision is documented if they decline ("opt-out" testing). A second test during the third trimester is recommended for pregnant individuals who are at high risk for HIV infection. Pregnant individuals with no prenatal care should be tested for HIV upon presenting to the labor and delivery unit (CDC, 2021c). Early screening allows for prompt confirmation of the HIV diagnosis and initiation of therapies to safeguard the individual's health and decrease the risk of perinatal transmission. Additionally, the rate of vertical transmission (maternal-to-child or MTCT) from pregnant HIV-positive pregnant individuals to their infant is reduced to less than 2% with use of antiretroviral regimens (Chilaka & Konje, 2021).

Screening for HIV can be done through several laboratory tests. The CDC (2021c) recommends initial testing with HIV-1/HIV-2 antigen/antibody combination assay. If this testing is repeatedly reactive a supplemental HIV-1/HIV-2 antibody differentiation assay should be performed. HIV-1 Western blot and HIV-1 IFA are no longer part of the recommended algorithm for confirmation of infection (CDC and Association of Public Health Laboratories, 2014). Advances in rapid HIV testing technology can allow for preliminary detection of HIV infection, often in less than 20 minutes. All preliminary reactive rapid tests should be confirmed with conventional laboratory assays (CDC, 2021c). The rapid HIV antigen/antibody immunoassay offers results within 45 minutes from a urine, saliva, or serum sample. False positives can occur, but the benefit is that the test can be performed at the POC.

Optimal care of the pregnant individual with HIV requires coordination between HIV specialists, maternity care providers, and supportive services (Department of Health and Human Services [HHS], Panel on Treatment of HIV During Pregnancy and Prevention of Perinatal Transmission, 2021). When HIV is diagnosed in pregnancy, it is recommended that antiretroviral therapy (ART) be started as soon as possible to prevent perinatal transmission. The medication therapy prevents transmission to the fetus by rapidly suppressing plasma HIV RNA below detectable levels. Pregnant individuals on established ART are encouraged to continue their medication regimen throughout their pregnancy to maintain viral suppression and minimize the development of drug resistance. Monitoring of HIV treatment response is done through viral load testing throughout pregnancy. At 36 weeks of gestation, this information is essential for the clinician and client to make the best decision regarding mode of birth (CDC and Association of Public Health Laboratories, 2014). The goal of therapy is to achieve and maintain a suppressed viral load.

There are over 24 antiretroviral drugs approved for use in HIV treatment, prescribed in various dosing schedules (HHS, Panel on Treatment of HIV During Pregnancy and Prevention of Perinatal Transmission, 2021). These drugs are divided into six categories, based on their mode of action: nucleoside/nucleotide reverse transcriptase inhibitors, non-nucleoside reverse transcriptase inhibitors, protease inhibitors, fusion inhibitors, CCR5 antagonists, and integrase inhibitors. Drugs are typically prescribed in combination. In general, the same dosing regimens are used in pregnant individuals as in other HIV-infected individuals (HHS, Panel on Treatment of HIV During Pregnancy and Prevention of Perinatal Transmission, 2021). An HIV-infected pregnant individual should make decisions about which ART drugs to take in conjunction with their HIV specialist after considering known and unknown benefits, harms, and risks of these drugs for themself and their baby.

Vaginal birth is possible for pregnant individuals with low viral loads (HIV RNA levels <50 copies/mL); however, cesarean birth should be considered if the viral loads are >400 (Chilaka & Konje, 2021). Decisions regarding route of birth are based on HIV RNA levels at the time of labor, as well as standard labor and birth considerations. Pregnant individuals are counseled that HIV infection can put them at higher risk of surgical complications of cesarean birth (HHS, Panel on Treatment of HIV During Pregnancy and Prevention of Perinatal Transmission, 2021).

HIV is found in breast milk, and thus, risk for transmission to a breastfed infant exists. There is an estimated risk of HIV transmission to the infant of 15–20% through breastfeeding if maternal and infant prophylaxis is not utilized (HHS, Panel on Treatment of HIV During Pregnancy and Prevention of Perinatal Transmission, 2021). The use of maternal ART throughout pregnancy can reduce but does not eliminate the risk of transmitting HIV to the child through breast milk. Therefore, breastfeeding is contraindicated where there is access to clean water and safe infant formula (HHS, Panel on Treatment of HIV During Pregnancy and Prevention of Perinatal Transmission, 2021).

Human Papillomavirus

HPV is the most common STI with high prevalence among individuals of reproductive age. Both high-risk and low-risk HPV types are prevalent among sexually active individuals. HPV is often subclinical and asymptomatic, although some may experience pruritis or pain associated with genital warts. High-risk HPV, the types associated with cervical cancer, are typically detectable only with cervical cytology or colposcopy.

Tiny abrasions in surface epithelium allow HPV to infect the basal layer of squamous epithelial cells. The squamocolumnar junction of the cervix and the oropharynx are also targets. There are five phases of the HPV life cycle: infection and uncoating, proliferation, genomic phase, viral synthesis, and shedding. Another possible phase is latency. After initial infection, the host immune system may induce a regression in the life cycle and the virus remains latent in the basal epithelium. Although nonsexual transmission is possible, the primary mechanism of infection is through sexual contact.

Approximately 40% of pregnant individuals harbor HPV DNA. Coinfection with multiple HPV strains is common (Pandey et al., 2019). Genital warts may appear and become larger and more numerous during pregnancy. This may be due to altered maternal immunity associated with pregnancy as well as high levels of estrogen and progesterone. Neonatal acquisition of HPV types associated with genital warts may result from aspiration of genital tract secretions during birth and may result in laryngeal papillomatosis.

There are contradictory data about the rate of vertical transmission, ranging from 1% to 80%. This is largely due to differences in study methodology. Most studies place the rate of transmission between 16% and 69% (Koskimaa et al., 2012). Several mechanisms of vertical transmission have been proposed but are not well understood. Prenatal transmission is suspected because infants have been born with condyloma and HPV DNA has been isolated from amniotic fluid prior to rupture of membranes.

Pregnancy Testing and Treatment

Generally, diagnosis of HPV types that cause genital warts is made through clinical observation of lesions. They are typically flesh-colored and may be flat or raised, or have a cauliflower-like appearance. Genital warts can proliferate and become friable during pregnancy. Treatment is not medically necessary during pregnancy, but may be desired; complete resolution may not be possible until after pregnancy due to changes in maternal immunity and the presence of increased estrogen. If treatment is desired, once weekly application of 80–90% trichloroacetic acid (TCA) or bichloroacetic acid (BCA) may clear lesions, especially in the second half of pregnancy. The acid is applied directly to the lesion until a frosted white appearance is obtained. Petroleum or lidocaine jelly can be applied to the surrounding healthy tissue to prevent injury to healthy tissue. Excessive acid application can be neutralized with soap or bicarbonate. Weekly treatments can be repeated until the lesions resolve. Podofilox, podophyllin, and sinecatechins are not appropriate for use in pregnancy and should be avoided. While the use of imiquimod appears to pose low risk, it should be avoided during pregnancy until additional data are available (CDC, 2021c). The presence of HPV at birth is not an indication for cesarean birth unless the lesions are obstructive, or if vaginal delivery would result in excessive bleeding.

Diagnosis of other types of HPV is made during cervical cytology or colposcopy. Guidelines for cervical cancer screening during pregnancy are the same as when not pregnant; pregnancy itself is not an indication for screening in the absence of meeting other criteria. Cytology and HPV test management algorithms may be different during pregnancy depending on result. Screening and management guidelines are frequently updated, and providers should make sure to stay current on these recommendations.

Since the introduction of the HPV vaccine, rates of cervical cancer have significantly decreased (Mix et al., 2021). The HPV vaccine is not recommended during pregnancy. Individuals who have initiated the HPV vaccine series should postpone completion until after birth (CDC, 2021c).

Hepatitis B

Sexual contact is the most common transmission pathway for hepatitis B in the United States, although in some areas of the world, maternal-child transmission is the primary pathway. Universal prenatal screening for hepatitis B infection and immunoprophylaxis have substantially reduced perinatal transmission and the subsequent development of chronic infection (US Preventive Services Task Force, 2019). All pregnant individuals should be offered screening for hepatitis B surface antigen (HBsAg), which indicates acute or chronic hepatitis B infection, at the first prenatal visit even if they have been tested or vaccinated before. Additional testing should be done at time of birth for populations at high risk for HBV infection. Hepatitis B vaccination is now part of routine childhood vaccinations, and many people of childbearing age will have already been vaccinated. Unvaccinated pregnant individuals who are at risk of hepatitis B exposure during pregnancy, such as those using injection drug users, having multiple sex partners, or living with infected individuals, should be offered the hepatitis B vaccine (CDC, 2021c). Pregnant people exposed to hepatitis B should be treated with hepatitis B immunoglobulin (HBIG) to reduce the chance of infection and fetal/newborn transmission. Prenatal transplacental transmission of the virus does occur and is implicated in immunoprophylaxis failure (Sirilert & Tongsong, 2021).

Hepatitis can be spread to a neonate during either a vaginal or cesarean birth. Babies infected with hepatitis B have a 90% chance of developing chronic hepatitis (CDC, 2020b). Infected newborns also have a high risk of carrying and spreading the disease. All infants born to people with hepatitis B should be given HBIG and all unaffected infants should also be given hepatitis B vaccine. Hepatitis is vaccine-preventable, and rates have declined dramatically with newborn vaccination programs.

However, recent data show a slight upward trend in hepatitis B in adults, driven by transmission through injection drug use (Kim & Kim, 2018).

Zika Virus

Zika virus is mentioned here because it can be transmitted sexually (CDC, 2019), although transmission via mosquito bite is the most common route of infection. Zika infection in pregnancy is associated with fetal microcephaly as well as spontaneous abortion, stillbirth, eye defects, hearing loss, impaired growth, and developmental delays. Individuals capable of reproduction who are considering childbearing in the near future are advised not to travel to areas with Zika. People with the capacity for pregnancy are advised to wait at least two months after possible exposure to conceive, and partners/sperm donors should wait at least six months after possible exposure. Recommended time delays vary based on travel history and sexual practices. The Zika virus remains detectable in semen for a variable and prolonged time; this should be considered when giving advice. Condoms are recommended for the prevention of transmission. Healthcare providers should continue to consult the CDC for guidance about families considering pregnancy in an area of a Zika outbreak. Zika virus is discussed more thoroughly in Chapter 55, *Infectious Diseases*.

Sexually Transmitted Parasitic Infection

Trichomoniasis

Trichomoniasis is a very common infection of the lower genital tract with the parasite *Trichomonas vaginalis*. Individuals may be asymptomatic or may present with intensely symptomatic vaginitis and profuse malodorous purulent discharge that is white, yellow, green, or frothy. Pruritis, burning, postcoital bleeding, urinary frequency, or dysuria may be present. The external genitalia and vagina may appear red, inflamed, and excoriated from scratching. The cervix may be friable, and petechiae may be observed. The pelvis and abdomen may be tender, and tender inguinal lymph nodes may also be noted.

Pregnant individuals who are symptomatic should be tested, and if positive should be treated. Repeat testing in three months is recommended due to the greater than 40% risk of reinfection or persistence in the pregnant population (Kim et al., 2020). However, the benefit of screening for trichomoniasis in asymptomatic pregnant individuals has not been established (CDC, 2021c). Diagnosing *T. vaginalis* can be challenging. While the NAAT assay vaginal culture is the preferred testing modality, test results take time (Kim et al., 2020). *T. vaginalis* can be detected on a saline slide through observation of motile organisms though this modality has poor sensitivity. *T. vaginalis* may be an incidental finding on a pap smear; however, this should not be considered diagnostic. Treatment for *T. vaginalis* should be considered once the infection is confirmed with a reliable diagnostic test. Most strains of *T. vaginalis* are susceptible to metronidazole. Recommended treatment is metronidazole 500 mg

2 times/day for seven days. This dosing regimen is appropriate at any stage of pregnancy (CDC, 2021c). The sexual partners of infected individuals should be screened for STIs and treated for trichomoniasis.

Recommended treatment for trichomoniasis in pregnancy

Metronidazole 500 mg orally 2 times/day for seven days

Source: CDC (2021c).

T. vaginalis is associated with adverse pregnancy outcomes, including prelabor rupture of membranes, PTB, and low birth weight, as well as respiratory and genital infections in the newborn. Vertical transmission is thought to occur in about 5% of pregnancies. Most cases of neonatal infection resolve within one month after birth without treatment.

Practice points for trichomoniasis

- Symptomatic trichomoniasis in pregnancy should be treated adequately.
- Metronidazole can be used in any trimester to treat trichomoniasis.
- Routine screening of asymptomatic pregnant women for trichomoniasis is not recommended.
- Partners should be treated; consider **expedited partner therapy (EPT)**.

Fungal Vaginitis

Vulvovaginal Candidiasis

Candidiasis is a common occurrence during pregnancy. Individuals may present with a thick, white vaginal discharge, dysuria, vaginal soreness, and pruritis. On exam, the vulva may appear edematous and red. Excoriation and fissures may also be present. Discharge may be scant or copious and adherent or may have a curdled appearance. Foul or fishy odor is not a defining characteristic of VVC; at times a distinctive yeast odor is noted. Diagnosis is made by microscopic observation of candidiasis hyphae and buds, which appear as long, translucent strands on a saline slide with 10% potassium hydroxide solution. In the absence of a concurrent bacterial infection, vaginal pH should be normal (less than 4.5). Candidiasis can also be cultured. It is important to distinguish candidiasis from the physiologic increase in vaginal secretions (leukorrhea) that is common during pregnancy. Recommended treatments are listed in the following box. Oral fluconazole has been shown to be associated with a statistically significant increased risk of spontaneous abortion compared to individuals with topical or no use of azoles (Molgaard-Nielsen et al., 2016).

Recommended treatments for candidiasis in pregnancy

- Clotrimazole 1% cream 5 g intravaginally daily for seven days
- Miconazole 1% cream 5 g intravaginally daily for seven days
- Terconazole 0.4% 5 g intravaginally daily for seven days

Source: CDC (2021c).

Candidiasis colonization rates during pregnancy are approximately 40%, roughly twice that of nonpregnant individuals. This may be due to increased levels of estrogen and progesterone. *Candida* itself is unlikely to be directly responsible for any poor pregnancy outcomes. Recent studies have shown that vaginal colonization with candidiasis is not associated with PTB and other adverse pregnancy outcomes (Schuster et al., 2020). The effect of *Candida* on vaginal flora may provide an indirect contribution to these adverse effects through its role in creating an environment conducive to the development of BV.

Practice points for VVC

- Symptomatic candidiasis in pregnancy should be treated adequately.
- Oral azole drugs should be avoided.
- Routine screening of asymptomatic pregnant people for candidiasis is not recommended.

Bacterial Vaginitis

Bacterial Vaginosis

BV is the most common lower genital tract disorder among both pregnant and nonpregnant individuals of reproductive age, affecting up to 30% of nonpregnant individuals and an estimated 6–20% of pregnant individuals (Owens et al., 2020). BV is associated with increased risk for acquiring STIs including HIV as well as the development of PID. It has also been implicated as a causal factor for PTB, prelabor rupture of membranes, and spontaneous abortion. Various factors have been associated with an increased risk of BV including multiple male sexual partners or any female sexual partners, new sex partners, not using condoms, douching, and HSV-2 infection (CDC, 2021c). Black women have a significantly higher risk of developing BV compared to White women. It is unclear as to the underlying cause behind this association; pathways being investigated include variations in the microbiome due to the chronic stress of racism (Murphy & Mitchell, 2016).

Pregnancy Testing and Treatment

In-office diagnosis can be made using Amsel's criteria. BV is clinically described as a homogenous grayish-white discharge, bacterial overgrowth, pH > 4.5, and an amine "fishy" odor

released when vaginal discharge is mixed with 10% potassium hydroxide solution (KOH). An additional criterion is the presence of "clue cells," with greater than 20% of vaginal epithelial cells with such a heavy coating of bacteria that the peripheral borders are obscured. A minimum of three of the four Amsel's criteria must be met to make a diagnosis of BV. Individuals symptomatic for BV may report an increase in white discharge with a strong "fishy" odor. These symptoms are often only noticeable or worsen after sexual activity.

Amsel's criteria

- An adherent and homogenous vaginal discharge
- Vaginal pH > 4.5
- Detection of clue cells (vaginal epithelial cells with such a heavy coating of bacteria that the edges are obscured) on saline slide
- An amine odor after the addition of potassium hydroxide (positive whiff test)

Gram-stain microscopic evaluation of vaginal secretions remains the gold standard for the diagnosis of BV, although use of Amsel's criteria is reliable and more common (Anderson et al., 2011). Characteristics of the microbial composition of the sample are made against the Nugent scoring system, (Table 56.3), and include the presence or relative absence of lactobacilli associated with vaginal health, plus the number of curved Gram-variable rods and *Bacteriodes* species morphotypes such as *Mobiluncus* spp., *Gardnerella vaginalis*, *Mycoplasma hominis*, and *Peptostreptococcus* spp. Cytology reports may suggest BV via comments such as "coccobacilli consistent with a shift in vaginal flora"; however, this is not a specific or sensitive test for BV. Organism-specific POC tests for BV, *Candida*, and *Trichomonas* are available and have higher sensitivity and specificity than in-office microscopic evaluation. These allow rapid differentiation of vaginitis, leading to prompt diagnosis and treatment.

Treatment for BV is recommended for all symptomatic pregnant individuals. BV has been associated with adverse pregnancy outcomes, including PTB, prelabor ruptured membranes, postpartum endometritis, PID, and possible spontaneous abortion (Owens et al., 2020). Antibiotic

Table 56.3 Nugent Scoring System for Gram-Stained Vaginal Smears

Score	*Lactobacillus* morphotypes	*Gardnerella* and *Bacteroides* spp. morphotypes	Curved Gram-variable rods
0	4+	0	0
1	3+	1+	1+
2	2+	2+	2+
3	1+	3+	3+
4	0	4+	4+

therapy has been shown to be an effective treatment for BV in pregnancy (Brocklehurst et al., 2013); see the following box. Treating BV with antibiotics was also shown to reduce the risk of late miscarriage, but not of PTB (Brocklehurst et al., 2013). The CDC (2021c) does not recommend treatment of sex partners or of asymptomatic pregnant individuals at low risk for PTB as there is no indication that it will reduce adverse outcomes of pregnancy. Routine screening for BV among pregnant people is not recommended.

Recommended treatments for bacterial vaginosis in pregnancy

- Metronidazole 500 mg orally 2 times/day for seven days
- Clindamycin 300 mg orally 2 times/day for seven days

Source: CDC (2021c).

BV: A Disturbance in the Vaginal Microbiome

The vagina is a unique microenvironment that is complex and dynamic. It can be relatively stable in some individuals and change quickly in others. Typically, there is a balance of *Lactobacillus acidophilus* and other endogenous microflora (Romm, 2018). Estrogen, pH balance, glycogen, and metabolic by-products of normal and pathogenic microbes contribute to the vaginal environment, influencing vulnerability to infections depending on the mix of elements. *Abnormal vaginal flora* is characterized by a lack of lactobacilli in the absence of other diagnostic criteria for BV or other infections such as chlamydia or gonorrhea. *Aerobic vaginitis* is the replacement of lactobacilli and infection of the parabasal cells by intestinal microflora such as *Escherichia coli,* enterococci, and group B *Streptococcus.* Aerobic vaginitis presents clinically as inflamed vaginal mucosa, sticky yellowish discharge, pH > 6, and a foul, not fishy, odor. Severe symptoms are rarely seen in pregnancy; however, less severe forms may be encountered. Both abnormal vaginal flora and aerobic vaginitis would have intermediate Nugent scores of 4–6 and meet some but not all Amsel criteria for diagnosis of BV. Symptomatic women should be considered for treatment.

BV has been associated with a variety of pregnancy complications, including PTB, spontaneous abortion, postpartum endometritis, and low infant birth weight (Owens et al., 2020); however, screening of all pregnant people for BV has not shown benefit in reduction of these issues and is not recommended. Symptomatic individuals and those at high risk for PTB should be screened and treatment offered if positive for BV. Treatment of BV can be safely administered at any time during pregnancy.

BV is often a chronic condition characterized by short-term relief of symptoms after appropriate antibiotic treatment, only to have bothersome symptoms return in weeks or months. Metronidazole efficiently kills anaerobic bacteria but not aerobic bacteria. Some cases of BV treatment failure may be due to a vaginal microbiome primarily composed of aerobic bacteria. This observation may explain why some studies have failed to demonstrate that metronidazole treatment of BV in pregnancy reduces PTB and prelabor rupture of membranes.

The vaginal microbiome often includes Gram-negative rods and cocci as well as several species of anaerobic and as yet unnamed bacteria (Chee et al., 2020). It is believed that a healthy vaginal floral composition is more than 95% lactobacilli. The vaginal microbiome is affected by hormonal changes throughout the reproductive years and during pregnancy. Hydrogen-peroxide-producing *Lactobacillus* species are important in maintaining an acidic environment that controls bacterial counts. BV is associated with a loss of lactic-acid-producing bacteria and an overgrowth of anaerobic bacteria.

There is limited knowledge of the fluctuations and composition of the vaginal microbiome. It is theorized that the protection that a healthy vaginal microbiome offers is due to a predominance of *Lactobacillus* species that produce lactic acid and various bacteriostatic and bactericidal compounds, and through competitive exclusion of other microorganisms (Chee et al., 2020).

Individuals will frequently turn to alternative and complementary therapies for vaginitis, most commonly for a self-diagnosed yeast infection (Romm, 2018). High-quality evidence is lacking for many of these regimens due to variations in dosing schedules and inconsistent composition of the compounds used; however, some therapies have a theoretical basis for effectiveness with little to no potential for harm. For example, oral or vaginal recolonization of lactobacilli with yogurt or probiotic capsules shows promise for the treatment of both candidiasis vaginitis and BV with little potential for harm (Romm, 2018). Equally important to support are lifestyle practices that promote rest, coping strategies to manage stress, and a nourishing diet with limited concentrated sugars; these strategies may help to restore balance and support healing of the vaginal microbiome.

BV practice points

- Screening all pregnant persons for BV has no benefit in reducing PTB.
- Individuals who are symptomatic or at increased risk of PTB should be screened.
- Mainstay treatment for BV is metronidazole or clindamycin.
- Condom use may be protective.
- People with BV should be counseled about the increased risk of contracting STIs.
- BV is not considered an STI but is most common in sexually active individuals.
- BV symptoms can be triggered by sexual activity, particularly vaginal intercourse.

Partner STI Treatment

Partner notification and treatment can reduce the risk of reinfection of pregnant individuals (Ferreira et al., 2013). The importance of partner notification should be discussed and specific community resources for partner testing and treatment provided. Encouraging individuals to bring their partners to the office to discuss diagnosis and treatment provides an opportunity for screening for STIs and counseling about the diagnosis, treatment, and prevention of reinfection.

For individuals who indicate that their partner is unlikely to seek treatment, the CDC (2021c) recommends the harm reduction strategy of EPT, which allows clinicians to give patients medications or prescriptions to distribute to their sexual partner(s). All sexual partners in the past 60 days, or the most recent sexual partner (if last contact was greater than 60 days), should be considered for treatment (Jamison et al., 2019). Through this effective healthcare practice, STI treatment is provided to sexual partners for infections such as chlamydia, gonorrhea, and trichomoniasis without diagnosis or counseling. The preferred approach to EPT is providing the patient with prepackaged doses of oral medications with instructions, medication warnings, and follow-up recommendations (CDC, 2021c). If prepackaged medication is not available, the clinician can provide multiple prescriptions to the patient, one for self-administration and one for partner(s).

EPT is legal in most states, but limited in others. Each state in which EPT is permissible issues guidance on the delivery of prescriptions. It is important for healthcare providers to be aware of state EPT rules and regulations (CDC, 2021b).

Legal Requirements for Reporting STI Diagnosis

Accurate and timely reporting of STI infections helps public health departments assess trends, notify partners, and allocate resources for the greatest impact. Reportable diseases vary somewhat from state to state. Syphilis, gonorrhea, chlamydia, HIV/AIDS, and chancroid are reportable in every state. Healthcare providers should be aware of reporting requirements where they practice. Local and state health departments are able to provide information on reporting requirements. STI reporting can be initiated by either the laboratory where the STI was identified or by the clinician receiving the STI diagnostic report (CDC, 2021c).

Psychosocial Impact of STI Diagnosis

Effects on the Individual

Sexual and reproductive health is an important part of a person's health and well-being which can be significantly threatened by the diagnosis of an STI. Diagnosis of STIs can have a profound impact on an individual's concept of self and how they relate to others in their social and familial networks (Haapa et al., 2018). It is not unusual for a person to be diagnosed for the first time with an STI during pregnancy, causing significant concern and guilt regarding fetal health.

STIs can differ in their characteristics. However, regardless of the nature of the infection, either bacterial, which can be cured with antibiotics, or viral, which may linger in the body for years or perhaps a lifetime, the impact of diagnosis may alter a person's self-image from that point forward (Haapa et al., 2018). Newer testing modalities such as serological testing for HSV-1 and HSV-2 and HPV DNA testing mean more individuals are being diagnosed with STIs without having symptoms. Additionally, the absence of symptoms and variable latency periods, sometimes lasting years, means that very little information can be given to individuals about when or how they contracted these infections. Surprise, denial, and confusion are common short-term reactions to STI diagnosis after serological testing in the absence of clinical symptoms. STI diagnosis can strongly impact an individual's sexuality and feeling of desirability. This can range from feelings of being unworthy of attention from intimate partners to complete cessation of sexual activity.

The stigma associated with contracting an STI is significant for many people (Cook & Dickens, 2014). Pregnant individuals and those with children may also express fear of transmitting the infection to their fetus or other children. For individuals pregnant when diagnosed, their primary concern may be preventing transmission to the fetus, and this remains true throughout pregnancy. Feelings of shock, denial, self-disgust, anxiety and fear of rejection by their partner, and concerns about future reproductive health are also common. Anger toward the individual believed to have infected them and feelings of guilt for possibly transmitting the infection to others are often present (Cook & Dickens, 2014). Disclosure of STI status may be fraught with anxiety and fear.

These emotional aspects of STI care should be addressed. Healthcare providers counseling newly diagnosed individuals can address the common nature of STIs to help reduce feelings of stigma and isolation. It is important that healthcare providers provide quality counseling, education, and support while encouraging people living with an STI to be active in their own care. Clarifying misinformation about STIs and providing resources for individuals to learn how to cope with infection are essential elements of care.

Discussing STI diagnosis

- Avoid using medical jargon.
- Acknowledge expressed emotions; be supportive.
- Tailor counseling to the individual's health literacy level.
- Take time to listen to the individual's questions and concerns.
- Provide consumer-friendly handouts or websites at an appropriate reading level.
- Be mindful of the amount of information given at the time of diagnosis.
- Ask the person to describe in their own words their understanding of the diagnosis to evaluate understanding.
- Use a respectful, caring, and sensitive approach.
- Provide access for follow-up questions.

Source: Adapted from: Bertram and Magnussen (2008).

STI Prevention within Relationships

Couples can demonstrate discordance between perception of monogamy and the practice of monogamy. Population studies suggest that up to 57% of married men and 35% of married women will have extradyadic sex (Conley et al., 2015). This lack of awareness can create a false perception of STI acquisition risk. Additionally, compliance with the practice of mutual monogamy is low. In the clinic setting, creating a safe place for couples to discuss STI diagnosis may help with disclosure and allow appropriate treatment and prevention strategies to be discussed.

There is little information available about STI transmission among cisgender women who have sex with cisgender women (WSW) during a pregnancy of one of the partners. It is likely that trichomonas, HSV, and HPV are exchanged between female sex partners. However, there is variation based on sexual practices. Oral sex may place WSW at higher risk for HSV-1 and BV has increased prevalence among WSW, but screening recommendations remain the same as for all pregnant people. Providers should familiarize themselves with healthy sex practices for WSW, such as cleaning and using barrier methods on shared sex toys, as well as barriers for digital, oral, genital, and anal sex if the partners are not monogamous or one has an infection. Counseling should be individualized accordingly.

Clinicians should remember that transgender men remain at risk for all STIs that affect the vulva, vagina, and cervix. Transgender men may have increased susceptibility to STIs due to frequently experienced stigma and barriers to care that negatively affect healthcare access (CDC, 2021c).

Individuals experiencing intimate partner violence (IPV) in pregnancy are at greater risk of contracting HIV or an STI through lack of control over sexual encounters and decreased ability to negotiate condom use. Pathways for this increase can also include having sex while intoxicated, or with multiple partners (Gonzalez-Guarda et al., 2021). Physical and psychological consequences of IPV, such as bruising or abrasions in the genital area or the down regulation of the immune system in response to stress, can decrease host resistance and facilitate HIV or STI infection.

The CDC (2021c) reports that prevalence rates of certain STIs, such as chlamydia and gonorrhea, are highest among adolescents and young adults. Adolescents and minors can consent for their own STI services in all 50 states. These services may include STI screening and treatment, HIV testing and treatment, and HPV vaccine. Adolescents seeking services should be provided sexuality education as part of their care. Adolescents should receive counseling regarding sexual behaviors, STI risk, and prevention methods such as correct and consistent condom use, minimizing the number of sex partners, and vaccinations (HPV and hepatitis B). In addition, all adolescents should receive specific counseling and information regarding HIV transmission, prevention, and testing (CDC, 2021c).

Counseling for adolescents diagnosed with STIs needs to include information about future susceptibility to reinfection or new infections. Young individuals may need support integrating condoms into sexual practices as well

as strengthening condom negotiation skills with their sexual partners, especially during pregnancy when there may be less perceived need for contraception (Hensel & Fortenberry, 2011). Pregnant adolescents are at high risk for STIs due to prevalence of condom nonuse and multiple sexual partners (Crosby & Bounse, 2012; Kann, 2016).

In addition to pre-exposure vaccination for HPV and hepatitis B, barrier methods including external and internal condoms and dental dams are essential components of STI prevention. Therefore, healthcare providers should regularly counsel and educate clients on the availability of vaccines and the use of barrier methods. In addition, providers must be adept at demonstrating correct use of barrier products. The healthcare provider should be familiar with and comfortable with advising patients and couples about methods of sexual satisfaction during pregnancy and postpartum that do not pose a risk of STI transmission. An often-overlooked barrier method of STI protection is the internal condom. The internal condom, also known as the female condom, covers the external genitalia as well as the vagina. It provides equivalent protection to the external or male condom, and when both are used together, effectiveness rates are enhanced (Wiyeh et al., 2020).

It is important that healthcare providers discuss HIV risk and prevention with all clients. In 2018, more than 38,000 people were newly diagnosed with HIV infections in the United States. The US Public Health Service and the CDC jointly recommend pre-exposure prophylaxis (PrEP) to all sexually active individuals (CDC, 2021a). Providers should counsel clients about both the benefits and the potential risks of PrEP use so that an informed decision can be made that is right for the client and their situation. PrEP is available in both oral and injectable forms. Correct and consistent utilization of PrEP has been strongly associated with protection from HIV infection (CDC, 2021c). As clinicians gather appropriate sexual history, they may identify individuals at greater risk for HIV infection, including those with multiple or new sexual partners, an STI during pregnancy, a partner who is HIV positive, a history of inconsistent or no condom use, incarceration, injection drug use, or living in an area with high prevalence (CDC, 2021c).

STI prevention strategies

- Clinicians should be comfortable counseling clients about risk reduction strategies.
- Both external and internal condoms reduce the risk of STI acquisition when used correctly.
- Clinicians should be comfortable with instructing individuals about the proper use of external and internal condoms.
- Penis models and pelvic models for demonstration of condom application should be available in the clinic setting.
- Clinicians should counsel on use of PrEP for HIV prevention.
- Clinicians should screen for IPV. Positive screen increases risk of STI acquisition.
- STI services should be culturally sensitive, confidential, and widely accessible.

Summary

Many STIs pose the risk of adverse pregnancy outcomes including spontaneous abortion, stillbirth, PTB, low birth weight, and ophthalmia neonatorum. Effective treatment and prevention are imperative to prevent these detrimental effects for both the pregnant individual and their fetus/newborn. Risk assessment for STIs should be initiated at the first prenatal visit, and screening protocols during prenatal care should follow current evidence. Drugs selected for treatment should be safe for the pregnant individual and their fetus, be efficacious, and be well tolerated. National guidelines for the management of STIs during pregnancy are produced and regularly updated by the CDC.

Resources for Healthcare Providers

CDC information on expedited partner therapy for STDs: https://www.cdc.gov/std/ept/default.htm

CDC treatment guidelines for STDs, including treatment during pregnancy: https://www.cdc.gov/std/treatment-guidelines/default.htm

Pre-Exposure Prophylaxis for the Prevention of HIV Infection in the United States—2021 Update: http://cdc.gov/hiv/pdf/risk/prep/cdc-hiv-prep-guidelines-2021.pdf

Resource for Patients and Partners

CDC Fact Sheets for Sexually Transmitted Diseases (STDs): https://www.cdc.gov/std/healthcomm/fact_sheets.htm

Planned Parenthood. STD Education and Prevention: https://www.plannedparenthood.org/learn/stds-hiv-safer-sex

STI Testing and Services Site Locator: https://gettested.cdc.gov

References

ACOG. (2020). Management of herpes in pregnancy. Practice bulletin no. 220. *Obstetrics & Gynecology*, *135*, e193–e202. https://doi.org/10.1097/AOG.0000000000003840

Adhikari, E. (2021). Syphilis in pregnancy. *Contemporary OB/GYN Journal*, *66*(1), 22–27.

Anderson, B., Zhao, Y., Andrews, W. W., Dudley, D. J., Sibai, B., Iams, J. D., Wapner, R. J., Varner, M. W., Caritis, S. N., O'Sullivan, M. J., & Eunice Kennedy Shriver National Institute of Child Health and Human Development (NICHD) Maternal-Fetal Medicine Units Network (MFMU). (2011). Effect of antibiotic exposure on Nugent score among pregnant women with and without bacterial vaginosis. *Obstetrics & Gynecology*, *117*(4), 844–849. https://doi.org/10.1097/AOG.0b013e318209dd57

Angel-Müller, E., Grillo-Ardila, C. F., Amaya-Guio, J., Torres-Montañez, N. A., & Vasquez-Velez, L. F. (2018). Point of care rapid test for diagnosis of syphilis infection in men and nonpregnant women. *The Cochrane Database of Systematic Reviews*, *5*, CD013036. https://doi.org/10.1002/14651858.CD013036

Bertram, C., & Magnussen, L. (2008). Informational needs and the experiences of women with abnormal Papanicolaou smears. *Journal of the American Academy of Nurse Practitioners*, *20*, 455–462.

Brocklehurst, P., Gordon, A., Heatley, E., & Milan, S. J. (2013). Antibiotics for treating bacterial vaginosis in pregnancy. *The Cochrane Database of Systematic Reviews*, *1*. https://doi.org/10.1002/14651858.CD000262.pub4

Centers for Disease Control and Prevention (CDC). (2019). *Zika Virus*. https://www.cdc.gov/zika/pregnancy/index.html

Centers for Disease Control and Prevention (CDC). (2020a). *Sexually transmitted disease surveillance 2020 – National overview-Syphilis*. https://www.cdc.gov/std/statistics/2020/overview.htm#Syphilis

Centers for Disease Control and Prevention (CDC). (2020b, January). *Protect your baby for life. When a pregnant woman has hepatitis B*. https://www.cdc.gov/hepatitis/hbv/pdfs/hepbperinatal-protectwhenpregnant.pdf

Centers for Disease Control and Prevention (CDC). (2020c, May 12). *Sexually transmitted diseases (STDs) – State statutory and regulatory language regarding prenatal syphilis screenings in the United States*. https://www.cdc.gov/std/treatment/syphilis-screenings.htm

Centers for Disease Control and Prevention (CDC). (2021a). *US Public Health Service: Preexposure prophylaxis for the prevention of HIV infection in the United States – 2021 Update: A clinical practice guideline*. https://www.cdc.gov/hiv/pdf/risk/prep/cdc-hiv-prep-guidelines-2021.pdf

Centers for Disease Control and Prevention (CDC). (2021b, April 19). *Legal status of expedited partner therapy*. https://www.cdc.gov/std/ept/legal/default.htm

Centers for Disease Control and Prevention (CDC). (2021c, July 23). *Morbidity and mortality weekly report – Sexually transmitted infections treatment guidelines*, *2021*, *70*(4). https://www.cdc.gov/std/treatment-guidelines/STI-Guidelines-2021.pdf

Centers for Disease Control and Prevention (CDC). (2021d, September 16). *Congenital syphilis – CDC fact sheet*. https://www.cdc.gov/std/syphilis/stdfact-congenital-syphilis.htm

Centers for Disease Control and Prevention (CDC) and Association of Public Health Laboratories. (2014). *Laboratory testing for the diagnosis of HIV infection: Updated recommendations*. https://doi.org/10.15620/cdc.23447

Chee, W. J. Y., Chew, S. Y., & Than, L. T. L. (2020). Vaginal microbiota and the potential of lactobacillus derivatives in maintaining vaginal health. *Microbial Cell Factories*, *19*(1), 1–24. https://doi.org/10.1186/s12934-020-01464-4

Chilaka, V. N., & Konje, J. C. (2021). HIV in pregnancy—an update. *European Journal of Obstetrics, Gynecology, and Reproductive Biology*, *256*, 484–491. https://doi.org/10.1016/j.ejogrb.2020.11.034

Clennon, E., Caughey, A. B., & Bullard, K. (2017). Obstetric outcomes complicated by chlamydia infection in all U.S. deliveries between 2011–2013. *Obstetrics & Gynecology*, *129*, S137.

Conley, T. D., Matsick, J. L., Moors, A. C., Ziegler, A., & Rubin, J. D. (2015). Re-examining the effectiveness of monogamy as an STI-preventive strategy. *Preventive Medicine*, *78*, 23–28. https://doi.org/10.1016/j.ypmed.2015.06.006

Cook, R. J., & Dickens, B. M. (2014). Reducing stigma in reproductive health. *International Journal of Gynecology & Obstetrics*, *125*(1), 89–92.

Crosby, R., & Bounse, S. (2012). Condom effectiveness: Where are we now? *Sexual Health*, *9*, 10–17.

Department of Health and Human Services: Panel on Treatment of HIV During Pregnancy and Prevention of Perinatal Transmission. (2021, December 30). *Recommendations for use of antiretroviral drugs during pregnancy and interventions to reduce perinatal HIV transmission in the United States*. https://clinicalinfo.hiv.gov/en/guidelines/perinatal/whats-new-guidelines

Ferreira, A., Young, T., Matthews, C., Zunza, M., & Low, N. (2013). Strategies for partner notification for sexually transmitted infections, including HIV. *The Cochrane Database of Systematic Reviews*, *10*. https://doi.org/10.1002/14651858.CD002843.pub2

Friedman, A. L., Uhrig, J., Poehlman, J., Scales, M., & Hogben, M. (2014). Promoting sexual health equity in the United States: Implications from exploratory research with African-American adults. *Health Education Research*, *29*(6), 993–1004. https://doi.org/10.1093/her/cyu003

Gaydos, C. A., Sheng, D., Pegany, R., Wendel, S. K., & Mani, S. B. (2017). Maternal syphilis: Variations in prenatal screening, treatment, and diagnosis of congenital syphilis. *Columbia Medical Review*, *1*(2), 20–29.

Gonzalez-Guarda, R. M., Williams, J. R., Williams, W., Lorenzo, D., & Carrington, C. (2021). Determinants of HIV and sexually transmitted infection testing and acquisition among female victims of intimate partner violence. *Journal of Interpersonal Violence*, *36*(13–14), NP7547–NP7566. https://doi.org/10.1177/0886260519827662

Haapa, T., Suominen, T., Paavilainen, E., & Kylmä, J. (2018). Experiences of living with a sexually transmitted disease: An integrative review. *Scandinavian Journal of Caring Sciences*, *32*(3), 999–1011. https://doi.org/10.1111/scs.12549

Hamilton, D. T., & Morris, M. (2015). The racial disparities in STI in the U.S.: Concurrency, STI prevalence, and heterogeneity in partner selection. *Epidemics*, *11*(2015), 56–61. https://doi.org/10.1016/j.epidem.2015.02.003

Hammad, W. A. B., & Konje, J. C. (2021). Herpes simplex virus infection in pregnancy–an update. *European Journal of Obstetrics & Gynecology and Reproductive Biology*, *259*, 38–45. https://doi.org/10.1016/j.ejogrb.2021.01.055

Hensel, D., & Fortenberry, D. (2011). Adolescent mothers' sexual, contraceptive, and emotional relationship content with the fathers of their children following a first diagnosis of sexually transmitted infection. *Journal of Adolescent Health*, *49*, 327–329.

Heumann, C. L., Quilter, L. A., Eastment, M. C., Heffron, R., & Hawes, S. E. (2017). Adverse birth outcomes and maternal *Neisseria gonorrhoeae* infection: A population-based cohort study in Washington state. *Sexually Transmitted Diseases*, *44*(5), 266–271.

Hogben, M., & Leichliter, J. S. (2008). Social determinants and sexually transmitted disease disparities. *Sexually Transmitted Diseases*, *35*(12 Suppl), S13–S18. https://doi.org/10.1097/OLQ.0b013e31818d3cad. PMID: 18936725

James, S. H., & Kimberlin, D. W. (2015). Neonatal herpes simplex virus infection. *Infectious Disease Clinics of North America*, *29*(3), 391–400.

Jamison, C. D., Coleman, J. S., & Mmeje, O. (2019). Improving women's health and combatting sexually transmitted infections through expedited partner therapy. *Obstetrics and Gynecology*, *133*(3), 416–422. https://doi.org/10.1097/AOG.0000000000003088

Kann, L. (2016). Youth risk behavior surveillance—United States, 2015. *MMWR. Surveillance Summaries*, *65*(6), 1–174.

Kim, B. H., & Kim, W. R. (2018). Epidemiology of hepatitis B virus infection in the United States. *Clinical Liver Disease*, *12*(1), 1. https://doi.org/10.1002/cld.732

Kim, T. G., Young, M. R., Goggins, E. R., Williams, R. E., Hogen-Esch, E., Workowski, K. A., Jamieson, D. J., & Haddad, L. B. (2020). Trichomonas vaginalis in pregnancy: Patterns and predictors of testing, infection, and treatment. *Obstetrics & Gynecology*, *135*(5), 1136–1144.https://doi.org/10.1097/AOG.0000000000003776.PMID: 32282605

Koskimaa, H., Waterboer, T., Pawlita, M., Grenman, S., Syrjanen, K., & Syrjanen, S. (2012). Human papillomavirus genotypes present in the oral mucosa of newborns and their concordance with maternal cervical human papillomavirus genotypes. *Journal of Pediatrics*, *160*(5), 837–843.

McNamara, M., & Yingling, C. (2020). The reemergence of syphilis: Clinical pearls for consideration. *Nursing Clinics*, *55*(3), 361–377. https://doi.org/10.1016/j.cnur.2020.06.009

Mix, J. M., Van Dyne, E. A., Saraiya, M., Hallowell, B. D., & Thomas, C. C. (2021). Assessing impact of HPV vaccination on cervical cancer incidence among women aged 15–29 years in the United States, 1999–2017: An ecologic study. *Cancer Epidemiology, Biomarkers & Prevention*, *30*(1), 30–37. https://doi.org/10.1158/1055-9965.EPI-20-0846

Molgaard-Nielsen, D., Svanstrom, H., Melbye, M., Hviid, A., & Pasternak, B. (2016). Association between use of oral fluconazole during pregnancy and risk of spontaneous abortion and stillbirth. *Journal of the American Medical Association*, *315*(1), 58–67.

Murphy, K., & Mitchell, C. M. (2016). The interplay of host immunity, environment and the risk of bacterial vaginosis and associated reproductive health outcomes. *The Journal of Infectious Diseases*, *214*(suppl_1), S29–S35.

Owens, D. K., Davidson, K. W., Krist, A. H., Barry, M. J., Cabana, M., Caughey, A. B., Donahue, K., Doubeni, C. A., Epling, J. W., Kubik, M., Ogedegbe, G., Pbert, L., Silverstein, M., Simon, M. A., Tseng, C., Wong, J. B., & US Preventive Services Task Force. (2020). Screening for bacterial vaginosis in pregnant persons to prevent preterm delivery: US preventive services task force recommendation statement. *JAMA*, *323*(13), 1286–1292. https://doi.org/10.1001/jama.2020.2684

Pandey, D., Soletti, V., Jain, G., Das, A., Prasada, K. S., Acharya, S., & Satyamoorthy, K. (2019). Human papillomavirus (HPV) infection in early pregnancy: Prevalence and implications. *Infectious Diseases in Obstetrics and Gynecology*, *2019*. https://doi.org/10.1155/2019/4376902

Rogan, S. C., & Beigi, R. H. (2019). Treatment of viral infections during pregnancy. *Clinics in Perinatology*, *46*(2), 235–256. https://doi.org/10.1016/j.clp.2019.02.009

Romm, A. (2018). *Botanical medicine for women's health* (2nd ed.). Elsevier Health Sciences.

Samies, N. L., & James, S. H. (2020). Prevention and treatment of neonatal herpes simplex virus infection. *Antiviral Research*, *176*, 104721. https://doi.org/10.1016/j.antiviral.2020.104721

Sampath, A., Maduro, G., & Schillinger, J. A. (2016). Infant deaths due to herpes simplex virus, congenital syphilis, and HIV in New York City. *Pediatrics*, *137*(4), 1–9.

Schmidt, R., Carson, P. J., & Jansen, R. J. (2019). Resurgence of syphilis in the United States: An assessment of contributing factors. *Infectious Diseases: Research and Treatment*, *12*, 1–9. https://doi.org/10.1177/1178633719883282

Schuster, H. J., de Jonghe, B. A., Limpens, J., Budding, A. E., & Painter, R. C. (2020). Asymptomatic vaginal *Candida* colonization and adverse pregnancy outcomes including preterm birth: A systematic review and meta-analysis. *American Journal of Obstetrics & Gynocology*, *2*(3). https://doi.org/10.1016/j.ajogmf.2020.100163

Sirilert, S., & Tongsong, T. (2021). Hepatitis B virus infection in pregnancy: Immunological response, natural course and pregnancy outcomes. *Journal of Clinical Medicine*, *10*(13), 2926. https://doi.org/10.3390/jcm10132926

Stephenson-Famy, A., & Gardella, C. (2014). Herpes simplex virus infection during pregnancy. *Obstetrics and Gynecology Clinics of North America*, *41*(4), 601–614.

Sutton, M. Y., Anachebe, N. F., Lee, R., & Skanes, H. (2021). Racial and ethnic disparities in reproductive health services and outcomes, 2020. *Obstetrics & Gynecology*, *137*(2), 225–233.

Tsimis, M. E., & Sheffield, J. S. (2017). Update on syphilis and pregnancy. *Birth Defects Research*, *109*(5), 347–352.

U.S. Preventive Services Task Force. (2019). Screening for hepatitis B virus infection in pregnant women: U.S. preventive services task force reaffirmation recommendation statement. *JAMA*, *322*(4), 349–354. https://doi.org/10.1001/jama.2019.9365

Westhoff, G., Little, S., & Caughey, A. (2011). Herpes simplex virus and pregnancy: A review of the management of antenatal and peripartum herpes infections. *Obstetrical & Gynecological Survey*, *66*(10), 629–638.

Wiyeh, A. B., Mome, R. K., Mahasha, P. W., Kongnyuy, E. J., & Wiysonge, C. S. (2020). Effectiveness of the female condom in preventing HIV and sexually transmitted infections: A systematic review and meta-analysis. *BMC Public Health*, *20*(1), 1–17. https://doi.org/10.1186/s12889-020-8384-7

Index

Note: Page numbers in *italic* denote figures, those in **bold** denote tables.

Prenatal and Postnatal Care: A Person-Centered Approach, Third Edition. Edited by Karen Trister Grace, Cindy L. Farley, Noelene K. Jeffers, and Tanya Tringali.
© 2024 John Wiley & Sons Ltd. Published 2024 by John Wiley & Sons Ltd.
Companion website: www.wiley.com/go/grace/prenatal